Preface

What is Immunosenescence?

The number of elderly people is steadily increasing in most countries. Concomitantly, the number of age-related diseases is unfortunately also increasing. One of the leading causes of death in the very elderly is infection, with cardio-vascular diseases and cancer less prevalent than in younger elderly. All three major pathologies are to some extent related to the immune system due to its well-known but still imperfectly investigated deregulation during aging.

Thus, the large amount of data accumulated during the last decade or more has allowed a better but still incomplete understanding of all the complex alterations affecting the immune system with aging. Although we do not know everything, we feel that it is important for the scientific community to become more acquainted with the corpus of knowledge recently generated in this domain, presented in a manner providing a critical evaluation of the current status of research. Many accepted ideas have changed during the last decade, such as the effect of aging on the innate immune system, antigen presentation, the cytokine imbalance and low grade inflammation. If not exactly a paradigm shift, the time seems ripe to present this critical evaluation and update of the state-of-the-art in these different areas. We perceive a great need to assemble this current knowledge in one volume by collecting contributions from the most eminent researchers in the field from all around the world. In this way, we aim to facilitate a synthesis of the different aspects of the disparate disciplines in ageing research to focus on immunosenescence for the first time (basic and clinical, molecular, cellular, biochemical, genetics). We hope this multidisciplinary approach from the aging, immunity and inflammation community will also be important for future innovative research in this domain.

Thus, this book will have as its main themes Aging, Immunity and Inflammation, with an emphasis on studies in humans. However, as data are not always available in this species, work in experimental animals will be also treated as appropriate. A large number of colleagues responded enthusiastically to our proposal and contributed with very high quality chapters. We begin with a description of Methods and models for studying immunosenescence. We continue with Cellular immunosenescence, treating most specifically T cells, B cells, neutrophils, antigen presenting cells and NK cells. We then proceed to mechanisms. In this context, receptor signaling, the role of mitochondrial activity, the proteasome, cytokine status and the neuro-endocrine-immune netweork are treated. The important but very challenging area of the Clinical relevance of immunosenescence for disease states is covered next by the individual treatment of infections, autoimmunity, cancer, metabolic syndrome, neurodegeneration and frailty. Finally, and even more challengingly, the last part of the book is devoted to possibilities for eventual intervention and modulation. We particularly emphasise nutritional aspects, lipids and experimental interventions. In this way we feel that we cover the whole range of areas from models, through basic molecular mechanisms to the clinical relevance and finally eventual modulation.

One of the main objectives of this book is to present in a systematic way our current knowledge in the field of the immunology related to aging. So do we now know what immunosenescence is? It is still difficult at answer this question, but we hope even the most specialist investigator in the field will find concepts and ideas within the book which will help him or her to approach an answer to this important question more closely than before. We would therefore sincerely like to hope that we have created an authoritative, innovative and thought-provoking book dedicated for the first time to this topic alone. We also like to hope that this volume will help to attract a new generation of researchers to the field of immunosenescence as an expanding and vital research arena.

Tamas Fulop
Claudio Franceschi
Katsuiku Hirokawa
Graham Pawelec

Quebec, Canada
Bologna, Italy
Tokyo, Japan
Tübingen, Germany

UNIVF
BIP

Handbook on Immunosenescence

Handbook on Immunosenescence

Basic Understanding and Clinical Applications

1

Editors

Tamas Fulop
University of Sherbrooke, Quebec, Canada

Claudio Franceschi
University of Bologna, Bologna, Italy

Katsuiku Hirokawa
Institute for Health and Life Sciences, Tokyo, Japan

Graham Pawelec
University of Tübingen, Tübingen, Germany

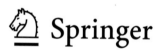 Springer

Editors

Tamas Fulop
Research Center on Aging
Division of Geriatrics
Dept. of Medicine, Faculty of Medicine
1036 Rue Belvedere
Sherbrooke J1H 4C4
Canada
tamas.fulop@usherbrooke.ca

Claudio Fraceschi
CIG Interdepartmental Center
"L. Galvani"
University of Bologna
Department of Experimental Pathology
Via San Giacomo 12
40126 Bologna
Italy
claudio.franceschi@unibo.it

Katsuiku Hirokawa
Institute for Health and Life Sciences
4-6-22 Kohinato
Tokyo
Bunkyo-ku
112-0006 Japan

Graham Pawelec
University of Tübingen
ZMF - Zentrum Med. Forschung
Abt. Transplant./ Immunologie
Waldhörnlestr. 22
72072 Tübingen
Germany
graham.pavelec@uni-tuebingen.de

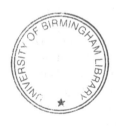

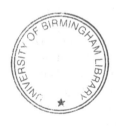
ISBN: 978-1-4020-9062-2   e-ISBN: 978-1-4020-9063-9

Library of Congress Control Number: 2008944075

Printed on acid-free paper

9 8 7 6 5 4 3 2 1

springer.com

Contents

Cellular Immunosenescence - B Cells

Cellular Immunosenescence - Neutrophils

Cellular Immunosenescence - Antigen Presenting Cells

Cellular Immunosenescence - NK and NKT Cells

Mechanisms - Cytokines

Mechanisms - Neuro-Endocrine-Immune Network

Mechanisms- Thymus

Mechanisms- Inflammation

Part IV: Clinical Relevance in Disease States-Infection

Contributors

A.I. Yashin
Center for Population Health and Aging, Duke University, Durham, USA

A.M. Robert
Université paris 5. Laboratoire de Recherche Ophtalmologique., 1 place du Parvis Notre Dame, 75181 Paris cedex 04, France

Agnieszka Brzezińska
Molecular Bases of Aging Laboratory, Nencki Institute of Experimental Biology, Polish Academy of Sciences, Pasteura 3, Warsaw Poland

Alan D. Roberts
Trudeau Institute, Saranac Lake, NY 12983, USA

Alessia Donnini
Laboratory of Tumour Immunology, INRCA Res. Dept., Via Birarelli 8, 60121 Ancona, Italy

Alexey A. Romanyukha
Institute of Numerical Mathematics, Russian Academy of Sciences, Moscow, Russia

Anders Wikby
Department of Natural Science and Biomedicine, School of Health Sciences, Jönköping University, Box 1026, 551 11 Jönköping, Sweden

Andrea Cossarizza
Chair of Immunology, Department of Biomedical Sciences, University of Modena and Reggio Emilia, Via Campi 287, Modena, 41100, Italy

Andrea Rossmann
Division of Experimental Pathophysiology and Immunology, Laboratory of Autoimmunity, Biocenter, Innsbruck Medical University, Fritz-Pregl-Strasse 3, A-6020-Innsbruck, Austria

Anis Larbi
Center for Medical Research, Section for Transplant-Immunology and Immuno-Hematology, Tuebingen Aging and Tumor Immunology group, University of Tuebingen Medical School, Waldhörnlestr. 22, D-72072 Tübingen, Germany

Ankmalika Gupta
Division of Basic and Clinical Immunology, University of California, Irvine, California

Ann Chidgey
Monash Immunology and Stem Cell Laboratories, Monash University, Clayton, Australia

Anna C. Phillips
School of Sport and Exercise Science, Birmingham University Medical School, Birmingham B15 2TT, UK

Anna Lang
Vaccine and Gene Therapy Institute, Department of Molecular Microbiology and Immunology and the Oregon National Primate Research Center, Oregon Health & Science University, Beaverton, OR 97006, USA

Anne Fletcher
Monash Immunology and Stem Cell Laboratories, Monash University, Clayton, Australia

Anshu Agrawal
Division of Basic and Clinical Immunology, University of California, Irvine, CA 92697, USA

Antonio Celada
Institute for Research in Biomedicine-University of Barcelona, Josep Samitier 1-5, 08028 Barcelona, Spain

Arianna Smorlesi
Laboratory of Tumour Immunology, INRCA Res. Dept., Via Birarelli 8, 60121 Ancona, Italy

Arie Ben Yehuda
University Hospital Kerem, The Department of Medicine at the Hadassah Ein, Jerusalem, Isreal

Barry W. Ritz
Drexel University, Department of Bioscience & Biotechnology, 118 Stratton Hall, 32nd and Chestnut Streets, Philadelphia, PA 19104, USA

Beatriz Sánchez-Correa
Immunology Unit, Department of Physiology, University of Extremadura, Cáceres, Spain

Bert E. Johansson
Innovation Sciences, Armonk, NY 10504, USA

Bertrand Friguet
Laboratoire de Biologie Cellulaire du Vieillissement, UMR 7079, Université Pierre et Marie Curie, 4 Place Jussieu, 75005 Paris, France

Blair Henderson
Division of Experimental Pathophysiology and Immunology, Laboratory of Autoimmunity, Biocenter, Innsbruck Medical University, Fritz-Pregl-Strasse 3, A-6020-Innsbruck, Austria

Bonnie B. Blomberg
Department of Microbiology and Immunology, University of Miami Miller School of Medicine, P.O. Box 016960 (R-138), Miami, FL 33101, USA

Boo Johansson
Institute of Gerontology, School of Health Sciences, Jönköping University, Box 1026, 551 11 Jönköping, Sweden, and Department of Psychology, Göteborg University, Box 500, 405 30 Göteborg, Sweden

Bruno Lesourd
EA 2431, Faculté de Médecine, 28 Place Henri Dunant, 63001 Clermont-Ferrand and Hôpital Nord du CHU de Clermont-Ferrand, BP 36, 63118 Cebazat, France

Claudio Franceschi
Department of Experimental Pathology, University of Bologna, Via San Giacomo 12, I-40126 Bologna, Italy; CIG-Interdepartmental Center "L. Galvani", University of Bologna, Via San Giacomo 12, I-40126 Bologna, Italy

Calogero Caruso
Gruppo di Studio sull'Immunosenescenza, Dipartimento di Biopatologia e Metodologie Biomediche, Università di Palermo, Corso Tukory 211, 90134 Palermo, Italy

Carl Fortin
Clinical research Center, Graduate Immunology Program, Division of Pulmonology, Department of Medicine, Faculty of Medicine, University of Sherbrooke, Sherbrooke, Quebec, Canada

Carlos Sebastián
Institute for Research in Biomedicine-University of Barcelona, Josep Samitier 1-5, 08028 Barcelona, Spain

Carmela Rita Balistreri
Gruppo di Studio sull'Immunosenescenza, Dipartimento di Biopatologia e Metodologie Biomediche, Università di Palermo, Corso Tukory 211, 90134 Palermo, Italy

Christina Mayerl
Division of Experimental Pathophysiology and Immunology, Laboratory of Autoimmunity, Biocenter, Innsbruck Medical University, Fritz-Pregl-Strasse 3, A-6020-Innsbruck, Austria

Christian R. Gomez
The Burn and Shock Trauma Institute and the Immunology and Aging Program; Department of Surgery; Loyola University Medical Center, 2160 South First Avenue, Maywood, IL 60153, USA; Facultad de Ciencias de la Salud, Universidad Diego Portales, Ejército 141, Santiago, Chile

Christopher A. Jolly
Division of Nutritional Sciences, The University of Texas, Austin, TX 78712, USA

Clarice Luz
LabVitrus, Rua Garibaldi, 659/502, Porto Alegre, RS 90035-050, Brazil

Claude Sportès
Experimental Transplantation & Immunology Branch, Center for Cancer Research, National Cancer Institute, National Institutes of Health, DHHS, Bethesda, MD, USA

Claudia Gravekamp
California Pacific Medical Center Research Institute, 475 Brannan Street, San Francisco, CA 94107, USA

Cornelia M. Weyand
Kathleen B. and Mason I. Lowance Center for Human Immunology, Department of Medicine, Emory University School of Medicine, Room 1003 Woodruff Memorial Research Building, 101 Woodruff Circle, Atlanta, GA, USA

Corona Alonso
Department of Immunology, Reina Sofia University Hospital, University of Córdoba, Corodoba, Spain

Cristina Bonorino
Faculdade de Biociências and Instituto de Pesquisas Biomédicas, Pontifícia Universidade Católica do Rio Grande do Sul (PUCRS), Av. Ipiranga 6690, 2° andar. P.O. Box 1429. Porto Alegre, RS 90.610-000, Brazil

Cristina Gatti
Laboratory of Tumour Immunology, INRCA Res. Dept., Via Birarelli 8, 60121 Ancona, Italy

Cristina M. Moriguchi Jeckel
Faculdade de Farmácia, PUCRS, Av. Ipiranga, 6681. Porto Alegre, RS 90619-900, Brazil

Daniela Frasca
Department of Microbiology and Immunology, University of Miami Miller School of Medicine, P.O. Box 016960 (R-138), Miami, FL 33101, USA; Graduate School of Cell Biology and Development, University of Rome La Sapienza, Rome, Italy

Daniela Monti
Department of Oncology and Experimental Pathology, University of Florence, Via Morgagni 50, Florence, Italy

David Bryder
Stem Cell Aging, Department of Experimental Medical Science, BMC D14, Lund University, 221 84 Lund, Sweden

David L. Lamar
Kathleen B. and Mason I. Lowance Center for Human Immunology, Department of Medicine, Emory University School of Medicine, Room 1003 Woodruff Memorial Research Building, 101 Woodruff Circle, Atlanta, GA, USA

David L. Woodland
Trudeau Institute, Saranac Lake, NY 12983, USA

Deborah K. Dunn-Walters
Department of Immunobiology, 2nd Floor, Borough Wing Guy's, King's and St. Thomas School of Medicine, King's College London, Guy's Hospital, Great Maze Pond, London SE1 9RT, UK

Delphine Sauce
Cellular Immunology laboratory, INSERM U543, Avenir Group, Hopital Pitie-Salpetriere, Université Pierre et Marie Curie-Paris, 91 Bd de l'Hopital, 75013 Paris, France

Dennis Taub
Clinical Immunology Section, Laboratory of Immunology, National Institute on Aging, National Institutes of Health, Baltimore MD 21224, USA

Domenico Lio
Gruppo di Studio sull'Immunosenescenza, Dipartimento di Biopatologia e Metodologie Biomediche, Università di Palermo, Corso Tukory 211, 90134 Palermo, Italy

Donna M. Murasko
Department of Bioscience and Biotechnology, Drexel University, Philadelphia, PA 19104, USA

Douglas E. Faunce
Department of Surgery and The Burn and Shock Trauma Institute; Department of Microbiology and Immunology; Loyola Aging and Immunology Program, Loyola University Medical Center, Stritch School of Medicine, Maywood, IL, USA

Elisa Cevenini
CIG-Interdepartmental Center "L. Galvani", University of Bologna, Via San
Giacomo 12, I-40126 Bologna, Italy

Elisa Nemes
Chair of Immunology, Department of Biomedical Sciences, University of Modena
and Reggio Emilia, Via Campi 287, Modena, 41100, Italy

Elissaveta Naumova
Central Laboratory of Clinical Immunology, University Hospital "Alexandrovska".
1. G. Sofiisky str., 1431 Sofia, Bulgaria

Elizabeth J. Kovacs
The Burn and Shock Trauma Institute and the Immunology and Aging Program;
Department of Surgery; Stritch School of Medicine, Loyola University Medical
Center, 2160 South First Avenue, Maywood, IL 60153, USA

Elizabeth M. Gardner
Department of Bioscience and Biotechnology, Drexel University, Philadelphia, PA
19104, USA; Department of Food Science and Human Nutrition, Michigan State
University, East Lansing, MI 48824, USA

Elke Richartz-Salzburger
Department of Psychiatry and Psychotherapy, University of Tübingen, Osiander-
strasse 24, DE-72076 Tübingen, Germany

Emilie Combet
Section of Medicine and Therapeutics, Western Infirmary, University of Glasgow,
Scotland

Enrico Lugli
Chair of Immunology, Department of Biomedical Sciences, University of Modena
and Reggio Emilia, Via Campi 287, Modena, 41100, Italy

Eric J. Yager
Trudeau Institute, Saranac Lake, NY 12983, USA

Eric T. Clambey
Integrated Department of Immunology, University of Colorado Health Sciences
Center, Denver, CO 80206, USA; Howard Hughes Medical Institute, National
Jewish Research & Medical Center, University of Colorado Health Sciences Center,
Denver, CO 80206, USA

Erika Roat
Chair of Immunology, Department of Biomedical Sciences, University of Modena
and Reggio Emilia, Via Campi 287, Modena, 41100, Italy

Erminia Mariani
Laboratorio di Immunologia e Genetica, Istituto di Ricerca Codivilla-Putti, IOR,
Via di Barbiano 1/10, 40136, Bologna, Italy

Esther Peralbo
Department of Immunology, Reina Sofia University Hospital, University of Córdoba, Spain

Eugenio Mocchegiani
Immunology Ctr., Section Nutrigenomic and Immunosenescence, Res. Dept. INRCA, Ancona, Italy

Ewa Bryl
Department of Pathophysiology, Medical University of Gdańsk, Poland

Ewa Sikora
Molecular Bases of Aging Laboratory, Nencki Institutew of Experimental Biology, Polish Academy of Sciences, Pasteura 3, Warsaw Poland

Flávia Ribeiro
Ageing and Tumour Immunology Group, University of Tübingen, Sektion Transplantionsimmunologie / Immunhämatologie, Waldhörnle Strasse 22, D- 72072 Tübingen, Germany

Florinda Listì
Gruppo di Studio sull'Immunosenescenza, Dipartimento di Biopatologia e Metodo-logie Biomediche, Università di Palermo, Corso Tukory 211, 90134 Palermo, Italy

Frances T. Hakim
Experimental Transplantation and Immunology Branch, Center for Cancer Research, National Cancer Institute, National Institutes of Health, DHHS, Bethesda, MD, USA

Gary Van Zant
Department of Internal Medicine, University of Kentucky, Lexington, Kentucky, USA

Georg Wick
Division of Experimental Pathophysiology and Immunology, Laboratory of Autoimmunity, Biocenter, Innsbruck Medical University, Fritz-Pregl-Strasse 3, A-6020-Innsbruck, Austria

George C. Wang
Division of Geriatric Medicine and Gerontology, Department of Medicine, Johns Hopkins University School of Medicine, 5505 Hopkins Bayview Circle, John R. Burton Pavilion, Baltimore, MD 21224, USA

Gilles Dupuis
Clinical research Center, Department of Biochemistry, Immunology Graduate Programme, Faculty of Medicine, University of Sherbrooke, Sherbrooke, Quebec, Canada

Giuseppina Candore
Gruppo di Studio sull'Immunosenescenza, Dipartimento di Biopatologia e Metodo-logie Biomediche, Università di Palermo, Corso Tukory 211, 90134 Palermo, Italy

Giuseppina Colonna-Romano
Gruppo di Studio sull'Immunosenescenza, Dipartimento di Biopatologia e Meto-
dologie Biomediche, Università di Palermo, Corso Tukory 211, 90134 Palermo,
Italy

Graham Pawelec
Center for Medical Research (ZMF); Tübingen Ageing and Tumour Immunology
Group, Center for Medical Research, University of Tübingen Medical School,
Waldhörnlestr. 22, D-72072 Tübingen, Germany

Hartmut Geiger
Division of Experimental Hematology and Cancer Biology, Cincinnati Children's
Hospital Medical Center and University of Cincinnati College of Medicine, Cincin-
nati, Ohio, USA

Haruyoshi Yamaza
Department of Investigative Pathology, Unit of Basic Medical Science, Graduate
School of Biomedical Sciences, Nagasaki University, Nagasaki, Japan

Hideto Tamura
Division of Hematology, Nippon Medical School, 1-1-5 Sendagi, Bunkyo-ku,
Tokyo 113-8603, Japan

Hui-Chen Hsu
Department of Medicine, 1825 University Blvd, SHELB 310; The University of
Alabama at Birmingham, Birmingham, Alabama 35294, USA

I. Maeve Rea
Department of Geriatric Medicine, Queens University of Belfast, Northern,
Ireland

Ian C. Brett
State University of New York, Stony Brook School of Medicine, Health Sciences
Center, L4, Stony Brook, NY 11794, USA

Inmaculada Gayoso
Department of Immunology, Reina Sofia University Hospital, University of
Córdoba, Spain

Isao Shimokawa
Department of Investigative Pathology, Unit of Basic Medical Science, Graduate
School of Biomedical Sciences, Nagasaki University, Nagasaki, Japan

Jacek M. Witkowski
Department of Pathophysiology, Medical University of Gdansk, Gdansk, Poland

Jacob E. Kohlmeier
Trudeau Institute, Saranac Lake, NY 12983, USA

Jan Strindhall
Department of Natural Science and Biomedicine, School of Health Sciences,
Jönköping University, Box 1026, 551 11 Jönköping, Sweden

Janet E. McElhaney
Geriatrics Research, University of British Columbia, Vancouver, Canada, and Center for Immunotherapy of Cancer and Infectious Diseases, University of Connecticut School of Medicine, Farmington, CT

Janet M. Lord
MRC Centre for Immune Regulation, Division of Immunity and Infection, Birmingham University Medical School, Birmingham B15 2TT, UK

Janko Nikolich-Zugich
Vaccine and Gene Therapy Institute, Department of Molecular Microbiology and Immunology and the Oregon National Primate Research Center, Oregon Health & Science University, Beaverton, OR 97006, USA

Jarrod Dudakov
Monash Immunology and Stem Cell Laboratories, Monash University, Clayton, Australia

Javier G. Casado
Immunology Unit, Department of Physiology, University of Extremadura, Cáceres, Spain

Jean L. Scholz
Department of Pathology and Laboratory Medicine, University of Pennsylvania School of Medicine, 36th and Hamilton Walk, Philadelphia, PA 19104-6082, USA

Jeff Leips
Department of Biological Sciences, 1000 Hilltop Circle, University of Maryland Baltimore County, Baltimore, MD, 21250, USA

Jens M. Nygren
Stem Cell Aging, Deptartment of Experimental Medical Science, BMC I13, Lund University, 221 84 Lund, Sweden

Jeremy Walston
Division of Geriatric Medicine and Gerontology, Department of Medicine, Johns Hopkins University School of Medicine, 5505 Hopkins Bayview Circle, John R. Burton Pavilion, Baltimore, MD 21224, USA

Jessica L. Palmer
Department of Surgery and The Burn and Shock Trauma Institute, Loyola University Medical Center, Stritch School of Medicine, Maywood, IL, USA

Jessica Reiseger
Monash Immunology and Stem Cell Laboratories, Monash University, Clayton, Australia

Jian Chen
Department of Medicine, 1825 University Blvd, SHELB 310; The University of Alabama at Birmingham, Birmingham, Alabama 35294, USA

John D. Mountz
Department of Medicine; Birmingham VA Medical Center, 1825 University Blvd, SHELB 310; The University of Alabama at Birmingham, Birmingham, Alabama 35294, USA

John W. Kappler
Integrated Department of Immunology, University of Colorado Health Sciences Center, Denver, CO 80206, USA; Howard Hughes Medical Institute, National Jewish Research & Medical Center, University of Colorado Health Sciences Center, Denver, CO 80206, USA; Departments of Medicine, University of Colorado Health Sciences Center, Denver, CO 80206, USA; Pharmacology, University of Colorado Health Sciences Center, Denver, CO 80206, USA

Jörg J. Goronzy
Kathleen B. and Mason I. Lowance Center for Human Immunology, Department of Medicine, Emory University School of Medicine, Room 1003 Woodruff Memorial Research Building, 101 Woodruff Circle, Atlanta, GA, USA

Jorge Lloberas
Institute for Research in Biomedicine-University of Barcelona, Josep Samitier 1-5, 08028 Barcelona, Spain

Joseph Lustgarten
Cancer Center Scottsdale, Mayo Clinic Arizona, 13400 East Shea Boulevard Scottsdale, AZ 85259, USA

Jürgen Kempf
Center for Medical Research (ZMF), University of Tübingen Medical School, Waldhörnlestr. 22, D-72072 Tübingen, Germany

Jyoti Misra Sen
Laboratory of Immunology, Clinical Immunology Section, National Institute on Aging, Intramural Research Program, National Institutes of Health, Baltimore, MD, USA

Kate L. Gibson
Department of Immunobiology, 2nd Floor, Borough Wing Guy's, King's and St. Thomas School of Medicine, King's College London, Guy's Hospital, Great Maze Pond, London SE1 9RT, UK

Katerina Vlahos
Monash Immunology and Stem Cell Laboratories, Monash University, Clayton, Australia

Katsuiku Hirokawa
Institute for Health and Life Sciences; Department of Comprehensive Pathology, Tokyo Medical & Dental University; Nakanosogo Hospital, Ascent Myogadani, Kohinata, Bunkyo-ku, Tokyo 112-0006, Japan

Kelly M. Hinkle
Department of Neuroscience, Mayo Clinic College of Medicine, Jacksonville, Florida, USA

Kenneth H. Ely
Trudeau Institute, Saranac Lake, NY 12983, USA

Kiyoyuki Ogata
Division of Hematology, Department of Medicine, Nippon Medical School, 1-1-5 Sendagi, Bunkyo-ku, Tokyo 113-8603, Japan

Ladislas Robert
Université paris 5. Laboratoire de Recherche Ophtalmologique., 1 place du Parvis Notre Dame, 75181 Paris cedex 04, France

Lara Gibellini
Chair of Immunology, Department of Biomedical Sciences, University of Modena and Reggio Emilia, Via Campi 287, Modena, 41100, Italy

Laura Bucci
Department of Experimental Pathology, University of Bologna, Via San Giacomo 12, I-40126 Bologna, Italy

Laura Celani
CIG-Interdepartmental Center "L. Galvani", University of Bologna, Via San Giacomo 12, I-40126 Bologna, Italy

Leonarda Troiano
Chair of Immunology, Department of Biomedical Sciences, University of Modena and Reggio Emilia, Via Campi 287, Modena, 41100, Italy

Letizia Scola
Gruppo di Studio sull'Immunosenescenza, Dipartimento di Biopatologia e Metodologie Biomediche, Università di Palermo, Corso Tukory 211, 90134 Palermo, Italy

Lia Ginaldi
Department of Internal Medicine and Public Health, University of L'Aquila, L'Aquila, Italy

Linda Bertoncelli
Chair of Immunology, Department of Biomedical Sciences, University of Modena and Reggio Emilia, Via Campi 287, Modena, 41100, Italy

Linda P. Fried
Division of Geriatric Medicine and Gerontology and Center on Aging and Health, Johns Hopkins University School of Medicine, Baltimore, Maryland, USA

Lothar Rink
Institute for Immunology, RWTH Aachen University Hospital, Pauwelsstr. 30, 52074 Aachen, Germany

Lucia P. Mengoli
Department of Internal Medicine and Public Health, University of L'Aquila, L'Aquila, Italy

M. Luisa Pita
Department of Immunology, Reina Sofia University Hospital, University of Córdoba, Spain

Marcello Pinti
Chair of Immunology, Department of Biomedical Sciences, University of Modena and Reggio Emilia, Via Campi 287, Modena, 41100, Italy

Marcia A. Blackman
Trudeau Institute, Saranac Lake, NY 12983, USA

Marco Malavolta
Immunology Ctr., Section Nutrigenomic and Immunosenescence, Res. Dept. INRCA, Ancona, Italy

Maria Paola Grimaldi
Gruppo di Studio sull'Immunosenescenza, Dipartimento di Biopatologia e Metodologie Biomediche, Università di Palermo, Corso Tukory 211, 90134 Palermo, Italy

Marilyn Armstrong
Department of Geriatric Medicine, Queens University Belfast, Belfast, Ireland, UK

Marius Wick
Department of Radiology, Innsbruck Medical University, Anichstrasse 35, A-6020 Innsbruck, Austria

Masanobu Kitagawa
Department of Comprehensive Pathology, Aging and Developmental Sciences, Graduate School, Tokyo Medical and Dental University, 1-5-45 Yushima, Bunkyo-ku, Tokyo 113-8519, Japan

Masanori Utsuyama
Institute for Health and Life Sciences; Department of Comprehensive Pathology, Tokyo Medical & Dental University, Ascent Myogadani 4F, 4-4-22, Kohinata, Bunkyo-ku, Tokyo 112-0006, Japan

Massimo De Martinis
Department of Internal Medicine and Public Health, University of L'Aquila, L'Aquila, Italy

Mauro Provinciali
Laboratory of Tumour Immunology, INRCA Res. Dept., Via Birarelli 8, 60121 Ancona, Italy

Maximilian Zeyda
Department Internal Medicine III, Medical University of Vienna, Währinger Gürtel 18-20, A-1090 Vienna, Austria

Michael P. Cancro
Department of Pathology and Laboratory Medicine, University of Pennsylvania School of Medicine, 36th and Hamilton Walk, Philadelphia, PA 19104-6082, USA

Milena Ivanova
Central Laboratory of Clinical Immunology, University Hospital "Alexandrovska". 1. G. Sofiisky str., 1431 Sofia, Bulgaria

Milena Nasi
Chair of Immunology, Department of Biomedical Sciences, University of Modena and Reggio Emilia, Via Campi 287, Modena, 41100, Italy

Miriam Capri
Department of Experimental Pathology, University of Bologna, Via San Giacomo 12, I-40126 Bologna, Italy; CIG-Interdepartmental Center "L. Galvani", University of Bologna, Via San Giacomo 12, I-40126 Bologna, Italy

Moisés E. Bauer
Faculdade de Biociências and Instituto de Pesquisas Biomédicas, Pontifícia Universidade Católica do Rio Grande do Sul (PUCRS), Av. Ipiranga 6690, 2° andar. P.O. Box 1429. Porto Alegre, RS 90.610-000, Brazil

Nan-Ping Weng
Laboratory of Immunology, National Institute on Aging, National Institutes of Health, Baltimore, MD, USA

Naozumi Ishimaru
Department of Oral Molecular Pathology, Institute of Health Biosciences, The University of Tokushima Graduate School, 3 Kuramotocho, Tokushima 770-8504, Japan

Natalie Seach
Monash Immunology and Stem Cell Laboratories, Monash University, Clayton, Australia

Niklas Koehler
Department of Psychiatry and Psychotherapy, University of Tübingen, Osiander-strasse 24, DE-72076 Tübingen, Germany

Noweeda Mirza
Cancer Center Scottsdale, Mayo Clinic Arizona, 13400 East Shea Boulevard Scottsdale, AZ 85259, USA

Olivier Lesur
Clinical research Center, Graduate Immunology Program, Division of Pulmonology, Department of Medicine, Faculty of Medicine, University of Sherbrooke, Sherbrooke, Quebec, Canada

Owen A. Ross
Department of Geriatric Medicine, Queens University Belfast, Belfast, Irelan d, UK; Department of Neuroscience, Mayo Clinic College of Medicine, Jacksonville, Florida, USA

Paul Moss
Institute for Cancer Studies, University of Birmingham, Vincent Drive, Birmingham B 15 2TT, UK

Pazit Beckerman
University Hospital Kerem, The Department of Medicine at the Hadassah Ein, Jerusalem, Isreal

Peter Uciechowski
Institute for Immunology, RWTH Aachen University Hospital, Pauwelsstr. 30, 52074 Aachen, Germany

Philippa Marrack
Integrated Department of Immunology, University of Colorado Health Sciences Center, Denver, CO 80206, USA; Howard Hughes Medical Institute, National Jewish Research & Medical Center, University of Colorado Health Sciences Center, Denver, CO 80206, USA; Departments of Medicine, University of Colorado Health Sciences Center, Denver, CO 80206, USA; Pharmacology, University of Colorado Health Sciences Center, Denver, CO 80206, USA; Biochemistry and Molecular Genetics, University of Colorado Health Sciences Center, Denver, CO 80206, USA

Piotr Trzonkowski
Laboratory of Experimental Transplantology, Department of Histology and Immunology, Medical University of Gdańsk, Ul. Dębinki 1, 80-211 Gdańsk, Poland

Qing Yu
Laboratory of Immunology, Clinical Immunology Section, National Institute on Aging, Intramural Research Program, National Institutes of Health, Baltimore, MD, USA

Rafael Solana
Department of Immunology, Reina Sofia University Hospital, University of Córdoba, Spain

Raquel Tarazona
Immunology Unit, Department of Physiology, University of Extremadura, Cáceres, Spain

Richard Aspinall
Department of Immunology, Imperial College London, Faculty of Investigative Sciences, Chelsea and Westminster Campus, 369 Fulham Road, London, UK

Richard Boyd
Monash Immunology and Stem Cell Laboratories, Monash University, Clayton, Australia

Richard L. Riley
Department of Microbiology and Immunology, University of Miami Miller School of Medicine, P.O. Box 016960 (R-138), Miami, FL 33101, USA

Rita B. Effros
Department of Pathology & Laboratory Medicine, David Geffen School of Medicine at UCLA, 10833 Le Conte Avenue, Los Angeles, CA 90095-1732, USA

Rita Ostan
Department of Oncology and Experimental Pathology, University of Florence, Via Morgagni 50, Florence, Italy

Roberta Ferraresi
Chair of Immunology, Department of Biomedical Sciences, University of Modena and Reggio Emilia, Via Campi 287, Modena, 41100, Italy

Sara Morgado
Immunology Unit, Department of Physiology, University of Extremadura, Cáceres, Spain

Sean X. Leng
Division of Geriatric Medicine and Gerontology and Center on Aging and Health, Johns Hopkins University School of Medicine, Baltimore, Maryland, USA

Sergey G. Rudnev
Institute of Numerical Mathematics, Russian Academy of Sciences, Moscow, Russia

Simona Neri
Laboratorio di Immunologia e Genetica, Istituto di Ricerca Codivilla-Putti, IOR, Via di Barbiano 1/10, 40136, Bologna, Italy

Sirisha Karri
Division of Nutritional Sciences, The University of Texas, Austin, TX 78712, USA

Sonya Vasto
Gruppo di Studio sull'Immunosenescenza, Dipartimento di Biopatologia e Metodologie Biomediche, Università di Palermo, Corso Tukory 211, 90134 Palermo, Italy

Stefano Salvioli
Department of Experimental Pathology, University of Bologna, Via San Giacomo 12, I-40126 Bologna, Italy; CIG-Interdepartmental Center "L. Galvani", University of Bologna, Via San Giacomo 12, I-40126 Bologna, Italy

Steven Castle
Geriatric Research Education and Clinical Center (GRECC) VA Greater Los Ange-
les Healthcare system, UCLA School of Medicine, 11301 Wilshire Boulvard, Los
Angeles, CA, 90073, USA

Sudhanshu Agrawal
Division of Basic and Clinical Immunology, University of California, Irvine, CA
92697, USA

Sudhir Gupta
Division of Basic and Clinical Immunology, University of California, Irvine, CA
92697, USA

Susan E. McNerlan
Department of Geriatric Medicine, Queens University Belfast, Belfast, Ireland,
UK

Takuya Chiba
Department of Investigative Pathology, Unit of Basic Medical Science, Graduate
School of Biomedical Sciences, Nagasaki University, Nagasaki, Japan

Tamas Fulop
Centre de recherche sur le vieillissement; Research Center on Aging, Department of
Medicine, Immunology Graduate Programme, Faculty of Medicine, University of
Sherbrooke, Sherbrooke, Quebec, Canada

Tatiana A. Sannikova
Institute of Numerical Mathematics, Russian Academy of Sciences, Moscow,
Russia

Thomas M. Stulnig
Department Internal Medicine III, Medical University of Vienna, Währinger Gürtel
18-20, A-1090 Vienna, Austria

Toshimitsu Komatsu
Department of Investigative Pathology, Unit of Basic Medical Science, Graduate
School of Biomedical Sciences, Nagasaki University, Nagasaki, Japan

Vanessa Nomellini
The Burn and Shock Trauma Institute and the Immunology and Aging Program;
Stritch School of Medicine, Loyola University Medical Center, 2160 South First
Avenue, Maywood, IL 60153, USA

Victor Appay
Cellular Immunology laboratory, INSERM U543, Avenir Group, Hopital Pitie-Sal-
petriere, Université Pierre et Marie Curie-Paris, 91 Bd de l'Hopital, 75013 Paris,
France

Wayne A. Mitchell
Department of Immunology, Imperial College London, Faculty of Investigative
Sciences, Chelsea and Westminster Campus, 369 Fulham Road, London, UK

Wiebke Arlt
Division of Medical Sciences, University of Birmingham, Birmingham B15 2TT, UK

William J. Quinn III
Department of Pathology and Laboratory Medicine, University of Pennsylvania School of Medicine, 36th and Hamilton Walk, Philadelphia, PA 19104-6082, USA

Yoshio Hayashi
Department of Oral Molecular Pathology, Institute of Health Biosciences, The University of Tokushima Graduate School, 3 Kuramotocho, Tokushima 770-8504, Japan

Yuko Kikuchi
Institute for Health and Life Sciences, Department of Comprehensive Pathology, Tokyo Medical & Dental University, Ascent Myogadani, Kohinata, Bunkyo-ku, Tokyo 112-0006, Japan

Part I
Methods and Models for Studying Immunosenescence

The Immune Risk Profile and Associated Parameters in Late Life: Lessons from the OCTO and NONA Longitudinal Studies

Anders Wikby, Jan Strindhall and Boo Johansson

Contents

Abstract: The OCTO Immune Longitudinal Study is a population-based study of ageing in a sample of 102 Swedish octogenarians with the aim to explore age changes of the immune system using a sample selected for good health. Data collection was performed in 1989, 1990, 1991 and 1997. An Immune Risk Profile (IRP) associated with increased mortality was characterized by high CD8+, low CD4+ T-cell counts and a poor T-cell proliferative response, inversion of the CD4/CD8 ratio and evidence of persistent cytomegalovirus infection was identified. The subsequent NONA Immune Longitudinal Study of 138 Swedish nonagenarians was performed in 1999, 2001, 2003, and 2005, not excluding individuals due to compromised health. The overall aim was to examine predictive factors for longevity and to further investigate in greater depth the immune risk profile identified in the OCTO Immune Study in the context of functional and disability parameters also examined

A. Wikby (✉) · J. Strindhall
Department of Natural Science and Biomedicine
School of Health Sciences
Jönköping University
Box 1026, 551 11 Jönköping, Sweden
Tel: +46-381-35101
Fax: + 46-381-36341
E-mail: anders.wikby@hhj.hj.se

B. Johansson
Institute of Gerontology, School of Health Sciences
Jönköping University, Box 1026, 551 11 Jönköping
Sweden, and Department of Psychology, Göteborg University
Box 500, 405 30 Göteborg, Sweden

T. Fulop et al. (eds.), *Handbook on Immunosenescence*,
DOI 10.1007/ 978-1-4020-9062-2_1, © Springer Science+Business Media B.V. 2009

in the NONA. The immune panel included the analysis of T-cell subsets, inflammatory markers, virus serology, cytokines, TCR clonotype mapping, and functional and phenotypic analysis of virus specific CD8+ cells by HLA/peptide multimers, in collaborations between participants of the EU funded T-CIA project.

The present chapter report findings from the longitudinal studies of Swedish octo-nonagenarians with focus on IRP and its associations with persistent virus infection, CD8+ T-cell differentiation, cytokines, cognitive functioning, inflammatory activity, virus specific CD8+ cells, CD8+ T-cell clonal expansions and longevity. It also reports on low grade inflammation processes of importance in predicting longevity in the very late life.

Keywords: Immune risk profiles • Immunosenescence • Longitudinal studies • T-cells

1 Introduction

The very old constitute the fastest growing age segment in developed countries. From a societal and population perspective, this demographic trend is also accompanied by an increase in the number of very old individuals with compromised health and significant requirements for service and health care. From a physiological perspective, the robustness of the immune system is particularly important in this age segment, considering the fact that the incidence of death due to infection diseases seems to continue to increase although mortality related to cardiovascular disease and cancer may level off in many populations (Vasto et al. 2007).

Immune studies of elderly populations, however, so far have mainly been conducted on individuals in their 60s and 70s. Few studies have focused on samples over 80 years and still fewer have employed longitudinal designs that allow studies of intra-individual change (Pawelec et al. 2005). In the Swedish OCTO and NONA Immune Longitudinal Studies (Wikby et al. 1994, 2002), we deliberately examined individuals in very late life because of the substantially elevated risk for compromised health, morbidity, and mortality. The overall aim was to provide better understanding of processes and mechanisms related to intra-individual change in various parts of the immune system regulation in very late life. An aim was also to identify presumptive predictors for subsequent mortality and clinical parameters related to the substantial morbidity/comorbidity observed in late life. From a clinical perspective detection of predictive markers may enable interventions that could assist in various improvements of quality of life for individuals in this rapidly growing age segment.

The OCTO Immune Longitudinal Study is a population-based study of ageing and the immune system in a sample of Swedish octogenarians (Wikby et al. 1994). It was started in 1989 in Jönköping, Sweden, as a collaboration between researchers at the Institute of Gerontology and the Department of Natural Science and Biomedicine, School of Health Sciences, Jönköping University, the Department of Microbiology, Hospital of Ryhov, Jönköping and the Department of Veterinary Science, Penn State University, USA and ended in 1997 when the vast majority participants were deceased. The subsequent NONA Immune Longitudinal Study of nonagenarians was initiated in 1999 to extend and refine findings from the OCTO Immune Longitudinal Study identifying an Immune Risk Profile (IRP) associated with an elevated mortality rate (Wikby et al. 2002). The NONA immune also became part of the EU supported programs *Immunology and Ageing in Europe, ImAginE,* (Pawelec, Caruso 2003) and *T cell immunity and ageing, T-CIA,* (Koch et al. 2005) creating collaborations between the NONA immune researchers and several European laboratories participating in these networks. The OCTO-NONA Immune Longitudinal Studies have investigated predictive factors for longevity with focus on immune risk profiles in a context of functional and disability health parameters of importance in late life. The present review summarizes some of the main findings and lessons learned from these studies.

2   Methodological Design and Sampling Considerations in Ageing Studies

2.1   Design Considerations

First we address the significant design and sampling considerations that directed our research. The two methods used in population-based studies of ageing are the cross-sectional and longitudinal designs (Wikby et al. 2003). The most common design is the cross-sectional, in which two or more age groups are compared at a single occasion. Age changes are typically inferred from the observed age differences in mean values. This design provides a procedure that is logistically easy and fast and less expensive than the longitudinal design. However, great caution is necessary in the interpretation of cross-sectional data since age differences may be confounded by the fact that birth-cohorts have been exposed to various environmental exposures and socio-cultural influences (Wikby et al. 2003; Pawelec 2006). Another confound that become more of an issue with age is that of selective mortality (Wikby et al. 2003). As a study population ages it becomes gradually more selected, since deaths do not occur at random. For example, if a high value in a variable is deleterious, death is likely to occur first in individuals with high values and last in individuals with low values. In a cross-sectional study an observed difference in mean values between age groups may be incorrectly interpreted as a real age change rather than as an effect of selective mortality. Many studies have characterized changes in the immune system with age, but a number of these have yielded conflicting results, partly due to the fact that the vast majority of these studies are cross-sectional (Wikby et al. 2003).

In a longitudinal design (Wikby et al. 2003) individuals are followed across time, usually with a number of years in between measurement occasions. This allows the detection of intra-individual change and minimizes many of the confounding artefacts likely to emerge in the cross-sectional design. Although the longitudinal design represents the superior alternative for conducting ageing research, the use of this design has been very limited, particularly in studies of the immune system. The main reason is that such studies are expensive and require considerable effort, financial support, and commitment of personnel. In addition, longitudinal studies require careful coordination, standardised procedures, and control of studied panels to avoid dropouts. A main caution to note in the use of a longitudinal design is the involvement of a possible confounding between age and time of measurement effects. Time of measurement confounding includes numerous factors, such as the motivation and interest of the participating subjects, experimenter effects including changes in personnel and their motivation, and in the methods, techniques and essays used across time. Many of these problems can be compensated for by including a younger group for comparisons across measurement occasions. The immune system changes that occur across times of measurement will then be negligible in the healthy young people compared to the very old. Also, restricted time periods between the measurements and the use of identical methods will prevent time of measurement effects.

2.2 Sampling Considerations

Advancing age is typically accompanied by an increased prevalence of compromised health and diseases (Jeune 2002). This is one of the primary problems in the selection and definition of a sample in population-based studies of ageing. To overcome this problem, most studies have used various selection schemes to exclude individuals with underlying diseases from participation in studies of the immune system. The stringent *SENIEUR* Protocol (Ligthart et al. 1984) represents an example of a widespread application of a set of exclusion criteria used to select individuals in good health, to be able to distinguish between age changes caused by *primary ageing* and *secondary ageing*, i.e. by diseases. Noteworthy, the exclusion of *non-SENIEUR* individuals will, however, result in a study of less than 10% of a population among individuals aged over 80 years and older (Pawelec et al. 2001). Another way to diminish confounding between primary ageing effects and disease has been to employ exclusion criteria tailored to the experimental situation (Hallgren et al. 1988), i.e. in immune studies to exclude individuals that have immune related diseases or who use drugs that affect the immune system. Such a strategy was used in the OCTO Immune Longitudinal Study but will also generate a select sample. In our case, about 50% in a population aged over 80 years were excluded (Wikby et al. 1994).

A way to overcome some of the selection problems is to examine a population-based sample, combined with careful continuous evaluation of individual health parameters (Nilsson et al. 2003). This was the approach taken in the NONA Immune Longitudinal Study. The clinical variables needed for the evaluation of individual health and morbidity are then of considerable value in the comparison of findings from the application of various protocols and in the categorization of individuals into subgroups according to their health status (Nilsson et al. 2003). Thus, the significance of a change in health status is included rather than excluded as an important consideration in these aging studies.

3 The OCTO and NONA Immune Longitudinal Studies

3.1 The OCTO Immune Study

The OCTO Immune Longitudinal Study was an integrated part of the OCTO Longitudinal Study of biobehavioral ageing, in Jönköping, Sweden. The municipality of Jönköping has 122 000 inhabitants and is situated in South-central part of Sweden. The aim of the OCTO immune was to explore age changes in the immune system in Swedish octogenarians relative to an array of medical, biobehavioral, and social variables (Wikby et al. 1994).

Census data was used to identify octogenarians living in Jönköping and born in 1897, 1899, 1901, and 1903. A non-proportional sample that composed of 100 persons in each of the birth-cohorts was recruited. From these 400 individuals, 324 were examined in the first wave in 1987/1988 of the OCTO study. The persons were then at the ages of 84, 86, 88, and 90 years old. At the second wave of the study, the OCTO Immune Longitudinal Study was initiated. Of the 324 examined at baseline of the OCTO, 96 were deceased before the start of the second wave of this study. Another 15 declined to participate, giving a total number of potential participants of 213 for the OCTO immune.

Exclusion criteria were set to diminish confound between ageing, disease, and medications and to secure reliable psychosocial self-reports. Potential candidates were included if they:

- Were noninstitutionalized
- Had normal cognition according to neuropsychological tests (Johansson et al. 1992)
- Were not on a drug regimen that may influence the immune system.

These exclusion criteria were similar to those of Hallgren et al. (1988). Of the potential 213 individuals, 110 met inclusion criteria. Of these, 102 individuals participated in the first wave. Sixty-nine individuals were available throughout the three waves in the longitudinal analysis and 23 participated in the longitudinal analysis over all four time-points, T1 (1989), T2 (1990), T3 (1991), and T4 (1997) (Table 1). Nonparticipation at the various measurement occasions was mainly due to mortality in the sample. Fourteen healthy middle-aged volunteers (39 years SD±5.8) of men and women working in the laboratories at Ryhov Hospital in Jönköping were included across the measurement occasions for comparative reasons.

A. Wikby et al.

Table 1   Characteristics of individuals included in the OCTO Immune Longitudinal Study

Occasion (Time)	Year	Number of individuals investigated	Age (years)	
			Mean	Range
1	1989	102	88	86–92
2	1990	83	89	87–93
3	1991	69	90	88–94
4	1997	23	95	94–100

The very old individuals were examined in their place of residence. Blood samples were drawn in the morning between 8:00 and 10:00 (a.m.). The following immune system parameters were investigated:

- Complete blood cell count
- Differential WBC count
- Antibody defined T and B cell surface molecules using three colour flow cytometry
- Proliferative response of PBMC using a mitogen stimulation assay with ConA in cell culture
- Interleukin 2 production
- Cytomegalovirus (CMV) and Herpes simplex serology.

3.2   The NONA Immune Study

Findings from the OCTO Immune Longitudinal Study constituted the background for the subsequent ongoing NONA Immune Longitudinal Study of nonagenarian individuals also living in the municipality of Jönköping (Wikby et al. 2002). The NONA immune is an integrated part of the NONA Longitudinal Study initiated to examine the disablement process in late life. The overall aim in the NONA immune is to examine predictive factors for longevity in the very old and to further investigate in greater depth the immune risk profile identified in the OCTO immune. The aim is also to consider immune data in the context of functional and disability parameters examined in the overall NONA. The overall study includes measurements of the following functional and disability domains:

- Physical and mental health
- Cognitive functioning
- Personal control/coping
- Social networks
- Provision of service
- Care and everyday functioning capacity.

The NONA immune examines a population-based random sample without excluding individuals due to compromised health, but to include a continuous evaluation of various individual health parameters (Nilsson et al. 2003). Individuals were drawn from the population (census) register of Jönköping. A nonproportional random sampling procedure was employed, including all individuals permanently residing in the municipality, with the goal to have individuals aged 86, 90, and 94 years old. The sampling frame was defined on the available census information in September 1999. As the number of available subjects in the oldest birth cohort was limited, a few subjects were also included from the birth cohorts of 1904 and 1906. Blood samples for the immune system analysis were drawn in 138 individuals, of whom 42 belonged to the oldest birth cohort, 47 were 90-years, and 49 86-years old. Data collections were made using two-year inter-occasion intervals in 1999, 2001, 2003, and 2005.

The mean age of the sample at baseline was 89.8 years with a total proportion of women of 70%. While about 60% of them lived in an ordinary housing, 40% resided in a sheltered housing or in institution. A comparison between individuals who participated in the in-person testing part of the NONA study ($n=157$), and those who accepted that blood was drawn ($n=138$), indicated no significant differences for demographics or overall ratings of physical and mental health. In the second wave, 61% of individuals participated, at the third 40%, and at the fourth only 22%. Nonparticipation at the various measurement occasions was mainly due to mortality. A younger group of 22 healthy middle-aged men and women working at the Ryhov Hospital in Jönköping participated (mean age 44.7, SD=8.9 at baseline) across measurement occasions for the sake of comparison. Characteristics of the individuals participating in the NONA Immune Longitudinal Study are summarised in Table 2.

Health was defined based on medical records and from clinical chemistry data, supplemented with information gathered in a health interview that focused on diagnosed illness, current symptoms, and use of medications (Nilsson et al. 2003). The neuropsychological battery used to identify cognitive impairment included the Mini-Mental State Examination (MMSE) and the Memory-In-Reality (MIR) test (Folstein et al. 1975, Johansson 1988/1989). MMSE is a screening device used in epidemiological studies to identify cognitive impairment. The MIR test comprises of a naming condition for 10 common real-life objects, followed by showing a three-dimensional model of an apartment. The participants are then asked to place the objects in the different rooms according to personal preferences. Following a distraction, a recall test is administered, followed by a recognition task for items not recalled. In the NONA Immune Longitudinal Study we used the following three

Table 2   Characteristics of the subjects participating in the NONA Immune Longitudinal Study

Occasion (year)	No. of subjects investigated	Proportion of women (%)	Age (years)	
			Mean	Range
1999	138	70	89.8	86–95
2001	84	69	91.6	88–97
2003	55	69	93.2	90–99
2005	31	81	94.7	92–101

cognitive status categories: 1) cognitive intact, 2) mild cognitive dysfunction or questionable cases (MCD, evidence of compromised memory/cognition, not fully meeting DMC-IV criteria for dementia, APA, 1994), and dementia (according to DMS-IV criteria, APA 1994). The two latter diagnostic categories were pooled under the category of "cognitive impairment" and compared with those rated as cognitively intact.

Subjects were examined in their place of residence by trained Registered Nurses with extensive experience of working with the elderly. The tests and interviews took about 3 hours, including breaks, for individuals who were able to participate in all parts. The blood samples were drawn in the morning between 09:00 and 10:00. The following immune and clinical components are studied in the NONA Immune Longitudinal Study:

- Complete blood cell count
- Differential WBC count
- Proteins, albumin, transthyretin, C-Reactive Protein, orosomucoid, haptoglobulin,
- IgG, IgM, IgA, urea, cystatinC, creatinine as indicators of malnutrition, inflammation or kidney disease
- Antibody defined T-cell surface molecules of T, NKT, NK cell populations, using three colour flow cytometry
- Secretion of cytokines, IL-2, IL-6, IL-10, interferon-gamma
- CMV, EBV and Herpes simplex serology
- MHC/peptide tetramers to analyze the number of CMV and EBV specific CD8+ cells
- TCR clonotype mapping with Denaturing Gradient Gel Electrophoresis (DGGE), including RNA extraction, cDNA synthesis and amplification by use of a primer panel amplifying the 24 BV region families covering a majority of TCR's. The resulting DNA fragments are separated by DGGE and expanded clones are identified as distinct bands on a gel (thorStraten et al. 1998).

4   Results and Discussion

4.1   The OCTO Immune Study

In the OCTO Immune Longitudinal Study we were able to identify an immune risk profile by multiple comparisons of individuals grouped by homogeneity of certain combinations of adaptive immune system parameters (Ferguson et al. 1995). These cluster analysis use profile similarities to group individuals when the number and nature of the groups are not known in advance, ideal in the exploration of complex systems like the immune system. The analysis was employed to determine groups based on immune functioning and T-cell subpopulations using the mitogen response to Concanavalin A, and the percentages of CD3, CD4, CD8, and CD19 positive cells. The groups identified by cluster analysis were then compared with respect to their impact on survival-non-survival by chi-square analysis. This analysis of immune data at baseline revealed an Immune Risk Profile (IRP) predictive of subsequent 2-year mortality (Ferguson et al. 1995). An IRP cluster, designated cluster 1, was characterized by immune parameters that consisted of high levels of CD8+ T-cells, low levels of CD4+ and CD19+ T-cells, and poor proliferative mitogen response to ConA (Table 3). No such association could be found using common methods for univariate analysis.

The result demonstrated that additional individuals developed the IRP by increases in the CD8+ cells as well as decreases in the CD4+ cells and CD4/CD8 ratio between baseline and a 2-year follow-up (Wikby et al. 1998). At that time the IRP individuals again were found to have increased subsequent 2-year mortality. Interestingly, we found that the IRP could be defined by using only the inverted CD4/CD8 ratio, since this sole marker was strongly associated with the IRP defined by the cluster of parameters (Wikby et al. 1998).

The results also showed that 31% individuals out of the 102 participating either had at baseline (16%) or developed (15%) an Immune Risk Profile during the 8-year longitudinal period of the study (Olsson et al. 2000). Noteworthy, individuals who belonged to the IRP category at baseline or moved into that category over the 8 years never moved out from this elevated mortality risk group (Olsson et al. 2000).

Although the significance for changes leading to a skewed CD4/CD8 ratio in the IRP was not well understood at the time of our initial exploration, the relationship observed between a reduced functional immune response and mortality had indeed been described in several previous studies. It was reported in humans that with age the lack of a response to three mitogens: the T-cell mitogens concanavalin A, phytohemagglutin, and the T-dependent B-cell mitogen, pokeweed, were associated with increased mortality (Murasko et al. 1987). In another study of individuals older than 80 years of age, it was found that anergic aged individuals had a 2-year mortality rate of 80% compared to 35% in those who were nonanergic (Roberts-Thomson et al. 1974). A third study examined the relation between anergy and all cause mortality in healthy individuals above 60 years of age (Wayne et al. 1990). The study showed that anergy, defined as a decreased delayed type hypersensitivity (DTH) response in a skin test to four common recall antigens, was associated with nonsurvival.

Since our study at baseline did not analyse subsets of CD4 and CD8 T-cells on the basis of other phenotypic markers, the changes in the CD4/CD8 balance in IRP individuals was not well characterized. In 2000 various subsets of CD4 and

Table 3 Statistical description of variables used in the formation of a three cluster solution

Cluster (n)	Mitogen response/DPM	CD3+/%	CD4+/%	CD8+/%	CD19+/%
1 (14)[a]	11077 (8413)[b]	62.6 (14.8)	30.8 (4.3)	43.3 (8.9)	5.5 (2.6)
2 (36)	16915 (11491)	75.6 (7.6)	47.9 (12.1)	26.5 (5.9)	8.4 (4.1)
3 (39)	29681 (14427)	54.5 (12.3)	42.4 (9.8)	20.5 (6.9)	12.5 (7.1)

[a] IRP cluster predicting non-survival
[b] Mean (SD)

CD8 were therefore included in the study (Olsson et al. 2000). The results indicated immune system changes that suggested a loss of T-cell homeostasis, as reflected by a substantial increase in the number of CD8 cells with parallel decrease in the number of CD4 cells in individuals with an inverted CD4/CD8 ratio. The changes were apparent in a number of T-cell subsets, with significant increases in the levels of CD8+CD28- cells, in particular, demonstrating that differentiated effector/memory CD8+ cells are disproportionately represented in this cell population. These cells has been shown by others have shortened telomers, suggesting an extensive history of replication (Effros 2007). Initially it was surprisingly found that these homeostatic T-cell changes associated with an inverted CD4/CD8 ratio was associated with persistent CMV infection, prevalent (90%) in the very old (Olsson et al. 2000). Importantly, our studies showed no evidence of a relationship of these T-cell changes and other viruses, Herpes simplex and Epstein Barr viruses, indicating an unique impact of CMV on the immune system. This result was unexpected since the carriage of CMV had long been considered to be quite harmless to individuals with a functional immune system. The finding thus suggested that the changes in the T-cell balance among IRP subjects at least partly is produced by the generation of CD8+ effector/memory cells against persistent CMV infection and subsequent homeostatic decreases in the CD4+ and CD4/CD8 ratio. This conclusion was supported by tetramer technology demonstrating significant expansions of CD8+ T-cells specific for the CMV_{NLV} peptide in HLA-A2 individuals to be associated with both age and the IRP (Ouyang et al. 2004).

4.2   The NONA Immune Study

Results from the OCTO Immune Longitudinal Study provided the basis for the subsequent Swedish NONA Immune Longitudinal Study (Wikby et al. 2002) and potentials to further advance and refine our knowledge about various predictive factors for longevity but still with special focus on the Immune Risk Profiles (IRP's). The NONA sample provided a broader set of functional and disability parameters, including morbidity, cognitive impairment and chronic viral infection, to be examined in relation to longitudinal changes in inflammatory parameters, the CD8+ T-cell phenotype and differentiation, and CD8+ T-cell clonal expansion.

4.2.1   Immune Parameters and Morbidity

Studies of the immune system in very old individuals are most commonly performed on highly selected samples by the use of selection protocols excluding individuals with conditions that influence the immune system (Nilsson et al. 2003). Among a great variety of protocols the SENIEUR protocol represent the most commonly used and accepted with a comprehensive set of health and laboratory criteria for sample selection aiming at the distinguishing between ageing per se and those associated with morbidity (Lighthart et al. 1984). Another selection protocol used in the studies of ageing and the immune system, used in the Swedish OCTO Immune Longitudinal Study, is that proposed by Hallgren et al (1988). This protocol excludes individuals with diseases and other conditions known to affect specifically the immune system to tailor the study to its particular purpose. In the NONA Immune Longitudinal Study a slightly modified SENIEUR and Hallgren protocol were used to characterize the sample according to health status (Nilsson et al. 2003). This permitted us to distinguish subgroups of very healthy, moderately healthy and frail individuals for various immune system parameter comparisons.

The modified SENIEUR protocol excluded 90.6% of the NONA immune sample at baseline, indicating that only 9.4% were rated as *very healthy*. The use of the original protocol, suggesting additional laboratory analysis for exclusion, would probably have excluded even more individuals, demonstrating the need for using less stringent criteria in studies of the immune system in later life to avoid studies of only highly selected, nonrepresentative samples. Thirty-eight (27.5%) participants, selected from those being not very healthy and defined as *moderately healthy*, met the criteria used in the previous OCTO Immune Longitudinal Study of not residing in an institution, not being demented, and not using medication known to affect the immune system. The remaining sample (63%) comprised *frail* individuals not meeting the above health criteria (Nilsson et al. 2003).

Applying the five most common exclusion criteria, cardiac insufficiency, medication, laboratory data, urea and malignancy, the modified SENIEUR protocol excluded 87% of the original sample (Nilsson et al. 2003). When the OCTO Immune protocol was applied, medications was found to be the most common criterion, excluding 43%, institutionalisation the second, excluding 39%, and cognitive dysfunction the third, excluding 14%. Among various diseases conditions cardiac insufficiency (51%), malignancy (15%), dementia (14%), chronic obstructive pulmonary disease (12%), diabetes mellitus (11%), rheumatoid arthritis (9%), hypothyroidism (6%) and pernicious anaemia (6%) constituted the eight most prevalent diagnoses. These figures demonstrate the considerable prevalence of morbidity and comorbidity in a representative sample of very old individuals (Nilsson et al. 2003).

A comparison of the number of T-cells across the subgroups of very healthy, moderately healthy and frail indicated no group differences for subsets characteristic of the immune risk profile, previously identified in octogenarians (Nilsson et al. 2003). Interestingly, the IRP might thus serve as a significant biomarker of ageing, independent of overall health status. This is further confirmed by results demonstrating that clusters of immune markers can predict longevity in noninbred mice independently of health conditions (Miller 2001).

4.2.2 Immune Risk Profile, Cognitive Impairment and Mortality

Prevalence and incidence of cognitive impairment and dementia become substantial in very old people. Studies have shown that compromised cognition is significantly related to proximity of death by a twofold increased mortality risk among demented octogenarians and nonagenarians (Johansson and Zarit 1997; Wilson et al. 2003). There is also considerable evidence suggesting interactions between the nervous and innate immune systems, in which cytokines have a central role as communicators (Wilson et al. 2003). Studies have suggested that higher levels of interleukin 6 (IL-6) are significantly associated with poorer cognitive function and predict future cognitive decline among the elderly (Marsland et al. 2006). In pathological conditions such as ischemia and Alzheimer's disease, microglia cells in the brain seem to respond to injury by producing increased levels of particularly the proinflammatory cytokines interleukin 1 (IL-1) and the multifunctional IL-6 (Tarkowski 2002).

Analysis of mortality in the very old NONA immune individuals (n=138) confirmed our previous findings in the OCTO Immune Longitudinal Study of an approximately twofold mortality rate in the 22 (16%) individuals with an IRP, i.e. showing a significantly higher relative 4-year mortality (77%) than those who were non-IRP individuals (43%), a finding suggesting that the IRP concept could be generalized to the more broadly defined NONA sample (Wikby et al. 2005). The findings was also in line with the Healthy Ageing Study in the Nottingham/Cambridge area in the UK in which it was found that an inverted CD4/CD8 ratio is predictive of nonsurvival in older adults (Huppert et al. 2003).

Our results also supported previous findings in samples of octogenarians and nonagenarians of a twofold elevated mortality risk in individuals with cognitive impairment (Wikby et al. 2005). Among the NONA Immune individuals (n=138), those who were categorized as cognitively impaired (29%) also showed a significantly higher 4-year mortality (75%) compared with cognitively intact individuals (39%). Moreover, the results showed that the two conditions of IRP and cognitive impairment independently predicted survival also when age, sex and various kinds of prevalent diseases and comorbidity were controlled for (Wikby et al. 2005). This provided further support for the previous findings that IRP constitute a major predictor of nonsurvival in very late life independently of morbidity. Only 9% of the NONA Immune individuals conformed to the SENIEUR criteria for optimal health (Nilsson et al. 2003).

4.2.3 Allostatic Load

The concept of allostatic load was proposed by McEwen and Stellar as a measure of dysfunctions across multiple physiological systems, suggesting that the cumulative dysfunctions may have more than an additive impact on overall health and survival (McEwen and Stellar 1993). Allostatic load derives from the concept of allostasis which in turn is derived from homeostasis (McEwen 2003). Allostasis, however, focus more specifically on the challenges upon the specific regulatory nervous, immune and endocrine systems in order to adapt to maintain balance though changes in various psychosocial or physical situations, like stress, in life (Karlamangla et al. 2002). Although such processes may be adaptive in the short term, they are likely to be damaging when becoming excessive in duration, frequency and magnitude (McEwen 2003). This line of thinking correspond to the growing interest to identify more comprehensive measures that incorporates multiple risk factors that may predict subsequent health and survival (Karlamangla et al. 2006).

In the NONA Immune Longitudinal Study we identified a small sample (n=8) with both IRP and compromised cognitive status at baseline (Wikby et al. 2005). A Kaplan-Meier survival analysis revealed that these individuals showed a significantly higher annual mortality rate (42%/year) compared with those with one of the conditions (15%/year) as well as with those having none (8.5%/year), corresponding to relative mortality rates of 5:2:2:1 (Fig. 1). These observed mortality effects indicates immune and central nervous system interactions, and were integrated into the general framework of allostatic load, since survival data suggested that the cumulative dysfunctions across the nervous and immune systems had more than an additive impact on survival (Wikby et al. 2005).

The allostatic load in IRP individuals with cognitive impairment was associated with changes in the levels of the cytokines IL-2 and IL-6 (Wikby et al. 2005). Cytokines in general are considered to have a central role in the mediations of allostasis by communications between the nervous, immune and endocrine systems (McEwen 2003). A suppression of the T-cellular function in IRP individuals is supported by our finding of poorer IL-2 responsiveness in those individuals compared with non-IRP's (Wikby et al. 2005). A further decline of this responsiveness in IRP individuals with cognitive impairment support the existence of an interaction between the nervous and peripheral immune system dysfunctions with a further down-regulation of the T-cellular response in these persons. Excessive increases in the plasma levels of the proinflammatory cytokine IL-6 did also represent changes characteristic of an allostatic load in the individuals and might have contributed to the T-cellular suppression by acting as an immunosuppressant via the hypothalamic-pituitary-adrenal axis (Wikby et al. 2005).

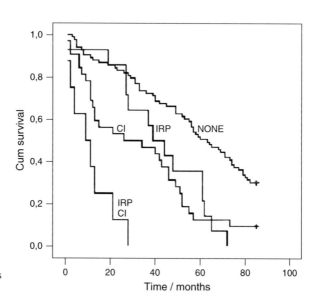

Fig. 1 Kaplan Meier survival curves for NONA individuals in subgroups created by IRP status combined with cognitive status. The subgroups were: "IRP, CI" (IRP, cognitively impaired); "CI" (cognitively impaired, non-IRP); "IRP" (IRP, cognitively intact); "NONE" (non-IRP, cognitively intact). Test for equality of survival distribution for the subgroups showed, $p<0.001$

4.2.4   IRP, T-cell Differentiation and Persistent Viral Infection

Baseline results also confirmed findings from the OCTO immune study that showed an association between the IRP and the prevalence of persistent CMV infection (Wikby et al. 2002). As for the OCTO immune study, the NONA study demonstrated a CD3+CD8+CD28-phenotype as markedly expanded for IRP and CMV-positive individuals. This led us to examine the T-cell differentiation in more detail, using the CD45RA+, CCR7+, CD27+ and CD28+ markers in a sequential model, suggesting a positive expression for naive cells, gradual losses of the markers in the various memory stages and negative expression for lately differentiated effector/memory cells (Appay et al. 2002, Akbar, Fletcher 2005). A final differentiation step occurs by reversion of CD45RO+ to CD45RA+ to obtain CD27-CD28-CCR7-CD45RA+ terminally differentiated cells of effector type (Wallace et al. 2004).

Our results suggested major decreases in the number of naive cells in the very old, changes that were even more pronounced in IRP individuals (Fig. 2). The results also showed significant increases in the number of CD8+CD27-CD28-CCR7-perforin+ effector/memory and effector cells in IRP individuals (Fig. 2) and since a majority of these cells also were CD45RA+, data confirmed that the IRP is strongly associated with increases in the number of terminally differentiated effector cells. Recent evidence suggests that increased proportions of terminally differentiated CD8+ cells possess characteristics of replicative senescence, including telomere shortening and apoptosis-resistance (Effros 2007). The inclusion of high proportions of senescent T-cells in the IRP may for the first time provide clinical confirmation of the Hayflick Limit theory of human ageing (Effros 2004). The clinical relevance for the prevalence of large amounts of senescent CD8+ T-cells has also been demonstrated by three independent studies performed on different elderly populations (Goronzy et al. 2001; Saurwein-Teissl et al. 2002; Trzonkowski et al. 2003. These studies showed consistently that a diminished antibody response to influenza vaccination is significantly associated with having high proportions of a population of CD8+ cells that lack expression of the costimulatory molecule CD28.

Evidence for a major impact of CMV in generating terminally differentiated CD8+ cells was demonstrated in the OCTO subjects by tetramer technology and was also confirmed in the NONA Immune Study (Reker-Hadrup et al. 2006). We found CMV_{NLV} specific expansions, mainly composed of terminally differentiated cells, in the range 1–20% of total CD8+ cells, similarly to findings in the OCTO Immune Study. Increases in the CMV_{NLV} percentages were associated with decreases in the IFN-γ responsiveness, suggesting that the accumulation of CMV-specific T-cells is a result of compensatory mechanisms to control CMV to balance the compromised functionality that occur with increasing age (Reker-Hadrup et al. 2006). Recent findings have indicated a failure in this control by indicating that the aged immune system is unable to control CMV and EBV, supporting the view that the expansion of virus-specific CD8+ T-cells might be due to increased herpes virus reactivation and replication (Stowe et al. 2007).

The NONA immune results also support the suggestion that besides CMV infection, persistent EBV infection plays a role as bystander associated with the

Fig. 2 Mean number of CD8+ T-cells (per µl) and subsets of CD8+ differentiation in IRP and non-IRP NONA individuals. Naïve cells were identified as CD8+CD45RA+CCR7+ cells, memory cells as CD8+CD28+CD27+ CD45RA-, CD8+CD28+ CD27-, CD8+CD28-CD27+ cells, and effector, effector/memory cells as CD8+CD28-CD27-CCR7- cells. The number of effector, effector/memory cells was significantly ($p<0.001$) higher in IRP individuals compared with non-IRP individuals

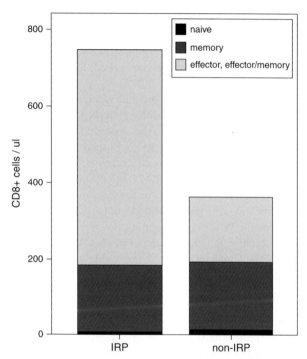

IRP (Wikby et al. 2005). IRP individuals were in all cases double sero-positive, suggesting that chronic viral load in the very old might contribute to the development of an IRP. Increased numbers of lately differentiated CD8+ cells, characteristic of the IRP, was also found particularly in double sero-positive individuals, to a less but significant extent in those being infected with CMV only, and to a low extent in individuals only infected with EBV (Wikby et al. 2005). In line with this we found significant expansions of EBV_{GLC} specific CD8+ cells; although their frequency was tenfold lower than for the CMV-specific cells (Ouyang et al. 2003).

4.2.5 TCR Clonotype Mapping

Clonal expansions have been detected in healthy old individuals and accumulating evidences suggest that that these expansions are associated with chronic antigen stress induced by persistent viral infections (Khan et al. 2002). We analysed the CD8+ T-cell clonal composition in NONA immune (n=39) and middle-aged (n=9) individuals using TCR clonotype mapping (Reker-Hadrup et al. 2006). The method combines RT-PCR and denaturing gel electrophoresis (DGGE) for rapid detection and characterization of T-cell clonal expansions by use of specific primers covering a vast majority of TCRBV 1–24 variable regions (thor Straten et al. 1998). With a polyclonal T-cell population a nondistinct smear in the denaturing gradient gel is seen while, in contrast, a population of clonally expanded TCR is seen as a distinct band. The clonal expansion were quantified by staining with anti-TCR-BV mAbs showing that for an individual CMV_{NLV} specific clone to be detected as expanded, the clone exceeds at least 1% of the CD8+ repertoire Reker-Hadrup et al. 2006).

The mean number of expanded clones was significantly higher in nonagenarians compared with the middle-aged (Fig. 3), suggesting a considerable impact of CD8+ clonal expansions in the very old (Reker-Hadrup et al. 2006). Importantly, these clonal expansions were also found to be stable across a two-year period of time. The results also showed a very strong association between the number of expansions and persistent CMV infection (Fig. 3), suggesting that a vast majority of CD8+ clonal expansions in the elderly are derived from CMV. Direct evidence for this was also demonstrated, since the sorting of CMV_{NLV} specific cells and subsequent TCR clonal mapping revealed that this specific T-cell population was oligoclonal with a mean number of six CMV related clone types (Reker-Hadrup et al. 2006). These results are comparable with findings showing that when a broad range of CMV epitopes was studied by tetramer technology, the aggregated percentages of the specific cells were more than 10% and as high as 50% of the total number of CD8+ cells (Moss and Khan 2004). Such substantial accumulations of CMV specific cells in a limited number of clones may reduce the available space for T-cells with other specificity, which may be lost through competition and result in a reduced clonal diversity and immune protection capability, particularly relevant for IRP's (Akbar and Fletcher 2005). A demonstration that clonal expansions of specific T-cells can compromise the response to other antigens by a mechanism through competition was given in mice (Messaoudi et al. 2004). The

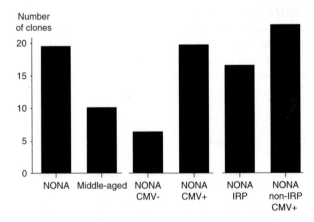

Fig. 3 The mean number of clonal expansions in the CD8+ repertoire determined by DGGE in subgroups of individuals. NONA individuals showed significantly ($p<0.01$) higher mean number (19.4, $n=39$) compared with middle-aged (10.1, $n=9$). CMV positive NONA individuals showed significantly ($p<0.001$) higher mean number (22.6, $n=31$) compared with CMV negative NONA individuals (7.4, $n=8$). CMV-positive NONA IRP individuals showed significantly ($p<0.05$) lower mean number (15.0, $n=8$) compared with non-IRP CMV+ individuals (25.2, $n=23$)

observations that infection with CMV can reduce prevailing levels of immunity to EBV (Khan et al. 2004) also support this hypothesis. Similarly to the CD8+ T-cell expansions, it has been shown for the CD4+ T-cells that the CMV-specific response expands considerably with age altering the CD4+ repertoire (Pourghey-sari et al. 2007), and that VZV-specific populations (Fletcher et al. 2005) are significantly decreased when CMV-specific CD4+ cells expand.

Surprisingly, however, we found that among sero-positive individuals, the IRP individuals showed a significantly lower number of expanded clones than the non-IRP's (Reker-Hadrup et al. 2006, Fig. 3). We also found that a decrease in clone numbers among IRP individuals was associated with increases in the inflammatory activity by elevated plasma IL-6 as well as with shorter survival times. This suggests that increased numbers of clonal expansions is beneficial to the individual, indicating an increased clonal expansion diversity and immune protection capability. It also support the hypothesis that when a critical point is reached, clonal exhaustion leads to shrinkage of the clonal expansion repertoire, detrimental to immune capabilities both for unrelated antigens and for CMV itself (Reker-Hadrup et al. 2006).

4.2.6 Low-Grade-Inflammation

There is considerable evidence of age-associated changes in immune capabilities resulting in increased morbidity and mortality due to altered function of the innate immune system (Krabbe et al. 2004). Low grade inflammation increases in the level of the inflammatory markers TNF-α, IL-6, and CRP and decreases in the levels of albumin in plasma have been shown to be significant predictors of mortality in population studies in the elderly (Evrin et al. 2005; Bruunsgaard et al. 2003; Reuben et al. 2002). Many studies have focused on the multi-factorial cytokine IL-6 and suggest that ageing independently of any particular disease is associated with two- to four-fold low grade increases in the plasma levels of this inflammatory mediator. Studies have shown that low-grade increases in IL-6 levels are related to increased amounts of fat tissue and loss of muscle mass, strength, functional capability and weight that occur with normal ageing. CRP is considered as a surrogate marker of IL-6, because CRP is produced by IL-6 induction in the liver (Krabbe et al. 2004). Increases in IL-6 are also associated with many age-related diseases such as cardiovascular disease, arthritis, osteoporosis and Type-2 diabetes (Forsey et al. 2003), which represent major morbidity classes and causes of death in the very old.

Using data from the second and third waves of the NONA immune study, we were able to confirm results from other studies that have demonstrated that ageing is associated with low-grade inflammation and that inflammatory markers are significant predictors of mortality in the very old (Wikby et al. 2006, Table 4). Logistic regression analysis also revealed that the IRP and low-grade inflammatory activity, defined by the marker IL-6, were independently predictive of 4-year survival, an outcome that remained when CRP and albumin were entered as covariates (Wikby et al. 2006). The independent main effect predicted 57% of nonsurvival

Table 4 Inflammatory parameters in plasma at Time 2 in very old individuals that had survived (survivors) and not survived (non-survivors) at Time 3 of the NONA Immune Longitudinal Study

Parameter	Survivor	Non-survivor	p<
IL-6 (pg/ml)	4.9 (61)[a]	9.2 (21)	0.001
CRP (mg/ml)	1.4 (60)[a]	3.6 (22)	0.05

[a] Median (n)

and, impressively, 97% of survival, showing that IRP and IL-6 are better predictors of survival than of subsequent mortality. These parameters are consequently strong candidates as significant markers of healthy ageing. IRP and IL-6 were predictive of mortality and not significantly affected by eight prevalent diseases, including Alzheimer's, cardiovascular disease and Type-2 diabetes, controlling for age and gender (Wikby et al. 2006). These results are in agreement with findings demonstrating that low-grade inflammation (Krabbe et al. 2004) and IRP (Nilsson et al. 2003) can predict mortality independently of disease and comorbidity. While the IRP reflects changes in the adaptive T-cell system primarily associated with lifelong persistent CMV infection, the increases in IL-6 seem to reflect innate immune system changes, including a wide range of alterations associated with overall devitalisation and frailty. This is supported by our findings of changes in the plasma levels with decreases in albumin and increases in acute-phase proteins (Wikby et al. 2006).

The above results may at first seem contradictory to our baseline findings of elevated IL-6 plasma levels specifically associated with cognitive impairment and mortality. This association was not seen at second wave follow-up (Wikby et al. 2006). However, cognitively impaired individuals who survived until the follow-up or who became incident cases were more likely to be in their early stages of the disease process compared with those who showed manifest cognitive impairment already at baseline with higher subsequent mortality rates. Thus, it is likely that sample composition variously reflect reasons for survival or selective mortality in late life (Pawelec et al. 2005).

A comparison of the inflammatory markers IL-6 and CRP at baseline, and two years later (wave 2) for IRP survivors and nonsurvivors four years after baseline, was performed in the NONA study. The result demonstrated only a minor inflammatory activity in the subgroups at baseline, indicating that the IRP is not associated with inflammation per se (Wikby et al. 2006). Increases in the inflammatory activity found between baseline and wave 2 among nonsurvivors, however, show that IRP individuals develop such an activity by increases in IL-6 and CRP in a terminal decline stage (Wikby et al. 2006). The results suggest a linkage between adaptive T-cell and innate immune system changes for IRP individuals that begins with acquisition of CMV infection in earlier life and is followed by an expansion and accumulation of senescent CD3+CD8+CD28-T-cells, the development of an IRP and finally an activation of the innate immune system in a terminal decline stage late in life (Wikby et al. 2006), including low-grade inflammatory processes with the secretion of proinflammatory cytokines like IL-6 and TNF-α (Zanni et al. 2003).

4.2.7   IRP Movement

In the NONA Immune Longitudinal study only 5 individuals (4%) moved into the category at risk by changes in the CD4/CD8 ratio, which was a significantly lower percentage as compared to the previous OCTO Immune Study (30%). Intriguingly and contrary to findings in the OCTO Immune Study, however, we have found that a few NONA individuals ($n=3$) actually moved out of the IRP category (Wikby et al. 2006). The changes found were associated with increases in IL-6, IL-10, neutrocytosis and lymphopenia, suggesting that IL-6 may induce an antiinflammatory rather than a proinflammatory effect in association with enhanced IL-10, neutrocytosis and lymphopenia to limit the potential injurious effects of sustained inflammation in these particular and rare individuals (Steensberg et al. 2003).

4.2.8   Longitudinal Changes

To follow a population of very old individuals over time in a longitudinal study offers unique opportunities to examine intraindividual changes as well as to test various factors predictive of longevity. Throughout the 20th century a remarkable increase in lifespan has taken place in humans and the increased number of centenarians in recent decades is considered to mainly be due to a dramatic decline in the mortality rate among those above 80-years of age (Jeune 2002), that is individuals exclusive focused upon in our studies. There is evidence that infectious disease become more important in the very old and that the immune system thus may be considered decisive for successful ageing and longevity in humans (Delarosa et al. 2006). In the NONA Immune

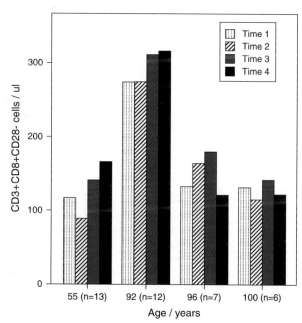

Fig. 4 Longitudinal data for the number of CD3+CD8+CD28- cells in subgroups of middle-aged and very old surviving through time 1 (1999), time 2 (2001), time 3 (2003) and time 4 (2005). Multivariate analysis of variance indicated significant differences between the age groups ($p<0.05$) with greater number of CD3+CD8+CD28-cells for the 92 year group as compared with other age groups. The analysis showed no significant change across time or group by time interaction effects

study, considering that the oldest cohort had become centenarians, commonly taken as a paradigm for "successful ageing" a question of significant interest was weather the "successfully aged" might be exceptional in their avoidance of the IRP.

Blood was drawn at baseline from 138 individuals with 42 belonging to the oldest 94-year old cohort, 47 to the 90-year cohort and 49 to the 86-year cohort. After 6 years, 99 individuals (72%) were deceased and another 8 declined to participate at this forth wave, giving a total number of 31 participants for the 6-year follow-up study. At baseline, 22 individuals resided in the IRP category and none of those had survived at 6-year follow-up. During the 6 year longitudinal study, five individuals developed an IRP by increases in the number of CD8+ and decreases in the number of CD4+ cells. Of these 4 were deceased at the 6-year follow-up, leaving only one individual with an IRP at 6-year follow-up (Strindhall et al. 2007).

At the 6-year follow-up, significant cross-sectional differences were found in the various T-cell subsets as well as in the CD4/CD8 ratio between age groups, differences not seen at baseline (Strindhall et al. 2007). The results suggest age-related changes but longitudinal data, however, revealed no significant changes at all across the 6-year period in any of the T-cell subsets (Figs. 4 and 5). These findings support the interpretation that the observed differences in the 6-year cross-sectional mean values are an effect of selective mortality. Individuals surviving until the age of 100 years did not display any T-cell changes associated with the Immune Risk Profile, i.e. they retain low numbers of CD8+CD28-cells and high CD4/CD8 ratio (Figs. 4 and 5), also predominant when these "successfully aged" people were younger, while among ten cases close to the CD4/CD8 cut-off of 1.00 (range 0.8–1.6), nine (including the one single IRP individual) belonged to the youngest age group (92 years old), and one to the 96 year old group (Strindhall et al. 2007). An effect of selective mortality is also

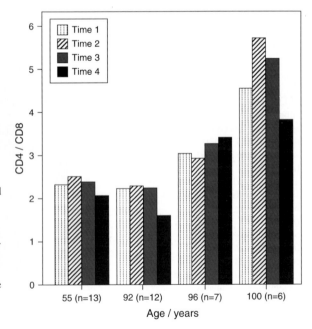

Fig. 5 Longitudinal data for the CD4/CD8 ratio in subgroups of middle-aged and very old surviving through time 1 (1999), time 2 (2001), time 3 (2003) and time 4 (2005). Multivariate analysis of variance indicated significant differences between the age groups ($p<0.05$) with the 96 and 100 year groups indicating higher ratio as compared with other age groups. The analysis showed no significant change across time or group by time interaction effects

supported by the fact that the prevalence of IRP decline from 16% at baseline to 3% at 6-year follow-up, when individuals in the NONA sample had become 95 years old on average.

The results also support the view that centenarians, although being "successfully survivors", they are not healthy (Jeune 2002). In the NONA Immune sample three quarters of the individuals were in fact classified as frail and at most 5% conformed to the SENIEUR criteria for being quite healthy (Wikby et al. 2006). The IRP, however, was shown to be predictive of mortality independently of the health status of the very old (Nilsson et al. 2003) and the absence of an IRP in centenarians therefore indicate a well preserved adaptive immune system, that helps to account for their survival in spite of substantial morbidity and co-morbidity.

5   Conclusions and Future Direction

Immunosenscence is the term used to describe the acquired dysfunctional immunity in old people and is characterized by changes in the T-lymphocyte system in particular. The changes become manifest as increasing numbers of lately differentiated T-cells that previously was exposed to antigens (memory and effector cells), and a decreasing number of cells being able to recognise and combat new antigens (naïve cells) that invade the human body (Akbar and Fletcher 2005). In the OCTO and NONA studies we have identified and examined a T-cellular IRP showing the above outlined characteristics of *immunosenscence*, i.e. the accumulation of dysfunctional terminally differentiated CD8+ cells with a CD3+CD8+CD27-CD28-CD45RA+CCR7-perforin+ phenotype and the depletion of the number of CD8+CCR7+CD45RA+ naïve cells (Wikby et al. 2005). Extensive analysis to search for associations between this IRP and various parameters including the psychosocial domains of physical and mental health, cognitive functioning, personal control/coping, social networks and everyday functioning capacity, clinical laboratory parameters, various diagnosed diseases and medication revealed that the IRP was associated only with evidence of persistent CMV infection (with EBV as a bystander). This result may indicate that CMV has a more insidious impact on the immune system than previously believed and also compared with other herpes viruses examined in these studies. The accumulation of large numbers of CMV-specific CD8+ T-cells as well as the finding that a majority of clonal expansions in the very old are associated with CMV has given additional information supporting the hypothesis that CMV greatly contribute to the development of an IRP and thus contributes to the development of *immunosenscence* in the elderly. Characteristics of the IRP identified in the OCTO and NONA studies are summarised in Table 5.

In the NONA Immune Longitudinal Study the IRP was studied in the context of low-grade inflammation, previously identified as a predictor of mortality in the old (Wikby et al. 2006). The IRP and low-grade inflammation were independently found to be main predictors of survival. This outcome was not significantly affected by individuals' health status, suggesting that the physiological ageing

Table 5   Characteristics of the Immune Risk Profile

Increased CD8+ and CD3+
Decreased CD4+ and CD19+
CD4/CD8 ratio < 1
Increased lately differentiated CD8+CD28-CD27- cells
Depletion of naïve CD8+CD45RA+CCR7+ cells
CMV-seropositivity
Clonal expansion of CD8+ cells carrying receptors for CMV
High proportion of dysfunctional cells among the CMV-specific CD8+ cells

processes of T-cell immunosenescence and low-grade inflammation are of crucial importance in late life survival (Wikby et al. 2006). The results also suggest a sequence of stages for IRP individuals (Fig. 6) that probably begins in early life with CMV infection, followed by the generation of large CD8+CD28-effector cell expansions to control lifelong persistent infection, homeostatic T-cell changes and a gradual change towards an IRP, that might be associated with a failure of the T-cell capability to control CMV. These individuals show decreased numbers of the CD8+ cell clonal expansions associated with increases in levels of plasma IL-6 and shorter survival, suggesting a stage in ageing where clonal exhaustion may lead to shrinkage of the clonal expansion repertoire detrimental to immune capabilities (Reker-Hadrup et al. 2006). It ends in a terminal decline stage with a low-grade inflammatory process that occurs in late life (Wikby et al. 2006,

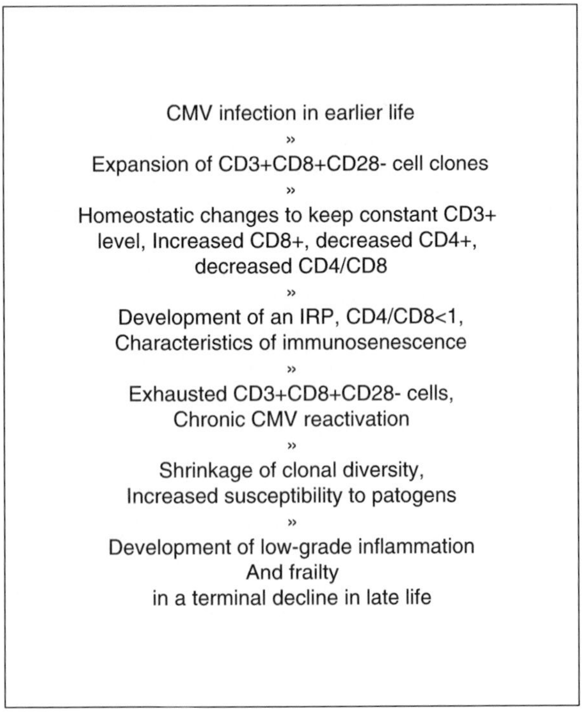

Fig. 6   Processes in a sequence of stages in the human life span of importance for late life survival in IRP individuals

The sequence is based on findings in the OCTO and NONA immune longitudinal studies and supports the inflamm-ageing hypothesis (Franceschi et al. 2000)

CMV infection in earlier life
»
Expansion of CD3+CD8+CD28- cell clones
»
Homeostatic changes to keep constant CD3+ level, Increased CD8+, decreased CD4+, decreased CD4/CD8
»
Development of an IRP, CD4/CD8<1, Characteristics of immunosenescence
»
Exhausted CD3+CD8+CD28- cells, Chronic CMV reactivation
»
Shrinkage of clonal diversity, Increased susceptibility to patogens
»
Development of low-grade inflammation And frailty in a terminal decline in late life

Fig. 6). This supports the inflamm-ageing hypothesis in human ageing suggesting that age-associated chronic inflammation causes frailty and that immunosenescence is driven by a chronic antigen load, associated with CMV infection, that induces a progressive expansion of compromised poorly functional CD8+CD28-effector T-cells (Franceschi et al. 2000; Fulop et al. 2005). The CD8+CD28-cells are able to secrete pro-inflammatory cytokines like IL-6 and TNF-a that may compensate for the defective T-cellular function, and/or amplify an ongoing inflammatory process (Zanni et al. 2003).

In future studies it will be important to investigate why only a certain fraction of CMV sero-positive individuals reside in or move into the category of risk. It is also urgent to further characterize those exceptional individuals that move out of the category of risk, allowing insight into clinical intervention approaches for those who remain in the IRP category until death. It is important to specifically study the phenomena of clonal expansion regarding frequencies and specificities of cells for various clones and to gain a better understanding of the nature of the link between CMV infection, phenotypic T-cell changes and changes in proinflammatory cytokines associated with the IRP. We should also study the relevance of the IRP more comprehensively in relation to age and gender. Future research also need to be multidisciplinary and include more detailed medical and biobehavioral evaluations of risk individuals to more fully understand the complex immune alterations that are associated with the major IRP marker.

Acknowledgment The authors acknowledge the considerable support from the EU project "T-cell immunity and ageing" T-CIA, contract no QLK6-CT-2002-02283, the Research Board in the County Council of Jönköping and the Research Council in the Southeast of Sweden (FORSS) for funding these projects. We also acknowledge Länsjukhuset Ryhov for provision of laboratory resources for the completion of these studies. The authors are also indebted to our coworkers Sture Löfgren, Bengt-Olof Nilsson, Jan Ernerudh, Jadwiga Olsson, and Per-Eric Evrin for their important contributions to these studies. We particularly would like to thank the nursing staff including Annica Andersson, Inga Boström, Gerd Martinsson, Agneta Carholt, Lene Ahlbäck, Lena Blom, Monica Janeblad, Gun Karlsson and Lena Svensson for their efforts in obtaining the blood samples used. We are particularly indebted to Frederick Ferguson, Roberta Valeski, Florence Confer, Margaret Kensinger, Penn State University, United States, and Andrea Tompa, Gunilla Isaksson, Inger Johansson, Cecilia Ottosson, Helen Olsson, Lisa Stark Jönköping, Sweden, for secretarial and technical assistence. We finally acknowledge Graham Pawelec, Qin Ouyang, University of Tubingen, Germany, Yvonne Barnett, Paul Hyland, Owen Ross and colleagues, University of Ulster, Northern Ireland, Julie Thompson, Unilever, UK, and Per thor Straten, Sine Reker-Hadrup, Tania Kollgaard and Tina Seremet, Danish Cancer Society, Copenhagen, Denmark, for successful cooperation.

References

Akbar AN, Fletcher JM (2005) Memory T-cell homeostasis and senescence during aging. Curr. Opin Immunol 17:480–485

Appay V, Dunbar PR, Callan M et al (2002) Memory CD8+ T-cells vary in differentiation phenotype in different persistent virus infections. Nat Med 8:379–385

Bruunsgaard H, Ladelund S, Pedersen AN, Schroll M, Jorgensen T, Pedersen BK (2003) Predicting death from tumour necrosis factor-alpha and interleukin-6 in 80-year-old people. Clin Exp Immunol 132:24–31

Delarosa O, Pawelec G, Peralbo E, Wikby A, Mariani E, Mocchegiani E, Tarazona R, Solana R (2006) Immunological biomarkers of ageing in man; changes in both innate and adaptive immunity are associated with health and longevity. Biogerontology 7:471–481

Effros R (2004) From Hayflick to Walford: the role of T-cell replicative senescence in human aging. Exp Gerontol 39:885–890

Effros RB (2007) Role of T-lymphocyte replicative senescence in vaccine efficacy. Vaccine 25:599–604

Evrin PE, Nilsson SE, Öberg T, Malmberg B (2005) Serum C-reactive protein in elderly men and women: association with mortality, morbidity and various biochemical values. Scand J Clin Lab Invest 65:23–31

Ferguson FG, Wikby A, Maxson P, Olsson J, Johansson B (1995) Immune parameters in a longitudinal study of a very old population of Swedish people: a comparison of survivors and nonsurvivors. J Gerontol Biol Sci 50A:B378–B382

Fletcher JM, Vukmanovic-Stejic M, Dunne PJ, Birch KE, Cook JE, Jackson SE, Salmon M, Rustin MH, Akbar AN (2005) Cytomegalovirus-specific CD4 +T-cells in healthy carriers are continuously driven to replicative exhaustion. J Immunol 175:8218–8225

Folstein MF, Folstein SE, McHugh PR (1975) "Mini-Mental State": a practical method for grading the cognitive state of patients for the clinician. J Psychiatr Res 12:189–198

Forsey RJ, Thompson JM, Ernerudh J, Hurst TL, Strindhall J, Johansson B, Nilsson BO, Wikby A (2003) Plasma cytokine profiles in elderly humans. Mech Ageing Dev 124:487–493

Franceschi C, Bonafe M, Valensin S, Olivieri F, De Luca M, Ottaviani E, De Benedictis G (2000) Inflamm-aging: an evolutionary perspective on immunosenescence. Ann NY Acad Sci 908:244–254

Fulop T, Larbi A, Wikby A, Mocchegiani E, Hirokawa K, Pawelec G (2005) Dysregulation of T-cell function in the elderly: scientific basis and clinical implications. Drugs Aging 22:589–603

Goronzy JJ, Fulbright JW, Crowson CS, Poland GA, O'Fallon WM, Weyand CM (2001) Value of immunological markers in predicting responsiveness to influenza vaccination in elderly individuals. J Virol 75:12182–12187

Hallgren HM, Bergh N, Rodysill KJ, O'Leary JJ (1988) Lymphocyte proliferative response to PHA and anti-CD3/Ti monoclonal antibodies, T-cell surface marker expression, and serum IL-2 receptor levels as biomarkers of age and health. Mech Ageing Dev 43:175–185

Huppert FA, Pinto EM, Morgan K, Brayne C (2003) Survival in a population sample is predicted by proportions of lymphocyte subsets. Mech Ageing Dev 124:449–451

Jeune B (2002) Living longer—but better? Aging Clin Exp Res 14:72–93

Johansson B (1988/89) The MIR—Memory in Reality Test. Stockholm, Sweden: Psykologiförlaget AB

Johansson B, Zarit SH, Berg S (1992) Changes in cognitive functioning of the oldest old. J Gerontol 47:P75–P80

Johansson B, Zarit SH (1997) Early cognitive markers of the incidence of dementia and mortality: a longitudinal population-based study of the oldest old. Int J Geriatr Psychiatry 12:53–59

Khan N, Shariff N, Cobbold M, Bruton R, Ainsworth, JA, Sinclair AJ, Nayak L, Moss PA (2002) Cytomegalovirus seropositivity drives the CD8 T-cell repertoire toward greater clonality in healthy elderly individuals. J Immunol 169:1984–1992

Khan N, Hislop A, Gudgeon N, Cobbold M, Khanna R, Nayak L, Rickinson AB, Moss PA (2004) Herpesvirus-specific CD8 T-cell immunity in old age: cytomegalovirus impairs the response to a coresident EBV infection. J Immunol 173:7481–7489

Karlamangla AS, Singer BH, McEwen BS, Rowe JW, Seeman TE (2002) Allostatic load as a predictor of functional decline: MacArthur studies of successful aging. J Clin Epidemiol 55:696–710

Karlamangla AS, Singer BH, Seeman TE (2006) Reduction in allostatic load in older adults is associated with lower all-cause mortality risk: MacArthur studies of successful aging. Psychosom Med 68:500–507

Koch S, Kempf J, Pawelec G (2005) T-CIA: investigating T-cells in aging. Sci Aging Knowledge Environ:pe21

Krabbe KS, Pedersen M, Bruunsgaard H (2004) Inflammatory mediators in the elderly. Exp Gerontol 39:687–699

Ligthart GJ, Corberand JX, Fournier C, Galanaud P, Hijmans W, Kennes B, Muller-Hermelink HK, Steinmann GG (1984) Admission criteria for immunogerontological studies in man: the SENIEUR protocol. Mech Ageing Dev 28:47–55

McEwen BS, Stellar E (1993) Stress and the individual: mechanisms leading to disease. Arch Intern Med 153:2093–2101

McEwen BS (2003) Interacting mediators of allostasis and allostatic load: towards an understanding of resilience in aging. Metabolism 52:10–16

Marsland AL, Petersen KL, Sathanoori R, Muldoon MF, Neumann SA, Ryan C, Flory JD, Manuck SB (2006) Interleukin-6 covaries inversely with cognitive performance among middle-aged community volunteers. Psychosom Med 68:895–903

Messaoudi I, Lemaoult J, Guevara-Patino JA, Metzner BM, Nikolich-Zugich J (2004) Age-related CD8 T-cell clonal expansions constrict CD8 T-cell repertoire and have the potential to impair immune defence. J Exp Med 200:1347–1358

Miller RA (2001) Biomarkers of aging: prediction of longevity by using age-sensitive T-cell subset determinations in a middle-aged, genetically heterogeneous mouse population. J Gerontol Biol Sci 56 A:B180–B186

Moss P, Khan N (2004) CD8+ T-cell immunity to cytomegalovirus. Human Immunol 65:456-464

Murasko DM, Weiner P, Kaye D (1987) Decline in mitogen induced proliferation of lymphocytes with increasing age. Clin Exp Immunol 70:440–448

Nilsson BO, Ernerudh J, Johansson B, Evrin P-E, Löfgren S, Ferguson F, Wikby A (2003) Morbidity does not influence the T-cell immune risk phenotype in the elderly: findings in the Swedish NONA Immune Study using sample selection protocols. Mech Ageing Dev 124:469–476

Olsson J, Wikby A, Johansson B, Löfgren S, Nilsson B-O, Ferguson F (2000) Age-related change in peripheral blood T-lymphocyte subpopulations and cytomegalovirus infection in the very old: the Swedish longitudinal OCTO immune study. Mech Ageing Dev 121:187–201

Ouyang Q, Wagner WM, Walter S, Muller CA, Wikby A, Aubert G, Klatt T, Stevanovic S, Dodi T, Pawelec G (2003). An age-related increase in the number of CD8+ T-cells carrying receptors for an immunodominant Epstein-Barr virus (EBV) epitope is counteracted by a decreased frequency of their antigen-specific responsiveness. Mech Ageing Dev 124:477–485

Ouyang Q, Wagner WM, Zheng W, Wikby A, Remarque EJ, Pawelec G (2004) Dysfunctional CMV-specific CD8+ T-cells accumulate in the elderly. Exp Gerontol 39:607–613

Pawelec G, Ferguson F, Wikby A (2001) The SENIEUR protocol after 16 years. Mech Ageing Dev 122:132–134

Pawelec G, Caruso C (2003) Immunology and ageing in Europe: ImAginE-ation in the EU. Mech Ageing Dev 124:357–360

Pawelec G, Akbar A, Caruso C, Grubeck-Loebenstein B, Solana R, Wikby A (2005) Human immunosenescence: is it infectious? Immunol Rev 205:257–268

Pawelec G (2006) Immunity and ageing in man. Exp Gerontol 41:1239–1242

Pourgheysari B, Khan N, Best D, Bruton R, Nayak L, Moss PA (2007) The CMV-specific CD4+ T-cell response expands with age and markedly alters the CD4+ T-cell repertoire. J Virol 81:7759–7765

Reker-Hadrup S, Strindhall J, Kollgaard T, Seremet T, Johansson B, Pawelec G, thor Straten P, Wikby A (2006) Longitudinal studies of clonally expanded CD8 T-cells reveal a repertoire shrinkage predicting mortality and an increased number of dysfunctional cytomegalovirus-specific T-cells in the very elderly. J Immunol 176:2645–2653

Reuben DB, Cheh AI, Harris TB, Ferrucci L, Rowe JW, Tracy RP, Seeman TE (2002) Peripheral blood markers of inflammation predict mortality and functional decline in high-functioning community-dwelling older persons. J Am Geriatr Soc 50:638–644

Roberts-Thomson IC, Whittingham S, Youngchaiyud U, Mackay IR (1974). Ageing, immune response and mortality. Lancet 2:368–370

Saurwein-Teissl M, Lung TL, Marx F, Gschösser C, Asch E, Blasko I, Parson W, Böck G, Schönitzer D, Trannoy E, Grubeck-Loebenstein B (2002) Lack of antibody production following immunization in old age: association with CD8+CD28-T-cell clonal expansions and an imbalance in the production of Th1 and Th2 cytokines. J Immunol 168:5893–5899

Steensberg A., Fischer CP, Keller C, Moller K, Pedersen BK (2003) IL-6 enhances plasma IL-1ra, IL-10, and cortisol in humans. Am J Physiol Endocrinol Metab 285:E433–E437

Stowe RP, Kozlova EV, Yetman DL, Walling DM, Goodwin JS, Glaser R (2007) Chronic herpesvirus reactivation occurs in aging. Exp Gerontol 42:563–570

Strindhall J, Nilsson BO, Löfgren S, Ernerudh J, Pawelec G, Johansson B, Wikby A (2007) No immune risk profile among individuals who reach 100 years of age: Findings from the Swedish NONA immune longitudinal study. Exp Gerontol 42:753–761

Tarkowski E (2002) Cytokines in dementias. Curr Drug Targets Inflamm Allergy 1:193–200

thor Straten P, Barfoed A, Seremet T, Saeterdal I, Zeuthen J, Guldberg P (1998) Detection and characterization of alpha-beta-T-cell clonality by denaturing gradient gel electrophoresis (DGGE). Biotechniques 25:244–250

Trzonkowski P, Mysliwska J, Szmit E, Wieckiewicz J, Lukaszuk K, Brydak LB, Machala M, Mysliwski A (2003) Associations between cytomegalovirus infection, enhanced proinflammatory response and low levels of antihemagglutinins during the antiinfluenza vaccination—an impact of immunosenescence. Vaccine 21:3826–3836

Wallace DL, Zhang Y, Ghattas H, Worth A, Irvine A, Bennett AR, Griffin GE, Beverley PC, Tough DF, Macallan DC (2004) Direct measurement of T-cell subset kinetics in vivo in elderly men and women. J Immunol 173;1787–1794

Wayne SJ, Rhyne RL, Garry PJ, Goodwin JS (1990) Cell-mediated immunity as a predictor of morbidity and mortality in subjects over 60. J Gerontol Med Sci 45:M45–M48

Vasto S, Colonna-Romano G, Larbi A, Wikby A, Caruso C, Pawelec G (2007) Role of persistent CMV infection in configuring T-cells immunity in the elderly. Immun Ageing 4:2

Wikby A, Johansson B, Ferguson F, Olsson J (1994) Age-related changes in immune parameters in a very old population of Swedish people: a longitudinal study. Exp Gerontol 29:531–541

Wikby A, Maxson P, Olsson J, Johansson B, Ferguson F (1998) Changes in CD8 and CD4 lymphocyte subsets, T-cell proliferation responses and nonsurvival in the very old: the Swedish longitudinal OCTO-immune study. Mech Ageing Dev 102:187–198

Wikby A, Johansson B, Olsson J, Löfgren S, Nilsson B-O, Ferguson F (2002) Expansions of peripheral blood CD8 T-lymphocyte subpopulations and an association with cytomegalovirus seropositivity in the elderly: the Swedish NONA immune study. Exp Gerontol 37:445–453

Wikby A, Johansson B, Ferguson F (2003) The OCTO and NONA immune longitudinal studies: a review of 11 years studies of Swedish very old humans. Adv Cell Aging Gerontol 13:1–16

Wikby A, Ferguson F, Forsey R, Thompson J, Strindhall J, Löfgren S, Nilsson B-O, Ernerudh J, Pawelec G, Johansson B (2005) An immune risk phenotype, cognitive impairment and survival in very late life: impact of allostatic load in Swedish octogenarian and nonagenarian humans. J Gerontol Biol Sci 60A:556–565

Wikby A, Nilsson BO, Forsey R, Thompson J, Strindhall J, Löfgren S, Ernerudh J, Pawelec G, Ferguson F, Johansson B (2006) The immune risk phenotype is associated with IL-6 in the terminal decline stage: findings from the Swedish NONA immune longitudinal study of very late life functioning. Mech Ageing Dev 127:695–704

Wilson CJ, Finch CE, Cohen HJ (2002) Cytokines and cognition: the case for a head-to-toe inflammation paradigm. J Am Geriatr Soc 50:2041–2056

Zanni F, Vescovini R, Biasini C, Fagnoni F, Zanlari L, Telera A, Di Pede P, Passeri G, Pedrazzoni M, Passeri M, Franceschi C, Sansoni P (2003) Marked increase with age of Type-1 cytokines within memory and effector/cytotoxic CD8+ T-cells in humans: a contribution to understand the relationship between inflammation and immunosenescence. Exp Gerontol 38:981–987

Lymphocytes Sub-Types and Functions in Centenarians as Models for Successful Ageing

Enrico Lugli, Leonarda Troiano, Marcello Pinti, Milena Nasi, Erika Roat, Roberta Ferraresi, Linda Bertoncelli, Lara Gibellini, Elisa Nemes and Andrea Cossarizza

Contents

Abstract: Several cell subsets participate to the immune response, and their close interplay is fundamental for the successful elimination of harmful pathogens. In addition, a tight regulation of the immune response has to occur in order to avoid excessive inflammation and potential autoreactivity towards self components. In the last years, the discovery and the characterization of new lymphocytes subsets, including regulatory T (Treg)-cells and Natural Killer T (NKT)-cells allowed a better understanding of how an effector immune response is induced and therefore down-modulated. During the ageing of the immune system, a process termed immunosenescence, these subsets undergo a profound remodelling, both in phenotype and function. In this chapter, we will describe the essential features of lymphocyte populations in centenarians and the differences that occur with unsuccessfully aged people.

A. Cossarizza (✉) · E. Lugli · L. Troiano · M. Pinti · M. Nasi · E. Roat · R. Ferraresi ·
L. Bertoncelli · L. Gibellini · E. Nemes
University of Modena and Reggio Emilia
Chair of Immunology, Department of Biomedical Sciences
Modena, 41100- Italy
Tel.: +39 059 2055415
Fax: +39 059 2055426
E-mail: cossarizza.andrea@unimore.it

T. Fulop et al. (eds.), *Handbook on Immunosenescence,*
DOI 10.1007/978-1-4020-9062-2_2, © Springer Science+Business Media B.V. 2009

1   Introduction

The progressive lengthening of the mean life span and the consequent growth of the elderly population has focused the attention of the scientific community on human longevity. Aging is a complex process characterized by a general decline in physiological function with an increasing morbidity and mortality. The specific causes of aging are not known. Several studies suggest an association between changes in immune function and longevity, and indicate that the deterioration of the immune function, termed "immunosenescence", could be the cause of the increased susceptibility to cancer, autoimmune and infectious diseases which characterize elderly. However, a common bias in the studies on immunosenescence has been the confusion between ageing and age-related diseases and the difficulty to study the immunology of the physiological ageing and not the immunology of the age-associated diseases. Centenarians have been proposed as model to study immunosenescence in physiological conditions, being exceptional individuals who have reached the extreme limit of human life escaping the major age-related diseases [1]. Many of them, the so called "healthy centenarians", have resulted free of diseases typical of ageing, such as cancer, dementia, diabetes, cardiovascular diseases and osteoporosis.

One of the most important characteristics of successful ageing is the ability to fight efficiently infective agents. An efficient immune response requires the coordinated action of several components, and is mainly due the presence of a consistent number of continuously renewed T- and B-cells that are equipped with a clonotypic receptor recognizing virtually every potential antigen. The immune system must have the ability to expand efficiently the adequate antigen-specific clone(s) and the ability of producing and maintaining memory cells that, during a following infection by a pathogen that has been recognized in the past, mount a more efficient response.

Immunosenescence is characterized not only by a simple deterioration of the functionality of the immune system, but also by a complex modification of several components. As a result, some immune parameters tend to diminish with ageing, while some others remain constant or even increase [1]. At the cellular level, features of immunosenescence are the constant decline in the number of naïve T-cells, the reduction of new B-cell precursors, and the tendency to expansion of T- and B-clones in the periphery, reflecting in a diminished capacity to recognize antigens [2, 3]. Indeed, at the molecular level, the expansion of antigen-specific clones is paralleled by a restriction of the T-cell repertoire, that defines the amplitude and diversity of the molecules that form the T-cell receptor (TCR) [4]. This is also accompanied by the restriction of the B-cell repertoire, and indeed the presence of clonal B-cell expansions that give origin to monoclonal gammopathies is relatively common in aged individuals, accompanied by a decline in peripheral blood B-cell count [5, 6].

2 An Overview on the Immune System

In order to cope with all possible antigens that can be encountered in the course of human life, T-cells have the capacity to generate theoretically 10^{15} different TCR, that form a really large T-cell repertoire. It has been estimated that, in a young healthy adult, about 10^8 different TCR are present in every moment [7]. T-cell compartment is generated and maintained by the production and output of new T-lymphocytes, naïve for their antigen, from the thymus. Such production tends to decline with age of about two orders of magnitude, and is considered the leading force of immunological ageing. Thymic activity is extremely efficient during childhood, but very low in the elderly. This is likely due to the fact that the immune system has to cope very early with an environment full of infectious agents, and thus has to be extremely strong and maximally functional in the first period of life, *i.e.*, during childhood.

In parallel with the decline of thymic acticvity, an increase in the number of circulating memory T-cells exists during ageing because of the differentiation and maturation of naïve T-cells, and/or the expansion and maintenance of memory cells that continuously encounter the same (persistent or recurrent) antigen. The contribution of these two components to the circulating T-cell pool changes with age. As thymic output declines (while the number of possible encounters with infective agents obviously increases with age), the relative importance of the reexpansion of "old" but experienced memory cells becomes more relevant than the differentiation of naïve T-cells. This age-related accumulation of memory cells can represent a response to the reduced number of naïve T-cells, required to fill the so-called "immunological space", or conversely a cumulative effect of the expansion of cells, likely due to persistent, subclinical infections [8–10]. It is not still clear which is the precise dynamics of the functional decline of the immune system, and at which age the generation of T-cells in the thymus is eventually exhausted. Some authors, based on the rate of reduction of the thymopoietic tissue, have estimated a complete loss of thymopoiesis at 105 years [11], but this estimation was clashed by the observation that active thymic tissue can be found even later [12]. Moreover, a recent study revealed the existence of a second organ that produces T-cells in mice, but this evidence still lacks in humans [13].

The pool of naïve T-cells can be maintained throughout life by a mechanism called "homeostatic proliferation", induced by cytokines such as interleukin (IL)-7 and IL-15. Small amounts of these molecules can maintain a small rate of T-cell proliferation, and thus keep the system alerted. After stimulation with these cytokines, naïve T-cells from elderly subjects can show a reduced capability to differentiate and proliferate. This seems to indicate that naïve T-cells that have undergone homeostatic proliferation are not fully functional, probably because an intrinsic reduction of their proliferative potential, and so a full immunological response cannot be generated [14].

The role of another key population, that of "naturally occurring" CD4+ regulatory T-cells (Treg), is currently under analysis. This is a population of T-cells with suppressor capacity, that regulate a wide variety of immune responses [15–18], including the activity of self-reactive T-cells that can potentially cause autoimmune disease. Treg exert their suppressive function in different manner, either by contact or production of inhibitory molecules, and preferentially express high levels of CD25 (the low affinity chain of the IL-2 receptor), the winged-helix family transcription factor forkhead box P3 (FoxP3) [18], the ectoenzymes CD39 and CD73 [19–21], and lack the interleukin-7 receptor α-chain (CD127) [22, 23]. Controversial data exist on the role and amount of this cell subset with age, and it is unclear whether and how these cells are altered, or in some way related to the immune dysfunction in the elderly [24]. It has been reported that the thymic output of Tregs may decrease when there is a significant loss of its capacity to generate new T-cells, and thus the homeostasis of Tregs has to be sustained by alternative pathways, i.e. the generation of Tregs in the periphery [25, 26]. Scanty data actually exist on this aspect of immune regulation, and further studies are needed.

The occurrence of modifications in the production and release of growth factors (such as G-CSF, SCF) or interleukins (such as IL-2, IL-7, IL-9, IL-13, IL-15) and chemokines (such as CXCL12, sCXCL10 and sCCL2) has been described either in the thymus or in the periphery, along with changes in the production of haematopoietic cells and other components, including cells forming the microenvironment where lymphocytes and monocytes are produced and activated. The cytokine network undergoes profound modifications with age, and several authors have shown the relevance of such a phenomenon [27–32].

Centenarians provide the best example of successful ageing and are an excellent model to understand the complex modifications of the aforementioned processes. They are exceptional individuals who have reached the age of 100 years in a relatively good state of health, from many points of view (cognitive, physical, endocrinological, biochemical and immunological) [33–35]. Studies on their immune system have revealed parameters that follow the degenerative trend often present in aged people (eg, reduction of B- and T-lymphocytes, reduction of proliferative capability), whereas other parameters are well preserved (natural killer cell activity, chemotaxis, phagocytosis) or even increased (production of proinflammatory cytokines) [33, 34]. In this chapter we will discuss the main features of lymphocyte subsets from centenarians in order to identify an "immunological signature" which is responsible for their difference with the entire elderly population.

3   B-cells in Centenarians

During ageing several changes in the B-cell compartment, in terms of new B-cell generation, homeostasis, repertoire and functionality, can occur. Peripheral B-cells and their progenitors can be classified in different subsets on the basis of phenotypic, anatomic and functional parameters. Most B-cells originate from bone marrow, where common lymphoid precursors are committed to specific lineage commitment, with rearrangement of immunoglobulin (Ig) genes and subsequent expression of surface IgM (sIgM). After B lineage commitment, cells rearrange the Ig heavy chain genes in a stage defined "pro-B-cell". Successful rearrangement initiates pre-B-cell stage, where cells express a pre-B-cell receptor (BCR) together with Igα and Igβ transmembrane signalling molecules. After a brief proliferation, the Ig light chain genes are rearranged, and cells express a complete surface receptor, defined as the BCR, characteristic of immature B-cells.

Immature B-cells complete their differentiation in the periphery, in a series of stages collectively defined as "transitional stages", classified as T1, T2 and T3 on the basis of surface expression markers. Cells that successfully complete differentiation join to peripheral pools; the large majority becomes mature follicular B-cells (the so-called B2-cells), which include precursors of primary antibody forming cells as well as memory cells, and represent more than 80% of B-lymphocytes [36]. Others cells join the marginal zone pool of lymph nodes, where they play a major role in response to T-cell independent antigens, or in the very early phase of T-cell dependent response. Even if the exact mechanism driving the differentiation in follicular or marginal zone B-cells is not fully clear, it is clear that BCR signal strength plays a crucial role in such a process [37, 38].

The last compartment of B-cells is formed by B1-cells (mostly CD5+), the first that appear during development, which is maintained by self renewal. B1-cells were originally identified as CD5+ B-cells participating in autoimmunity, and sharing similarities with those causing human chronic lymphocytic leukaemia [39, 40]. In humans, B1-cells are normally about 1–5% of the total B-cells, and are found in a variety of tissues including the spleen, peritoneal cavity, pleural cavity and intestines. B1-cells can be further divided in B1a or B1b using surface markers CD19, CD45 (B220), and CD5. B1a-cells are CD19+, CD45+ and expresses high levels of CD5, while B1b are CD19+, CD45+ and express low to almost-absent levels of CD5 [41].

Concerning naïve and memory B-cell subpopulations, a series of studies have shown that human B-cell subpopulations can be distinguished on the basis of CD27 expression and have striking characteristic features [42–45]. In particular, it is possible to identify three main subsets: CD19+, IgD+, CD27- (naïve B-cells), CD19+, IgD+, CD27+ (memory cells that underwent somatic hypermutation, and express high affinity IgM), and CD19+, IgD-, CD27+ (memory cells that switched Ig class) [44, 45].

The expression of CD27 on B-cells increases gradually with age: cord blood B-cells do not express CD27, whereas approximately 40% of adult peripheral blood B-cells are CD27+ [46, 47]. These two subpopulations are different: indeed, CD27+ B-cells are large cells with abundant cytoplasm, whereas CD27- B-cells are smaller and have a scanty cytoplasm [48].

Studies on the B-cell compartment in centenarians were not as accurate as those regarding T-cells. As in the case of T-cells, it is widely accepted that the maintenance and renewal of the B-cell pools are subjected to a complex network of homeostatic processes which undergoes to substantial modifications with ageing. During the

'90s, several studies have shown a significant modification in the pattern of B-cells subpopulations (reviewed in [33, 34]). It was shown that the proportion of B-cells in the peripheral blood usually decreases in elderly persons, including centenarians [6]. Moreover, age-related increase of the serum level of immunoglobulin classes (IgG and IgA but not IgM) and IgG subclasses (IgG1, 2 and 3, but not IgG4) was detected [49].

Conversely, less attention was paid to modifications of the B-cell compartment during ageing, and only a few studies have analyzed B-cells subsets in centenarians [50–52]. These studies have shown an age-dependent decrease in the absolute number of CD5+ and CD40+ B-cells, and a slight, even if not significant decrease of CD19+, CD27+ cells. The changes in absolute counts were mainly due to the decrease of the absolute number of B-cells. The percentage of CD19+, CD27+ B-cells increased significantly with age, reflecting increase in memory cells and decrease in naïve B-cells; centenarians did not escape from this trend. It was observed that the percentage of IgD+, CD27+ memory cells increases until 30–40 years, and then declines, with a secondary deficiency in IgM production in elderly subjects. The shift observed towards memory cells, as in the case of T-cells, can mirror the continuous exposure to foreign antigens throughout life [50, 51].

Similar results were obtained by other authors, who analyzed changes in B-cells with ageing, in a population of healthy subjects 21-99 years old, and demonstrated a rapid increase in the absolute number of memory B-cells (either IgD+ or IgD-) in the first three decades of life, and then a slight decrease of IgD-, CD27+ B-cells, and a marked decrease of IgD+, CD27+ elements. Concerning the percentage of these subset among B cells, CD27+ B cells increase during childhood and adulthood and then decline, the most marked decline regarding IgD+, CD27+ cells. The percentage of naïve B-cells increased with age. Again, extremely old people fit perfectly the trend observed in "normal" people [52]. Functional studies have shown that memory B-cells in the elderly have remarkable diminished production of Igs after stimulation, and that induction of plasma cell differentiation was decreased in elderly persons compared with that in adults [52]. These observations are in complete agreement with the reduction of clonotypic response to new antigens, accompanied by the progressive expansion of monoclonal B-lymphocytes observed in the elderly and the consequent increase in monoclonal immunoglobulin (MIg).

MIgs are known to appear with a high frequency during ageing and indeed about 20% of elderly humans have serum MIg; there are direct evidences that, in the mouse model, cells producing MIg derive from expansion of single clones [53]. About 1% of elderly subjects transform these alterations into myeloma, and perhaps chronic lymphocytic leukaemia, a lymphoid malignancy that appears with a relative frequency in advanced age [54]. The shift in the specificity of antibodies from foreign to autoantigens observed with ageing is mirrored by the specificities of serum MIg, according to data indicating that approximately 50% of MIg reacts with autoantigens [55]. Indirect evidence from studies performed in mice suggests that cells that secrete MIg derive from the CD5+ B-cell population, even if also CD5- monoclonal B-lymphocytes can be present in humans [56].

Such modifications of B-cell subsets with ageing, and in particular the progressive increase in memory B-cells and the reduced capability to cope with new antigens, as well as with recurrent encounters with the same antigen, is clearly reflected in deep changes in the production of antibodies. The concentration of natural and antigen-induced antibodies specific for foreign antigens decline with age, as well as specific antibody responses to almost all vaccines [57]. Despite this defect in the antibody response to foreign antigens, the level of serum Ig does not decline during ageing [57], a paradox that can be explained by an age-dependent increased serum concentration of autoantibodies [58]. Thus, ageing is associated with alterations in the B-cell repertoire with respect to the ratio of antibodies specific for the nominal versus self antigen. The autoantibodies detected at increased concentrations in the serum of elderly people are specific for autoantigens such as DNA, immunoglobulins, thyroglobulin, and are found at high concentrations in patients with systemic lupus erythematosis, rheumatoid arthritis or hypothyroidism. However, it is interesting to note that centenarians are characterized by a striking absence of organ specific autoantibodies, whereas nonorgan specific autoantibodies increase in healthy aged donors, as well as in centenarians [6, 33, 34, 59].

The serum concentration of IgM, IgA and IgG also increases with age [60] although the concentration of IgD decreases in elderly people, including centenarians [61]. The preferential loss during ageing of IgG and high affinity antibody, the most protective antibodies against bacterial and viral diseases, can be related to the increased susceptibility and severity of infections and a lower efficacy of vaccines in elderly people.

4   General Features of T-cells in Centenarians

The fine analysis of the phenotype of peripheral T-lymphocytes is crucial for a better comprehension of the T-cell homeostasis during ageing. Not only this allows to determine T-cell dynamics, but also to deeply investigate the role of specific T-cell subsets. One of the most age-related changes within the T-cell population is the progressive accumulation of memory cells in spite of the naïve T-cell pool [62–65]. It is to note that in the past years several studies, including ours, have used the expression of CD45 isoforms, CD45RA and CD45R0, to define naïve/unprimed and memory/experienced T-cells, respectively [62]. As a consequence, it was reported that a well preserved number of naïve T-cells can be still present in people with advanced age, included centenarians [33, 62]. Few years later the publication of such studies it was shown that CD45RA+ cell population was quite heterogeneous, includes terminally differentiated T-cells, and that several different memory subsets are present in the peripheral blood, which can be recognized by the simultaneous use of anti-CD45RA, anti-CCR7 and anti-CD62L monoclonal antibodies [66]. Interestingly, a particular subset of memory cells, the so-called TEMRA (T effector memory RA+) subset, more frequent in the CD8+ than in the CD4+ compartment, is formed by terminally differentiated memory cells that are capable of reexpressing the CD45RA

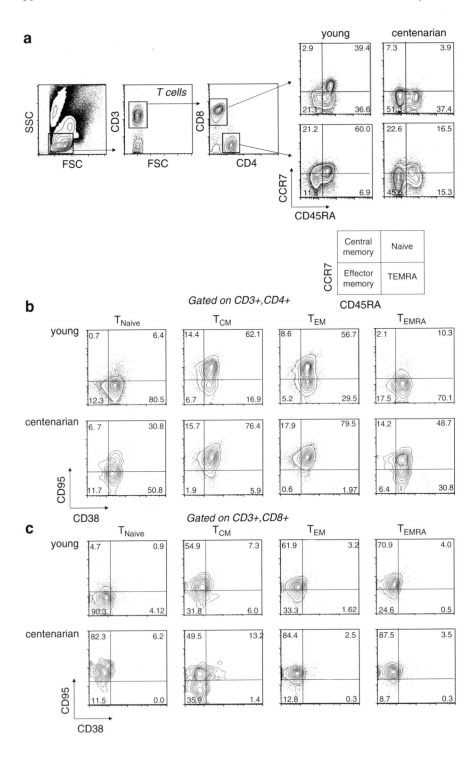

isoform, but are incapable of recirculating in secondary lymphoid organs. These CD45RA+ revertant cells have been definitely demonstrated to behave as memory cells [67].

The advent of polychromatic flow cytometry (PFC) has increased the capacity to analyze several antigens in the same cell and, as a consequence, has allowed a better definition of T-cell differentiation state. As evidenced in Figs. 1 and 2, multiple subsets can be identified in the peripheral blood by the simultaneous analysis of differentiation (i.e. CD45RA, CCR7, CD95), activation (i.e. CD38) and survival (i.e. CD127) markers. PFC led to demonstrate that the use of only one or two markers is not sufficient for the definition of naïve T-cell [68, 69]. PFC has been recently used by our group to analyze T-cell differentiation in centenarians, and we have found that in these subjects true naïve T-cells are extremely rare [70]. Indeed, a small proportion of CD4+ and CD8+ T-cells coexpress CD45RA and CCR7 [71], but further analysis of these "naïve" T-cells reveals that most of them also express CD95 (typically present on memory cells). Several questions still await an answer, such as where do these cells come from and where are they going (in terms of which lymphoid site is their final destination), do they represent an intermediate subset between naïve and memory cells, or are they terminal effector cells with the capability to recirculate to lymphnodes and spleen. It is to note that, in the elderly, the majority of CD45RA+ cells lack the costimulatory molecules CD27 and CD28 [64, 72], express CD57 and KLRG1 [73, 74] and produces IFN-γ upon stimulation [64], suggesting that these cells are part of the memory pool.

Both repeated exposure to antigens for more than a century and reduced thymopoiesis can account for the striking accumulation of memory T-cells in centenarians. It has been estimated that thymopoiesis declines over 80% after the age of 60 years and minimal or no thymic activity can be predicted after 100 years, due to the progressive loss of thymic epithelial space [75]. T-cell receptor rearrangement excision circles (TRECs), which are indicative of thymic activity [76], are practically undetectable in these subjects, although in our experience about 15% of centenarians (4 out of 25) displayed detectable levels of TREC+ lymphocytes [71]. It is thus likely that external factors such as the activity of homeostatic cytokines could contribute to the maintanance of the few naïve T-cells in old age [75]. However, competition with memory cells for those factors could compromise naïve T-cell survival and maintenance (see below).

IL-7 and IL-15 have been widely described as important cytokines for the regulation of T-cell homeostasis [77]. In particular, IL-7 plays a pivotal role in determin-

Fig. 1 Polychromatic flow cytometric analysis of peripheral blood T-cells from a centenarian and a young donor (23 years old) (**a**) Lymphocytes were first gated on the basis of forward (FSC) and side (SSC) scatter, then T-cell subsets were selected by gating on CD3+, CD4+ or CD3+, CD8+ cells. Further analysis of the expression of CD45RA and CCR7 allowed the identification of naïve (TN: CD45RA+, CCR7+), central memory (TCM: CD45RA-,CCR7+), effector memory (TEM: CD45RA-,CCR7-) and CD45RA+ terminal effector (TEMRA: CD45RA+, CCR7-) cells (b, c) Analysis of the expression of CD38 and CD95 in naïve and memory subsets of (b) CD4+ and (c) CD8+ T lymphocytes. Numbers indicate the percentages of the population identified by anti-CD38 and anti-CD95 mAbs

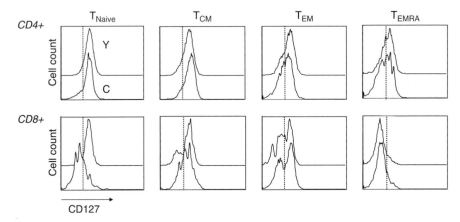

Fig. 2 Analysis of CD127 expression on naïve and memory subsets of CD4+ (upper panels) and CD8+ (lower panels) T-cells In each panel, upper histogram indicates CD127 expression in a young donor (Y), while lower panels are referred to a centenarian (C)

ing the survival of naïve T-cells and their proliferation in lymphopenic conditions. For naïve cells, IL-15 seems to be less important, since IL-15$^{-/-}$ and IL-15R$\alpha^{-/-}$ mice display only slightly reduced levels of naïve CD8+ T-cells, which could be due to modest defects in thymic production, or to effects on the survival and/or proliferation of naïve CD8+ T-cells [77–79]. It is noteworthy that CD4+ T-cells, which express higher levels of IL-7Rα than CD8+ T-cells, appear to be more dependent on survival signals mediated by IL-7 signals. IL-7 is also important for the maintenance of memory CD4+ T-cells while memory CD8+ T-cells mainly rely on IL-15 signals. Recently it has been reported that CD8+ T$_{EMRA}$ cells from elderly subjects (>65 years old) display altered expression of CD127 and reduced responsiveness to IL-7 in vitro [80]. Differently, we recently demonstrated that centenarians do not undergo a remodeling of the IL-7/IL-7 receptor system, as it is in the elderly, suggesting an active role for this cytokine in very old age [71]. We found that plasma IL-7 levels were unmodified throughout life, and the same was observed for CD127, both at the mRNA and protein level [71]. However, more detailed analysis of T-cell subsets by PFC revealed that slight modifications regarding CD127 expression can be found in certain subsets after analysis of T-cell flow cytometric profile by novel bioinformatic approaches (see below) [70].

IL-15 may also play a role in regulating T-cell homeostasis in centenarians. IL-15 level is increased in these subjects [81] and may itself contribute to the accumulation of memory cells. IL-15 has also a potent capacity to induce peripheral T-cell expansion and, together with IL-7, may compensate loss of thymic activity by driving homeostatic turnover. The idea that aged subjects are characterized by a higher T-cell turnover than young subjects is supported by several experimental evidences: i) old people have nearly twice Ki67+ T-cells in the periphery in comparison to young donors [82]; ii) studies using the deuterated glucose technique revealed an accelerated turnover of the CD8+,CD45RA+ subset in the elderly population [83]; these cells, that in old people are probably part of the so-called T$_{EMRA}$ subset, can be generated, at least in vitro, by the proliferation of central memory T (T_{CM}) cells in response to hoemostatic cytokines rather than by the direct expansion of T_{EMRA} cells themselves [84]; iii) TREC+ cells, which are not only influenced by thimic activity but also by the rate of immune activation and proliferation occurring in the periphery, are undetectable in most centenarians [71]. As a consequence, it is possible to speculate that the expanded memory pool, which is a predominant feature of centenarians, may compete with naïve T-cells for IL-7 and IL-15 availability, thus limiting naïve T-cell survival and proliferation.

5   T-cell Function in Centenarians

There is large agreement that T-cell function is in part compromised during ageing, and it affects both CD4+ and CD8+ T-cells at the level of antigen-specific immunity [85]. These alterations regard many aspects of cellular function such as proliferation, intracellular signalling, cytokine production and effector function.

CD4+ T-cells display age-related reduced helper capability. Studies in aged mice revealed that effector CD4+ T-cells generated from naïve CD4+ T-cells are characterized by a reduced expression of differentiation and activation markers such as the CD40 ligand (CD154) and CD25 [86, 87]. As a consequence, reduced B-cells response was observed due to a defective helper activity [87], which is mainly ascribed to reduced IL-2 production [86]. Decreased production of IL-2 and impaired response to this cytokine have been documented in aged humans as well. However, altered production and utilization of this cytokine can be potentiated by exposing cells from aged donors to low frequency-pulsed electromagnetic fields, suggesting that these altereations are reversible and can be positively modulated [88].

Age-related defects in naïve CD4+ T-cells are likely due to the chronologic age of the CD4+ T-cells rather than to the chronologic age of the individual [14]. In fact, newly generated naïve CD4+ T-cells in old mice exhibit normal effector function *ex vivo* and *in vivo*. These data indicate that long-term maintenance of the naïve T-cell pool by homeostatic mechanisms may result in the alteration of T-cell activity. On the other side, restoring or boosting thymic activity may help in reducing immune defects in the elderly.

In addition to IL-2, alterations in the production of several cytokines have been detected such as decreased production of IL-4 by CD4+ T-cells from aged mice after stimulation with anti-CD3 antibody [89], or increased production of TNF-α from aged humans after stimulation with PMA/ionomycin [90]. By contrast, the production of TNF-α was not modified in centenarians [90]. Increased inflammation exerted by CD4+ T-cells could reflect the proinflammatory status which is often observed in the elderly but not in centenarians [10].

Reduced effector function has also been observed for CD8+ T-cells by analyzing antigen-specific immune responses. For example, CMV-specific CD8+ T-cells from >65 year old people are highly expanded in CMV carriers but they are impaired in IFN-γ and IL-10 production after CMV stimulation [91]. By contrast, secretion of IFN-γ was observed after stimulation with mitogens. Surface receptor analysis revealed a highly differentiated effector-memory (CD45RA- CCR7-) or terminal effector (CD45RA+ CCR7-) phenotype and lack of CD28 and CD27 molecules but high levels of the KLRG-1 receptor, which is associated to end-stage differentiation and apoptosis resistance [91]. The same authors reported that CMV-specific CD8+ T-cells from HLA-A2+ centenarians were not so highly expanded and displayed lower KLRG-1 expression, suggesting earlier differentiation and normal mechanisms of apoptosis [91]. However, other authors reported that CMV-specific CD8+ T-cells for a HLA-B7-restricted epitope can occur at very high frequency in centenarians as well [92]. Differently, EBV-specific CD8+ T-cells response remains constant with ageing but it is interesting to note that in CMV-seronegative donors, the response to EBV increases significantly with age [93].

Modifications in the proliferation of peripheral blood lymphocytes (PBLs) from centenarians have been detected but they were not unidirectional. In fact, full capability of PBL proliferation has been observed in response to anti-CD3 antibody, pokewood mitogen and phorbol esters, while proliferation in response to PHA, IL-2, autologous and allogenic mixed lymphocyte reaction is reduced [94]. However, it is to be noted that, after PHA stimulation, PBLs from centenarians showed a delayed peak of thymidine incorporation but the overall thymidine incorporation was comparable to that of young donors [95]. Analysis of telomeres revealed an inverse correlation between age and telomere length, indicating that centenarians do not escape the phenomenon of telomere erosion. Interestingly, in fibroblasts from centenarians telomere length is indistinguishable from those from young donors [96, 97]. Thus the general idea is that lymphocyte proliferation in centenarians is in part preserved. As defects in the production of and response to IL-2 have been proven in human ageing, by contrast lymphocytes from centenarians are fully capable of binding IL-2 [33]. IL-2 could certainly sustain lymphocyte proliferation but it remains to be determined whether IL-2 production is critically modified in these subjects. Genetic analysis of the IL-2 promoter revealed that the IL-2 high-producer genotype is less frequent in centenarians than in young people [98]. These data contrast with what has been reported above but it is to be noted that an increase of IL-2 production characterizes the Alzheimer's disease serum profile. Moreover, people carrying the IL-2 low-producer genotype have a lower CD8 cell count in comparison to those carrying the IL-2 high-producer genotype. These data together suggest that the genetic background could not be a bystander factor in determining the so-called "immune risk phenotype" (IRP). Longitudinal studies identified the IRP phenotype as a composition of parameters which includes CMV seropositivity, a CD4:CD8 T-cell ratio of <1 due to increased CD8+ T-cells, an expansion of CD8+ CD28- T-cells with features of terminally differentiated T-cells, the presence of CD8+ T-cell clonal expansions, and elevated levels of proinflammatory cytokines in serum [99–101]. It has been also demonstrated that the IRP strongly influences the survival of people above the age of 80 [99, 100].

CD8+ T-cell clonal expansion is very common in aged people and has been also reported in animals [102]. In humans, a strong correlation exists between age and the incidence of CD8+ T-cell clonal expansions, with one-third of adults over the age of 65 years developing CD8+ clonal expansions [103]. However, the occurrence of such a high number of monoclonal CD8+ T-cells does not seem to be pathological since CD8+ T-cell lymphomas do not develop in these subjects, suggesting that CD8+ T-cell clonal expansion is still under homeostatic control. Antigen may play a predominant role in the occurrence and maintenance of this phenomenon. In particular, CMV infection seems to drive CD8+ T-cell clonal expansion. By using MHC tetramers bearing CMV antigen, authors found that a T-cell clone specific for a single CMV antigen can account for a high proportion of the entire CD8+ T-cell pool in the elderly population [93, 104]; however, at the moment, it is still unclear whether this occurs also in the centenarian cohort [91, 92]. Persistent CMV infection is thought to actively contribute in the definition of the IRP; however, little is known on how CMV strongly influence subjects' survival in advanced age and how clonal expansion of CMV-specific CD8+ T-cells is driven, as these subjects did not display any reactivation of CMV infection [92]. Some authors hypothesized that such a high oligoclonal expansion of CMV-specific T-cells in the elderly population may shape the T-cell repertoire, fill the immunological space and compete for survival and growth factors [105]. For this reason, memory CD8+ T-cells specific for other antigens than CMV could be impaired [93] or lost through competition, resulting in the exposure of elderly people to otherwise silent infections.

Compared with a sample of very old, the prevalence of IRP and the associated increase of CMV specific T-cells might decline in a sample of centenarians by selective mortality, because survival in those aged 80–95 years occurs preferably in the non-IRP individuals [10].

6 Regulatory T-cells in Centenarians

It was supposed, since many years, that effector immune response should be tightly regulated in order to avoid excessive inflammation and, subsequently, tissue damage. This hypothesis and further experimental evidences suggested the existence of a subset of cells involved in the suppression of the immune response. Extensive research in the past decades led to the identification of suppressor T-cells as subsets of the CD4+ T-cell lineage. In particular, in 1995, Sakaguchi and colleagues reported that "activated" CD4+ CD25+ T-cells, now defined naturally-occurring regulatory T (Treg) cells, were able to maintain immunologic self-tolerance [106] while, in 1997, Roncarolo and colleagues identified an inducible subset of CD4+ T-cells capable of suppressor function [107]. These cells, therefore defined Type-1 T-regulatory cells 1 (Tr1), differed from Treg cells because they were not naturally present in the circulation but could be induced by prolonged treatment with IL-10 in vitro and responded after recognition of cognate antigen [107]. Further research confirmed that Treg cells originated from the thymus and constitute a different lineage from Tr1 cells and conventional CD4+ T-cells [108]. Treg cells constitutively express the forkhead box transcription factor FoxP3, which acts as a key control gene of their development and function [109]. Differently, Tr1-cells and other subsets of suppressor/regulatory T-cells later identified, such T-helper Type-3 (T_H3) cells, are inducible and can develop from conventional CD4+ T-cells when exposed to specific stimulatory conditions such as the blockade of costimulatory signals, deactivating cytokines or different drugs [110].

Naturally occurring Treg cells constitute the 1-8% of total CD4+ cells in healthy adults. This large imprecision in the determination of their number could be due to the different criteria used for their identification (defined either CD4+, CD25[high] or CD4+, CD25[high], FoxP3+) or to the limited number of subjects studied. In fact, the definition of Treg cells solely based on the expression of high levels of CD25 (CD4+, CD25[high]) could overestimate their number, since the CD25 antigen is also upregulated in activated T-cells. This raises several doubts on the reliability of CD25 as a unique marker of CD4+ Treg cells, expecially in the contest of chronic immune activation, such as HIV infection, autoimmune diseases and ageing itself, where an increased number of activated T-cells in the peripheral blood has been described [33]. Additional markers, possibly in combination and in the same cells, should be investigated for this purpose, such as FoxP3 [109], CD127 [22, 23] or CD39 and CD71 [19–21].

Whether the amount of Treg cells in peripheral blood is dependent on age is still a matter of debate. Many independent groups studied large cohort of subjects and positive correlations between age and the number of Treg cells were reported or not [24]. However, people with advanced age (>80 years) were considered only in a few studies and none of them were centenarians. Thus, up to now, no data are present on the number and function of Treg cells and other regulatory T-cell subsets in centenarians. Adding to this, controversial data are available on the influence of the ageing process on the function of Treg cells. A study reported the decline in the suppressive function of Treg cells by almost 90% with age over 50 years [111], but others reported equivalent function of Treg cells between young and old donors [112, 113].

Animal studies suggest that phenotipic and functional modifications can occur in this subset with ageing. In aged mice, high accumulation of CD4+, CD25+, FoxP3+ Treg cells has been observed in the spleen [114, 115] and lymph nodes [114], and these cells retained suppressive capability [114, 115]. Removing these cells by anti-CD25 monoclonal antibodies restored effector CTL response and anti-tumour immunity [114]. However, major suppressor activity was found in a subset of CD4+, CD25- cells [116], which have been later demonstrated to harbour intracellular FoxP3 [115]. Thus, it is possible that other subsets rather than only CD4+, CD25[high] cells are able to regulate effector responses. It remains to be determined whether these CD25- suppressor cells were CD25[high] Treg cells in origin, or have been generated from conventional CD4+ T-cells under particular conditions of stimulation. In any case, further experiments, including the analysis of multiple Treg markers together with functional studies, are required to clarify the role of the ageing process on this CD4+ lineage.

7 γδ T-cells in Centenarians

In addition to conventional αβ T-cells in blood and in peripheral tissues, a second subset of T-cells bearing a different T-cell receptor, composed of γ and δ chains, can be identified. These γδ T-cells represent only 5% of total T-cells in peripheral blood but are enriched in many organs containing epithelia such as skin, lung, intestine, and genitourinary tract [117]. Since multiple γ and δ genes are available, different combinations of γ and δ chains are possible, thus generating different families of γδ T-cells. Intriguingly, γδ T-cells in different epithelial tissues use distinct Vγ/Vδ chains; for example, in the intestinal epithelium and lamina propria, γδ T-cells, which represent 30% and 5% of total T-cells, respectively, are mostly Vγ8/Vδ1, while in the peripheral blood Vγ9/Vδ2 are found [117]. These data suggest that different subsets of γδ T-cells may recognize specific antigens and may play different roles during the immune response.

Despite a strong similarity with conventional αβ T-cells dictated by the presence of a TCR and αβ surface markers, γδ T-cells exhibit cytolitic activity by a major histocompatibility complex (MHC) antigen-unrestricted mechanism [118]. Thus, γδ T-cells are not activated by peptides presented by antigen-presenting cells (APC) but by nonpeptidic compounds of low molecular weight and cell-cell contact is needed for γδ T-cell activation to occur [117, 119, 120]. So far, their most potent activator is (E)-4-hydroxy-3-methyl-but-2-enyl pyrophosphate (HMB-PP), an intermediate of the microbial nonmevalonate pathway of isopentenyl pyrophosphate (IPP) biosynthesis [121, 122]. Other ligands than phosphoantigens can be recognized by γδ T-cells, including MHC-class I like molecules, such as T10 and T22 in mice and MICA and MICB in humans, and an ATP synthase F1-apolipoprotein A-I (AS-ApoA-I) complex [123]. The role of these cells in immunity is still to be clarified but γδ T-cell response is nowadays considered foundamental in tumor surveillance and in infectious diseases.

In several microbial infections in humans, such as tularemia, salmonellosis, brucellosis and ehrlichiosis, γδ T-cells are expanded up to 48-97% of total T-cells [124]. Increased levels of circulating γδ T-cells have been also described in infections with protozoal parasites (malaria, toxoplasmosis, leishmaniasis) and mycobacteria (*M. avium* and *M. tuberculosis*) [124]. Recent studies in nonhuman primate models concerning the major subset of γδ T-cells, *i.e.,* that expressing the Vγ9/Vδ2 TCR, revealed that γδ T-cells may play an active role during the early phases of the immune response [125]. In macaques, the expansion of γδ T-cells was detected 2–3 weeks after inoculation of *M. Bovis* BCG, and was observed in the lung and intestine, but not in lymphoid organs [125]. Accumulation of γδ T-cells at infection sites but not in lymph nodes has been also described in murine infections. Moreover, γδ T-cells specific for the murine MHC class Ib molecule T22 harboured Vγ4 and Vγ1 in the spleen and Vγ7 in the gut epithelium [126]. These data together suggest that this lymphocyte population acts locally in a tissue-specific, and not antigen-specific, manner and is excluded from secondary lymphoid organs.

However, contrasting data have been reported. CCR7 and CD62L receptors, which are able to mediate the homing to secondary lymphoid tissues, are not expressed on the majority of Vγ9/Vδ2 T-cells. The phenotype of these cells resembles that of conventional effector T-cells, *i.e.* CD45RA-, CD45R0+, CD27-, CD11a[bright] [127], which are preferentially localized to nonlymphoid tissues [128]. However, upon activation with cognate ligand, γδ T-cells can acquire an APC phenotype, by inducing the expression of HLA-DR, CD80 and CD86 costimulatory molecules together with CCR7. These cells are able to present antigens to conventional αβ T-cells, thereby activating the adaptive immune response [117, 129].

Due to the difficulty to obtain specimens from different anatomic sites, the majority of studies conducted in humans concerns peripheral blood γδ T-cells. Recent data reported a prominent role of these lymphocytes in regulating intestinal homeostasis [120], and thus it would be interesting to check whether this sort of protection is maintained in the elderly or, if altered, could be responsible for immune pathologies of the gastro-intestinal tract.

Different subsets of γδ T-cells are affected by age in a different way. In fact, while the absolute number and percentage of Vδ2 T-cells progressively diminishes with age, that of Vδ1 remains rather constant throughout life [130, 131]. This obviously leads to a subversion in the Vδ2/ Vδ1 *ratio*, that is more prominent in centenarians than in old donors, despite the total γδ T-cell count does not differ between the two groups [130]. Ageing did not change the proportion of γδ T-cells as regards to αβ CD3+ T-cells, suggesting common mechanisms of depletion [130]. It is thus possible that thymic involution and peripheral expansion may play a role in regulating the homeostatis of γδ T-cells. However, these aspects need further elucidation.

Interestingly, γδ T-cells were not impaired in their cytolitic potential in old age, despite an age-dependent decrease in proliferative capability in response to isopentenyl diphosphate (IPP), which was completely ascribed to the Vδ2 subset [130]. Increased production of TNF-α, but not IFN-γ, by γδ T-cells has been observed in centenarians in comparison to young donors [130]; moreover, γδ T-cells from centenarians displayed higher tendency to undergo apoptosis after treatment with TNF-α and anti-CD95 monoclonal antibody [131]. Higher percentage of CD95+ γδ T-cells in centenarians may reflect the accumulation of effector memory-like T-cells, which are known to be highly sensitive to activation-induced cell death mediated by signals passing through CD95/Fas. Milder alterations in the γδ T-cell population have also been described in old people [130, 131]. This suggests that a progressive loss of γδ T-cell activity is observed with age and, as for αβ T-cells, centenarians do not escape this phenomenon.

Whether γδ T-cells play a role during immune responses in old age is still a matter of debate. Many papers confirmed a continued, protective role of this subset in adult animals [132, 133], including humans [134–136] but recent studies in mice revealed a largely redundant role in the presence of a fully mature and expanded αβ T-cell compartment [137].

Sex-dependent phenotypic and functional differences have been described in γδ T-cells. In particular, the number of V>9/V>2 cells and their effector capacity remain constant with age in females, while drop in males [138]. It would be interesting to confirm these data in old people and centenarians in order to determine whether this cell subtype could influence the female predominance in the centenarian population.

8 NK-cells in Centenarians

NK-cells are lymphocytes that can recognize and kill virus-infected as well tumor cells without antigen-presentation or MHC-restriction. NK and T-cells share a common precursor, that expresses FcγRIII, but can develop independently of the presence of the thymus, as shown in athymic mice [139]. NK-cells do not rearrange immunoglobulin (Ig) or T-cell receptor (TCR) genes and therefore neither Ig nor the TCR/CD3 complex is expressed at the cell surface, except for the ζ chain [140]. In humans, these cells are characterized by the expression of CD56, an isoform of the neural cell adhesion molecule (N-CAM), CD16, the low-affinity IgG Fc receptor (FcgRIII-A), CD57, an oligosaccharide antigenic determinant, and CD2, an adhesion molecule that appears to be correlated with the acquisition of Fas ligand-mediated cytotoxicity [141]. They also express inhibitory receptors that interact with MHC class I molecules and prevent unwanted destruction of the target cells. Thus the function of NK-cells results from a balance between activating and inhibitory signals delivered by specific membrane receptors and NK cell activation requires the interaction of activating NK receptors with their ligands on the targets and also the lack of inhibitory signals initiated by the interaction of NK inhibitory receptors with target MHC class I molecules.

They can kill target cells by the secretion of specialized lysosomes, containing pore-forming protein perforins [142], or by the induction of programmed cell-death pathways [143]. Some cytokines (such as IL-2, IL-12, IL-15, IL-18 and IFN-α/β) can induce NK cell proliferation and activation, migration and production of IFN-γ, TNF-α and GM-CSF (for review see [144]). NK-cells can produce also cytokines and chemokines that directly participate in the elimination of pathogens or activate other cellular components of immunity.

Several alterations have been described in NK cell function with ageing both in animals and humans. In humans, the different selection criteria of the elderly populations have produced contrasting data. Some authors reported a decrease in cytotoxic function of the circulating NK-cells of elderly subjects [145] which is associated with an increased incidence of infectious diseases [146, 147]. Indeed, there is an increase of mortality risk of 3 times in people more than 85 years with low numbers of NK-cells respect those with high NK cell numbers [148]. Several pathologies usually associated with ageing are associated with low NK cell activity in the elderly, such as atherosclerosis [149]. On the contrary, high NK cytotoxicity is associated with lower incidence of infections of the respiratory tract and with a better development of protective antibody in response to influenza vaccination [150].

Indeed, in centenarians, NK cell number, as revealed by analysis of CD56 expression on PBMCs, and functionality are not modified in comparison to young donors while a partial loss of NK cell cytotoxic activity can be found in middle-age subjects, despite the CD57+ and CD16+ populations, which are capable of rapid cytotoxic activity, increased as in centenarians [151]. Further studies revealed a preferential expansion of the terminally differentiated CD56^{dim}CD16+ subset while minor modifications were found in the CD56^{bright}CD16- subset [152].

Whereas NK cell activation mediated by CD16 is not affected by aging [144, 148, 149, 153], poor data exist on the function of other NK receptors and probably other NK activating or inhibitory receptors are defective in the elderly. It was reported that the expression of HLA-specific killer receptors is not significantly affected in NK-cells from elderly [154], but more recent studies have shown that NK-cells display an age-related increase in KIR expression and a reciprocal decrease in CD94/ NKG2A expression, although the CD94/NKG2A inhibitory signaling pathway is intact [153].

The killing activity mediated by perforins is not modified in people with advanced age and no significant decrement of these molecules has been observed in NK-cells from young and old donors [155]. Interestingly, a greater decline of perforin expression is present in elderly men if compared to elderly women [156]. This could be a further element to understand the typically higher percentage of females among centenarians [157].

NK-cell activity and phenotype can be affected by the differential presence of cytokines between the young and the old population, as well as centenarians. In fact, a reduced production of cytokines involved in NK-cell activation, i.e, IL-2, IL-12, IFN-α and IFN-γ, is observed with increased age [158]. Accordingly, IFN-γ secretion by NK-cells in response to IL-2 [159] and chemokine secretion in response to IL-12 or IL-2 decrease in elderly [160]. In aged mice and humans the response of NK-cells to IFN-α/β is decreased and could be related to the delay in virus clearance observed in aged mice [159]. The decrease of NK-cell secretion could lead to an impaired adaptive immune response that could contribute to age-related diseases.

The functionality of the immune system is strongly influenced by the presence of certain hormones in a circuit that is called "neuroendocrine immune system" [161], which undergoes profound remodelling with increasing age [162]. NK-cells, as other immune cells, express some hormone receptors on their surface. As a consequence, certain hormones of the hypothalamic–pituitary–gonadal axis as well as thyroid hormones, dehydroepiandrosterone (DHEA), insulin-like growth factor (IGF)-1, melatonin or insulin regulate their function. Moccheggiani *et al.* showed that hormonal treatments with T3, T4, melatonin, GH or IGF-1 in old mice can restore NK-cell cytotoxicity and IL-2 and IFN-γ production [163, 164]. In healthy nonagenarians and centenarians, NK cell number and/or cytolytic activity was positively associated with serum levels of vitamin D, while T3 and i-PTH hormones were associated only with NK-cell number, suggesting a positive role of these molecules in regulating NK-cell homeostasis [165]. Preserved NK-cell functionality in these subjects, *i.e.,* NK-cell cytotoxicity and IFN-γ production, was also associated with good zinc ion bioavailability which, by contrast, is reduced in old animals and humans, but not in centenarians [165–167].

9 NKT-cells in Centenarians

The term "NKT" includes more than one subset of T-lymphocytes that have different phenotype, functional capacities and tissue distribution and that express NK-associated receptors (NKR) [168], historically CD161 in humans [169] and NK1.1 in mice [170].

The large number of studies regards the so-called "classical" or "invariant" NKT-cells (iNKT) expressing a semi-invariant T-cell receptors (TCR), characterized in most cases by Vα14/Vβ8.2 in mice [171] and by Vα24/Vβ11 in humans [172, 173]. iNKT-cells TCR can recognize CD1d (a monomorphic class Ib molecole) [174] and bind endogenous glycosphingolipids and α-glycuronosylceramide (present on the microbial cell wall), suggesting a role in the protection from bacteria that are not detected by classical pattern recognition receptors [175–178].

iNKT-cells can be divided at least in three subset on the basis of the expression of CD4 or CD8 coreceptor and on their cytokine production. iNKT-cells that express CD4+ produce Th1 and Th2 cytokines, while CD4- NKT-cells primarily produce Th1 cytokines. CD4- NKT-cells can be further divided into CD4-CD8- (double negative; DN) and CD8+ NKT-cells, which predominantly express the CD8αα dimer instead of the CD8αβ form present on conventional cytotoxic T lymphocytes [179–181]. Indeed, it has been shown that iNKT-cells express CD45RO but lack CD62L. It was hypothesized that this effector memory phenotype probably derives from the endogenous self ligands recognition [182]. A minority of iNKT-cells are classified as central memory (CCR7+CD45RO+), while most Vα24CD4+ and CD4- NKT-cells could be defined as effector memory cells (CCR7-CD45RO+)[183].

There is evidence that CD1-restricted NKT-cells represents a thymus-dependent population. They are absent in nude mice, do not develop in thymectomized mice and first appear in the thymus slightly later than most other T-cell subsets. There is also convincing evidence that NKT-cells segregate from conventional T-cells at the stage of double positive (CD4+CD8+, DP) thymocyte in the thymic cortex [184]. Indeed, it seems that they acquire a relative resistance to activation-induced apoptosis in the late stage of intrathymic development [185].

iNKT-cells play an important role in host defense and immunoregulation, including the prevention of tumor development and metastasis, suppression of allergic responses and protection against viruses, parasites, bacteria and their products [171, 173, 186]. The most striking property of NKT-cells is their capacity to secrete large amounts of cytokines (IFN-γ, IL-4, IL-2, IL-5, IL-10, IL-13, GM-CSF and TNF-α) within minutes after TCR stimulation. Activation of NKT-cells also leads to upregulation of CD40L, resulting in IL-12 production by dendritic cells upon CD40 triggering [187]. Upon TCR engagement, NKT-cells have cytotoxic activities through the release of perforins and granzymes and by the expression of membrane-bound members of the TNF family (such as FasL) [188]. Activation of NKT-cells leads to subsequent activation of other cells, such as NK-cells, B cells, DC, macrophages, and conventional T-cells in mice as well as humans [189, 190]. Thus, they can affect the acquired immune system by activating pathogen-specific

CD4 Th1 cells as well as CD8 T-cells, suggesting an important role in conferring protection against microbial pathogens, like malaria. Moreover, they have been shown to play a crucial role in interfering with the initiation, growth and metastatic spread of tumours. NKT-cell-derived Th2 cytokines, such as IL-4, can downregulate immune responses and have been shown to contribute to protection against the development of autoimmune diseases (reviewed in [191]). Consequently, NKT-cell activation results in a cascade of immune reactions, providing a possible explanation for their regulatory effects.

Human iNKT-cells can be identified either by their invariant TCR formed by Vα24 and Vβ11 gene segments, or by CD1d-tetramers loaded with α-galactosylceramide (α-GalCer), a marine sponge-derived glycolipid able to selectively activate iNKT-cells in a CD1d-dependent manner [171, 192]. In human peripheral blood, however, classical CD1d-restricted NKT-cells are typically less than 0.1%.

Besides iNKT-cells, a different subset of conventional CD1d-independent α/β T-cell, called "NKT-like" or "nonclassical NKT"-cells, can express several NKR, such as CD16, CD56, CD57, CD161, CD94, NKG2A. The majority of NKT-like-cells likely belongs to nonclassical subpopulation and are mostly CD8+. The nonclassical NKT-cells can account for 5-20% of total T-cells in human peripheral blood [193, 194].

A limited number of studies investigated the role of peripheral blood NKT-cells in aged people. Studies on iNKT frequency in peripheral blood of centenarians from Okinawa were performed by Miyaji et al. who analyzed the so-called "extrathymic T-cells", characterized by the expression of CD3 and CD56 or CD57. They found a higher frequency of these cells compared to middle-aged subjects but no differences were detected between males and females [194]. Thus, these authors confirmed that the proportion and the absolute number of NKT-cells (CD56+ or CD57+ T-cells expressing Vα24+) were highly increased in the blood of centenarians, along with the proportion of IFNγ-producing cells among NKT-cells [166].

Other studies showed an effect of age on the homeostasis and function of circulating NKT-cells but elderly subjects rather than centenarians were considered. DelaRosa et al. found a decreased percentage of Vα24+ T-cells in elderly when compared with young controls and, within Vα24+ T-cells, a significant increase in the percentage of Vα24+CD4−CD8+ T-cells, while the percentage of Vα24+ within CD3+CD28+ was similar [195]. In accordance with that study, an age-related decrease in the percentage and absolute count of Vα24+Vβ11+ iNKT-cells has been shown in healthy individuals, although their functional capacity to respond to α-GalCer was not altered [196]. Indeed, a decline of 3.4% per year was evaluated in Vα24+Vβ11+ iNKT-cells with age [197], which involved both their absolute levels and their proportion as to the total T-cell compartment. In addition, they found a gender-related difference in the frequency of circulating iNKT-cells, that was lower in males than in females, and decreased faster with age in the formers than in the latters [197]. Similar results were obtained by Peralbo et al. who also reported a decreased proliferative potential of Vα24+Vβ11+ iNKT-cells in reponse to α-GalCer in healthy elderly compared to young subjects [198]. A decrease in the frequency of iNKT-cells in the elderly has been also reported by Jing et al. which was also associated with an alteration in the iNKT-cell subset compositions, that is an increase in the proportion of the CD4(+) subset and a decrease in the proportion of the CD4/CD8 DN subset [199]. In addition, iNKT-cells from aged people produced predominantly Th2 rather than Th1 cytokines [199].

Whereas iNKT-cells are characterized by the expression of a semi-invariant TCR that interact with CD1d loaded with glycolipids, "NKT-like" T-cells are NKR-expressing conventional T-lymphocytes which display an oligoclonal TCR repertoire able to recognize classical MHC molecules loaded with peptides [200]. Most of NKT-like cells have an effector memory phenotype and contain high levels of perforin and granzymes [201]. NKR-expressing T-cells expand with aging and centenarians do not escape this phenomenon, as revealed by the increased expression of CD56 on T-cells [151].

Little is known about the function of NKT-like cells but the general belief is that their accumulation is primarily driven by a chronic inflammatory environment, as it is in the elderly population as well as in patients with persistent viral infections, rheumatic diseases and autoimmune diseases, in which a chronic stimulation of the immune system occurs [201]. In particular, the expansion of NKT-like cells accompanies the loss of CD28 expression on T-cells after antigenic stimulation in vitro and is associated with the accumation of CD28^{null} T-cells *in vivo* [202].

In summary, several studies have demonstrated age-related effects on iNKT-cells, a diminished proliferative functionality, a shift from Th1 to Th2 response and a modification in the iNKT subset ratio. However, only one study investigated the frequency of these cells in centenarians.

All these findings may contribute to highlight the role of NKT in the general deterioration of the immune response in the elderly. Considering the importance of these cells in the recognition and elimination of Gram-negative bacteria [178], these defects could be involved in the increased morbidity and mortality due to bacterial infection associated to ageing. The age-dependent alterations in NKT-cells might also reflect the thymic involution, as conventional T-lymphocytes [203–205]. Molling *et al.* suggested that iNKT-cells decrease could affect an efficient tumor immunosurveillance in aged donors, representing a risk factor for tumour development [197]. Furthermore age-dependent alterations in iNKT cytokine production might contribute to the dysregulation of the cytokine network shown in the aged people [206, 207].

10   Bioinformatics Tools for the Analysis of Cellular Dynamics in Centenarians

As described above, a huge number of lymphocytes subsets exists in human peripheral blood. The fine analysis of these subtypes is of extreme importance for a better understanding of the cellular dynamics during physiological processes such as the ageing of the immune system. So far, the simultaneous analysis of multiple parameters at the level of single cell can only be performed by polychromatic flow cytometry [208, 209]. A huge amount of data can be generated by such a technology which is, however, difficult to manage. In fact, several functional different populations can be identified by combining the positive and negative expression of each antigen (typically 2^n, where n is the number of parameters analyzed). Thus, using 8 fluorochromes coupled to 8 different monoclonal antibodies, it is thus possible to identify 256 lymphocyte subpopulations in 100 µL of blood.

T-cells from centenarians were recently studied by 8-colour flow cytometry in our laboratory. By combining the expression of CD45RA, CCR7, CD127 (IL-7rα), CD95 and CD38 (whose expression can be further distinguished between *dim* and *bright*), we were able to identify up to 48 subpopulations both for CD4+ and CD8+ T-cells (Fig. 1). In order to uncover subtle differences among the three groups of subjects under investigation (20 years old donors, middle aged and centenarians) that otherwise could be missed by classical approaches, we used global approaches based on the Cluster Analysis (CA) and on the Principal Component Analysis (PCA), which are often used for microarray experiments [70]. In particular, the former is able to generate groups or "clusters" of variables on the basis of their similarities and differences, while the latter allows the dimensionality of a multidimensional dataset to be reduced, in order to obtain a new system of coordinates, *i.e.* the principal components. In this ideal space, subjects are plotted by considering all the variables, *i.e.* the T-cell subsets generated by boolean combination. These analyzes revealed that, in centenarians, CD4+ T-cells can be highly heterogeneous since it was not possible to cluster centenarians on the basis of the CD4+ T-cell flow cytometric profile. PCA of CD4+ T-cell subsets revealed the expansion of either CD95+ central memory or effector memory cells where the expression of CD127 could be retained or not. A different behavior was observed for CD8+ T-cells, where a striking expression of terminally differentiated effector (CD45RA+, CCR7-) T-cells with a preferential CD95+, CD127-, CD38- phenotype was detected. More detailed analysis by using different approaches for data pretreatment, such as data scaling, revealed that, for instance, that the same memory subset from young donors and centenarians differentially express CD127. These data thus suggest that, while the production of IL-7 remains constant throughout life [71], T-cells subsets from centenarians could be differentially regulated in terms of peripheral homeostasis [14, 80, 105, 210].

These approaches are very useful to identify cellular dynamics during the ageing process and to identify minimal difference among different ages or clinical conditions. More detailed analysis, in particular in larger cohorts, will reasonably lead to the identification of specific subsets with a possible protective role towards diseases of various origins.

11   Concluding Remarks and Future Directions

We have described some crucial modifications occurring in different lymphocyte subsets with ageing, and underlined that centenarians display some special features that are not shared by the entire elderly populations. Whether these components, rather than genetic or environmental determinants, are responsible for reaching such an advanced age still remains to be determined. It is however general opinion that all of the aforementioned factors act in synergy. Until now, many studies investigated whether the function of a specific subset is maintained or modified in these individuals, but data are lacking on the interplay among different lymphocyte populations.

An efficient immune response is the result of the tight cooperation of many cell types, and the disfunction of one of them can lead to the persistence of the antigen (or the pathogen), and to the onset of a chronic inflammatory enviroment. Thus, it is needed to uncover specific interactions among cell types by using more global approaches such as systems biology, genome-wide analysis and bioinformatics. A complete and detailed picture of the immune system of centenarians can reveal potential targets for therapy and vaccination in the elderly.

References

1. Franceschi C, Cossarizza A (1995) Introduction: the reshaping of the immune system with age. Int Rev Immunol, 12:1–4s
2. Allman D, Miller JP (2005) B-cell development and receptor diversity during aging. Curr Opin Immunol, 17:463–467
3. Linton PJ, Dorshkind K (2004) Age-related changes in lymphocyte development and function. Nat Immunol, 5:133–139
4. Wack A, Cossarizza A, Heltai S, Barbieri D, D'Addato S, Fransceschi C, Dellabona P, Casorati G (1998) Age-related modifications of the human alphabeta T-cell repertoire due to different clonal expansions in the CD4+ and CD8+ subsets. Int Immunol, 10:1281–1288
5. Crawford J, Eye MK, Cohen HJ (1987) Evaluation of monoclonal gammopathies in the "well" elderly. Am J Med, 82:39–45
6. Mariotti S, Sansoni P, Barbesino G, Caturegli P, Monti D, Cossarizza A, Giacomelli T, Passeri G, Fagiolo U, Pinchera A, et al (1992) Thyroid and other organ-specific autoantibodies in healthy centenarians. Lancet, 339:1506–1508
7. Goronzy JJ, Weyand CM (2005) T-cell development and receptor diversity during aging. Curr Opin Immunol, 17:468–475
8. Franceschi C, Valensin S, Fagnoni F, Barbi C, Bonafe M (1999) Biomarkers of immunosenescence within an evolutionary perspective: the challenge of heterogeneity and the role of antigenic load. Exp Gerontol, 34:911–921
9. Franceschi C, Bonafe M, Valensin S (2000) Human immunosenescence: the prevailing of innate immunity, the failing of clonotypic immunity, and the filling of immunological space. Vaccine, 18:1717–1720
10. Pawelec G, Akbar A, Caruso C, Solana R, Grubeck-Loebenstein B, Wikby A (2005) Human immunosenescence: is it infectious? Immunol Rev, 205:257–268
11. George AJ, Ritter MA (1996) Thymic involution with ageing: obsolescence or good housekeeping? Immunol Today, 17:267–272
12. Steinmann GG, Klaus B, Muller-Hermelink HK (1985) The involution of the ageing human thymic epithelium is independent of puberty. A morphometric study. Scand J Immunol, 22:563–575
13. Terszowski G, Muller SM, Bleul CC, Blum C, Schirmbeck R, Reimann J, Pasquier LD, Amagai T, Boehm T, Rodewald HR (2006) Evidence for a functional second thymus in mice. Science, 312:284–287
14. Swain S, Clise-Dwyer K, Haynes L (2005) Homeostasis and the age-associated defect of CD4 T-cells. Semin Immunol, 17:370–377

15. Kronenberg M, Rudensky A (2005) Regulation of immunity by self-reactive T-cells. Nature, 435:598–604
16. Sakaguchi S (2005) Naturally arising Foxp3-expressing CD25+CD4+ regulatory T-cells in immunological tolerance to self and non-self. Nat Immunol, 6:345–352
17. von Boehmer H (2005) Mechanisms of suppression by suppressor T-cells. Nat Immunol, 6:338–344
18. Ziegler SF (2006) FOXP3: of mice and men. Annu Rev Immunol, 24:209–226
19. Borsellino G, Kleinewietfeld M, Di Mitri D, Sternjak A, Diamantini A, Giometto R, Hopner S, Centonze D, Bernardi G, Dell'Acqua ML, Rossini PM, Battistini L, Rotzschke O, Falk K (2007) Expression of ectonucleotidase CD39 by Foxp3+ Treg cells: hydrolysis of extracellular ATP and immune suppression. Blood, 110:1225–1232
20. Bopp T, Becker C, Klein M, Klein-Hessling S, Palmetshofer A, Serfling E, Heib V, Becker M, Kubach J, Schmitt S, Stoll S, Schild H, Staege MS, Stassen M, Jonuleit H, Schmitt E (2007) Cyclic adenosine monophosphate is a key component of regulatory T-cell-mediated suppression. J Exp Med, 204:1303–1310
21. Deaglio S, Dwyer KM, Gao W, Friedman D, Usheva A, Erat A, Chen JF, Enjyoji K, Linden J, Oukka M, Kuchroo VK, Strom TB, Robson SC (2007) Adenosine generation catalyzed by CD39 and CD73 expressed on regulatory T-cells mediates immune suppression. J Exp Med, 204:1257–1265
22. Seddiki N, Santner-Nanan B, Martinson J, Zaunders J, Sasson S, Landay A, Solomon M, Selby W, Alexander SI, Nanan R, Kelleher A, Fazekas de St Groth B (2006) Expression of interleukin (IL)-2 and IL-7 receptors discriminates between human regulatory and activated T-cells. J Exp Med, 203:1693–1700
23. Liu W, Putnam AL, Xu-Yu Z, Szot GL, Lee MR, Zhu S, Gottlieb PA, Kapranov P, Gingeras TR, Fazekas de St Groth B, Clayberger C, Soper DM, Ziegler SF, Bluestone JA (2006) CD127 expression inversely correlates with FoxP3 and suppressive function of human CD4+ T reg cells. J Exp Med, 203:1701–1711
24. Dejaco C, Duftner C, Schirmer M (2006) Are regulatory T-cells linked with aging? Exp Gerontol, 41:339–345
25. Apostolou I, von Boehmer H (2004) In vivo instruction of suppressor commitment in naive T-cells. J Exp Med, 199:1401–1408
26. Kretschmer K, Apostolou I, Hawiger D, Khazaie K, Nussenzweig MC, von Boehmer H (2005) Inducing and expanding regulatory T-cell populations by foreign antigen. Nat Immunol, 6:1219–1227
27. Antonelli A, Rotondi M, Fallahi P, Ferrari SM, Paolicchi A, Romagnani P, Serio M, Ferrannini E (2006) Increase of CXC chemokine CXCL10 and CC chemokine CCL2 serum levels in normal ageing. Cytokine, 34:32–38
28. Begley L, Monteleon C, Shah RB, Macdonald JW, Macoska JA (2005) CXCL12 overexpression and secretion by aging fibroblasts enhance human prostate epithelial proliferation in vitro. Aging Cell, 4:291–298
29. Fagiolo U, Cossarizza A, Santacaterina S, Ortolani C, Monti D, Paganelli R, Franceschi C (1992) Increased cytokine production by peripheral blood mononuclear cells from healthy elderly people. Ann N Y Acad Sci, 663:490–493
30. Fagiolo U, Cossarizza A, Scala E, Fanales-Belasio E, Ortolani C, Cozzi E, Monti D, Franceschi C, Paganelli R (1993) Increased cytokine production in mononuclear cells of healthy elderly people. Eur J Immunol, 23:2375–2378
31. Gerli R, Monti D, Bistoni O, Mazzone AM, Peri G, Cossarizza A, Di Gioacchino M, Cesarotti ME, Doni A, Mantovani A, Franceschi C, Paganelli R (2000) Chemokines, sTNF-Rs and sCD30 serum levels in healthy aged people and centenarians. Mech Ageing Dev, 121:37–46
32. Sempowski GD, Hale LP, Sundy JS, Massey JM, Koup RA, Douek DC, Patel DD, Haynes BF (2000) Leukemia inhibitory factor, oncostatin M, IL-6, and stem cell factor mRNA expression in human thymus increases with age and is associated with thymic atrophy. J Immunol, 164:2180–2187

33. Cossarizza A, Ortolani C, Monti D, Franceschi C (1997) Cytometric analysis of immunose-nescence. Cytometry, 27:297–313
34. Franceschi C, Monti D, Sansoni P, Cossarizza A (1995) The immunology of exceptional individuals: the lesson of centenarians. Immunol Today, 16:12–16
35. Paolisso G, Barbieri M, Bonafe M, Franceschi C (2000) Metabolic age modelling: the lesson from centenarians. Eur J Clin Invest, 30:888–894
36. Cancro MP (2005) B-cells and aging: gauging the interplay of generative, selective, and homeostatic events. Immunol Rev, 205:48–59
37. Lopes-Carvalho T, Foote J, Kearney JF (2005) Marginal zone B-cells in lymphocyte activa-tion and regulation. Curr Opin Immunol, 17:244–250
38. Pillai S, Cariappa A, Moran ST (2005) Marginal zone B cells. Annu Rev Immunol, 23:161–196
39. Boumsell L, Bernard A, Lepage V, Degos L, Lemerle J, Dausset J (1978) Some chronic lym-phocytic leukemia cells bearing surface immunoglobulins share determinants with T-cells. Eur J Immunol, 8:900–904
40. Hayakawa K, Hardy RR, Parks DR, Herzenberg LA (1983) The "Ly-1 B" cell subpopulation in normal immunodefective, and autoimmune mice. J Exp Med, 157:202–218
41. Berland R, Wortis HH (2002) Origins and functions of B-1 cells with notes on the role of CD5. Annu Rev Immunol, 20:253–300
42. Maurer D, Holter W, Majdic O, Fischer GF, Knapp W (1990) CD27 expression by a distinct subpopulation of human B-lymphocytes. Eur J Immunol, 20:2679–2684
43. Maurer D, Fischer GF, Fae I, Majdic O, Stuhlmeier K, Von Jeney N, Holter W, Knapp W (1992) IgM and IgG but not cytokine secretion is restricted to the CD27+ B-lymphocyte subset. J Immunol, 148:3700–3705
44. Agematsu K (2000) Memory B-cells and CD27. Histol Histopathol, 15:573–576
45. Agematsu K, Hokibara S, Nagumo H, Komiyama A (2000) CD27: a memory B-cell marker. Immunol Today, 21:204–206
46. Agematsu K, Kobata T, Sugita K, Freeman GJ, Beckmann MP, Schlossman SF, Morimoto C (1994)_ Role of CD27 in T-cell immune response. Analysis by recombinant soluble CD27. J Immunol, 153:1421–1429
47. Agematsu K, Nagumo H, Yang FC, Nakazawa T, Fukushima K, Ito S, Sugita K, Mori T, Kobata T, Morimoto C, Komiyama A (1997) B-cell subpopulations separated by CD27 and crucial collaboration of CD27+ B-cells and helper T-cells in immunoglobulin production. Eur J Immunol, 27:2073–2079
48. Shi Y, Agematsu K, Ochs HD, Sugane K (2003) Functional analysis of human memory B-cell subpopulations: IgD+CD27+ B-cells are crucial in secondary immune response by producing high affinity IgM. Clin Immunol, 108:128–137
49. Paganelli R, Quinti I, Fagiolo U, Cossarizza A, Ortolani C, Guerra E, Sansoni P, Pucillo LP, Scala E, Cozzi E, et al (1992) Changes in circulating B cells and immunoglobulin classes and subclasses in a healthy aged population. Clin Exp Immunol, 90:351–354.
50. Colonna-Romano G, Aquino A, Bulati M, Di Lorenzo G, Listi F, Vitello S, Lio D, Candore G, Clesi G, Caruso C (2006) Memory B-cell subpopulations in the aged. Rejuvenation Res, 9:149–152
51. Colonna-Romano G, Bulati M, Aquino A, Scialabba G, Candore G, Lio D, Motta M, Mala-guarnera M, Caruso C (2003) B-cells in the aged: CD27, CD5, and CD40 expression. Mech Ageing Dev, 124:389–393
52. Shi Y, Yamazaki T, Okubo Y, Uehara Y, Sugane K, Agematsu K (2005) Regulation of aged humoral immune defense against pneumococcal bacteria by IgM memory B-cell. J Immunol, 175:3262–3267
53. LeMaoult J, Manavalan JS, Dyall R, Szabo P, Nikolic-Zugic J, Weksler ME (1999) Cellular basis of B-cell clonal populations in old mice. J Immunol, 162:6384–6391
54. Kyle RA, Rajkumar SV (1999) Monoclonal gammopathies of undetermined significance. Hematol Oncol Clin North Am, 13:1181–1202

55. Merlini G, Farhangi M, Osserman EF (1986) Monoclonal immunoglobulins with antibody activity in myeloma, macroglobulinemia and related plasma cell dyscrasias. Semin Oncol, 13:350–365

56. Ghia P, Prato G, Scielzo C, Stella S, Geuna M, Guida G, Caligaris-Cappio F (2004) Monoclonal CD5+ and CD5- B-lymphocyte expansions are frequent in the peripheral blood of the elderly. Blood, 103:2337–2342

57. Schwab R, Walters CA, Weksler ME (1989) Host defense mechanisms and aging. Semin Oncol, 16:20–27

58. Rowley MJ, Buchanan H, Mackay IR (1968) Reciprocal change with age in antibody to extrinsic and intrinsic antigens. Lancet, 2:24–26

59. Hallgren HM, Buckley CE 3rd, Gilbertsen VA, et al (1973) Lymphocyte phytohemagglutinin responsiveness, immunoglobulins and autoantibodies in aging humans. J Immunol, 111:1101–1107

60. De Greef GE, Van Tol MJ, Van Den Berg JW, Van Staalduinen GJ, Janssen CJ, Radl J, Hijmans W. (1992) Serum immunoglobulin class and IgG subclass levels and the occurrence of homogeneous immunoglobulins during the course of ageing in humans. Mech Ageing Dev, 66:29–44

61. Listi F, Candore G, Modica MA, Russo M, Di Lorenzo G, Esposito-Pellitteri M, Colonna-Romano G, Aquino A, Bulati M, Lio D, Franceschi C, Caruso C (2006) A study of serum immunoglobulin levels in elderly persons that provides new insights into B-cell immunosenescence. Ann N Y Acad Sci, 1089:487–495

62. Cossarizza A, Ortolani C, Paganelli R Barbieri D, Monti D, Sansoni P, Fagiolo U, Castellani G, Bersani F, Londei M, Franceschi C (1996) CD45 isoforms expression on CD4+ and CD8 +T-cells throughout life, from newborns to centenarians: implications for T-cell memory. Mech Ageing Dev, 86:173–195

63. Miller RA (1996) The aging immune system: primer and prospectus. Science, 273:70–74

64. Nociari MM, Telford W, Russo C (1999) Postthymic development of CD28–CD8+ T-cell subset: age-associated expansion and shift from memory to naive phenotype. J Immunol, 162:3327–3335

65. Okumura M, Fujii Y, Takeuchi Y, Inada K, Nakahara K, Matsuda H (1993) Age-related accumulation of LFA-1high cells in a CD8+CD45RAhigh T-cell population. Eur J Immunol, 23:1057–1063

66. Sallusto F, Lenig D, Forster R, Lipp M, Lanzavecchia A (1999) Two subsets of memory T lymphocytes with distinct homing potentials and effector functions. Nature, 401:708–712

67. Lanzavecchia A, Sallusto F (2005) Understanding the generation and function of memory T-cell subsets. Curr Opin Immunol, 17:326–332

68. Fagnoni FF, Vescovini R, Passeri G, Bologna G, Pedrazzoni M, Lavagetto G, Casti A, Franceschi C, Passeri M, Sansoni P (2000) Shortage of circulating naive CD8(+) T-cells provides new insights on immunodeficiency in aging. Blood, 95:2860–2868

69. De Rosa SC, Herzenberg LA, Roederer M (2001) 11–color, 13-parameter flow cytometry: identification of human naive T-cells by phenotype, function, and T-cell receptor diversity. Nat Med, 7:245–248

70. Lugli E, Pinti M, Nasi M, Troiano L, Ferraresi R, Mussi C, Salvioli G, Patsekin V, Robinson JP, Durante C, Cocchi M, Cossarizza A (2007) Subject classification obtained by cluster analysis and principal component analysis applied to flow cytometric data. Cytometry A, 71:334–344

71. Nasi M, Troiano L, Lugli E, Pinti M, Ferraresi R, Monterastelli E, Mussi C, Salvioli G, Franceschi C, Cossarizza A (2006) Thymic output and functionality of the IL-7/IL-7 receptor system in centenarians: implications for the neolymphogenesis at the limit of human life. Aging Cell, 5:167–175

72. Hamann D, Kostense S, Wolthers KC, Otto SA, Baars PA, Miedema F, van Lier RA (1999) Evidence that human CD8+CD45RA+CD27– cells are induced by antigen and evolve through extensive rounds of division. Int Immunol, 11:1027–1033

73. Merino J, Martinez-Gonzalez MA, Rubio M, Inoges S, Sanchez-Ibarrola A, Subira ML (1998) Progressive decrease of CD8high+ CD28+ CD57- cells with ageing. Clin Exp Immunol, 112:48–51

74. Ouyang Q, Wagner WM, Voehringer D, Wikby A, Klatt T, Walter S, Muller CA, Pircher H, Pawelec G (2003) Age-associated accumulation of CMV-specific CD8+ T-cells expressing the inhibitory killer cell lectin-like receptor G1 (KLRG1). Exp Gerontol, 38:911–920

75. Haynes BF, Markert ML, Sempowski GD, Patel DD, Hale LP (2000) The role of the thymus in immune reconstitution in aging, bone marrow transplantation, and HIV-1 infection. Annu Rev Immunol, 18:529–560

76. Douek DC, McFarland RD, Keiser PH, Gage EA, Massey JM, Haynes BF, Polis MA, Haase AT, Feinberg MB, Sullivan JL, Jamieson BD, Zack JA, Picker LJ, Koup RA (1998) Changes in thymic function with age and during the treatment of HIV infection. Nature, 396:690–695

77. Ma A, Koka R, Burkett P (2006) Diverse functions of IL-2, IL-15, and IL-7 in lymphoid homeostasis. Annu Rev Immunol, 24:657–679

78. Lodolce JP, Boone DL, Chai S, Swain RE, Dassopoulos T, Trettin S, Ma A (1998) IL-15 receptor maintains lymphoid homeostasis by supporting lymphocyte homing and proliferation. Immunity, 9:669–676

79. Kennedy MK, Glaccum M, Brown SN, Butz EA, Viney JL, Embers M, Matsuki N, Charrier K, Sedger L, Willis CR, Brasel K, Morrissey PJ, Stocking K, Schuh JC, Joyce S, Peschon JJ (2000) Reversible defects in natural killer and memory CD8 T-cell lineages in interleukin 15-deficient mice. J Exp Med, 191:771–780

80. Kim HR, Hong MS, Dan JM, Kang I (2006) Altered IL-7Ralpha expression with aging and the potential implications of IL-7 therapy on CD8+ T-cell immune responses. Blood, 107:2855–2862

81. Gangemi S, Basile G, Monti D, Merendino RA, Di Pasquale G, Bisignano U, Nicita-Mauro V, Franceschi C (2005) Age-related modifications in circulating IL-15 levels in humans. Mediators Inflamm, :245–247

82. Naylor K, Li G, Vallejo AN, Lee WW, Koetz K, Bryl E, Witkowski J, Fulbright J, Weyand CM, Goronzy JJ (2005) The influence of age on T-cell generation and TCR diversity. J Immunol, 174:7446–7452

83. Wallace DL, Zhang Y, Ghattas H, Worth A, Irvine A, Bennett AR, Griffin GE, Beverley PC, Tough DF, Macallan DC (2004) Direct measurement of T-cell subset kinetics in vivo in elderly men and women. J Immunol, 173:1787–1794

84. Geginat J, Lanzavecchia A, Sallusto F (2003) Proliferation and differentiation potential of human CD8+ memory T-cell subsets in response to antigen or homeostatic cytokines. Blood, 101:4260–4266

85. Weng NP (2006) Aging of the immune system: how much can the adaptive immune system adapt? Immunity, 24:495–499

86. Haynes L, Linton PJ, Eaton SM, Tonkonogy SL, Swain SL (1999) Interleukin 2, but not other common gamma chain-binding cytokines, can reverse the defect in generation of CD4 effector T-cells from naive T-cells of aged mice. J Exp Med, 190:1013–1024

87. Eaton SM, Burns EM, Kusser K, Randall TD, Haynes L (2004) Age-related defects in CD4 T-cell cognate helper function lead to reductions in humoral responses. J Exp Med, 200:1613–1622

88. Cossarizza A, Monti D, Bersani F, Paganelli R, Montagnani G, Cadossi R, Cantini M, Franceschi C (1989) Extremely low frequency pulsed electromagnetic fields increase interleukin-2 (IL-2) utilization and IL-2 receptor expression in mitogen-stimulated human lymphocytes from old subjects. FEBS Lett, 248:141–144

89. Witkowski JM, Li SP, Gorgas G, Miller RA (1994) Extrusion of the P glycoprotein substrate rhodamine-123 distinguishes CD4 memory T-cell subsets that differ in IL-2-driven IL-4 production. J Immunol, 153:658–665

90. Sandmand M, Bruunsgaard H, Kemp K, Andersen-Ranberg K, Schroll M, Jeune B (2003) High circulating levels of tumor necrosis factor-alpha in centenarians are not associated with increased production in T-lymphocytes. Gerontology, 49:155–160

91. Koch S, Solana R, Dela Rosa O, Pawelec G (2006) Human cytomegalovirus infection and T-cell immunosenescence: a mini review. Mech Ageing Dev, 127:538–543

92. Vescovini R, Telera A, Fagnoni FF, Biasini C, Medici MC, Valcavi P, di Pede P, Lucchini G, Zanlari L, Passeri G, Zanni F, Chezzi C, Franceschi C, Sansoni P (2004) Different contribution of EBV and CMV infections in very long-term carriers to age-related alterations of CD8+ T-cells. Exp Gerontol, 39:1233–1243

93. Khan N, Hislop A, Gudgeon N, Cobbold M, Khanna R, Nayak L, Rickinson AB, Moss PA (2004) Herpesvirus-specific CD8 T-cell immunity in old age: cytomegalovirus impairs the response to a coresident EBV infection. J Immunol, 173:7481–7489

94. Sansoni P, Fagnoni F, Vescovini R, Mazzola M, Brianti V, Bologna G, Nigro E, Lavagetto G, Cossarizza A, Monti D, Franceschi C, Passeri M (1997) T lymphocyte proliferative capability to defined stimuli and costimulatory CD28 pathway is not impaired in healthy centenarians. Mech Ageing Dev, 96:127–136

95. Franceschi C, Monti D, Cossarizza A, Fagnoni F, Passeri G, Sansoni P (1991) Aging, longevity, and cancer: studies in Down's syndrome and centenarians. Ann N Y Acad Sci, 621:428–440.

96. Bellavia D, Frada G, Di Franco P, Feo S, Franceschi C, Sansoni P, Brai M (1999) C4, BF, C3 allele distribution and complement activity in healthy aged people and centenarians. A Biol Sci Med Sci, 54:B150–B153

97. Mondello C, Petropoulou C, Monti D, Gonos ES, Franceschi C, Nuzzo F (1999) Telomere length in fibroblasts and blood cells from healthy centenarians. Exp Cell Res, 248:234–242

98. Scola L, Candore G, Colonna-Romano G, Crivello A, Forte GI, Paolisso G, Franceschi C, Lio D, Caruso C (2005) Study of the association with -330T/G IL-2 in a population of centenarians from centre and south Italy. Biogerontology, 6:425–429

99. Olsson J, Wikby A, Johansson B, Lofgren S, Nilsson BO, Ferguson FG (2000) Age-related change in peripheral blood T-lymphocyte subpopulations and cytomegalovirus infection in the very old: the Swedish longitudinal OCTO immune study. Mech Ageing Dev, 121:187–201

100. Wikby A, Johansson B, Olsson J, Lofgren S, Nilsson BO, Ferguson F (2002) Expansions of peripheral blood CD8 T-lymphocyte subpopulations and an association with cytomegalovirus seropositivity in the elderly: the Swedish NONA immune study. Exp Gerontol, 37:445–453

101. Wikby A, Ferguson F, Forsey R, Thompson J, Strindhall J, Lofgren S, Nilsson BO, Ernerudh J, Pawelec G, Johansson B (2005) An immune risk phenotype, cognitive impairment, and survival in very late life: impact of allostatic load in Swedish octogenarian and nonagenarian humans. J Gerontol A Biol Sci Med Sci, 60:556–565

102. Callahan JE, Kappler JW, Marrack P (1993) Unexpected expansions of CD8-bearing cells in old mice. J Immunol, 151:6657–6669

103. Clambey ET, van Dyk LF, Kappler JW, Marrack P (2005) Non-malignant clonal expansions of CD8+ memory T-cells in aged individuals. Immunol Rev, 205:170–189

104. Ouyang Q, Wagner WM, Wikby A, Walter S, Aubert G, Dodi AI, Travers P, Pawelec G (2003) Large numbers of dysfunctional CD8+ T lymphocytes bearing receptors for a single dominant CMV epitope in the very old. J Clin Immunol, 23:247–257

105. Akbar AN, Fletcher JM (2005) Memory T-cell homeostasis and senescence during aging. Curr Opin Immunol, 17:480–485.

106. Sakaguchi S, Sakaguchi N, Asano M, Itoh M, Toda M (1995) Immunologic self-tolerance maintained by activated T-cells expressing IL-2 receptor alpha-chains (CD25). Breakdown of a single mechanism of self-tolerance causes various autoimmune diseases. J Immunol, 155:1151–1164

107. Groux H, O'Garra A, Bigler M, Rouleau M, Antonenko S, de Vries JE, Roncarolo MG (1997) A CD4 +T-cell subset inhibits antigen-specific T-cell responses and prevents colitis. Nature, 389:737–742

108. Kim JM, Rudensky A (2006) The role of the transcription factor Foxp3 in the development of regulatory T-cells. Immunol Rev, 212:86–98

109. Zheng Y, Rudensky AY (2007) Foxp3 in control of the regulatory T-cell lineage. Nat Immunol, 8:457–462

110. Bluestone JA, Abbas AK (2003) Natural versus adaptive regulatory T-cells. Nat Rev Immunol, 3:253–257

111. Tsaknaridis L, Spencer L, Culbertson N, Hicks K, LaTocha D, Chou YK, Whitham RH, Bakke A, Jones RE, Offner H, Bourdette DN, Vandenbark AA (2003) Functional assay for human CD4+CD25+ Treg cells reveals an age-dependent loss of suppressive activity. J Neurosci Res, 74:296–308

112. Gregg R, Smith CM, Clark FJ, Dunnion D, Khan N, Chakraverty R, Nayak L, Moss PA (2005) The number of human peripheral blood CD4+ CD25high regulatory T-cells increases with age. Clin Exp Immunol, 140:540–546

113. Trzonkowski P, Szmit E, Mysliwska J, Mysliwski A (2006) CD4+CD25+ T regulatory cells inhibit cytotoxic activity of CTL and NK-cells in humans-impact of immunosenescence. Clin Immunol, 119:307–316

114. Sharma S, Dominguez AL, Lustgarten J (2006) High accumulation of T regulatory cells prevents the activation of immune responses in aged animals. J Immunol, 177:8348–8355

115. Nishioka T, Shimizu J, Iida R, Yamazaki S, Sakaguchi S (2006) CD4+CD25+Foxp3+ T-cells and CD4+CD25-Foxp3+ T-cells in aged mice. J Immunol, 176:6586–6593

116. Shimizu J, Moriizumi E (2003) CD4+CD25- T-cells in aged mice are hyporesponsive and exhibit suppressive activity. J Immunol, 170:1675–1682

117. Moser B, Eberl M (2007) gammadelta T-cells: novel initiators of adaptive immunity. Immunol Rev, 215:89–102

118. Morita CT, Mariuzza RA, Brenner MB (2000) Antigen recognition by human gamma delta T-cells: pattern recognition by the adaptive immune system. Springer Semin Immunopathol, 22:191–217

119. Hayday AC (2000) [gamma][delta] cells: a right time and a right place for a conserved third way of protection. Annu Rev Immunol, 18:975–1026

120. Nanno M, Shiohara T, Yamamoto H, Kawakami K, Ishikawa H (2007) gammadelta T-cells: firefighters or fire boosters in the front lines of inflammatory responses. Immunol Rev, 215:103–113

121. Hintz M, Reichenberg A, Altincicek B, Bahr U, Gschwind RM, Kollas AK, Beck E, Wiesner J, Eberl M, Jomaa H (2001) Identification of (E)-4-hydroxy-3-methyl-but-2-enyl pyrophosphate as a major activator for human gammadelta T-cells in Escherichia coli. FEBS Lett, 509:317–322

122. Reichenberg A, Hintz M, Kletschek Y, Kuhl T, Haug C, Engel R, Moll J, Ostrovsky DN, Jomaa H, Eberl M (2003) Replacing the pyrophosphate group of HMB-PP by a diphosphonate function abrogates Its potential to activate human gammadelta T-cells but does not lead to competitive antagonism. Bioorg Med Chem Lett, 13:1257–1260

123. Scotet E, Martinez LO, Grant E, Barbaras R, Jeno P, Guiraud M, Monsarrat B, Saulquin X, Maillet S, Esteve JP, Lopez F, Perret B, Collet X, Bonneville M, Champagne E (2005) Tumor recognition following Vgamma9Vdelta2 T-cell receptor interactions with a surface F1-ATPase-related structure and apolipoprotein A-I. Immunity, 22:71–80

124. Chen ZW, Letvin NL (2003) Vgamma2Vdelta2+ T-cells and anti-microbial immune responses. Microbes Infect, 5:491–498

125. Shen Y, Zhou D, Qiu L, Lai X, Simon M, Shen L, Kou Z, Wang Q, Jiang L, Estep J, Hunt R, Clagett M, Sehgal PK, Li Y, Zeng X, Morita CT, Brenner MB, Letvin NL, Chen ZW (2002) Adaptive immune response of Vgamma2Vdelta2+ T-cells during mycobacterial infections. Science, 295:2255–2258

126. Shin S, El-Diwany R, Schaffert S, Adams EJ, Garcia KC, Pereira P, Chien YH (2005) Antigen recognition determinants of gammadelta T-cell receptors. Science, 308:252–255

127. De Rosa SC, Andrus JP, Perfetto SP, Mantovani JJ, Herzenberg LA, Roederer M (2004) Ontogeny of gamma delta T-cells in humans. J Immunol, 172:1637–1645

128. Masopust D, Vezys V, Marzo AL, Lefrancois L (2001) Preferential localization of effector memory cells in nonlymphoid tissue. Science, 291:2413–2417

129. Brandes M, Willimann K, Moser B (2005) Professional antigen-presentation function by human gammadelta T-Cells. Science, 309:264–268

130. Argentati K, Re F, Donnini A, Tucci MG, Franceschi C, Bartozzi B, Bernardini G, Provinciali M (2002) Numerical and functional alterations of circulating gammadelta T lymphocytes in aged people and centenarians. J Leukoc Biol, 72:65–71

131. Colonna-Romano G, Aquino A, Bulati M, Lio D, Candore G, Oddo G, Scialabba G, Vitello S, Caruso C (2004) Impairment of gamma/delta T lymphocytes in elderly: implications for immunosenescence. Exp Gerontol, 39:1439–1446

132. Girardi M, Oppenheim DE, Steele CR, Lewis JM, Glusac E, Filler R, Hobby P, Sutton B, Tigelaar RE, Hayday AC (2001) Regulation of cutaneous malignancy by gammadelta T-cells. Science, 294:605–609

133. Groh V, Steinle A, Bauer S, Spies T (1998) Recognition of stress-induced MHC molecules by intestinal epithelial gammadelta T-cells. Science, 279:1737–1740

134. Dechanet J, Merville P, Lim A, Retiere C, Pitard V, Lafarge X, Michelson S, Meric C, Hallet MM, Kourilsky P, Potaux L, Bonneville M, Moreau JF (1999) Implication of gammadelta T-cells in the human immune response to cytomegalovirus. J Clin Invest, 103:1437–1449

135. Sciammas R, Bluestone JA (1999) TCRgammadelta cells and viruses. Microbes Infect, 1:203–212

136. Dieli F, Troye-Blomberg M, Farouk SE, Sireci G, Salerno A (2001) Biology of gammadelta T-cells in tuberculosis and malaria. Curr Mol Med, 1:437–446

137. Ramsburg E, Tigelaar R, Craft J, Hayday A (2003) Age-dependent requirement for gammadelta T-cells in the primary but not secondary protective immune response against an intestinal parasite. J Exp Med, 198:1403–1414

138. Caccamo N, Dieli F, Wesch D, Jomaa H, Eberl M (2006) Sex-specific phenotypical and functional differences in peripheral human Vgamma9/Vdelta2 T-cells. J Leukoc Biol, 79:663–666

139. Budzynski W, Radzikowski C (1994) Cytotoxic cells in immunodeficient athymic mice. Immunopharmacol Immunotoxicol, 16:319–346

140. Lanier LL, Yu G, Phillips JH (1989) Coassociation of CD3 zeta with a receptor (CD16) for IgG Fc on human natural killer cells. Nature, 342:803–805

141. Nakazawa T, Agematsu K, Yabuhara A (1997) Later development of Fas ligand-mediated cytotoxicity as compared with granule-mediated cytotoxicity during the maturation of natural killer cells. Immunology, 92:180–187

142. Griffiths GM (2003) Endocytosing the death sentence. J Cell Biol, 160:155–156

143. Trapani JA (1998) Dual mechanisms of apoptosis induction by cytotoxic lymphocytes. Int Rev Cytol, 182:111–192

144. Solana R, Mariani E (2000) NK and NK/T-cells in human senescence. Vaccine, 18:1613–1620

145. Kutza J, Murasko DM (1994) Effects of aging on natural killer cell activity and activation by interleukin-2 and IFN-alpha. Cell Immunol, 155:195–204

146. Ogata K, Yokose N, Tamura H, An E, Nakamura K, Dan K, Nomura T (1997) Natural killer cells in the late decades of human life. Clin Immunol Immunopathol, 84:269–275

147. Ogata K, An E, Shioi Y, Nakamura K, Luo S, Yokose N, Minami S, Dan K (2001) Association between natural killer cell activity and infection in immunologically normal elderly people. Clin Exp Immunol, 124:392–397

148. Pawelec G, Solana R, Remarque E, Mariani E (1998) Impact of aging on innate immunity. J Leukoc Biol, 64:703–712

149. Bruunsgaard H, Pedersen AN, Schroll M, Skinhoj P, Pedersen BK (2001) Decreased natural killer cell activity is associated with atherosclerosis in elderly humans. Exp Gerontol, 37:127–136

150. Mysliwska J, Trzonkowski P, Szmit E, Brydak LB, Machala M, Mysliwski A (2004) Immunomodulating effect of influenza vaccination in the elderly differing in health status. Exp Gerontol, 39:1447–1458

151. Sansoni P, Cossarizza A, Brianti V, Fagnoni F, Snelli G, Monti D, Marcato A, Passeri G, Ortolani C, Forti E, et al (1993) Lymphocyte subsets and natural killer cell activity in healthy old people and centenarians. Blood, 82:2767–2773

152. Borrego F, Alonso MC, Galiani MD, Carracedo J, Ramirez R, Ostos B, Pena J, Solana R (1999) NK phenotypic markers and IL2 response in NK-cells from elderly people. Exp Gerontol, 34:253–265

153. Lutz CT, Moore MB, Bradley S, Shelton BJ, Lutgendorf SK (2005) Reciprocal age related change in natural killer cell receptors for MHC class I. Mech Ageing Dev, 126:722–731

154. Mariani E, Monaco MC, Cattini L, Sinoppi M, Facchini A (1994) Distribution and lytic activity of NK cell subsets in the elderly. Mech Ageing Dev, 76:177–187

155. Mariani E, Sgobbi S, Meneghetti A, Tadolini M, Tarozzi A, Sinoppi M, Cattini L, Facchini A (1996) Perforins in human cytolytic cells: the effect of age. Mech Ageing Dev, 92:195–209

156. Rukavina D, Laskarin G, Rubesa G, Strbo N, Bedenicki I, Manestar D, Glavas M, Christmas SE, Podack ER (1998) Age-related decline of perforin expression in human cytotoxic T lymphocytes and natural killer cells. Blood, 92:2410–2420

157. Franceschi C, Motta L, Valensin S, Rapisarda R, Franzone A, Berardelli M, Motta M, Monti D, Bonafe M, Ferrucci L, Deiana L, Pes GM, Carru C, Desole MS, Barbi C, Sartoni G, Gemelli C, Lescai F, Olivieri F, Marchegiani F, Cardelli M, Cavallone L, Gueresi P, Cossarizza A, Troiano L, Pini G, Sansoni P, Passeri G, Lisa R, Spazzafumo L, Amadio L, Giunta S, Stecconi R, Morresi R, Viticchi C, Mattace R, De Benedictis G, Baggio G (2000) Do men and women follow different trajectories to reach extreme longevity? Italian Multicenter Study on Centenarians (IMUSCE). Aging (Milano), 12:77–84

158. Rink L, Cakman I, Kirchner H (1998) Altered cytokine production in the elderly. Mech Ageing Dev, 102:199–209

159. Murasko DM, Jiang J (2005) Response of aged mice to primary virus infections. Immunol Rev, 205:285–296

160. Mariani E, Meneghetti A, Neri S, Ravaglia G, Forti P, Cattini L, Facchini A (2002) Chemokine production by natural killer cells from nonagenarians. Eur J Immunol, 32:1524–1529

161. Kelley KW, Weigent DA, Kooijman R (2007) Protein hormones and immunity. Brain Behav Immun, 21:384–392

162. Straub RH, Cutolo M (2001) Involvement of the hypothalamic--pituitary--adrenal/gonadal axis and the peripheral nervous system in rheumatoid arthritis: viewpoint based on a systemic pathogenetic role. Arthritis Rheum, 44:493–507

163. Mocchegiani E, Giacconi R, Muti E, Rogo C, Bracci M, Muzzioli M, Cipriano C, Malavolta M (2004) Zinc, immune plasticity, aging, and successful aging: role of metallothionein. Ann N Y Acad Sci, 1019:127–134

164. Mocchegiani E, Malavolta M (2004) NK and NKT cell functions in immunosenescence. Aging Cell, 3:177–184

165. Mariani E, Ravaglia G, Forti P, Meneghetti A, Tarozzi A, Maioli F, Boschi F, Pratelli L, Pizzoferrato A, Piras F, Facchini A (1999) Vitamin D, thyroid hormones and muscle mass influence natural killer (NK) innate immunity in healthy nonagenarians and centenarians. Clin Exp Immunol, 116:19–27

166. Miyaji C, Watanabe H, Toma H, Akisaka M, Tomiyama K, Sato Y, Abo T (2000) Functional alteration of granulocytes, NK-cells, and natural killer T-cells in centenarians. Hum Immunol, 61:908–916

167. Mocchegiani E, Muzzioli M, Giacconi R, Cipriano C, Gasparini N, Franceschi C, Gaetti R, Cavalieri E, Suzuki H (2003) Metallothioneins/PARP-1/IL-6 interplay on natural killer cell activity in elderly: parallelism with nonagenarians and old infected humans. Effect of zinc supply. Mech Ageing Dev, 124:459–468

168. Porcelli S, Yockey CE, Brenner MB, Balk SP (1993) Analysis of T-cell antigen receptor (TCR) expression by human peripheral blood CD4-8- alpha/beta T-cells demonstrates preferential use of several V beta genes and an invariant TCR alpha chain. J Exp Med, 178:1–16
169. Davodeau F, Peyrat MA, Necker A, Dominici R, Blanchard F, Leget C, Gaschet J, Costa P, Jacques Y, Godard A, Vie H, Poggi A, Romagne F, Bonneville M (1997) Close phenotypic and functional similarities between human and murine alphabeta T-cells expressing invariant TCR alpha-chains. J Immunol, 158:5603–5611
170. Makino Y, Kanno R, Ito T, Higashino K, Taniguchi M (1995) Predominant expression of invariant V alpha 14+ TCR alpha chain in NK1.1+ T-cell populations. Int Immunol, 7:1157–1161
171. Taniguchi M, Harada M, Kojo S, Nakayama T, Wakao H (2003) The regulatory role of Valpha14 NKT-cells in innate and acquired immune response. Annu Rev Immunol, 21:483–513
172. Prussin C, Foster B (1997) TCR V alpha 24 and V beta 11 coexpression defines a human NK1 T-cell analog containing a unique Th0 subpopulation. J Immunol, 159:5862–5870
173. Brigl M, Brenner MB (2004) CD1: antigen presentation and T-cell function. Annu Rev Immunol, 22:817–890
174. Bendelac A, Rivera MN, Park SH, et al (1997) Mouse CD1-specific NK1 T-cells: development, specificity, and function. Annu Rev Immunol, 15:535–562
175. Zhou D, Mattner J, Cantu C, 3rd, Schrantz N, Yin N, Gao Y, Sagiv Y, Hudspeth K, Wu YP, Yamashita T, Teneberg S, Wang D, Proia RL, Levery SB, Savage PB, Teyton L, Bendelac A (2004) Lysosomal glycosphingolipid recognition by NKT-cells. Science, 306:1786–1789
176. Kinjo Y, Wu D, Kim G, Xing GW, Poles MA, Ho DD, Tsuji M, Kawahara K, Wong CH, Kronenberg M (2005) Recognition of bacterial glycosphingolipids by natural killer T-cells. Nature, 434:520–525
177. Zajonc DM, Maricic I, Wu D, Halder R, Roy K, Wong CH, Kumar V, Wilson IA (2005) Structural basis for CD1d presentation of a sulfatide derived from myelin and its implications for autoimmunity. J Exp Med, 202:1517–1526
178. Mattner J, Debord KL, Ismail N, Goff RD, Cantu C, 3rd, Zhou D, Saint-Mezard P, Wang V, Gao Y, Yin N, Hoebe K, Schneewind O, Walker D, Beutler B, Teyton L, Savage PB, Bendelac A (2005) Exogenous and endogenous glycolipid antigens activate NKT-cells during microbial infections. Nature, 434:525–529
179. Kim CH, Butcher EC, Johnston B (2002) Distinct subsets of human Valpha24-invariant NKT-cells: cytokine responses and chemokine receptor expression. Trends Immunol, 23:516–519
180. Lee PT, Benlagha K, Teyton L, Bendelac A (2002) Distinct functional lineages of human V(alpha)24 natural killer T-cells. J Exp Med, 195:637–641
181. Gumperz JE, Miyake S, Yamamura T, Brenner MB (2002) Functionally distinct subsets of CD1d-restricted natural killer T-cells revealed by CD1d tetramer staining. J Exp Meds, 195:625–636
182. D'Andrea A, Goux D, De Lalla C, Koezuka Y, Montagna D, Moretta A, Dellabona P, Casorati G, Abrignani S (2000) Neonatal invariant Valpha24+ NKT lymphocytes are activated memory cells. Eur J Immunol, 30:1544–1550
183. Sandberg JK, Bhardwaj N, Nixon DF (2003) Dominant effector memory characteristics, capacity for dynamic adaptive expansion, and sex bias in the innate Valpha24 NKT cell compartment. Eur J Immunol, 33:588–596
184. Godfrey DI, Berzins SP (2007) Control points in NKT-cell development. Nat Rev Immunol, 7:505–518
185. Seino K, Taniguchi M (2004) Functional roles of NKT cell in the immune system. Front Biosci, 9:2577–2587
186. Godfrey DI, Kronenberg M (2004) Going both ways: immune regulation via CD1d-dependent NKT-cells. J Clin Invest, 114:1379–1388
187. Kitamura H, Iwakabe K, Yahata T, Nishimura S, Ohta A, Ohmi Y, Sato M, Takeda K, Okumura K, Van Kaer L, Kawano T, Taniguchi M, Nishimura T (1999) The natural killer T

(NKT) cell ligand alpha-galactosylceramide demonstrates its immunopotentiating effect by inducing interleukin (IL)-12 production by dendritic cells and IL-12 receptor expression on NKT-cells. J Exp Med, 189:1121–1128

188. Kawano T, Nakayama T, Kamada N, Kaneko Y, Harada M, Ogura N, Akutsu Y, Motohashi S, Iizasa T, Endo H, Fujisawa T, Shinkai H, Taniguchi M (1999) Antitumor cytotoxicity mediated by ligand-activated human V alpha24 NKT-cells. Cancer Res, 59:5102–5105

189. Nieda M, Okai M, Tazbirkova A, Lin H, Yamaura A, Ide K, Abraham R, Juji T, Macfarlane DJ, Nicol AJ (2004) Therapeutic activation of Valpha24+Vbeta11+ NKT-cells in human subjects results in highly coordinated secondary activation of acquired and innate immunity. Blood, 103:383–389

190. Kronenberg M (2005) Toward an understanding of NKT cell biology: progress and paradoxes. Annu Rev Immunol, 23:877–900

191. Linsen L, Somers V, Stinissen P (2005) Immunoregulation of autoimmunity by natural killer T-cells. Hum Immunol, 66:1193–1202

192. MacDonald HR (2002) Development and selection of NKT-cells. Curr Opin Immunol, 14:250–254

193. McNerlan SE, Rea IM, Alexander HD, Morris TC (1998) Changes in natural killer cells, the CD57CD8 subset, and related cytokines in healthy aging. J Clin Immunol, 18:31–38

194. Miyaji C, Watanabe H, Minagawa M, Toma H, Kawamura T, Nohara Y, Nozaki H, Sato Y, Abo T (1997) Numerical and functional characteristics of lymphocyte subsets in centenarians. J Clin Immunol, 17:420–429

195. DelaRosa O, Tarazona R, Casado JG, Alonso C, Ostos B, Pena J, Solana R (2002) Valpha24+ NKT-cells are decreased in elderly humans. Exp Gerontol, 37:213–217

196. Crough T, Purdie DM, Okai M, Maksoud A, Nieda M, Nicol AJ (2004) Modulation of human Valpha24(+)Vbeta11(+) NKT-cells by age, malignancy and conventional anticancer therapies. Br J Cancer, 91:1880–1886

197. Molling JW, Kolgen W, Van Der Vliet HJ, Boomsma MF, Kruizenga H, Smorenburg CH, Molenkamp BG, Langendijk JA, Leemans CR, von Blomberg BM, Scheper RJ, Van Den Eertwegh AJ (2005) Peripheral blood IFN-gamma-secreting Valpha24+Vbeta11+ NKT cell numbers are decreased in cancer patients independent of tumor type or tumor load. Int J Cancer, 116:87–93

198. Peralbo E, Delarosa O, Gayoso I, Pita ML, Tarazona R, Solana R (2006) Decreased frequency and proliferative response of invariant Valpha24Vbeta11 natural killer T (iNKT) cells in healthy elderly. Biogerontology, 7:483–492

199. Jing Y, Gravenstein S, Rao Chaganty N, Chen N, Lyerly KH, Joyce S, Deng Y (2007) Aging is associated with a rapid decline in frequency, alterations in subset composition, and enhanced Th2 response in CD1d-restricted NKT-cells from human peripheral blood. Exp Gerontol

200. Godfrey DI, MacDonald HR, Kronenberg M, Smyth MJ, Van Kaer L (2004) NKT-cells: what's in a name? Nat Rev Immunol, 4:231–237

201. Tarazona R, DelaRosa O, Alonso C, Ostos B, Espejo J, Pena J, Solana R (2000) Increased expression of NK cell markers on T-lymphocytes in aging and chronic activation of the immune system reflects the accumulation of effector/senescent T-cells. Mech Ageing Dev, 121:77–88

202. Abedin S, Michel JJ, Lemster B, Vallejo AN (2005) Diversity of NKR expression in aging T-cells and in T-cells of the aged: the new frontier into the exploration of protective immunity in the elderly. Exp Gerontol, 40:537–548

203. Berzins SP, Uldrich AP, Pellicci DG, McNab F, Hayakawa Y, Smyth MJ, Godfrey DI (2004) Parallels and distinctions between T and NKT cell development in the thymus. Immunol Cell Biol, 82:269–275

204. Benlagha K, Wei DG, Veiga J, Teyton L, Bendelac A (2005) Characterization of the early stages of thymic NKT cell development. J Exp Med, 202:485–492

205. Egawa T, Eberl G, Taniuchi I, Benlagha K, Geissmann F, Hennighausen L, Bendelac A, Littman DR (2005) Genetic evidence supporting selection of the Valpha14i NKT cell lineage from double-positive thymocyte precursors. Immunity, 22:705–716

206. Forsey RJ, Thompson JM, Ernerudh J, Hurst TL, Strindhall J, Johansson B, Nilsson BO, Wikby A (2003) Plasma cytokine profiles in elderly humans. Mech Ageing Dev, 124:487–493
207. De Martinis M, Modesti M, Ginaldi L (2004) Phenotypic and functional changes of circulating monocytes and polymorphonuclear leucocytes from elderly persons. Immunol Cell Biol, 82:415–420
208. Perfetto SP, Chattopadhyay PK, Roederer M (2004) Seventeen-colour flow cytometry: unravelling the immune system. Nat Rev Immunol, 4:648–655
209. Lugli E, Troiano L, Cossarizza A. Investigating T cells by polychromatic flow cytometry. T cell protocols:Second edition, Vol. 54. G. De Libero Ed. Humana Press, 2009 (in press)
210. Clambey ET, Kappler JW, Marrack P (2007) CD8 T-cell clonal expansions & aging: a heterogeneous phenomenon with a common outcome. *Exp Gerontol*, 42:407–411

Mouse Models and Genetics of Immunosenescence

Qing Yu, Jyoti Misra Sen and Dennis Taub

Contents

Abstract: Age-related changes in the immune system result in deterioration in the ability of elderly human beings to develop immunity after vaccination and to respond to infections. Thereby the quality of longer lifespan enjoyed by modern man is significantly compromised. Furthermore, higher mortality in the elderly from infections, autoimmune disease and cancer is associated with decline in the immune function. The use of rodent models has yielded critical knowledge of mechanisms by which immune cells develop and function. In this chapter, we focus on several mouse models that have provided significant data on the changes in immune system with advancing age. A greater understanding of many of the age-related changes in immune function, recently defined as immunosenescence, may provide important insight into the development of clinical strategies and interventions for the maintenance of adequate immune system as human beings age.

Keywords: Immune system • Thymic involution • Immune aging • Mouse models • Immunosenescence

1   Introduction

In mammals, adaptive immunity complements the more primitive innate immunity resulting in a more comprehensive protection from infection and neoplasms. Cells of the adaptive immune system, T-cells and B-cells are activated by the antigenic stimulation provided by the pathogen in combination with various growth factors and

D. Taub (✉) · Q. Yu · J. Misra Sen
Laboratory of Immunology
Clinical Immunology Section
National Institute of Ageing
Intramural Research Program
National Institute of Health
Baltimore, MD 21224-6825, USA
Tel: 410-558-8159; Fax: 410-558-8284
E-mail: taubd@grc.nia.nih.gov

T. Fulop et al. (eds.), *Handbook on Immunosenescence,*
DOI 10.1007/ 978-1-4020-9062-2_3, © Springer Science+Business Media B.V. 2009

immunomodulatory molecules of the innate immune system (e.g., cytokines). The mammalian immune system undergoes significant changes throughout the animal's lifespan. Aging has been associated with immunological changes (immunosenescence) including thymic involution, lower number of naive T-cells, decrease in several cell immune functions and increase in others, and poor vaccination response to new antigens. At each stage of immune development over a lifespan, complex changes have been observed involving multiple cell types and molecular events, making it unlikely that we will be able attribute the age-related changes to a single gene or signalling pathway. Therefore, it has become imperative to understand not only the development and function of individual cell types that participate in normal immune responses and age-associated immunosenescence but also the interactions between various cells and signalling mediators and growth factors.

Many of the early efforts to examine age-associated immune dysfunction have centered on possible loss or alterations in the number of circulating lymphocytes, more specifically T-cells (Taub and Longo 2005). The focus on T-cells makes sense given the fact that T-cells are produced by the thymus, which is known to involute with advancing age resulting in a significant loss in its capability to generate new T-cells for export into the peripheral T-cell pool. Interestingly, this age-associated loss in thymic output does not result in any significant change in the total peripheral number of T-cells. It is believed that peripheral T-cell numbers with aging are maintained by a homeostatic compensatory process involving the peripheral thymus-independent expansion of mature T-cells. Given that T-cells have a limited replicative lifespan, the continued proliferation of T-cells with age is believed to lead to an accumulation of replicative-senescent T-cells possessing a diminished capacity to respond to new or recall antigens and activation stimuli. This homeostatic expansion of peripheral T-cells results in a significantly limited T-cell receptor (TCR) repertoire with age (Taub and Longo 2005). Moreover, while a number of additional age-associated alterations including effects on TCR and growth factor signaling, loss of bone marrow and thymic activity and output, alterations in cytokine and hormone expression and deficits in accessory cell function have been reported, the literature contains a number of contradictory findings describing age-related alterations in immune function suggesting significant variability in the immune aging process. Such variability hinders the identification of a central factor(s) responsible for the loss of immune function. Therefore, with the involvement of so many distinct processes within the aging immune system, the development of potential therapeutic interventions and strategies to reverse the aging process and rejuvenate the immune system has been hindered. Given that the loss in thymic function is one of the earliest and most consistent steps in the progression to immune dysfunction, strategies that target the involuting thymus are the focus of many interventions with the specific goal to reverse thymic atrophy and restore thymopoiesis and T-cell export. Increases in the numbers of new and functional T-cells in the circulating pool may extend and expand the peripheral T-cell repertoire as well as the individual's ability to mount a response to new or recall antigens.

In addition to the age-associated decline in T-cell function, the number of B-cells generated also decline with age resulting in a paucity of naive B-cells. Diminished immune responses to novel antigens in the elderly are the cumulative effect of fewer newly generated naïve T- and B-cells and a decline in B-cell function and proliferative capacity. This decline in B-cell generation results from the deterioration of the hematopoietic stem cells (HSC) as well as the inability of the older bone marrow environment to support lymphopoiesis. This has lead to increasing interest in the study of HSCs and the local lymphoid environment and their ability to survive, expand and mature during the aging process. Moreover, apart from age-associated defects observed in the adaptive immune system, a number of immunological defects have also been observed in cells of the innate immune system including dendritic cells (DCs), natural killer (NK) cells, monocytes and macrophages, neutrophils, eosinophil, basophil and mast cells. The innate immune system forms the first line of defence in a host with phagocytes (macrophage, DC, granulocytes) engulfing microbes and particulate antigens, killing microbes and tumor cells and presenting processed antigens to T-cells. Defects in many of the established functions of innate immune cells have been reported (Taub and Longo 2005). Thus, it would appear that aging has an impact on many of the immune cell subsets and together may impact our ability to respond to antigens, microbial challenges and tumors with advancing age. Thus, increasing our understanding of the potential mechanisms believed responsible for age-related immunosenescence should yield valuable insight into the development and optimization of interventional strategies aimed at restoring thymic and bone marrow function and boosting the responsiveness of adaptive and innate cell subsets.

Animal models are commonly utilized in aging research to obtain data on specific tissue and organ systems that are difficult to obtain directly from humans. In addition, given the significantly shorter life span of animals and ethical issues with performing certain treatments in human volunteers or patients, it is much easier to examine the impact of genetic, hormonal, nutritional and physiological changes in these models than in humans. For example, one can easily examine the impact of caloric restriction in mice and rats over their 2–3 year life span compared to similar studies in human, which would be nearly impossible to perform from birth to death. Moreover, in mice, various genes can be manipulated and modified to generate gene hyper-expressing or deficient animals to examine the influence of a single gene pathway on life span or various physiological functions. A number of animal model systems have been established examining the age-associated defects in immune function and specific pathways that have been shown to be altered, accelerated and/or influenced by normal or pathological aging. These immunosenescence models include mice with alterations in telomerase activity, tumor suppressor function, oxidative stress, hormone expression and various other molecules associated with immune development and differentiation as well as longevity. A number of unique findings have been made in these models regarding basic immune function and the relationship between various pathways associated with longevity and immune function. Many of these models can be divided into several categories including those mouse models demonstrating a shorter life span, an extended lifespan and little to no significant differences in life expectancy. In this chapter, we have reviewed and consolidated the available data on many of these established mouse model systems that have been utilized to study alterations in innate and adaptive immune function and their relationship to age-related immunosenescence and clonal exhaustion.

2   Mouse Models Demonstrating a Shorter Life Span

A. Klotho Mice. Klotho gene is the first gene to be documented that accelerates aging and shortens life span upon disruption and extends life span when overexpressed (Kuro-o et al. 1997; Kurosu et al. 2005). The Klotho protein is a 130kD single-pass transmembrane protein, but the extracellular fraction of the protein is shed and secreted into the blood and body fluids and thus it is now believed to function as a hormone or cytokine. The Klotho protein inhibits intracellular insulin and IGF-1 signalling, which is a major mechanism for Klotho's effect on preventing aging (Kurosu et al. 2005). Klotho mice, which bear an insertional mutation of Klotho gene, have demonstrated various disorders resembling human aging as well as a significantly shortened life span (Kuro-o et al. 1997). Klotho mice have dramatically accelerated age-related thymic atrophy (Kuro-o et al. 1997) and significantly accelerated age-related decline in B-lymphopoiesis (Okada et al. 2000). The defective B-lymphopoiesis is not cell autonomous and thus Klotho may exert its effect by influencing hematopoietic microenvironment, which includes IL-7 gene expression by bone marrow stromal cells (Okada et al. 2000).

B. Senescence-accelerated Mouse (SAM). The SAM series were generated in 1980s from the breeding of AKR/J mice when the researchers found that certain litters of mice had an accelerated senescence in an inherited manner. To date, the SAM series includes nine SAMP strains with accelerated aging and three SAMR strains with normal aging, and each SAMP mouse shows various strain-specific and age-associated phenotypes (Higuchi, 1997; Hosono et al., 1997; Takeda et al., 1991; Takeda et al., 1981). The genetic changes in SAMP mice await extensive investigations, although alterations in the expression of apolipoprotein A-II (Apo A-II) has been identified in these strains (Higuchi 1997). SAMP mice demonstrate age-associated early decline in various immune functions, including decline of antibody production to T-independent antigens and NK cell activity; decline in antibody response to T-dependent antigens as a result of impaired T helper cell activity for antibody response and early onset of autoantibody production (Haruna et al. 1995; Hosokawa et al. 1987a; Hosokawa et al. 1987b; Hosono et al. 1997; Yoshioka et al. 1993).

C. Terc Deficient Mice. Telomerase is the protein complex that synthesizes telomeres and thus preventing telomere shortening during cell division and the consequent chromosomal instability and cell cycle arrest or apoptosis. Telomerase consists of two basic components, telomerase reverse transcriptase (Tert) and telomerase RNA component (Terc), which provides the RNA template for the telomeric DNA repeats (Collins 2000; Nugent and Lundblad 1998). Mice that are deficient for Terc are initially normal, but after 5–6 generations both females and males are sterile and demonstrate certain premature aging phenotypes and shorter life spans (Blasco et al. 1997; Lee et al. 1998). These mice also exhibit an impaired ability to regenerate hematopoietic cells after ablation of these cells by 5-FU, decreased antibody responses and germinal center formation to a T-dependent antigen and reduced T and B-cell proliferation after activation in vitro. These results confirm that telomere shortening can influence immunoresponsiveness, although the precise mechanisms by which this occurs remains unknown (Herrera et al., 2000; Lee et al., 1998).

D. Tumor Suppressor Mouse Models. A number of genes that are involved in tumor suppression, DNA repair and cell cycle checkpoint also regulate aging and life span. The direct studies on effect of tumor suppressor P53 have been hampered by the early onset of tumor in p53[-/-] mice and failure of embryonic development in mice overexpressing p53 (Donehower et al. 1992; Tyner et al. 2002). However, mice expressing two types of truncated forms of p53, p24 and p44 (that bestow enhanced activity to endogenous full-length p53), show early onset of aging, a range of aging phenotypes and significantly decreased life span (Maier et al. 2004; Tyner et al. 2002). Disruption of Wip1, Brca1, Atm, Ku86, K70 or XPD all lead to shortened life span by modulating p53 activity (Barlow et al. 1996; Cao et al. 2003; Choi et al. 2002; de Boer et al. 2002; Li et al. 2007; Vogel et al. 1999). In p53[-/-] mice, apart from the development of thymic lymphoma, peripheral CD4+ T-cells demonstrate traits of immune senescence such as accumulation of memory type cells and defective proliferative response upon activation (Clarke et al. 1993; Donehower et al. 1992; Lowe et al. 1993; Ohkusu-Tsukada et al. 1999). In mice deficient for Wip1, a serine/threonine phosphatase that inhibits p53 activity, T-cell and B-cell proliferation response to mitogen stimulation is reduced and the immune system also manifest some other changes indicating of immune senescence (Choi et al. 2002). In Ku86[-/-], K70[-/-] and Atm[-/-] mice, development of T- and/or B-cells are severely impaired due to the critical requirement of these genes for recombination of antigen receptor genes and the incidence of lymphoma development is dramatically increased, both of which prevent a thorough study of the effect of these genes on immune aging (Gu et al. 1997; Li et al. 1998; Li et al. 2007; Matei et al. 2007; Matei et al. 2006; Nussenzweig et al. 1996; Zhu et al. 1996). The development and aging of the immune system in other interesting aging models, p53[+/m] mice, p44-Tg mice and TTD (XPD[-/-]) mice remains to be thoroughly investigated.

E. Reactive Oxygen Models. Reactive oxygen species (ROS) are involved in pathology of aging and cancer and therefore molecules that provide defences against oxidative stress and ROS are important in preventing aging. Peroxiredoxin is a family of small antioxidant proteins that scavenge peroxide and play a role in the cellular response to ROS. Peroxiredoxin-1[-/-] mice have a shorter life span due to hemolytic anemia and develop several types of cancer including T- and B-cell lymphomas (Neumann et al. 2003). The mice have impaired innate immune systems with decreased number of NK-cells that express activation receptor Ly49D and decreased NK-cell cytolytic activity as well as reduced NK-enhancing activity in RBCs. The impaired NK-cell activity may be one of the factors responsible for increased tumor development in these mice (Neumann et al. 2003).

F. Hormonal Models. Growth hormone/insulin-like growth factor 1 (GH/IGF-1) signalling pathway has long been associated with the aging process and has been demonstrated to negatively affect life span, primarily by decreasing cellular antioxidative capacity and increasing cell apoptosis (Bartke 2005; Everitt 2003; Quarrie and Riabowol 2004). Transgenic mice expressing GH demonstrate various

Table 1 Mouse Models Demonstrating a Shorter Life Span

Strain name (reference)	Molecular description	Immune system	References (immune system)
Klotho mice (Kuro-o et al. 1997)	Mice with an insertional mutation of Klotho gene Novel membrane protein and aging suppressor, 20–40% sequence homology to bacteria and plant β-glucosidases and mammalian lactase glycosylceramidase. Function as a hormone and inhibits insulin and IGF1 signaling Multiple disorders resembling human aging Life span: decreased significantly	Significantly accelerated thymic atrophy with thymus normal early after birth but barely detectable at 6–9 weeks of age Markedly decreased B-cells in bone marrow, spleen and blood Reduced IL-7 responsive B-cell precursors Decreased IL-7 gene expression in bone marrow stromal cells but injection of IL-7 does not rescue the defective B-lymphopoiesis HSCs have normal capacity of B-lymphopoiesis in vitro and in normal hosts Normal B-cell development in neonates and young KO mice before 2 weeks of age that have no aging phenotypes	(Kuro-o et al. 1997) (Okada et al. 2000)
SAMP mice (Takeda et al. 1991) (Takeda et al. 1981)	Senescence-accelerated mice, naturally occurring mutant mice (AKR/J background) Accelerated aging Life span: decreased by 27%	Age-associated early decline in immune function Early onset of regression in Ab production to T-independent Ag (DNP-Ficoll) and NK-cell activity Profound defect in Ab response to T-dependent Ag (sRBC), due to the impaired T-helper-cell activity for Ab response Early decline of stimulatory activity in DCs and B-cells Earlier production of autoantibodies against DNA and collagen Type II Some cellular immuneresponses, such as mix lymphocyte reaction, CTL response and DTH reaction are normal	(Hosono et al. 1997) (Hosokawa et al. 1987a) (Hosokawa et al. 1987b) (Yoshioka et al. 1993) (Haruna et al. 1995)

Table 1 (continued)

Strain name (reference)	Molecular description	Immune system	References (immune system)
TERC⁻/⁻(mTR⁻/⁻) (Blasco et al. 1997)	Target knockout of telomerase RNA template (mTR) Later generation TERC⁻/⁻ mice have shorter life span and some phenotypes of accelerated aging	Normal initial development of lymphocytes and other hematopoietic lineages, impaired ability to regenerate hematopoietic populations after 5-FU treatment Reduced proliferative response of T- and B-cells in vitro Decreased T-cell dependent humoral response in vivo, including decreased Ab response and germinal center formation	(Herrera et al. 2000) (Lee et al. 1998)
P53⁻/⁻mice (Donehower et al. 1992)	Target knockout of P53 gene Tumor suppressor, induces DNA repair, cell cycle arrest and apoptosis Increased incidence of early death, mostly not due to tumor	Thymocyte development initially normal, but develop thymic lymphoma Thymocytes and B-cells are resistant to DNA damage induced apoptosis Accelerated aging of immune system Accelerated age-related accumulation of memory like CD4 T-cells Increased cytokine production and decreased proliferation of CD4 T-cells upon activation in adult mice	(Donehower et al. 1992) (Clarke et al. 1993) (Lowe et al. 1993) (Ohkusu-Tsukada et al. 1999)
P53⁺/ᵐmice (Tyner et al. 2002)	Transgenic mice expressing N-terminus truncated P53 protein Early onset of various aging phenotypes. Effects dependent on wild-type P53 Life span decreased by 17–19%	Significantly enhanced age-associated lymphoid atrophy	(Tyner et al. 2002)

Table 1 (continued)

Strain name (reference)	Molecular description	Immune system	References (immune system)
pL53 mice (Tyner et al. 2002)	Transgenic mice expressing temperature sensitive mutant P53 protein Early onset of aging phenotypes Life span: not documented		
P44-Tg mice (Maier et al. 2004)	Transgenic mice expressing P44, the shorter isoform of P53 Early onset of aging phenotypes Life span: decreased by 40–50%		
Wip1⁻/⁻ mice (Choi et al. 2002)	Knockout of Wip1 (wild-type P53-induced phosphatase1) Serine/threonine phosphatase induced in a P53-dependent manner by DNA damaging agents. Inhibits P53 activity by inhibiting P38 phosphorylation Life span: dramatically decreased in males	Enhanced susceptibility to pathogens Increased inflammation and skin ulcerations Abnormal lymphoid histopathology Decreased T-cell and B-cell proliferative response to mitogenic stimuli	(Choi et al. 2002)
Brca-1⁻/⁻P53⁺/⁻ (Cao et al. 2003)	Targeted knockout of Brca-1 gene plus heterozygote knockout of P53 gene. Protein that has been implicated in many normal cellular functions such as DNA repair, transcriptional regulation, cell-cycle checkpoint control Brca-1⁻/⁻ mice are embryonic lethal, Brca-1⁻/⁻ P53⁺/⁻ mice are viable but show dramatic aging phenotypes and significantly shorter life span compared to P53⁺/⁻ mice		

Table 1 (continued)

Strain name (reference)	Molecular description	Immune system	References (immune system)
Atm⁻/⁻ mice (Barlow et al. 1996)	Target knockout of Atm (ataxia-telangiectasia mutated) Protein kinase that coordinates DNA damage monitoring and repair pathways. Phosphorylates and activates effectors that mediate cell-cycle checkpoint responses Life span: death before 4.5 month due to thymic lymphomas	Decreased generation and survival of DP thymocytes undergoing TCRα gene recombination Severely reduced number of mature CD4+ and CD8+ single positive thymocytes Develop aggressive thymic lymphoma, causing death before 4.5 months	(Barlow et al. 1996)(Matei et al. 2007)(Matei et al. 2006)
Ku86⁻/⁻ mice (Vogel et al., 1999) (Li et al., 2007)	Target knockout of Ku86 Important component of DNA-dependent protein kinase (DNA-PK) that's required for repairing DNA double-strand break (DSB) by nonhomologous end-joining (NHEJ) Early onset of senescence in multiple tissues and organs Life span: decreased by 61–66%	Severe immune deficiency due to early arrest of T- and B-cell development, resulting from failure in VDJ recombination Early onset of age-associated acute and chronic immune reactions in multiple organs, sometimes resulting in sepsis	(Zhu et al. 1996)(Nussenzweig et al. 1996)
Ku70⁻/⁻ mice (Li et al. 2007)	Target knockout of Ku70 Important component of DNA-dependent protein kinase (DNA-PK) that's required for repairing DNA double-strand break (DSB) by nonhomologous end-joining (NHEJ) Early onset of senescence in multiple tissues and organs Life span: decreased by 66%	Deficiency of mature B-cells or serum immunoglobulin Severely decreased thymocytes and peripheral T-cells due to severe impairment in VDJ recombination Significant incidence of CD4+CD8+ Significant incidence of CD4+CD8+ thymic lymphoma and disseminated T-cell lymphomas at a mean age of 6 months	(Gu et al. 1997)(Li et al. 1998)

Table 1 (continued)

Strain name (reference)	Molecular description	Immune system	References (immune system)
TTD mice (de Boer et al., 2002)	Target mutation of XPD gene DNA helicase involved in DNA repair and transcription Exhibit many premature aging symptoms Life span: decreased by >50%	Lower NK-cell activity reported in TTD patients	(Mariani et al. 1992)
GH-Tg mice (Palmiter et al. 1992) (Selden et al. 1989) (McGrane et al. 1988) (Bartke 2003)	Transgenic mice expressing growth hormone (GH) under mouse metallothionein I (MT) promoter or rat PEPCK (phosphoenolpyruvate carboxykinase) promoter Transgenic GH is expressed in multiple tissues, such as liver and kidney Exhibit multiple premature aging symptoms Life span: significantly decreased	Increased numbers of migrating cells in laminin-coated transwells Increased CXC chemokine ligand 12 (CXCL12)-driven migration Increased recent thymic emigrants in lymph nodes	(Smaniotto et al. 2005)
Peroxiredoxin⁻/⁻ mice (Neumann et al. 2003)	Target knockout of peroxiredoxin Small antioxidant proteins, scavenge peroxide and are involved in cellular response to reactive oxygen species (ROS) Life span: significantly decreased	Decreased NK cell cytolytic activity, decreased frequency of NK-cells expressing activation receptor Ly49D Significantly reduced NK-enhancing activity in RBCs from KO mice Development of B- and T-cell lymphomas	(Neumann et al. 2003)

premature aging phenotypes and have drastically decreased life span (Bartke 2003; McGrane et al. 1988; Palmiter et al. 1992; Selden et al. 1989). The development and aging of the immune system in these mice remain poorly studied and await more detailed examination.

3   Mouse Models Demonstrating an Extended Life Span

A. Caloric Restriction Models. Caloric restriction (CR) (limiting food intake without causing nutritional deficiencies) has been the most potent environmental factor that results in consistent extension of life span. The mechanisms responsible for the effect of CR include reducing oxidative damage, lowering GH/IGF level and triggering an innate beneficial response to low-level stressors (Masoro 1996; Merry 2000; Quarrie and Riabowol 2004; Sohal and Weindruch 1996; Weindruch and Walford 1982). CR is also the most extensively studied factor that leads to potent and consistent delay or prevention of immune senescence processes. CR results in delay or reversal of age-related reduction in naïve T-cells, decline of T-cell proliferative response to mitogens and decline in anti-viral immune response, increase in occurrence of tumor and autoimmune diseases and increase in production of inflammatory cytokines (Chen et al. 1998; Effros et al. 1991; Hobbs et al. 1993; Hursting et al. 2003; Spaulding et al. 1997a; Spaulding et al. 1997b; Walford et al. 1973; Weindruch and Walford 1982). Together, these data suggest that overall the immune system benefits from CR. However, in vivo immune responses to pathogens have not been studied to determine if infected CR mice fare better than age-matched mice on ad libitum diets. These studies will provide critical support to the hypothesis that CR benefits immune function.

B. Hormonal Models. A large group of mouse models that have extended life span involve reduced pituitary GH/IGF-1 function (Quarrie and Riabowol 2004). Among these models, the Ames dwarf and Snell dwarf mice have mutate Prop1 gene and Pit1 gene, respectively, both of which result in lowered GH/IGF-1 levels that account for both an extended life span and dwarfism (Bartke et al. 2001; Brown-Borg et al. 1996; Flurkey et al. 2001). Little mice have mutation in Ghrhr gene that encodes GH-releasing hormone receptor and the Laron mice have targeted mutation in growth hormone receptor (GHR) and GH binding protein. The p66shc$^{-/-}$ mice lack the downstream effector of GH/IGF-1 signaling and the IGF-1R$^{-/-}$ mice lack the receptor for IGF-1 (Coschigano et al. 2000; Flurkey et al. 2001; Holzenberger et al. 2003; Lupu et al. 2001; Migliaccio et al. 1999; Zhou et al. 1997). All of these mice have demonstrated extended life spans presumably due to their defective GH/IGF-1 axis. The studies on immune function in these animals are much less extensive than that done with CR mice and many results remain controversial. Among them, the immune senescence of Snell dwarf mice has been the more thoroughly investigated and results show that multiple immune senescence processes are delayed or reversed in these mice (Flurkey et al. 2001; Taub and Longo 2005). These include

Table 2 Mouse Models Demonstrating a Longer Life Span

Strain name	Molecular description	Immune system	References
Klotho-Tg mice (Kurosu et al., 2005)	Transgenic mice expressing Klotho gene under the control of human elongation factor 1α Life span: increased by 20–30% in male, and around 19% in female		(Chen et al. 1998) (Walford et al. 1973) (Weindruch and Walford 1982)
CR mice (Masoro 1996) (Merry 2000) (Sohal, Weindruch 1996) (Weindruch, Walford 1982)	Mice with caloric restriction (limiting food intake without causing nutritional deficiencies) Life span: significantly increased	Delayed or reversed immune senescence, which include age-associated decrease in naïve CD4+ and CD8+ T-cells, decline in T-cell proliferation to mitogenic stimuli, increase in incidence of tumor and autoimmune disease, decrease in anti-viral immunity, increase in production of inflammatory cytokines	(Hursting et al. 2003) (Effros et al. 1991) (Hobbs et al. 1993) (Spaulding et al. 1997a) (Spaulding et al. 1997b)
Ames Mice (Brown-Borg et al. 1996) (Bartke et al. 2001)	Mutation of Prop1 gene Transcription factor in embryonic development of anterior pituitary Life span: increased by 40–50%	Decreased thymocyte numbers	(Duquesnoy 1972)
Snell mice (Brown-Borg et al. 1996)	Mutation of Pit1 gene Pituitary-specific transcription factor Life span: increased by 40–50%	Delayed or reversed immune senescence The age related increase in splenic memory CD4+ T-cells and memory CD8+ T-cells is almost completely prevented, so is the increase in CD4+ and CD8+ T-cells that express cell surface P-glycoprotein The age related decrease in CD4+ and CD8+ T-cell function reflected by IL-2 production and generation of cytotoxic effectors is also near completely prevented	(Flurkey et al. 2001)

Table 2 (continued)

Strain name	Molecular description	Immune system	References
Little mice (Flurkey et al. 2001) (Lupu et al. 2001)	Recessive mutation of Ghrhr (GH-releasing hormone receptor) Life span: increased by 23–25% when maintained on low fat diet		
Laron Mice (Zhou et al. 1997) (Coschigano et al. 2000)	Target knockout of GHR (growth hormone receptor) and GHBP (GH binding protein) Life span: increased by 37–55%		
p66shc⁻/⁻ mice (Migliaccio et al. 1999)	Target knockout of P66shc Downstream effector of IGF-1R Life span: increased by 30%	T-cells are less susceptible to apoptogenic stimuli, and have enhanced proliferation in response to TCR stimulation in vitro	(Pacini et al. 2004)
IGF-1R⁻/⁻ mice (Holzenberger et al. 2003)	Heterozygous for the IGF-1R gene (IGF-1R⁻/⁻ is lethal) Life span: increased by 26% overall, 33% in female, 16% in male mice and not statistically significant	Decreased T-cell-independent B-cell response by in vivo assay	(Kelley et al. 1998)
TRX-Tg mice (Mitsui et al. 2002)	Transgenic mice expressing thioredoxin driven by human β-actin promoter Small thiol-mediated redox-active protein Enhanced resistance to a variety of oxidative stresses Life span: increased by 35%	Tg mice sustain the Th1 skewed status of Th1/Th2 balance during aging, in contrast to the gradual polarization to Th2 in WT mice Tg macrophages retain the phenotype of reductive macrophages with the ability to produce IL-12, and produce increased amount of NO and reduced amount of IL-6 and IL-10 during aging	(Murata et al. 2002)
FIR-KO mice (Bluher et al. 2003)	Conditional knockout of insulin receptor (IR) in adipose tissues Life span: increased by 18%		
uPA-Tg mice (Miskin, Masos 1997)	Transgenic mice expressing uPA (urokinase-type plasminogen activator) in the brain Reduced food consumption, body size and weight Life span: increased by 16%		

an age-related increase in memory T-cells and a decrease in IL-2 production and generation of cytotoxic CD8+ T-effector-cells (Flurkey et al. 2001).

4 Mouse Models Demonstrating a Normal or Undocumented Life Spans

A. Wnt-β-catenin-TCF signaling models. Wnt-β-catenin-T Cell Factor (TCF) signalling pathway has been shown to regulate thymic involution. TCF-1$^{-/-}$ mice have decreased thymocyte cellularity as early as during embryonic development, resulting from impairment at early stages of thymocyte development (Verbeek et al. 1995). In these mice, thymic involution becomes increasingly severe with age such that by 6 months of T-cells are essentially depleted (Schilham et al. 1998). Mice expressing stabilized form of β-catenin, a partner of TCF-1 for activating target gene transcription, also show enhanced thymic involution with decreased number of all thymocyte subpopulations (Xu and Sen 2003). Thus, increased Wnt signalling, as seen in transgenic mice expressing β-catenin, or decreased Wnt signalling documented in TCF-1-deficienct mice both promote thymic involution. While the precise molecular mechanisms involved in these processes remains under investigation, a balanced Wnt-β-catenin-TCF signalling pathway appears to be essential to maintain thymic function.

B. Ghrelin Infusion and Knockout Mouse Models. Recent studies have demonstrated important roles of Ghrelin in promoting thymopoiesis during aging (Dixit et al. 2007). Ghrelin is a peptide hormone mainly produced by enteroendocrine cells in the stomach in response to negative energy balance. Ghrelin binds to the GH secretagogue receptor (GHS-R) and stimulates growth hormone (GH) secretion from the pituitary. Both ghrelin and GHS-R are expressed by resting and activated human T-cells and exert anti-inflammatory effects on immune cells and systemically in mice (Dixit et al. 2004; Dixit and Taub 2005). Ghrelin and GHS-R expression declines within the thymus with age (Dixit et al. 2007). Mice deficient for ghrelin or GHS-R demonstrate enhanced age-associated thymic involution and decreased numbers of lymphoid progenitor cells in the bone marrow and thymus. Conversely, infusion of ghrelin into old mice significantly improves age-associated changes in thymic cellularity, the number of ETP, CLP, LSK and RTE and improves the TCR diversity of peripheral T-cells (Dixit et al. 2007). Thus, ghrelin emerges as an important factor to promote thymopoiesis during aging.

C. Cytokine Models. Cytokines, particularly IL-7, have been found to be associated with preventing age related thymic involution. IL-7, produced mainly by thymic and bone marrow stromal cells, is a critical trophic factor for both T- and B-cell progenitors, and deficiency of IL-7, its receptors (IL-7Rα and γ$_c$) and its downstream signalling molecule Jak3 all lead to severe defects in early T- and B-cell development and thus thymic involution and lymphopenia. IL-7 mRNA levels in the thymus decreases 15-fold by 22 months of age (Alves et al. 1995; Andrew and Aspinall 2002; Ortman et al. 2002). Effect of IL-7 administration on

Table 3 Mouse Models Demonstrating Normal or Undocumented Life Span

Strain name	Molecular description	Immune system	References
TCF-/- mice	Target knockout of TCF-1 Transcription factor downstream of Wnt signalling pathway, binds DNA and forms a complex with β-catenin which activates gene transcription	Dramatically decreased thymic cellularity starting from embryonic stage and throughout life; incomplete block at DN1, DN2 and ISP stage of thymocyte development in young mice and complete block at DN1 stage in older mice	(Verbeek et al. 1995) (Schilham et al. 1998)
CAT-Tg mice	Transgenic mice expression stabilized β-catenin under proximal Lck promoter Mediator of Wnt signalling pathway, pairs with TCF-1/LEF-1 to activate gene transcription	Enhanced thymic involution Decreased number of all the thymic subpopulations No drastic reduction in splenic T-cells	(Xu and Sen 2003)
Ghrelin-/-mice	Target knockout of Ghrelin Peptide hormone mainly produced by stomach Also expressed by thymocytes and T-cells	Enhanced age-associated thymic involution with reduced thymopoiesis Infusion of ghrelin into old mice significantly improves age-associated changes in thymic cellularity, number of ETP, CLP, LSK and RTE and improves the TCR diversity of peripheral T-cells	(Dixit et al. 2004; Dixit and Taub 2005; Dixit et al. 2007)
GHS-R-/- mice	Target knockout of GHS-R (growth hormone secretagogue receptor) G-protein coupled receptor, receptor for Ghrelin	Enhanced age-associated thymic involution with reduced thymopoiesis and diminution of bone marrow and peripheral LSK hematopoietic stem cell population	(Dixit et al. 2004) (Dixit and Taub 2005) (Dixit et al. 2007)
Lurcher mice	LC mutation, autosomal semidominant mutation of glutamate receptor (GluRδ2) gene Selectively expressed on Purkinje cells and LC mutation causes their apoptosis by a high glutamate concentration LC/LC mice die early after birth	LC/+ mice show significant reduction of DP thymocytes and thymic involution by 3 month of age due to enhanced cell death, while peripheral T-cell number is normal compared to control mice	(Mandakova et al. 2005) (Mandakova et al. 2003) (Mandakova et al. 2003)

Table 3 (continued)

Strain name	Molecular description	Immune system	References
Dnmt1^{-/-} mice	Target knockout of Dnmt1 (DNA methyltransferase 1) Enzyme responsible for maintaining DNA methylation through mitosis	Delayed immune senescence, reflected by significantly delayed age-associated increase in memory-like CD4 T-cells, decline of CD4 T-cell proliferative response and IL-2 production Delayed development of autoimmunity	(Yung et al. 2001)
IL-7^{-/-}	Target knockout of IL-7	Severe T- and B-cell lymphopenia resulting from severe impairment of early T- and B-cell development	(von Freeden-Jeffry et al. 1995) (Moore et al. 1996)
IL-7Rα^{-/-} **γc**^{-/-} **mice**	Target knockout of IL-7 receptor alpha (α) chain and the common gamma (γ) chain	Severe T- and B-cell lymphopenia resulting from severe impairment of early T- and B-cell development	(Peschon et al. 1994) (Akashi et al. 1998) (Cao et al. 1995)
Jak3^{-/-} **mice**	Target knockout of Jak3 Jak family Tyrosine kinase mediating IL-7 receptor signal	Severe T- and B-cell lymphopenia resulting from severe impairment of early T- and B-cell development Severe defects in NK-cell development	(Nosaka et al. 1995) (Thomis et al. 1995) (Baird et al. 2000)
Lck-IL-7-Tg mice	Transgenic mice expressing IL-7 under proximal lck promoter	Low level IL-7 expression: increased thymocyte number, increased DP and SP thymocyte number Medium level IL-7 expression: no significant changes in thymocyte number High level IL-7 expression: decreased thymocyte number due to impaired proliferation of DN thymocytes	(El Kassar et al. 2004)
IL-7Rα-Tg mice	Transgenic mice expressing IL-7Rα under human CD2 promoter	Normal thymocyte number at birth, rapid decline in thymocyte number with age	(Munitic et al. 2004)

Table 3 (continued)

Strain name	Molecular description	Immune system	References
IL-12β⁻/⁻ mice	Target knockout of IL-12β IL-12 p40 subunit is produced by APCs and regulates function of T-cells and NK-cells.	Accelerated thymic involution due to increased thymocyte apoptosis Accelerated degeneration of thymic structures with decreased cortex/medulla ratio No defect in thymocyte development in young mice No age-associated decrease in IL-12 level produced by APCs in normal mice	(Hsu et al. 2005; Li et al. 2004)
CD11c-Bcl-2-Tg mice	Transgenic mice expressing human BCL-2 under CD11c promoter, in DC cells	Increased frequencies and numbers of DCs, increased turnover/survival (longevity) of DCs Enhanced humoral and cellular immune response in vivo, including enhanced IgG production, T-cell proliferation and cytotoxic activity	(Nopora and Brocker 2002)
CD2-Fas-Tg mice	Transgenic mice expressing Fas under CD2 promoter, in T-cells. Surface molecule that is critical for apoptosis and stimulation during T-cell development	Prevent age-associated decrease in ligand-induced apoptosis and proliferation as well as changes in IL-2, IL-10 and IFNγ production in T-cells; decrease in density of cell surface lipid raft elements possibly influencing cell death or activation	(Zhou et al. 1995)

thymopoiesis and thymic output has been controversial because some reports did not demonstrate significant effects (Fry and Mackall 2002), while others showed that IL-7 increases recent thymic emigrants in periphery without enhanced thymic function and restores immunity in athymic T-cell-depleted hosts (Chu et al. 2004; Fry et al. 2001; Mackall et al. 2001). IL-12, produced mainly by dendritic cells, is another factor that's required for preventing thymic involution during aging process. Aged IL-12$\beta^{-/-}$ mice, but not young IL-12$\beta^{-/-}$ mice, demonstrate accelerated thymic involution compared to age-matched wild type mice. IL-12 enhances the proliferation of thymocytes from aged IL-12$\beta^{-/-}$ and wild type mice in response to IL-2 and IL-7. Thus, IL-12 enhances IL-7 and IL-2 signalling in thymocytes from aged mice and thus may compensate for the age-associated reduction in IL-7 and IL-2 expression and signal, and thereby inhibiting thymic involution in older mice (Hsu et al. 2005). Thus, cytokines can enhance T-cell generation as well as regulate thymic function and peripheral T-cell activity. Additional work is required to define challenges in administrating cytokines to therapeutically enhance T-cell output in older humans.

5   Conclusions

The selection of an animal model for aging or immunosenescence research is dependent on the specific cells, pathways and interventions being considered or studies by an investigator and how such models may physiologically relate to normative aging and immune function. The loss or gain of immune function in a transgenic, knockout or mutant mouse does not necessarily reflect the physiological role of the manipulated molecules within a normal immune response. However, such manipulation does permit one to examine the impact of a pathway or system on life span, aging, immunity and immune development and interactions between various organ systems. Information from these animals can then lead to further examination under physiological conditions and eventually to the development of strategies to manipulate these same systems for possible therapeutic benefit. To date, only a few systems have been examined in the context of aging and much more work is needed. Many of the model systems discussed in this chapter have provided valuable new information on both aging and age-associated immunosenescence, which have lead investigators to initiate more detailed studies on specific molecules and signalling systems as well as the development of additional mouse models to further examine the interrelationships and interactions between these various ligand and signalling pathways. Moreover, some of these studies have even lead to the development of clinical trials in human subjects, such as in several hormonal administration trials. With the completion of the human genome project, we can expect the development of many additional mouse models and our need to understand the role of these molecules in the context of aging, age-related pathologies and immunosenescence will be required.

Acknowledgments This research was supported in part by the Intramural Research Program of the National Institute on Aging, National Institutes of Health.

References

Akashi K, Kondo M, Weissman IL (1998) Role of interleukin-7 in T-cell development from hematopoietic stem cells. Immunol Rev 165:13–28

Alves LA, Campos de Carvalho AC, Cirne Lima EO, Rocha e Souza, CM, Dardenne M, Spray DC, Savino W (1995) Functional gap junctions in thymic epithelial cells are formed by connexin 43. Eur J Immunol 25:431–437

Andrew D, Aspinall R (2002) Age-associated thymic atrophy is linked to a decline in IL-7 production. Exp Gerontol 37:455–463

Baird AM, Lucas JA, Berg LJ (2000) A profound deficiency in thymic progenitor cells in mice lacking Jak3. J Immunol 165:3680–3688

Barlow C, Hirotsune S, Paylor R, Liyanage M, Eckhaus M, Collins F, Shiloh Y, Crawley JN, Ried T, Tagle D, Wynshaw-Boris A (1996) Atm-deficient mice: a paradigm of ataxia telangiectasia. Cell 86:159–171

Bartke A (2003) Can growth hormone (GH) accelerate aging? Evidence from GH-transgenic mice. Neuroendocrinology 78:210–216

Bartke A (2005) Minireview: role of the growth hormone/insulin-like growth factor system in mammalian aging. Endocrinology 146:3718–3723

Bartke A, Wright JC, Mattison JA, Ingram DK, Miller RA, Roth GS (2001) Extending the lifespan of long-lived mice. Nature 414:412

Blasco MA, Lee HW, Hande MP, Samper E, Lansdorp PM, DePinho RA, Greider CW (1997) Telomere shortening and tumor formation by mouse cells lacking telomerase RNA. Cell 91:25–34

Bluher M, Kahn BB, Kahn CR (2003) Extended longevity in mice lacking the insulin receptor in adipose tissue. Science 299:572–574

Brown-Borg HM, Borg KE, Meliska CJ Bartke A (1996) Dwarf mice and the ageing process. Nature 384:33

Cao L, Li W, Kim S, Brodie SG, Deng CX (2003) Senescence, aging, and malignant transformation mediated by P53 in mice lacking the Brca1 full-length isoform. Genes Dev 17:201–213

Cao X, Shores EW, Hu-Li J, Anver MR, Kelsall BL, Russell SM, Drago J, Noguchi M, Grinberg A, Bloom ET et al (1995) Defective lymphoid development in mice lacking expression of the common cytokine receptor gamma chain. Immunity 2: 223–238

Chen J, Astle CM, Harrison DE (1998) Delayed immune aging in diet-restricted B6CBAT6 F1 mice is associated with preservation of naive T-cells. J Gerontol A Biol Sci Med Sci 53:B330-B337; discussion B338–B339

Choi J, Nannenga B, Demidov ON, Bulavin DV, Cooney A, Brayton C, Zhang Y, Mbawuike IN, Bradley A, Appella E, Donehower LA (2002) Mice deficient for the wild-type P53-induced phosphatase gene (Wip1) exhibit defects in reproductive organs, immune function, and cell cycle control. Mol Cell Biol 22:1094–1105

Chu YW, Memon SA, Sharrow SO, Hakim FT, Eckhaus M, Lucas PJ, Gress RE (2004) Exogenous IL-7 increases recent thymic emigrants in peripheral lymphoid tissue without enhanced thymic function. Blood 104:1110–1119

Clarke AR, Purdie CA, Harrison DJ, Morris RG, Bird CC, Hooper ML, Wyllie AH (1993) Thymocyte apoptosis induced by P53-dependent and independent pathways. Nature 362:849–852

Collins K (2000) Mammalian telomeres and telomerase. Curr Opin Cell Biol 12:378–383

Coschigano KT, Clemmons D, Bellush LL, Kopchick JJ (2000) Assessment of growth parameters and life span of GHR/BP gene-disrupted mice. Endocrinology 141:2608–2613 de Boer J, Andressoo JO, de Wit J, Huijmans J, Beems RB, van Steeg H, Weeda G, Van Der Horst GT, van Leeuwen W, Themmen AP, et al. (2002) Premature aging in mice deficient in DNA repair and transcription. Science 296:1276–1279

Dixit VD, Schaffer EM, Pyle RS, Collins GD, Sakthivel SK, Palaniappan R, Lillard JW Jr, Taub DD (2004) Ghrelin inhibits leptin- and activation-induced proinflammatory cytokine expression by human monocytes and T-cells. J Clin Invest 114:57–66

Dixit VD, Taub DD (2005) Ghrelin and immunity: a young player in an old field. Exp Gerontol 40:900–910

Dixit VD, Yang H, Sun Y, Weeraratna AT, Youm YH, Smith RG, Taub DD (2007) Ghrelin promotes thymopoiesis during aging. J Clin Invest

Donehower LA, Harvey M, Slagle BL, McArthur MJ, Montgomery CA Jr, Butel JS, Bradley A (1992) Mice deficient for P53 are developmentally normal but susceptible to spontaneous tumours. Nature 356:215–221

Duquesnoy RJ (1972) Immunodeficiency of the thymus-dependent system of the Ames dwarf mouse. J Immunol 108:1578–1590

Effros RB, Walford RL, Weindruch R, Mitcheltree C (1991) Influences of dietary restriction on immunity to influenza in aged mice. J Gerontol 46:B142-B147

El Kassar, N Lucas, PJ Klug, DB, Zamisch M, Merchant M, Bare CV, Choudhury B, Sharrow SO, Richie E, Mackall CL, Gress RE (2004) A dose effect of IL-7 on thymocyte development. Blood 104:1419–1427

Everitt AV (2003) Food restriction, pituitary hormones and ageing. Biogerontology 4:47–50

Flurkey K, Papaconstantinou J, Miller RA, Harrison DE (2001) Lifespan extension and delayed immune and collagen aging in mutant mice with defects in growth hormone production. Proc Natl Acad Sci U S A 98:6736–6741

Fry TJ, Christensen BL, Komschlies KL, Gress RE, Mackall CL (2001) Interleukin-7 restores immunity in athymic T-cell-depleted hosts. Blood 97:1525–1533

Fry TJ, Mackall CL (2002) Current concepts of thymic aging. Springer Semin Immunopathol 24:7–22

Gu Y, Seidl KJ, Rathbun GA, Zhu C, Manis JP, Van Der Stoep N, Davidson L, Cheng HL, Sekiguchi JM, Frank K et al (1997) Growth retardation and leaky SCID phenotype of Ku70-deficient mice. Immunity 7:653–665

Haruna H, Inaba M, Inaba K, Taketani S, Sugiura K, Fukuba Y, Doi H, Toki J, Tokunaga R, Ikehara S (1995) Abnormalities of B-cells and dendritic cells in SAMP1 mice. Eur J Immunol 25:1319–1325

Herrera E, Martinez AC, Blasco MA (2000) Impaired germinal center reaction in mice with short telomeres. Embo J 19:472–481

Higuchi K (1997) Genetic characterization of senescence-accelerated mouse (SAM). Exp Gerontol 32:129–138

Hobbs MV, Weigle WO, Noonan DJ, Torbett BE, McEvilly RJ, Koch RJ, Cardenas GJ, Ernst DN (1993) Patterns of cytokine gene expression by CD4+ T-cells from young and old mice. J Immunol 150:3602–3614

Holzenberger M, Dupont J, Ducos B, Leneuve P, Geloen A, Even PC, Cervera P, Le Bouc Y (2003) IGF-1 receptor regulates lifespan and resistance to oxidative stress in mice. Nature 421:182–187

Hosokawa T, Hosono M, Hanada K, Aoike A, Kawai K, Takeda T (1987a) Immune responses in newly developed short-lived SAM mice. Selectively impaired T-helper cell activity in in vitro antibody response. Immunology 62:425–429

Hosokawa T, Hosono M, Higuchi K, Aoike A, Kawai K, Takeda T (1987b) Immune responses in newly developed short-lived SAM mice. I. Age-associated early decline in immune activities of cultured spleen cells. Immunology 62:419–423

Hosono M, Hanada K, Toichi E, Naiki H, Higuchi K, Hosokawa T (1997) Immune abnormality in relation to nonimmune diseases in SAM mice. Exp Gerontol 32:181–195

Hsu HC, Li L, Zhang HG, Mountz JD (2005) Genetic regulation of thymic involution. Mech Ageing Dev 126:87–97

Hursting SD, Lavigne JA, Berrigan D, Perkins SN, Barrett JC (2003) Calorie restriction, aging, and cancer prevention: mechanisms of action and applicability to humans. Annu Rev Med 54:131–152

Kelley KW, Meier WA, Minshall C, Schacher DH, Liu Q, VanHoy R, Burgess W, Dantzer R (1998) Insulin growth factor-I inhibits apoptosis in hematopoietic progenitor cells. Implications in thymic aging. Ann NY Acad Sci 840:518–524

Kuro-o M, Matsumura Y, Aizawa H, Kawaguchi H, Suga T, Utsugi T, Ohyama Y, Kurabayashi M, Kaname T, Kume E et al (1997) Mutation of the mouse klotho gene leads to a syndrome resembling ageing. Nature 390:45–51

Kurosu H, Yamamoto M, Clark J D, Pastor JV, Nandi A, Gurnani P, McGuinness OP, Chikuda H, Yamaguchi M, Kawaguchi H et al (2005) Suppression of aging in mice by the hormone Klotho. Science 309:1829–1833

Lee HW, Blasco MA, Gottlieb GJ, Horner JW 2nd, Greider CW, DePinho RA (1998) Essential role of mouse telomerase in highly proliferative organs. Nature 392:569–574

Li GC, Ouyang H, Li X, Nagasawa H, Little JB, Chen DJ, Ling CC, Fuks Z, Cordon-Cardo C (1998) Ku70: a candidate tumor suppressor gene for murine T-cell lymphoma. Mol Cell 2:1–8

Li H, Vogel H, Holcomb VB, Gu Y, Hasty P (2007) Deletion of either Ku70, Ku80 or both causes early aging without substantially increased cancer. Mol Cell Biol

Li L, Hsu HC, Stockard CR, Yang P, Zhou J, Wu Q, Grizzle WE, Mountz JD (2004) IL-12 inhibits thymic involution by enhancing IL-7- and IL-2-induced thymocyte proliferation. J Immunol 172:2909–2916

Lowe SW, Schmitt EM, Smith SW, Osborne BA, Jacks T (1993) P53 is required for radiation-induced apoptosis in mouse thymocytes. Nature 362:847–849

Lupu F, Terwilliger JD, Lee K, Segre GV, Efstratiadis A (2001). Roles of growth hormone and insulin-like growth factor 1 in mouse postnatal growth. Dev Biol 229:141–162

Mackall CL, Fry TJ, Bare C, Morgan P, Galbraith A, Gress RE (2001) IL-7 increases both thymic-dependent and thymic-independent T-cell regeneration after bone marrow transplantation. Blood 97:1491–1497

Maier B, Gluba W, Bernier B, Turner T, Mohammad K, Guise T, Sutherland A, Thorner M, Scrable H (2004) Modulation of mammalian life span by the short isoform of P53. Genes Dev 18:306–319

Mandakova P, Sinkora J, Sima P, Vozeh F (2005) Reduced primary T-lymphopoiesis in 3-month-old lurcher mice: sign of premature ageing of thymus? Neuroimmunomodulation 12:348–356

Mandakova P, Virtova M, Sima P, Beranova M, Slipka J (2003) Congenitally determined neurode-generation "Lurcher" induces morphofunctional changes of thymus. Folia Microbiol (Praha) 48:394–398

Mariani E, Facchini A, Honorati MC, Lalli E, Berardesca E, Ghetti P, Marinoni S, Nuzzo F, Ast-aldi Ricotti GC, Stefanini M (1992) Immune defects in families and patients with xeroderma pigmentosum and trichothiodystrophy. Clin Exp Immunol 88:376–382

Masoro EJ (1996) Possible mechanisms underlying the antiaging actions of caloric restriction. Toxicol Pathol 24:738–741

Matei I R, Gladdy RA, Nutter LM, Canty A, Guidos CJ, Danska JS (2007) ATM deficiency disrupts Tcra locus integrity and the maturation of CD4+CD8+ thymocytes. Blood 109:1887–1896

Matei IR, Guidos CJ, Danska JS (2006) ATM-dependent DNA damage surveillance in T-cell development and leukemogenesis: the DSB connection. Immunol Rev 209:142–158

McGrane MM, de Vente J, Yun J, Bloom J, Park E, Wynshaw-Boris A, Wagner T, Rottman F M, Hanson RW (1988) Tissue-specific expression and dietary regulation of a chimeric phosphoenolpyruvate carboxykinase/bovine growth hormone gene in transgenic mice. J Biol Chem 263:11443–11451

Merry BJ (2000) Calorie restriction and age-related oxidative stress. Ann NY Acad Sci 908:180–198

Migliaccio E, Giorgio M, Mele S, Pelicci G, Reboldi P, Pandolfi PP, Lanfrancone L, Pelicci PG (1999) The p66shc adaptor protein controls oxidative stress response and life span in mammals. Nature 402:309–313

Miskin R, Masos T (1997) Transgenic mice overexpressing urokinase-type plasminogen activator in the brain exhibit reduced food consumption, body weight and size, and increased longevity. J Gerontol A Biol Sci Med Sci 52:B118–B124

Mitsui A, Hamuro J, Nakamura H, Kondo N, Hirabayashi Y, Ishizaki-Koizumi S, Hirakawa T, Inoue T, and Yodoi J (2002) Overexpression of human thioredoxin in transgenic mice controls oxidative stress and life span. Antioxid Redox Signal 4:693–696

Moore TA, von Freeden-Jeffry U, Murray R, Zlotnik A (1996) Inhibition of gamma delta T-cell development and early thymocyte maturation in IL-7/mice. J Immunol 157:2366-2373

Munitic I, Williams JA, Yang Y, Dong B, Lucas PJ, El Kassar N, Gress RE, Ashwell JD (2004) Dynamic regulation of IL-7 receptor expression is required for normal thymopoiesis. Blood 104:4165–4172

Murata Y, Amao M, Yoneda J, Hamuro J (2002) Intracellular thiol redox status of macrophages directs the Th1 skewing in thioredoxin transgenic mice during aging. Mol Immunol 38:747–757

Neumann CA, Krause DS, Carman CV, Das S, Dubey DP, Abraham JL, Bronson RT, Fujiwara Y, Orkin SH, Van Etten RA (2003) Essential role for the peroxiredoxin Prdx1 in erythrocyte antioxidant defence and tumour suppression. Nature 424:561–565

Nopora A, Brocker T (2002) Bcl-2 controls dendritic cell longevity in vivo. J Immunol 169:3006–3014

Nosaka T, van Deursen JM, Tripp RA, Thierfelder WE, Witthuhn BA, McMickle AP, Doherty PC, Grosveld GC, Ihle JN (1995) Defective lymphoid development in mice lacking Jak3. Science 270:800–802

Nugent CI, Lundblad V (1998) The telomerase reverse transcriptase: components and regulation. Genes Dev 12:1073–1085

Nussenzweig A, Chen C, da Costa Soares V, Sanchez M, Sokol K, Nussenzweig MC, Li GC (1996) Requirement for Ku80 in growth and immunoglobulin V(D)J recombination. Nature 382:551–555

Ohkusu-Tsukada K, Tsukada T, Isobe K (1999) Accelerated development and aging of the immune system in P53-deficient mice. J Immunol 163:1966–1972

Okada S, Yoshida T, Hong Z, Ishii G, Hatano M, Kuro, O M, Nabeshima Y, Nabeshima Y, Tokuhisa T (2000) Impairment of B-lymphopoiesis in precocious aging (klotho) mice. Int Immunol 12:861–871

Ortman CL, Dittmar KA, Witte PL, Le PT (2002) Molecular characterization of the mouse involuted thymus: aberrations in expression of transcription regulators in thymocyte and epithelial compartments. Int Immunol 14:813–822

Pacini S, Pellegrini M, Migliaccio E, Patrussi L, Ulivieri C, Ventura A, Carraro F, Naldini A, Lanfrancone L, Pelicci P, Baldari CT (2004) P66SHC promotes apoptosis and antagonizes mitogenic signaling in T-cells. Mol Cell Biol 24:1747–1757

Palmiter RD, Brinster RL, Hammer RE, Trumbauer ME, Rosenfeld MG, Birnberg NC, Evans RM (1992) Dramatic growth of mice that develop from eggs microinjected with metallothionein-growth hormone fusion genes (1982). Biotechnol J 24:429–433

Peschon JJ, Morrissey PJ, Grabstein KH, Ramsdell FJ, Maraskovsky E, Gliniak BC, Park LS, Ziegler SF, Williams DE, Ware CB et al (1994) Early lymphocyte expansion is severely impaired in interleukin 7 receptor-deficient mice. J Exp Med 180:1955–1960

Quarrie JK, Riabowol KT (2004) Murine models of life span extension. Sci Aging Knowledge Environ 2004:re5

Schilham MW, Wilson A, Moerer P, Benaissa-Trouw BJ, Cumano A, Clevers HC (1998) Critical involvement of Tcf-1 in expansion of thymocytes. J Immunol 161:3984–3991

Selden RF, Yun JS, Moore DD, Rowe ME, Malia MA, Wagner TE, Goodman HM (1989) Glucocorticoid regulation of human growth hormone expression in transgenic mice and transiently transfected cells. J Endocrinol 122:49–60

Smaniotto S, de Mello-Coelho V, Villa-Verde DM, Pleau JM, Postel-Vinay MC, Dardenne M, Savino W (2005) Growth hormone modulates thymocyte development in vivo through a combined action of laminin and CXC chemokine ligand 12. Endocrinology 146:3005–3017

Sohal RS, Weindruch R (1996) Oxidative stress, caloric restriction, and aging. Science 273:59–63

Spaulding CC, Walford RL, Effros RB (1997a) The accumulation of nonreplicative, nonfunctional, senescent T-cells with age is avoided in calorically restricted mice by an enhancement of T-cell apoptosis. Mech Ageing Dev 93:25–33

Spaulding CC, Walford RL, Effros RB (1997b) Calorie restriction inhibits the age-related dysregulation of the cytokines TNF-alpha and IL-6 in C3B10RF1 mice. Mech Ageing Dev 93:87–94

Takeda T, Hosokawa M, Higuchi K (1991) Senescence-accelerated mouse (SAM): a novel murine model of accelerated senescence. J Am Geriatr Soc 39:911–919

Takeda T, Hosokawa M, Takeshita S, Irino M, Higuchi K, Matsushita T, Tomita Y, Yasuhira K, Hamamoto H, Shimizu K et al (1981) A new murine model of accelerated senescence. Mech Ageing Dev 17:183–194

Taub DD, Longo DL (2005) Insights into thymic aging and regeneration. Immunol Rev 205:72–93

Thomis DC, Gurniak CB, Tivol E, Sharpe AH, Berg LJ (1995) Defects in B-lymphocyte maturation and T-lymphocyte activation in mice lacking Jak3. Science 270:794–797

Tyner SD, Venkatachalam S, Choi J, Jones S, Ghebranious N, Igelmann H, Lu X, Soron G, Cooper B, Brayton C et al (2002) P53 mutant mice that display early ageing-associated phenotypes. Nature 415:45–53

Verbeek S, Izon D, Hofhuis F, Robanus-Maandag E, te Riele H, van de Wetering M, Oosterwegel M, Wilson A, MacDonald HR, Clevers H (1995) An HMG-box-containing T-cell factor required for thymocyte differentiation. Nature 374:70–74

Vogel H, Lim DS, Karsenty G, Finegold M, Hasty P (1999) Deletion of Ku86 causes early onset of senescence in mice. Proc Natl Acad Sci U S A 96:10770–10775

von Freeden-Jeffry U, Vieira P, Lucian LA, McNeil T, Burdach SE, Murray R (1995) Lymphopenia in interleukin (IL)-7 gene-deleted mice identifies IL-7 as a nonredundant cytokine. J Exp Med 181:1519–1526

Walford RL, Liu RK, Gerbase-Delima M, Mathies M, Smith GS (1973) Longterm dietary restriction and immune function in mice: response to sheep red blood cells and to mitogenic agents. Mech Ageing Dev 2:447–454

Weindruch R, Walford RL (1982) Dietary restriction in mice beginning at 1 year of age: effect on life-span and spontaneous cancer incidence. Science 215:1415–1418

Xu Y, Sen J (2003) Beta-catenin expression in thymocytes accelerates thymic involution. Eur J Immunol 33:12–18

Yoshioka H, Yoshida H, Usui T, Sung M, Ko K, Takeuchi E, Kita T, Sugiyama T (1993) Spontaneous development of anti-collagen type II antibodies with NTA, and anti-DNA antibodies in senescence-accelerated mice. Autoimmunity 14:215–220

Yung R, Ray D, Eisenbraun JK, Deng C, Attwood J, Eisenbraun MD, Johnson K, Miller RA, Hanash S, Richardson B (2001) Unexpected effects of a heterozygous dnmt1 null mutation on age-dependent DNA hypomethylation and autoimmunity. J Gerontol A Biol Sci Med Sci 56: B268–B276

Zhou T, Edwards CK 3rd, Mountz JD (1995) Prevention of age-related T-cell apoptosis defect in CD2-fas-transgenic mice. J Exp Med 182:129–137

Zhou Y, Xu BC, Maheshwari HG, He L, Reed M, Lozykowski M, Okada S, Cataldo L, Coschigamo K, Wagner TE et al (1997) A mammalian model for Laron syndrome produced by targeted disruption of the mouse growth hormone receptor/binding protein gene (the Laron mouse). Proc Natl Acad Sci U S A 94:13215–13220

Zhu C, Bogue MA, Lim DS, Hasty P, Roth DB (1996) Ku86-deficient mice exhibit severe combined immunodeficiency and defective processing of V(D)J recombination intermediates. Cell 86:379–389

Insect Models of Immunosenescence

Jeff Leips

Contents

Abstract: For the past few decades invertebrates have been used extensively as models for understanding the general process of senescence (see reviews by Partridge and Gems 2002; Grotewiel et al. 2005; Keller and Jemielity 2006; Houthoofd and Vanfleteren 2007) and since the 1920's as models for understanding the genes, signaling pathways and cellular processes involved in innate immunity (Brey 1998). These two fields of study have begun to merge as invertebrate models, chiefly terrestrial insects, are increasingly being used to understand both the causes and consequences of age-related changes in immunocompetence. Invertebrates are ideally suited for such studies as they generally have short generation times, short life spans and can be raised in large numbers which improves statistical power for detecting the effects of genetic and environmental influences on functional measures of the immune response. In addition, recently completed genome sequences of invertebrates (e.g., *Caenorhabditis elegans*: C. elegans Sequencing Consortium 1998; *Drosophila melanogaster:* Adams et al. 2000; *Anopheles gambiae*: Holt et al. 2002: *Bombyx mori:* Xia et al. 2004) reveal that many of the genes regulating the innate immune response have homologous genes in vertebrates. Molecular genetic studies have also revealed extensive homology between invertebrates and vertebrates in the signaling pathways that are activated to fight infection (Hoffmann and Reichhart 2002). Thus, the use of invertebrate models is likely to contribute a great deal to our

J. Leips (✉)
Department of Biological Sciences
1000 Hilltop Circle
University of Maryland Baltimore County
Baltimore, Maryland, 21250
Fax: 410-455-3875
Tel: 410-455-2238
E-mail: leips@umbc.edu

T. Fulop et al. (eds.), *Handbook on Immunosenescence,*
DOI 10.1007/978-1-4020-9062-2_4, © Springer Science+Business Media B.V. 2009

understanding of the genetic influences on immunosenescence in a wide range of organisms, including humans.

Keywords: Immune response • survival • bacterial clearance • *Toll* • IMD • JNK • phenoloxidase • phagocytosis • encapsulation • hemocyte • aging

1   Introduction

One complication in translating what we learn about immunosenescence in invertebrates to vertebrate organisms is that invertebrates rely solely on an innate immune response and lack the components of the adaptive immune system found in vertebrates. While there is some evidence to suggest that invertebrates have immunological memory (Sadd and Schmid-Hempel 2006; Pham et al. 2007), this ability is not well understood. Our current understanding suggests that immunological memory in invertebrates results from remodulation of existing cells to enhance their ability to phagocytize previously encountered pathogens. As such, this is fundamentally different from immunological memory that stems from the use of the B- and T-cells of the adaptive component of the immune response. Looked at in another way however, the lack of the adaptive component of the immune response can be considered an advantage because it allows us to examine the effect of age on the innate immune response without the complications of interactions between the adaptive and innate immune systems. Given the similarity among organisms in the many components of the innate immune response, studies of immunosenescence in invertebrates are likely to provide insight into the effect of aging in the innate immune system in all metazoans, including humans.

This chapter begins with a brief review of the immune system of invertebrates, drawn largely from information on the invertebrate with the most extensively studied immune response, *Drosophila melanogaster.* Those wishing to explore this topic further should consult the many excellent reviews on this topic (e.g., Hoffmann et al. 1996; Tzou et al. 2002; Hultmark 2003; Kurz and Ewbank 2003; Brennan and Anderson 2004; Cerenius and Söderhäll 2004; Christophides et al. 2004; Loker et al. 2004; Gravato-Nobre and Hodgkin 2005; Kim and Ausubel 2005; Mylonakis and Aballay 2005; Schmid-Hempel 2005; Evans et al. 2006; Lemaitre and Hoffmann 2007; Royet and Dziarski 2007; Uvell and Engström 2007). The next section summarizes what we have learned about age related changes in the immune system in invertebrates and includes a discussion of the various techniques used to study this phenomenon. The final section outlines some future directions for the use of invertebrates as models of immunosenescence, highlighting both the challenges and the promise that these organisms provide for a more complete understanding of the causes and consequences of age-related deterioration of the innate immune function.

2   Invertebrate Immunity

There are three general components of the innate immune system shared by most invertebrates: i) a wound response which involves proteolytic cascades and melanization to limit the spread of infection and kill pathogens, ii) cellular responses which involve phagocytosis and/or encapsulation of the invading organism, and iii) local and systemic synthesis and secretion of antimicrobial proteins. Age-related deterioration in any of these components is likely to reduce the effectiveness of the immune system.

2.1   Immune Response Activation

The immune response is typically induced following recognition of nonself by the host. In most invertebrates pathogen recognition is accomplished by pattern recognition receptors circulating in the hemolymph or embedded in the cell membranes of hemocytes (Khush and Lemaitre 2000; Hoffmann and Reichhart 2002 Hultmark 2003; Leulier et al. 2003; Royet and Dziarski 2007). These receptors recognize and bind evolutionarily conserved molecular structures that are unique to the surfaces of different types of microorganisms such as the peptidoglycan components of gram-positive and gram-negative bacteria, β-1,3 glycan in fungi, and phosphoglycan of parasites (Kimbrell and Beutler 2001; Janeway and Medzhitov 2002; Hultmark 2003). Invertebrates produce several classes of these pattern recognition receptors such as peptidoglycan receptor proteins (Royet and Dziarski 2007) and C-type lectins (Nicholas et al. 2004; Ao et al. 2007; O'Rourke et al. 2007), many of which have shared homology with vertebrate receptors (Kang et al. 1998; Khush and Lemaitre 2000; Chaput and Boneca 2007; Griffiths et al. 2007). This shared homology suggests that the general strategies for pathogen recognition are evolutionarily conserved.

In most invertebrates studied to date, the binding of recognition receptors to pathogens initiates a series of proteolytic cascades that result in coagulation of blood and in many species the localized production of melanin (Hoffmann and Reichhart 2002; Cerenius and Söderhäll 2004; Theopold et al. 2004). Interestingly, C. elegans is an exception in this case as genes regulating the proteolytic pathway leading to melanization in other invertebrates do not appear to have homologues in the worm genome (Ewbank 2002). Binding of these receptors also initiates signaling pathways to produce antimicrobial peptides (discussed below). The melanization reaction requires the activation of phenoloxidase by prophenoloxidase enzymes which typically reside within particular cell types (the names of these cells vary depending on the organism, Lavine and Strand 2002) and are released following cell disruption. Release of prophenoloxidase enzymes initiates a series of reactions leading to production of melanin (Cerenius and Söderhäll 2004). Deposition of melanin at wound sites contributes to wound healing and the toxic reactive compounds produced during melanin formation are thought to act as disinfectants (Bogdan et al. 2000; Nappi and Ottaviani 2000; Nappi et al. 2000; Cerenius and Söderhäll 2004).

2.2   Cellular Response

The cellular immune responses consist of phagocytosis (engulfment of small pathogens by single cells), nodulation (binding of multiple cells to bacterial aggregations),
encapsulation (binding of cells to form a capsule surrounding foreign bodies too large
to be phagocytized), and participation in clot formation at wound sites (Lavine and
Strand 2002). While phagocytic cells appear to be present in most invertebrates, hemocytes of *C. elegans* do not appear to have phagocytic capabilities (Ewbank 2002). In
Drosophila, three blood cell types are recognized that participate in various aspects of
the immune response: plasmatocytes, crystal cells and lamellocytes (Meister 2004).
Plasmatocytes are the phagocytic cells, comprising the largest fraction of the hemocytes in larvae (> 95%, Williams 2007) and are the only blood cell type in adults.
Crystal cells are smaller cells containing enzymes for initiation of the phenoloxidase cascade. Encapsulation and nodulation of particles too large to be phagocytized
appears to be a unique feature of invertebrates and cell types most often involved in
these cell aggregates are plasmatocytes and granulocytes (Jiravanichpaisal et al. 2006).
In *Drosophila* encapsulation is carried out only in larvae by lamellocytes which are
produced by the differentiation of larval plasmatocytes (Evans et al. 2003).

  Phagocytosis involves a complex set of cellular changes involving binding of
the pathogen, reorganization of the plasma membrane, induction of cytoskeletal
changes and processing of the ingested organism by the phagosome. The use of
model genetic organisms, primarily *Drosophila*, combined with large scale genomic
studies are beginning to reveal the genes that regulate this process (e.g., Wu et al.
2001, Brennan et al. 2007). Several families of receptor proteins have been implicated as important for the first step in this process, the binding of plasmatocytes to
microorganisms. Known receptor families include the *Drosophila* homologue of the
mammalian CD36 family of scavenger proteins (Philips et al. 2005), genes in the
scavenger receptor class C Type-1 family (Rämet et al. 2001), peptidoglycan receptor proteins (Rämet et al. 2002), proteins with EGF-like repeats (*Eater*: Kocks et al.
2005; *Nimrod*: Kurucz et al. 2007), integrins (Moita et al. 2006) and *Dscam*, a protein
with an immunoglobulin domain (Watson et al. 2005; Dong et al. 2006). *Dscam* is
of particular interest as this gene has four alternatively spliced exons, different combinations of which can result in the production of over 18,000 different transcripts
in *Drosophila* (Watson et al. 2005) and over 30,000 transcripts in *Anopheles* (Dong
et al. 2006). This potentially allows recognition and discrimination of a wide diversity of pathogens and may even provide a mechanism for immunological memory
in invertebrates. Hundreds of genes appear to be required for internalization and
processing of microorganisms as has been revealed by genome wide RNAi analysis
(Rämet et al. 2002; Philips et al. 2005; Agaisse et al. 2005; Stroschein-Stevenson
et al. 2006) and combined proteomic and RNAi analyses (Stuart et al. 2007). A great
deal of research remains to be done to understand how this complex genetic network
is organized to regulate phagocytosis.

  Invertebrates also produce complement type proteins that act as opsonins to
enhance phagocytosis. In the mosquito *Anopheles gambiae,* a circulating thiol-ester

protein (aTEP-1) binds to gram-positive and gram-negative bacteria and stimulates phagocytosis by blood cells (Levashina et al. 2001). The *Drosophila* genome encodes at least four TEP-like genes, three of which are up-regulated after immune-challenge, and one of which seems to be up-regulated by the JAK/STAT signaling pathway (Lagueux et al. 2000; De Gregorio et al. 2001; Agaisse and Perrimon 2004). Proteins encoded by the TEP genes have significant similarity with vertebrate complement proteins of the C3/α_2-macroglobulin superfamily (Levashina et al. 2001, Nonaka and Yoshizaki 2004). This lends support to the idea that the general function of these proteins to promote phagocytosis has been conserved during evolution.

2.3   Humoral Response

The third component of the immune response is the humoral response which results in the local and systemic production of antimicrobial peptides (AMPs). In *Drosophila*, the systemic response of AMPs primarily results from two signaling pathways that regulate NF-κB transcription factors in the cells of insect fat bodies (the functional equivalent of the mammalian liver). Comparative genomic studies have shown these pathways to be generally conserved in most insects (Christophides et al. 2002; Evans et al. 2006; Luna et al. 2006; Cheng et al. 2007). In addition, functional genetic studies and genomic sequence comparisons indicate that the genes regulating the intracellular steps in these pathways are remarkably similar to those regulating the innate immune response in mammals (Hoffmann and Reichhart 2002; Minakhina and Steward 2006).

In *Drosophila*, two pathways regulate the production of up to 20 different AMPs, the *Toll* pathway and the immune deficiency (IMD) pathway (Lemaitre and Hoffmann 2007). The *Toll* pathway, which is similar to the mammalian toll-like receptor (TL-R) signaling pathway, is activated through the binding of the growth factor-like cytokine Spätzle to the *Toll* receptor. *Toll* is a transmembrane receptor first identified as a necessary component for dorsal-ventral patterning (Wu and Anderson 1997). Signaling through this pathway results in the translocation of the transcription factors DIF and Dorsal to the nucleus and upregulation of AMPs such as drosomycin and defensin which act directly on fungi and gram-positive bacteria respectively. The IMD pathway, which exhibits similarity to the mammalian tumor necrosis factor receptor (TNF-R) pathway, is thought to be regulated by the binding of a transmembrane peptidoglycan receptor protein (PGRP-LC) to gram-negative bacteria (Gottar et al. 2002; Choe et al. 2005; Tanji and Ip 2005). Signaling through this pathway results in the translocation of the NF-κB transcription factor Relish to the nucleus and subsequent expression of a number of AMPs generally targeting gram-negative bacteria, although some downstream targets of both pathways are effective against gram-negative and gram-positive bacteria. Recent evidence also suggests that signaling through the IMD pathway also activates the Jun N-terminal kinase (JNK) pathway which contributes to the production of AMPs by the fat body (Delaney et al. 2006). Although the *Toll* pathway is triggered primarily by infection from fungi and gram-positive bacteria (Ligoxygakis et al. 2002; Lemaitre et al. 1996) and the IMD pathway primarily triggered by gram-negative bacteria, it has been known for quite some time that there is cross talk between these pathways and this provides some level of redundancy in the immune response to infection by these organisms (Lemaitre et al. 1997). A recent model developed by Delaney et al. (2006) proposes that this cross talk results in part from the activation of the JNK pathway whereby the downstream transcription factors of the JNK pathway upregulate AMPs normally targeted by the transcription factors of the *Toll* and IMD pathways. *Toll* and IMD have also been shown to act synergistically, jointly contributing to the upregulation of representative target genes of both of these pathways. This synergism appears to result from the fact that the transcription factors of each pathway can bind to different domains of the promotor regions of these target genes leading to higher levels of expression than expected by the additive effect of each pathway when considered alone (Tanji et al. 2007).

While the fat body of most insects is the primary tissue involved in the systemic response to infection, epithelial surfaces of the epidermis, gut, reproductive system and respiratory tract are also responsible for the constitutive and inducible production of antimicrobial agents to limit microbial growth (Brey et al. 1993; Tzou et al. 2000; Ha et al. 2005; Pinheiro and Ellar 2006, Shapira et al. 2006). Interestingly, production of AMPs at wound or infection sites does not rely solely on the activation of NF-κB pathways, but instead on tissue specific transcription factors and local production of reactive oxygen species (Ferrandon et al. 1998; Ryu et al. 2004; Han et al. 2004; Ryu et al. 2006).

Much of the work in invertebrates has focused on understanding the immune response to bacterial and fungal pathogens; however there is a great deal of recent interest in understanding the immune response to viruses. A major mechanism thought to regulate the response to viral infection is by RNA interference (RNAi), an evolutionarily conserved mechanism for silencing the translation of RNA (Meister and Tuschl 2004). Functional genetic analysis in both *Drosophila* and *C. elegans* indicates that this is also a conserved and effective way to fight viral infection (Schott et al. 2005; Wilkins et al. 2005; Cherry and Silverman 2005; Fritz et al. 2006; van Rij et al. 2006). In addition, expression studies of *Drosophila* artificially infected with the Drosophila X Virus suggest that the *Toll* and JAK/STAT pathways are also involved in mediating an immune response to viral infection (Dostert et al. 2005; Zambon et al. 2005).

3   Invertebrates as Models of Immunosenescence

Many different aspects of immunosenescence have been measured in invertebrates including assessment of the age-specific ability to clear and survive infection and measurements of functional changes in the components of the immune response. Age-specific survival measurements have been obtained either by pricking individuals with a septic needle (Burger et al. 2007), microinjecting individuals with a

standard concentration of bacteria (Adamo et al. 2001; Hillyer et al. 2005), or exposing individuals of different ages to a pathogen (Laws et al. 2004). Typically a large
number of individuals of each age group are infected and the subsequent number
of deaths scored daily to identify differences in mortality rates following infection.
Age-specific abilities to clear bacterial infections are carried out by either pricking
or microinjecting individuals of different ages with a standard concentration of bacteria, allowing 24–48 hrs for individuals to clear the infection, and then homogeniz-
ing or perfusing individuals and plating aliquots of the solution on agar plates (Kim
et al. 2001; Hillyer et al. 2005; Lesser et al. 2006). The resulting number of colony
forming units on the plate is an estimate of the ability of that individual to clear the
infection. Both age-specific survival and clearance assays provide no functional
information on the causes of age-specific changes in the immune response. Functional changes in age-specific components of the immune system that have been
measured include age-related changes in expression of immune response genes following infection (Hillyer et al. 2005; Zerofsky et al. 2005), age-specific changes in
hemocyte counts (Adamo et al. 2001; Doums et al. 2002; Amdam et al. 2004, 2005;
Hillyer et al. 2005), age-specific phagocytic ability of hemocytes (Hillyer et al.
2005), age-specific phenoloxidase activity (Adamo et al. 2001), age-specific encapsulation and melanization ability (Doums et al. 2002) and even age-specific changes
in the quantity of fat (used as an indicator of the size of the fat body, the major site of
lipid storage and the tissue most responsible for secretion of antimicrobial peptides,
Doums et al. 2002).

   While it is clear from these studies that the ability to survive and clear a bacterial infection declines with age, the data so far indicate that the underlying causes
of immunosenescence differs among species. Adamo et al. (2001) studied various
indicators of immunosenescence using a population of crickets, *Gryllus texensis*,
that had been collected in the wild but maintained for several generations in the laboratory. They measured sex-specific changes in phenoloxidase (PO) activity (based
on an in-vitro enzyme assay with cricket hemolymph that measures the rate of conversion of L-dopa to quinone), counts of hemocyte numbers and survival following
injection of *Serratia marcescens* at four ages spanning prereproductive maturity to
4 weeks of age. Males and females were similar in the various immune response
indicators up to the age at which males began to display sexual behavior. Sexually mature males had lower phenoloxidase activity and higher mortality following
infection compared with younger males and same aged females. This was interpreted by the authors as males trading off immunity for reproduction although the
functional connection between PO activity and mating behavior is unclear. The relationship between PO activity and survival following infection was weak however,
as 2 week old females had higher PO activity compared to earlier and later ages,
but exhibited higher mortality following infection compared with prereproductive
ages. The authors speculate allocation of energy toward reproduction offsets the
increased protection that would have resulted from higher PO activity, producing
a trade-off between reproduction and survival following infection. This hypothesis
could potentially be tested with age-matched virgins to minimize the survival cost
of reproduction. Unlike PO activity, there was no age-specific change in hemocyte

number and no correlation between hemocyte number and the ability individuals to survive infection at any age. Both males and females had a reduced ability to survive infection with increasing age but were also more likely to die from a sham injection of saline with age. This increase in mortality following sham injection suggests that older individuals may have a reduced ability to withstand the stress imposed by the injection and also possibly a reduced ability to repair a wound site.

An interesting contrast is provided by the work of Hillyer et al. (2005) on the mosquito, *Aedes aegypti*. This study examined age-associated changes in a number of traits including changes in hemocyte numbers, the phagocytic ability of cells, the production of antimicrobial peptides, the ability to clear infection and mortality during the first five days following eclosion. They observed age-related reductions in hemocyte number, a reduction in the ability to clear an artificial injection of bacteria, and an increase in mortality rates following infection. They found no change in the production of antimicrobial proteins following infection at different ages and no decline in the phagocytic ability of hemocytes with age. In this case, age-specific decline in clearance ability and the age-specific increase in mortality rates following infection may be largely explained by a decline in hemocyte number with age. As mosquitoes, like most insects, are not known to produce new hemocytes as adults (either by hematopoiesis or by mitosis, Hillyer et al. 2005) the rate of change in immunocompetence with age may largely depend on the total number of blood cells produced during the larval and pupal periods and the age-specific rate of loss of hemocytes as adults. These conclusions are of course based on observation of correlated changes with age and the causal relationship between hemocyte number and age-specific immunocompetence needs to be further tested. One caveat with this study is that the age-associated changes observed may not reflect senescence per se, as this species can live between 2 weeks to over a month in the laboratory. Further assessment of immune function at later ages, perhaps concurrently with other indicators of senescence such as age specific mortality rates will determine if the interrelationship between immunocompetence and hemocyte number is consistent as the organism ages.

3.1   Implications for Social Influences on Immunosenescence

Comparisons of different species of social insects reveal the potential for age-specific hormonal control of immunosenescence. Doums et al. (2002) implanted workers of two different species of bumblebees (*Bombus terrestris* and *Bombus lucorum*) with nylon filaments at two different ages to measure the age-specific ability to encapsulate and melanize a foreign object. Encapsulation and melanization ability declined in both species with age. In an effort to provide a physiological explanation they measured age-specific changes in the size of the fat body and the number of circulating hemocytes in one species, *Bombus terrestris,* and found only a slight reduction in the size of the fat body and no change in hemocyte number with age. Their conclusion was that the age-related decline in encapsulation and melanization ability could not be attributed to changes in hemocyte number and the size of the fat body. Of course, this leaves open a number of possibilities yet to be explored to explain their results including age-related changes in the phagocytic ability of the hemocytes. Using a different species of hymenoptera, the honey bee *Apis mellifera*, Amdam et al. (2004) found that immunosenescence is cued by a change in social status as hive workers shift to foragers when they reach 18–28 days old (Winston 1987). This change in social status from hive bee to forager leads to higher levels of juvenile hormone (JH), a reduction in vitellogenin production, a decrease in hemocyte numbers and an increase in the number of pycnotic hemocytes which are not phagocytic. As vitellogenin is an important carrier of zinc the increased pycnosis in hemocytes probably results from low zinc availability. Phagocytic ability of the nonpycnotic cells did not change with age. Interestingly, when foragers are forced to revert to hive duties, juvenile hormone titers are reduced leading to an increase in vitellogenin, increased hemocyte numbers and a reduced number of pycnotic cells (Amdam et al. 2005). The source of these new hemocytes is unclear but may result from hematopoiesis, cell division or mobilization of previously sessile cells. Thus, immunosenescence in this aspect of the cellular component of the immune response in honeybees appears to be under social control and so is reversible, at least temporarily. The fact that *Bombus* do not exhibit age-specific changes in hemocyte number while *Apis* does, may reflect the different social biology of these organisms. *Apis* have a very defined schedule of changing tasks and social status as they age, while *Bombus* are much less regimented, performing both hive and foraging duties for their entire life. As such, JH titres in *Bombus* adults may not change in the manner seen in *Apis* and so the resultant change in hemocyte number is not seen in this organism. A comparative study using these species, and indeed other social invertebrates, in which similar immune response traits are examined with age (combined with changes in survival and clearance ability following infection) would elucidate the general importance of social behavior and hormonal influences in regulating immunosenescence.

3.2 Genetic Basis for Immunosenescence

While the studies discussed above are aimed at understanding the cellular and physiological causes of immunosenescence another set of studies has aimed at understanding the potential genetic contributions to age-related changes in immunocompetence. Kim et al. 2001 were the first to document the existence of an age-related decline in the immune response in an invertebrate system. They used *Drosophila melanogaster* to test the effect of age on the ability to clear an infection of *E. coli*. They used a wild type strain and a strain containing a mutation in *xanthine dehydrogenase* (*XDH*), a gene that influences the production of uric acid, a scavenger of reactive oxygen species and so is a candidate gene for aging. Reactive oxygen species and nitric oxide levels were substantially higher in the mutants and mutants had a significantly higher rate of mortality compared to wild type flies. Interestingly, in the wild type strain they found a dramatic reduction in their ability to clear bacterial infection as the flies aged, with approximately 60% reduction in this ability from 2–80 days of age. Flies with the mutation were extremely limited in their ability to clear infection and did not show any age-related decline. This is may be due to the fact that the immune response of mutant flies had very little scope for an age-specific decline in immune-response as infection levels were over 25 times higher in mutants than in wild type flies at all ages. Their results suggest that generation of high levels of reactive oxygen is deleterious to all physiological systems, including the immune response. It does not imply that *XDH* directly plays a role in regulating the immune-response or immunosenescence in *Drosophila*.

As the term immunosenescence itself implies age-specific changes in immune function, studies of age-related changes in gene expression are more likely to be useful for understanding genetic influences on immunosenescence than studies using mutants. Microarray studies of flies and mammals have identified a number of age-related changes in the expression of immune response genes a consequence of general aging. In fact, genes known to be involved in the immune-response exhibit some of the most dramatic changes in gene expression with age compared to genes involved in other processes such as metabolism, and growth regulation (Pletcher et al. 2002; Seroude et al. 2002; Landis et al. 2004). Of interest is that immune response genes are typically upregulated with increasing age. This likely reflects a higher pathogen load in older individuals (as demonstrated in *Drosophila* by Ren et al. 2007) and not the age-related deterioration in the control of transcription in general. Another possibility is that older individuals are hyperresponsive to pathogens, and as a consequence show higher levels of transcription following infection compared with younger individuals. This last hypothesis was tested in the experiment described below.

Zerofsky et al. 2005 used changes in transcript levels of the antimicrobial peptide diptericin following artificial infection at different ages as an indicator of age-specific immune function. In their study virgin females of different ages were infected by pricking the cuticle with a needle containing a mixture of bacteria (*E. coli* and *Micrococcus luteus*) that were either live or killed. They found that older females had higher background levels of diptericin than younger females before the artificial infection, reflecting the findings of microarray studies on aging flies. They also found that when flies are infected with live bacteria older females had a higher and more sustained level of diptericin transcription than younger flies. The authors interpreted this as an indication that older flies were less able to clear the infection and so continually maintained production of high levels of diptericin. Unfortunately the bacterial load was not measured in old and young flies and so this conclusion awaits confirmation. When infected with killed bacteria, younger females had higher and more sustained production of diptericin than older flies. Older flies upregulated diptericin production during the first six hours following infection, matching the production of the young flies, but then diptericin transcripts gradually declined. These results suggest that older individuals are not hyperresponsive to infection. Combining the results of this study with observation of higher transcript levels of immune response genes in older flies implies that older flies carry higher pathogen loads and so have elevated transcription of immune response genes.

The nematode *Caenorhabditis elegans* is an emerging invertebrate model for studying evolutionarily conserved responses to infection (Kurz and Ewbank 2003) and recent work has begun to identify some interrelationship between immunocompetence and longevity. The utility of *C. elegans* for understanding the cellular and physiological processes of immunosenescence may be limited by the fact that many components of the innate immune system common in other invertebrates are missing in this species. As discussed above however, there may be a limited number of such features that are generally responsible for immunosenescence across taxa, even within species. However, given the genetic utility of this species, understanding the genetic basis of immunosenescence in this organism may provide key insights not provided by other insect models. It is clear that *C. elegans* experience higher age-specific mortality when exposed to pathogens (Kurz et al. 2003; Laws et al. 2004). While there is some indication of a connection between genes regulating the immune response and longevity in *C. elegans* (Kurz and Tan 2004; Troemel et al. 2006) additional research is necessary to determine if these same genes act to influence immunosenescence.

3.3 Understanding Natural Genetic Variation Underlying Immunosenescence

In a seminal paper Lazzaro et al. (2004) found that natural populations harbor extensive genetically based variation in the ability to clear infection and indentified single nucleotide polymorphisms in candidate genes associated with this variation. This study has opened up an exciting new direction to identify genes that regulate age-specific changes in immunocompetence. Lesser et al. (2006) used a modified assay developed by McKean and Nunney (2001) to demonstrate a genetic basis for age-related changes in immunocompetence. Using twenty five genetically distinct lines derived from a natural population of *Drosophila* they found that only five lines exhibited an age-related decline in clearance ability (measured at 1 and 4 weeks of age) while eleven lines showed an improved ability to clear an infection with age. The clearance ability of the remaining nine were unaffected by age. They also found no genetic correlation in the ability clear the infection between the two ages. This lack of a genetic correlation in immunocompetence across ages suggests that different genes are responsible for producing the phenotypic variation in clearance ability at different ages. Identification of the genes controlling these age-related changes in the ability to clear infection is an important priority.

4   Future Directions

As highlighted above, many of the age-related changes in the components of innate immunity appear to be species-specific. This undoubtedly reflects the evolutionary divergence in the innate immune system among lineages, the different nature of infective agents faced by these organisms in their particular ecological setting, and also differences among species in the strength of selection to maintain immune function with age. As invertebrates have only recently been used as models to explore the causes and consequences of immunosenescence, perhaps more generalities will be revealed as more species are examined. Much could be gained by a systematic study of age-related changes in key components of the immune response in closely related taxa to establish the extent to which changes in particular components of the immune system (e.g., hemocyte count, phagocytic ability) are unique to particular lineages and which might be generally conserved across taxa. Shared features of the innate immune response that show age-specific decline in function among invertebrates are those most likely to be shared across broader taxonomic groups including vertebrates.

An exciting future goal is to use a combination of techniques for assessing age-specific changes in the immune response in invertebrates to gain a more wholistic view of the mechanisms that underlie immunosenescence. These should include assessing the concentration and identity of pathogen recognition proteins, the levels and killing ability of antimicrobial peptides, measurements of hemocyte numbers and age-specific phagocytic ability. Combining these measurements with age-specific abilities to survive and clear infection will provide the key to understanding which components of the immune response change with age and which have functional consequences for the survival and fitness of the organism.

Shirasu-Hiza and Schneider (2007) have also suggested that we pay more attention to physiological changes in other aspects of the host following infection to identify the causes of mortality when it occurs. As they point out, when humans get sick we measure many physiological indicators that reflect their health and which ultimately contribute to the ability of the individual to survive the infection. They rightly suggest that we expand our understanding of the pathology of infection to monitor changes in aspects of organisms that are not necessarily part of the immune response when experiments are done on model organisms. Additional traits that may be influential include changes in feeding or reproductive behaviors, changes in energy allocation to storage or reproduction, and changes in basic metabolic processes like respiration and the rate and quality of waste produced. As these behavioral, life history and metabolic processes normally change with age, understanding the interrelationship between these physiological characteristics and immunocompetence in the aging organism will provide a more complete understanding of age-related changes in the pathology of infections.

Finally, technological advances are likely to greatly facilitate our understanding of the genetic contribution to age related changes in immunosenescence. Whole genome microarray and proteomic studies are likely to reveal a number of genes that exhibit age-related transcriptional changes prior to and following infection. The key to interpreting these data and identification of important genes will be to directly test the effect of changes in transcript and/or protein expression with functional tests of immunocompetence. This is perhaps where the real advantage of using invertebrate model systems like *Drosophila* lies. During the past decade there have been a number of tools developed to control the expression of candidate genes in an age—and tissue—and even cell type specific manner in both *Drosophila* and *C. elegans* (e.g., Roman et al. 2001; McGuire et al. 2004; Johnson et al. 2005; Dietzl et al. 2007; Qadota et al. 2007). Controlled up- and down-regulation of candidate genes at different ages prior to and following infection, combined with measurements of survival, bacterial clearance efficiency, or the efficacy of particular components of the immune response (e.g., phagocytic ability) will allow direct tests of the importance of candidate gene expression on age-specific immune function.

Genetic mapping techniques such as quantitative trait loci (QTL) mapping have proven useful for identifying genomic regions that contribute to natural variation in age-specific phenotypes (e.g., Leips et al. 2006) and continued development of these techniques should allow us to rapidly identify the actual genes that contribute to age-specific changes in immune response (Lai et al. 2007). In addition, as age-specific transcriptional controls are likely to contribute to age-specific immunocompetence, the continued use and improvement of expression QTL mapping methods (e.g., Alberts et al. 2007; Jia and Zu 2007) holds great promise for identifying the genes that regulate age-specific expression of those genes that directly contribute to immunosenescence.

Acknowledgment   I am grateful to Tashauna Felix and Adrienne Starks for thoughtful discussions of immunosenescence. Also, I owe a great deal of thanks to Tashauna Felix, Mary Kaminski, Adrienne Starks and Louisa Wu for their critical comments on this manuscript. This work was supported by a research grant from the National Institutes of Health (NHLBI R01HL080812).

References

Adams MD et al (2000) The genome sequence of *Drosophila melanogaster.* Science 287: 2185–2195

Adamo SA, Jensen M, Younger M (2001) Changes in lifetime immunocompetence in male and female *Gryllus texensis* (formerly *G. integer*): trade-offs between immunity and reproduction. Anim Behav 62:417–425

Adamo SA (2004) Estimating disease resistance in insects: phenoloxidase and lysozyme-like activity and disease resistance in the cricket *Gryllus texensis.* J Insect Physiol 50:209–216

Agaisse H, Perrimon N (2004) The roles of JAK/STAT signaling in *Drosophila* immune responses. Immunol Rev 198:72–82

Agaisse H, Burrack LS, Philips JA, Rubin EJ, Perrimon N, Higgins DE (2005) Genome-wide RNAi screen for host factors required for intracellular bacterial infection. Science 309:1248–1251

Alberts R, Terpstra P, Li Y, Breitling R, Nap JP, Jansen RC (2007) Sequence polymorphisms cause many false cis eQTLs. PLoS Biol 2:e622

Amdam GV, Simões ZLP, Hagen A, Norberg K, Schrøder K, Øyvind M, Kirkwood TBL, Omholt SW (2004) Hormonal control of the yolk precursor vitellogenin regulates immune function and longevity in honeybees. Exp Gerontol 39:767–773

Amdam GV, Aase ALTO, Seehuus S-C, Fondrk MK, Norberg K, Hartfelder K (2005) Social reversal of immunosenescence in honey bee workers. Exp Gerontol 40:939–947

Ao J, Ling E, Yu XQ (2007) *Drosophila* C-type lectins enhance cellular encapsulation. Mol Immunol 44:2541–2548

Bogdan C, Rollinghoff M, Diefenbach A (2000) Reactive oxygen and reactive nitrogen intermediates in innate and specific immunity. Curr Opin Immunol 12:64–76

Brennan CA, Anderson KV (2004) *Drosophila*: the genetics of innate immune recognition and response. Annu Rev Immunol 22:457–483

Brennan CA, Delaney JR, Schneider DS, Anderson KV (2007) Psidin is required in Drosophila blood cells for both phagocytic degradation and immune activation of the fat body. Curr Biol 17:67–72

Brey PT, Lee WJ, Yamakawa M, Koizumi Y, Perrot S, Francois M, Ashida M (1993) Role of the integument in insect immunity: epicuticular abrasion and induction of cecropin synthesis in cuticular epithelial cells. Proc Natl Acad Sci 90:6275–6279

Brey PT (1998) The contributions of the Pasteur school of insect immunity. In: Brey PT, Hultmark D (eds) Molecular mechanisms of immune response in insects. Chapman and Hall, London, pp 1–39

Burger JMS, Hwangbo DS, Corby-Harris V, Promislow DEL (2007) The functional costs and benefits of dietary restriction in *Drosophila*. Aging Cell 6:63–71

C elegans sequencing consortium (1998) Genome sequence of the nematode *C. elegans*: a platform for investigating biology. Science 282:2012–2018

Cerenius L, Söderhäll K (2004) The prophenoloxidase-activating system in invertebrates. Immunol Rev 198:116–126

Chaput C, Boneca IG (2007) Peptidoglycan detection by mammals and flies. Microbes Infect 9:637–647

Cheng TC, Zhang YL, Liu C, Xu PZ, Gao ZH, Xia QY, Xiang ZH (2007) Identification and analysis of Toll-related genes in the domesticated silkworm, *Bombyx mori*. Dev Comp Immunol 32:464–475

Cherry S, Silverman N (2006) Host-pathogen interactions in *Drosophila*: new tricks from an old friend. Nat Immunol 7:911–917

Choe KM, Lee H, Anderson KV (2005) *Drosophila* peptidoglycan recognition protein LC (PGRP-LC) acts as a signal-transducing innate immune receptor. Proc Natl Acad Sci 102:1122–1126

Christophides GK, Zbodnov E, Barillas-Mury C, Birney E, Blandin S, Blass C, Brey PT, Collins FH, Danielli A, Dimopoulos G, Hetru C, Ngo T, Hoa B, Hoffmann JA, Kanzok SM, Letunic I, Levashina EA, Loukeris TG, Lycett G, Meister S, Michel K, Moita LF, Müller HM, Osta MA, Paskewitz SM, Reichhart JM, Rzhetsky A, Troxler L, Vernick KD, Vlachou D, Volz J, von Mering C, Xu J, Zheng L, Bork P, Kafatos KC (2002) Immunity-related genes and gene families in *Anopheles gambiae*. Science 298:159–165

Christophides GK, Vlachou D, Kafatos FC (2004) Comparative and functional genomics of the innate immune system in the malaria vector, *Anopheles* gambiae. Immunol Rev 198:127–148

De Gregorio E, Spellman PT, Rubin GM, Lemaitre B (2001) Genome-wide analysis of the *Drosophila* immune response by using oligonucleotide microarrays. Proc Natl Acad Sci 98:12590–12595

Delaney JR, Stöven S, Uvell H, Anderson KV, Engström Y, Mlodzik M (2006) Cooperative control of *Drosophila* immune responses by the JNK and NF-κB signaling pathways. EMBO J 25:3068–3077

Dietzl G, Chen D, Schnorrer F, Su KC, Barinova Y, Fellner M, Gasser B, Kinsey K, Oppel S, Scheiblauer S, Couto A, Marra V, Keleman K, Dickson BJ (2007) A genome-wide transgenic RNAi library for conditional gene inactivation in *Drosophila*. Nature 448:151–156

Dong Y, Taylor HE, Dimopoulos G (2006) AgDscam, a hypervariable immunoglobulin domain-containing receptor of the *Anopheles gambiae* innate immune system. PLoS Biol 4:e229

Dostert C, Jouanguy E, Irving P, Troxler L, Galiana-Arnoux D, Hetru C, Hoffmann JA, Imler JL (2005) The Jak-STAT signaling pathway is required but not sufficient for the antiviral response of *Drosophila*. Nat Immunol 6:946–953

Doums C, Moret Y, Benelli E, Schmid-Hempel P (2002) Senescence of immune defence in *Bombus* workers. Ecol Entomol 27:138–144

Evans CJ, Hartenstein V, Banerjee U (2003) Thicker than blood: conserved mechanisms in *Drosophila* vertebrate hematopoiesis. Dev Cell 5:673–690

Evans JD, Aronstein K, Chen YP, Hetru C, Imler JL, Jiang H, Kanos M, Thompson GJ, Zou Z, Hultmark D (2006) Immune pathways and defense mechanisms in honey bees *Apis mellifera*. Insect Mol Biol 15:645–656

Ewbank JJ (2002) Tackling both sides of the host-pathogen equation with *Caenorhabditis elegans*. Microbes Infect 4:247–256

Ferrandon D, Jung AC, Criqui M-C, Lemaitre B, Uttenweiler-Joseph S, Michaut L, Reichhart J-M, Hoffmann JA (1998) A drosomycin-GFP reporter transgene reveals a local immune response in *Drosophila* that is not dependent on the *Toll* pathway. EMBO J 17:1217–1227

Fritz JH, Girardin SE, Philpott DJ (2006) Innate immune defense through RNA interference. Sci STKE (339):pe27

Gottar M, Gobert V, Michel T, Belvin M, Duyk G, Hoffmann JA, Ferrandon D, Royet J (2002) The *Drosophila* immune response against Gram-negative bacteria is mediated by a peptidoglycan recognition protein. Nature 416:640–644

Grotowiel MS, Martin I, Bhandari P, Cook-Wiens E (2005) Functional senescence in *Drosophila melanogaster*. Ageing Res Rev 4:372–397

Gravato-Nobre MJ, Hodgkin J (2005) *Ca_enorhabditis elegans* as a model for innate immunity to pathogens. Cell Microbiol 7:741–751

Griffiths M, Neal JW, Gasque P (2007) Innate immunity and protective neuroinflammation: new emphasis on the role of neuroimmune regulatory proteins. Int Rev Neurobiol 82:29–55

Ha EM, Oh CT, Bae YS, Lee WJ (2005) A direct role for dual oxidase in *Drosophila* gut immunity. Science 310:847–850

Han SH, Ryu JH, Oh CT, Nam KB, Nam HJ, Jang IH, Brey PT, Lee WJ (2004) The moleskin gene product is essential for Caudal-mediated constitutive antifungal Drosomycin gene expression in *Drosophila* epithelia. Insect Mol Biol 13:323–327

Hillyer JF, Schmidt SL, Fuchs JF, Boyle JP, Christensen BM (2005) Age-associated mortality in immune challenged mosquitoes *Aedes aegypti* correlates with a decrease in haemocyte numbers. Cell Microbiol 7:39–51

Hoffmann JA, Reichhart JM, Hetru C (1996) Innate immunity in higher insects. Curr Opin Immunol 8:8–13

Hoffmann JA, Reichhart JM (2002) *Drosophila* innate immunity: an evolutionary perspective. Nat Immunol 3:121–126

Holt et al (2002) The genome sequence of the malaria mosquito *Anopheles gambiae*. Science 298:129–149

Houthoofd K, Vanfleteren JR (2007) Public and private mechanisms of life extension in *Caenorhabditis elegans*. Mol Genet Genomics 277:601–617

Hultmark D (2003) *Drosophila* immunity: paths and patterns. Curr Opin Immunol 15:12–19

Janeway CA, Medzhitov R (2002) Innate immune recognition. Annu Rev Immunol 20:197–216

Jia Z, Xu S (2007) Mapping quantitative trait loci for expression abundance. Genetics 176: 611–623

Jiravanichpaisal P, Lee BL, Söderhäll K (2006) Cell-mediated immunity in arthropods: hematopoiesis, coagulation, melanization and opsonization. Immunology 211:213–236

Johnson NM, Behm CA, Trowell SC (2005) Heritable and inducible gene knockdown in C. *elegans using* Wormgate and the ORFeome. Gene 359:26–34

Kang D, Liu G, Lundström A, Gelius E, Steiner H (1998) A peptidoglycan recognition protein in innate immunity conserved from insects to humans. Proc Natl Acad Sci 95:10078–10082

Keller L, Jemielity S (2006) Social insects as a model to study the molecular basis of aging. Exp Gerontol 41:553–556

Khush RS, Lemaitre B (2000) Genes that fight infection: what the *Drosophila* genome says about animal immunity. Trends Genet 16: 442–449

Kim DH, Ausubel FM (2005) Evolutionary perspectives on innate immunity from the study of *Caenorhabditis elegans*. Curr Opin Immunol 17:4–10

Kim YS, Nam HJ, Chung HY, Kim ND, Ryu JH, Lee WJ, Arking R, Yoo MA (2001) Role of *xanthine dehydrogenase* and aging on the innate immune response of *Drosophila*. J Amer Aging Assoc. 24:187-194

Kimbrell DA, Beutler B (2001) The evolution and genetics of innate immunity. Nat Rev Genet 2:256–267

Kocks C, Cho JH, Nehme N, Ulvila J, Pearson AM, Meister M, Strom C, Conto,SL, Hetru C, Stuart LM, Stehle T, Hoffmann JA, Reichhart JM, Ferrandon D, Rämet M, Ezekowitz RA (2005) *Eater*, a transmembrane protein mediating phagocytosis of bacterial pathogens in *Drosophila*. Cell 123:335–346

Kurucz E, Márkus R, Zsámboki J et al (2007) *Nimrod*, a putative phagocytosis receptor with EGF repeats in *Drosophila* plasmatocytes. Curr Biol 17:649–54

Kurz CL, Ewbank JJ (2003) *Caenorhabditis elegans:* an emerging genetic model for the study of innate immunity. Nat Rev Genet 4:380–390

Kurz CL, Chauvet S, Andres E, Aurouze M, Vallet I, Michel GP, Uh M, Celli J, Filloux A, De Bentzmann, S, Steinmetz I, Hoffmann JA, Finlay BB, Gorvel JP, Ferrandon D, Ewbank JJ (2003) Virulence factors of the human opportunistic pathogen *Serratia marcescens* identified by in vivo screening. EMBO J 22:1451–1460

Kurz CL, Tan MW (2004) Regulation of aging and innate immunity in C. *elegans*. 3:185–193

Lagueux M, Perrodou E, Levashina EA, Capovilla M, Hoffmann JA (2000) Constitutive expression of a complement-like protein in *Toll* and JAK gain-of-function mutants of *Drosophila*. Proc Natl Acad Sci 97:11427–11432

Lai CQ, Leips J, Zou W, Roberts JF, Wollenberg KR, Parnell LD, Zeng ZB, Ordovas JM, Mackay TF (2007) Speed-mapping quantitative trait loci using microarrays. Nat Methods 4:839–841

Landis GN, Abdueva D, Skvortsov D, Yang J, Rabin BE, Carrick J, Tavare S, Tower J (2004) Similar gene expression patterns characterize aging and oxidative stress in *Drosophila melanogaster*. Proc Natl Acad Sci 101:7663–7668

Lavine MD, Strand MR (2002) Insect hemocytes and their role in immunity. Insect Biochem Mol Biol 32:1295–1309

Laws TR, Harding SV, Smith MP, Atkins TP, Titball RW (2004) Age influences resistance of *Caenorhabditis elegans* to killing by pathogenic bacteria. FEMS Microbiol Lett 234:281–287

Lazzaro BP, Sceurman BK, Clark AG (2004) Genetic basis of natural variation in *D. melanogaster* antibacterial immunity. Science 303:1873–1876

Leips J, Gilligan P, Mackay TF (2006) Quantitative trait loci with age-specific effects on fecundity in *Drosophila melanogaster*. Genetics 172:1595–1605

Lemaitre B, Nicolas E, Michaut L, Reichhart JM, Hoffmann JA (1996) The dorsoventral regulatory gene cassette spatzle/*Toll*/cactus controls the potent antifungal response in *Drosophila* adults. Cell 86:973–983

Lemaitre B, Reichhart JM, Hoffmann JA (1997) *Drosophila* host defense: differential induction of antimicrobial peptide genes after infection by various classes of microorganisms. Proc Natl Acad Sci 94:14614–14619

Lemaitre B, Hoffmann J (2007) The host defense of *Drosophila melanogaster*. Annu Rev Immunol 25:697–743

Lesser KJ, Paiusi IC, Leips J (2006) Naturally occurring genetic variation in the age-specific immune response of *Drosophila melanogaster*. Aging Cell 5:293–295

Levashina EA, Moita LF, Blandin S, Vriend G, Lagueux M, Kafatos FC (2001) Conserved role of a complement-like protein in phagocytosis revealed by the dsRNA knockout in cultured cells of the mosquito, *Anopheles gambiae*. Cell 104:709–718

Ligoxygakis P, Pelte N, Hoffmann JA, Reichhart J-M (2002) Activation of *Drosophila Toll* during fungal infection by a blood serpine protease. Science 297:114–116

Loker ES, Adema CM, Zhang S-M, Kepler TB (2004) Invertebrate immune systems — not homogenous, not simple, not well understood. Immunol Rev 198:10–24

Leulier F, Parquet C, Pili-Floury S, Ryu JH, Caroff M, Lee W-J, Mengin-Lecreulx D, Lemaitre B (2003) The *Drosophila* immune system detects bacteria through specific peptidoglycan recognition. Nat Immunol 4:478–84

Luna C, Hoa NT, Lin H, Zhang L, Nguyen HL, Kanzok SM, Zheng L (2006) Expression of immune responsive genes in cell lines from two different Anopheline species. Insect Mol Biol 15:721–729

McGuire SE, Roman G, Davis RL (2004) Gene expression systems in *Drosophila*: a synthesis of time and space. Trends Genet 20:384–391

McKean KA, Nunney L (2001) Increased sexual activity reduces male immune function in *Drosophila melanogaster*. Proc Natl Acad Sci 98:7904–7909

Meister M (2004) Blood cells of *Drosophila*: cell lineages and role in host defense. Curr Opin Immunol 16:10–15

Meister G, Tuschl T (2004) Mechanisms of gene silencing by double stranded RNA. Nature 431:343–349

Minakhina S, Steward R (2006) Nuclear factor-kappa B-pathways in *Drosophila*. Oncogene 25:6749–6757

Moita LF, Vriend G, Mahairaki V, Louis C, Kafatos FC (2006) Integrins of *Anopheles gambiae* and a putative role of a new beta integrin, BINT2, in phagocytosis of *E. coli*. Insect Biochem Mol Biol 36:282–290

Mylonakis E, Aballay A (2005) Worms and flies as genetically tractable animal models to study host-pathogen interactions. Infect Immun 73:3833–3841

Nappi AJ, Ottaviani E (2000) Cytotoxicity and cytotoxic molecules in invertebrates. Bioessays 22:469–480

Nappi AJ, Vass E, Frey F, Carton Y (2000) Nitric oxide involvement in *Drosophila* immunity. Nitric Oxide 4:423–430

Nicholas HR, Hodgkin J (2004) Responses to infection and possible recognition strategies in the innate immune system of *Caenorhabditis elegans*. Mol Immunol 41:479–493

Nonaka M, Yoshizaki F (2004) Evolution of the complement system. Mol Immunol 40:897–902

O'Rourke D, Baban D, Demidova M, Mott R, Hodgkin J (2007) Genomic clusters, putative pathogen recognition molecules, and antimicrobial genes are induced by infection of *C. elegans* with *M. nematophilum*. Genome Res 16:1005–1016

Partridge L, Gems D (2002) Mechanisms of ageing: public or private? Nat Rev Genet 3:165–175

Pham LN, Dionne MS, Sirasu-Hiza M, Schneider DS (2007) A specific primed immune response in *Drosophila* is dependent on phagocytes. PLoS Pathog 3:e26 doi:10.1371/journal.ppat.0030026

Philips JA, Rubin EJ, Perrimon N (2005) *Drosophila* RNAi screen reveals CD36 family member required for mycobacterial infection. Science 309:1251–1253

Pinheiro VB, Ellar DJ (2006) How to kill a mocking bug? Cell Microbiol 8:545–557

Pletcher SD, Macdonald SJ, Marguerie R, Certa U, Stearns SC, Goldstein DB, Partridge L (2002) Genome-wide transcript profiles in aging and calorically restricted *Drosophila melanogaster*. Curr Biol 12:712–723

Qadota H, Inoue M, Hikita T, Koppen M, Hardin JD, Amano M, Moerman DG, Kaibuchi K (2007) Establishment of a tissue-specific RNAi system in *C. elegans*. Gene 400:166–173

Rämet M, Pearson A, Manfruelli P, Li X, Koziel H, Göbel V, Chung E, Kreiger M, Ezekowitz RA (2001) *Drosophila* scavenger receptor CI is a pattern recognition receptor for bacteria. Immunity 15:1027–1038

Rämet M, Manfruelli P, Pearson A, Mathey-Prevot G, Ezekowitz RA (2002) Functional genomic analysis of phagocytosis and identification of a *Drosophila* receptor for *E. coli*. Nature 416:644–648

Ren C, Webster P, Finkel SE, Tower J (2007) Increased internal and external bacterial load during *Drosophila* aging without life-span trade off. Cell Metab 6:144–152

Roman G, Endo K, Zong L, Davis RL (2001) P{Switch}, a system for spatial and temporal control of gene expression in *Drosophila melanogaster*. Proc Natl Acad Sci 98:12602–12607

Royet J, Dziarski R (2007) Peptidoglycan recognition proteins: pleiotropic sensors and effectors of antimicrobial defenses. Nat Rev Microbiol 5:264–277

Ryu JH, Nam KB, Oh CT, Nam HJ, Kim SH, Yoon JH, Seong JK, Yoo MA, Jang IH, Brey PT, Lee WJ (2004) The homeobox gene *Caudal* regulates constitutive local expression of antimicrobial genes in *Drosophila* epithelia. Mol Cell Biol 24:172–185

Ryu JH, Ha EM, Oh CT, Seol JH, Brey PT, Jin I, Lee DG, Kim J, Lee D, Lee WJ (2006) An essential complementary role of NF-κB pathway to microbial oxidants in *Drosophila* gut immunity. EMBO J 25:3693–3701

Sadd BM, Schmid-Hempel P (2006) Insect immunity shows specificity in protection upon secondary pathogen exposure. Curr Biol 1206–1210

Schmid-Hempel P (2005) Evolutionary ecology of insect immune defenses. Annu Rev Entomol 50:529–551

Schott DH, Cureton DK, Whelan SP, Hunter CP (2005) An antiviral role for the RNA interference machinery in *Caenorhabditis elegans*. Proc Natl Acad Sci 102:18420–18424

Seroude L, Brummel T, Kapahi P, Benzer S (2002) Spatio-temporal analysis of gene expression during aging in *Drosophila melanogaster*. Aging Cell 1:47–56

Shapira M, Hamlin BJ, Rong J, Chen K, Ronen M, Tan MW (2006) A conserved role for a GATA transcription factor in regulating epithelial innate immune responses. Proc Natl Acad Sci 103:14086–14091

Shirasu-Hiza MM, Schneider DS (2007) Confronting physiology: how do infected flies die? Cell Microbiol 9:2775–2783

Stroschein-Stevenson SL, Foley E, O'Farrell PH, Johnson AD (2006) Identification of *Drosophila* gene products required for phagocytosis of *Candida albicans*. PLoS Biol 4:e4

Stuart LM, Boulais J, Charriere GM, Hennessy EJ, Brunet S, Jutras I, Goyette G, Rondeau C, Letarte S, Huang H, Ye P, Morales F, Kocks C, Bader JS, Desjardins M, Ezekowitz RA (2007) A systems biology analysis of the *Drosophila* phagosome. Nature 445:95–101

Tanji T, Ip YT (2005) Regulators of the Toll and IMD pathways in the *Drosophila* immune response. Trends Immunol 26:193–198

Tanji T, Hu X, Weber ANR, Ip T (2007) *Toll* and IMD pathways synergistically activate innate immune response in *Drosophila melanogaster*. Mol Cell Biol 27:4578–4588

Theopold U, Schmidt O, Söderhall K, Dushay MS (2004) Coagulation in arthropods: defense, wound closure and healing. Trends Immunol 25:289–294

Troemel ER, Chu SW, Reinke V, Lee SS, Ausubel FM, Kim DH (2006) (p38) MAPK regulates expression of immune response genes and contributes to longevity in *C. elegans*. PLoS Genet 2:e183 doi:101371/journal.pgen.0020183

Tzou P, Ohresser S, Ferrandon D, Capovilla M, Reichhart J-M, Lemaitre B, Hoffmann JA, Imler JL (2000) Tissue-specific inducible expression of antimicrobial peptide genes in *Drosophila* surface epithelia. Immunity 13:737–748

Tzou P, De Gregorio E, Lemaitre B (2002) How *Drosophila* combats microbial infection: a model to study innate immunity and host-pathogen interactions. Curr Opin Microbiol 5:102–110

Uvell H, Engström Y (2007) A multilayered defense against infection: combinatorial control of insect immune genes. Trends Genet 23:342–349

van Rij RP, Saleh MC, Berry B, Foo C, Houk A, Antoniewski C, Andino R (2006) The RNA silencing endonuclease *Argonaute* 2 mediates specific antiviral immunity in *Drosophila melanogaster*. Genes Dev 20:2985–2995

Watson FL, Püttmann-Holgado R, Thomas F, Lamar DL, Hughes M, Kondo M, Rebel VI, Schmucker D (2005) Extensive diversity of Ig-superfamily proteins in the immune system of insects. Science 309:1874–1878

Wilkins C, Dishongh R, Moore SC, Whitt MA, Chow M, Machaca K (2005) RNA interference is an antiviral defense mechanism in *Caenorhabditis elegans*. Nature 436:1044–1047

Williams MJ (2007) *Drosophila* hemopoiesis and cellular immunity. J Immunol 178:4711–4715

Winston ML (1987) The biology of the honey bee. Harvard University Press, Cambridge, Massachussetts

Wu LP, Anderson KV (1997) Related signaling networks in *Drosophila* that control dorsoventral patterning in the embryo and the immune response. Cold Spring Harb Symp Quant Biol 62:97–103

Wu LP, Choe KM, Lu Y, Anderson KV (2001) *Drosophila* immunity: Genes on the third chromosome required for the response to bacterial infection. Genetics 159:189–199

Xia et al (2004) A draft sequence for the genome of the domesticated silkworm (*Bombyx mori*). Science 306:1937–1940

Zambon RA, Nandukumar M, Vakharia VN, Wu LP (2005) The *Toll* pathway is important for an antiviral response in Drosophila. Proc Natl Acad Sci 102:7257–7262

Zerofsky M, Harel E, Silverman N, Tatar M (2005) Aging of the innate immune response in *Drosophila melanogaster*. Aging Cell 4:103–108

Clonal Culture Models of T-cell Senescence

Graham Pawelec, Jürgen Kempf and Anis Larbi

Contents

Abstract: Studying human T-cell senescence is mostly limited to investigations on peripheral blood ex vivo or on cultured cells in vitro. In both cases, single cell analysis is challenging and many age-associated alterations described are the result of changes in the proportions of the ever-increasing numbers of different T-cell subsets rather than changes to the cells per se. One model avoiding this problem utilises monoclonal populations cultured long-term in vitro. Such T-cell clones (TCC) can be maintained without oncogenic transformation by intermittent antigen restimulation in the presence of growth factors. However, TCC possess finite lifespans (which vary greatly from clone to clone). This TCC model can be used to investigate many aspects of the processes of clonal expansion and contraction essential for adaptive immunity, including biomarker discovery at the genomic, proteomic and functional levels, and to test interventions of possible clinical utility. This chapter describes techniques for the production and maintenance of human TCC in vitro, the impact of culture conditions and oxygen levels on lifespan, and the application of genomic and proteomic analyses in this model.

Keywords: Chronic antigenic stress • Immunosenescence • In vitro culture model • Physiological oxygen level • T-cell clones

G. Pawelec (✉) · J. Kempf · A. Larbi
Center for Medical Research (ZMF)
University of Tübingen Medical School, Waldhörnlestr. 22
D-72072 Tübingen, Germany
Fax: ++49 7071 8884679
Tel.: ++49 7071 253211
E-mail: graham.pawelec@uni-tuebingen.de

T. Fulop et al. (eds.), *Handbook on Immunosenescence,*
DOI 10.1007/ 978-1-4020-9062-2_5, © Springer Science+Business Media B.V. 2009

1   Introduction

Long-term propagation of human T-cells became possible after the discovery of "T-cell growth factor", enabling single T-cells to be isolated and cultured for extended (Gillis et al. 1978) but not indefinite periods (Effros and Pawelec 1997). All TCC culture systems relied on the presence of "feeder cells" to facilitate T-cell growth via ill-defined mechanisms of cell contact and cytokine secretion. Nowadays, T-cells can be cultured with defined factors such as the common γ-chain cytokines IL 2, IL 7 and IL 15, together with nanoparticles presenting antibodies to stimulatory surface molecules, commonly the T-cell receptor (TCR) CD3 component and the costimulatory receptor CD28, or together with TCR-cognate antigen and antigen presenting cells (APC) or particles. Notwithstanding all these variations, the basic principles remain the same: to propagate T-cells in vitro it is necessary to provide them not only with exogenous growth factors but also to stimulate them intermittently via their cell surface receptors, most usually the TCR. TCC cultured in this way provide a model for reactivity against antigens which cannot be eliminated by the immune system, i.e. certain parasites, viruses and commonly cancer. When confronted with acute infection, adaptive immunity develops effector responses to clear the antigen; thereafter, excess effector cells are purged from the system and memory cells retained for any future challenges. However, antigens from persistent viruses, notably Herpes viruses, as well as immunogenic cancers, are not cleared, but continuously stimulate specific T-cells. The number of different, mostly CMV-specific, T-cell clonal expansions quantified in vivo first increases and then decreases with age; in the very elderly, the number of remaining clones correlates closely with residual survival time (Hadrup et al. 2006). Thus, chronic antigenic stress (mostly CMV antigens in this case) causes clonal exhaustion and attrition, with clinical consequences. We hypothesize that similar phenomena can occur in younger people harbouring different sources of chronic antigen, especially cancer (Pawelec et al. 2006). The process of T-cell clonal expansion and eventual attrition can be modelled in vitro in tissue culture. We can hope to learn how to modulate this process in vivo by improving and studying the model in vitro.

2   T-cell Cloning

As with fibroblasts, early data on T-cells suggested that clonal lifespan in culture was influenced by age of the donor from whom the starting population was obtained. Thus, clones derived from neonates averaged a larger number of population doublings (PD), than those from adults, especially the elderly (McCarron et al. 1987). Our own more extensive results, collected over many years from multiple cloning experiments, do not support this finding. Individual TCC do have very varied lifespans, but the overall patterns for T-cells of quite different origins and donors of different ages are remarkably similar, as we have previously reported (Pawelec et al. 2002); thus, clonable T-cells from a centenarian or from a young adult behave similarly, implying that the former have not been functionally compromised. This is consistent with the main age-associated alteration in human T-cells being the changed distribution of T-cell subsets, reflected most prominently in the decreased proportion of naïve cells and the increased proportion of memory cells of different subtypes.

The process of clonal attrition is striking in this in vitro model (Table 1). After 20 PD, representing a clone size of 10^6 cells, about half of the clones originally obtained in each experiment have already been lost. By 30 PD, another half of these is lost, so that only one quarter of the originally clonable cells is still present. By 40 PD (which now represents a very large clone size of 10^{12} cells, at least theoretically if no daughter cells ever die at each cell division), although more clones have been lost, 15% of the original starting clonal population does still remain. These results reflect a steady attrition of T-cell diversity at the clonal level, but with retention of something like 5% of the original CD4 repertoire up to 40 PD and with retention of very rare clones for much longer (some at least to 70 PD). Although difficult to establish, similar clonal attrition probably occurs in vivo as well, at least in infectious mononucleosis, perhaps with quite similar distributions of clonal longevities (Maini et al. 1999). Similar considerations concerning cells from other sources predict that any T-cell, if clonable under these conditions, will behave in a very similar way to any other. This is borne out by the finding that T-cells generated in situ from CD34+ hematopoietic progenitors and those from cancer patients do not manifest greater or lesser average and maximum longevities, respectively (Table 1).

Table 1 Longevities of human T-cell clones under standard culture conditions

Origin	%CE	Clones/ Expts	Percentage of clones reaching:			Max. longevity
			20 PD	30 PD	40 PD	
CD3 (young)	47	1355/15	47	24	15	70
CD3 (old)	52	298/7	48	26	16	77
CD3 (cent)	38	52/3	41	23	17	80
CD3 (CML)	49	35/1	60	35	14	51
CD34 (periph)	55	533/6	31	17	6	60
CD34 (cord)	43	94/2	29	15	5	57

CE, cloning efficiency (calculated from percentage of wells positive in cloning plates). Longevity is expressed as a percentage of established clones (ie. those counted as positive in calculating the CE) which survive to 20, 30 or 40 PD. Origins: CD34+, positively-selected hematopoietic stem cells from peripheral or cord blood; CD3+, normal peripheral T cells; young, apparently healthy donors under 30 yr.; old, healthy donors over 85 yr.; cent, centenarians; CML, a middle-aged donor with chronic myelogenous leukemia in chronic phase treated with interferon.

3   Changes in Behavior over the TCC Life Cycle

The 15–35% of TCC surviving for prolonged periods can be followed longitudinally over their finite lifespans regarding surface molecule expression, activation, signal transduction, cytokine secretion, cytotoxicity, and many other parameters. A typical growth curve of such a clone is shown in Fig. 1 (in this case, a CD4+ clone derived from an octogenarian donor). Growth is well-maintained until 40–50 PD, after which it slows, and the clone is lost at around 55 PD. This slow-down and demise is caused by increasing susceptibility to CD4+ TCC to apoptosis caused by activation-induced cell death, rather than changes to cell division rate. Age-associated alterations discovered in this way over the lifespan of the TCC can be used to screen for similar changes ex vivo in order to validate biomarkers of immune ageing, and they can also be used to test interventions in vitro aimed at preventing or reversing deleterious changes.

3.1   Changes of Surface Phenotype and Function

Bearing in mind the constraints of the cloning procedure, "early passage" TCC will have already undergone at least 22 or 23 PD before sufficient cells are available for analysis and further propagation of the clone, but as mentioned above, at this point there is still a good representation of the original repertoire. TCC can be

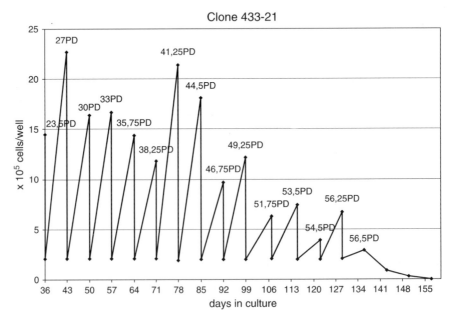

Fig. 1 Growth characteristics of TCC 433-21, showing days in culture plotted against the number of cells per culture well and giving the CPD estimated at each subculture

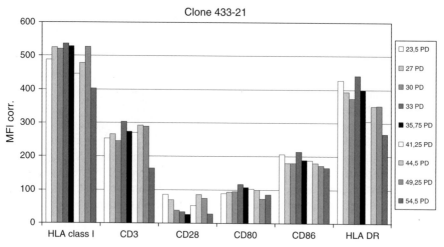

Fig. 2 Surface marker expression of TCC 433-21 giving the CPD estimated at each subculture

analyzed by flow cytometry for changes to expression of an ever-increasing number of monoclonal antibody-defined cell surface molecules, many with important known functions for T-cell responses. A common but not universal age-associated reduction in the level of expression of the costimulatory receptor CD28 has been documented (Pawelec et al. 1997), whereas the level of TCR remains more stable (Fig. 2). This suggests that these cells retain the ability to recognise and respond to antigen but may lack full costimulation, which may contribute to the changes observed in the patterns of cytokines secreted, commonly resulting in decreased levels of IL 2 and increased levels of IL 10 (Pawelec et al. 1997). When comparing the growth curve and the surface marker expression of the same clone, there was a correlation between CD28 expression and the capacity of the clone to grow. CD28 expression is decreasing from 27 to 35 PD and is then re-expressed and finally lost at the end-stage of the clone's lifespan (Fig. 2). This perfectly correlated with the number of cells obtained at each PD (Fig. 1). Nonetheless, other factors certainly play a role in the varied age-associated changes seen in different individual clones. Because T-cell functions are triggered by intracellular signaling via a multitude of surface receptors in addition to the TCR and CD28, any alterations impinging on the membrane (early events) through the cytoplasm (intermediate events) to the nucleus (late events) will influence the final outcome of each encounter with APC for each individual T-cell. This suggests that stochastic events may drive heterogeneity within clonally expanding T-cell populations, a hypothesis for which some evidence does exist.

4   Genomic and Proteomic Analysis

We recently undertook a first global gene expression analysis of early and late passage TCC derived from an octogenarian donor, one of which is shown in Fig. 1. This screening approach allows the hypothesis-free identification of potentially important age-associated changes which can be usefully followed up at the protein and functional levels. Array analysis has thus revealed a wide range of differentially expressed genes, including those encoding proteins involved in signal transduction, inflammation, apoptosis, and other processes implicated in senescence (Mazzatti et al. 2007b). Of particular note may be the age–associated upregulation of genes encoding various proinflammatory molecules, considered an important factor in physiological ageing and development of frailty. A similar approach applied at the proteome level may also assist in the discovery of biomarkers of relevance in vivo. Thus, using SELDI-Tof-MS protein profiling, we have identified several protein/peptide peaks which could be associated with T-cell senescence (Mazzatti et al. 2007a). One protein identified through this analysis, profilin-1, hitherto unsuspected in the context of senescence, has important roles in cellular survival, cell division, cytoskeleton remodeling and motility, and may contribute to immunosenescence or possibly cellular senescence in general.

5   Interventions

5.1   Culture Conditions

Interventions that we have tested in the in vitro longitudinal T-cell ageing system described here include culturing TCC in different cytokine cocktails, supplementing with factors such as zinc, attempting to block apoptosis in various ways, and culturing in lower levels of oxygen. The basic culture conditions have remained the same: use of an excess of feeder cells usually consisting of irradiated PBMC pooled from many different healthy donors, culture medium containing human serum or more recently serum free (X-Vivo 15, Lonza, Basel, Switzerland), and a source of growth factors. Briefly, of the many different variants that we have tested, relatively few have had much impact on the growth characteristics and longevities of the TCC. One of these, neutralisation with antibodies of the TNF-α secreted into the culture medium by essentially all TCC, resulted in an increased cumulative PD (CPD) of 10-15 PD (Pawelec et al. 2006). This can translate to a very large number of cells at later passages, and could be used in vivo, since agents that neutralise TNF are licensed for use in humans in diseases such as rheumatoid arthritis. The only other manipulation which has had an impact on TCC longevity, also increasing CPD by 5-15 PD, is to culture the cells in a more physiological level of oxygen, as described in the next section.

5.2   Physiological Oxygen

All of the above-mentioned studies, and indeed most cell culture experiments in any context, are performed at 37°C in humidified incubators gassed with 5% CO_2

but otherwise containing air. This equates to a hyperoxic environment with 20% O_2, not applicable in vivo. We are therefore embarking on experiments in which TCC are cultured in lower oxygen environments. Earlier experiments using 4 different TCC suggested that oxidative DNA damage measured in TCC by a modified Comet assay increased with increasing PD in culture in air. Reducing the oxygen level to 5% led to a marked reduction in accumulated oxidative DNA damage, but contrary to expectations did not lead to an increased longevity of the TCC (Duggan et al. 2004). However, more recent experiments reducing the level of oxygen further to 2% suggest that while some TCC do not show increased longevity under 2% compared to 20% oxygen, the majority does (Fig. 3). Changes in expression of inducible heat shock proteins and other parameters parallel the growth and signal transduction modulations observed in TCC cultured in what we believe approximates a more "physiological" oxygen tension than air. Thus, the interpretation of data derived from the usual type of in vitro culture in air must be treated with caution, and ideally experiments repeated at lower oxygen levels not only in the context of TCC but essentially all other culture-based systems.

5.3 Telomerase Induction

Expanded TCC loss of CD28 expression is associated with reduced telomerase activity and thus telomere length. Transferring the human telomerase reverse tran-

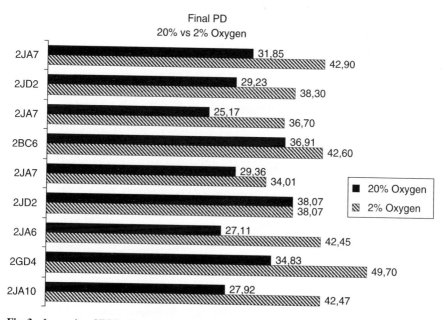

Fig. 3 Longevity of TCC cultured in air or at 2% oxygen. CPD are given for each of 9 individual TCC

scriptase (TERT) gene into T-lymphocytes can increase their lifespan (Rufer et al. 2001). T-cell clones with high levels of telomerase maintained or increased their telomere lengths for extended periods of time. Thus, enforced telomerase expression can increase T-cell longevity.

5.4 Autoantigen-specific T-cell Cloning

The cloning of autoreactive T-cells is more difficult. On early attempts to do so, we concluded that factors other than cytokines including IL 2, IL 4 and IL 7 were required for the expansion of these cells. Mannering et al., recently used CFSE-stained cells, a known cell tracker dye used to assess proliferative capacity of cells, to pre-select responding clones. After stimulation with the auto-antigen acid decarboxylase-65 for 7 days, propidium iodide-negative CD4+CFSE^{dim} cells could be cloned. The cytokine cocktail included IL 2, IL 4 and IL 7 but also IL 15 (5 ng/ml). This resulted in a cloning efficiency averaging from 10 to 15%. IL 15 may therefore be the crucial factor (Mannering et al. 2005).

6 Conclusions

Human T-cell clones can be maintained for extended but finite periods without transformation in tissue culture but eventually cease proliferating at time points up to the Hayflick limit. This remains the case even when known inhibitory factors such as TNF-α are neutralized and when more physiological oxygen tensions are applied, which can increase lifespan but not indefinitely. Only enforced expression of telomerase may greatly extend the lifespan, but this probably also fails to immortalize the cells. The changes which can be investigated longitudinally over the lifespan of the TCC and which reflect in vivo alterations make this a good model for studying human T-cell immunosenescence.

Acknowledgments We thank Ms A. Rehbein and K. Hähnel for maintaining the TCC and Dr. H. Eltschig for use of the low oxygen work station. Some of the work of the authors mentioned here was most recently supported by the Deutsche Forschungsgemeinschaft (DFG SFB 685-B4; DFG Pa 361/11-1) and the European Commission (QLK6-2002-02283, T-CIA; LSHC-CT-2004-503306, ENACT; LSHG-CT-2007-036894, LifeSpan).

References

Duggan O, Hyland P, Annett K, Freeburn R, Barnett C, Pawelec G, Barnett Y (2004) Effects of a reduced oxygen tension culture system on human T cell clones as a function of in vitro age. Exp Gerontol 39:525–530

Effros RB, Pawelec G (1997) Replicative senescence of T cells: does the Hayflick Limit lead to immune exhaustion? Immunol Today 18:450–454

Gillis S, Baker PE, Ruscetti FW, Smith KA (1978) Long-term culture of human antigen-specific cytotoxic T-cell lines. J Exp Med 148:1093–1098

Hadrup SR, Strindhall J, Kollgaard T, Seremet T, Johansson B, Pawelec G, Straten PT, Wikby A (2006) Longitudinal studies of clonally expanded CD8 T cells reveal a repertoire shrinkage predicting mortality and an increased number of dysfunctional cytomegalovirus-specific T cells in the very elderly. J Immunol 176:2645–2653

Maini MK, Soares MV, Zilch CF, Akbar AN, Beverley PC (1999) Virus-induced CD8+ T cell clonal expansion is associated with telomerase up-regulation and telomere length preservation: a mechanism for rescue from replicative senescence. J Immunol 162:4521–4526

Mannering SI, Dromey JA, Morris JS, Thearle DJ, Jensen KP, Harrison LC (2005) An efficient method for cloning human autoantigen-specific T cells. J Immunol Methods 298:8–392

Mazzatti DJ, Pawelec G, LongdinR, Powell JR, Forsey RJ (2007a) SELDI-TOF-MS ProteinChip array profiling of T-cell clones propagated in long-term culture identifies human profilin-1 as a potential bio-marker of immunosenescence. Proteome Sci 5:7

Mazzatti DJ, White A, Forsey RJ, Powell JR, Pawelec G (2007b) Gene expression changes in long-term culture of T-cell clones: genomic effects of chronic antigenic stress in aging and immunosenescence. Aging Cell 6:155–163

McCarron M, Osborne Y, Story CJ, Dempsey JL, Turner DR, Morley AA (1987) Effect of age on lymphocyte proliferation. Mech Ageing Dev 41:211–218

Pawelec G, Barnett Y, Mariani E, Solana R (2002) Human CD4+ T cell clone longevity in tissue culture: lack of influence of donor age or cell origin. Exp Gerontol 37:265–269

Pawelec G, Koch S, Griesemann H, Rehbein A, Hahnel K, Gouttefangeas C (2006) Immunosenescence, suppression and tumour progression. Cancer Immunol Immunother 55:981–986

Pawelec G, Rehbein A, Haehnel K, Merl A, Adibzadeh M (1997) Human T-cell clones in long-term culture as a model of immunosenescence. Immunol Rev 160:31–42

Rufer N, Migliaccio M, Antonchuk J, Humphries RK, Roosnek E, Lansdorp PM (2001) Transfer of the human telomerase reverse transcriptase (TERT) gene into T lymphocytes results in extension of replicative potential. Blood 98:597–603

Mouse Models of Influenza

Ian C. Brett and Bert E. Johansson

Contents

Abstract: Influenza is an enveloped, segmented negative sense RNA virus capable of infecting epithelial cells lining the human respiratory tract. Influenza A and B are important causes of disease in humans. Transmitted via aerosol, the virus possesses two major surface, hemagglutinin (HA) and neuraminidase (NA). HA has binding specificity for sialic acid, and allows viral attachment and entry into the cell. NA cleaves sialic acid residues off glycoproteins or mucoproteins, which aids new progenitor virions in eluting from the cell. The primary method of reducing influenza disease burden has been through vaccination.

Keywords: Influenza • murine • pulmonary titers

1   Introduction

Many different animal models of influenza infection have been used throughout the years, including ferret, mouse, rabbit and swine. However, the mouse is the preferred model for infection because of its ease of breeding, handling and relative low-cost. Importantly the mouse model can be a good predictor of the human response to

I. C. Brett (✉)
State University of New York, Stony Brook School of Medicine, Health Sciences Center,
L4, Stony Brook, NY 11794, USA
Fax: +1-631-632-1555
E-mail: ian.brett@hsc.stonybrook.edu

B. E. Johansson
Innovation Sciences, Armonk, NY 10504
E-mail: bertjoh@pol.net

T. Fulop et al. (eds.), *Handbook on Immunosenescence*,
DOI 10.1007/978-1-4020-9062-2_6, © Springer Science+Business Media B.V. 2009

infection and vaccination. Mouse models have been useful in developing and testing vaccine formulations and pharmacological treatments, as well understanding the pathogenesis of the virus and the dynamics of the host antiviral response. Recent studies have sought to delineate the changes in response to influenza infection or vaccination with age. Studying vaccine efficacy and immune responses in this population is especially important given that the elderly typically show decreased immune response and vaccine efficacy.

This chapter will cover the most widely used mouse strains, discuss gene knock-out models, host response to infection and practical aspects of experiments involving mice to provide a starting point for new investigators interested in utilizing mouse models for studying influenza.

2   Inbred Mouse Strains

Investigators requiring mice for research can choose subjects from a large number of inbred and random-bred lines. As part of selecting the ideal murine strain for an experiment, the investigator must choose the genetic state that makes the model a valid representation of the target population. This may include, but is not limited to: selection of histocompatiblity antigens (H2 haplotype), T-helper 1 or 2 skewing of the immune response, or predilections for particular disease states (Table-1). An inbred line consists of a population of great genetic homogeneity, and experiments performed within such a population can test the treatment variability, which in the haphazardly bred mouse might be confounded with genetic variability.

The development of inbred lines of mice in biological research is equivalent to the development of measurement standards and the preparation of reagent and

Table 1   Common Mouse Strains used in Influenza Studies

Strain	Source	H2 Haplotype	Comments
BALB/c	221 (BALB/cJ); 235 (BALB/cByJ) inbred generations	d	Th_2 Skewed; nonaggressive strain; very large reticuloendothelial system
C57BL/6	226 inbred generations	b	Th_1 skewed; High mammary tumor incidence; high mortality in chloroform exposure; low erythrocyte & leukocyte counts; poor LPS response; aggressive strain
Nude (*nu*)	BALB/c-*nu*/+97 inbred generations	d	T-cell deficient, intact B-cell immune system
Nude (*nu*)	C57BL/*lac-nu*+ (B6. Cg-*Foxn1nu*/J)51 congenic generations	b	As above
Swiss Webster	-	outbred	-

Adapted from: Altman PI, Katz DD (1979). Inbred and Genetically Defined Strains of Laboratory Mice; Part 1: Mouse and Rat. Federation of American Societies for Experimental Biology. [1] Source data from Jackson Laboratories Website [22].

analytical grade chemicals and serological reagents. The "reagent grade" animal, the result of carefully controlled inbreeding, permits design and repetition of experiments requiring fine discrimination within an animal species. The inbred mouse line is a population of animals that has attained homozygosis at nearly every locus through the use of a mating system that reduces the number of genetically dissimilar ancestors [44]. Traditionally, the most common practice is rigid brother-sister mating over many generations.

The history of the inbred laboratory mammal is actually the history of the use of the mouse in cancer studies. In order to attain repeatable and controlled systems for studying factors affecting tumor transplantation and for providing insight into why cancer develops, Little and Tyzzer [36] began to breed mice to obtain the necessary genetic homogeneity. Many of the early inbred strains of mice originated from a small number of stocks [12]. This relatively restricted gene pool accounts for the similarities and differences in the classic inbred lines. The history of each inbred mouse line is included in the listing of *Standardized Nomenclature of Inbred Strains of Mice* [54] published regularly. We strongly recommend that the most recent publication of the list of inbred strains be consulted.

The *inbreeding coefficient*, F, is a useful theoretical measurement of the progress of inbreeding, which has retained its usefulness with the experimental use of transgenic animals. It is defined as the probability that both alleles at a locus are identical by descent. It therefore indicates the proportionate decrease of heterozygous loci in the inbred individual relative to those in a representative individual of the starting population. F increases at different rates, depending on the amount of ancestry shared by the mated individuals. F should be used with caution, it is a theoretical value calculated from a pedigree, and not only does it ignore mutational effects, it also ignores effects of selection favoring heterozygotes [12, 53]. Once inbred lines are established, they can be genetically manipulated to establish yet other strains with special attributes for genetic analysis and control. Namely, these are: the *congenic* lines, the *coisogenic* lines, and the *recombinant-inbred* line. A *congenic* line is an inbred line genetically identical to an already established inbred strain except for a short chromosomal segment that bears a distinctive gene of interest. The congenic line is created by crossing the established inbred strain with an individual mouse bearing the distinctive gene of interest; a gene introduced either by breeding or molecular biological techniques. By repeatedly crossing selected carriers of the distinctive gene back to the established inbred strain, in time all introduced genes except the distinctive gene and closely linked genes will have been purged [53]. The locus at which the distinctive gene resides is known as the *differential* locus, the linked genes carried along on the introduced segment are called *passenger* genes, and the original established inbred strain is termed the *partner* or *background* strain. Congenic lines are used (i) to compare effects of genes without the interference of genes in the background, (ii) to easily identify, by the congenic line in which they are carried, individual genes that have similar phenotypic effects, such as histocompatablity genes, and (iii) to assist in linkage studies. In contrast, to the congenic line, a *coisogenic* line is one that differs from its partner strain at a single locus, as a result of a mutation, random or introduced, in an established inbred line. A *recombinant-inbred* (RI) strain is derived from a cross of two already established highly inbred strains (the progenitor strains), followed by systematic inbreeding as for any other inbred strain. This procedure, with no conscious selection pressure applied, allows the reassortment and fixation of genes from the two progenitor lines [12, 53].

Inbred mice lack the genetic and phenotypic variation seen in outbred mouse populations. The H2 allele is the region that codes for the major histocompatibility complex (MHC), the proteins responsible for processing and presenting processed antigen peptides to T-cells for immune system activation. There are several H2 alleles in circulation in mouse populations, but inbred mice only possess one of these alleles (*e.*g., BALB/c has the H2^d allele). These alleles may vary in the number of different MHC proteins that can be expressed by an organism, or by variation in the protein sequence of amino acids in the cleft that binds and presents processed peptide. However, studies in inbred mice strains infected with *Rickettsia* [2] and murine cytomegalovirus (MCMV) [38] failed to establish a clear role for H2 haplotype in determining susceptibility or resistance to these pathogens. It is likely that several alleles persisted in the population because having the ability to bind a greater number of antigens or having the ability to bind certain antigens conferred some evolutionary advantage to the mouse and allowed persistence of these genes. Therefore, the use of inbred mice homozygous at this locus may skew the results of experiments in an unanticipated manner by artificially restricting the number or type of antigens that can be processed and/or presented by the organism's immune system. Conversely, experimental results may be better than seen in a genetically diverse population. One must be careful in interpreting results and extending generalizations to genetically diverse populations.

3   Specific Inbred Strains

BALB/c is the most common inbred mouse strain used in influenza vaccine studies, developed by HJ Bagg in 1913 (*Bagg alb*ino). Many substrains of the original BALB/c mouse are now in general use (e.g., BALB/cJ and BALB/cByJ). The substrains share a high degree of genetic identity, but do differ at least one locus [46] and have behavioral and breeding dissimilarities [21]. BALB/c mice have a skewed Th2 immune response; characterized by CD4+ cell expression of IL-4, IL-5, IL-6 and IL-10, cytokines that correspond to activation of the humoral response to infection. IFN-γ and IL-2 correspond to the cell-mediated response. Several studies have demonstrated the BALB/c mouse's skewed Th2 immune response to infection with various pathogens or vaccination [18, 20, 38]. With respect to influenza infection and vaccination, primary infection or primary immunization with different vaccines [20, 16] causes a Th1 immune response in this mouse model, whereas a secondary response to vaccine [16, 55] induces a Th2 type immune response.

The *C57BL/6* mouse is opposite of its BALB/c cousin. This mouse is much more aggressive than the comparatively docile BALB/c. The immune response is skewed toward a Th1 response, which explains the phenotype of resistance to pathogens such as HSV-1, Sendai virus, *Leishmania* and *Rickettsia* [2, 6, 18, 45]. Though this strain has been used to study influenza infection and vaccination, it is usually used experimentally in conjunction with BALB/c mice as a comparison [3].

Nude mice are substrains of BALB/c and C57BL/6 mice homozygous for the *nu* allele carried on chromosome 11, which contains a nucleotide deletion in the *Foxn1* gene. This results in an athymic and hairless animal [19]. The *Foxn1* gene encodes a transcription factor (Forkhead Box) controlling development of the thymic epithelium, important for providing the correct environment for T-cell education [11]. The advantage of an athymic animal model is the ability to study immune responses that require T-cell participation. Sullivan et al. [54] studied infection with A/PR/8/34 (H1N1) found that nude mice had a lower rate of sero-conversion and lower geometric mean titers to virus challenge, indicating that to mount an effective humoral immune response, an intact T-cell immune system is required. However, the mean time to death for nude mice was increased versus BALB/c mice, suggesting that the immunopathology seen in animal models is due in part to Type-1 cell-mediated immunity.

4   Outbred mice

The advantage of using outbred mice for experiments involving infection or vaccine testing is, outbred mice are genetically and phenotypically dissimilar, and therefore a more heterogeneous population. Theoretically, experimental results from studies in such a population may better represent actual results of similar studies in humans. Studies directly comparing influenza infection in outbred models to inbred models are lacking, but studies performed with other pathogens provide data to elucidate differences and similarities of immune responses. Outbred mice have been used for the biological characterization of flavivirus *Alfuy* infection [39], *Coxsackievirus B4 E2* viral spread post-infection [23], Sendai virus infection [45], *Neospora caninum* infection [49] anthrax vaccine studies [14], and a DNA-based FMDV (foot and mouth disease virus) vaccine [4]. In another case [5], outbred mice failed to mount an immune response to vaccination with a plasmid expressing F1 antigen from *Yersinia,* while BALB/c mice demonstrated a robust antibody response. The arsenal of outbred mouse strains to choose from is extensive, however, the Swiss-Webster mouse, its derivative the ICR mouse, are the most used for influenza infection and vaccine studies, though CD-1 and NIH/S mice have been used as well.

Typically, differences between inbred and outbred models were seen in susceptibility or resistance to infection or in response to vaccination, indicating that genetic heterogeneity, likely at multiple loci, is an important consideration for these types of studies. Therefore, based on all studies mentioned in this section, knowledge of the model chosen for study is essential, and extrapolation of experimental results must be done with extreme caution, and may not be possible in all cases.

5 Transgenic Animals

A transgenic animal is one that carries a foreign gene that has been deliberately inserted into its genome. The foreign gene is constructed using recombinant DNA methodology. In addition to a structural gene, the DNA usually includes other sequences to enable it to be incorporated into the DNA of the host and to be expressed correctly by the cells of the host. Transgenic mice have provided the tools for exploring many biological questions. Two methods of producing transgenic mice are widely used:

1. *The Embryonic Stem Cell Method (Method "1"):* Embryonic stem cells (ES cells) are harvested from the inner cell mass (ICM) of mouse blastocysts. They can be grown in culture and retain their full potential to produce all the cells of the mature animal, including its gametes.
2. *The Pronucleus Method (Method "2"):* Harvest freshly fertilized eggs before the sperm head has become a pronucleus, then inject the male pronucleus with your DNA. When the pronuclei have fused to form the diploid zygote nucleus, allow the zygote to divide by mitosis to form a 2-cell embryo. These embryos are then implanted in a pseudopregnant foster. Every cell in the offspring will contain the gene of interest.

5.1 Random vs. Targeted Gene Insertion

The early vectors used for gene insertion could, and did, place the gene (from one to 200 copies of it) anywhere in the genome. However, if you know some of the DNA sequence flanking a particular gene, it is possible to design vectors that replace that gene. The replacement gene can be one that restores function in a mutant animal or knocks out the function of a particular locus.

If the replacement gene is nonfunctional (a "null" allele), mating of the heterozygous transgenic mice will produce a strain of "knockout mice" homozygous for the nonfunctional gene (both copies of the gene at that locus have been "knocked out").

Knockout mice are valuable tools for discovering the function(s) of genes for which mutant strains were not previously available. Two generalizations have emerged from examining knockout mice:

1. Knockout mice are often surprisingly unaffected by their deficiency. Many genes turn out not to be indispensable. The mouse genome appears to have sufficient redundancy to compensate for a single missing pair of alleles.
2. Most genes are pleiotropic. They are expressed in different tissues in different ways and at different times in development.

6 Experimentally Infecting Mice with Influenza Virus

6.1 Viral Adaptation to Growth in a Mouse

Investigators utilizing murine models to study influenza virus must select or adapt an influenza viral strain suitable to address the experimental question. That is to say, does the murine model system and the infection induced accurately mimic real world phenomenon? In designing such experiments the investigator must address two questions: 1) Does the selected viral strain infect the mouse in a manner that is similar to a human infection in penetrance, viral replication, and replication kinetics? 2) Is the immunity engendered by an experimental vaccine or pharmacologic activity of a drug in the mouse mimic that in the human model? Investigators should be aware that the various immunogenic components of the influenza virus induce very different types of immunity easily reflected in a mouse model system. A more detailed discussion of the immune response to influenza virus can be found in reference [31]. Briefly, antibodies to HA neutralize viral infectivity [26]; antibody to the viral NA [26] and M2 [37] proteins are infection-permissive across a broad range of antibody levels (ie, no reduction in the number of infected subjects) but result in the reduction of pulmonary virus titers below a pathogenic threshold. Antibodies to M1 and NP can be found in the sera of animals immunized with whole virus vaccines, purified protein preparations and after infection. These studies failed to demonstrate a significant role for these antibodies in the amelioration of disease [25]. Despite evidence that live and inactivated influenza vaccines induce cross-reactive T-cells in humans [34] and mice [41], reinfection with homologous or heterotypic virus occurs. The level of anti-influenza CTLs correlates with the rate of viral clearance but not alter susceptibility to infection or subsequent infection [41].

Adaptation of influenza virus by serial passage in new host invariably results in the selection of mutants better equipped to replicate and spread within the new host. Most influenza virus strains grow readily in the mouse lung or murine tissue culture; thus influenza viruses, which are inherently cytolytic, adapt or become more damaging to the animal host not by changes in capacity to infect (which they already must possess) but by mutational changes that permit attainment of higher titers in the host. A common feature of adaptation of both influenza A and B viruses to the mouse has been the emergence of virus characterized by a more rapid growth rate [56, 35] and the capacity to reach higher concentrations in the lung [50]. Adaptation has been studied in the laboratory for many years. Changes in viral phenotype have been noted concomitant with sequential passage of virus in mice [8, 9, 40]. Serial passage of influenza A viruses in the mouse lung has been associated with antigenic changes [15], increased resistance to mucoprotein inhibitor, and changed sensitivity of viral HA to thermal inactivation [31]. Co-variation of these phenotypic changes with attainment of mouse lung virulence has not been unequivocally established. Whether adaptation comprises a complex series of mutational events or primarily entails selection of preexisting viral variants is not clear. Mouse-adapted virus is characterized by both a faster growth rate and the capacity to attain higher titers in the lung [13]; indicating that both selection of preexisting mouse lung replication mutants and their subsequent mutation occur.

There have been several studies examining the specific mutations and in which viral genes that confer a mouse-adapted phenotype. Adaptation of human influenza virus to mice by serial passage results in the selection of highly virulent variants that have acquired mutations in multiple genes [8, 9, 40]. Analyses of the genetic basis for virulence by using reassortants that possess mixtures of genes from virulent and avirulent strains have identified various groupings of genes, which in aggregate implicate all eight genome segments [9]. Brown et al. [9] demonstrated in H3N2 virus that a group of 11 mutations convert an avirulent virus to a virulent variant. Thirteen of the 14 amino acid substitutions (93%) detected among clonal isolates were likely instrumental in adaptation because of their positive selection, location in functional regions, and or independent occurrence in other virulent influenza viruses. Mutations in virulent variants repeatedly involved nuclear localization signals and sites of protein and RNA interaction, implicating them as novel modulators of virulence. Mouse-adapted variants with the same HA mutations possessed different pH optima of fusion, indicating that other viral genes can modulate HA fusion activity. Experimental adaptation resulted in the selection of three mutations that were in common with the virulent human H5N1 isolate A/HK/156/97 [9]. Similarly, adaptation of the A/FM/1/47 H1N1 strain to mice resulted in selection of a variant with increased virulence. Complete sequence analysis identified mutations in the PB1, PB2, HA, NA, and M1 genes; all five mutations were shown to control virulence but also the replicative capacity in the mouse. The HA, NA and M1 mutations increased yield in all three hosts whereas in combination the PB1 and PB2 mutations were host restrictive changing the virus to a mouse specific strain. However, the HA mutation increased virulence largely independent of increased growth indicating a change in pathological properties [8]. Serial passage of an initially avirulent influenza B virus, B/Memphis/12/97, resulted in the selection of a variant that was lethal in mice. Sequencing data suggested one change in the C-terminal domain of the M1 protein, an asparagine to a serine at position 221, was responsible for acquisition of virulence and lethality [40].

6.2   Practical Experimental Points

Viral strains suitable for adaptation to the mouse can be derived from wild-type [50–52], classic reassortant virus [24, 28–30] or products of reverse genetics [57]. Use of each method has distinct advantages and disadvantages. Use of wild-type strains can be a quick, simple and allows for opportunities to mimic wild-type antigenic exposures from both the internal and surface antigens. However, adapting the strain to mouse may prove laborious, difficult to standardize and low-yield growth in embryonated chick eggs may limit experimental choices. Whereas, use of the classic reassortant and reverse genetic techniques offers the advantage of placing the surface glycoproteins,

HA and NA of a wild-type strain onto a background of internal proteins derived from A/PR/8/34 (H1N1) virus, as done annually, in the production of conventional inactivated influenza vaccine. A/PR/8/34 has an optimal growth temperature of 39°C -the average body temperature of a BALB/c mouse [1], is permissive to growth in a variety of experimentally useful tissue culture cell-lines including Madin-Darby Canine Kidney (MDCK) [31] and there are many commercially available serologic and immunologic reagents compatible with this system. The disadvantage of reassortants and reverse genetics is the need to expand the virus in embryonated chicken eggs to obtain sufficient virus to do the experiment. Passage in chicken eggs leads to deadaptation to the mouse [24, 28– 30]. A reverse genetics plasmid kit containing genes encoding influenza internal proteins from a mouse adapted strain is not available; therefore viral products of reverse genetics will require adaptation passages.

Traditionally, influenza virus has been adapted to increased penetrance or viral growth by sequential passage of virus in mouse lungs [9, 31, 50], with limited passage for expansion in embryonated chicken eggs, which may select for virus less adapted to growth in the mouse lung [24, 50–52]. Passage in MDCK selects for and preserves mouse-adapted characteristics. However, the total amount of virus produced in tissue culture is less than in eggs. Both methods require purification of virions from the growth medium; simple centrifugation and sucrose gradient centrifugation can produce usable high yields of infectious virus [48]. There are commercially available affinity chromatographic methods. Irrespective of the selection method chosen for passing the virus close attention must be paid to dilution (concentration) of virus used in passage studies. Successful adaptation to the mouse lung can be achieved with a wide range of varying viral concentrations and multiplicity of infections (*moi*). Too low of a *moi* may be insufficient for productive infection, to high of a concentration may result in multiplicity interference. Often prior to an experiment the optimal range of viral dilutions is unknown therefore titration of the virus in mice using several dilutions is warranted. In both reassortment and selection of viral strains, one must be cognizant of the enormous mutation rate of influenza (and other RNA viruses) and their apparent requirement for high *moi* for maintaining fitness in a given host system [33, 43]. In other words, either the introduction of populations limited in genetic diversity or the attempt to clone high titer virus by limiting dilution may lead to the establishment of a less fit virus. If such a virus is then maintained by high dilution passage, it will never regain adapted vigor. This phenomenon is known as a genetic "bottleneck" or "Muller's ratchet" [10]. In our laboratory, we have observed the loss of rapid growth and viral titer in mice if passed too early at high dilution. The practical lessons are: pass at sequential low dilutions early; then after sufficient dilutions and passages to escape unwanted nonadapted genes, passage should be maintained at a dilution sufficient to assure a reasonable gene pool. If using A/PR/8/34 reassortants this is in the range of 10^{-4} to 10^{-5} egg infectious dose (EID_{50}). In general, following infection with influenza virus in the mouse peak viral replication is at 3–4 days post inoculation and peak pulmonary lesions are seen on day 7 postinoculation [28–31, 51, 52, 57]. Although, there are viral strains that can peak earlier, it is our opinion that any mortality among the mice prior to day 3 should be examined by assaying the lungs in a tissue culture based plaque assay.

6.3 Experimental Techniques for Infecting Mice with Influenza Virus

Influenza virus has been used to infect mice via several routes of entry including intracerebral inoculation [42, 47], discussion will be limited to the most common techniques: intranasal instillation and aerosol exposure.

Intranasal instillation: Mice should be lightly anesthetized with Metofane anesthesia (Mallinckrodt Veterinarian) or another non-ether, non-chloroform based anesthetic agent. Light anesthesia should induce a state where the animal is not in distress and is mildly hyperpneic. The animal should be firmly held behind its neck and in one hand between the thumb and forefinger, the tail can be held by the investigator's fifth digit. With the animal held supine, 50 µl of live virus or phosphate-buffered saline can be instilled intranasally by pipette or syringe [17, 24, 51, 52]. A range of viral dilutions is recommended.

Aerosol exposure: Shulman and Kilbourne described a technique [24, 50–52] utilizing a retired autoclave. By the use of air pumps the interior of the autoclave could be maintained at a steady negative pressure relative to the room. Dilutions of virus could be aerosolized under positive pressure via an air pump. The aerosolizing devices are delicate, fragile and expensive, which in part contributes to the popularity of intranasal instillation. No mouse-to-mouse transmission has been observed [24, 51, 52].

6.4 Measurement of Endpoints of Infection

When initiating an experimental protocol decisions regarding how endpoint of infection will be measured should be made *a priori*. The options are: measure virus pulmonary titers in plaque assay [32] or by PCR [57] at specific time points; calculation of mouse infectious dose 50 (MID_{50}), monitor mortality/lethality to calculate a lethal dose 50 (LD_{50}) [9, 50]; measure weight loss and recovery [27]. Serologic studies (e.g., antibody titers to HA, NA or other viral antigens) and cellular immunologic studies (e.g., B-cell, T-helper and CTL assays) can be easily included [28–30]. Briefly, these assays are:

1. *Mouse Infectious dose (MID)* is a measure of the amount of infectious virus in a given sample, not the number of virions but a functional assay of infectious capacity. MID_{50} is the calculated dilution of a viral preparation that is expected to infect 50% of the mice inoculated. Usually stated as units of MID_{50} i.e., 1 MID_{50}; 100 MID_{50}. For example if a 10^{-5} dilution infected 50% of the mice exposed then the MID_{50} is 10^5; 100 MID_{50} would be a 10^{-3} dilution. The same concept is true for EID_{50} and $TCID_{50}$.

2. *Mortality-lethality* is a measure of how many and when animals die post exposure. A *Lethal dose* (LD) is often used, as with MID, a lethal dose 50 (LD_{50}),

a dilution of virus inducing an infection lethal to 50% of the animals exposed can be calculated. Relative risk (RR) and odds ratios (OR) can be extracted from these data.

3. *Mean pulmonary titer (mPVT)* can be directly measured in hemagglutination assay of lung preparation, or to increase sensitivity, HA assay can performed after lung preparations are inoculated into chicken eggs. Tissue culture assays allow calculation of *viral plaque forming units (PFU)*. In monolayer cell cultures maintained under agar, it can be shown that influenza-virus induced plaques usually are initiated by single virions [31]. Therefore, counting the number of plaques in a given dilution of lung preparation provides an estimation of the pulmonary viral load [7].

4. *Pulmonary lesion/plaques* lungs can be removed from infected animals on day 7 post exposure and the distinct plum colored pulmonary lesions induced by influenza cytopathology can be measured and counted.

5. *Weight gain/loss* is a sensitive measure of illness in the murine model for influenza. Infected animals become less active, eat and drink less in the context of increased metabolic demands of an acute illness. Daily weighing accurately detects weight loss and recovery. Weight loss and lack of recovery are good predictors of mortality [27].

7 Conclusion

The murine model for the study of influenza is well established. Although the mouse is not an exact mimic of avian, equine or human influenza knowledge of the systems experimental strengths and flaws can produce valid and reliable data.

References

1. Altman PL, Katz DD (eds) (1979) Inbred and genetically defined strains of laboratory animals; Part 1: mouse and rat. Federation of American Societies for Experimental Biology. Bethesda
2. Anderson GW, Osterman JV (1980) Host defenses in experimental Rickettsialpox: genetics of natural resistance to infection. Infect Immun 28(1):132–136
3. Asanuma H, Fujihashi K, Miyakoshi T, Yoshikawa T, Fujita-Yamaguchi Y, Kojima N, Nakata M, Suzuki Y, Tamura S, Kurata T, Sata T (2007) Long- and short-time immunological memory in different strains of mice given nasally an adjuvant-combined nasal influenza vaccine. Vaccine doi:10.1016/j.vaccine.2007.06.060
4. Borrego B, Fernandez-Pacheco P, Ganges L, Domenech N, Fernandez-Borges N, Sobrino F, Rodríguez F (2006) DNA vaccines expressing B- and T-cell epitopes can protect mice from FMDV infection in the absence of specific humoral responses. Vaccine 24:3889–3899
5. Brandler P, Saikh KU, Heath D, Friedlander A, Ulrich RG (1998) Weak anamnestic responses of inbred mice to *Yersinia* F1 genetic vaccine are overcome by boosting with F1 polypeptide while outbred mice remain nonresponsive. J Immunol 161:4195–4200

6. Brenner GJ, Cohen N, Moynihan JA (1994) Similar immune response to nonlethal infection with Herpes Simplex Virus-1 in sensitive (BALB/c) and resistant (C57BL/6) strains of mice. Cell Immunol 157:510–524

7. Brett IC, Johansson BE (2005) Immunization against influenza A virus: comparison of conventional inactivated, live-attenuated and recombinant baculovirus produced purified hemagglutinin and neuraminidase vaccines in a murine model system. Virology 339:273–280

8. Brown EG, Bailly JE (1999) Genetic analysis of mouse-adapted influenza A virus identifies roles for the NA, PB1, and PB2 genes in virulence. *Virus Res* 61(1):63–76

9. Brown EG, Liu H, Kit LC, Baird S Nesrallah M (2001) Pattern of mutation in the genome of influenza A virus on adaptation to increased virulence in the mouse lung: identification of functional themes. Proc Natl Acad Sci U S A 98(12):6883–6888

10. Clarke DK, Duarte EA, Moya A, Elena SF, Domingo E, Holland J (1993) Genetic bottlenecks and population passages cause profound fitness differences in RNA viruses. J Virol 67(1):222–228

11. Coffer PJ, Burgering BMT (2004) Forkhead-Box transcription factors and their role in the immune system. Nat Rev Immunol 4:889–899

12. Crow JF (2002) CC Little, Cancer and inbred mice. Genetics 161:1357–1361

13. Davenport FM (1954) The inequality of potential influenza virus for adaptation to mice. J Exp Med 72:485

14. Flick-Smith HC, Waters EL, Walker NJ, Miller J, Stagg AJ, Green M, Williamson ED (2005) Mouse model characterization for anthrax vaccine development: comparison of one inbred and one outbred mouse strain. Microb Pathog 38:33–40

15. Gitelman AK, Kaverian NV, Kharitonenkov IG, Rudneva IA, Zhadnov VM (1984) Changes in antigenic specificity of influenza virus hemagglutinin in the course of adaptation to mice. Virology 134:230

16. Hauge S, Madhun AS, Cox RJ, Brokstad KA, Haaheim LR (2007) A comparison of the humoral and cellular immune responses at different immunological sites after split influenza virus vaccination in mice. Scand J Immunol 65:14–21

17. Hedrich H (ed) (2006) *Laboratory mouse handbook*. American Association for Laboratory Animal Science, 4th ed. Academic Press, New York

18. Heinzel FP, Sadick MD, Mutha SS Locksley RM (1991) Production of interferon-γ, interleukin 2, interleukin 4, and interleukin 10 by CD4+ lymphocytes *in vivo* during healing and progressive murine leishmaniasis. Proc Natl Acad Sci U S A 88:7011–7015

19. Holub M (1989) *Immunology of nude mice*. CRC Press, Boca Raton

20. Hovden AO, Cox RJ, Haaheim LR (2005) Whole influenza virus vaccine is more immunogenic than split influenza virus vaccine and induces primarily an IgG2a response in BALB/c mice. Scand J Immunol 62:36–44

21. Jackson Laboratories, Inc. Jax Lab Notes No. 430 (1987). http://jaxmice.jax.org/library/notes/430a.html (Accessed 8/25/07)

22. Jackson Laboratories website, http://www.jax.org/index.html (Accessed 8/26/07)

23. Jaïdane H, Gharbi J, Lobert P, Lucas B, Hiar R, Ben M'Hadheb M, Brilot F, Geenen V, Aouni M, Hober D (2006) Prolonged viral RNA detection in blood and lymphoid tissues from *Coxsackievirus B4 E2* orally-inoculated *Swiss* mice. Microbiol Immunol 50(12):971–974

24. Johansson BE, Kilbourne ED (1991) Comparative long-term effects in a mouse model system of influenza whole virus vaccine and purified neuraminidase vaccine followed by sequential infections. J Infect Dis 162:800–808

25. Johansson BE, Kilbourne ED (1996) Immunization with dissociated neuraminidase, matrix, and nucleoproteins from influenza A virus eliminates cognate help and antigenic competition. Virology 225:136

26. Johansson BE, Bucher DJ, Kilbourne E (1989) Purified influenza virus hemagglutinin and neuraminidase are equivalent in stimulation of antibody response but induce contrasting types of immunity to infection. J Virol 63:1239

27. Johansson BE, Grajower B, Kilbourne ED (1993) Infection permissive immunization with influenza virus neuraminidase prevents weight loss of infected mice. Vaccine 10:1037

28. Johansson BE, Moran TM, Kilbourne ED (1987) Antigen-presenting B-cells and helper T-cells cooperatively mediate intravirionic antigenic competition between influenza A virus surface glycoproteins. Proc Natl Acad Sci U S A 84:6869

29. Johansson BE, Moran TM, Bona CA, Kilbourne ED (1987). Immunologic response to influenza virus neuraminidase is influenced by prior experience with the associated viral hemagglutinin: III. Reduced generation of neuraminidase-specific helper T-cells in hemagglutinin primed mice. J Immunol 139:2015

30. Johansson BE, Moran TM, Bona CA,, Popple SW, Kilbourne ED (1987) Immunologic response to influenza virus neuraminidase is influenced by prior experience with the associated viral hemagglutinin: II. Sequential infection of mice simulates human experience. J Immunol 139:2010

31. Kilbourne ED (1987). *Influenza* (1st ed) Plenum Medical Book Co., New York

32. Kilbourne ED, Laver W, Schulman JL, Webster R (1968) Antiviral activity of antiserum specific for an influenza virus neuraminidase. I. in vitro effects. J. Virol 2:281

33. Lamb R, Choppin P (1983) Gene structure and replication of influenza virus. Virology 81:382

34. Lawson C, Bennink J, Restifo N, Yewdell J,, Murphy BR (1994) Primary pulmonary cytotoxic T-lymphocytes induced by immunization with a vaccinia virus recombinant expressing influenza A virus nucleoprotein peptide do not protect mice against challenge. J Virol 68:3505

35. Ledinko N (1956) An analysis of the process of influenza virus B of recent human origin to the mouse lung. J Gen Microbiol 15:47

36. Little CC, Tyzzer EE (1916) Further experimental studies on the inheritance of susceptibility to a transplantable carcinoma (JA) of the Japanese waltzing mouse. J Med Res 33:393–427

37. Liu W, Li H, Chen Y-H (2003) N-terminus of M2 protein could induce antibodies with inhibitory activity against influenza virus replication. FEMS Immunol Med Microbiol 35:141

38. Lloyd ML, Nikolovski S, Lawson MA, Shellam GR (2007) Innate antiviral resistance influences the efficacy of a recombinant murine cytomegalovirus immunocontraceptive vaccine. Vaccine 25:679–690

39. May FJ, Lobigs M, Lee E, Gendle D, Mackenzie JS, Broom AK, Conlan JV, Hall RA (2006) Biologic, antigenic and phylogenetic charactherization of the flavivirus Alfuy. J Gen Virol 87:329–337

40. McCullers JA, Hoffmann E, Huber VC, Nickerson AD (2005) A single amino acid change in the C-terminal domain of the matrix protein M1 of influenza B virus confers mouse adaptation and virulence Virology 336(2):318

41. McMicheal A, Grotch F, Cullen P,, Askonas B, Webster R (1981) The human cytotoxic T-cell response to influenza vaccination. Clin Exp Immunol 43:276

42. Miyoshi K, Wolf A, Harter DH,, Duffy PE, Gamhoa ET, Hsu KC (1973) Murine influenza virus encephalomyelitis. I. Neuropathological and immunofluorescence findings. J Neuropathol Exp Neurol 32:51–71

43. Neuman G, Kawaoka Y (2006) Host range restriction and pathogenicity in the context of influenza pandemic. Emerg Infect Dis 12(6):881–886

44. Paigen K (2003) One hundred years of mouse genetics: an intellectual history. I. The classical period (1902–1980). Genetics 163(1):1–7

45. Parker JC, Whiteman MD, Richter CB (1978) Susceptibility of inbred and outbred mouse strains to Sendai virus and prevalence of infection in laboratory rodents. Infect Immun 19(1):123–130

46. Potter M (ed) (1985) *The BALB/c mouse: Genetics and immunology.* Curr Top Microbiol Immunol (122) Springer-Verlag, Berlin, New York

47. Rainacher M, Bonin J, Narayan O, Scholtissek C (1983) Pathogenesis of neurovirulent influenza A virus infection in mice. Route of entry of virus into brain determines infection of different populations of cells. Lab Invest 49:686–692

48. Reimer CB, Baker RS, van Frank RM,, Newlin TE, Cline GB, Anderson NG (1967) Purification of large quantities of influenza virus by density gradient centrifugation. J Virol 1(6):1207–1216

49. Rettinger C, Leclipteux T, De Meerschman, F Focant C, Losson B (2004) Survival, immune responses and tissue cyst production in outbred (Swiss white) and inbred (CBA/Ca) strains of mice experimentally infected with *Neospora caninum* tachyzoites. Vet Res 35:225–232
50. Schulman JL (1970) Effects of immunity on transmission of influenza: Experimental studies. Prog Med Virol 12:128
51. Schulman JL, Kilbourne ED (1963) Experimental transmission of influenza virus infection in mice. I. Period of transmissibility. J Exp Med 118:257–266
52. Schulman JL, Kilbourne ED (1963) Experimental transmission of influenza virus infection in mice. II. Some factors affecting the incidence of transmitted infection. J Exp Med 118:267–275
53. Staats J (1985) Standardized nomenclature for inbred strains of mice: eighth listing. Cancer Res 45(3):945–977
54. Sullivan JL, Mayner RE, Barry DW, Ennis FA (1976) Influenza virus infection in nude mice. J Infect Dis 133(1):91–94
55. Szyszko E, Brokstad K, Cox RJ,,Hovden AO, Madhun S, Haaheim LR (2006) Impact of influenza vaccine formulation with a detailed analysis of the cytokine response. Scand J Immuno 64:467–475
56. Wang CI (1948) The relation of infectious and hemagglutinin titers to the adaptation of influenza virus to the mouse. J Exp Med 88:515
57. Webby R, Hoffmann E, Webster R (2004) Molecular constraints to interspecies transmission of viral pathogens. Nat Med 10(12):S77–S81
58. Wyde PR, Couch RB, Mackler BF, Cate TR, Levy BM (1977) Effects of low- and high-passage influenza virus infection in normal and nude mice. Infect Immun 15(1):221–229

A Transgenic Dwarf Rat Strain as a Tool for the Study of Immunosenescence in Aging Rats and the Effect of Calorie Restriction

Isao Shimokawa, Masanori Utsuyama, Toshimitsu Komatsu,
Haruyoshi Yamaza and Takuya Chiba

Contents

Abstract: Immunosenescence or dysregulation of the immune system may accelerate the aging process and shorten the lifespan in animals. Calorie restriction, a well-known nutritional intervention for longevity in laboratory animals, retards immunosenescence and modulates the immunosystem. These effects of CR could contribute partly to extending the lifespan. A transgenic (Tg) dwarf rat strain, in which the growth hormone (GH) axis is selectively suppressed, lived longer and exhibited several phenotypes similar to those in CR rats, suggesting an important role for the GH axis in the effect of CR. Here, we describe the longevity, pathology, thymic and splenic lymphocyte subpopulations and response to endotoxin in Tg rats in comparison with CR rats. The findings support the importance of the GH axis in the effect of CR on the immune system and, in particular, longevity. The Tg rats could be a useful tool to better understand the molecular mechanisms underlying the antiaging effect of CR.

I. Shimokawa (✉) · T. Komatsu · H. Yamaza · T. Chiba
Department of Investigative Pathology, Unit of Basic Medical Science
Graduate School of Biomedical Sciences, Nagasaki University
12-4 Sakamoto I-chome, Nagasaki City 852-8523, Japan
Tel.: +81-95-819-7051, Fax: +81-95-819-7052
E-mail: shimo@nagasaki-u.ac.jp

M.Utsuyama
Department of Pathology and Immunology
Aging and Developmental Sciences,
Tokyo Medical and Dental University Graduate School

T. Fulop et al. (eds.), *Handbook on Immunosenescence*,
DOI 10.1007/978-1-4020-9062-2_7, © Springer Science+Business Media B.V. 2009

1 Introduction

Innate and acquired immunity is important for animals not only to protect against infection of microorganisms but also to inhibit a number of diseases including cancers, which are prevalent in aged animals. The immune system is, however, a 'double-edged sword' as the inflammatory hypothesis of aging presumes [1]. Aging-related dysregulation of the immune system could accelerate the aging process and shorten the lifespan of animals by activating proinflammatory processes that lead to excess generation of reactive oxygen and nitrogen species that potentially injure cellular components.

Restriction of food intake with supplying essential nutrients for survival in laboratory animals, referred to as calorie restriction (CR), reduces morbidity and mortality [2]. This effect has been called 'anti-aging' because many laboratories also confirmed retardation or inhibition of the pathophysiological aging processes by CR, an effect first reported by McCay et al [3]. Although proper modulation of the immune system could be one of the main mechanisms by which CR affects aging and longevity in animals, our knowledge is incomplete.

Another line of studies in the biomedical gerontology have found that a single gene, if spontaneously mutated or genetically engineered, could prolong the lifespan of organisms. Although this evidence was initially limited to invertebrates, over 10 genes are now reported in laboratory rodents (Fig. 1). Many of these longevity genes are clustered into the signaling pathway of GH and subsequently insulin-like growth factor (IGF)-1 or insulin. Attenuation of these signaling pathways favors longevity. The GH-IGF-1/insulin pathway is important for understanding the mechanism underlying the effect of CR, because CR is also known to reduce plasma levels of IGF-1 and insulin in laboratory animals [4, 5]. Because GH and IGF-1 are known to modulate the immune system [6], we may hypothesize that CR exhibits the antiaging effect through suppression of the GH-IGF-1/insulin axis and thus modulating immune system.

In this study, we describe some traits of the transgenic dwarf (Tg) rat strain that we established as an aging research model [7, 8], in comparison with CR rats. Published data have indicated that Tg rats fed ad libitum had phenotypes similar to wild-type CR rats for body weight, food intake, fat content, glucose tolerance, insulin sensitivity, and adiopokines such as adiponectin and leptin [8-10]. Although, at present, the immunological findings of Tg rats are limited, this rat model could provide knowledge on the relevance of immunosenecence to aging and longevity. Similarily, data on immunosenescence in other longevity models are limited and, thus, future analyses of the immune system in these models are needed to explore the role for each gene or gene product in immunosenescence and aging.

2 Animal Husbandry and General Data

2.1 Transgenic Dwarf Rats and Husbandy

The Tg rats, with a genetic background of Jcl:Wistar (Japan Clea, Inc., Tokyo, Japan), were produced from founders created by introducing fusion genes into rat embryos [11]. The transgene consisted of four copies of thyroid hormone response

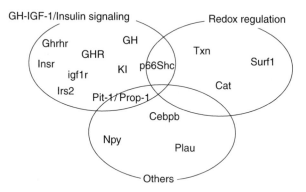

Fig. 1 Longevity genes in rodents. Genes that extend the lifespan of mice or rats, if spontaneously mutated or genetically engineered, are listed. The genes can be classified into three categories; genes that are associated with the GH-IGF-1/ insulin signaling pathway, redox regulation and other genes, although these categories are not mutually exclusive. *Prop-1* (spontaneously mutated mice for paired like homeodomain factor 1 gene; [15]): *Pit-1* (spontaneously mutated mice for POU domain, class 1, transcription factor 1 gene; [32]: *p66Shc* (knockout mice of src homology 2 domain-containing transforming protein C1 gene; [22]: *Ghrhr* (spontaneously mutated mice for growth hormone releasing hormone receptor gene; [32]: *GHR* (knockout mice for growth hormone (GH) receptor gene; [16]: *GH* (over-expression rats for antisense GH gene; [7]: *igf1r* (knockdown mice for insulin-like growth factor I receptor gene: [23]: *Insr* (mice for adipocyte-specific disruption of the insulin receptor gene; [33]): *Txn* (Overexpression mice for human thioredoxin gene: [34]): *Cat* (Mitochondria-specific overexpression mice for human catalase gene; [35]): *Plau* (brain-specific over-expression mice for urokinase type of plasminogen activator: [36]): *Npy* (overexpression rats for neuropeptide Y gene; [37]): *Cebpb* (knock-in mice for CCAAT/enhancer binding protein (C/EBP) beta gene; [38]): *Kl* (overexpression mice for klotho gene; [39]): Irs2 (whole body or brain-specific knockout mice for insulin receptor substrate 2 gene; [40]): *Surf1* (knockout mice for surfeit gene 1; [41])

elements, rat GH promoter, and antisense cDNA sequence for rat GH. The rat GH antisense gene was expressed in the pituitary gland of Tg rats as early as 3 weeks of age. Reverse transcription PCR analyses in Tg rats at 6 months of age confirmed that antisense GH-mRNA was expressed in the pituitary gland, spleen, and thymus, but not in the lungs, liver, heart, kidneys, and testis [7].

F1 hybrid rats were also generated at our laboratory animal center by mating female W rats with male Tg rats to moderate the reduced level of suppression of the GH-IGF-1 axis; the animals were referred to as tg/tg, tg/–, and –/– regarding the presence of the transgene.

At 4 weeks of age, weanling male rats were transferred to a barrier facility, housed separately, and maintained under specific-pathogen-free conditions. The animal husbandry is reported in detail elsewhere [7, 8]. Briefly, rats were provided a standard diet and tap water throughout the experiment (the AL group). The CR regimen in each rat group was initiated at 6 weeks of age. Rats in the CR group were provided 30% less food of the AL group by feeding them with two portions of food every other day 30 min before the lights were turned off.

Table 1 Characteristics of Tg and CR rats at 6 months of age

	(-/-)		(tg/-)		(tg/tg)	
	AL	CR	AL	CR	AL	CR
Body weight (g)	478.9 (34.1)	342.0 (16.9)*	316.6 (32.1)#	226.2 (15.4)*/#	199.1 (8.9)#	124.4 (10.5)*/#
Food intake (g/day)	21.6 (3.5)	15.9	17.0 (2.2)#	11.7	11.2 (1.3)#	7.9
Blood glucose (mg/dl)	126 (34)	112 (12)	106 (18)	90 (16)	106 (17)	n/a
Serum insulin (ng/ml)	102 (49)	15 (10)*	22 (18)#	20 (26)	21 (19)#	n/a
Plasma IGF-1 (ng/ml)	1094 (119)	864 (79) *	627 (90) #	346 (40)*/#	266 (23)#	170 (11)*/#
Plasma GH (ng/ml)	157.3 (55.0)	178.3 (26.7)	172.1 (44.1)	129.6 (35.9)	142.8 (33.9)	126.0 (46.0)
Pituitary GH-mRNA	1.00 (0.25)	0.81 (0.15)	0.34 (0.10)#	n/a	n/a	n/a

Values represent the mean (standard deviation) of 3–6 rats. (–/–); wild type rats. (tg/–); transgenic hemizygotic rats. (tg/tg); transgenic homozygotic rats. AL; ad libitum feeding rats. CR; 30% calorie-restricted rats. * $p < 0.05$ versus (vs) group AL in each rat group. #, $p < 0.05$ vs (–/–) of each diet group.

2.2   Characteristics of Tg and CR Rats at 6-Months of Age

The body weight and food intake in the AL condition decreased comparatively in tg/– and tg/tg rats, gene-dose dependently (Table 1). Following the 30% CR regimen for each AL group, the CR group showed 30~40% reduction in the body weight compared with the respective AL group. It should be noted that both the body weight and food intake in (tg/–)-AL rats were similar to those in (–/–)-CR rats for the first 24 months in the lifespan study [8].

Blood glucose levels under non-fasting conditions were slightly reduced in (tg/–)-AL and (tg/tg)-AL rats, while not significantly different between (tg/–)-AL and (tg/tg)-AL rats. CR also reduced the blood glucose level. The serum insulin level was significantly lower in (tg/–)-AL and (tg/tg)-AL. CR in (–/–) rats led to a significant reduction in the insulin level; there was no additional decrease by CR in (tg/–) and (tg/tg) rats.

The plasma IGF-1 concentration, an index for the degree of suppression of GH-IGF-1 signaling, decreased by 40% in (tg/–)-AL rats and by 75% in (tg/tg)-AL rats compared with (–/–)-AL rats. CR in each rat group further decreased the IGF-1 level; the level in (–/–)-CR rats was reduced to 80% of the level of (–/–)-AL rats. Thus the level was slightly lower in (tg/–)-AL rats than (–/–)-CR rats. The pituitary GH-mRNA level was also reduced by 20 and 66% in (–/–)-CR and (tg/–)-AL rats, respectively.

2.3   Longevity and Pathology

The lifespan at the 25th percentile point was increased by 10 and 11% in (tg/–)-AL and (–/–)-CR rats, as compared to (–/–)-AL rats (Figure 2); however, it was reduced

Table 2 Probable causes of death in Tg and CR rats

	(–/–)		(tg/–)		(tg/tg)	
	AL	CR	AL	CR	AL	CR
Total	30	26	30	30	39	17
Neoplastic (subtotal)	15	18	22	14	37*	11
Leukemia/lymphoma	0	1	2	3	21#	8
Pituitary adenoma	5	8	11	2#	1	0
Others	10	9	9	9	15	3
Non-neoplastic (subtotal)	15	8	8	16	2	6

Data represent the number of rats. The proportion of each category or disease was analyzed by χ^2 test or Fisher's exact test. * $p < 0.05$ versus (–/–)-AL rats. # $p < 0.05$ versus (tg/–)-AL rats.

by 9% in (tg/tg)-AL rats. Postmortem examination indicated that 50% of (tg/tg)-AL rats died of leukemia (Table 2); in contrast, only a few (tg/–) and (–/–) rats suffered from the disease. Furthermore, pituitary adenoma was less frequently in the cause of death in (tg/tg) rats. Our previous analysis indicated that moderate suppression of GH increased lifespan mostly due to the delay or inhibition of non-neoplastic causes; the effect on neoplastic causes was minor [7, 12].

Most of the rats that were considered to die of leukemia showed hepatosplenom-egaly. Microscopic analysis and immunohistochemistry with an antibody for NK cells indicated that most of the cases were mononuclear large cell leukemia, which is frequently observed in inbread F344/N rats [13, 14]. Because this type of leukemia is not commonly observed in outbread Wistar rats and that the tg/tg rats were expanded from a pair of founder Tg rats, it is likely that this specific type of leukemia become tangible during the inbreeding process in (tg/tg) rats. Conditional survival analysis was performed to determine if the leukemic death was eliminated (Figure 2). However, the survival did not exceed that in (–/–)-AL rats.

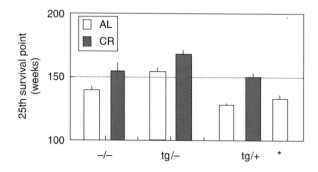

Fig. 2 Lifespan of transgenic dwarf rats: the effect of calorie restriction. Each bar represents the age (weeks) of 25th percentile survival point of lifespan (+ standard error). –/–, wild type rats. tg/–, hemizygotes for the transgene. tg/tg, homozygotes for the transgene. AL, a group of rats fed ad libitum. CR, 30% calorie-restricted rats. N = 30 for each group at the start of the study, with the exception of the (tg/tg)-AL group (N = 55) and (tg/tg)-CR group (N = 35). Survival data is described in more detail elsewhere [7, 8], except for the (tg/tg)-CR group. * Conditional survival if leukemia was excluded from the causes of death, i.e., leukemic death was considered to be the same censorship as random sacrifice of rats. The details of the procedure for the conditional survival are described elsewhere [42]

Thus, our data in dwarf rats suggest that moderate (but not severe) suppression of GH contributes to lifespan extension. This finding contrasts with those in long-lived mice whose GH signaling is almost deficient [15, 16].

CR increased the lifespan in all rat groups. Although CR decreased the plasma IGF-1 level in each rat group compared with the corresponding AL group, the reduced IGF-1 level alone is unlikely to contribute to the extended lifespan. As described above, the lifespan in (tg/tg)-AL rats was shorter than that in (tg/–)-CR rats, even if leukemic death was eliminated, while the plasma IGF-1 level was similar between the groups. Therefore, CR could have a GH-IGF-1 independent mechanism(s) for lifespan extension.

3   Subpopulation of Thymic and Splenic Lymphocytes

3.1   Thymic Lymphocyte Subpopulation

The weight of the thymus at 6 months of age did not differ significantly between rats or between diet groups, when normalized for body weight (Table 3). Flow cytometric analysis of thymocytes prepared from the 6-month-old rats illustrated that only double negative (DN; CD4– & CD8–) cells tended to increase in (tg/–) and (tg/tg) rats, particularly in (tg/–)-CR rats. However, there was no significant difference in double positive (DP; CD4+ & CD8+), CD4-single positive (SP4), or CD8-single positive (SP8) subpopulations among rats or between diet groups. Thus, the present data suggest that the suppression of GH or CR does not significantly affect the composition of thymocytes at least in the 6-month-old male rats.

The present data in Tg rats are in accord with the dwarf mice models in which pituitary GH, PRL, TSH are deficient or IGF-1-null mice, or hypophysectomized mice demonstrating no statistical difference in thymocyte subsets between the hormone-deficient mice and their normal littermates [6]. Neither GH nor IGF-1 is required for primary lymphopoiesis. However, possible aging-related changes in thymic cell subpopulations and functions in Tg rats need to be analyzed in future studies.

3.2   Splenic Lymphocyte Subpopulation and Mitogenic Response

The weights of the spleen did not differ between the rat groups when normalized for body weight (Table 4); the normalized weight was reduced by 4–9% by CR. The proportion of T-cells (CD3+/CD45R–) did not differ among rat groups, while it was slightly increased by CR, particularly in (–/–) rats. The B cell population (CD3–/CD45R+) was lower in (tg/tg) rats; CR significantly decreased the B cell population. Subsequently, the T/B cell ratio did not differ among rat groups, although it was increased in the CR group, particularly in (–/–) and (tg/tg) rats. The NK cell

Table 3 Subpopulation of thymocytes in the transgenic and calorie-restricted rats at 6 months of age

	(–/–)		(tg/–)		(tg/tg)		
	AL	CR	AL	CR	AL	CR	2-f ANOVA
Thymus	40.4 (4.4)	47.0 (4.8)	51.5 (6.6)	39.0 (6.6)	43.0 (3.2)	33.3 (1.4)	
DN	2.8 (0.4)	3.0 (0.6)	3.2 (0.7)	6.1 (0.6)*/#	4.5 (1.1)	4.4 (0.6)	Genotype effect, $p = 0.0508$
DP	73.6 (1.5)	75.7 (2.4)	76.4 (2.0)	72.9 (2.4)	76.5 (3.8)	75.2 (1.0)	
SP4	20.3 (3.0)	18.1 (1.4)	17.7 (1.5)	18.0 (2.0)	16.2 (2.4)	17.4 (1.3)	
SP8	3.3 (0.3)	3.2 (0.5)	2.7 (0.3)	3.0 (0.3)	2.8 (0.5)	3.1 (2.3)	

Values represent the means (standard error) of 5 or 6 rats. Thymus (mg/100g body weight); DN, DP, SP4, SP8 (% of total thymocytes). (–/–); wild type rats. (tg/–); transgenic hemizygotic rats. (tg/tg); transgenic homozygotic rats. AL; ad libitum feeding rats. CR; 30% calorie-restricted rats. * $p < 0.05$ versus (vs) the AL group in each genotype. # $p < 0.05$ vs (–/–) in each diet group.

(CD3–/NKR+) population and activity were decreased in (tg/tg)-AL rats compared with (–/–)-AL rats. The proportion of NK cell but not the activity of NK cells was increased in the CR group.

The naive T-cell (CD4+, OX22+) population was greatest in the following order; (tg/tg), (tg/–), and (–/–) rats. Memory T-cell (CD4+, OX22–) population was slightly reduced in (tg/tg) rats. CR also increased the proportion of naive T-cells, particularly in the (–/–) rats.

The mitogenic response of splenic cells, examined by the response to phytohemagglutinin (PHA), concanavalin (CON) A, and anti-CD3 antibodies did not differ significantly among groups (Table 5); responses to PHA and ConA tended to increase in CR groups.

Thus, it can be summarized as follows: 1) that reduction of GH does not affect the T and B lymphocyte populations except NK cells, 2) severe suppression of GH decreases the cell number and activity of NK cells, 3) CR increases the T-cell fraction and decreases B cells in splenic cells, 4) CR restores the NK cell function that was reduced by severe suppression of GH, 5) reduction of GH does not affect the proliferative response of splenic lymphocytes to stimulants, while CR tends to enhance this response.

Although our analysis is limited to 6-month-old rats, our results suggest that CR and suppression of GH affect the development of secondary lymphoid organs. The aged immune system is characterized by a decrease in T-cell function caused by an increase in the fraction of memory T-cells that are less capable of responding to mitogens or novel antigen stimulation [17, 18]; in contrast, the number or proportion of naive T-cells declines. Thus, we can speculate that the increased proportion of naive T-cells in the CR group and (tg/–)-AL rats is attributable in part to the prolonged lifespan. The restored NK cell activity and/or increased T-cell fraction by CR in (tg/tg) rats might also contribute to the extended lifespan in short-lived (tg/tg) rats, because these innate immune functions have important roles for the prevention of cancers [19].

Our analysis suggests that CR and moderate GH suppression exert similar beneficial effects on immune function, while severe suppression of GH may produce some adverse effects.

Table 4 Subpopulations of splenic lymphocytes

	(-/-) AL	(-/-) CR	(tg/-) AL	(tg/-) CR	(tg/tg) AL	(tg/tg) CR	2-f ANOVA
Spleen (g)/ 100 g Body weight	0.19 (0.04)	0.19 (0.02)	0.20 (0.01)	0.18 (0.01)	0.19 (0.01)	0.17 (0.01)	CR effect, p = 0.0477
CD3+ (%)	40.5 (4.2)	49.2 (1.7)*	44.3 (2.2)	42.2 (1.8)#	40.8 (1.7)	45.7 (1.6)	CR effect, p = 0.0449
CD45R+ (%)	45.1 (4.0)	34.7 (2.9)*	42.7 (2.1)	39.1 (3.1)	39.2 (1.4)	29.7 (1.2)*	GH effect, p = 0.0341 CR effect, p = 0.0007
T/B cell ratio	0.97 (0.22)	1.50 (0.18)*	1.06 (0.10)	1.13 (0.12)	1.06 (0.08)	1.55 (0.08)*	CR effect, p = 0.0024
Naïve T (%)	13.5 (1.1)	18.2 (1.0)*	18.0 (0.6)#	21.0 (1.1)	21.1 (1.4)#	23.9 (2.4)#	GH effect, p = 0.0003 CR effect, p = 0.0049
Memory T (%)	15.9 (0.4)	15.4 (0.7)	15.9 (1.0)	13.8 (0.4)*	12.9 (0.9)#	12.2 (0.5)#	GH effect, p = 0.0003 CR effect, p = 0.0573
N/M ratio	0.85 (0.08)	1.20 (0.09)	1.15 (0.08)	1.52 (0.06)*	1.68 (0.15)#	1.99 (0.22)#	GH effect, p < 0.0001 CR effect, p = 0.0031
NKR+/CD3- (%)	7.5 (0.7)	7.8 (0.6)	7.0 (0.5)	9.7 (0.8)*	5.8 (0.2)	9.9 (1.0)*/#	CR effect, p = 0.0002 GH x CR interaction, p = 0.0285
NK cell activity (%)	37.7 (3.6)	36.2 (3.0)	34.8 (3.3)	35.9 (3.9)	27.1 (1.0)#	35.3 (3.9)	

Values represent the means (standard error) of 5 or 6 rats. (-/-); wild type rats. (tg/-); transgenic hemizygotic rats. (tg/tg); transgenic homozygotic rats. AL; ad libitum feeding rats. CR; 30% calorie-restricted rats. * $p < 0.05$ versus (vs) group AL in each rat group. #, $p < 0.05$ vs (-/-) group AL in corresponding diet group.

Table 5 Proliferative response of splenic cells

	(–/–)		(tg/–)		(tg/tg)		
	AL	CR	AL	CR	AL	CR	2-f ANOVA
PHA	2.69 (0.81)	4.87 (1.62)	4.57 (0.99)	6.11 (1.41)	2.96 (0.71)	6.43 (1.97)	CR effect, p = 0.0285
ConA	7.12 (0.4)	8.88 (1.49)	7.01 (0.78)	9.58 (1.15)	6.97 (0.69)	11.02 (2.68)	CR effect, p = 0.0276
aCD3	4.63 (0.62)	4.41 (0.72)	5.34 (0.95)	6.21 (0.95)	4.16 (0.66)	6.27 (1.51)	
LPS	5.09 (0.45)	5.12 (0.42)	3.88 (0.53)	6.01 (0.83)*	4.40 (0.34)	5.13 (1.26)	

Values represent the means (standard error) of 5 or 6 rats. Proliferative response (stimulation index) of splenic cells to PHA, ConA, antibody to CD3 (aCD3), and lipopolysaccharide (LPS) was evaluated as previously reported {Utsuyama, 1997 #103}. (–/–); wild type rats. (tg/–); transgenic hemizygotic rats. (tg/tg); transgenic homozygotic rats. AL; ad libitum feeding rats. CR; 30% calorie-restricted rats. * $p < 0.05$ versus (vs) the AL group in each genotype.

4 Response to LPS-induced Inflammatory Challenge

CR protects laboratory rodents against a variety of stressors including inflammatory and toxic agents [20]. Many stressors damage cellular components through an increase in reactive oxygen and nitrogen species, i.e., oxidative stress, which are thought to cause or accelerate aging and diseases. Thus, resistance to stressors could be one of the essential mechanisms underlying the retardation of aging and prolonging the lifespan of organisms. Indeed, embryonic or skin fibroblasts prepared from long-lived mouse models have been shown to resist oxidative stress induced by UV light, hydrogen peroxide, paraquat, or heavy metals [21]. Some of the mice models also exhibit higher survival rates after paraquat administration [22, 23].

We analyzed the acute phase response of 6-month-old Tg and CR rats to lipopolysaccharide (LPS), a component of Gram-negative bacteria that elicits inflammatory processes. LPS initiates a cascade of cytokine mediators, i.e., successive waves of increments of the plasma concentrations of tumor necrosis factor (TNF)-α, interleukin (IL)-1, and IL-6 [24]. The initial step of activation of cytokines subsequently augments secretion and synthesis of interferon (IFN)-γ, an incremental increase in nitric oxide (NO) by induction of iNOS and platelet-activating factor in the plasma, and increased synthesis of acute phase reactants. In the activation cascade, monocytes and macrophages are functionally enhanced to eliminate invading bacteria; however, these processes also result in endothelial cell injuries, which, in turn triggers the coagulation process, and finally lead to hypoperfusion and ischemic injuries in peripheral tissues.

The procedure of LPS-induced inflammatory challenge was described in more detail elsewhere [25]. Briefly, a low dose of LPS (1.6 mg/kg body weight) administered intraperitoneally significantly increased the blood AST (aspartate aminotransferase) level, an indicator of tissue injury, at 4 and 8 h in control

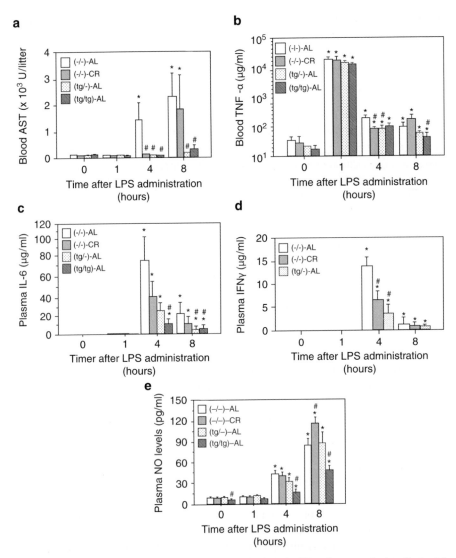

Fig. 3 (a-e) Response to LPS-induced inflammatory stress in CR and transgenic dwarf rats at 6 months of age. Values represent means + SE of 3–8 rats. * p < 0.05 versus 0 h in each rat group; # p < 0.05 versus (–/–)-AL rats at each time point. Blood or plasma samples were prepared for the following enzyme, cytokines, and nitric oxide assays (refer to Tsuchiya T et al [23] for further details) a) Blood levels of aspartate aminotransferase (AST), an index of tissue injuries after LPS administration. b) Tumor necrosis factor (TNF)-α, c) Interleukin (IL)-6, d) Interferon (IFN)-γ e) Nitric oxide (NO)

(–/–)-AL rats (Fig 3a). CR delayed the incremental increase in blood AST. In (tg/–)-AL and (tg/tg) rats, there was no significant increase. These findings indicate that either moderate or severe suppression of GH diminishes tissue injuries due to LPS challenge. This effect seems to be stronger than that of CR. Since the degree of suppression of the GH-IGF-1 axis, indicated by the plasma concentration of IGF-1, was greater in (tg/–)-AL rats than in (–/–)-CR rats, the levels of AST correlated with the GH-IGF-1 levels.

The blood TNF-α did not differ between (–/–)-AL and (–/–)-CR rats at 1 h (Fig 3b); however, the TNF-α level at 1 h was low in (tg/–)-AL and (tg/tg)-AL rats. IL-6 was significantly increased at 4 h and reduced at 8 h (Fig 3c). This level was lower in the following order; (tg/tg)-AL, (tg/–)-AL, (–/–)-CR, and (–/–)-AL rats. The peak values of plasma INF-γ at 4 h was lower in the following order; (tg/–)-AL, (–/–)-CR, and (–/–)-AL rats (data for (tg/tg)-AL rats are not available), the finding was comparable to those of AST and IL-6. The level of NO was gradually increased between 0 and 8 h (Fig 3d). The level at 8 h was highest in (–/–)-CR rats and similar between (–/–)-AL and (tg/–)-AL rats, although the level was lowest in (tg/tg)-AL rats. These findings suggest that the suppression of GH attenuates the LPS-induced cytokine activating cascade and minimizes tissue injuries, and that CR also diminishes tissue injuries probably, in part, through the same mechanism, because CR modestly suppressed the GH-IGF-1 axis. The difference in severity of tissue injuries between the rat groups seemed to correlate with the degree of suppression of GH-IGF-1 axis. CR, however, could affect the LPS-initiated inflammatory cascade and related tissue injuries differently, because the NO level at 8 h was significantly higher in (–/–)-CR rats than in (–/–)-AL and (tg/–)-AL rats.

Previous studies indicate that GH primes phagocytes for an increased production of reactive oxygen intermediates [26, 27]. GH potentiates the biological activities of entotoxin, i.e., lethality, in the rat [28]. However, IGF-1 did not induce this effect, indicating that the enhancement of endotoxin effects by GH is via an IGF-1-independent pathway [29]. Priming rats by GH induced a further increased response to serum IFN-γ but not TNF-α to subsequent entotoxin challenge, suggesting that INF-γ rather than TNF-α is likely to be involved in this process [29]. In other words, the suppression of GH diminishes the propagation of the inflammatory cascade downstream of TNF-α and minimizes tissue injuries. In this context, we can conclude that lower levels of GH favors longevity in animals via minimization of activation of monocytes and macrophages that are provoked by inflammation at the molecular levels during the aging process.

The diminution of inflammatory cascade could sometimes be harmful in organisms particularly regarding the elimination of invading bacteria. GH-treated animals release more superoxide and TNF-α in response to the appropriate trigger stimuli and ingest Listeria monocytogenes better than macrophages from untreated animals [30, 31]. GH has also been shown to protect hypopituitary animals from lethal Salmonella typhimurium infections [31]. In nature, infectious challenges by microorganisms are frequent and, thus, enhanced innate immunity could be beneficial to increase survival, even if the enhanced immunity also damages host tissues and cells. Therefore, there could be optimal levels of the strength of innate immunity in animals to protect infectious agents but minimize host–tissue damage, depending on their living conditions.

5 Conclusion

If the GH levels in commercially available rats are set as control values, moderate suppression of GH favors longevity and exhibits few demerits in the immune system. Severe suppression of GH may have some adverse effects on innate immunity, e.g., the diminished NK cell activity and the attenuated cytokine activation cascade that may decrease survival probability under usual living conditions where animals are often exposed to a variety of infection agents. In other words, there could be optimal levels for GH to maximize survival of organisms, depending on living conditions. Under SPF conditions in the laboratory, the demerits of severe suppression of GH are masked and only the merit, minimization of host-tissue injuries caused by the self-defense system, is emphasized.

Tg and CR rats exhibited similar trends regarding the selected immune functions, suggesting that the GH signaling could mediate the effect of CR in part. In this sense, the Tg rat is an intriguing animal model to better understand the roles of the GH axis in the aging process and the anti-aging effect of CR. Because our analysis on the immune system in Tg rats is limited, future studies are required to further understand the role of immunosenescene in the aging process and the anti-aging effect of CR.

References

1. Chung HY, Sung B, Jung KJ, et al (2006) The molecular inflammatory process in aging. Antioxid Redox Signal 8:572–581
2. Masoro E J (2005) Overview of caloric restriction and ageing. Mech Ageing Dev 126:913–922
3. Mccay CM, Crowell MF, Maynard LA (1989) The effect of retarded growth upon the length of life span and upon the ultimate body size, (1935). Nutrition 5:155–171; discussion 172
4. Masoro EJ, Mccarter R J, Katz M S, et al (1992) Dietary restriction alters characteristics of glucose fuel use. J Gerontol 47:B202–B208
5. Breese CR, Ingram RL, Sonntag W E (1991) Influence of age and long-term dietary restriction on plasma insulin-like growth factor-1 (IGF-1), IGF-1 gene expression, and IGF-1 binding proteins. J Gerontol 46:B180–B187
6. Dorshkind K, Horseman ND (2000) The roles of prolactin, growth hormone, insulin-like growth factor-I, and thyroid hormones in lymphocyte development and function: insights from genetic models of hormone and hormone receptor deficiency. Endocr Rev 21:292–312
7. Shimokawa I, Higami Y, Utsuyama M, et al (2002) Life span extension by reduction in growth hormone-insulin-like growth factor-1 axis in a transgenic rat model. Am J Pathol 160:2259–2265
8. Shimokawa I, Higami Y, Tsuchiya T, et al (2003) Life span extension by reduction of the growth hormone-insulin-like growth factor-1 axis: relation to caloric restriction. Faseb J 17:1108–1109
9. Yamaza H, Komatsu T, Chiba T, et al (2004) A transgenic dwarf rat model as a tool for the study of calorie restriction and aging. Exp Gerontol 39:269–272
10. Yamaza H, Komatsu T, To K, et al (2007) Involvement of insulin-like growth factor-1 in the effect of caloric restriction: regulation of plasma adiponectin and leptin. J Gerontol A Biol Sci Med Sci 62:27–33

11. Matsumoto K, Kakidani H, Takahashi A, et al (1993) Growth retardation in rats whose growth hormone gene expression was suppressed by antisense RNA transgene. Mol Reprod Dev 36:53–58

12. Shimokawa I (2006) A transgenic mini rat strain as a tool for studying aging and calorie restriction, in handbook of models for human aging, P.M. Conn (ed), Elsevier Academic Press: Burlington, MA p 367–378

13. Tanaka S, Tamaya N, Matsuzawa K, et al (2000) Differences in survivability among F344 rats. Exp Anim 49:141–145

14. Ward J M, Reynolds C W (1983) Large granular lymphocyte leukemia. A heterogeneous lymphocytic leukemia in F344 rats. Am J Pathol 111:1–10

15. Brown-Borg H M, Borg K E, Meliska C J, et al (1996) Dwarf mice and the ageing process. Nature 384:33

16. Coschigano K T, Clemmons D, Bellush LL, et al (2000) Assessment of growth parameters and life span of GHR/BP gene-disrupted mice. Endocrinology 141:2608–2613

17. Aw D, Silva AB, Palmer DB (2007) Immunosenescence: emerging challenges for an ageing population. Immunology 120:435–446

18. Chen J, Astle CM, Harrison DE (1998) Delayed immune aging in diet-restricted B6CBAT6 F1 mice is associated with preservation of naive T-cells. J Gerontol A Biol Sci Med Sci 53: B330–B337; discussion B338–B339

19. Wallace ME, Smyth MJ (2005) The role of natural killer cells in tumor control—effectors and regulators of adaptive immunity. Springer Semin Immunopathol 27:49–64

20. Masoro E J (1998) Hormesis and the antiaging action of dietary restriction. Exp Gerontol 33:61–66

21. Murakami S (2006) Stress resistance in long-lived mouse models. Exp Gerontol

22. Migliaccio E, Giorgio M, Mele S, et al (1999) The p66shc adaptor protein controls oxidative stress response and life span in mammals. Nature 402:309–313

23. Holzenberger M, Dupont J, Ducos B, et al (2003) IGF-1 receptor regulates lifespan and resistance to oxidative stress in mice. Nature 421:182–187

24. Van Amersfoort ES, Van Berkel TJ, Kuiper J (2003) Receptors, mediators, and mechanisms involved in bacterial sepsis and septic shock. Clin Microbiol Rev 16:379–414

25. Tsuchiya T, Higami Y, Komatsu T, et al (2005) Acute stress response in calorie-restricted rats to lipopolysaccharide-induced inflammation. Mech Ageing Dev 126:568–579

26. Warwick-Davies J, Lowrie DB, Cole PJ (1995) Growth hormone is a human macrophage activating factor. Priming of human monocytes for enhanced release of H2O2. J Immunol 154:1909–918

27. Fu YK, Arkins S, Wang BS, et al (1991) A novel role of growth hormone and insulin-like growth factor-I. Priming neutrophils for superoxide anion secretion. J Immunol 146:1602–1608

28. Liao W, Rudling M, Angelin B (1996) Growth hormone potentiates the in vivo biological activities of endotoxin in the rat. Eur J Clin Invest 26:254–258

29. Liao W, Rudling M, Angelin B (1997) Contrasting effects of growth hormone and insulin-like growth factor I on the biological activities of endotoxin in the rat. Endocrinology 138:289–295

30. Edwards CK 3rd, Ghiasuddin SM, Schepper JM, et al (1988) A newly defined property of somatotropin: priming of macrophages for production of superoxide anion. Science 239:769–771

31. Edwards CK 3rd, Ghiasuddin SM, Yunger LM, et al (1992) In vivo administration of recombinant growth hormone or gamma interferon activities macrophages: enhanced resistance to experimental Salmonella typhimurium infection is correlated with generation of reactive oxygen intermediates. Infect Immun 60:2514–2521

32. Flurkey K, Papaconstantinou J, Miller RA, et al (2001) Lifespan extension and delayed immune and collagen aging in mutant mice with defects in growth hormone production. Proc Natl Acad Sci U S A 98:6736–6741

33. Bluher M, Kahn BB, Kahn C R (2003) Extended longevity in mice lacking the insulin receptor in adipose tissue. Science 299:572–574

34. Mitsui A, Hamuro J, Nakamura H, et al (2002) Overexpression of human thioredoxin in transgenic mice controls oxidative stress and life span. Antioxid Redox Signal 4:693–696
35. Schriner SE, Linford NJ, Martin GM, et al (2005) Extension of murine life span by overexpression of catalase targeted to mitochondria. Science 308:1909–1911
36. Miskin R, Masos T (1997) Transgenic mice overexpressing urokinase-type plasminogen activator in the brain exhibit reduced food consumption, body weight and size, and increased longevity. J Gerontol A Biol Sci Med Sci 52:B118–B124
37. Michalkiewicz M, Knestaut KM, Bytchkova EY, et al (2003) Hypotension and reduced catecholamines in neuropeptide Y transgenic rats. Hypertension 41:1056–1062
38. Chiu CH, Lin WD, Huang SY, et al (2004) Effect of a C/EBP gene replacement on mitochondrial biogenesis in fat cells. Genes Dev 18:1970–1975
39. Kurosu H, Yamamoto M, Clark JD, et al (2005) Suppression of aging in mice by the hormone Klotho. Science 309:1829–1833
40. Taguchi A, Wartschow LM, White MF (2007) Brain IRS2 signaling coordinates life span and nutrient homeostasis. Science 317:369–372
41. Dell'agnello C, Leo S, Agostino A, et al (2007) Increased longevity and refractoriness to Ca(2+)-dependent neurodegeneration in Surf1 knockout mice. Hum Mol Genet 16:431–44
42. Shimokawa I, Yu BP, Masoro EJ (1991) Influence of diet on fatal neoplastic disease in male Fischer 344 rats. J Gerontol Biol Sci 46:B228–B232

Mathematical Modeling of Immunosenescence: Scenarios, Processes and Limitations

A.A. Romanyukha, S.G. Rudnev, T.A. Sannikova and A.I. Yashin

Contents

Abstract: Mathematical modeling of immunosenescence is the new area of research emerging at the interface of the immunology, gerontology, and mathematics. In this paper we outline basic variables important for modeling aging immunity. We discuss the role of evolution in shaping pattern of aging in the immune system of modern humans. We investigate mathematical models of postnatal changes in the population of peripheral T-cells, effects of the antigenic load during development on the body growth, and contribution of immunosenescence to the old age increase in the risk of death from respiratory infections.

Keywords: Antigenic load • aging immunity • mortality from infections • body growth • population of T-cells

1 Introduction

There are two types of mathematical models applied to the life science problems. The objectives and methodology used in these models differ substantially. The first type of models deals with the problems of analysis and interpretation of the results

A.A. Romanyukha (✉) · S.G. Rudnev · T.A. Sannikova
Institute of Numerical Mathematics
Russian Academy of Sciences, Moscow, Russia

A.I. Yashin
Center for Population Health and Aging
Duke University, Durham, USA

T. Fulop et al. (eds.), *Handbook on Immunosenescence,*
DOI 10.1007/ 978-1-4020-9062-2_8, © Springer Science+Business Media B.V. 2009

of a certain experimental study, or a series of such studies. The main objective of such modeling is the quantification of sensitivity of the phenomenon to changes in various factors. The results of modeling contribute to better understanding the roles of factors and mechanisms in the processes under study. The focus of the second type of models is systematization of knowledge and data in order to develop systemic view, obtain integral description of the results of heterogeneous experimental studies, and check consistency of such description with existing theories. The models of the second type deal with the description of the phenomenon: they assimilate results of different experiments, test their mutual compatibility, and correspondence to existing theories. Such models are an effective means of testing accumulated knowledge and can be used to predict effects of exposure to external factors on functioning of living systems, or changes in characteristics of the organism itself.

2 Modeling Immunosenescence

In this study we will investigate properties of the first type models of aging immunity. Such modeling is a relatively new area of research, emerging at the interface of immunology, gerontology, and mathematics. It studies regularities of aging related decline in functioning of the components of the immune system, as well as dynamic interaction among them during the aging process. To describe such nonlinear multi-dimensional aging related changes in the immune defense mechanism the dynamic mathematical and computer modeling of these phenomena is needed. An important step in such modeling is the selection of variables or "units" of the immunosenescence. These units suppose to reflect the basic features and processes of aging immunity. These variables include:

- The characteristics of the lymphocytes' aging (telomere length, the ability to respond to the antigenic and cytokine signals, intercellular cooperation;
- Population-wide characteristics of lymphocytes and other immune system cells (proportion of naïve and memory cells, the proportion of the various lymphocyte subpopulations, antigenic repertoire of lymphocytes);
- The characteristics of activity of the immune system (rate of lymphocyte formation in thymus and the bone marrow, the amount of active parenchyma in the lymphoid organs, the rate of lymphoid proliferation processes);
- The characteristics of the state of the organism (frequency and severity of infectious disease, activity of inflammatory process, probability of death and/or decrease of reproduction due to the deficiency of immune protection).

2.1 The Immune Life Histories

Thus, the units of immunosenescence should relate lymphocytes' characteristics to the processes developing in the aging body. These include infection, inflammation, tissue and organ aging, fertility and life span. These variables should relate the dynamics of lymphocyte populations and characteristics of individual fitness. The age trajectories of these interrelated variables comprise the immune life history (McDade 2003). We will consider age-related changes in the: naïve cells concentration; memory cells concentration; replicative potential of lymphocyte subpopulations; antigen repertoire of lymphocytes; rate of the influx of immune cells from the thymus and bone marrow; incidence of infectious and, maybe, cardiovascular diseases; individual inflammatory status; antigenic load. All values, except the latter are characteristics of the immune system. The antigenic load is a measure of pressure of external and internal conditions at the immune system.

2.1.1 Antigenic Load

We define the antigenic load as the rate of the inflow of the alien, or modified antigens into the lymphoid tissue. The activity of the immune system and its rate of aging depend significantly on the level of antigenic load, because it affects the rate of division of the lymphocytes and their mortality risk. The antigenic load consists of the two components: alien antigens and modified self-antigens. Alien antigens may arrive from the external environment and reproducing in the host. They may also be located in the host and reproducing in certain circumstances.

The rate of inflow of infectious and noninfectious antigens from the environment must be proportional to the consumption of nutrients and the oxygen. Because such consumption is directly connected to the metabolic rate, it is reasonable to hypothesize that the level of external antigenic load is proportional to the metabolic rate.

A large proportion of modified self-antigens are formed due to action of free radicals; the rate of their formation is proportional to the metabolic rate as well. So we will assume that the rate of generation of self-antigens is proportional to the metabolic rate. Therefore, the total antigenic load largely depends on the intensity of metabolism.

The level of infectious component of the antigenic load is strongly influenced by the two factors, weakly dependent on the metabolic rate: the density of infectious microorganisms in the environment and the effectiveness of the immunity. Obviously, the high density of microorganisms in the environment increases the frequency of infections and, hence, the antigenic load also increases. On the other hand, in the presence of many memory cells, the infectious antigenic load will loosely depend on the microbial density or metabolic rate.

2.1.2 Antigenic Load and Immunosenescence

The intensity of metabolism declines with age. The effectiveness of the immune protection also varies with age: the frequency of infectious diseases is highest in the childhood, lowest in the intermediate age and increases in the old ages. Specific characteristics of the antigenic load affect the development of the immune system, its aging rate, and, hence, individual fitness. Consequently, many properties of the aging immunity, observed in modern humans, are formed by evolution during many thousands of years in the past. The principal objectives of the immune system are to ensure survival to reproductive age and provide maximum protection against infections during the reproductive period.

148

A.A. Romanyukha et al.

Fig. 1 Hypothetical
scheme of life-long antigenic
load dynamics for primitive
(—), and contemporary man
(— —), AL—antigenic load
(in arbitrary units)

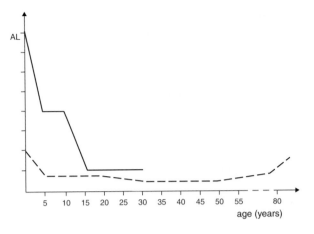

age (years)

An important mechanism for ensuring effective protection involves adaptive immunity based on production of the immune memory cells. The more memory cell is formed after the primary immune response, and the longer they live; the more protected is the body from secondary infections of this type. Since the resources of the immune system are limited, there is a competition between the naïve cells and memory cells. The memory cells provide effective protection from a few known pathogens in current and future situations. The naïve cells are supposed to provide future protection from all possible pathogens. If the life expectancy is large and emergence of the new diseases is a likely scenario, it is beneficial to maintain more naïve cells and have active thymus, with less effective protection against endemic pathogens. In case of short life and low rate of emergence of the new diseases it is more profitable for an organism to produce less naïve lymphocytes and make higher investment to the memory cells. Thus, the fundamental property of the immunosenescence is its evolutionary coadaptation with antigenic load and other life history characteristics of the aging human organisms.

Figure 1 shows a hypothetical dynamics of antigenic load during life of primitive and modern man. It is important to understand how the immune system, evolutionary adjusted to the living conditions of primitive man, adapts to current environmental and living conditions. The main difference between the curves 1 and 2 involves significant reduction of the infectious burden, especially at the beginning of life and an increase of life expectancy in modern humans[1].

2.2 Scenarios of Immunosenescence

The differences in the current and prehistoric antigenic loads affect process of immunosenescence. The age related changes in the immune system of a primitive human were formed by high infectious load in the first years of life, where the immunity learning period is included in the child's growth interval. Short life and the relative isolation

---

[1] When creating the Fig. 1 we have assumed that the antigenic load of the modern humans is approximately equal to load by their self-modified antigens, and the antigenic load of the primitive humans was about an order of magnitude larger than of the modern ones.

from the new pathogens defined the replacement rate of the naïve cells by the memory cells, the rate of reduction of the naive lymphocytes production, the rate of reduction of replicative capacity of the memory cells with age. An exposure to the antigens during the growth period ensured training of the immunity for survivors, efficient use of the body resources and protection against antigens during the reproductive period.

Note that the high infant mortality rate observed in the past may indicate substantial variability in the antigenic load among survivors. Such scenario of developing immunity can be called **forced immunomaturation**. The essence of this scenario is the accelerated maturation and learning of the immune system. Reducing the antigenic load at this scenario improves the immunity condition in middle age. In modern conditions external antigenic load has much less impact on the aging immunity. The age decline of immunity is determined by the changes in the stem cell properties, lack of naive cells, a narrow repertoire of the memory cells, and reduced replicative ability of the memory cells. Thus, in modern conditions immunosenescence is largely defined by traits selected during the evolution of immunity (early decline of naive cell production, reduction of their replicative ability, etc.) as well as by traits depending on general properties of aging body (the aging of stem cell pool, increase of the self-modified antigen generation rate, etc.). Such scenario of age related changes in immunity can be called **inertial immunosenescence.** An important feature of this aging scenario is that the decline in the antigenic load, or slowing down of thymus involution has little impact on immunity in the older ages.

In this case in order to improve the immune function a combined influence on the immune system such as the rejuvenation of stem cells, thymus function enhancement, accelerated elimination of the old memory and naive cells, and accelerated immunity learning through vaccination is required. This procedure will be accompanied by a temporary decrease in the immune protection. Therefore, this process can not be conducted on the background of a strong decline in immunity, the optimal age is the border between medium and older age.In fact this is a repetition of immunity development and learning period in its reduced form. It can be assumed that in some individuals such events can occur as a result of natural events (starvation, severe stress, etc.).Hypothetical version of immune life history with such periodic recovering of the immune system can be called the **reciprocating immunorejuvenation** scenario.

2.3 Constraints of Adaptation

The adaptation responses develop in the presence of explicit or implicit limitations on the rate and the magnitude of physiological processes involved in such adaptations. For example, the total number of immune system cells should not change significantly during the adulthood. This restriction results in diminishing the memory cell life time, when the production rate of the naive cells by the thymus increases. An example of implicit limitation of the immune system adaptation is the need to coordinate the growth of the body size, growth of the immune system mass, and the rate of the immunity learning. If the new antigens presentation will delay an increase in the body mass the homeostatic proliferation of lymphocytes may lead to undesirable distortions in the immune cells' repertoire.

Mathematical modeling is a convenient method for studying such problems. Below we will consider examples of the use of mathematical models to study aging related changes in the immune system. They include postnatal changes in the population of peripheral T-cells, effects of the antigenic load during development on the body growth, and contribution of immunosenescence to the old age increase in the risk of death from respiratory infections.

First we investigate how the basic immunosenescence processes such as thymus decay, shortening of telomeres in the newly forming naive T-lymphocytes and shrinking of the peripheral lymphoid tissues interact depending on the antigenic load.

For description of these processes, we propose a mathematical model (1). It describes the balance of influx and usage of T-cells and their replicative potential. The model equations are based on two main assumptions:

- the T-lymphocyte concentration in the peripheral lymphoid tissue must be maintained constant;
- the naive cells are superior to the memory cells in the competition for free space in the lymphoid tissue.

Based on these assumptions, we construct a model describing the age dynamics of the following variables:

$N^*(t)$, rate of naive T-cells influx in IPLT at the age t (cell/day);
$V(t)$, volume of IPLT at the age t, (ml);
$P^*(t)$, length of telomere repeats in naive T-cells produced at the age t, (bp/cell);
$N(t)$, concentration of nai've T-cells in IPLT at the age t, (cell/ml);
$M(t)$, concentration of memory T-cells in IPLT at the age of t (cell/ml);
$PN(t)$, average length of telomere repeats in naive T-cell at the age t (bp/cell);
$PM(t)$, average length of telomere repeats in memory T-cell at thew age t (bp/cell);
Function $L(t)$ describes total antigenic load at the age t (g/day).

The mathematical model of age-related changes in peripheral T-cell population is represented by the system of the following seven ordinary differential equations:

$$\frac{dN^*}{dt} = -k_T N^*,$$

$$\frac{dN}{dt} = \frac{N^*}{V} - \alpha_1 \frac{L}{V} N - \mu_N N - \frac{dV}{dt}\frac{N}{V},$$

$$\frac{dP_N}{dt} = (P^* - P_N)\frac{N^*}{NV},$$

$$\frac{dM}{dt} = \rho_1\alpha_1 \frac{L}{V} N + \rho_2\alpha_2 \frac{L}{V} M + \mu_M (C^* - N - M) - \frac{dV}{dt}\frac{M}{V},$$

$$\frac{dP_M}{dt} = \rho_1\alpha_1 \frac{L}{V}(P_N - \lambda_N - P_M)\frac{N}{M} - (\rho_2 + 1)\alpha_2\lambda_M \frac{L}{V}.$$

$$\frac{dV}{dt} = -k_V V,$$

$$\frac{dP^*}{dt} = -k_p P^* \tag{1}$$

For simplicity, we assume that the antigenic load remains constant throughout life, but the production rate of naive T-lymphocytes and the volume of peripheral lymphoid tissues decrease with constant relative rate. However, developed model is flexible enough to investigate more complicated scenarios.

Numerical experiments with this model revealed some interesting dependencies: the lengthy production of naive T-lymphocytes strengthens the immune protection in advanced ages, but relatively weakens immunity in middle age because it reduces maintenance resources and duration of immune memory. The calculations also showed that an important factor in ensuring the immune protection in advanced ages is slowing of the stem cell aging.

These results allowed for addressing the question on how the body growth processes affect the aging of immunity.

3 Modeling Postnatal Changes in the Population of Peripheral T-cells

The most apparent changes in the population of peripheral T-cells in humans occur in childhood (Rufer et al. 1999; Zeichner et al. 1999), when the relative rate of body growth and the infection morbidity are maximal. These changes are accompanied by the early onset of thymus atrophy—a primary lymphoid organ, in which the development of bone marrow-derived progenitors into mature T-cells takes place (Steinmann et al. 1985) (Fig. 2). Such atrophy substantially restricts the ability of adults to produce naive T-cells, which, in turn, affects the strength and efficiency of adaptive immune response. An expansion of intact peripheral lymphoid tissue (IPLT) at early age by memory cells affects the immune system learning capacity at later ages. Therefore, when studying the immune system aging, it is important to take the conditions and regularities of the development of this system early in life into account.

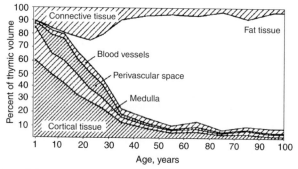

Fig. 2 Involution of thymus (Steinmann et al. 1985). After the age of 1, the volume of thymus remains relatively constant. The division of thymic precursor T-cells takes place primarily in cortical tissue

3.1   The Extended Model

We address these issues using the extended mathematical model of age-related changes in population of peripheral T-cells suggested by Romanyukha and Yashin (2003). The extended model adds one equation on age-related changes in body mass to the system of equations specified in (Romanyukha and Yashin 2003), and exploits the new fundamental assumption that the value of antigenic load is proportional to the intensity of basal metabolism. The resulting model allows for describing development of adaptive immunity during all postnatal life, including childhood. The dependence of basal metabolism on body mass is described using the Kleiber's 3/4 power scaling law (Kleiber 1932; West, Brown 2005).

Taking into account the above considerations, the mathematical model of age-related changes in population of peripheral T-cells can be written in the form:

$$\frac{dN^*}{dt} = -k_T N^*,$$

$$\frac{dN}{dt} = \frac{N^*}{V} - \alpha_1 \frac{L}{V} N - \mu_N N - \frac{dV}{dt}\frac{N}{V},$$

$$\frac{dM}{dt} = \rho_1 \alpha_1 \frac{L}{V} N + \rho_2 \alpha_2 \frac{L}{V} M + \mu_M (C^* - N - M) - \frac{dV}{dt}\frac{M}{V},$$

$$\frac{dP^*}{dt} = -\left(\frac{\bar{k}_P}{m}\frac{dm}{dt} + k_P\right) P^*,$$

$$\frac{dP_N}{dt} = (P^* - P_N)\frac{N^*}{NV},$$

$$\frac{dP_M}{dt} = \rho_1 \alpha_1 (P_N - P_M - \lambda_N)\frac{L}{V}\frac{N}{M} - (\rho_2 + 1)\alpha_2 \lambda_M \frac{L}{V},$$

$$\frac{dV}{dt} = \alpha_3 \frac{L}{V}\frac{dm}{dt} - k_V V,$$

$$\frac{dm}{dt} = \alpha_4 m^{3/4} - k_m m.$$

$$(2)$$

Here the variable t corresponds to individual's age; $N^*(t)$ is the rate of naive T-cells influx from thymus into IPLT; $N(t)$ is the concentration of naive T-cells in the IPLT; $M(t)$ is the concentration of the memory T-cells in the IPLT; $P^*(t)$ is the length of telomeres in naive T-cells leaving thymus at the age t; $P_N(t)$ is the length of telomeres in the naive T-cells; $P_M(t)$ is the length of telomeres in the memory T cells, $V(t)$ is the volume of the IPLT; $m(t)$ is the body mass. Rapid telomere shortening in the stem cells during the first years of life entails similar changes in telomeres' length of the newly produced naive T-cells in the thymus (Rufer et al. 1999). We assume that the corresponding rate is proportional to the relative increase in the body mass. So, the rate parameter in the equation for P^* can be written as a function of age: $k_P(t) = \bar{k}_P(dm/dt)/m + k_P$ where k_P is taken from the original model of Romanyukha and Yashin (2003). We assume also that the rate of the early IPLT expansion is proportional to specific anti-

Fig. 3 The sequence of the model parameters adjustment

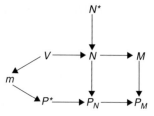

genic load (L/V) and the rate of body mass change. Initial conditions correspond to the age of birth:

$$N^*(0) = N_0^*, \quad N(0) = C^*, \quad M(0) = M_0^*, \quad P^*(0) = P_0^*,$$
$$P_N(0) = P_N^0, \quad P_M(0) = P_M^0, \quad V(0) = V_0, \quad m(0) = m_0. \tag{3}$$

The sequence of model parameters adjustment is shown in Fig. 3 Using this scheme, we constructed initial estimates of model parameters (Table 1).

Table 1 Initial parameters' estimates and initial conditions for simulation of age related changes in population of peripheral T-cells

Parameter	Physical meaning	Dimension	Value
α_1	Rate constant of naive T-cells stimulation	ml/g	1.5×10^4
α_2	Rate constant of memory T-cells stimulation	ml/g	1.5×10^4
α_3	Rate constant of the intact peripheral lymphoid tissue (IPLT) growth	ml²×day/g	3×10^7
α_4	Rate constant of body mass growth	$g^{1/4}$/day	2.5×10^{-2}
α_5	Parameter which relates antigen load and basal metabolic rate	$g^{1/4}$/day	2.8×10^{-10}
μ_N	Rate constant of natural death rate for naive T-cells	1/day	1.3×10^{-4}
μ_M	Rate constant of competitive death (or homeostatic proliferation) for memory T-cells	1/day	0.07
α_1	Number of memory T-cells produced by one naïve cell	—	100
α_2	Number of memory T-cells produced by one memory cell	—	1.1
λ_N	Length of telomere repeats lost during transformation of naïve T-cells to memory cell	base pairs (bp)	1400
λ_M	Length of telomere repeats lost during self-replication of memory cells	bp	500
C^*	Low limit for normal concentration of memory T-cells in intact lymphoid tissue	cell/ml	2.5×10^9
k_T	Rate of diminishing of naïve T-cells production with age	1/day	1.1×10^{-4}
k_V	Relative rate of reduction of the IPLT volume with age	1/day	2.7×10^{-5}
$\bar{k}_p$	Relative rate of the telomere repeats reduction in the progenitor of naïve cells	bp/day	1×10^{-5}
k_p	Relative rate of accelerated telomere shortening in the progenitor of naïve T-cells in early childhood	bp/day	0.07
k_m	Rate parameter in the equation for body mass	1/day	1.5×10^{-3}
N_0^*	Rate of naive T-cells release from thymus at birth	cell/day	8×10^8
N^0	Concentration of naïve T-cells in the IPLT at birth	cell/ml	2.5×10^9
M^0	Concentration of memory T-cells in the IPLT at birth	cell/ml	2.5×10^7
P_0^*	Average length of telomeres in naive T-cells leaving thymus at birth	bp	10370
P_N^0	Average length of telomeres in naive T-cells in the IPLT at birth	bp	10370
P_M^0	Average length of telomeres in memory T-cells at birth	bp	8970
V_0	Volume of intact lymphoid tissue at birth	ml	150
m_0	Body mass at birth	g	3500

3.2 Parameters' Estimation

The level of agreement between the model and data was characterized by the value of the least-squares function for the log-transformed data and model solutions.

$$F(\alpha) = \sum_{i,j} \left(\lg \left| \frac{x^i(t_j, \alpha)}{X_j^i} \right| \right)^2$$

Here, α is the vector of model parameters, $x^i(t_j, \alpha)$ is the value of the i th component of model solution at age t_j, and X_j^i is the corresponding data. The solution of the constrained minimization problem of the function $F(\alpha)$ obtained on a subset of model parameters is shown as dotted lines on Fig. 4. It was obtained using differential evolution (DE) algorithm (Storn, Price 1997). The refined parameters are shown in Table 2. One can see from Fig. 4 that the model satisfactorily describes the data on age-related changes in T-cell populations at the entire interval of aging except for the initial age interval.

During the first 6 months of life, the immune defense is provided mainly by maternal antibodies though it was shown recently that the mature T-cell immune response against viral and macroparasitic infections may occur even in the prenatal conditions (King et al. 2002; Marchant et al. 2003; Hazenberg et al. 2004). Along with an increase in the volume of thymus, the total number of peripheral T-cells and the volume of the IPLT grow rapidly. Between ages of 0.5 and 6 years the number of lymphocytes in the body remains relatively stable and then increases, approaching a maximum at the age of 20 years (Valentin 2002). At the initial age interval a rapid decline in the length of telomeres of the newly produced T-cells in the thymus takes place (Rufer et al. 1999). These data were not fit well by the model (Fig. 4). In order to investigate the dynamics of relative antigen load and also of naïve T-cells division, we considered a refined model using explicit log-linear functions for N^*, P^* and V at the corresponding initial age intervals.

Table 2 The results of sequential parameters' estimation for modeling age related changes in population of peripheral T-cells. Permissible boundaries for the model parameters are shown as XVmin and XVmax. The values of the residual function F are shown in the last row

Parameter	XVmin	XVmax	Initial estimate	Refined estimate		
				1	2	3
N^*_0	4×10^8	10^9	8×10^8	8.34×10^8		
k_T	8×10^{-5}	2×10^{-4}	1.1×10^{-4}	1.06×10^{-4}		
α_4	0.01	0.04	0.025		0.023	
k_p	5×10^{-5}	2×10^{-5}	10^{-5}		1.3×10^{-5}	
k_P	0.01	0.1	0.07		0.06	
α_3	10^7	5×10^7	3×10^7		2.8×10^7	
α_1	5×10^3	5×10^4	1.5×10^4			10^5
μ_N	10^{-4}	10^{-2}	1.3×10^{-4}			5×10^{-5}
ρ_1	10	1000	100			2000
ρ_2	1	100	1.1			324
μ_M	0.001	0.1	0.07			8.7
F			0.32	0.28	0.26	0.25

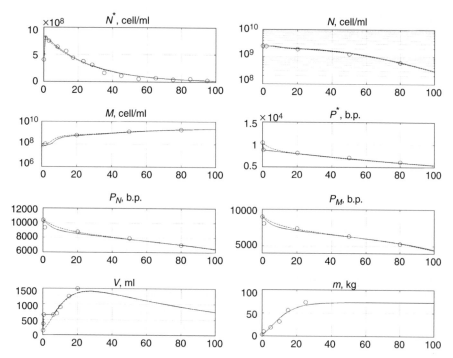

Fig. 4 Solution to the refined model system (solid lines). Dotted lines represent the solution to the initial model. Along the x-axis is age (years). The data are shown as open circles

The solution of the refined model is shown in Fig. 4 as solid lines. Because of the absence of parameters in the equation for P_N, it is interesting to see that the good agreement between P^* and the data turned out to be insufficient for the precise description of the telomeres' length in the naïve T-cells (P_N) early in life. One possible explanation involves the effect of the naive T-cells' *homeostatic proliferation* (Unutmaz et al. 1994). Such proliferation results in increased telomere shortening in the naive T-cells as compared with the rate induced by telomere shortage in the stem and/or precursor T-cells, and, hence, can be accounted for in the equation for P_N. One can see from the Fig. 4 that the rate of homeostatic proliferation of the naive T-cells is comparable with the rate of their production in thymus. Similar results were obtained in Hazenberg et al. (2000, 2004); Ye, Kirschner (2002); Dutilh, DeBoer (2003) when modeling data on the T-cell receptor excision circles (TREC) kinetics.

Figure 5 shows the dynamics of specific antigenic load L/V for the refined and initial models. The refined model is characterized by significantly smaller values of L/V at early ages. This can be interpreted as an initial "reserve" of the immune system owing to fast initial increase in the volume of the IPLT.

An important part of the antigenic load L is represented by the infection load, related to the impact of *multiplying* antigens. At present, it is difficult to obtain quantitative estimates of the relative contribution of the infection load to the total antigenic

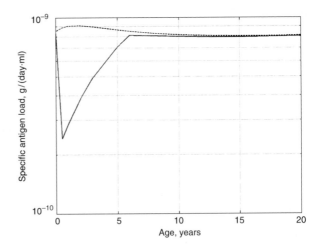

Fig. 5 Specific antigen load L/V as a function of age for refined (solid line) and initial models (dotted line)

load. However, the evidence is accumulating that this contribution can be significant. The results of simulation of the impact of the HIV infection on the rate of T-cell population aging suggest 2 to 8-fold increase in the fraction of divided naive T-cells, and, hence, of the total antigenic load (Hazenberg et al. 2000; Sannikova et al. 2004).

The magnitude of infectious pathogens growth in human body in case of acute infections vary from 10^5–10^6 for bacterial pneumonia (Romanyukha, Rudnev 2001) to 10^{10}–10^{11} for viral infections, such as influenza A, or hepatitis B (Marchuk et al. 1991; Bocharov, Romanyukha 1994).

We assume here that the total antigenic load L depends linearly from basal metabolic rate. The high rate of infection diseases in the childhood imply a significant excess of the value of L at this age compared to the value determined by the basal metabolic rate. One can assume that this "initial reserve" of the immune system is, in fact, "consumed" by the infection load. As a result, the specific antigenic load, L/V, can be significantly *higher* than the values suggested by the refined model (continuous line on Fig. 5). The comparison of graphs in Fig. 5 suggests that the initial reserve of the immune system early in life allows for 2–4-fold increase in the total antigenic load above the values permitted by the basal metabolic rate.

4 Immune System Development and Body Growth

The increasing body of evidence from animal and human studies supports the idea on the existence of trade-off between immune defense and organism's growth. For example, the data from gnotobiological studies show that the infection of germ-free chicken impairs body growth by 15–30% (Lochmiller, Deerenberg 2000). Primary immunodeficiencies in humans can also lead to growth impairment and even growth failure (Bjorkander et al. 1984). This holds true for the HIV infection, depending on the extent of the viral load (Arpadi et al. 2000) which, presumably, reflects a rising energy deficit caused by the gradual increase in the antigenic load.

The suggested model allows for evaluation of possible consequences of such a trade-off. For this, we assumed a linear dependence of the body growth from the antigenic load: $\alpha_4 = a - b\alpha_5$, where α_4 is the rate constant of the body growth, and α_5 is the parameter, which relates antigenic load and basal metabolic rate. The parameter a in this formula characterizes a maximal rate of body growth attained in the absence of antigenic load, and b describes the detrimental effect of antigenic load on the body growth.

For illustrative purposes, based on the results of modeling the effects of HIV infection on the rate of immune system aging (Hazenberg et al. 2004; Sannikova et al. 2004), we assumed that the arrest of the body growth takes place when the value of antigenic load is 10-fold greater than normal. From this assumption, the values of a and b were determined. The results of calculations suggest the presence of stabilizing effect of the body growth on the immune system development: the antigenic load up to 1.5 times higher than normal insignificantly affects the dynamics of model variables except for the rate of body mass change and the stationary level of the body mass in the adulthood (changes from 73 kg to 60 kg). Further increase in the antigenic load results in a more pronounced effect on the immune system development with the remarkable effect on the volume of the IPLT at the adult age. Counter-intuitively, both an increase and decrease in the antigenic load result in the detrimental effect on the "adult" values of the volume of the IPLT with mild unidirectional effect on the dynamics of the naïve and memory cells and in the opposite effect on the telomeres' lengths. A decrease in the antigenic load results in the increased level of the adult body mass with a maximum of 115 kg in the absence of the antigenic load (Fig. 6).

The results presented in Fig. 7 show an increasing effect of antigenic load on body mass with age.

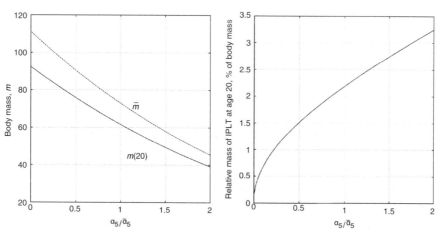

Fig. 6 The influence of antigenic load on body mass at age 20 (left panel), and on the relative mass of the IPLT (right panel)

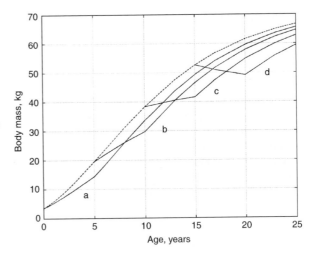

Fig. 7 The influence of 2-fold increase in antigen load at the age intervals (a) [0, 5 years], (b) [5, 10 years], (c) [10, 15 years] and (d) [15, 20 years] respectively, on the dynamics of body mass. The normal age-related changes of body mass are shown as dotted line

5 Model of Age-related Risk of Death from Respiratory Infections

Preliminary analysis revealed that mortality rates from pneumonia and other respiratory infections follow certain regularity pattern in different human populations (Sannikova 2007). The principal traits of the pattern are relatively high mortality level during infancy and early childhood, very low during the reproductive period, exponential (or faster) increase after age 50. Since such an increase takes place despite the presence of the modern health care systems we suppose that the aging of the T-cell immunity is responsible for the steep growth of pneumonia mortality curve at advanced ages.

We develop a mathematical model establishing the relationship between age-related changes in the peripheral T-cells population and mortality caused by respiratory infections (Fig. 8).

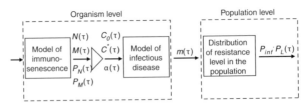

Fig. 8 The relationship between age-related changes in the peripheral T-cells population and increasing risk of death from infectious disease. The proliferative capacity of the T-cells decreases with age, which results in deceleration of lymphocyte proliferation during the immune response. So, the severity of the disease increases with increasing age. The higher the disease severity, the higher the risk of the lethal outcome

The model of age-related risk of death from respiratory infections consists of three component models: a model of age-related changes in peripheral T-cells population (1), a model of infectious disease (Marchuk 1997) and a relationship between disease severity and risk of death. Numerical solution of the system (1) yields the sets of immune characteristics (such as the concentration of naive and memory T-cells and their replicative capacity) for each age. These characteristics are used in the second model, the model of infectious disease, to determine the value of the lymphocyte concentration at the beginning of disease and the rate of immune response. This model makes it possible to simulate the course of unified infectious disease for each set of immune characteristics or, in other words, for each age. Disease severity is defined as a maximum of target tissue damage in the course of the disease.

The third model is a function of the distribution of the resistance to infections in the population. Infection resistance is defined as a probability of recovery at a certain value of target tissue damage (disease severity). As an output of the model we have risk assessment of lethal outcome in the course of the disease. To estimate the probability of death from certain diseases during a time interval (e.g., during 1 year) we multiply the risk of lethal outcome in the course of the disease by the probability of becoming infected during the age interval under consideration.

5.1   Relationship Between Disease Severity and the Risk of Death

We define the infection resistance *Res* as a probability of recovery from the disease having the severity value S. Then, the probability of the lethal outcome is $p_L = 1 - Res$. Further, we assume that this characteristic is normally distributed in the population. Hence, the probability of the lethal outcome p_L at the severity value S could be represented as the corresponding distribution function

The values of the parameter were estimated based on the clinical observations. Thus, by means of the model of infectious disease and expression (3), a relationship between age-related changes in the T-cells population and the risk of death could be established.

$$p_L(S) = \Phi(S) = \int_0^S \frac{1}{\sigma\sqrt{2\pi}} e^{-\frac{(t-a)^2}{2\sigma^2}} dt \tag{3}$$

5.2   Results of Simulation

The WHO data on pneumonia mortality in Austria, Italy, Portugal, the United Kingdom, the USA, and Japan in 1999 are represented by symbols in Fig. 9. The prob-

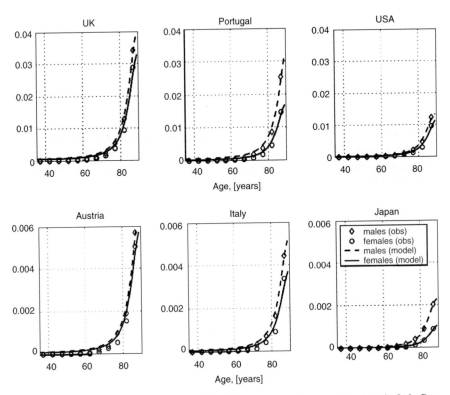

Fig. 9 Pneumonia mortality (probability of death from pneumonia per year) in Austria, Italy, Portugal, United Kingdom, USA, and Japan in 1999. WHO data are represented by symbols, results of simulation by lines

ability of death from pneumonia in the age group 80–84 in the UK is 27 times higher than in Japan and 10 times higher than in Italy.

We assume that these populations experience different antigenic load throughout adult life. This can be related to differences in climatic and ecological conditions, modes of living, and national cuisines. We fit the model of age-related risk of death from respiratory infections to the data. The results of the simulations are represented by the solid and dashed lines in Fig. 9. There is good agreement between the model and the data sets for medium and large values of the death rate. For small values (age group 35–39), the estimated risk of death is higher than observed.

To provide a good fit, two parameters of the model were estimated for every population: the value of the antigenic load and the frequency of pneumonia (Fig. 10). The differences in age-specific mortality between countries are mainly described by variations in the frequency of pneumonia. Males in Japan and in the US have higher estimate of the antigenic load than in other countries under consideration. The higher rate of immunosenescence in the male populations of these countries

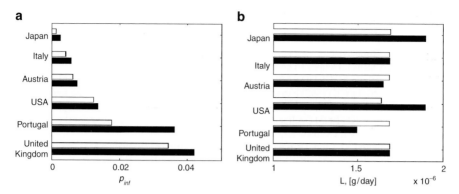

Fig. 10 Parameter estimates of environmental conditions which influenced immunosenescence in the populations under consideration. (a) frequency of pneumonia and (b) antigenic load. Black bars correspond to males; white bars to females

may also be related to the dynamic and stressful mode of living (Epel et al. 2004; Segerstrom, Miller 2004).

6 Conclusion

The proposed model describes the relation between immunosenescence and demographic aging. The initial values of variables in the model (1) correspond to the population average. In the case of availability of the clinical measurements, the proposed model can be transformed into the individualized risk model, which makes it possible to predict consequences of individual interventions. There is growing body of evidence that modification of the immune state by vaccination, antiviral and hormonal therapies, stem cell transplantation, and, possibly, by regulation of telomerase activity (Bodnar 1998), could slow down processes associated with immunosenescence. Mathematical modeling is a convenient tool for testing such intervention strategies.

Acknowledgment The research of AY was supported by P01-AG-008761, 5R01AG027019-02, and 5R01AG028259-02 grants from the National Institute on Aging (NIA), USA. The authors thank Jim Vaupel, for the opportunity to complete this research using facilities of Max Planck Institute for Demographic Research in Rostock, Germany.

References

Arpadi SM, Cuff PA, Kotler DP, Wang J, Bamji M, Lange M, Pierson RN, Matthews DE (2000) Growth velocity, fat-free mass and energy intake are inversely related to viral load in HIV-infected children. J Nutr 130:2498–2502

Bjorkander J, Bake B, Hanson LA (1984) Primary hypogammaglobulinaemia: impaired lung function and body growth with delayed diagnosis and inadequate treatment. Eur J Respir Dis 65:529–536

Bocharov GA, Romanyukha AA (1994) Mathematical model of antiviral immune response III. Influenza A virus infection. J Theor Biol 167:323–360

Bodnar AG, Ouellette M, Frolkis M, Holt SE, Chiu C-P, Morin GB, Harley CB, Shay J W, Lichtsteiner S, Wright WE (1998) Extension of life-span by introduction of telomerase into normal human cells. Science 279:349–352

Dutilh BE, De Boer RJ (2003) Decline in excision circles requires homeostatic renewal or homeostatic death of naive T-cells. J Theor Biol 224:351–358

Epel E S, Blackburn E H, Lin J, Dhabhar F S, Adler N E, Morrow J D, Cawthon R M (2004) Accelerated telomere shortening in response to life stress. PNAS 101:17312–17315

Hazenberg MD, Cohen Stuart JWT, Otto SA, Borleffs JCC, Boucher CAB, de Boer RJ, Miedema F, Hamann D (2000) T-cell division in human immunodeficiency virus (HIV)-1 infection is mainly due to immune activation: a longitudinal analysis in patients before and during highly active antiretroviral therapy (HAART). Blood 95:249–255

Hazenberg MD, Otto SA, van Rossum AMC, Schrerpbier HJ, de Groot R, Kuijpers TW, Lange JMA, Hamann D, de Boer RJ, Borghans JAM, Miedema F (2004) Establishment of the CD4+ T-cell pool in healthy children and untreated children infected with HIV-1. Blood 104:3513–3519

King CL, Malhotra I, Wamachi A et al (2002) Acquired immune responses to Plasmodium falciparum merozoite surface protein-1 in the human fetus. J Immunol 168;356–364

Kleiber M (1932) Body size and metabolism. Hilgardia 6:315–353

Lochmiller RL, Deerenberg C (2000) Trade-offs in evolutionary immunology: just what is the cost of immunity? OIKOS 88:7–98

Marchant A, Appay V, Van Der Sande M et al (2003) Mature CD8(+) T lymphocyte response to viral infection during fetal life. J Clin Invest 111:1747–1755

Marchuk G (1997) Mathematical modelling of immune response in infectious diseases. Kluwer Academic Publishers, Dordrecht

Marchuk GI, Petrov RV, Romanyukha AA, Bocharov GA (1991) Mathematical model of antiviral immune response. I. Data analysis, generalized picture construction and parameters evaluation for hepatitis B. J Theor Biol 151:P1–40

McDade TW (2003) Life history theory and the immune system: steps toward a human ecological immunology. Yearbook of physical anthropology 46:100–125

Romanyukha AA, Rudnev SG (2001) A variational principle for modeling infection immunity by the example of pneumonia. Math Modelling 13:P65–84 (in Russian)

Romanyukha AA, Yashin AI (2003) Age related changes in population of peripheral T-cells: towards a model of immunosenescence. Mech Ageing Dev 124:P433–443

Rufer N, Brümmendorf TH, Kolvraa S, Bischoff C, Christensen K, Wadsworth L, Schulzer M, Lansdorp PM (1999) Telomere fluorescense measurements in granulocytes and T-lymphocyte subsets point to a high turnover of hematopoietic stem cells and memory T-cells in early childhood. J Exp Med 190:157–167

Sannikova TE (2007) Analysis of infectious mortality by means of the individualized risk model. ECMTB05 conference proceedings "Mathematical modeling of biological systems, volume II", A Deutsch et al (ed) Birkhäuser, Boston, pp 169–181

Sannikova TE, Rudnev SG, Romanyukha AA, Yashin AI (2004) Immune system aging may be affected by HIV infection: mathematical model of immunosenescence. Russ J Numer Anal Math Modelling 19:315–329

Segerstrom S C, Miller G E (2004) Psychological stress and the human immune system: a metaanalytic study of 30 years of inquiry. Psychol Bull 130:601–630

Steinmann GG, Klaus B, Müller-Hermelink HK (1985) The involution of the ageing human thymic epithelium is independent of puberty. A morphometric study. Scand J Immunol 22:563–575

Storn R, Price K (1997) Differential evolution—a simple and efficient heuristic for global optimization over continuous spaces. J Global Optim 11:341–359

Unutmaz D, Pileri P, Abrignani S (1994) Antigen-independent activation of naive and memory resting T-cells by a cytokine combination. J Exp Med 180:1159–1164

Valentin J (2002) Basic anatomical and physiological data for use in radiological protection: reference values. ICRP Publication 89. Ann ICRP 32:1–277

West JB, Brown JH (2005) The origin of allometric scaling laws in biology from genomes to ecosystems: towards a quantitative unifying theory of biological structure and organization. J Exp Biol 208:1575–1592

Ye P, Kirschner DE (2002) Reevaluation of T-cell receptor excision circles as a measure of human recent thymic emigrants. J Immunol 169:4968–4979

Zeichner SL. Palumbo P, Feng Y, Xiao X, Gee D, Sleasman J, Goodenow M, Biggar R, Dimitrov D (1999) Rapid telomere shortening in children. Blood 93:2824–2830

Part II
Cellular Immunosenescene - T Cells

Age, T-cell Homeostasis, and T-cell Diversity in Humans

David L. Lamar, Cornelia M. Weyand and Jörg J. Goronzy

Contents

1   Introduction

A fundamental feature of mammalian adaptive immunity is the highly diverse pool of antigen receptors found on lymphocytes. The T-cell receptor and the surface immunoglobulin on B cells facilitate the recognition of foreign structures found on tumors and pathogens that have overwhelmed the defenses of the innate immune system. Because pathogen encounters and neoplasic transformations are inherently unpredictable, an immense lymphocyte receptor repertoire is required to meet all of the possible challenges an organism will face. In young humans, the daily production of naïve B cells from the bone marrow and T cells from the thymus steadily

J. J. Goronzy (✉) · C. M. Weyand · D. L. Lamar
The Kathleen B. and Mason I. Lowance Center for Human Immunology
Department of Medicine
Emory University School of Medicine
Room 1003 Woodruff Memorial Research Building
101 Woodruff Circle, Atlanta, GA
Tel.: (404) 727-7310
Fax: (404) 727-7371
E-mail: jgoronz@emory.edu

T. Fulop et al. (eds.), *Handbook on Immunosenescence*,
DOI 10.1007/978-1-4020-9062-2_9, © Springer Science+Business Media B.V. 2009

injects the lymphocyte pool with new antigen receptors. Unfortunately, as humans age functional thymic tissue gradually involutes and is replaced by fat. In parallel, the daily production of new naïve T cells declines such that no meaningful thymic T-cell production occurs after the age of fifty. Thus, the T-cell repertoire of an adult human must be maintained for decades in the absence of a replenishing source. Although homeostatic mechanisms are remarkably successful at maintaining the T-cell repertoire for many years, obvious changes begin to emerge with advanced age. Most strikingly, the naïve CD4 T cells that remain after the age of 65 undergo a sudden and dramatic collapse of T-cell receptor diversity. Naïve CD8 T cells may experience an earlier and more gradual diversity loss, although direct evidence for this is not yet available. A steadily expanding memory population maintains total T-cell numbers despite the decline in naïve T cells. Among these memory cells, an increasing percentage acquires a terminally differentiated phenotype character-ized by abnormal expression of regulatory receptors and resistance to apoptosis. Oligoclonal populations accumulate after a lifetime of repeated challenges such as chronic infections, leading to a contracted memory repertoire. Although the con-sequences of repertoire contraction are not yet known, this phenomenon may have important implications for the health of the ever growing elderly population.

This review will first delineate the developmental steps that lead to a diverse naïve T-cell repertoire followed by a discussion of the homeostatic mechanisms required to maintain T cells in the periphery after thymic involution. Some of the techniques employed to monitor thymic decline, peripheral homeostasis, and reper-toire integrity will be highlighted throughout. Finally, the impact of aging on main-taining a diverse repertoire with stable representation of functional T-cell subsets will be discussed.

2   T-cell Generation

2.1   T-cell Progenitors

Being highly dynamic and in constant turnover, the T-cell system is dependent on the generation of new T cells. T cells derive from self-renewing, pluripotent hemat-opoietic stem cells (HSC), the ancestors of all blood cells. Early lineage commit-ments occur in the bone marrow, but final T-cell differentiation and generation of T-cell diversity is entirely dependent on a functional thymus. HSC first develop into multipotent progenitors capable of becoming both myeloid and lymphoid cells. Additional differentiation leads to the common lymphoid progenitor cells which can become T cells, B cells, and NK cells. Little is known about the exact T-cell progenitor that exits the bone marrow and is destined to enter the thymus [1]. CD34, a marker of HSC in the bone marrow, is expressed on circulating cells with strong in vitro T-cell potential [2]. Intrathymic multipotent precursors also initially express CD34 suggesting that T-cell precursors come from the circulating CD34+ popula-tion [3]. Within the thymus, committed T-cell precursors are thought to differentiate from CD34$^+$ cells that have acquired CD1a expression [4]. Additionally, expression of the Notch1 receptor and signaling apparatus, which are required for T- versus B-cell lineage commitment, are likely characteristics of intrathymic T-cell precursors [5]. Whatever the true characteristics of circulating and intrathymic T-cell progenitors are, T-cell generation is dependent on a continual supply of potential thymocytes entering the thymus for further maturation.

2.2   Generation of T-cell Receptor Diversity

The effectiveness of the human adaptive immune system requires a diverse array of antigen receptors on lymphocytes. In both B and T cells, this diversity arises from the somatic rearrangement of gene segments encoding each subunit of the antigen receptor and the combination of these uniquely encoded subunits to make a complete receptor. For the T cell, this process occurs in the thymus and results in the expression of a single T-cell receptor (TCR) consisting of two rearranged receptor subunits. The vast majority of T-cells express receptor chains encoded by the TCRA and TCRB loci and are called $\alpha\beta$ T-cells. The remaining T-cells (2–14% of peripheral T-cells [6]) are called $\gamma\delta$ T cells and have TCR encoded by the TCRG and TCRD loci. This discussion will focus only on $\alpha\beta$ T cells.

To appreciate what T-cell diversity generation entails, the remainder of this section will detail the intrathymic events that transform genetically homogeneous and undifferentiated thymocytes into mature naïve CD4 and CD8 T cells displaying genetically and structurally diverse TCR. The mature TCR is a heterodimer composed of two Type-I membrane-spanning subunits called the α- and β-chains [7]. Each chain has two Ig-like domains and a short transmembrane region. The membrane-proximal Ig-like domains are called constant domains because they are nearly identical on all $\alpha\beta$ T cells. The membrane-distal Ig-like domains differ from T cell to T cell and are called variable domains. They are responsible for antigen recognition and are the basis for the immense diversity necessary to respond to the full array of potential pathogens encountered by naïve T cells.

A schematic representation of TCR genes is depicted in Fig. 1. Early thymocytes do not express any TCR, and both alleles of each TCR gene are fully intact. These CD34$^+$CD1a$^+$ thymocytes also lack the TCR coreceptors CD4 and CD8 and are thus known as double negative thymocytes. In humans, unlike in mice, before TCR rearrangement begins, thymocytes will express CD4 alone or both CD4 and CD8 in some cases [8]. The first step towards expression of a functional TCR is expression of RAG1 and RAG2 by thymocytes [9]. These proteins are essential for somatic recombination, and once they are expressed, the TCRB locus begins to rearrange. The diversity (D_β) and joining (J_β) gene segments are the first to be combined, followed by joining of a variable (V_β) segment to the D_β-J_β junction. The particular segments included are stochastically chosen and the order of segment joining is dictated by recombination signal sequences flanking the gene segments (reviewed in [10]). During recombination, the enzyme terminal deoxyribonucleotidyl trans-

a TCRβ Chain Rearrangement

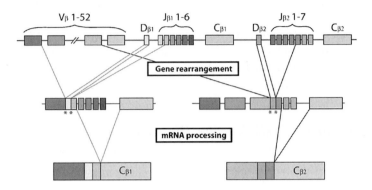

b TCRα Chain Rearrangement

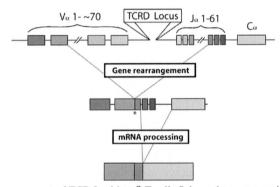

Fig. 1 Rearrangement of TCR Loci in αβ T cells Schematic representations of TCR gene rearrangement and mRNA processing to yield mature TCR chains (gene segments are not to scale). (a) The TCRB locus on chromosome 7 rearranges first. (b) The TCRA locus on chromosome 14 rearranges after successful β-chain rearrangement and expression. The TCRD locus lies within the TCRA locus and is deleted when TCRA rearrangement occurs. * indicates sites of terminal deoxyribonucleotidyl transferase-mediated generation of junctional diversity

ferase (TdT) facilitates the random addition and subtraction of a variable number of nucleotides at segment junctions [11]. This imprecise joining, termed junctional diversity, is an important source of variable domain sequence diversity for both TCR chains. As depicted in Fig. 1, the TCRB locus has two C_β gene segments. A failed attempt to rearrange the locus using the $C_{\beta 1}$ gene segment can be followed by an attempt to use the $C_{\beta 2}$ locus on the same chromosome. When the TCRB locus is successfully rearranged, the resulting protein will be expressed at the surface in complex with the pre-Tα-chain, an invariant surrogate required for β-chain expression [12]. Expression of this pre-TCR signals completion of β-chain rearrangement. At this time, RAG1/2 expression ceases, preventing further rearrangement of the second TCRB allele and ensuring that all T cells express a single β-chain [4].

An additional consequence of successful TCRB rearrangement and pre-TCR expression is a massive proliferation of β-chain$^+$ thymocytes before TCRA rearrangement. By expanding at this stage, each unique successful β-chain rearrangement can be combined with many different α-chains, thereby dramatically enhancing the total TCR repertoire. It is estimated that roughly 10 divisions occur between β-chain expression and TCRA rearrangement, resulting in ~1000 thymocytes with the same β-chain [13]. This number is much higher than the number of distinct α-chains paired with a single β-chain in mature peripheral T cells because only 10% percent of β-chain$^+$ thymocytes will successfully rearrange the TCRA locus and survive positive and negative selection. After expansion, β-chain$^+$ thymocytes reexpress the RAG proteins and TCRA gene rearrangement begins [9]. TCRB and TCRA gene rearrangements proceed by the same mechanism with a few distinctions. Whereas the β-chain variable domains are comprised of V, D, and J segments, the TCRA locus only has V and J segments. Unlike β-chain rearrangement, a cell without a successful α-chain rearrangement can continue rearranging by joining upstream V_α segments to downstream J_α segments until a competent chain is formed [14]. Additionally, surface expression of a rearranged α-chain, in complex with the β-chain, does not silence RAG1/2 expression. Instead, RAG1/2 expression ceases after positive selection (discussed below), which signals completion of TCR gene rearrangement [15]. A consequence of prolonged RAG1/2 expression during TCRA rearrangement is the possible coexpression of more than one α-chain on each T-cell [14]. It is likely, however, that only TCR containing the positively selected α-chain allele will interact with MHC-peptide complexes in the periphery during an immune response.

2.3 Positive Selection and Negative Selection

Thymocytes with successfully rearranged TCR will only emerge from the thymus as CD4 or CD8 naïve T cells if they survive positive and negative selection. These selection processes require interactions between the TCR on thymocytes and the MHC class I and II molecules on bone marrow-derived cells and specialized epithelial cells within the thymus. Because a functional T-cell response requires recognition of pathogenic peptides presented in complex with MHC molecules, only TCR capable of making stable contacts with MHC are useful additions to the T-cell repertoire. Thymocytes must receive signals through the TCR to avoid death by neglect (positive selection), which is the fate of about 90% of all TCR$^+$ thymocytes [16]. The requirement for positive selection ensures the elimination of TCR least likely to contribute to an immune response. Additionally, an excessively high affinity interaction will lead to the death of the T cell and removal of that cell's TCR from the repertoire (negative selection). Because only self-peptides are presented on MHC molecules in the thymus, negative selection removes T cells with potentially autoreactive TCR. About half of the remaining 10% of TCR$^+$ thymocytes are removed by negative selection [16]. Survivors of both positive and negative selection exit the thymus as mature T cells expressing a TCR that may recognize an epitope from potential pathogens.

In addition to ensuring that a T cell expresses a fully functional yet self-tolerant TCR, intrathymic TCR:MHC interactions dictate a key determinant of each thymocyte's future function: the choice of CD4 versus CD8 coreceptor expression [16]. A mature T cell whose TCR interacts with MHC class I molecules during positive selection will express CD8. Alternatively, if positive selection occurs against MHC class II molecules, the resulting mature T cell will express CD4.

2.4 How Diverse is the Human T-cell Repertoire?

As stated above, all receptor diversity in the T-cell pool is generated by somatic gene rearrangement during thymocyte maturation. By examining the key sources of this diversity, a theoretical upper limit of distinct $\alpha\beta$ TCR has been estimated [7]. Three main factors contribute to the diversity of the TCR repertoire: the inclusion of a single V, D, and J gene segment (V and J only for the α-chain) in the variable domain of each TCR chain, the random addition and subtraction of nucleotides at the junction of combined gene segments (junctional diversity), and the pairing of one rearranged α-chain with one rearranged β-chain to yield a complete TCR. There are ~70 V_α and 61 J_α gene segments which when combined would yield 4,270 different α-chains if all combinations are productive. The 52 V_β, 2 D_β, and 13 J_β gene segments could potentially combine to form 1,352 different β-chains. Without accounting for junctional diversity, 5.8 million different TCR could be generated by combining one α-chain with one β-chain. Estimates suggest that junctional diversity may increase TCR diversity by a factor of 2×10^{11} to a total of 10^{18} potential unique TCR. This estimate is an overstatement of the true repertoire potential because many V_α-J_α and V_β-D_β-J_β combinations result in nonsense frame shifts and not all α-β-chain combinations can be expressed. Even with a more modest estimate, it is clear that the receptor repertoire of any individual, whose total T-cell compartment contains only ~3×10^{11} cells, represents only a minute fraction of the potential diversity.

A variety of techniques used to measure diversity (discussed below) estimate that the T-cell repertoire consists of about 10^8 different TCR in young humans. If TCR were all equally represented, the clonal size of T cells bearing the same receptor would be about 1,000. In reality, certain clones are more abundant than others, and the receptor repertoire differs among the different functional T-cell subsets. Naïve cells, which represent about 50% of total CD4 and CD8 T cells [17–19] in young humans, harbor the majority of total TCR diversity. An assessment of TCR repertoire within CD4 T cells in young donors revealed that memory cells have only 5–10% of the β-chain diversity of naïve cells [19]. As, each β-chain in the memory population is generally paired with a single α-chain, this translates to only 1% of the total naïve $\alpha\beta$ TCR diversity.

Because an organism cannot predict which pathogens will be encountered by the immune system, it is beneficial that naïve lymphocyte antigen receptors are highly diverse. Naturally, the receptor repertoire in the memory compartment can only be, and is only required to be, as diverse as the epitopes against which a primary response has already been raised. However, in addition to receptor diversity, memory T cells comprise several different functional populations. The paradigm of the memory T-cell life-cycle dictates that the cells remaining after the contraction phase of a primary immune response will be either central memory or effector memory cells [20]. Central memory cells, defined as CD45RA$^-$ and CCR7$^+$, reside in lymphoid tissues such as the spleen and lymph nodes. Effector memory cells, defined as CD45RA$^-$ and CCR7$^-$, are found in peripheral sites where antigen exposure is most likely, such as the skin, lungs, and GI tract.

In addition to distinct homing patterns, central and effector memory T cells respond differently upon antigen reexposure [21]. While both memory subsets are much more sensitive to TCR stimulation than naïve T cells, effector memory cells have an even lower activation threshold. Consistent with their localization at the frontlines of antigen exposure, effector memory cells are quickly and potently triggered to produce effector cytokines such as IFN-γ, a key molecule in a strong immune response. Conversely, central memory cells likely reencounter antigen only after it has been delivered to lymphoid tissue and presented on antigen-presenting cells. After stimulation, these cells produce high amounts of IL-2 which promote expansion of activated T cells. Several studies in mice suggest that central memory cells differentiate into effector memory cells, thereby enhancing the current immune response and seeding the periphery for future exposures [22, 23]. A third memory subset, the terminally differentiated effector cell (known as CD45RA effector cells), is defined by reversion of effector memory cells to CD45RA positivity while still lacking CCR7 [24]. These cells are much more common in the CD8 compartment and are characterized by potent cytotoxicity, resistance to apoptosis, and weak proliferative potential. As we will discuss later, CD45RA effector cells accumulate with age and may result in altered functionality of memory responses in the elderly.

2.5 Techniques for Assessing Diversity

Before discussing the mechanism of diversity maintenance and the TCR repertoire changes that occur with age, we will discuss the techniques used to estimate human TCR diversity. The staggering array of unique TCR gene rearrangements in peripheral T cells makes direct measurement of diversity a challenge. Only gross changes in repertoire, such as large clonal expansions or the loss of entire V$_\beta$ families, can be detected using the following low sensitivity methods. Flow cytometry allows detection of differences in V$_\beta$ family usage among various T-cell compartments or age ranges [25]. However, even a severe loss of repertoire diversity that affected the different V$_\beta$ families similarly would be missed by this method. TCR clonotyping, which utilizes V$_\beta$-C$_\beta$ or V$_\alpha$-C$_\alpha$ specific PCR and denaturing gradient gel electrophoresis, relies on the existence of clonal expansions large enough to dominate the PCR products of entire V$_\beta$ families [26]. Similarly, the "immunoscope" method (see below) uses PCR to detect large expansions within V_β families [27]. While this technique is only slightly more sensitive than clonotyping, immunoscoping is a useful tool to estimate total T-cell diversity when combined with sequencing [28].

More direct assessments of TCR repertoire all use a common approach: isolate and characterize a small subset of sequences and extrapolate their frequencies, based on parameters such as V_β frequency and possible $\alpha\beta$ combinations, to the whole T-cell pool. Wagner et al. examined repertoire diversity using TCR-specific probes and limiting dilution of CD4 T cells [29]. Using primers specific for two V_β-J_β combinations ($V_\beta 8$-$J_\beta 1S4$ and $V_\beta 18$-$J_\beta 2S5$), representative samples of β-chain gene sequences from CD4 T cells of several donors were obtained. Specific biotinylated probes complementary to the TCR N-D-N region (this region is highly variable and includes the junctional nucleotides that flank the D gene segment) were then generated. In a subsequent step, a second sample of CD4 T cells from the same donor was screened for the presence of these sequences in a limiting dilution system. cDNA was isolated from replicates of serially diluted T cells ranging from 10^5 to 5×10^6 cells, amplified by PCR with the appropriate V_β-J_β primer set and hybridized with the labeled probes specific for the isolated TCR sequences. This method determines the frequency of each specific β-chain sequence in the entire T-cell pool and allows for an estimate of the total diversity. Studies using this method [19, 29] have estimated that a given β-chain obtained from naïve CD4 T cells is present with a median frequency of <1 in 2×10^7 T cells in healthy young and middle-aged adult humans, i.e., the human naïve CD4 T-cell compartment encompasses around 20 million different TCR β-chains. Because the sensitivity of the limiting dilution system is less than 100%, this estimate represents the upper range.

The "immunoscope" technique, mentioned above as a method to detect T-cell clonal expansions [27], has been exploited to estimate human $\alpha\beta$ TCR diversity. As with the limiting dilution assay of Wagner, et al. [29], this technique requires PCR amplification across the β-chain N-D-N region followed by sequencing. Previously, it was observed that the lengths of rearranged TCRB transcripts between constant sequences flanking the N-D-N region follow a Gaussian distribution. The span of sizes results from the stochastic addition and subtraction of nucleotides during the joining of gene segments [11]. Electrophoretic separation of PCR products amplified from a heterogeneous T-cell cDNA pool reveals a laddering of discrete bands separated by a gel distance corresponding to 3 nucleotides/1 codon. A graphical depiction of intensities of these bands reveals 6–8 peaks, with the most intense central peak corresponding to an N-D-N region length of 8–10 amino acids. A non-Gaussian spectrum results when one or a few TCR clones are overrepresented.

It has been shown that, when normally distributed, the intensity of each peak is proportional to the diversity of specific TCR sequences present in the peak. To estimate total human β-chain diversity, Arstila, et al. isolated a single band from the separation of $V_\beta 18$-$J_\beta 1.4$ PCR products and identified all TCR variants by sequencing [28]. The total number of $V_\beta 18$–$J_\beta 1.4$ sequences was extrapolated based on the intensity of the sequenced band and total β-chain diversity was extrapolated from the frequency of $V_\beta 18$ and $J_\beta 1.4$ positive T cells in the individuals used for the study. After repeating this procedure for several donors and other V_β-J_β segments, the authors arrived at a minimal estimate of 1.3×10^6 different TCR β-chains.

2.6   Thymic Decline with Age

The anatomy of the thymus is expressly suited to allow for the maturation of new T cells with a staggering array of unique TCR. The thymus is the sole organ where naïve T cells are produced and diversity can be generated or refreshed. Consequently, thymic integrity plays a key role in T-cell repertoire maintenance over the many decades of a human life. In the following section, we will discuss how aging affects the thymus and its ability to provide a steady supply of new naïve T cells and, therefore, new TCR clonotypes.

The thymic architecture consists of the thymic epithelial space and the perivascular space (reviewed in [30]). Thymopoiesis occurs entirely within the thymic epithelial space which includes the cortical and medullary epithelial cells and bone marrow-derived antigen-presenting cells required for positive and negative selection. The perivascular space is located within the thymic capsule and is separated from the thymic epithelial space by a basement membrane. The cellular component of the perivascular space consists of fibroblasts, lymphoid cells, and a few adipocytes and is notable for the absence of thymocytes. The classical description of thymic anatomy, consisting mostly of thymic epithelial space with only a small contribution from perivascular space, applies only to very young human thymi. As early as age 2, the thymic epithelial space begins to decline with a compensatory enlargement of the perivascular space by adipocytosis. Although total thymic mass remains constant, the loss of thymic epithelial space results in a steady decrease of new T-cell production after adolescence.

Numerous studies have observed decreased thymopoiesis with age. The most common techniques for evaluating thymic output involve quantifying the number of recent thymic emigrants in the peripheral blood. In the absence of a reliable surface marker for recent thymic emigrants, many groups have resorted to the detection of TCR excision circles (TREC) which are DNA remnants of TCR gene rearrangements. During thymocyte maturation, chromosomal DNA within the TCR loci is broken and religated to join V or D gene segments with J gene segments and V segments with D-J gene segments. In each case, the DNA sequence between the joined gene segments is excised from the chromosome and the cleaved ends of the deleted sequence are ligated together resulting in a TREC. The correlation of TREC with thymic output follows from the fact that, with each cell division, chromosomal DNA is replicated while TREC DNA is not [31]. After excision of a TREC during TCR gene rearrangement, subsequent mitotic events will dilute the TREC/cell ratio because only a single descendent of the original thymocyte, regardless of the number of future divisions, will retain the TREC. The stability of TREC in the absence of division has been debated, and the persisting TREC with aging may therefore derive from nondividing cells rather than from recent thymic emigrants.

Each TREC represents a single gene rearrangement event, and each step in the TCR rearrangement process can lead to the formation of a different TREC. TREC resulting from the V, D, and J segment-joining events are unique to the particular segments joined and are, therefore, rare in the total population and not useful for a global assessment of recent thymic emigrants. A fortuitous requirement for the successful rearrangement of the TCRA locus is the deletion of the TCRD locus which is found between the TCRA V and J segments (see Fig. 1b). TCRD deletion requires the joining of two genetic elements flanking the delta locus, δRec and ψJα [32]. The resulting TREC (sjTREC) contains a δRec-ψJα signal joint that is identical for all TCRD deletion events. When the TCRA gene is subsequently rearranged, the δRec-ψJα coding joint will be included in the resulting TREC (cjTREC) regardless of which TCRA segments are joined (diagrammed in [33]). Although either of these TREC can be used for estimating αβ T-cell production, the sjTREC is the more common choice because the δRec-ψJα coding joint can still remain on the incompletely rearranged chromosome in 5% of αβ T cells [33]. An additional advantage of TCRD TREC, which are produced late in TCR rearrangement, is that only 3–4 divisions occur between TCRD deletion and full TCR rearrangement [34]. Thus, δRec-ψJα TREC are minimally diluted in newly matured αβ T cells.

Regardless of which TREC is used to assess recent thymic emigrants, thymic function comparisons can be made among donors of various ages. Multiple studies suggest that thymic production steadily declines with age [34–36]. This decline occurs at the rate of about 3% per year, which is the same rate estimated for the loss of thymic epithelial space with age [37, 38]. TCR rearrangement in thymocytes occurs normally regardless of age, generating a diverse Vβ repertoire [39]. Additionally, newly generated T cells in individuals up to at least age 50 perform as well as young T cells in in vitro assays. Therefore, it is thought that while total thymic epithelial space and consequently new naïve T-cell production declines with age, T-cell production in the remaining tissue is qualitatively intact [30]. Quantitatively, however, the thymus is unable to provide a meaningful supply of new naïve T cells after middle age as evidenced by the small numbers of peripheral TREC. Additionally, the ability to reconstitute the T-cell compartment following ablative bone marrow transplantation decreases steadily with age. In fact, patients in their fifties fail to return to pretreatment cell numbers even 2 years after transplant [40].

TREC levels in T cells are used as an indirect surrogate of thymic T-cell output and many papers treat TREC⁺ naïve T cells as recent thymic emigrants. However, it has been noted that the interpretation of TREC measurements is more complicated [33]. Indeed, decreased thymic output results in dilution of the TREC/cell ratio over time; so does homeostatic proliferation or death of existing TREC⁺ T cells. For this reason, TREC measurements tend to overestimate thymic output and interpretations should take into account the kinetics of T-cell turnover. Recently, one group has proposed a new marker for recent thymic emigrants that may help resolve the potential ambiguity of TREC dilution. Kimmig et al. reported that CD31 positivity on CD45RA⁺RO⁻ naïve T cells correlated strongly with the presence of sjTREC [41]. Conversely, CD45RA⁺RO⁻CD31⁻ T cells, although functionally and phenotypically naïve, have almost no TREC. The authors suggest that recent thymic emigrants lose CD31 expression upon antigen-induced or homeostatic proliferation, an idea that is supported by the loss of CD31 by in vitro culture. An examination of the percentage of CD4 T cells with a CD45RA⁺CD45RO⁻CD31⁺ phenotype with age revealed a steady decline similar to that seen when TREC are examined. It remains to be seen whether CD31 will become a widely used marker for recent thymic emigrants, but the results of Kimmig and colleagues lend credence to the TREC-based findings that thymic production of new naïve T cells declines with age.

3 Maintenance of Diversity

In the absence of foreign antigen, all peripheral T-cell pools experience a steady-state turnover characterized by cell loss (to attrition, death, or phenotypic shift) and compensatory proliferation. In order to maintain the original diversity of recent thymic emigrants, death and replacement of naïve T cells must be completely random so as not to preferentially deplete or replace T cells of certain specificities. An additional requirement for maintaining diversity is that each clonal population expressing a given TCR is of an adequate size to ensure that normal cell death will not eliminate a TCR from the repertoire. The latter requirement is met by proliferation of thymocytes bearing a functionally rearranged TCR before and shortly after mature naïve T cells exit the thymus. Fully random steady-state turnover of peripheral T cells is much more difficult to achieve. In the context of thymic export of new naïve T cells, this problem is not likely to result in a compromised repertoire. However, the severe and early decline of thymic production of T cells seen in humans suggests that peripheral homeostatic mechanisms are crucial for life-long TCR diversity.

Maintenance of the TCR repertoire is a balance between factors that introduce or preserve diversity and those that pose a threat (see Fig. 5). Naïve and memory T cells share some of these factors. For both cell types, the thymus is the ultimate source of new diversity; however, the proximal source of diversity in the memory compartment is activation and differentiation of naïve cells in response to antigen. Therefore, establishment of the memory repertoire depends both on the initial naïve repertoire and the history of antigen exposure. T-cell activation against a novel antigen, while seeding the memory compartment after contraction of the primary response, represents an important threat to naïve T-cell diversity. Normal daily turnover leads to loss of T cells, and potentially TCR, from all compartments. Assuming an adequate initial clonal size, homeostatic proliferation of remaining T cells will replace lost cells and maintain normal compartment sizes. While total T-cell numbers can easily be maintained by replacement proliferation, it is unlikely that all TCR clones are lost and replaced with equal kinetics. Consequently, over many years of homeostatic maintenance, the TCR representation, for both memory and naïve cells, is at risk of skewing and contraction.

3.1 Assessment of T-cell Turnover

A crucial component to T-cell homeostasis, and therefore maintenance of T-cell heterogeneity, is cell turnover. The persistence of a T-cell clone with a given TCR depends on proliferation of existing cells in the face decreased thymic output and daily cell loss. It is important to understand the power and the limitations of the techniques used to examine T-cell kinetics and turnover in humans before reviewing the available data.

3.1.1 Ki67 Staining

One easy method for assessing the fraction of proliferating cells within a lymphocyte population is by intracellular staining for Ki67. Ki67 is a nuclear antigen expressed in the G_1, S, G_2, and M phases of proliferating cells. Its absence in resting G_0 cells makes it a good marker of cycling cells [42]. Using standard flow cytometric identification of intracellular antigens [43], a panel of antibodies can be designed to assess the proportion of proliferating cells within T-cell subsets at a given time. This method has been used to estimate the T-cell turnover rates in several contexts, including HIV and aging [19, 44, 45]. The accuracy of Ki67 staining has been confirmed by more advanced metabolic labeling techniques (see below) that simultaneously assess proliferation and loss from a population. While these newer techniques provide a more complete picture of T-cell kinetics, Ki67 staining remains a useful method for immediate ex vivo assessment of proliferation within peripheral blood subsets.

3.1.2 Deuterated Glucose or Water Incorporation

To obtain direct in vivo measures of human T-cell kinetics, several studies have utilized deuterated glucose or water [46–49]. Each of these methods allows for the labeling and monitoring of dividing cells because glucose and water contribute molecules to the biosynthesis of DNA. Consequently, in the presence of these deuterated substances, a certain percentage of molecules in newly synthesized DNA will be labeled with deuterium, ^2H [47, 48]. After a defined administration period, the ^2H source is discontinued and blood samples are taken at several time points to determine the ^2H content in the DNA of cell types of interest. Measurements made before and soon after delivery of labeled glucose or water are used to determine the percentage of cells that proliferate during the administration period. Further measurements made at multiple later time points allow for calculation of the loss rates and half-lives of the isolated cell subsets.

Because deuterated glucose and water are neither radioactive nor a mutagenic threat, they are useful tools for in vivo studies of human T-cell kinetics. The use of ^2H_2O is the more recent of the two labeling methods and, as described by Neese, et al. [48], has financial, feasibility, and experimental advantages over deuterated glucose. For example, deuterated water can simply be added to normal drinking water whereas glucose must be administered intravenously. Without the need for expensive supervised infusion, deuterated water can be delivered over a longer period of time which is beneficial for examining low turnover cell types such as naïve T cells.

3.2   T-cell Homeostatic Mechanisms

In light of the well-documented steady decline in thymic production of new naïve T cells with age, the kinetics and mechanisms of T-cell survival and turnover are vital for maintenance of a diverse and functional adaptive immune system. Using techniques described above, direct estimates of replacement rates and half-lives of human T-cell subsets have been made in vivo. Examination of T-cell kinetics in young adult humans by deuterated glucose [46] revealed that about 0.59 and 0.45% of naïve (CD45RA$^+$) CD4 and CD8 T cells, respectively, proliferate each day. These figures translate to a replacement time of 118 and 145 days, respectively. CD45RO$^+$ memory T cells divide much more frequently than naïve cells. 2.65% of CD4 and 5.09% of CD8 memory T cells proliferate each day, which corresponds to replacement times of 26 and 14 days, respectively. Additional studies by the same group [49, 50] and Ki67 staining of CD4 T-cell subsets by our group [19, 29] confirmed these estimates. Extrapolations from these data suggest that a total of 4×10^9 T cells are produced by peripheral expansion each day [46]. As total T-cell numbers remain stable over time, a comparable loss of T cells also must occur each day. Without a constant supply of new naïve T cells from the thymus, and keeping in mind the requirement of fully random replacement of T cells to maintain a complete TCR repertoire, this extensive daily turnover poses a potential threat to TCR diversity in adults.

3.2.1   Naïve T-cell Homeostasis

In a young, healthy human, the normal daily turnover of naïve T cells is replaced with new T-cell production by the thymus and by proliferation of existing naïve T cells. Our examination of neonatal T-cell kinetics showed that about 10% of daily naïve T-cell production in infants comes from the thymus [45]. Other estimates based on modeling suggest that, at the age of twenty-five, about 20% of the peripheral naïve T-cell pool is populated directly from the thymus [51]. Therefore, even in individuals with an intact thymus, peripheral expansion is the major source of circulating naïve cells. As long as the thymus continues injecting new TCR into the naïve pool, extensive homeostatic proliferation does not threaten receptor diversity. However, as thymic involution proceeds, the burden of maintaining the naïve pool increasingly lies with homeostatic mechanisms. In fact, by age 55, the thymus contributes, at maximum, 5% of the peripheral naïve T cells [51] and probably much less.

   Mounting evidence suggests that survival and proliferative maintenance of human T cells in the periphery depend on both TCR- and cytokine-delivered signals. In the absence of exogenous antigen, TCR:MHC interactions in the periphery are analogous to those that mediate positive selection in the thymus; namely, a self-peptide conjugated with the appropriate MHC allele acts as a ligand to provide a survival signal to T cells with a TCR that binds with sufficient affinity. Studies in mice do indeed suggest that peripheral naïve T cells are lost in mice lacking MHC molecules. CD4

T cells are vastly reduced in animals lacking MHC class II [52, 53] and similarly, adoptively transferred CD8 T cells will only persist in mice that express MHC class I [54, 55]. For CD8 T cells, it has been shown that the peripheral MHC requirement extends to the exact class I allele against which the T cell was positively selected in the thymus [54]. Additional studies show that peripheral T cells rely on TCR-generated signals not only for survival but for homeostatic expansion [56, 57].

The role and requirement for a TCR-generated signal to maintain T-cell homeostasis has implications regarding the long-term integrity of the TCR repertoire in the context of dwindling thymic output. If homeostatic responses depend on the strength of the TCR:MHC interaction, it is necessarily the case that some TCR will more readily receive survival or expansion signals. An obvious consequence of this scenario is nonrandom TCR maintenance and/or proliferation and, therefore, repertoire skewing. Because a given TCR's affinity for a self-peptide:MHC complex is unlikely to predict a strong response to a pathogen peptide:MHC complex, the skewed repertoire generated by self-antigen-driven homeostatic proliferation would not only deplete T-cell clonal diversity but would do so without promoting enhanced protection.

Fortunately, antigen-independent stimuli delivered by cytokines also play an important role in peripheral T-cell maintenance. Extensive work in the mouse, and more recently in the human, has established that cytokines signaling via the common γ-chain (which include IL-2, IL-4, IL-7, IL-15, and IL-21) play a key role in peripheral T-cell maintenance and expansion [58]. While the cytokine requirements for homeostasis differ among the various T-cell subsets and with regard to the particular function examined, IL-7 and IL-15 seem to be the most important. In mice, naïve T cells, in addition to TCR:MHC interactions, require IL-7 for steady-state survival in vivo. Although other molecules are likely involved, studies in mice [59] and humans point to upregulation of the antiapoptotic protein Bcl-2 as a mechanism for cytokine-mediated T-cell survival [60].

Homeostatic expansion of peripheral T cells is controlled by the same general mechanisms that mediate survival. Steady-state naïve T-cell turnover, as discussed above, is quite low compared to memory T cells. This implies that memory cells have a stronger proliferative response to the required signals. While this may be true, naïve T cells are capable of a robust expansion in lymphopenic situations [61]. From these studies it can be argued that, while naïve T-cell survival and proliferation require the same TCR- and cytokine-mediated signals, space in the compartment is also necessary for homeostatic expansion. In the steady state, the characteristic naïve and memory T-cell replacement rates [46] may be a direct response to fill compartmental space made available by attrition or cell death.

4 Aging and the Loss of T-cell Heterogeneity

Given that thymic production is the only source of new naïve T cells, and that very little meaningful thymic output remains after early adulthood, one may expect dramatic changes in the peripheral T-cell pool with age. In fact, some obvious changes occur while other features remain intact. Total T-cell numbers decrease only slightly

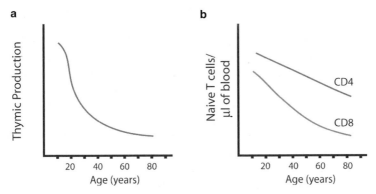

Fig. 2 Naive T-cell Production and Maintenance with Age (a) Schematic representation of loss of thymic production of naive T cells with age. (b) Schematic representation of loss of peripheral naive T cells with age

with age, exhibiting a steady but shallow decline throughout adulthood [17]. Although the maintenance of T-cell numbers is remarkable considering negligible thymic output, the composition of peripheral T cells in the elderly becomes increasingly distinct from young individuals. A consistent and striking finding is the significant loss of naïve cells with age (depicted in Fig. 2). About 50% of young adult T cells are naïve compared to about 35% in 70-year-olds [17]. Remarkably, this naïve loss is much more pronounced for CD8 T cells than for CD4 T cells. In fact, by the age of 70, the percentage of naïve CD8 T cells is consistently around 10%. In contrast, naïve CD4 T cells still make up about 40% of total CD4 T cells [17, 19, 62]. At ages beyond 70, naïve CD4 T cells continue to decline at a steady rate

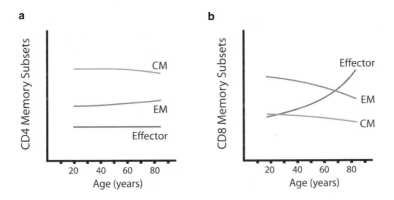

Fig. 3 Changes in Memory T-cell Subsets with Age (a) Schematic representation of changes within CD4 memory T-cell subsets with age. (b) Schematic representation of changes within CD8 memory T-cell subsets with age. CM, central memory; EM, effector memory; Effector, CD45RA+ effector memory

whereas naïve CD8 T cells drop to single digit percentages and are virtually gone in individuals who reach 100 [17].

Naturally, with declining naïve T-cell numbers in the context of only slightly reduced total T-cell numbers, the percentage of memory T cells increases with age. In addition, it is clear that memory populations are also qualitatively different in the elderly (depicted in Fig. 3). As appears to be the case for most features of T-cell aging, the CD8 memory T-cell pool experiences a more striking transformation than does the CD4 memory T-cell pool. In young adults, about half of the CD8 memory T-cells have an effector memory phenotype [18, 63]. The remaining half is split equally between central memory and CD45RA effector cells. Throughout adulthood, these proportions shift in favor of CD45RA effector cells which, by the mid-seventies, represent over 50% of all memory CD8 T cells [63]. Because the memory pool as a whole is increased, this translates into more than a 4-fold increase in the absolute numbers of circulating CD8+ CD45RA effector cells. Even central and effector CD8 memory T-cell subsets in the elderly, while comprising a decreased percentage of total CD8 memory T cells, are increased in absolute numbers relative to young adults. Within the CD4 memory T-cell population, aging does not have a significant effect on subset distribution [63]. However, as total memory cells are increased, the absolute numbers of each subset within the CD4 memory T-cell population does increase with age.

A well-established feature of memory T-cell aging is the loss of the costimulatory molecule CD28 [64]. Additional molecules have been identified whose patterns of expression changes with age. Interestingly, many of these molecules, like CD28, are immunoregulatory receptors that might alter the ability of T cells to respond to antigen. Similar to the effects of age on memory T-cell subset distribution, CD8 T cells more readily exhibit these changes than do CD4 T cells. For example, up to 70% of CD8 T cells have lost CD28 by age 80, compared to a maximum of 25% of CD4 cells [63]. Similarly, CD85j, an inhibitory receptor for most classical and nonclassical MHC class I molecules [65], is dramatically increased on memory CD8 T cells in the elderly [63]. This acquisition, which in CD8 T cells is as robust as the loss of CD28, occurs on only a very small subset of CD4 T cells. The distinct behaviors of aging CD4 and CD8 T cells, which are also seen in nonhuman primates [66], extends to more artificial human settings as well; long-term in vitro culture of T cells, which mimics aging in many molecular respects, induces characteristic changes much more readily in CD8 T cells [63].

4.1   TCR Repertoire Loss with Age

In light of thymic decline and the steady decrease in naïve T cells with age, it is important to know whether the naïve TCR repertoire undergoes a similar contraction. Our lab developed a technique (described above) to estimate TCR β-chain frequency in an individual. Two studies of naïve CD4 T cells [19, 29] using this method revealed that, in young individuals, the median frequency of T cells bearing a given β-chain is <1 in 20 million. This predicts a total β-chain repertoire of 20 million in naïve CD4 T cells. This value is an upper estimate due to the suboptimal sensitivity of the limiting dilution system used. Arstila, et al. used the immunoscope technique, which should underestimate true diversity, to arrive at a figure of 1–2 million different β-chains in naïve CD4 T cells in the young [28]. The actual value is probably in between this and our estimate.

How does the naïve CD4 TCR repertoire change with age? Remarkably, in spite of little to no thymic output, β-chain sequences from individuals up to the age of 65 are present in frequencies similar to those of 20-year-olds. Not only do the most infrequent β-chains represent over 60% of the tested sequences, resulting in the same median frequency of <1 in 20 million, the 60- to 65-year-old donors do not have an increase in overrepresented β-chain sequences; only 20% of tested sequences in both age groups are more frequent than 1 in 1 million. These findings indicate that homeostatic mechanisms effectively maintain the naïve repertoire through age 65 even without significant input of new T cells from the thymus.

When individuals in their late seventies are examined, a dramatic change in naïve CD4 T-cell repertoire maintenance is revealed. Whereas in younger individuals, about 60–70% of β-chain sequences examined are less frequent than 1 in 5 million, nearly 100% of β-chain sequences from 75- to 80-year-old individuals are more frequent than 1 in 1 million. In fact, the majority of sequences are present at a frequency greater than 1 in 200,000. Thus, in a single decade, 99% of the β-chain repertoire is lost. A similarly dramatic repertoire collapse is seen in the memory compartment of CD4 T cells in the elderly (depicted in Fig. 4). This may reflect a generalized break down in T-cell homeostatic mechanisms at advanced age.

While a similar examination of the naïve CD8 T-cell repertoire in the elderly has not been done, indirect evidence suggests that diversity loss occurs earlier and more steadily in CD8 T cells. As discussed above, the loss of naïve CD8 T cells is more severe than for CD4 T cells (see Fig. 2). The corresponding homeostatic pressure to counteract this loss may proceed without preservation of the TCR repertoire. Indeed, CD8 T-cell clonal expansions emerge early in life and continue to accumulate with age [67]. As depicted in Fig. 4b, clonal expansions are much less common and occur later in life with the CD4 T-cell compartment [68]. While many

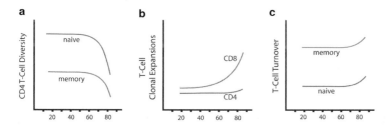

Fig. 4   Changes in T-cell Heterogeneity and Turnover with Age (a) Schematic representation of CD4 TCR repertoire collapse after age 65. (b) Schematic representation of accumulation of CD4 and CD8 T-cell clonal expansions with age. (c) Schematic representation of increased peripheral T-cell turnover late in life

expanded clones come from the memory compartment, naïve TCR clones may each respond differently to increased homeostatic stimuli, and unbalanced proliferation may compromise the diversity of the dwindling naïve compartment. Future studies that directly assess naïve CD8 T-cell diversity are needed to more fully appreciate the consequences of age on the naïve T-cell pool.

In the absence of new thymic T-cell production, naïve CD4 TCR diversity is maintained until the seventh decade of life. Similarly, the naïve CD8 T-cell population, while experiencing a steadier decline in numbers and probably diversity, is remarkably stable for many years after thymic involution. Why, after years of successful repertoire preservation, does this maintenance begin to fail? One possibility is that, with a minimal influx of new T cells from the thymus, peripheral homeostatic mechanisms are capable of maintaining a diverse repertoire [69]. In this case, the collapse of naïve diversity after age [65] may follow the *absolute* end of thymic production, thereby overwhelming homeostatic mechanisms.

Alternatively, evidence from humans and nonhuman primates points to a failure of homeostasis late in life. For both human naïve CD4 T cells [19] and rhesus macaque naïve CD4 and CD8 T cells [70], T-cell turnover significantly increased in old individuals (depicted for humans in Fig. 4c). In macaques, the increases proliferation seems to be a reaction to increased cell loss. In fact, animals with the smallest naïve compartments experience the most dramatic cell turnover. As the authors suggest [70], declining naïve T-cell numbers trigger a compensatory, yet inadequate, proliferation to refill the compartment. This stimulus exacerbates the problem by shifting naïve cells to a memory phenotype, thereby further depleting naïve numbers. Thus, the very mechanism for preserving the naïve population may contribute to its ultimate demise by creating a feedback loop that overwhelms the homeostatic capacity of elderly individuals. The factors leading to declining T-cell diversity in the elderly are depicted in Fig. 5.

5   Implications of Diversity Loss

A wide array of unique TCR within the naïve T-cell compartment is necessary to protect against an unpredictable and diverse antigen pool. Without a naïve response, many ubiquitous and benign infections would be deadly. Emerging neoplastic cells, whose presence would normally be detected by naïve T cells, could survive for the time required to accumulate the additional mutations needed for malignancy. Effective vaccinations require the long-lived memory cells that remain following activation and expansion of naïve T cells specific for the target antigen. Additionally, existing T-cell memory, from past infections or vaccines, must persist to prevent reactivation of chronic infections or reinfection by a familiar pathogen. It seems clear that the elderly, who face a steady decline in naïve T-cells and a dramatic collapse of naïve and memory T-cell repertoire diversity late in life, should respond poorly to challenges requiring full T-cell function. Although infections, cancer, and poor vaccine responses disproportionately affect the very old, it is difficult to assess

a. 20-year-old adult

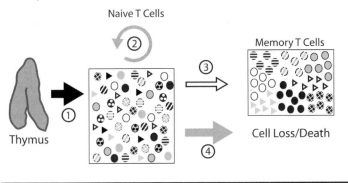

b. 80-year-old adult

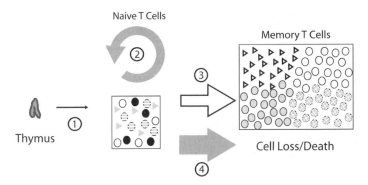

Fig. 5 Determinants of Naive T-cell Diversity (a) Young adult human. 1- A steady supply of new naive T cells continually adds to TCR repertoire. 2- Existing naive T cells proliferate in response to daily cell loss. 3- Exposure to antigen shifts naive clones to the memory compartment. 4- Naive T cells are lost to cell death or attrition. (b) Elderly adult human. 1- Thymus no longer contributes new naive T cells. 2- Declining naive T-cell numbers result in severe homeostatic pressure to proliferate. 3- In addition to antigen exposure, naive T cells shift to memory phenotype because of excessive homeostatic expansion. 4- Naive T-cell death is accelerated due to exhaustion from strong proliferative pressures. Black arrows—promotes diversity of naive TCR repertoire; Black-outlined arrows—depletes naive TCR repertoire; gray arrows—can have neutral and/or detrimental effects on naive TCR repertoire

how much of this is due to a loss of TCR diversity. Several examples of decreased T-cell repertoire in mice and humans hint at the importance of a diverse response.

Many natural and experimentally manipulated genetic backgrounds in mice result in contracted T-cell repertoires. These settings have been used to assess how reduced TCR availability affects immune responses. NZW mice and strains with the tcr^a haplotype (e.g. C57L) lack certain elements of the TCRB locus [NZW: deletion of $C_{\beta1}$, $D_{\beta2}$, and all $J_{\beta2}$ segments (71); tcr^a: deletion of five V_β segments and altered $V_\beta10$ sequence (72)] resulting in a 50–60% reduction in potential TCR. T cells from these mice exhibit reduced ex vivo responsiveness after immunization against some, but not all, tested antigens. TdT-deficient mice are unable to diversify D-J, V-J, and V-DJ junctions during TCR gene rearrangement resulting in a ~90% repertoire contraction. Interestingly, these mice are fully protected from lymphocytic choriomeningitis virus and Sendai virus infections [73]. Although other challenges have not been examined, it is clear that a limited repertoire is capable of enough cross-reactivity to control certain pathogens.

Gene targeting of TCR loci reduces TCR diversity even more dramatically than deletion of the TdT enzyme. For example, all T cells from the TCR OT-1β transgenic mouse express the same TCR β-chain (specific for an OVA peptide when expressed with the OT-1α-chain) and, therefore, all TCR diversity results from TCRA gene rearrangement. In the context of this dramatic repertoire contraction (>98%), these mice are unable to reject allogeneic bone marrow [74]. Other experiments using a different TCR β-chain transgenic strain have shown that some antigen-specific responses are not absent, merely different [75]. After immunization with the bacteriophage protein cl, splenic T cells from both TCR β chain transgenic mice and wild-type littermates responded ex vivo to the cl protein. When challenged with peptides derived from cl, wild-type splenocytes responded most strongly to the peptide known to be immunodominant. In contrast, transgenic mice responded more strongly to a different peptide that yielded no response in wild-type splenocytes. Interestingly, both strains of mice were equally capable of a strong response to both peptides when the peptide, rather than whole cl protein, was the immunizing antigen. Therefore, it seems the severe repertoire contraction in these TCR β-chain transgenic mice created a shift of immunodominance without creating a "hole" in the repertoire. That is to say, T cells from these mice *can* respond well to the classical immunodominant peptide but, when faced with the full protein antigen, expand more readily against a different peptide.

From the above examples, it is clear that the requirement for TCR diversity in the mouse is context dependent. This is most likely true for humans too, although direct examination of repertoire contraction in humans is more difficult. A single patient with a partial X-linked severe combined immunodeficiency (Xid) reversion has provided a rare glimpse at the in vivo consequences of TCR contraction in humans. Although family and clinical history and gene sequencing suggested the patient had Xid, a disease caused by the genetic lack of a functional cytokine common γ-chain [76], he had a nearly full-sized T-cell compartment [77]. The Xid mutation usually blocks T-cell development by preventing IL-2 signaling. In this patient, a compensating somatic mutation in the common γ-chain gene occurred in a single T-cell precursor allowing descendants of this cell to undergo normal thymic development. Immunoscope analysis at age 3 revealed that extensive post-thymic expansion of an estimated 25,000 distinct TCR clones managed to fill the T-cell compartment [78]. In vitro challenge of T cells with a variety of antigens revealed blunted responsiveness. While some in vivo T-cell functions, such as a skin test for the BCG vaccine, were intact, it is unclear if these responses would be protective in the face of a pathogen challenge [78]. Subsequent follow-up has not been reported, and it remains to be seen if this patient will be at increased risk of immune deficiency in the future.

An in vivo Hepatitis C virus study in chimpanzees revealed a setting where the antigen-specific CD8 T-cell repertoire predicted the outcome of infection [79]. A cohort of animals were all inoculated with an identical strain of virus and followed. Some animals exhibited a diverse array of TCR antigen-binding domains within virus-specific T cells while other responses were more homogeneous. Those animals with a narrow repertoire among responding T cells were more likely to carry viral escape mutants and to never clear the infection. This homogeneity preceded viral escape and persisted after a response was mounted to the new mutants. Presumably, animals with more diverse responses were able to respond to viral mutations as they arose, thus preventing expansion of novel epitopes. These findings highlight the contribution of TCR diversity to a flexible immune response capable of adapting to pathogens that evolve during an infection.

Indirect evidence from studies of human aging suggests that age-related repertoire collapse may indeed have detrimental effects on survival. A longitudinal examination of octogenarians in Sweden revealed an "immune risk phenotype" (IRP) that predicted 2-year mortality. Individuals with the IRP, which was originally defined as inversion of the CD4:CD8 ratio (normal is >1; IRP is <1) and decreased in vitro T-cell proliferation, were more likely to die within the 2-year follow-up period compared to non-IRP individuals [80]. Additionally, the prevalence of the IRP doubled from 16 to 32% over the 2 years. A subsequent study showed that a decreased CD4: CD8 ratio alone is an adequate marker of the IRP and its accompanying increased mortality risk [81]. Importantly, as the proportion of CD8 cells increases, the contribution to total CD8 T cells comes from fewer and fewer clonotypes [26]. Thus, in this elderly population, the individuals with the least diverse CD8 populations were more likely to die during the 2-year study period. While the direct cause of increased mortality is unknown, this correlation is consistent with other studies linking CD8 clonal expansions to decreased EBV [82] and influenza responses [83, 84].

Interestingly, a more recent report following the nonagenarians found that those individuals who reach the age of 100 are free from the IRP and have T cells more similar to middle-aged individuals than even the younger-elderly [85]). For example, the CD4:CD8 ratios of centenarians are not only >1 but are consistently more CD4-heavy than even individuals in their early nineties. Additionally, centenarians had fewer CD8$^+$CD28$^-$ T cells, by absolute numbers and as percent of total CD8 T cells, than younger-elderly. As the authors suggest, the collective characteristics of the centenarian population obviously excludes those individuals who have died and, therefore, may represent features of "successful aging." For this reason, a longitudinal examination of T-cell repertoires in the very old may contribute to our understanding of the requirement of TCR diversity for longevity. Can TCR diversity within various T-cell compartments predict mortality as successfully as the IRP? Do the successfully-aged exhibit the dramatic collapse of the naïve CD4 repertoire that we have found in individuals after age 75? Answers to questions like these will help clarify the true in vivo importance of declining TCR diversity with age.

References

1. Bhandoola A, H von Boehmer, HT Petrie, JC Zuniga-Pflucker (2007) Commitment and developmental potential of extrathymic and intrathymic T-cell precursors: plenty to choose from. Immunity 26:678–689
2. Blom B, P Res, E Noteboom, K. Weijer, H Spits (1997) Prethymic CD34+ progenitors capable of developing into T cells are not committed to the T-cell lineage. J Immunol 158:3571–3577
3. Galy A, S Verma, A Barcena, H Spits (1993) Precursors of CD3+CD4+CD8+ cells in the human thymus are defined by expression of CD34. Delineation of early events in human thymic development. J Exp Med 178:391–401
4. Blom B, MC Verschuren, MH Heemskerk, AQ Bakker, EJ van Gastel-Mol, IL Wolvers-Tettero, JJ van Dongen, H Spits (1999) TCR gene rearrangements and expression of the pre-T-cell receptor complex during human T-cell differentiation. Blood 93:3033–3043
5. Pui JC, D Allman, L Xu, S DeRocco, FG Karnell, S Bakkour, JY Lee, T Kadesch, RR Hardy, JC Aster, WS Pear (1999) Notch1 expression in early lymphopoiesis influences B versus T lineage determination. Immunity 11:299–308
6. van Dongen JJ, WM Comans-Bitter, L Wolvers-Tettero, J Borst (1990) Development of human T-lymphocytes and their thymus-dependency. Thymus 16:207–234
7. Davis MM, PJ Bjorkman (1988) T-cell antigen receptor genes and T-cell recognition. Nature 334:395–402
8. Spits H (2002) Development of alphabeta T cells in the human thymus. Nat Rev 2:760–772
9. Wilson A, W Held, HR MacDonald (1994) Two waves of recombinase gene expression in developing thymocytes. J Exp Med 179:1355–1360
10. Krangel MS (2003) Gene segment selection in V(D)J recombination: accessibility and beyond. Nat Immunol 4:624–630
11. Benedict CL, S Gilfillan, TH Thai, JF Kearney (2000) Terminal deoxynucleotidyl transferase and repertoire development. Immunol Rev 175:150–157
12. von Boehmer H (2005) Unique features of the pre-T-cell receptor alpha-chain: not just a surrogate. Nat Rev 5:571–577
13. Trigueros C, AR Ramiro, YR Carrasco, VG de Yebenes, JP Albar, ML Toribio (1998) Identification of a late stage of small noncycling pTalpha—pre-T cells as immediate precursors of T-cell receptor alpha/beta+ thymocytes. J Exp Med 188:1401–1412
14. Petrie HT, F Livak, DG Schatz, A Strasser, IN Crispe, K Shortman (1993) Multiple rearrangements in T-cell receptor alpha chain genes maximize the production of useful thymocytes. J Exp Med 178:615–622
15. Brandle D, C Muller, T Rulicke, H Hengartner, H Pircher (1992) Engagement of the T-cell receptor during positive selection in the thymus down-regulates RAG-1 expression. Proc Natl Acad Sci U S A 89:9529–9533
16. Palmer E 2003 Negative selection—clearing out the bad apples from the T-cell repertoire. Nat Rev 3:383–391
17. Fagnoni FF, R Vescovini, G Passeri, G Bologna, M Pedrazzoni, G Lavagetto, A Casti, C Franceschi, M Passeri, P Sansoni (2000) Shortage of circulating naive CD8(+) T cells provides new insights on immunodeficiency in aging. Blood 95:2860–2868
18. Hong MS, JM Dan, JY Choi, I Kang (2004) Age-associated changes in the frequency of naive, memory and effector CD8+ T cells. Mech Ageing Dev 125:615–618
19. Naylor K, G Li, AN Vallejo, WW Lee, K Koetz, E Bryl, J Witkowski, J Fulbright, CM Weyand, JJ Goronzy (2005) The influence of age on T-cell generation and TCR diversity. J Immunol 174:7446–7452
20. Sallusto F, D Lenig, R Forster, M Lipp, A Lanzavecchia (1999) Two subsets of memory T-lymphocytes with distinct homing potentials and effector functions. Nature 401:708–712
21. Lanzavecchia A, F Sallusto (2000) Dynamics of T-lymphocyte responses: intermediates, effectors, and memory cells. Science (New York, N.Y) 290:92–97

22. Jacob J, D Baltimore (1999) Modelling T-cell memory by genetic marking of memory T cells in vivo. Nature 399:593–597
23. Opferman JT, BT Ober, PG Ashton-Rickardt (1999) Linear differentiation of cytotoxic effectors into memory T-lymphocytes. Science (New York, N.Y) 283:1745–1748
24. Faint JM, NE Annels, SJ Curnow, P Shields, D Pilling, A D Hislop, L Wu, AN Akbar, CD Buckley, PA Moss, DH Adams, A B Rickinson, M Salmon (2001) Memory T cells constitute a subset of the human CD8+CD45RA+ pool with distinct phenotypic and migratory characteristics. J Immunol 167:212–220
25. Van Den Beemd R, PP Boor, EG van Lochem, WC Hop, AW Langerak, IL Wolvers-Tettero, H Hooijkaas, JJ van Dongen (2000) Flow cytometric analysis of the Vbeta repertoire in healthy controls. Cytometry 40:336–345
26. Hadrup SR, J Strindhall, T Kollgaard, T Seremet, B Johansson, G Pawelec, P thor Straten, A Wikby (2006) Longitudinal studies of clonally expanded CD8 T cells reveal a repertoire shrinkage predicting mortality and an increased number of dysfunctional cytomegalovirus-specific T cells in the very elderly. J Immunol 176:2645–2653
27. Even J, A Lim, I Puisieux, L Ferradini, PY Dietrich, A Toubert, T Hercend, F Triebel, C Pannetier, P Kourilsky (1995) T-cell repertoires in healthy and diseased human tissues analysed by T-cell receptor beta-chain CDR3 size determination: evidence for oligoclonal expansions in tumours and inflammatory diseases. Res Immunol 146:65–80
28. Arstila T P, A Casrouge, V Baron, J Even, J Kanellopoulos, P Kourilsky (1999) A direct estimate of the human alphabeta T-cell receptor diversity. Science New York, N.Y 286:958–961
29. Wagner UG, K Koetz, CM Weyand, JJ Goronzy (1998) Perturbation of the T-cell repertoire in rheumatoid arthritis. Proc Natl Acad Sci U S A 95:14447–14452
30. Taub DD, DL Longo (2005) Insights into thymic aging and regeneration. Immunol Rev 205:72–93
31. Livak F, DG Schatz (1996) T-cell receptor alpha locus V(D)J recombination by-products are abundant in thymocytes and mature T cells. Mol Cell Biol 16:609–618
32. de Villartay JP, RD Hockett, D Coran, SJ Korsmeyer, DI Cohen (1988) Deletion of the human T-cell receptor delta-gene by a site-specific recombination. Nature 335:170–174
33. Hazenberg MD, MC Verschuren, D Hamann, F Miedema, JJ van Dongen (2001) T-cell receptor excision circles as markers for recent thymic emigrants: basic aspects, technical approach, and guidelines for interpretation. J Mol Med (Berlin, Germany) 79:631–640
34. Douek DC, RD McFarland, PH Keiser, EA Gage, JM Massey, BF Haynes, MA Polis, AT Haase, MB Feinberg, JL Sullivan, BD Jamieson, JA Zack, LJ Picker, R A Koup (1998) Changes in thymic function with age and during the treatment of HIV infection. Nature 396:690–695
35. Koetz K, E Bryl, K Spickschen, WM O'Fallon, JJ Goronzy, CM Weyand (2000) T-cell homeostasis in patients with rheumatoid arthritis. Proc Natl Acad Sci U S A 97:9203–9208
36. Poulin JF, MN Viswanathan, JM Harris, KV Komanduri, E Wieder, N Ringuette, M Jenkins, J M McCune, R P Sekaly (1999) Direct evidence for thymic function in adult humans. J Exp Med 190:479–486
37. Flores KG, J Li, GD Sempowski, BF Haynes, L P Hale (1999) Analysis of the human thymic perivascular space during aging. J Clin Invest 104:1031–1039
38. Steinmann GG, B Klaus, HK Muller-Hermelink (1985) The involution of the ageing human thymic epithelium is independent of puberty. A morphometric study. Scand J Immunol 22:563–575
39. Jamieson BD, DC Douek, S Killian, LE Hultin, DD Scripture-Adams, JV Giorgi, D Marelli, R A Koup, J A Zack (1999) Generation of functional thymocytes in the human adult. Immunity 10:569–575
40. Hakim FT, SA Memon, R Cepeda, EC Jones, CK Chow, C Kasten-Sportes, J Odom, BA Vance, BL Christensen, CL Mackall, RE Gress (2005) Age-dependent incidence, time course, and consequences of thymic renewal in adults. J Clin Invest 115:930–939
41. Kimmig S, G K Przybylski, CA Schmidt, KLaurisch, B Mowes, A Radbruch, A Thiel (2002) Two subsets of naive T-helper cells with distinct T-cell receptor excision circle content in human adult peripheral blood. J Exp Med 195:789–794

42. Gerdes J, H Lemke, H Baisch, HH Wacker, U Schwab, H Stein (1984) Cell cycle analysis of a cell proliferation-associated human nuclear antigen defined by the monoclonal antibody Ki-67. J Immunol 133:1710–1715

43. Betts MR, JM Brenchley, DA Price, SC De Rosa, DC Douek, M Roederer, RA Koup (2003) Sensitive and viable identification of antigen-specific CD8+ T cells by a flow cytometric assay for degranulation. J Immunol Methods 281:65–78

44. Hazenberg MD, JW Stuart, SA Otto, JC Borleffs, CA Boucher, RJ de Boer, F Miedema, D Hamann (2000) T-cell division in human immunodeficiency virus (HIV)-1 infection is mainly due to immune activation: a longitudinal analysis in patients before and during highly active antiretroviral therapy (HAART). Blood 95:249–255

45. Schonland SO, JK Zimmer, CM Lopez-Benitez, T Widmann, KD Ramin, JJ Goronzy, CM Weyand (2003) Homeostatic control of T-cell generation in neonates. Blood 102:1428–1434

46. Macallan DC, B Asquith, AJ Irvine, DL Wallace, A Worth, H Ghattas, Y Zhang, GE Griffin, DF Tough, P C Beverley (2003) Measurement and modeling of human T-cell kinetics. Eur J Immunol 33:2316–2326

47. Macallan DC, CA Fullerton, RA Neese, K Haddock, SS Park, MK Hellerstein (1998) Measurement of cell proliferation by labeling of DNA with stable isotope-labeled glucose: studies in vitro, in animals, and in humans. Proc Natl Acad Sci U S A 95:708–713

48. Neese RA, LM Misell, S Turner, A Chu, J Kim, D Cesar, R Hoh, F Antelo, A Strawford, JM McCune, M Christiansen, MK Hellerstein (2002) Measurement in vivo of proliferation rates of slow turnover cells by 2H2O labeling of the deoxyribose moiety of DNA. Proc Natl Acad Sci U S A 99:15345–15350

49. Wallace DL, Y Zhang, H Ghattas, A Worth, A Irvine, AR Bennett, GE Griffin, PC Beverley, DF Tough, DC Macallan. (2004) Direct measurement of T-cell subset kinetics in vivo in elderly men and women. J Immunol 173:1787–1794

50. Hellerstein M, MB Hanley, D Cesar, S Siler, C Papageorgopoulos, E Wieder, D Schmidt, R Hoh, R Neese, D Macallan, S Deeks, JM McCune (1999) Directly measured kinetics of circulating T-lymphocytes in normal and HIV-1-infected humans. Nat Med 5:83–89

51. Murray JM, GR Kaufmann, PD Hodgkin, SR Lewin, AD Kelleher, MP Davenport, JJ Zaunders (2003) Naive T cells are maintained by thymic output in early ages but by proliferation without phenotypic change after age twenty. Immunol Cell Biol 81:487–495

52. Brocker T (1997) Survival of mature CD4 T-lymphocytes is dependent on major histocompatibility complex class II-expressing dendritic cells. J Exp Med 186:1223–1232

53. Kirberg J, A Berns, H von Boehmer (1997) Peripheral T-cell survival requires continual ligation of the T-cell receptor to major histocompatibility complex-encoded molecules. J Exp Med 186:1269–1275

54. Tanchot C, FA Lemonnier, B Perarnau, AA Freitas, B Rocha (1997) Differential requirements for survival and proliferation of CD8 naive or memory T cells. Science (New York, N.Y) 276:2057–2062

55. Murali-Krishna K, LL Lau, S Sambhara, F Lemonnier, J Altman, R Ahmed (1999) Persistence of memory CD8 T cells in MHC class I-deficient mice. Science (New York, N.Y) 286:1377–1381

56. Ge Q, VP Rao, BK Cho, HN Eisen, J Chen (2001) Dependence of lymphopenia-induced T-cell proliferation on the abundance of peptide/ MHC epitopes and strength of their interaction with T-cell receptors. Proc Natl Acad Sci U S A 98:1728–1733

57. Wang Q, J Strong, N Killeen (2001) Homeostatic competition among T cells revealed by conditional inactivation of the mouse Cd4 gene. J Exp Med 194:1721–1730

58. Jameson SC (2002) Maintaining the norm: T-cell homeostasis. Nat Rev 2:547–556

59. Tan JT, E Dudl, E LeRoy, R Murray, J Sprent, KI Weinberg, C D Surh (2001) IL-7 is critical for homeostatic proliferation and survival of naive T cells. Proc Natl Acad Sci U S A 98:8732–8737

60. Geginat J, A Lanzavecchia, F Sallusto (2003) Proliferation and differentiation potential of human CD8+ memory T-cell subsets in response to antigen or homeostatic cytokines. Blood 101:4260–4266

61. Hazenberg MD, SA Otto, JW Cohen Stuart, MC Verschuren, JC Borleffs, CA Boucher, RA Coutinho, JM Lange, TF Rinke deWit, A Tsegaye, JJ van Dongen, D Hamann, RJ de Boer, F Miedema (2000) Increased cell division but not thymic dysfunction rapidly affects the T-cell receptor excision circle content of the naive T-cell population in HIV-1 infection. Nat Med 6:1036–1042

62. Goronzy JJ, WW Lee, CM Weyand (2007) Aging and T-cell diversity. Exp Gerontol 42:400–406

63. Czesnikiewicz-Guzik M, WW Lee, D Cui, Y Hiruma, DL Lamar, ZZ Yang, JG Ouslander, C M Weyand, JJ Goronzy (2008) T-cell subset-specific susceptibility to aging. Clin Immunol 127:107-118

64. Effros RB, N Boucher, V Porter, X Zhu, C Spaulding, RL Walford, M Kronenberg, D Cohen, F Schachter (1994) Decline in CD28+ T cells in centenarians and in long-term T-cell cultures: a possible cause for both in vivo and in vitro immunosenescence. Exp Gerontol 29:601–609

65. Colonna M, F Navarro, T Bellon, M Llano, P Garcia, J Samaridis, L Angman, M Cella, M Lopez-Botet (1997) A common inhibitory receptor for major histocompatibility complex class I molecules on human lymphoid and myelomonocytic cells. J Exp Med 186:1809–1818

66. Jankovic V, I Messaoudi, J Nikolich-Zugich (2003) Phenotypic and functional T-cell aging in rhesus macaques (Macaca mulatta): differential behavior of CD4 and CD8 subsets. Blood 102:3244–3251

67. Ricalton NS, C Roberton, JM Norris, M Rewers, RF Hamman, BL Kotzin (1998) Prevalence of CD8+ T-cell expansions in relation to age in healthy individuals. J Gerontol 53: B196–B203

68. Wack A, A Cossarizza, S Heltai, D Barbieri, S D'Addato, C Franceschi, P Dellabona, G Casorati (1998) Age-related modifications of the human alphabeta T-cell repertoire due to different clonal expansions in the CD4+ and CD8+ subsets. Int Immunol 10:1281–1288

69. Goronzy JJ, CM Weyand (2005) T-cell development and receptor diversity during aging. Curr Opin Immunol 17:468–475

70. Cicin-Sain L, I Messaoudi, B Park, N Currier, S Planer, M Fischer, S Tackitt, D Nikolich-Zugich, A Legasse, MK Axthelm, LJ Picker, M Mori, J Nikolich-Zugich (2007) Dramatic increase in naive T-cell turnover is linked to loss of naive T cells from old primates. Proc Natl Acad Sci U S A 104:19960–19965

71. Kotzin BL, VL Barr, E. Palmer (1985) A large deletion within the T-cell receptor beta-chain gene complex in New Zealand white mice. Science (New York, N.Y) 229:167–171

72. Nanda NK, R Apple, E Sercarz (1991) Limitations in plasticity of the T-cell receptor repertoire. Proc Natl Acad Sci U S A 88:9503–9507

73. Gilfillan S, A Dierich, M Lemeur, C Benoist, D Mathis (1993) Mice lacking TdT: mature animals with an immature lymphocyte repertoire. Science (New York, N.Y) 261:1175–1178

74. Kikly K, G Dennert (1992) Evidence for a role for T-cell receptors (TCR) in the effector phase of acute bone marrow graft rejection. TCR V beta 5 transgenic mice lack effector cells able to cause graft rejection. J Immunol 149:3489–3494

75. Perkins DL, YS Wang, D Fruman, JG Seidman, IJ Rimm (1991) Immunodominance is altered in T-cell receptor (beta-chain) transgenic mice without the generation of a hole in the repertoire. J Immunol 146:2960–2964

76. Noguchi M, H Yi, HM Rosenblatt, AH Filipovich, S Adelstein, WS Modi, OW McBride, W J Leonard (1993) Interleukin-2 receptor gamma chain mutation results in X-linked severe combined immunodeficiency in humans. Cell 73:147–157

77. Stephan V, V Wahn, F Le Deist, U Dirksen, B Broker, I Muller-Fleckenstein, G Horneff, H Schroten, A Fischer, G de Saint Basile (1996) Atypical X-linked severe combined immunodeficiency due to possible spontaneous reversion of the genetic defect in T cells. N Engl J Med 335:1563–1567

78. Bousso P, V Wahn, I Douagi, G Horneff, C Pannetier, F Le Deist, F Zepp, T Niehues, P Kourilsky, A Fischer, G de Saint Basile (2000) Diversity, functionality, and stability of the T-cell repertoire derived in vivo from a single human T-cell precursor. Proc Natl Acad Sci U S A 97:274–278

79. Meyer-Olson D, NH Shoukry, KW Brady, H Kim, DP Olson, K Hartman, AK Shintani, CM Walker, SA Kalams (2004) Limited T-cell receptor diversity of HCV-specific T-cell responses is associated with CTL escape. J Exp Med 200:307–319

80. Ferguson FG, A Wikby, P Maxson, J Olsson, B Johansson (1995) Immune parameters in a longitudinal study of a very old population of Swedish people: a comparison between survivors and nonsurvivors. J Gerontol 50:B378–B382

81. Wikby A, P Maxson, J Olsson, B Johansson, FG Ferguson (1998) Changes in CD8 and CD4 lymphocyte subsets, T-cell proliferation responses and non-survival in the very old: the Swedish longitudinal OCTO-immune study. Mech Ageing Dev 102:187–198

82. Khan N, A Hislop, N Gudgeon, M Cobbold, R Khanna, L Nayak, A B Rickinson, PA Moss (2004) Herpesvirus-specific CD8 T-cell immunity in old age: cytomegalovirus impairs the response to a coresident EBV infection. J Immunol 173:7481–7489

83. Goronzy JJ, JW Fulbright, CS Crowson, GA Poland, W. M. O'Fallon, and CM Weyand. (2001) Value of immunological markers in predicting responsiveness to influenza vaccination in elderly individuals. J Virol 75:12182–12187

84. Trzonkowski P, J Mysliwska, E Szmit, J Wieckiewicz, K Lukaszuk, LB Brydak, M Machala, A Mysliwski (2003) Association between cytomegalovirus infection, enhanced proinflammatory response and low level of anti-hemagglutinins during the anti-influenza vaccination—an impact of immunosenescence. Vaccine 21:3826–3836

85. Strindhall J, BO Nilsson, S Lofgren, J Ernerudh, G Pawelec, B Johansson, A Wikby (2007) No immune risk profile among individuals who reach 100 years of age: findings from the Swedish NONA immune longitudinal study. Exp Gerontol 42:753–761

The Role of T-regulatory Cells in Immune Senescence

Paul Moss

Contents

1   Introduction

T-regulatory cells have come to dominate immunology over the last decade [1]. The ability of cellular components of the immune system to suppress immune function was noticed more than 20 years ago and was recognized by a number of highly cited publications [2]. However, the lack of a specific phenotype for these cells, and an inability to document precise physiological mechanisms for their action, limited their investigation by detailed experimental study. The pioneering work of Sakaguchi and colleagues reestablished regulatory cells and has generated a field of research that extends into all areas of clinical immunology, including immune senescence [3].

At first sight, the concept that the immune system must require some form of cellular control of immune activation is surely no surprise. There are very few physiological systems that can proceed without any form of feedback mechanism and it is now appreciated that there are many different subsets of regulatory cells involved in immune haemostasis. By far the most widely recognized is a CD4+ T-cell population that expresses high levels of CD25. The CD4+CD25+ subset has become the prototypic "T-regulatory" cell in both murine and human studies and has provided the basis for many thousands of publications. However, the fact that CD25 is also expressed on all activated effector T-cells has lead to the quest for a "third marker" that will provide a more definitive and unique phenotype for the regulatory population. Several of these molecules have been suggested over recent years, including

P. Moss (✉)
Institute for Cancer Studies
University of Birmingham, Vincent Drive
Birmingham B15 2TT, UK
E-mail: p.moss@bham.ac.uk

T. Fulop et al. (eds.), *Handbook on Immunosenescence*,
DOI 10.1007/978-1-4020-9062-2_10, © Springer Science+Business Media B.V. 2009

GITR and low expression of CD127. However, it is the transcription factor FOXP3 that has emerged as the most reliable marker for this functional subset [4, 5] (Fig. 1). FOXP3 is a member of an important family of transcription factors that are involved in processes such as language development and which seem to have a central role in development of developmental functions. This is supported by observations in mice deficient in FOXP3 gene function, which develop an autoimmune condition secondary to unregulated immune responses. Even more compelling are the findings in rare human individuals that were born without FOXP3 function and suffer from an unusual syndrome of autoimmune disease dominated by inflammation of endocrine organs. Although there is some evidence that FOXP3 may be up-regulated on activation of effector T-cells in humans, most authors now agree that this marker is a valid and reliable marker of functional regulatory phenotype across both species. Unfortunately, one concern with the use of FOXP3 is that its detection requires the permeabilisation of cells and therefore renders cells unviable for further downstream analysis. For this reason, a surface membrane phenotype which would allow for the cloning and isolation of regulatory cells would provide a significant boost to this area of research. In 2006 low level expression of CD127 emerged as a good marker of FoxP3 expression in regulatory CD4+ T-cells [6, 7]. CD39 is the most recently evaluated phenotypic marker and is positively associated with FoxP3 expression [8].

The mechanism of action of T-regulatory cells remains the subject of active investigation and it is perhaps fair to say that no consensus has emerged on this topic. Some regulatory populations appear to secrete immunosuppressive cytokines such as IL10 or TGFβ but these properties are not documented in all subsets. Cytotoxic activity has also being observed in some experiments. The target cells for T-regulatory function are also uncertain, as it appears that regulatory cells can act both at the level of antigen presenting cells, and therefore modulate induction of immune responses, as well as act directly on effector cells.

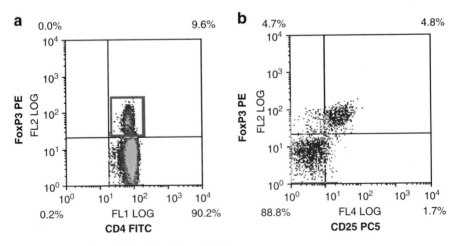

Fig. 1 Phenotypic analysis of regulatory T cells
a. The characteristic phenotype is of CD4+FoxP3+ cells. b. FoxP3 expression correlates with high expression of CD25.

2 The Origin of T-regulatory Cells: Thymically-derived or Generated in the Periphery?

Much has been made of the concept that most regulatory cells are derived by a discrete developmental pathway within the thymus which leads to a committed population of "natural" regulatory cells which never have the capacity to act as typical effector populations. Whilst much of this work has, necessarily, been performed in murine models, it has been much more difficult to determine that this is the case within human individuals. Interestingly, studies from both young and aged mice have shown that CD4+ FoxP3+ T-cells are found in both cohorts with some evidence of increased production during ageing. This raises the question as to whether CD4+ FoxP3+ T-cells continue to be produced by the human thymus throughout life. At first sight this might be considered unlikely given the well documented process of thymic involution that occurs during healthy human ageing, although it should be appreciated that the deterioration in naïve T-cell output is much more marked for the CD8+ population in comparison to CD4+ subsets. The reason for this last observation has never been entirely explained and could conceivably be partly explained by some contribution of ongoing CD4+ regulatory production.

However, it is also now clear that T-regulatory cells can be induced within the peripheral immune system by derivation from naïve or effector CD25- T-cell populations [9] (Fig. 2). The conditions that give rise to the generation of regulatory

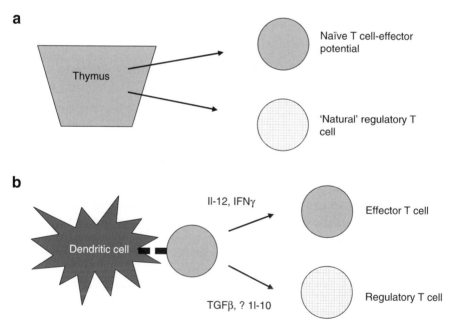

Fig. 2 Model for generation of T regulatory cells
Regulatory cells might arise from (a) a discrete pathway of differentiation through the thymus or (b) be induced from naïve T cell populations during T cell priming.

cells have not been entirely resolved, but are likely to involve microenvironmental signals including the presence of immunosuppressive molecules such as TGFβ and Il-10 at the time of dendritic cell priming of T-cell effector molecules [10]. When present during the first 3 days of T-cell priming the presence of TGFβ can induce FoxP3 expression in up to 90% of responding T-cells and this expression can be sustained for long periods of time in at least a subset of this population [11]. This mechanism of T-regulatory cell production is likely to become increasingly important during ageing of human populations. Given the longevity of humans and the well characterized involution of thymic function that occurs, it would appear highly unlikely that a discrete pathway of thymic maturation could provide the only source of T-regulatory cell production in adult life. Moreover, recent evidence has emerged to suggest that the turnover of T-regulatory cells is actually surprisingly short and that these cells are a highly proliferative population with short telomeres and great susceptibility to apoptosis [12]. Taken together, this evidence does strongly suggest that the peripheral production of T-regulatory cells within the immune system is a powerful factor in their generation. The site of origin of regulatory cell induction is also likely to be important in the functional properties of the mature cell as evidence is accumulating that extrathymic maturation is associated with impaired proliferative potential [13].

The number of CD4+ regulatory cells within the human immune system is variable depending both on the precise definition of such cells, the age of the individual and any underlying disease processes. Typically, between 2 and 5% CD4+ T-cells will express a CD25+ or FoxP3+ phenotype and further studies are required to show whether these numbers are influenced by any genetic or environmental factors.

3 T-regulatory Cell Populations During Healthy Ageing

An important question in relation to immune senescence is how the number and function of T-regulatory cells is influenced by physiological ageing, both in humans and in murine models. T-regulatory function certainly appears to be required throughout life and depletion of FoxP3+ T-cells in mice leads to a breakdown of self-tolerance at all ages [14]. Within murine systems, a number of investigators have shown an apparent increase in the number of CD4+ FoxP3+ T-cells in aged mice. CD4+FoxP3+ T-cell numbers can increase early in murine development with the BDC2.5NOD mouse showing an increase between the age of 6 and 18 weeks. However a 4 month old mouse is not aged in terms of the natural murine lifespan so this observation has limited relevance to studies of immune senescence. Zhao et al. studied Balb/c mice that were over 20 months of age and therefore represented a physiologically aged cohort [15]. In a comprehensive study they showed that the number of CD4+CD25+FoxP3+ T-cells increased with age in virtually all lymphoid compartments. However, the regulatory function of these cells did show some deficiencies in comparison to cells from young mice. In particular there was reduced inhibition of cytokine production by effector cells despite comparable suppression of proliferation. It is interesting that the proportion of natural T-regulatory cells within the thymus can also increase during ageing suggesting that this mechanism may continue to make a contribution to peripheral accumulation [16]. Thymic-regulatory cells from elderly mice were able to suppress effector T-cells from young animals with similar efficiency to regulatory cells from younger mice. However, their ability to suppress effector cells from elderly mice was impaired indicating some functional differences between cells from young and older animals.

Sakaguchi's group has also addressed accumulation of T-regulatory cells during murine ageing and identified only a marginal increase in natural CD4+CD25+FoxP3+ T-cells. In contrast, increased levels of FoxP3 expression were seen in the CD4+CD25- population and identified a population with hyporesponsive function [17]. Their interpretation was that decreased immune function during ageing was primarily a reflection of a decrease in effector cell function rather than regulatory cell accumulation [18]. Comparable findings have been demonstrated in human subjects.

A number of studies are now addressing the number and function of T-regulatory cells in adult human populations. Our own data published in 2005 used CD4+CD25^{high}+CD45RO+ membrane phenotype as a marker of regulatory cell function [19]. Somewhat to our surprise at that time, we observed a significant increase in the regulatory T-cell population during ageing. In addition, we showed that the functional activity of these populations was also maintained during the ageing process with equivalent suppressor activity to that seen in young patients on a cell for cell basis. There are a number of methods by which T-regulatory function may be assessed, but suppression of interferon-γ cytokine production by effector T-cells in coculture experiments is one of the most reliable and sensitive methods. Suppression of proliferation of effector cells in antigenic stimulation or allogenic mixed lymphocyte cultures can also be a valuable test.

Other investigators have also addressed the question of T-regulatory cell numbers in human ageing [20, 21] and have demonstrated that CD4+ FoxP3+ T-cells are seen to increase during ageing [22]. This is reassuring as it indicates that the more contemporary phenotype of regulatory cells, namely FoxP3 expression, can also be used to corroborate the increase in regulatory cells with ageing. Despite this, some evidence continues to suggest that functional activity is not equivalent in older subjects [23].

An important question that needs to be addressed in T-regulatory cell biology is the degree of coexpression of FoxP3 and CD25 on CD4 regulatory populations. In particular, CD25- T-cells expressing FoxP3 are observed in a number of clinical settings and may be related to the use of immune-suppression, ongoing chronic activation, or potentially immune senescence. There have been few studies to address this within humans although within murine systems an increase in CD25- FoxP3+ regulatory cells with ageing has been observed. In general, the evidence seems to suggest that FoxP3 is the more reliable marker of functional regulatory activity and the expression of CD25 therefore becomes less significant. CD25 is the high affinity receptor for interleukin 2 and its physiological role in T-regulatory functions has never been completely explained. Some authors have suggested that CD4+ CD25+

T-cells act as a "sink" for cytokine production and thereby act to limit cellular proliferation within the microenvironment but this proposal has not yet received substantial and confirmatory support.

The accumulation of regulatory cells with ageing does suggest that there may be increased generation of regulatory cells within the peripheral immune system in association with ageing. The mechanisms that may underlie this are unknown but differences have been reported between signalling processes in dendritic cells from young and old donors [24]. Reduced phosphorylation of AKT within DC in response to cell stimulation may be one reflection of differential signalling responses in these cells from elderly donors.

As with effector populations, T-regulatory cells can be divided into naïve and memory subsets based on their expression of CD45 isoforms. Naive regulatory populations characterized by CD45RA expression are predominant in infants but are still detectable in adult subjects [25]. The extent to which these remain in elderly donors with immune senescence has yet to be studied.

4   Regulatory T-cell Populations within the CD8+ T-cell Repertoire

In contrast to the extensive investigation of CD4+ regulatory T-cells there has been much less study of regulatory populations on cells within the CD8+ population. Suppressor T-cells have been described for many years and their phenotype appears to be dominated by lack of expression of the CD28 costimulatory molecule whereas expression of FoxP3 on CD8 has been poorly characterized. Naive CD8+ T-cell numbers decline dramatically with age to be replaced by accumulation of effector populations and this homeostatic instability may contribute to the differential structure of CD4 and CD8 T-cell pools [26].

A complexity is that FoxP3 may be expressed transiently after T-cell activation of effector T-cells although this induction does not lead to acquisition of complete regulatory function [27]. CD8+ populations that do express FoxP3 have been reported in a number of clinical scenarios [28, 29] but their functional role, and relevance to ageing, has not yet been addressed.

5   The Potential Contribution of T-regulatory Cells to Immune Senescence

One area in which there has been disappointing progress in T-regulatory biology has been confirmation of the antigenic specificity of these populations. Great debate continues to address the issue as to whether effector CD4+ T-cells and CD4+ regulatory cells recognize the same population of antigenic determinants or display specificity against discrete epitopes which may themselves play a role in determining the physiological direction of T-cell differentiation [30]. T-regulatory cells do appear to have specificity for self-epitopes and in this regard overlap at least partially with a population of potentially self reactive effector cells [31]. The former hypothesis gains considerable import from use of T-cell receptor transgenic models in which alteration of environmental conditions can lead to the generation of T-regulatory or T-effector cells with the same T-cell receptor expression. It had been believed that T-regulatory cells may represent a population with uniquely high affinity for self-antigen but such experiments suggest that critical determinants during T-cell priming maybe more important in determining the nature of T-cell differentiation after antigen priming.

Despite this, it has been widely reported that, although T-regulatory cells may require antigenic stimulation for activity, their activity, once triggered, is non-specific in nature and therefore can act to suppress bystander populations. In this regard, it is entirely possible that individuals who accumulate large populations of T-regulatory cells can be subject to some form of generalized immune suppression which may impact on their ability to mount effective immune responses against infectious agents or, potentially, tumour cells. There is great interest in studying the number and function of T-regulatory cells in patients with active malignant disease and a number of trials and animal models, either targeting CD25 or CTLA4, are now addressing how suppressional manipulation of T-regulatory cell function may serve to increase antigen-specific T-cell immune responses against transformed tissue [32, 33]. Some of these studies are already providing encouraging clinical responses but, perhaps not surprisingly, such treatments can often unleash powerful autoimmune phenomena with unusual antigenic specificities, including hypophysitis or hepatitis [34].

The question therefore needs to be addressed as to whether the increase in T-regulatory cells that is observed during healthy ageing contributes directly to immune senescence in this population [35]. In contrast, despite an increase in absolute numbers the suggestion that regulatory cell function may be impaired in ageing might also be relevant to the increase in autoimmune disease with age. To date there has been little experimentation which has allowed any detailed interpretation of this concept. However, Trzonkowski et al. have shown that the accumulation of regulatory cells that is observed with ageing is directly associated with impaired activity of CD8+ and NK-cells [21]. When effector cells were purified away from regulatory populations they regained their natural level of activity whereas add-back of regulatory populations led to reestablishment of impaired function. Within the murine system it should be possible to deplete these populations and assess T-cell immunity in mice of different ages and these experiments are eagerly awaited. Sharma et al. have shown that the accumulation of regulatory T-cells in aged Balb/c mice is directly responsible for the inability of older animals to reject tumour tissue [36]. Encouragingly, depletion of regulatory T-cells with an anti-CD25 antibody was able to reverse this deficiency.

Within the human system, such experiments are clearly much more difficult to devise but there is surely enough evidence now to make this an important clinical aim. Useful information is likely to be gleaned from the increasing number of early phase trials of T-regulatory modulation in both malignant and infectious disease which will reveal something regarding contribution of T-regulatory cells to immune senescence. Therapeutic manipulation of T-reg numbers will prove a difficult challenge but the use of agents such as interleukin-7 may modulate the nature of thymic output [37]. Granulocyte colony stimulating factor (G-CSF) administration leads to increased recruitment of regulatory cells through activation of tolerogenic plasmacytoid dendritic cells [38] and this cytokine axis might therefore offer scope for intervention. Adrenergic innervation of the thymus has been postulated to play a role in thymic involution and pharmacological blockade leads to increased T-regulatory cell production [39]. One interesting question will be the relative serum level and tissue availability of TGFβ during ageing as this may play an important role in the peripheral accumulation of regulatory cells.

6 Conclusion

In conclusion, T-regulatory cells are emerging as the most intensively studied population of cells within the human immune system at the current time. As such, it is not surprising that they are now being addressed in relation to immune senescence, itself one of the most important areas of clinical immunology. Initial data suggests that regulatory cell numbers are indeed increased in healthy elderly individuals, and that the functional properties of these cells are also maintained. Although more needs to be discovered regarding the antigenic specificity and functional activity of these cells, it is likely that manipulation of T-regulatory cell function could represent a novel form of immunotherapeutic intervention in elderly individuals. Whether or not it will be possible to limit regulatory cell function without an associated increase in autoimmunity is currently unknown. Such clinical intervention is likely only to be possible when much greater understanding is made of the natural physiological role of these cells in immune responses.

References

1. Banham AH, FM Powrie, E Suri-Payer (2006) FOXP3+ regulatory T-cells: current controversies and future perspectives. Eur J Immunol 36(11):p. 2832–2836
2. Dorf ME, B Benacerraf (1984) Suppressor cells and immuno-regulation. Annu Rev Immunol 2:p. 127–157
3. Sakaguchi S, et al (1995) Immunologic self-tolerance maintained by activated T-cells expressing IL-2 receptor alpha-chains (CD25). Breakdown of a single mechanism of self-tolerance causes various autoimmune diseases. J Immunol 155(3):p. 1151–1164
4. Hori S, T Nomura, S Sakaguchi (2003) Control of regulatory T-cell development by the transcription factor Foxp3. Science 299(5609):p. 1057–1061
5. Fontenot JD, MA Gavin, AY Rudensky (2003) Foxp3 programs the development and function of CD4+CD25+ regulatory T-cells. Nat Immunol 4(4):p. 330–336

6. Seddiki N, et al (2006) Expression of interleukin (IL)-2 and IL-7 receptors discriminates between human regulatory and activated T-cells. J Exp Med 203(7):p. 1693–1700

7. Liu W, et al (2006) CD127 expression inversely correlates with FoxP3 and suppressive function of human CD4 +T-reg cells. J Exp Med 203(7):p. 1701–1711

8. Borsellino G, et al (2007) Expression of ectonucleotidase CD39 by Foxp3+ Treg-cells: hydrolysis of extracellular ATP and immune suppression. Blood 110(4):p. 1225–1232

9. Walker MR, et al (2003) Induction of FoxP3 and acquisition of T-regulatory activity by stimulated human CD4+CD25- T-cells. J Clin Invest 112(9):p. 1437–1443

10. Zheng SG, et al (2004) Natural and induced CD4+CD25+ cells educate CD4+CD25- cells to develop suppressive activity: the role of IL-2, TGF-beta, and IL-10. J Immunol 172(9):p. 5213–5221

11. Selvaraj RK, TL Geiger (2007) A kinetic and dynamic analysis of Foxp3 induced in T cells by TGF-beta. J Immunol 179(2):p. 11 following 1390

12. Vukmanovic-Stejic M, et al (2006) Human CD4+ CD25hi Foxp3+ regulatory T-cells are derived by rapid turnover of memory populations in vivo. J Clin Invest 116(9):p. 2423–2433

13. Blais ME, et al (2008) Why T-cells of thymic versus extrathymic origin are functionally different. J Immunol 180(4):p. 2299–2312

14. Kim JM, JP Rasmussen, AY Rudensky (2007) Regulatory T-cells prevent catastrophic autoimmunity throughout the lifespan of mice. Nat Immunol 8(2):p. 191–197

15. Zhao L, et al (2007) Changes of CD4+CD25+Foxp3+ regulatory T-cells in aged Balb/c mice. J Leukoc Biol 81(6):p. 1386–1394

16. Kozlowska E, et al (2007) Age-related changes in the occurrence and characteristics of thymic CD4(+) CD25(+) T-cells in mice. Immunology 122(3):p. 445–453

17. Nishioka T, et al (2006) CD4+CD25+Foxp3+ T-cells and CD4+CD25-Foxp3+ T-cells in aged mice. J Immunol 176(11):p. 6586–6593

18. Shimizu J, E Moriizumi (2003) CD4+CD25- T-cells in aged mice are hyporesponsive and exhibit suppressive activity. J Immunol 170(4):p. 1675–1682

19. Gregg R, et al (2005) The number of human peripheral blood CD4+ CD25high regulatory T-cells increases with age. Clin Exp Immunol 140(3):p. 540–546

20. Bryl E, JM Witkowski (2004) Decreased proliferative capability of CD4(+) cells of elderly people is associated with faster loss of activation-related antigens and accumulation of regulatory T-cells. Exp Gerontol 39(4):p. 587–95

21. Trzonkowski P, et al (2006) CD4+CD25+ T-regulatory cells inhibit cytotoxic activity of CTL and NK-cells in humans-impact of immunosenescence. Clin Immunol 119(3):p. 307–316

22. Rosenkranz D, et al (2007) Higher frequency of regulatory T-cells in the elderly and increased suppressive activity in neurodegeneration. J Neuroimmunol 188(1–2):p. 117–127

23. Tsaknaridis L, et al (2003) Functional assay for human CD4+CD25+ Treg-cells reveals an age-dependent loss of suppressive activity. J Neurosci Res 74(2):p. 296–308

24. Agrawal A, et al (2007) Altered innate immune functioning of dendritic cells in elderly humans: a role of phosphoinositide 3-kinase-signaling pathway. J Immunol 178(11):p. 6912–6922

25. Seddiki N, et al (2006) Persistence of naive CD45RA+ regulatory T-cells in adult life. Blood 107(7):p. 2830–2838

26. Czesnikiewicz-Guzik M, et al (2008) T-cell subset-specific susceptibility to aging. Clin Immunol

27. Allan SE, et al (2007) Activation-induced FOXP3 in human T-effector cells does not suppress proliferation or cytokine production. Int Immunol 19(4):p. 345–354

28. Kiniwa Y, et al (2007) CD8+ Foxp3+ regulatory T-cells mediate immuno-suppression in prostate cancer. Clin Cancer Res 13(23):p. 6947–6958

29. Meloni F, et al (2006) Foxp3 expressing CD4+ CD25+ and CD8+CD28- T-regulatory cells in the peripheral blood of patients with lung cancer and pleural mesothelioma. Hum Immunol 67(1–2):p. 1–12

30. Pacholczyk R, et al (2006) Origin and T-cell receptor diversity of Foxp3+CD4+CD25+ T-cells. Immunity 25(2):p. 249–259

31. Hsieh CS, et al (2006) An intersection between the self-reactive regulatory and nonregulatory T-cell receptor repertoires. Nat Immunol 7(4):p. 401–410
32. Rudge G, et al (2007) Infiltration of a mesothelioma by IFN-gamma-producing cells and tumor rejection after depletion of regulatory T-cells. J Immunol 178(7):p. 4089–4096
33. Chaput N, et al (2007) Regulatory T-cells prevent CD8 T-cell maturation by inhibiting CD4 Th-cells at tumor sites. J Immunol 179(8):p. 4969–4978
34. Hodi FS, et al (2008) Immunologic and clinical effects of antibody blockade of cytotoxic T-lymphocyte-associated antigen-4 in previously vaccinated cancer patients. Proc Natl Acad Sci U S A
35. Dejaco C, C Duftner, M Schirmer (2006) Are regulatory T-cells linked with aging? Exp Gerontol 41(4):p. 339–345
36. Sharma S, AL Dominguez, J Lustgarten (2006) High accumulation of T-regulatory cells prevents the activation of immune responses in aged animals. J Immunol 177(12):p. 8348–8355
37. Aspinall R (2006) T-cell development, ageing and Interleukin-7. Mech Ageing Dev 127(6):p. 572–578
38. Kared H, et al (2005) Treatment with granulocyte colony-stimulating factor prevents diabetes in NOD mice by recruiting plasmacytoid dendritic cells and functional CD4(+)CD25(+) regulatory T-cells. Diabetes 54(1):p. 78–84
39. Pesic V, et al (2007) Long-term beta-adrenergic receptor blockade increases levels of the most mature thymocyte subsets in aged rats. Int Immunopharmacol 7(5):p. 674–686

Age-related Changes in Subpopulations of Peripheral Blood Lymphocytes in Healthy Japanese Population

Masanori Utsuyama, Yuko Kikuchi, Masanobu Kitagawa and Katsuiku Hirokawa

Contents

Abstract: Peripheral blood mononuclear cells were obtained from healthy Japanese individuals ranging in age from 20 to 90 years old and analyzed by using three color flow cytometer with regards to the number and percentage of various lymphocytes. In addition, we assessed the proliferative capacity of T-cells in the presence of an anti-CD3 monoclonal antibody and the amount of cytokines produced in the supernatant.

The results showed that an age-related decline was observed in the numbers of CD3+ T-cells, CD8+ T-cells, naive T-cells, CD8+CD28+ T-cells, and B-cells and in the proliferative capacity of T-cells. The rate of decline in these immunological parameters except for the number of CD8+ T-cells was steeper in males than in females ($p<0.05$). An age-related increase was observed in the number of CD4+ T-cells, memory T-cells, and NK-cells and in the CD4/CD8 ratio The rate of increase of these immunological parameters was steeper in females than in males ($p<0.05$). The T-cell proliferation index (TCPI), which was calculated based on T-cell proliferative activity and the number of T-cells, showed an age-related decline. The rate of decline in the TCPI was again steeper in males than in females ($p<0.05$). The score of immunological vigor calculated using 5 T-cells parameters also declined with age, and the rate of decline was steeper in males than in females ($p<0.05$). The

K. Hirokawa (✉)
Institute for Health and Life Sciences
Ascent Myogadani 4F
4-6-22, Kohinata, Bunkyo-ku
Tokyo 112-0006, Japan
Tel: 81-3-6820-6139
E-mail: hirokawa@h-ls.jp

T. Fulop et al. (eds.), *Handbook on Immunosenescence*,
DOI 10.1007/ 978-1-4020-9062-2_11, © Springer Science+Business Media B.V. 2009

present study has confirmed the age-related changes in immunological parameters reported in literature. In addition, we found that a statistically significant difference was observed between males and females in some immunological parameters such as the number of T-cells and TCPI. The slower rate of decline in the immunological parameters studied in females than in males may be consistent with the fact that women survive for longer period of time than men.

1 Introduction

Immunological functions are known to decline with age in many animal models and humans (Linton and Dorshkind 2004; Utsuyama et al. 1992; Hirokawa et al. 2006). Understanding the level of immunological functions at an individual level is clinically important, since the immunological decline is accompanied by various diseases such as infections, cancer and vascular diseases.

Accumulating evidences mainly obtained from animal models have shown that age-related immunological decline mainly occurs in T-cell dependent immune functions, and is mainly caused by thymic involution that begins in the early phase of life (Hirokawa et al. 2006).

In humans, data regarding immunological functions are mainly obtained from blood serum and blood cells. Serum contains immunoglobulins, complements and cytokines. The levels of IgG and IgA in serum show a trend of increase with age (Suzuki et al. 1984). The level of complements does not change remarkably with age. The level of cytokines in healthy people is generally low. In contrast, the level of white blood cells (WBC) changes remarkably during disease and also with aging. WBC comprises granulocytes, lymphocytes and monocytes. There are various subpopulations of lymphocytes with different functions. Data regarding the age-related changes in lymphocytes and their functions are not sufficiently available as yet.

The purpose of this study is to provide immunological data on peripheral blood lymphocytes obtained from 162 male and 194 female healthy volunteers, ranging in age from 20 to 90 years. Our study discusses the age-related changes in subpopulations of peripheral blood lymphocytes from both immunological and gerontological viewpoints.

2 Materials and Methods

Blood specimens: Two milliliters of blood was taken in a tube containing ethylenediaminetetraacetic acid (EDTA-2K) for hematological analysis performed using a PENTRA80 analyzer (Horiba, Kyoto, Japan). Eight milliliters of blood was taken in a cell preparation tube (vacutainer, 362761, Becton Dickinson (BD), NJ) for collecting mononuclear cells and was used for immunological analyses.

Subjects: Healthy volunteers were selected based on clinical records and laboratory examinations. None of the blood donors were suffering from neoplastic or autoimmune disease; further, none were receiving any medications that could

Table 1 Number of male and female subjects

Age	20 – 29	30 – 39	40 – 49	50 – 59	60 – 69	70 – 79	80 –	Total
Male	13	23	35	37	29	22	3	162
Female	44	32	36	34	18	26	4	194

influence immune functions. Routine laboratory examinations of the serum were performed to examine the liver and kidney functions. A total of 162 males and 194 females were examined in the present study. Table 1 shows the number of male and female subjects and their ages.

Flow cytometry: Mononuclear cells that were obtained from the peripheral blood, as described above, were stained with a combination of 2 or 3 monoclonal antibodies (mAbs) conjugated with 2 or 3 chromophores. A fluorescence-activated cell sorting flow cytometer (FACScan BD) was employed in the present study.

Monoclonal antibodies: The antibodies used were fluorescein isothiocyanate (FITC) conjugated anti-CD4, FITC-conjugated anti-CD20 and FITC-conjugated anti-CD16; phycoerythrin (RD1) conjugated anti-CD3, RD1-conjugated anti-CD8 and RD1-conjugated anti-CD25; phycoerythrin-Texas Red (ECD) conjugated anti-CD45RA and ECD-conjugated anti-CD3; phycoerythrin-cyanin 5.1 (PC5) conjugated anti-CD28: phycoerythrin (PE) conjugated anti-CD56. Those mAbs were purchased from Beckman Coulter. The following combinations of mAbs were used: CD3-RD1/CD20-FITC, CD4-FITC/CD8-RD1/CD45RA-ECD, CD4-FITC/CD8-RD1/CD28-PC5, CD56-PE/CD16-FITC, CD3-ECD/CD4-FITC/CD25-RD1.

Proliferative response of T-cells: The proliferative response of T-cells to anti-CD3 mAb (ORTHOCLONE OKT3, ORTHO BIOTEC, NJ) was assessed according to MTS method (Cell Titer 96 Aqueous One Solution Cell Proliferation Assay (Promega Co., WI)).

Assays were performed in microplates (3860-096, Asahi Glass Co. Japan). The cells (1×10^5) in 0.2 ml of RPMI 1640 medium supplemented with 5% fetal bovine serum (FBS) were stimulated with immobilized anti-CD3 mAb (Orthoclone OKT3, Ortho Biotec, NJ). The plates were then placed in a 5% CO_2 incubator for 72 hrs. After incubation for 68 hrs, 40 μl of MTS solution (Cell Titer 96 Aqueous One Solution Cell Proliferation Assay (Promega Co., WI)) was added into each well and absorbance at 490nm was recorded with a spectrophotometric plate reader; this value was used for determining the relative magnitude of T-cell proliferation.

T-cells proliferation index (TCPI) and immunological age (IA): TCPI was calculated by the following equation.

TCPI = T-cell proliferative activity × (T-cell number/1000)

In this equation, T-cell proliferative activity was obtained as optical density (OD_{490}) ranging between 0.95 and 2.0 by the abovementioned MTS method. The TCPI and age showed a statistically significant correlation: TCPI = −0.0174 x (Age)+ 2.5348 (Fig. 5c and 5d). Using this equation, it is possible to calculate age by assigning a value to TCPI. The age calculated by this equation was referred to as immunological age (IA).

Scoring and grading of immunological functions: The values of immune parameters were standardized by assigning scores of 3 (high level), 2 (moderate level) and 1

Table 2 Scoring and grading of immunological vigor

Scoring		
SIV-7 7 parameters	SIV-5 5 parameters	Grading
21	15	Grade V Sufficiently high
20 ~ 18	14 ~ 13	Grade IV Safety zone
17 ~ 14	12 ~ 10	Grade III Observation zone
13 ~ 10	9 ~ 7	Grade II Warning zone
9 ~ 7	6 ~ 5	Grade I Critical zone

(low level) according to the data base obtained from 300 healthy people. After standardization, the scores of different types of immune parameters were summed and the numerical value obtained for each individual was termed the score of immunological vigor (SIV). These scores were then classified into 5 grades, as shown in Table 2.

SIV-7 comprises 7 parameters that are number of T cells, TCPI, CD4/CD8 ratio, number of naïve T cells, naïve/memory ratio, number of B cells and number of NK cells. SIV-5 comprise 5 T cell-related parameters that T cells, TCPI, CD4/CD8 ratio, number of naïve T cells and naïve/memory T cells ratio.

Assessment of cytokine production: Assays were performed in microplates (3860-024, Asahi Glass Co. Japan). Cells (1×10^6) in 1.5 ml of RPMI 1640 supplemented with 10% FBS were stimulated with immobilized anti-CD3 mAb (Orthoclone OKT3, Ortho Biotec, NJ). Culture supernatant were collected at 48 hrs and stored at -80°C until use. A flow cytomix kit (BMS810FF, Bender MedSystems, Austria) was employed for the evaluation of cytokines (Interleukin (IL)-1β, IL2, IL-4, IL5, IL-6, IL-8, IL-10, IL-12/p70, interferon (IFN) γ, tumor necrosis factor (TNF) α, TNFβ and the assessment was performed using a FACScan analyzer.

Statistical Analysis: All statistical analyses were performed using StatView software. Statistical significance was defined as $p < 0.05$. Gender difference was examined by SMA analysis.

3   Results

3.1   Number of Whole WBCs, Red Blood Cells and Lymphocytes in the Blood

The number of red blood cells (RBC) showed a significant age-related decrease ($p < 0.001$) in males and a declining trend with age in females ($p=0.9535$) (Fig. 1a and 1b) (Table 3). The difference between males and females with regard to the age-related decline in the number of RBC was statistically significant ($p < 0.001$). Although an age-related decline was observed in males, but not in females, the absolute level of RBC was higher in males than in females regardless of age.

The number of WBCs including granulocytes, lymphocytes and monocytes showed a declining trend with age in both males ($p=0.0824$) and females ($p=0.2588$); no statistically significant difference was observed between males and females in this regard (Fig. 1c and 1d) (Table 3).

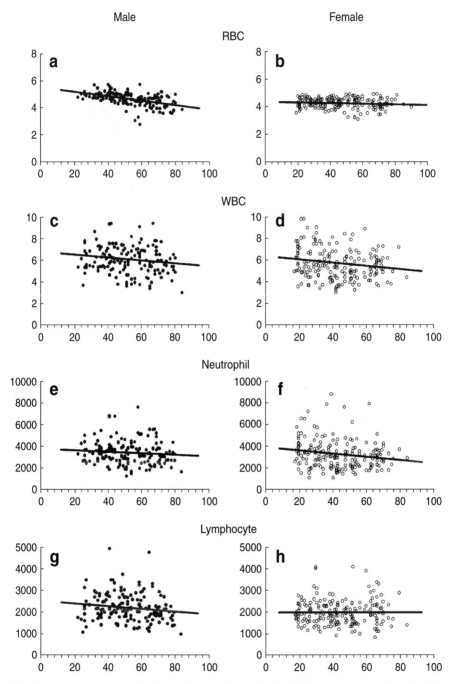

Fig. 1 Age related changes in the number of red blood cells (RBC) in males (a) and females (b), white blood cells (WBCs) in males (c) and females (d), neutrophils in males (e) and females (f), and lymphocytes in males (g) and females (h)

Table 3 Results of regression analysis on age and immunological parameters

	Male (N=162)			Female (N=194)			SMA[§] analysis
	Regression curve	R*	p value	Regression curve	R*	p value	
RBC	−0.017x + 5.544	0.517	<0.0001	−0.0002x + 4.264	0.004	0.9535	0.001
Lymphocytes[#]	−6.430x + 2526	0.149	0.0593	+1.038x + 1934	0.031	0.6637	0.015
T-cells[#]	−6.150x + 1791	0.186	0.0176	−2.390x + 1508	0.111	0.1249	0.049
CD4[+] T-cells[#]	+0.024x + 903.3	0.001	0.9897	+1.962x + 769.6	0.116	0.1075	0.005
CD8[+] T-cells[#]	−4.564x + 719.3	0.286	0.0002	−4.048x + 649.6	0.306	<0.0001	NS
CD4/CD8 ratio	+0.027x + 0.839	0.316	<0.0001	+0.029x + 0.898	0.452	<0.0001	0.003
Naïve T-cells[#]	−1.365x + 471.3	0.089	0.2615	−0.598x + 439.5	0.055	0.4470	0.004
Memory T-cells[#]	+1.392x + 431.8	0.113	0.1531	+2.557x + 330.1	0.253	<0.0001	NS
Naïve / Memory ratio	−0.005x + 1.081	0.159	<0.0001	−0.007x + 1.356	0.258	0.0003	NS
MTS (OD$_{490}$)	−0.006x + 1.629	0.314	<0.0001	−0.004x + 1.544	0.224	0.0017	NS
Proliferation Index	−0.016x + 2.817	0.289	0.0002	−0.008x + 2.306	0.190	0.0080	0.010
SIV[##] (5 items)	−0.036x + 14.01	0.262	0.0008	−0.035x + 14.07	0.334	<0.0001	0.012
B-cells[#]	−1.844x + 266.0	0.167	0.0336	−0.444x + 148.8	0.103	0.1525	0.001
NK-cells[#]	+1.787x + 368.6	0.103	0.1935	+3.208x + 218.5	0.269	0.0002	0.001
[$]CD8[+]CD28[+] cells[#]	−6.089x + 597.0	0.543	<0.0001	−4.136x + 476.9	0.477	<0.0001	0.038
WBC[#]	−0.014x + 6.801	0.137	0.0824	−0.007x + 6.118	0.082	0.2558	NS
Neutrophils[#]	−6.942x + 3719	0.097	0.2178	−8.535x + 3729	0.116	0.1063	NS
SIV[##] (7 items)	−0.039x + 19.65	0.270	0.0005	−0.032x + 19.17	0.264	0.0002	NS
[$$]Regulatory T-cells[#]	+0.042x + 46.01	0.026	0.7502	+0.132x + 36.32	0.100	0.1818	NS

#: Number / mm^3 . *: R, Correlation coefficient. §: SMA Standardized Major Axis Test,

##: SIV: Scoring of immunological vigor

$: Number of CD8[+] CD28[+] cells was obtained from 107 males and 103 females.

$$: Number of regulatory T-cells (CD4[+] CD25[+]) was obtained from 154 males and 181 females.

The number of neutrophils showed a decreasing trend with age in both males (p=0.2178) and females (p=0.1063); no significant difference was observed between males and females (Fig. 1e and 1f) (Table 3).

The number of lymphocytes showed a decreasing trend with age in males (p=0.0593) and an increasing trend with age in females (p=0.1249); statistically significant difference was observed in the age-related change between males and females (p=0.015) (Fig. 1g and 1h) (Table 3).

3.2 Flow Cytometric Analysis

(a) CD3⁺ T-cells.

The number of CD3⁺ T-cells showed a statistically significant decrease with age in males (p =0.0186), and a decreasing trend with age in females (p =0.1249). The difference in the age-related change in the number of CD3⁺T-cells between males and females was statistically significant (p=0.049) (Fig. 2a and 2b) (Table 3).

(b) CD4⁺ T-cells.

The number of CD4⁺ T-cells showed an increasing trend with age in both males (p=0.9897) and females (p=0.1075). This trend was greater in females than in males, and the difference between males and females with regard to this trend was statistically significant (p=0.005) (Fig. 2c and 2d) (Table 3).

(c) CD8⁺T-cells.

The number of CD8⁺T-cells showed an age-related decrease in both males ($p < 0.0002$) and females ($p < 0.0001$), but no difference was observed between males and females with regard to this decrease (Fig. 2e and 2f) (Table 3).

(d) The ratio of CD4⁺ T-cells to CD8⁺ T-cells (CD4/CD8 ratio).

The CD4/CD8 ratio increased with age in both males (p <0.0001) and females ($p < 0.0001$), and this increase was significantly greater in females than in males ($p < 0.003$) (Fig.2g and 2h) (Table 3).

(e) CD8⁺CD28⁺ T-cells.

The number of CD8⁺CD28⁺ T-cells showed an age-related decrease in both males (p <0.0001) and females (p <0.0001) (Fig. 3a and 3b), and the rate of this decline was more pronounced in males (-6.089) and in females (-4.136) ($p < 0.003$) (Table 3).

(f) CD4⁺CD45RA⁺ naïve T-cells.

The number of CD4⁺CD45RA⁺ naïve T-cells showed a decreasing trend with age in both males (p=0.2615) and females (p=0.4470) (Fig.3c and 3d). This decreasing trend was greater in males than in females, and the difference between males and females was statistically significant (p=0.004).

(g) CD4⁺CD45RO⁺ memory T-cells.

The number of CD4⁺CD45RO⁺ memory T-cells showed an increasing trend with age in males (p=0.1531), and an age-related increase in females (p=0.0001) ($p < 0.0001$) (Fig. 3e and 3f). In this case, there is no significant gender difference (Table 3).

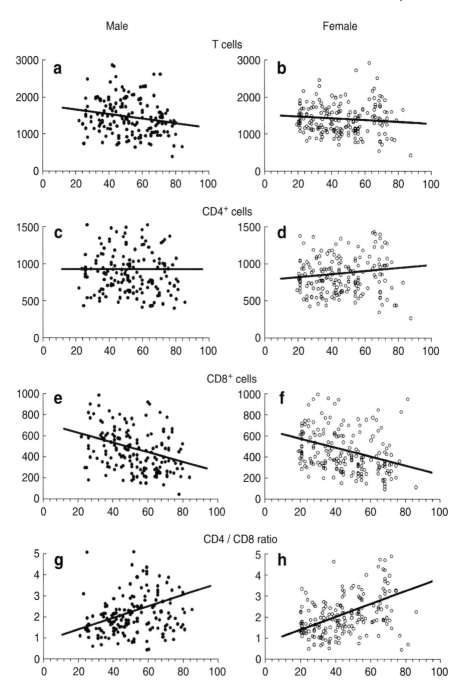

Fig. 2   Age related changes in the number of T-cells in males (a) and females (b), CD4+ T-cells in males (c) and females (d), CD8+ T-cells in males (e) and females (f), and the CD4/CD8 ratio in males (g) and females (h)

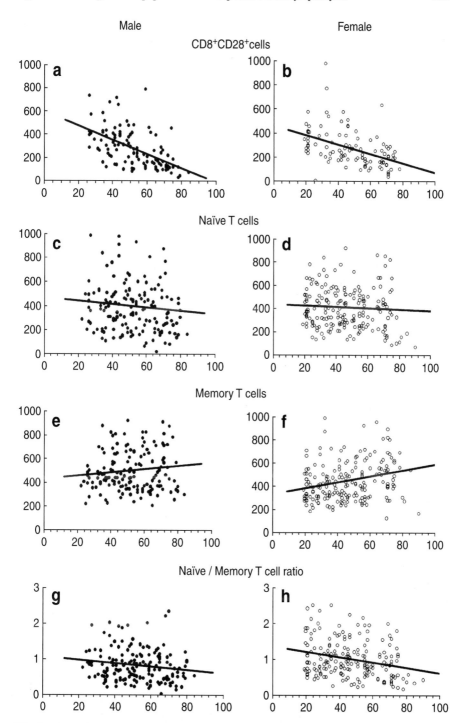

Fig. 3 Age related changes in the number of CD8+CD28+ T-cells in males (a) and females (b), naive T-cells in males (c) and females (d), memory T-cells in males (e) and females (f), and native to memory T-cells (N/M) ratio in males (g) and females (h)

(h) Ratio of naïve to memory T-cells.

The naïve to memory T-cells (N/M) ratio showed an age-related decrease in both males (p <0.0001) and females (p <0.0003), and this decrease was statistically significant (Fig. 3g and 3h). However, no significant gender difference was observed (Table 3).

(i) CD4+CD25+ T-cells.

The number of CD4+CD25+ T-cells showed an increasing trend with age in both males (0.7502) and females (0.1818) (Fig. 4a and 4b), but this increase was statistically not significant. Further, no gender difference was observed (Table 3).

(j) CD20+ B-cells.

The number of CD20+ B-cells showed a decrease with age in males (p < 0.05) and showed a decreasing trend with age in females (p =0.15) (Fig. 4c and 4d); no statistically significant difference was observed between males and females with regard to this decrease (p < 0.001) (Table 3).

(k) CD56+CD16+ NK-cells.

The number of CD56+CD16+ NK-cells showed an age-related increase in females (p <0.0002) and an increasing trend with age in males (p=0.19) (Fig. 4e and 4f). A statistically significant gender difference was observed (p <0.001) (Table 3).

3.3 Proliferative Response of T-cells

(a) Proliferative response of T-cells by anti-CD3 monoclonal antibody (MTS-OD$_{490}$).

The proliferative response of T-cells was measured by MTS method and was expressed as OD$_{490}$. It showed an age-related decrease in both males (p<0.0001) and females (p<0.002) (Fig. 5a and 5b), but no gender difference was observed.

(b) T-cell proliferation index (TCPI).

The TCPI showed an age-related decrease in both males (p < 0.0002) and females (p <0.008) (Fig. 5c and 5d). The decrease was more pronounced in males than in females (p < 0.01) (Table 3).

(c) Correlation between CD8+CD28+ T-cells and T-cell proliferative response (MTS-OD$_{490}$).

The number of CD8+CD28+ T-cells and MTS-OD$_{490}$ showed an age-related decease in both males and females; this decrease was statistically significant. It is interesting to note that a good correlation was observed between the number of CD8+CD28+ T-cells and MTS-OD$_{490}$ (Fig. 4g and 4h).

3.4 Scoring of Immunological Vigor (SIV)

(a) SIV-7.

SIV-7 was calculated based on 7 parameters: T-cells number, TCPI, CD4/CD8 ratio, naïve T-cell number, naive/memory T-cells ratio, B-cell number and NK-cell number.

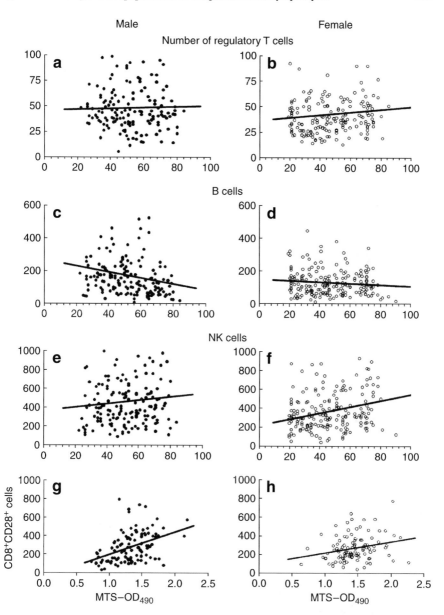

Fig. 4 Age related changes in the number of regulatory T-cells in males (a) and females (b), B-cells (WBC) in males (c) and females (d), NK-cells in males (e) and females (f), and the correlation between the number of CD8⁺CD28⁺ T-cells and the T-cell proliferative response (MTS-OD490) in males (g) and females (h)

SIV-7 showed an age-related decrease in both males ($p < 0.0005$) and females ($p < 0.0002$) (Fig. 5e and 5f). No gender difference was observed (Table 3).

(b) SIV-5.

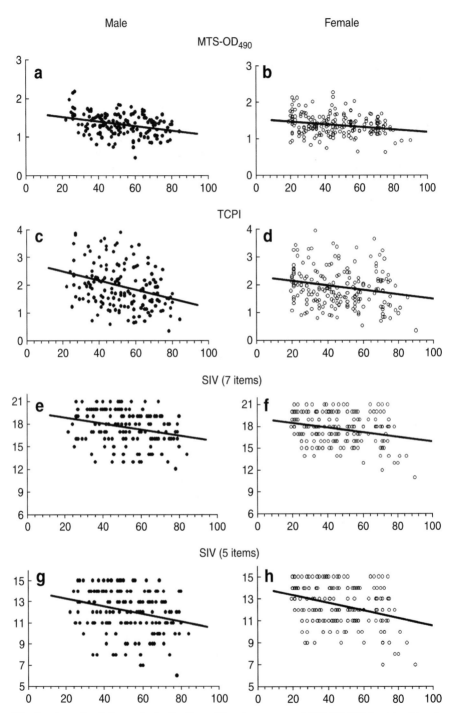

Fig. 5 Age-related change in the T-cells proliferative response (MTS-OD490) in males (a) and females (b), T-cell proliferation index (TCPI) in males (c) and females (d), score of immunological vigor (SIV)-7 in males (e) and females (f), and SIV-5 (T-cell immune score) in males (g) and females (h)

Table 4 Regression analysis on cytokine productions and age in males and females

	Males (N=64)			Females (N=49)			SAM[#]
	Regression curve	R*	p value	Regression curve	R*	p value	analysis
IFNγ	-10.29x + 0.227	2951	0.0707	-5.95x + 2823	0.123	0.3969	NS
IL-1β	-20.72x + 0.276	2553	0.0272	-17.27x + 2857	0.170	0.2419	NS
IL-2	-2.498x + 0.129	307	0.3477	-4.188x + 360	0.243	0.1077	NS
IL-4	-0.021x + 0.020	18.8	0.8853	+0.063x + 11.1	0.083	0.6010	NS
IL-5	+0.694x + 0.099	50.9	0.4468	+0.068x + 53.0	0.022	0.8880	NS
IL-6	-72.72x + 0.248	7713	0.0482	-36.90x + 9470	0.076	0.6054	p=0.010
IL-8	+ 4.94x + 0.133	2291	0.2939	+ 5.34x + 2073	0.150	0.3025	NS
IL-10	- 9.05x + 0.175	1282	0.1655	- 1.78x + 742	0.063	0.6656	p=0.004
TNFα	-144.5x + 0.192	24500	0.1411	-185.5x + 28125	0.251	0.1003	NS
TNFβ	-10.02x + 0.378	974	0.0017	- 3.48x + 596	0.222	0.1284	p=0.012

*R: Correlation coefficient. [#] SMA: Standardized Major Axis Test. NS: Not significant.

SIV-5 was calculated by using 5 parameters: T-cells number, TCPI, CD4/CD8 ratio, naïve T-cell number, and naive/memory T-cells ratio; SIV-5 is sometimes termed as T-cell immune score.

The T-cell immune score showed an age-related decrease in both males ($p < 0.001$) and females ($p < 0.0001$) (Fig. 5g and 5h). A more pronounced decrease was observed in males than in female ($p <0.02$) (Table 3).

3.5   Cytokine Production

In the present study, lymphocytes were cultured in vitro in the presence of immobilized anti-CD3 mAb and the cytokines produced in the supernatant were assessed as described previously. The subjects for cytokine production comprised 64 males and 49 females; this sample size was not adequate for statistical analysis. This preliminary examination has revealed that an age related decrease in the levels of IFNγ, IL-1β, IL-2, IL-4, IL-5, IL-6, IL-10, TNFα and TNFβ in both male and female subjects. In contrast, an age-related increase was observed in IL-8 (Table 4).

3.6   Difference in Gender

Table 3 lists the regression curves calculated for the data described above, and the significance of gender difference was examined by standardized major axis test (SMA) analysis.

The rate of decrease in the number of T-cells, naïve T-cells, and CD8+CD28+ cells; T-cell proliferation index (TCPI), SIV-5 parameters was slower in females than in males. Further, this difference was statistically significant ($p <0.05 – 0.003$). The

Table 5 Gender difference in people over 60 years old

	Male over 60 years N=54	Female over 60 years N=48
T-cells (number/mm³)	1365 ± 53	1395 ± 73
CD4⁺ T cells (number/mm³)	910 ± 59	961 ± 55
T-cell proliferation index	1.72 ± 0.11	1.87 ± 0.12
SIV-5 (T-cell immune score)	11.6 ± 0.3	11.7 ± 0.3
CD8⁺CD28⁺ (number/mm³)	181 ± 19	200 ± 20

rate of increase in the number of CD4$^+$ T-cells was greater in females than in males and a statistically significant difference was observed between males and females (p < 0.005). In other words, the slower rate of decline or the greater rate of increase in these parameters may indicate that the immunological functions are relatively well preserved in elderly females than in elderly males; this finding may be consistent with the fact that women survive for longer periods than men. Table 5 shows the values of these immunological parameters in elderly males and females over 60 years of age. All parameters show higher values in elderly females than in males; however, the difference is statistically not significant because of the small sample size.

4   Discussion

In 1992, we reported age-related change in subpopulations of lymphocytes in healthy subjects ranging in age from 6 to 102 years (Utsuyama et al. 1992). In the present study, we confirmed most of the results presented in our previous report; i.e., an age-related decrease in CD3$^+$ T-cells, more pronounced decrease in CD8$^+$ T-cells than in CD4$^+$ T-cells, an age-related increase in CD4/CD8 ratio, a decrease in the number of naïve T-cells with a concomitant increase in memory T-cells, a decrease in B-cells and an increase in NK-cells.

In the present study, we examined the proliferative activity of T-cells and confirmed that it gradually declines with advancing age. In addition, we developed a new parameter, T-cell proliferation index (TCPI), which is calculated by using the proliferative activity and the number of T-cells. TCPI was also observed to significantly decrease with age.

It is interesting to note that the rate of decline in the studied parameters differed with gender. The rate of decline in the number of T-cells calculated by the regression curve was -6.150 in males and -2.390 in females. The rate of decline in TCPI was -0.016 in males and -0.008 in females. This gender difference in the T-cells and TCPI vales was statistically significant (Table 3). A relatively gradual decrease in the studied parameters in females than in males may be consistent with the fact that women survive for longer period than men in Japan.

A low number of CD8$^+$CD28- T-cells and high CD4/CD8 ratio are associated with populations that survive until the age of 100 years (Strindhall et al. 2007). Susceptibility to influenza infection in older adults is associated with an increased population of CD8$^+$CD28- T-cells (Xie, McElhaney 2007). In this respect, we confirmed that the number of CD8$^+$CD28$^+$ cells decreased with age and this decrease was associated with a decrease in the T-cell proliferative response ($MTS\text{-}OD_{490}$); i.e., the rate of decline was significantly slower in females than in males.

The absolute number of total B-lymphocytes increases about 3-fold from the base line in the first year of life and progressively decreases until adult age (Veneri et al. 2007). We further confirmed that the number of B-cells continued to gradually decrease throughout the life and decline was significantly steeper in males than in females.

It is still not clear whether the age-related increase in the prevalence of $CD4^+CD25$(high) regulatory T-cells (TREGs) is responsible for immune dysfunction in the elderly (Dejaco et al. 2006). In this respect, we found that the number of TREGs showed an increasing trend with age.

An age-related increase was observed in the number of NK-cells and this rate of increase was significantly steeper in females than in males. In this respect, Lee et al. (1996) reported that higher percentage of NK-cells in the Asian population than in Caucasian subjects.

Olsson et al. (2000) reported that a decrease in the CD4/CD8 ratio was an important indicator of the immune risk phenotype (IRP). In the present survey, a contrasting feature was observed between $CD4^+$T-cells and $CD8^+$T-cells. The number of $CD4^+$ T-cells was relatively steady level or showed an increasing trend with age, while the number of $CD8^+$ T-cells significantly decreased with age; therefore, the CD4/CD8 ratio showed a distinct age-related increase. Higher percentage and number of $CD8^+$ T-cells and a decreased CD4/CD8 ratio was observed in the Saudi male population compared with Caucasian controls (Shababuddin 1995). Hence, racial difference should be considered in this case.

Anti-CD3 stimulation of T-lymphocytes significantly increased IL-8 production and this increase was more evident in the nonagenarian subjects (Mariani E et al. 2001). Centenarians showed high level of IL-8, indicating that an increased level of IL-8 is related to longevity (Wieczorowska-Tobis et al. 2006). These reports were consistent with the result of the present study indicating an age-related increase in IL-8.

Individuals who are genetically predisposed to produce high level of IL-6 have a reduced capacity to reach the extreme limits of the human lifespan. On the other hand, a high IL-10 producing genotype is observed among centenarians (Caruso C et al. 2004). These results were partly consistent with those of the present study, which showed that both IL-6 and IL-10 decreased with age. In future studies, an adequate sample size should be selected for analysis of cytokine production.

References

Caruso C, Lio D, Cavallone L, Franceschi C (2004) Aging, longevity, inflammation and cancer. Ann N Y Acad Sci 1028:1–13

Dejaco C, Duftner C, Schirmer M (2006) Are regulatory T cells linked with aging? Exp Gerontol 41:339–45

Hirokawa K, Utsuyama M, Makinodan T (2006) Immunity and ageing. In: Principles and practice of geriatric medicine, 4th edition (eds Pathy MSJ, Sinclair AJ, Morley JE) John Wiley & Sons, Ltd. pp 19–36

Lee B, Yap HK, Chew FT et al (1996) Age- and sex-related changes in lymphocyte subpopulations of healthy Asian subjects: from birth to adulthood. Cytometry 26:8–15

Linton PJ Dorshkind K (2004) Age-related changes in lymphocytes development and function. Nat Immunol 5:133–139

Mariani E et al (2001) Different IL-8 production by T and NK lymphocytes in elderly subjects. Mech Ageing Dev 122:1383–395

Olsson J et al (2000) Age-related change in peripheral blood T-lymphocyte subpopulations and cytomegalovirus infection in the very old: the Swedish longitudinal OCTO immune study. Mech Ageing Dev 121:187–201

Peralbo E Alonso C, Solana R (2007) Invariant NKT and NKT-like lymphocytes: two different T cell subsets that are differentially affected by ageing. Exp Gerontol 42:703–708

Shahabuddin S (1995) Quantitative differences in CD8+ lymphocytes, CD4/CD8 ratio, NK cells, and HLA-DR(+)-activated T cells of racially different male populations. Clin Immunol Immunop 75:168–170

Strindhall J et al (2007) No immune risk profiles among individuals who reach 100 years of age: findings form Swedish NONA immune longitudinal study. Exp Gerontol 42:753–761

Utsuyama M et al (1992) Differential age-change of CD4+CD45RA+ and CD4+CD29+ T cells subsets in human peripheral blood. Mech Ageing Dev 63:57–66

Wieczorowska-Tobis K et al (2006) Can an increased level of circulating IL-8 be a predictor of human longevity? Med Sci Monit 12:CR118–CR121

Veneri D et al (2007) Changes of human B and B-1a peripheral blood lymphocytes with age. Hematol 12:337–341

Xie D, McElhaney JE (2007) Lower GrB+CD62Lhigh CD8 TCM effector lymphocyte response to influenza virus in older adults is associated with increased CD28null CD8+ T lymphocytes. Mech Ageing Dev 128:392–400

Age-associated T-cell Clonal Expansions (TCE) in vivo—Implications for Pathogen Resistance

Cellular Immunosenescence – T cells

Janko Nikolich-Žugich and Anna Lang

Contents

Abbreviations

pMHC	peptide MHC complex
RTE	recent thymic emigrants
SPF	specific pathogen-free
TCE	T-cell clonal expansions

Abstract: Age-related T-cell clonal expansions (TCE) are an incompletely understood disturbance in T-cell homeostasis found frequently in old humans and experimental animals. These accumulations of CD8 T-cells have the potential to distort T-cell population balance and reduce T-cell repertoire diversity above and beyond the changes seen in the aging of T-cell pool in the absence of TCE. This chapter discusses our current knowledge of the role of these expansions in health and disease, with a special focus on their influence upon immune defense against infectious diseases.

Keywords: Ageing • Clonal expansions • Homeostasis • Infectious diseases • T-cells

J. Nikolich-Žugich (✉) · A. Lang
Department of Immunobiology and the Arizona Center on Aging
University of Arizona college of Medicine
Tucson, AZ 85719, USA
Phone: +1-520-626-6065
Fax: +1-520-626-2100
E-mail: nikolich@arizona.edu

T. Fulop et al. (eds.), *Handbook on Immunosenescence*,
DOI 10.1007/ 978-1-4020-9062-2_12, © Springer Science+Business Media B.V. 2009

1   Introduction

As was extensively discussed in other chapters of this handbook, immunosenescence encompasses a number of diverse age-related cellular and extracellular milieu changes that affect cells and molecules of the immune and inflammatory system. The very definition of immunosenescence, however, operationally includes not only the decline of immunity with age by itself, but also its most important clinical manifestation, the increased susceptibility to infection and decreased immunosurveillance of cancer. Other factors can contribute to the increased exposure to infectious diseases and increased colonization with infectious pathogens (e.g., reduced barrier function of skin and mucosal membranes) with age, and multiple factors certainly strongly contribute to the age-related increase in incidence of cancer. However, it is clear that the inability to mount rapid and vigorous immune defense once an infectious invasion (and, likely, detectable malignant transformation) had occurred lies at the heart of many of the clinical manifestations of immunosenescence. Due to the involvement of numerous other nonimmunological factors in the age-related increase of cancer-related morbidity and mortality, this review will solely deal with infectious diseases.

It has long been known that aging is accompanied by an increase in mortality and morbidity from a number of common respiratory infections such as influenza (20,000–40,000 annual deaths in the USA alone) (Bender 2003; Betts and Treanor 2000; Couch et al. 1986; Glezen and Couch 2003; High 2004; Yoshikawa 2000), pneumococcal pneumonia (Bender 2003; High et al. 2005; Yoshikawa 2000) and RSV (Glezen and Couch 2003; High et al. 2005; Yoshikawa 2000), and urinary infections (Bender 2003; Hazelett et al. 2006). Moreover, this vulnerability extends to dangerous established pathogens such as variola (Hanna 1913) as well as the newly emerging pathogens that disproportionally affect the elderly such as the West Nile virus (Murray et al. 2006) the Severe Acute Respiratory Syndrome-causing Coronavirus (SARS-CoV) (Chan et al. 2007; Leung et al. 2004) and others.

Several types of age-related defects in the immune function can contribute to this increased susceptibility to infection, including defects in innate immunity, antigen uptake, processing and presentation, provision of second and third signals to the adaptive immune system and impaired humoral immunity, all of which are competently covered in other chapters of this handbook. However, T-cells have been known to exhibit some of the most pronounced age-related defects (Miller 1996), and intervention to correct these defects resulted in successful correction of the immune function in a number of cases (Effros et al. 1991; Haynes et al. 2004; Haynes et al. 1999; Messaoudi et al. 2006a). These defects can be grossly divided into cell-autonomous defects, which affect T-cells regardless of age-related or compensatory alterations that affect other components of the immune system and which can be detected in assays where T-cells are the only component of the immune system affected by aging; and age-related changes in the T-cell population balance, which mostly involve the initial loss of naïve T-cells and the compensatory, reactive changes aimed to maintain T-cell homeostasis in the face of this loss.

This chapter will focus upon the latter changes, given that other aspects of T-cell dysfunction will be covered in other chapters of this volume. Moreover, we will discuss the impact of a specific type of age-related T-cell disturbances, T-cell clonal expansions (TCE) (Callahan et al. 1993; Hingorani et al. 1993a; Posnett et al. 1994), upon immune defense and pathogen resistance, highlighting the extent and the limits of our current knowledge, and the tasks and problems that need to be solved before we can fully understand and treat these disturbances.

2 T-cell Homeostasis and Development of T-cell Clonal Expansions (TCE)

The current evidence strongly suggests that the involution of the thymus and the decline in production of new naïve T-cells are the initiating factors behind the generation of at least some TCE (Messaoudi et al. 2006b), whereas latent persistent viral infections may be the perpetrators driving other types of TCE (Pawelec et al. 2004). Moreover, homeostatic mechanisms that are activated as a consequence of naïve T-cell loss may themselves participate in the onset and/or maintenance of TCE (Messaoudi et al. 2006b, 2006c). Therefore, at the risk of being redundant, we will very briefly review thymic T-cell production, involution, latent persistent infections and T-cell homeostasis. For a more detailed review of these topics, the reader is encouraged to read sections of this handbook devoted to thymic involution, as well as the recent volume of Seminars in Immunology devoted to T-cell rejuvenation (Nikolich-Žugich 2007; Zuniga-Pflucker and van den Brink 2007).

2.1 Homeostatic Maintenance of T–cell Subsets

T-cell homeostasis is defined here as maintenance of naïve and memory T-cell pool numbers and diversity and the ability to restore these numbers and diversity following antigenic (Ag) challenge. T-cell homeostasis is regulated by the response of T-cells to environmental trophic and survival signals and by the presence and availability of such signals. The most important and best understood of these signals are the common γ-chain cytokines (most notably IL-7, IL-15 and IL-2) and self-peptide: MHC (pMHC) complexes. The contribution of each of these signals to homeostatic maintenance varies depending on the T-cell subset.

Following maturation and selection in the thymus, new T-cells are released into the periphery as recent thymic emigrants (RTEs) (Scollay et al. 1980). Release of RTEs bearing a variety of randomly rearranged TCRs ensures the diversity of the peripheral T-cell pool. Once released from the thymus, the RTE join the naïve T-cell pool. Naïve T-cells have no preset life spans and are maintained by IL-7 and trophic signals from interaction of their TCR with self-p:MHC complexes (rev. in (Lee and Surh 2005). When these two signals are present, naïve T-cells are believed to be able to survive indefinitely, based upon the results of serial transfer experiments (Sprent et al. 1991). Murine RTE proliferate faster than naïve peripheral T-cells in the first three weeks after export, perhaps in order to maximize naïve T-cell diversity, before they equilibrate with other naïve T-cells (Berzins et al. 1998). Naïve T-cells display very low levels of spontaneous (or homeostatic) cycling in vivo. Homeostatic cycling is greatly increased in lymphopenia, where T-cells sense a signal, most likely provided by an excess of unused IL-7 and IL-15 (Surh and Sprent 2002). Under lymphopenic conditions T-cells undergo Ag-independent homeostatic proliferative expansion (HPE), in a seeming attempt to fill the empty compartment (Fry and Mackall 2005; Surh et al. 2006). Unlike naïve T-cells, memory T-cells do not require specific p: MHC contact for survival. Instead, their survival is dependent on continued homeostatic proliferation, driven mainly by IL-15, or by IL-7 in the absence of IL-15. Memory cells cycle and self-renew in vivo significantly (up to four times) faster than naïve T-cells and also exhibit faster proliferation during lymphopenia (Surh et al. 2006). It is likely that there may be other, presently unknown pathways regulating T-cell homeostasis, some of which could include energy metabolism regulation (Frauwirth and Thompson 2004).

The above described homeostatic mechanisms function to maintain a balanced and diverse T-cell pool. Over lifetime this means regulating the process of Ag-driven expansion of naïve T-cells, their contraction, and selection and maintenance of memory T-cells. The role of the homeostatic mechanisms is to balance the composition of the T-cell pool so that it contains both naïve precursors with diverse TCRs, as well as Ag-experienced memory T-cells, as both of these subsets are crucial for the health of the host. The homeostatic forces work very efficiently in adult mice housed under specific pathogen free (SPF) conditions, as evidenced by remarkably similar size and diversity of the T-cell pool among individual mice of the same strain. However, maintenance of homeostasis becomes more complicated in the face of constant encounters with new acute pathogens, long-term interactions with persistent pathogens and the aging-associated defects, all of which are discussed below.

2.2   Disruption of T-cell Homeostasis in Ageing

Thymic involution begins soon after birth in humans and quickly after puberty in mice, which results in decreased RTE output (Haynes et al. 2000; Hirokawa and Utsuyama 1984). Thus, 22-mo-old mice receive less than 10% of RTE compared to young adult mice (Hale et al. 2006; Heng et al. 2005). Even in old age the thymus continues to produce RTE proportionally to its overall cellularity, but as the cellularity itself decreases, so does the output (Gruver et al. 2007; Hale et al. 2006). The cause of thymic involution is discussed in more detail elsewhere in this volume. From the standpoint of this chapter, thymic involution presents a challenge for the homeostatic mechanisms, which strive to maintain the size and diversity of the peripheral T-cell pool in the face of decreased influx of diverse new T-cells.

Despite the fact that thymus involution begins early in life, it is only in old age that homeostatic mechanisms falter and allow dysbalance amongst T-cell subsets.

A marked difference between the adult and old lymphocyte T-cell compartment is an age-related decrease in representation of naïve phenotype T-cells and concomitant increase in frequency and numbers of memory phenotype T-cells. The exact mechanisms leading to this population shift were not formally dissected, but are believed to likely involve a combination of 1) decrease in naïve T-cell production, 2) their conversion into effector or memory cells as a result of encounters with pathogens, and 3) changes in the environment, including the availability of homeostatic cytokines (IL-7, IL-15, IL-2). For example, IL-2 production by CD4 T-cells is decreased in old mice(Gillis et al. 1981; Miller and Stutman 1981; Thoman and Weigle 1981). Less is known about age-related changes in IL-7 or IL-15 levels or the expression and function of their receptors on different T-cell subsets. In addition, the naïve T-cell pool could be indirectly affected by a growing pool of memory T-cells that may compete with naïve T-cells. Considering that there is some overlap in the use of survival and maintenance cytokines by these two pools, particularly in case of IL-7(Fry, Mackall 2005; Tan et al. 2002), it is possible that the two are not always independently regulated, particularly in aging where there is many fewer naïve T-cells. Thus, if naïve T-cells continue to decrease in number, this may lead to an excess of survival and maintenance cytokines which normally would have been consumed by naïve T-cells. This could trigger homeostatic proliferative expansion (HPE) of the remaining naïve T-cells and drive their conversion to memory-phenotype. This was demonstrated in mice under lymphopenic conditions (Cho et al. 2000; Goldrath et al. 2000), and strongly suggestive results were also obtained in aging monkeys (Cicin-Sain et al. 2007) and humans (Naylor et al. 2005).

2.3   T-cell Clonal Expansions (TCE)

One of the hallmarks of immune aging is loss of TCR repertoire diversity (rev. in (Nikolich-Žugich 2005)), due in large part to the dominance of memory T-cells over the naïve ones. However, on top of that reduction, the CD8 T-cell compartment often shows additional loss of diversity, in the form of large, often clonal expansions of T-cells bearing the same TCR, named T-cell clonal expansions (TCE) (Callahan et al. 1993; Hingorani et al. 1993b; Posnett et al. 1994). Development of TCEs has been documented across mammalian species, including rodents, nonhuman primates, and humans, with fractions between 30 and 60% of individuals surveyed exhibiting one or more age-associated TCE (rev. in (Nikolich-Žugich, Messaoudi 2005). More on the biology of TCE can be found in the excellent review by Clambey and Marrack elsewhere in this book. However, for the purpose of this chapter, it is most pertinent to classify TCE into at least two types with respect to the mechanism of their generation and/or maintenance. Large Ag-independent TCE (AI-TCE) are thought to arise and/or be maintained independently of antigenic stimulation, due to age-related changes in perceiving homeostatic signals. This is based upon: (i) activation marker expression on these cells, which dominantly exhibit central memory phenotype, with no evidence of recent or repeated antigen-driven activation (Callahan et al. 1993; Ku et al. 2001; Messaoudi et al. 2006c); (ii) cytokine receptor, specifically IL-7R and IL-15R, expression, which is higher on these cells compared to other memory or naïve T-cells (Messaoudi et al. 2006c); (iii) the ability of these cells to proliferate upon adoptive transfer (Ku et al. 2001), with a constant rate regardless of whether the recipient is lymphopenic or not (Messaoudi et al. 2006c); and (iv) the ability of manipulations that induce lymphopenia to increase the incidence and accelerate the onset of development of AI-TCE (Messaoudi et al. 2006b). While these results have been obtained in mice, there is evidence that similar fundamental principles are at work in primates, including humans (Cicin-Sain et al. 2007; Naylor et al. 2005). In contrast, TCE that have general characteristics consistent with the response to antigen, also called Ag-reactive TCE (AR-TCE), were linked to latent persistent herpesviral infections in mice (Holtappels et al. 2000; Karrer et al. 2003; Podlech et al. 2000) and humans (Almanzar et al. 2005; Fletcher et al. 2005; Ouyang et al. 2003c; Pawelec et al. 2004). Broad discussion of these virus-related abnormalities is also presented in other chapters of this handbook.

TCE can occupy up to 90% of the total murine and up to 50% of the human memory CD8 T-cell pool. TCE themselves are not malignant and do not affect the overall size of the CD8 T-cell pool (there is no increase in total T-cell numbers in individuals carrying TCE). However, TCE do disturb T-cell homeostasis and diversity (Callahan et al. 1993; LeMaoult et al. 2000; Posnett et al. 1994) and a drastic disturbance of this type can be expected to impair the ability to mount T-cell responses. While T-cell responses are plastic, with a significant reserve that allows T-cells to respond to pathogens despite loss of much of the repertoire, this plasticity is not unlimited (rev. in (Nikolich-Žugich et al. 2004). However, we still do not have precise quantitative understanding of limits of T-cell diversity necessary to mount protective responses against pathogenic challenge, an issue highly relevant from the standpoint of evaluating the impact of TCE upon immune defense.

3 Impact of TCE on Pathogen Resistance—the Mouse Model

The most important question related to the presence of TCE is related to their impact upon the health of the organism. One could envision several possibilities in that regard. First, TCE could be neutral and not impact the overall health or the immune defense of the old organism. While this possibility is intellectually unexciting, it is likely that many TCE coexist with the state of health based on their high incidence in asymptomatic individuals (Hingorani et al. 1993b; Posnett et al. 1994). Indeed, it is likely that a TCE needs to grow to a certain size before it becomes a problem for its bearer. Second, TCE could affect other components of the organism, without impacting immune defense. While this is possible, this scenario had not been documented so far and will not be further discussed here. Third, TCE could have an active effect, whereby they would secrete cytokines and other short-acting mediators that could alter the function of other components of the immune (and other) systems in the body. This would be akin to the functional shift seen in replicatively senescent fibroblasts, which upon cessation of replication drastically change their secretory properties and have the potential to alter extracellular matrix, neovascularization and other microenvironmental properties (rev. in (Campisi 2002). At the present, there is some evidence in support of this possibility (Ortiz-Suarez and Miller 2002; Ortiz-Suarez and Miller 2003), but more precise studies at the level of isolated, highly purified TCE are needed. Moreover, the impact of the observed changes upon pathogen resistance remains untested.

Finally, the role of TCE could be passive, but nevertheless negative. Under that scenario, which was invoked by immunologists before (Callahan et al. 1993; Hingorani et al. 1993a; Posnett 1994 #1976), and which will be discussed in more detail as it currently appears the most likely, these accumulating T-cell clones would constrict the repertoire and reduce the useful T-cell repertoire that defends us against new infection. Mechanistically, this would most likely occur by these cells gaining a survival/maintenance advantage over other T-cells in the body. The fact that TCE which occur spontaneously in SPF mice express high levels of IL-7Rα and IL-2/15Rβ (Messaoudi et al. 2006c) is consistent with the possibility that TCE operate as IL-7 and/or IL-15 "cytokine sinks", taking them slowly away from other T-cells. Consistent with that, we (Lang et al. submitted) and others (Ely et al., 2007) have recently found that often TCE can arise from the pool of cells that respond(ed) to prior acute or latent infection. Of interest, once these cells begin to significantly expand in old age, they tend to acquire high levels of IL-7 and IL-15 receptors (Lang et al. submitted), raising the possibility that the "cytokine sink" may be the unifying mechanism by which both "spontaneous" and antigen-specific large TCE constrict the remainder of useful T-cell repertoire. In fact, it is likely that the "spontaneous" TCE designation simply covers up the fact that we don't know the original antigen that was recognized by these cells, and that may be irrelevant if indeed these cells primarily respond to cytokines once they become TCE.

In order for a TCE to have a demonstrably negative effect upon immune defense via TCR repertoire constriction, such a TCE needs to sufficiently erode the numbers and diversity of other T cells needed to respond to a new pathogen. Numerous studies have shown that manipulations which take away up to half or more of TCR diversity are reasonably compatible with T-cell responsiveness (rev. in (Nikolich-Žugich et al. 2004). However, in other models losses of this or greater magnitude have been shown to impair responsiveness to certain antigens (rev in. (Nikolich-Žugich et al. 2004) and references therein). In terms of the impact of TCE upon the residual diversity of aged naïve T- cells in relationship to immune defense against infectious diseases, it is important to consider the overall diversity and overall numbers of T-cells involved in a typical response to a pathogen. Exciting new studies with direct measuring of precursor T-cell frequencies concur that on the average a hundred, and in some cases as few as 15-20 CD4 or CD8 T-cells may be responding to a single epitope (Badovinac et al. 2007; Moon et al. 2007). Even if this is an underestimation, reducing that number by 90%, or even by half, due to the presence of a TCE, certainly has the potential to diminish and cripple the response to epitopes where few T-cell precursors exist. This low responsiveness would be further compounded by an already diminished overall reserve of naïve T-cells in aging, as well as by the blunted T-cell signaling (Tamir et al. 2000). On the other hand, most pathogens present multiple epitopes to the immune system, and even if one accounts for immunodominance, usually a handful of epitopes are available for T-cell stimulation. Moreover, in many cases other arms of the immune system will synergize to provide protection even if T-cell responses are diminished. Thus, for a TCE to impact pathogen resistance, T-cells have to provide primary and nonredundant protection against that pathogen, the pathogen should have few, rather than many, immunodominant and protective epitopes and frequency of T-cells specific for these epitopes should be low. In the one case where the impact of TCE upon immune defense was tested (Messaoudi et al. 2004), most, if not all, of the above conditions were met. In that study, resistance to herpes simplex virus (HSV-1) was studied in B6 mice, where an octamer derived from the glycoprotein B accounts for > 90% of the total CD8 T-cell response (Dyall et al. 2000; Messaoudi 2001 #1644; Wallace et al. 1999). Moreover, the response itself is highly restricted with regard to TCRV region utilization (with Vβ10 and 8 contributing >80% of the response (Cose et al. 1995)). Old animals with and without TCE were challenged with HSV and magnitude and functional characteristics of the response measured. It was found that TCE could impair the generation of productive responses in a selective manner. So, when an animal contained a large TCE which expressed Vβ10 and 8, it was unable to mount a response to HSV gB, whereas TCE expressing other TCR Vβ segments did not impair responsiveness beyond the reduction seen due to age in a littermate control group (Messaoudi et al. 2004). These results were somewhat puzzling and suggested that TCE preferentially competed out against the T-cells bearing the same TCRVβ segment. This could be explained, for example, if TCRVβ residues conserved within the Vβ family but differing between Vβ families (e.g. CDR1 & 2 and "framework" parts of CDR3) were important in contacting self-pMHC complexes in the course of trophic interactions needed for T-cell maintenance, so that a TCE would compete out naïve T-cells of the same TCRVβ family. Such a mechanism remains to be substantiated. Nevertheless, the above study (Messaoudi et al. 2004) does show that TCE can potentially impair protective immunity.

While the above experiments were performed with spontaneously arising TCE, which were most likely AI-TCE, there is no reason to believe that a similar situation may not exist with AR-TCE as well. Our group is in the process of testing this possibility. Another unaddressed question relates to the impact of TCE upon memory responses. Memory T-cells are more difficult to compete out than naïve T-cells, possibly due to their ability for self-renewal and relative resistance to apoptosis. Perhaps the most pertinent question is whether TCE can affect the response to latent and/or chronic persistent pathogens, where a large fraction of the immune system is periodically or continuously stimulated by these pathogens. At the present, this issue remains unresolved.

4 Impact of TCE on Pathogen Resistance—Evidence from Humans

In reviewing the known impact of TCEs on pathogen resistance, one needs to distinguish between two parameters: 1) correlation of presence of TCE with presence of other immunological factors known to impair immune responses, and 2) direct evidence for impact of TCE on pathogen resistance. The occurrence of TCEs has been well documented in patients and in a variety of animal models, so we shall first review that scenario. One should bear in mind, however, that it is often difficult to distinguish the specific effect of TCE from the effects of old age-associated defects in antipathogen immunity, since in most cases TCEs are detected only in advanced age. It is therefore most appropriate to evaluate TCE as a superimposing, possibly aggravating factor that may, or may not, further impair protective immunity in an already suboptimal setting of an old organism.

Some TCEs have known antigenic specificity. Two types of conclusions on the effects of these TCEs on pathogen resistance can be drawn: 1) effect upon resistance to the pathogen the TCE is specific for, and 2) effect upon resistance to unrelated pathogens. In humans, the most commonly documented cases of TCEs of known specificity involve memory CD8 T-cells specific for CMV (rev. in (Pawelec et al. 2004)) and, to a lesser extent, EBV (Ouyang et al. 2003b). Original studies documented the presence of CD28⁻ CD8⁺ TCEs in elderly patients (Hingorani et al. 1993b; Posnett et al. 1994). With the advent of tetramers and intracellular cytokine staining techniques that allowed enumeration of Ag-specific T-cells, it was shown that the CD28- CD8 T-cell expansions were frequently specific for CMV and were clonal or oligoclonal in nature (Ouyang et al. 2002). Moreover, longitudinal studies in the Swedish elderly cohorts concluded that CMV seropositivity, together with an array of additional immune characteristics such as the inverted CD4:CD8 ratio and poor proliferative responses of T-cells to mitogens, constitute an immune risk phenotype (IRP, discussed in detail elsewhere in this book) (Wikby et al. 2005), which predicted mortality within 2 years in octogenerians of the Swedish cohort (Hadrup et al. 2006). It will be important to reproduce these results in genetically diverse populations of the elderly, particularly in light of early reports that the elderly from West Sicily may not show the same effect (Colonna-Romano et al. 2007). Moreover, it is not clear exactly how the presence of CMV-specific TCE might affect pathogen resistance, in isolation from the other IRP-associated defects, highlighting one of the problems inherent to the otherwise highly informative human longitudinal studies.

At the present, there is some evidence that CMV-specific T-cells may themselves be compromised as a direct result of development of TCE. Several studies demonstrated accumulation of dysfunctional CMV-specific memory CD8 T-cells in the elderly (Ouyang et al. 2003a; Ouyang et al. 2003c; Ouyang et al. 2004). In addition, the large CMV-specific memory cell population expressed a marker of replicative senescence, KLRG-1, and its expression correlated with decreased production of IFNγ upon antigenic stimulation (Ouyang et al. 2004). The key question is whether this leads to inability to mount an adequate functional response to viral reactivation, permitting viral replication above the subclinical level normally associated with

CMV seropositivity. In that regard, one study (Stowe et al. 2007) demonstrated the presence of CMV and EBV DNA in urine (CMV) and blood (EBV) of elderly patients, as opposed to the seropositive adults, implying some loss of control of viral reactivation in the elderly. Consistent with that explanation, these authors also found elevated expression of lytic and latent EBV genes in blood of elderly but not adult seropositive patients (Stowe et al. 2007). It is possible that accumulation of dysfunctional CMV- or EBV-specific TCE, which were unable to control the virus, may be the reason for increase in viral reactivation in aging. However, in that study, the elderly actually had an elevated frequency of IFNγ-producing CMV- and EBV-specific memory CD8 T-cells, making the hypothesis unlikely. Moreover, CMV-mediated disease does not seem to be associated with aging in the absence of iatrogenic or acquired immune suppression, suggesting that a manifest loss of CMV control does not occur in the elderly. Further studies are needed to decisively address the role of accumulation of dysfunctional CMV-specific TCEs on the persistent latent Herpes virus control in old age.

A separate issue is whether CMV-specific TCE affect immunity to other infections in humans, and how. There is some evidence that presence of CMV-specific TCE is associated with lower frequency of memory CD8 T-cells specific for coresident EBV infection (Khan et al. 2004). This study did not examine whether control of latent EBV in patients with large CMV-specific TCE is impaired. While one could speculate that the T-cell response, and therefore immunity to EBV will be compromised in patients with large CMV-specific TCE similar to the results seen in mice with the effect of spontaneous TCE upon HSV immunity (Messaoudi et al. 2004), the mechanism by which these TCE affect the size of the EBV memory CD8 T-cell pool is currently unknown.

Since many of the TCEs identified in humans are specific for CMV, it was proposed that CMV is the main driver behind generation of TCEs (Pawelec et al. 2004). While this may be the case, evidence from murine studies suggests that virus-specific TCE can also develop independently from ongoing antigenic stimulation. Ely et al. (Ely et al. 2007) detected presence of TCE specific for Sendai virus and flu in old mice that had been infected as adults. Similarly, we have found that old mice infected with WNV at a young age developed expansions of virus-specific memory CD8 T-cells in old age (A Lang et al. submitted). In a different infection model, we found that following localized (ocular) HSV-1 infection, mice develop expansions of HSV-specific memory CD8 T-cells once they reach old age. This process was unlikely to be caused by viral reactivation, as mice treated continuously with antiviral drugs also developed these age-associated T-cell expansions. At present, only a small number of these antigen-independent age-associated expansions were confirmed to be clonal, with oligoclonality being seen more often (A Lang et al. submitted). Unlike is the case with CMV-specific TCEs, the T-cell expansions that developed independently from ongoing antigenic stimulation were fully functional, showing excellent correlation of percentage of tetramer⁺ and IFNγ⁺ cells (A Lang et al. submitted). Therefore, it is not likely that development of TCEs by this mechanism will affect immunity to the cognate pathogen. Additional studies will be required to determine whether TCEs can develop from preexisting memory CD8 T-cells specific for nonpersisting pathogens in elderly humans, as they do in old mice.

Are these TCE impairing productive immunity in humans? Of interest, the number of influenza-specific memory CD8 T-cells was shown to decline with age in humans (Goronzy et al. 2001). This phenomenon was independent of the patients' CMV status. In another study of success of flu vaccination in CMV-seropositive patients, CMV seropositivity correlated with impaired response to vaccination (Saurwein-Teissl et al. 2002). However, the authors did not delineate whether this correlates best to the presence of TCE, to the overall decrease in number of naïve cells or to proliferative/replicative senescence, and, as with most clinical studies, the mechanism responsible for this outcome has not been resolved. Therefore, the presence of TCE could be one of the useful biomarkers predicting poor outcome of flu vaccination (Goronzy et al. 2001; Saurwein-Teissl et al. 2002), or perhaps even general immunological vulnerability, but that requires further and rigorous verification in larger and heterogeneous populations of human subjects.

5   Concluding Remarks, Challenges and Questions

It follows from the above discussion that much remains to be learned about the biology of TCE and their precise impact upon resistance to infectious diseases. Drawing generalized conclusions about the impact of TCEs on pathogen resistance from the available data is often difficult, since they come from a number of different experimental models. At present we do not know how closely the mechanisms of generation of TCEs and their subsequent effects on pathogen resistance compare between them. However, the models and the reagents that are currently available provide good tools to systematically address the questions that still remain regarding the impact of TCEs on immunity. In particular, new quantitative tools are becoming available allowing us to precisely dissect the breadth and the reserve of T-cell receptor repertoire and the size of precursor populations specific for immunodominant epitopes of various pathogens, and that should allow us to quantitatively evaluate to what extent is TCR repertoire constricted by different types of TCE, and to determine what type of intervention (many of which are now in clinical trials (Zuniga-Pflucker, van den Brink 2007)) could be applied in individual situations.

Overall, the most important practical issues related to TCE and the infectious diseases of the elderly are:

1. Which groups of elderly are at an increased risk of infection and which are not? Are TCE a risk factor in that regard?
2. For those groups that are at risk, can they be helped with the existing vaccines or do they need alternate ways of immunostimulation? Can TCE be removed or shrunken?
3. If immunostimulation is to be attempted in a targeted manner, which modes of immunostimulation are the most efficacious? Different vaccination regimens, additional costimulation or cytokine treatments?

4. For those where immunostimulation may be insufficient, is T-cell rejuvenation the best option?

Answering these questions will undoubtedly be rewarding for scientists and physicians,as well as to the growing populations of elderly around the world.

References

Almanzar G, Schwaiger S, Jenewein B, Keller M, Herndler-Brandstetter D, Wurzner R, Schonitzer D, Grubeck-Loebenstein B (2005) Long-term Cytomegalovirus infection leads to significant changes in the composition of the CD8 T-cell repertoire, which may be the basis for an imbalance in the cytokine production profile in elderly persons. J Virol 79:3675–3683

Badovinac VP, Haring JS, Harty JT (2007) Initial T cell receptor transgenic cell precursor frequency dictates critical aspects of the CD8(+) T cell response to infection. Immunity 26:827–841

Bender B S (2003). Infectious disease risk in the elderly. Immunol Allergy Clin North Am 23: 57–64 vi

Berzins SP, Boyd RL, Miller JFAP (1998) The role of the thymus and recent thymic migrants in the maintenance of the adult peripheral lymphocyte pool. J Exp Med 187:1839–1848

Betts RF, Treanor JJ (2000) Approaches to improved influenza vaccination. Vaccine 18:1690–1695

Callahan JE, Kappler JW, Marrack P (1993) Unexpected expansions of CD8-bearing cells in old mice. J Immunol 151:6657–6669

Campisi J (2002) Between scylla and charybdis: p53 links tumor suppression and aging. Mech Ageing Dev 123:567–573

Chan JC, Tsui EL, Wong VC (2007) Prognostication in severe acute respiratory syndrome: a retrospective time-course analysis of 1312 laboratory-confirmed patients in Hong Kong. Respirology 12:531–542

Cho BK, Rao VP, Ge Q, Eisen HN, Chen J (2000) Homeostasis-stimulated proliferation drives naive T cells to differentiate directly into memory T cells. J Exp Med 192:549–556

Cicin-Sain L, Messaoudi I, Park B, Currier N, Planer S, Fischer M, Tackitt S, Nikolich-Žugich D, Legasse A, Axthelm MK, et al (2007) Dramatic increase in naive T cell turnover is linked to loss of naive T cells from old primates. Proc Natl Acad Sci U S A 104:19960–19965

Colonna-Romano G, Akbar AN, Aquino A, Bulati M, Candore G, Lio D, Ammatuna P, Fletcher JM, Caruso C, Pawelec G (2007) Impact of CMV and EBV seropositivity on CD8 T lymphocytes in an old population from West-Sicily. Exp Gerontol 42:995–1002

Cose SC, Kelly JM, Carbone FR (1995) Characterization of a diverse primary herpes simplex virus type 1 gB-specific cytotoxic T-cell response showing a preferential V beta bias. J Virol 69:5849–5852

Couch RB, Kasel JA, Glezen WP, Cate TR, Six HR, Taber LH, Frank AL, Greenberg SB, Zahradnik JM, Keitel WA (1986) Influenza: its control in persons and populations. J Infect Dis 153:431–440

Dyall R, Messaoudi I, Janetzki S, Nikolic-Žugic J (2000) MHC polymorphism can enrich the cell repertoire of the species by shifts in intrathymic selection. J Immunol 164:1695–1698

Effros RB, Walford RL, Weindruch R, Mitcheltree C (1991) Influences of dietary restriction on immunity to influenza in aged mice. J Geronto l46:B142–B147

Ely KH, Ahmed M, Kohlmeier JE, Roberts AD, Wittmer S T, Blackman MA, Woodland DL (2007) Antigen-specific CD8+ T cell clonal expansions develop from memory T cell pools established by acute respiratory virus infections. J Immunol 179:3535–3542

Fletcher JM, Vukmanovic-Stejic M, Dunne PJ, Birch KE, Cook JE, Jackson SE, Salmon M, Rustin MH, Akbar AN (2005) Cytomegalovirus-specific CD4+ T cells in healthy carriers are continuously driven to replicative exhaustion. J Immunol 175:8218–8225

Frauwirth KA, Thompson CB (2004) Regulation of T lymphocyte metabolism. J Immunol 172:4661–4665

Fry TJ, Mackall CL (2005) The many faces of IL-7: from lymphopoiesis to peripheral T cell maintenance. J Immunol 174:6571–6576

Gillis S, Kozak R, Durante M, Weksler M E (1981) Immunological studies of aging. Decreased roduction of and response to T cell growth factor by lymphocytes from aged humans. J Clin Invest 67:937–942

Glezen WP, Couch RB (2003) Estimating deaths due to influenza and respiratory syncytial virus. Jama 289:2500; author reply 2500–2502

Goldrath AW, Bogatzki LY, Bevan MJ (2000) Naive T cells transiently acquire a memory-like phenotype during homeostasis-driven proliferation. J Exp Med 192:557–564

Goronzy J, Fulbright J, Crowson, C, et al. (2001) Value of immunological markers in predicting responsiveness to influenza vaccination in elderly individuals. JVirol 75:12182–12187

Gruver AL, Hudson LL, Sempowski GD (2007) Immunosenescence of ageing. J Pathol 211:144–156

Hadrup SR, Strindhall J, Kollgaard T, Seremet T, Johansson B, Pawelec G, thor Straten P, Wikby A (2006) Longitudinal studies of clonally expanded CD8 T cells reveal a repertoire shrinkage predicting mortality and an increased number of dysfunctional cytomegalovirus-specific T cells in the very elderly. J Immunol 176:2645–2653

Hale JS, Boursalian TE, Turk GL, Fink PJ (2006) Thymic output in aged mice. Proc Natl Acad Sci U S A 103:8447–8452

Hanna W (1913) Studies in small-pox and vaccination. Rev Med Virol 4:201–209

Haynes BF, Sempowski GD, Wells AF, Hale LP (2000) The human thymus during aging. Immunol Res 22, 253-261

Haynes L, Eaton SM, Burns EM, Rincon M, Swain SL (2004) Inflammatory cytokines overcome age-related defects in CD4 T cell responses in vivo. J Immunol 172:5194–5199

Haynes L, Linton PJ, Eaton SM, Tonkonogy SL, Swain SL (1999) Interleukin 2, but not other common gamma chain-binding cytokines, can reverse the defect in generation of CD4 effector T cells from naive T cells of aged mice. J Exp Med 190:1013–1024

Hazelett SE, Tsai M, Gareri M, Allen K (2006) The association between indwelling urinary catheter use in the elderly and urinary tract infection in acute care. BMC Geriatr 6:15

Heng TS, Goldberg GL, Gray DH, Sutherland JS, Chidgey AP, Boyd RL (2005) Effects of castration on thymocyte development in two different models of thymic involution. J Immunol 175:2982–2993

High KP (2004) Infection as a cause of age-related morbidity and mortality. Ageing Res Rev 3:1–14

High KP, Bradley S, Loeb M, Palmer R, Quagliarello V, Yoshikawa T (2005) A new paradigm for clinical investigation of infectious syndromes in older adults: assessment of functional status as a risk factor and outcome measure. Clin Infect Dis 40:114–122

Hingorani R, Choi I-H, Akolka P, Gulwani-Akolkar B, Pergolizzi R, Silver J, Gregersen PK (1993a) Clonal predominance of T cell receptors within the CD8+ CD45RO+ subset in normal human subjects. J Immunol 151:5762–5769

Hingorani RC, H Akolka, P, Gulwani-Akolkar B, Pergolizzi R, Silver J, Gregersen PK (1993b) Clonal predominance of T cell receptors within the CD8+ CD45RO+ subset in normal human subjects. J Immunol 151:5762

Hirokawa K, Utsuyama M (1984) The effect of sequential multiple grafting of syngeneic newborn thymus on the immune functions and life expectancy of aging mice. Mech Ageing Dev 28:111–121

Holtappels R, Pahl-Seibert MF, Thomas D, Reddehase MJ (2000) Enrichment of immediate-early 1 (m123/pp89) peptide-specific CD8 T cells in a pulmonary CD62L(lo) memory-effector cell pool during latent murine cytomegalovirus infection of the lungs. J Virol 74:11495–11503

Karrer U, Sierro S, Wagner M, Oxenius A, Hengel H, Koszinowski UH, Phillips RE, Klenerman P (2003) Memory inflation: continuous accumulation of antiviral CD8+ T cells over time. J Immunol 170:2022–2029

Khan N, Hislop A, Gudgeon N, Cobbold M, Khanna R, Nayak L, Rickinson AB, Moss, PA (2004) Herpesvirus-specific CD8 T cell immunity in old age: cytomegalovirus impairs the response to a coresident EBV infection. J Immunol 173:7481–7489.

Ku CC, Kappler J, Marrack P (2001) The Growth of Very Large CD8+ T cell Clones in Older Mice is Controlled by Cytokines. Journal of Immunology166:2186–2193

Lee SK, Surh CD (2005) Role of interleukin-7 in bone and T-cell homeostasis. Immunol Rev 208:169–180

LeMaoult J, Messaoudi I, Manavalan JS, Potvin H, Nikolich-Žugich D, Dyall R, Szabo P, Weksler M E, Nikolich-Žugich J (2000) Age-related dysregulation in CD8 T cell homeostasis: kinetics of a diversity loss. J Immuno 165:2367–2373

Leung GM, Hedley AJ, Ho LM, Chau P, Wong IO, Thach TQ, Ghani AC, Donnelly CA, Fraser C, Riley S, et al. (2004) The epidemiology of severe acute respiratory syndrome in the 2003 Hong Kong epidemic: an analysis of all 1755 patients. Ann Intern Med 141:662–673

Messaoudi I, Lemaoult J, Guevara-Patino JA, Metzner BM, Nikolich-Žugich J (2004) Age-related CD8 T cell clonal expansions constrict CD8 T cell repertoire and have the potential to impair immune defense. J Exp Med 200:1347–1358

Messaoudi I, Warner J, Fischer M, Park B, Hill B, Mattison J, Lane MA, Roth GS, Ingram DK, Picker LJ, et al. (2006a) Delay of T cell senescence by caloric restriction in aged long-lived nonhuman primates. Proc Natl Acad Sci U S A 103:19448–19453

Messaoudi I, Warner J, Nikolich-Žugich D, Fischer M, Nikolich-Žugich J (2006b) Molecular, cellular, and antigen requirements for development of age-associated T cell clonal expansions in vivo. J Immunol 176:301–308

Messaoudi I, Warner J, Nikolich-Žugich J (2006c) Age-related CD8+ T cell clonal expansions express elevated levels of CD122 and CD127 and display defects in perceiving homeostatic signals. J Immunol 177:2784–2792

Miller RA (1996) The aging immune system: primer and prospectus. Science 273:70–74

Miller RA, Stutman O (1981) Decline, in aging mice, of the anti-2,4,6-trinitrophenyl (TNP) cytotoxic T cell response attributable to loss of Lyt-2-, interleukin 2-producing helper cell function. Eur J Immunol 11:751–756

Moon JJ, Chu HH, Pepper M, McSorley SJ, Jameson SC, Kedl RM, Jenkins MK (2007) Naive CD4(+) T cell frequency varies for different epitopes and predicts repertoire diversity and response magnitude. Immunity 27:203–213

Murray K, Baraniuk S, Resnick M, Arafat R, Kilborn C, Cain K, Shallenberger R, York TL, Martinez D, Hellums JS, et al (2006) Risk factors for encephalitis and death from West Nile virus infection. Epidemiol Infect 134:1325–1332

Naylor K, Li G, Vallejo AN, Lee WW, Koetz K, Bryl E, Witkowski J, Fulbright J, Weyand C M, Goronzy JJ (2005) The influence of age on T cell generation and TCR diversity. J Immunol 174:7446–7452

Nikolich-Žugich J (2005) T cell aging: naive but not young. J Exp Med 201:837–840

Nikolich-Žugich J (2007) Non-human primate models of T-cell reconstitution. Semin Immunol 19:310–317

Nikolich-Žugich J, Messaoudi I (2005) Mice and flies and monkeys too: caloric restriction rejuvenates the aging immune system of non-human primates. Exp Gerontol 40:884–893

Nikolich-Žugich J, Slifka MK, Messaoudi I (2004) The many important facets of T-cell repertoire diversity. Nat Rev Immunol 4:123–132

Ortiz-Suarez A, Miller R A (2002) A subset of CD8 memory T cells from old mice have high levels of CD28 and produce IFNg1. Clin Immunol 104:282–292

Ortiz-Suarez A, Miller RA (2003) Antigen-Independent Expansion of CD28hi CD8 Cells From Aged Mice: Cytokine Requirements and Signal Transduction Pathways. J Gerontol ABiol Sci 58A:11063–11073

Ouyang Q, Wagner WM, Voehringer D, Wikby A, Klatt T, Walter S, Muller CA, Pircher H, Pawelec G (2003a) Age-associated accumulation of CMV-specific CD8+ T cells expressing the inhibitory killer cell lectin-like receptor G1 (KLRG1). Exp Gerontol 38:911–920

Ouyang Q, Wagner WM, Walter S, Muller CA, Wikby A, Aubert G, Klatt T, Stevanovic S, Dodi T, Pawelec G (2003b) An age-related increase in the number of CD8+ T cells carrying receptors for an immunodominant Epstein-Barr virus (EBV) epitope is counteracted by a decreased frequency of their antigen-specific responsiveness. Mech Ageing Dev 124:477–485

Ouyang Q, Wagner WM, Wikby A, Remarque E, Pawelec G (2002) Compromised interferon gamma (IFN-gamma) production in the elderly to both acute and latent viral antigen stimulation: contribution to the immune risk phenotype? Eur Cytokine Netw 13:392–394

Ouyang Q, Wagner WM, Wikby A, Walter S, Aubert G, Dodi AI, Travers P, Pawelec G (2003c) Large numbers of dysfunctional CD8+ T lymphocytes bearing receptors for a single dominant CMV epitope in the very old. J Clin Immunol 23:247–257

Ouyang Q, Wagner WM, Zheng W, Wikby A, Remarque EJ, Pawelec G (2004) Dysfunctional CMV-specific CD8(+) T cells accumulate in the elderly. Exp Gerontol 39:607–613

Pawelec G, Akbar A, Caruso C, Effros R, Grubeck-Loebenstein B, Wikby A (2004) Is immunosenescence infectious? Trends Immunol 25:406–410

Podlech J, Holtappels R, Pahl-Seibert MF, Steffens HP, Reddehase MJ (2000) Murine model of interstitial cytomegalovirus pneumonia in syngeneic bone marrow transplantation: persistence of protective pulmonary CD8-T-cell infiltrates after clearance of acute infection. J Virol 74:7496–7507

Posnett DN, Sinha S, Kabak S, Russo C (1994) Clonal populations of T cells in normal elderly humans: the T cell equivalent to "benign monoclonal gammapathy". J Exp Med 179:609–617

Saurwein-Teissl M, Lung T, Marx F, Gschösser C, Asch E, Blasko I, Parson W, Bäck G, Schönitzer D, Trannoy E, Grubeck-Loebenstein B (2002) Lack of antibody production following immunization in old age: association with CD8+CD28- T cell clonal expansions and an imbalance in the production of Th1 and Th2 cytokines1. J Immunol 168:5893–5899

Scollay R, Butcher E, Weissman I (1980) Thymus migration: quantitative studies on the rate of migration of cells from the thymus to the periphery in mice. Eur J Immunol 10:210

Sprent J, Schaefer M, Hurd M, Surh C D, Ron Y (1991) Mature murine B and T cells transferred to SCID mice can survive indefinitely and many maintain a virgin phenotype. J Exp Med 174:717–728

Stowe RP, Kozlova EV, Yetman DL, Walling DM, Goodwin JS, Glaser R (2007) Chronic herpesvirus reactivation occurs in aging. Exp Gerontol 42:563–570

Surh CD, Boyman O, Purton JF, Sprent J (2006) Homeostasis of memory T cells. Immunol Rev 211:154–163

Surh CD, Sprent J (2002) Regulation of naive and memory T-cell homeostasis. Microbes Infect 4:51–56

Tamir A, Eisenbraun MD, Garcia GG, Miller RA (2000) Age-dependent alterations in the assembly of signal transduction complexes at the site of T cell/APC interaction. J Immunol 165:1243–1251

Tan J, Ernst B, Kieper W, LeRoy E, Sprent J, Surh C (2002) Interleukin (IL)-15 and IL-7 jointly regulate homeostatic proliferation of memory phenotype CD8+ cells but are not required for memory phenotype CD4 +cells. J Exp Med 195:1523–1532

Thoman ML, Weigle W O (1981) Lymphokines and aging: interleukin-2 production and activity in aged animals. J Immunol 127:2102–2106

Wallace ME, Keating R, Heath WR, Carbone FR (1999) The cytotoxic T-cell response to herpes simplex virus type 1 infection of C57BL/6 mice is almost entirely directed against a single immunodominant determinant. J Virol 73:7619–7626

Wikby A, Ferguson F, Forsey R, Thompson J, Strindhall J, Lofgren S, Nilsson B O, Ernerudh J, Pawelec G, Johansson B (2005) An immune risk phenotype, cognitive impairment, and survival in very late life: impact of allostatic load in Swedish octogenarian and nonagenarian humans. J Gerontol A Biol Sci Med Sci 60:556–565

Yoshikawa TT (2000) Epidemiology and unique aspects of aging and infectious diseases. Clin Infect Dis 30:931–933

Zuniga-Pflucker JC, Van Den Brink MR (2007) Giving T cells a chance to come back. Semin Immunol 19:279

T-cell Cycle and Immunosenescence: Role of Aging in the T-cell Proliferative Behaviour and Status Quo Maintenance

Jacek M. Witkowski

Contents

Organismal aging is affecting the performance of the immune system of mammals (including human one, being the topic of this chapter), and usually is associated with decreased ability to built adequate immune response to new and even cognate antigenic challenges on one side, and with reported increased frequency of autoimmune reactivity against own antigens [34, 61, 64] (but see the chapter by Ewa Bryl and JMW in this volume). Common manifestations of this immunological impairment are thus increased susceptibility (and more difficult curability) of infectious diseases (which in the old age become one of the most important killers despite the achievements of modern "western" medicine), as well as increased frequencies of at least certain malignancies.

The pool of T-lymphocytes, getting their name from its intrathymic period of maturation and selection after exiting the bone marrow and prior to settling in the peripheral lymphatic organs, is a variable, multifunctional and multi-phenotype group of not-so-similar cells. There is—of course—the basic subdivision into the "T-helper" or CD4$^+$ and "T cytotoxic/suppressor" CD8$^+$ lymphocytes, but this is by far a simplification. Thus, within each of the abovementioned, one would encounter first the subpopulations differing in their "life history" prior to the moment of analysis. Among them, the cells that are still "fresh" from the thymus, or had never yet encountered the antigenic epitope for which their T-cell receptors or TCRs were selected, are rightly called the naïve or virgin T-lymphocytes, while those that are a result of such an encounter would be further subdivided into the—relatively short-lived—effector lymphocytes and the supposedly long-lived memory cells (but see below on the lifespan of naïve and memory T-cells). Within the latter, a further subdivision exists that allows the distinction of so called central and effector memory cells. These subpopulations can be relatively easily detected and quantified with the use of monoclonal antibodies recognizing their specific antigens (e.g. CD45RA, CD45R0, CD62L, CCR7 and many others, as described in all current immunology

J. M. Witkowski (✉)
Department of Pathophysiology
Medical University of Gdansk
Poland

T. Fulop et al. (eds.), *Handbook on Immunosenescence,*
DOI 10.1007/ 978-1-4020-9062-2_13, © Springer Science+Business Media B.V. 2009

textbooks) and flow cytometry, in the samples of peripheral blood, and—when an animal (usually mouse) model is studied, also in other lymphatic organs and bone marrow.

All these cell types function with one major goal: to survey the organism in search of alien moieties that are or may become damaging to the integrity of the organism, and to develop specific ways of their neutralization and elimination (called adoptive immunity), regardless from their origin, which may obviously be extra- and intra-organismal. To achieve this goal, the T-lymphocytes must properly **interact with each other** within the general, and, as sketched above, already complex "family", by means of either direct contact or secreted mediators (cytokines). The scheme of these interactions is depicted in Fig. 1. Their function towards this goal is not standing alone; contrarily, in order to perform adequately (i.e., to eliminate or otherwise neutralize the alien antigen or cell) T-lymphocytes must interact with, influence and be influenced by other cell types, including the broad family of antigen-presenting cells (professional APCs, requiring the MHC (or HLA) Class II to interact with the CD4$^+$ cells) on one side, and the two remaining groups of lymphocytes—the NK- and B-cells—on the other. One has to remember however, that the above does NOT constitute all contacts and interactions of the T-cells. Thus, practically every cell may influence the behavior of CD8$^+$ lymphocytes via its HLA Class I molecules and epitopes anchored onto them; cells belonging to the players in the inflammatory process (especially, but not exclusively, all forms of macrophages) would affect the T-cells by secreting the "pro-inflammatory" cytokines (e.g., IL-1, IL-6 or TNF) that are known to trigger specific receptors on these cells. Finally, T-lymphocytes contain receptors (and relevant intracellular signalling pathways) able to react to the plethora of other biologically important mediators that may appear in the organism under stress, exercise, injury and on many other instances; these would include first of all neuromediators generated by the central nervous system and hormones (Fig. 1). Through these integrative systems of the organism the lymphocytes get knowledge about its status and about external factors that might require their activity. Any and all of these interactions might be (and, according to the current knowledge mostly are) affected by the aging process.

Now, the effectiveness of an immune response, understood as the quickness and completeness of the neutralization/removal of potentially dangerous antigen is therefore **dependent on the two major, related factors. The first** is the availability of adequate numbers of the cells that can react to the antigenic challenge. They would have appropriate, broad repertoire of the TCR/CD3 complexes and accessory molecules (including first of all the CD4 or CD8 and CD28 in right numbers on their surface, and the intracellular machinery of signal transduction, protein synthesis, DNA replication, cell division etc. in good working order. **The second** stems from the first and is the ability of a T-cell population to temporarily increase numbers of effector T-cells, whose role is to neutralize the invading antigen directly or with the help of cytokine-driven NK killer cells or antibody-producing B-lymphocytes, and which should then quickly get stopped by regulatory/suppressive T-cells and ultimately disappear by the Activation-Induced Cell Death (AICD) being a form of apoptosis (see the chapter by Ewa Sikora in this volume). This second

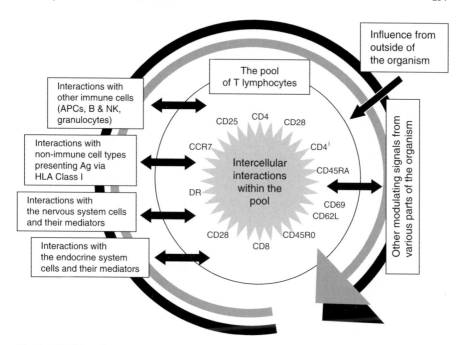

Fig. 1 The idea of T-cells' pool interactions within the broader organismal network, requiring proper numbers and functionalities of all members

utmost important factor ascertaining the optimal immune response is therefore the process, called **T-cell proliferation**.

The above is of course the basic tenet of current immunology. However, what perspires as important for our consideration of aging-related changes in the performance of the immune system, is the need to maintain the right **proportions and numbers** of all of the abovementioned cellular (sub)populations in order to keep the whole system optimally effective (please mark "optimally", which does not mean "maximally" and might mean the difference between the immunity and the autoimmunity). As mentioned above, direct intercellular contacts and humoral signals form the two ways various cells of the immune system communicate with each other and with other cell types. For these "means of communication" to be optimally effective and lead to the goal being the antigen neutralization, the communicating cells have to be in proximity to each other and in adequate numbers, which is maintained by effective proliferation (multiplication) of various T-cell subpopulations responding to an antigenic challenge. It is commonly accepted that both the proportions as well as absolute numbers of various subpopulations of the human T-cell pool change with advancing age which may be at least one of the reasons for decreased overall performance of the system in the elderly.

Thus, T-lymphocyte pool appears as a component of a very complex, dynamic, (and by far not fully understood) web or network of interactions, where the signals conveying information may be either direct intercellular contacts or cellular (secreted) molecules. Each and every component of this network may undergo aging- and/or pathology-associated changes, affecting its functions and—among other—its interactions with the immune system and with the T-cells in particular. It is a very hard task to understand, how in fact aging *"as such"* is affecting the (T) cells of the immune system (example: a whatever subpopulation of T-cells drawn from an old organism might be absolutely normal and do not functionally differ from the same population drawn from a young organism; however, at the moment of sampling, the nervous (or say, hormonal) system in the old organism could have failed to secrete some mediator or hormone and this lack would affect the T-cell under study leading to an observed different reactivity, when compared with these from a young individual). Therefore in practically all current studies such broad analysis of multivariable status of organisms, from which the immune cells are drawn, is not performed and it is assumed that whatever "extra-T-cell" influences may affect the T-cells of an old individual they would integrate and be relatively similar through the healthy elderly cohort (yet different from the healthy young cohort, as a matter of course). Thus, the result of any test comparing the immune cells' function in the healthy young and elderly bear the burden (and thus—doubts) of our lack of general knowledge about the individual's status preceding the experiment.

While trying to understand the complexity of the T-cell system as a part of the (more general) immune system, its interactions and interrelations (both within the system and with the other ones (Fig. 1)) and, especially, any changes in its function related to advancing age and the process of aging, one has to be very aware of a basic difference between the immune systems of human beings and of model laboratory animals. The latter, usually germ-free or at least "specific pathogen-free" mice, have their immune systems all but dormant until the experimenter challenges them in vivo or in vitro (with possible exception of newly transformed neoplasm cells, that may form an unpredicted source of antigens even under such conditions). On the other hand, our own immune cells are not only on constant alert, but, in fact, constantly in-fight (although not all of them at the same time, of course!); our environment (the air we breathe, the foods and drinks, other members of our species, our pets and farm animals etc.) is full of antigens, both those already known to the immune (memory) cells and the new ones, challenging the naïve T-cell pool.

Within the abovementioned network pervading the organism, the T-cells will dwell only in certain locations or microenvironments, providing for them the relevant survival and sometimes mitogenic signals; these locations can be collectively called the "T-cell niche" (Fig. 2), even if it is already known that different T-cell subpopulations would require different sets of these survival-and-proliferative signals and thus will rather live in a few partially overlapping "niches". A very good example here is the memory T-cell niche, which had recently been shown to be defined by the ligands belonging to the TNF family and in fact differentiating between the CD8[+] memory and CD4[+] memory "subniches" [74].

Thus, the T-cell niche (being, in fact, a sum of all "T-cell subpopulations' niches") in a human organism is never static. Both the proportions and the absolute numbers of various T-cell (sub)populations are homeostatically maintained throughout most of our adult life, in order to keep this niche (consisting of the T-cell compartments in

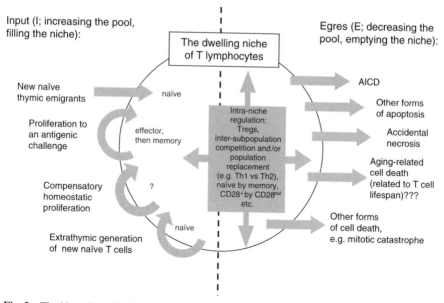

Input (I; increasing the pool, filling the niche):

The dwelling niche of T lymphocytes

Egres (E; decreasing the pool, emptying the niche):

New naïve thymic emigrants

naïve

Proliferation to an antigenic challenge

effector, then memory

Compensatory homeostatic proliferation

?

Intra-niche regulation: Tregs, inter-subpopulation competition and/or population replacement (e.g. Th1 vs Th2), naïve by memory, CD28+ by CD28nul etc.

naïve

Extrathymic generation of new naïve T cells

AICD

Other forms of apoptosis

Accidental necrosis

Aging-related cell death (related to T cell lifespan)???

Other forms of cell death, e.g. mitotic catastrophe

Fig. 2   The idea of T-cell niche homeostasis; I = E

the lymphatic organs, bone marrow and circulating lymphocytes, although the latter can also be considered a "common sink" or corridor for all of the relevant "niches", where members of different ones may meet and interact) relatively constant in volume, yet ready to respond to any antigenic challenge with enough effectiveness to keep the organism healthy (or, at least, to ascertain its survival when confronted by a pathogen). These **homeostatic regulators (homeostats)** consist of the mechanisms leading on one hand to fast and concerted accumulation of all the required effector cells (the "input" side in the Figs. 2 and 3), but containing various ways the T-cell may die (apoptosis, necrosis etc., the "egres" side in the Figs. 2 and 3), including the production of regulatory T-cells with one or another type of suppressive activity against their activated sisters on the other (see below and the chapters by K Hirokawa and by P Moss in this volume for more detail on T-cell homeostasis and regulatory T-cells respectively).

One of the most important questions for our understanding what happens with our T-cells when we age was interesting gerontologists for many years and it is still not answered yet. Why—knowing that our immune system is impaired and generally loosing its functionality when we age—we do not observe major decrease in its volume—in the peripheral blood lymphocytosis for example, or in the palpable volume of the lymph nodes in the old individuals? In other words: what keeps the T-cell niche in an active equilibrium over our young and middle age, i.e., what homeostats play the major role(s) in the process, and how they change when we get old? Let us consider the general situation in the T-cell niche (Fig. 2.). The mechanisms increasing the volume of the niche(s) (the "input" side in the Fig. 2.) can be divided into intrinsic and extrinsic to the niche-dwelling cells itself. Those

intrinsic to the in-niche T-cells themselves will mostly depend on the antigenic (or, in vitro—also mitogenic) challenge. They will consist of: **ability to recognize the stimulatory signal** (an antigen, in vitro also mitogens) from environmental noise, which requires proper diversity and numbers of the TCR/CD3 complexes, **ability to distinguish the signal as "requiring response"** which requires proper MHC/HLA context, availability of other (costimulator) molecules (especially CD28) interacting with the antigen-presenting cells, adequate numbers (surface densities) of these, and the **ability to properly respond to incoming signals** which requires functional signal transduction mechanisms (starting from the proper numbers of relevant T-cell surface receptors), functional gene activation and transcription machinery, functional protein synthesis apparatus. Within this proper response lays, of course, the **ability to divide** (proliferate, i.e., undergo productive mitosis, leading to the generation of viable daughter (effector) cells), which requires adequately functional cellular machinery directly involved in the processes of error-free DNA replication, and in its separation into newly formed nuclei of the daughter cells.

The mechanisms **extrinsic to the in-niche T-lymphocytes** would contain **influx of new, naïve T**-cells generated in the thymus or extra-thymically, **T-cell survival signals,** which may be generated in the niche or outside (these include IL-2 and other growth factors) and, possibly, also the hypothetical and currently mostly unknown **factors that govern the development and size of the microenvironment** creating the niche stroma. One has also to bear in mind the postulated homeostatic proliferation of the T-cells—one that supposedly provides new naïve T-cells even after the cessation of thymic lymphopoiesis; it can probably also increase or at least sustain the numbers of the memory cells (possibly *ex definitione* also without antigenic stimulation) and thus would get more and more importance with advancing age (see below).

Considering the mechanisms decreasing the volume of the niche(s) or the eliminators of "surplus" (or temporary surplus) T-cells (the "egres" side in the Fig. 2), one would have to list first those intrinsic to the activation process, i.e., any form of Activation Induced Cell Death (AICD). This is a major safety valve against uncontrolled overproduction or protracted dwelling of activated T-lymphocytes in the niche, which could—and sometimes does—result in either autoimmunity or transformation into leukaemic growth, that eliminates practically all no-more-necessary effectors. Apparently, the AICD occurs only or mostly at the early G1A phase of the cell cycle [43]. Other forms of apoptosis will constitute another negative homeostat—like the one related to lack of growth- or survival-promoting factors, or that induced by irreparable (or not repaired soon enough) DNA damage. These would not be limited to any specific phase of the cell cycle.

Another somewhat similar way of elimination of the T-cells will be the **mitotic catastrophe**—when all the signals and processes are in order until the moment of mitosis, where "something" goes wrong and proper separation of genetic material does not occur; however, in case of normal human lymphocytes, this way of cellular dying is not yet well understood or even proven [82].

The T-cell (similarly to other 300+ cell types of our of organism) my also die by other means, not directly related to their physiological function. First of all, they may die by **accidental necrosis**—when the intracellular compensatory (homeo-static) mechanisms fail when confronted with—for example—a metabolic toxin, lack of oxygen, or (admittedly very unlike for lymphocytes) mechanical damage.

And finally, what should be of an utmost interest considering the topic of this chapter and the entire book, it is possible that **T-cells die "of old age"** i.e., because they had aged so much that their intracellular homeostats cannot support life anymore. This last possibility bears with it another question, that about the actual lifespan of human lymphocytes. Are they short-lived (on the scale of days) and rapidly replaced? Are they long-lived and—when not confronted with an antigenic challenge—is their lifespan comparable to that of the organisms (i.e., measured in many years for human beings)? This question, obviously of an utmost importance for understanding the balance within the T-cell niche, is not so easy to answer. In order to know the actual (or maximal) lifespan of any T-cells' subpopulation, one would have to mark it somehow at the beginning of the individuals' life and then observe how long these marked cells would stay present in the organism under study. In fact, such analysis has been performed both for mice and for humans. In the former, it is possible to draw and isolate the lymphocytes, mark them with a stable fluorescent tag (for example the carboxyfluorescein diacetate succinimidyl ester (CFSE)), reinject in the animal and then seek the fluorescent cells in the blood or lymphatic organ of the animal after at least many months, which correspond to a substantial portion of the animals' life [46]. The fluorochrome is found not only to be a stable marker of the tagged cell, but also to be proportionally, arithmetically diluted into its daughter cells; i.e., if the CFSE-tagged cell divided once, their daughters would contain ½ of the fluorescent signal, their daughters 1/4th etc. Thus, if after some time we would still see the cells with the fluorescent signal exceeding ½ of the original, we must assume they did not divide since the tagging operation, so their lifespan has to be at least equal to the period between the tagging and the observation. For murine T-cells it was shown to exceed on average half a year, which for most mice strains is about 1/4th of their typical lifespan. This constitutes a proof that at least some murine T-cells may live for a major portion of the animal's life and, possibly, their lifespan would be similar to the lifespan of the mouse.

The same is much more difficult in humans—for obvious reasons we cannot tag and observe our own cells that way. Also, one has to be careful to distinguish between the proliferative lifespan of a T cell—i.e., how long it and its progeny of the same clone would stay in the organism—and the lifespan of a T-cell "as such"—i.e., how long a nondividing T-cell can stay alive and "clog the niche". A dreadful event in recent history actually did the human cell tagging for us. In 1945, citizens of two Japanese cities were exposed to extremely high radiation of atom bombs. Many of those, who survived the holocaust, exhibited various mutations and changes in their genetic material, frequently leading to the development of malignancy (including the leukemias). However, in some of them a special type of chromosomal mutation can be demonstrated; this one leads to the appearance of circular chromosomes and other chromosomal mutation, precluding the symmetrical division of such T-cells [40, 41]. Thus, putting the two together: if the cell with this mutation was generated in 1945 and it can still be detected today, it must be more than 60 years old; in fact, these are the maximal estimates of the human lymphocyte lifespan based on this singular phenomenon [53–55].

Newer data, utilizing other approaches for establishing the maximal (or average) lifespan of human T-cells are more confounding and yield much smaller values, from a few days or weeks in the case of naïve, to at most a couple of years for the memory T-cells [5, 47, 48] (albeit some papers state that the memory T-cells do not differ or have a shorter lifespan [87]. However, these tests, marking the cells for example with deuterated (^{2}H)-glucose, do NOT actually "see" the marked cells throughout their life, but estimate average lifespans based on incorporation of the ^{2}H-glucose deuterium in the DNA; thus it is rather an average than a maximal lifespan that they estimate. Another popular way of assessing the T-cell clone lifespan is by the estimation of number of population doubling in vitro and then multiplying it by the time required for a single population doubling. This is of course the T-cell proliferative lifespan, not the maximal (or even average) time any single T-lymphocyte may live when undisturbed in an organism. This type of study yields the average lifespan for human memory cells about 15 years and their maximal lifespan of about 35 years [1]. More recent data from the in vitro cultivated T-cell clones show that hey can perform close to 100 population doublings, which would extend their maximal lifespan to that close to observed for T-cells of the A-bomb victims [62, 63]. Concluding, at least some T-cells may stay alive for a long time even if not dividing and thus "clog the niche";—i.e., limit the available space for the progeny of the still-reactive lymphocytes.

As long as the two processes (i.e., production and/or influx of new T-cells and the removal of the T-lymphocytes that are no more needed) are in relative balance, the niche "volume" or total numbers of included T-cells will stay more or less stable (even if the properties (phenotype) of the cells filling it will change, the quantity will be homeostatically maintained). This seems to be true for the fate of T-cell niche in the healthy young individuals (Fig. 3a). Still, all the time one has to be aware that the above description is general (using the keyword "T-cells" rather than alluding to separate subpopulations of these) and that so far there are not much data regarding the behaviour of any single T-cell subpopulation as a niche-filler. One consideration that must be made here and that would impact on the overall reactivity of the T-cell system in the aged (but would not in fact change much the total numbers of T-cells in the niche) would be the slow replacement of many very diversified variants of the T-cell receptor TCR (deciding on the ability of T-cells to react to multitude of previously unknown antigens) by much fewer numbers of these, leading to the phenomenon described as TCR repertoire contraction and resulting in vastly reduced ability of T-cells of even healthy elderly to recognize and react to new antigenic challenges [60].

However, as the organism/individual ages, these homeostats seem to become more and more impaired, as we know from the observational and experimental evidence accumulated so far.

Based on the early studies of the ability of T-cells of old mice and elderly people to proliferate in vitro to mitogenic challenge, it was long ago established that their overall proliferative capacity is significantly dwindling with advancing age. It

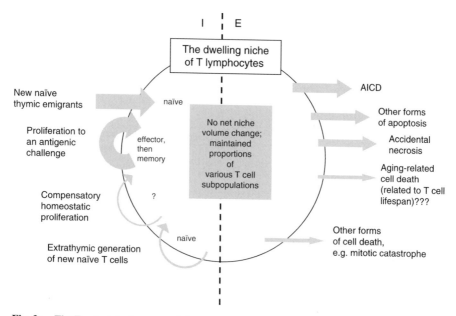

Fig. 3a The T-cell niche homeostasis in young adults: I ≈ E

has been shown many times both for the T-cells of old mice as well as for human peripheral blood lymphocytes (for the review see for example [33, 61]). T-cells of old organisms incorporate less ³H-thymidine when stimulated in vitro with either immobilized anti-CD3/anti-CD28 or with plant mitogens (like phytohaemagglutinin or concanavalin A) or with the "membrane-bypassing" cocktail of calcium ionophore ionomycin and phorbol ester. Also, when their ability to double their numbers in vitro is calculated, it is significantly, much lower than that of young cells. Both these parameters tell us that the general, T-cell population-wide ability to respond to relevant stimuli is decreased in the T-cells of old individuals (reviewed in [20 33]). The net result should be the reduction of the T-cell niche volume/cellularity (Fig. 3b).

One of the problem a researcher of T-cell aging encounters when studying the field is the T-cell phenotypic shift occurring in the elderly. The best known forms of this remodeling are the naïve-to-memory shift and the accumulation of T-cells deprived of CD28 costimulatory molecule [9, 24, 28]. The first, naïve-to-memory shift (or accumulation of phenotypically memory T-cells at the expense of naïve ones) is intuitively obvious: given relatively constant T-cell niche volume and many years of exposure to environmental antigens and pathogens, our adaptive immune system must produce many variants of memory cells left behind after each antigenic challenge, that will take the niche space [16]. In addition, we know for many decades that the main if not sole provider of new naïve T-cells in our youth, the thymus, is grossly reducing its output after the puberty (even if we know now, that it does NOT stop working then; in fact, naïve T-cells and the thymic hormones are

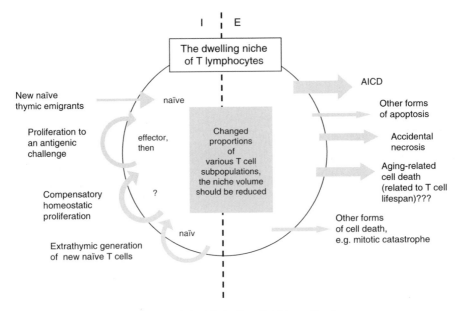

Fig. 3b The T-cell niche homeostasis in elderly: I << E (old paradigm)

produced still when we are approaching old age) [15, 59]. At the very old age the thymus is apparently no more the source of new, naïve T-lymphocytes, yet even in the very old people we can still detect some of them [59, 65]. This leads to the conclusion that either they are the survivors from our youth or middle age (but see the discussion on the T-cell lifespan in this chapter!) or they are maturing from the bone marrow precursors without the need of the thymic microenvironment (extra-thymically). The data showing decreased numbers of new thymic emigrants containing the TCR gene rearrangement excision circles or TRECS suggest that in the very old (centenarians) such cells are practically absent [59] which would rather support the first possibility. The question how it in fact is and another—whether these naïve T-cells that appear in the elderly are still fully functional (for instance, can they still divide as dynamically as the naïve T-cells of young individuals when challenged)—remains unanswered so far.

A related factor is that the proportion of T-cells that do not enter division cycle upon stimulation (nonzero even in the young individuals) is vastly increasing among T-cells of old people. These lymphocytes are presumably proliferatively senescent, i.e. post-mitotic and unable to divide anymore. However, it is not known as yet, whether they in fact only "stay there" and "clog the niche", or are they still able to perform some other, nonproliferative functions, like the cytotoxic or regulatory (cytokine- or contact-related) activities. One of the possibilities is that they could be devoid of certain essential molecule (or signalling pathway) necessary for initiation of proliferation; an important candidate here could be the major costimulator molecule of the T-cells, the CD28.

Accumulation of the CD28^{nul} subpopulation in both the CD4$^+$ and CD8$^+$ lymphocyte populations was found to accompany even healthy aging [9, 21, 24, 88, 92]. Certain studies demonstrated that these CD28^{nul} cells have many features ascribed to the aging T-cell population, including the decreased proliferative capability measured by ^{3}H-TdR incorporation [9, 13, 18, 19, 22, 23, 92], contracted T-cell repertoire [78, 89] (see also the chapter by J. Goronzy in this volume) and modified cytokine production [2, 26, 76]. Thus it was assumed that their accumulation might be responsible for the impaired functioning of the T-cell pool in the elderly. However, while CD28^{nul} cells may form even more than 50% of all circulating CD8$^+$ lymphocytes they rarely exceed 10% of the CD4$^+$ cells in a healthy elderly individual [9, 11, 21, 24, 88, 92]. Thus, their accumulation cannot be considered the culprit for grossly decreased proliferation rate of either CD4$^+$ or even CD8$^+$ lymphocytes (even in the latter population, the decrease in 3H-thymidine incorporation is by far more than 50% when we compare cells from young and elderly individuals). Interestingly, even the relatively high accumulation of CD8$^+$CD28^{nul} lymphocytes in the elderly cannot be responsible for decreased proliferative capacity of the CD8$^+$ population in old people; it was recently found (using the flow cytometric DCT technique utilizing the supravital staining of proliferating cells with the fluorescein derivative, CFSE) that in fact, these CD8$^+$CD28^{nul} cells do proliferate more and more with advancing age and, when drawn from the blood of oldest old, they can make in vitro many divisions [14]. This was also shown for t he CD4$^+$CD28^{nul} cells, albeit the latter seem to be less proliferatively active in the elderly than their CD8$^+$ counterparts [12]. Thus, overall effect of accumulation of CD28^{nul} cells on the status of the T-cell pool in the aged (at least for its CD4$^+$ compartment) cannot be that much, unless they would be functional regulators/suppressors. This latter possibility is tempting, however until now (mid-2007) it had not been sufficiently documented, despite showing at least some cytotoxic abilities in them [52, 56, 58].

On the other hand, the existence and potential importance of the CD28^{nul} cells (at least within the CD4$^+$ population of human lymphocytes) may be just the tip of an iceberg, with the most of it metaphorically containing the CD4$^+$ cells with lowered numbers of CD28 molecules on their surfaces, but not lacking them altogether. In fact, we were able to show some transcriptive activity of the CD28 gene by RT-PCR even in the notorious CD4$^+$CD28^{nul} clones, which suggests that the actual range of CD28 expression level on the human CD4$^+$ lymphocytes might be from near-zero to whatever maximum (Witkowski, unpublished). We have shown before that this is the case: CD4$^+$ lymphocytes of healthy elderly people express on average fewer CD28 molecules per cell than those from healthy young people [12, 93]. This observation is similar to that obtained for the CD4$^+$ lymphocytes of rheumatoid arthritis (RA) patients, considered to show the phenotype of accelerated aging [11]. Decreased numbers of CD28 on elderly CD4$^+$ cells expectedly have their consequence, the CD28 being known as a major costimulatory molecule for these cells. Using advanced DCT technique we were able to show that the CD28 molecules' number inversely correlates with the time, required by the T-cell to exit the resting G_0 phase and to enter their first division upon stimulation [12, 93].

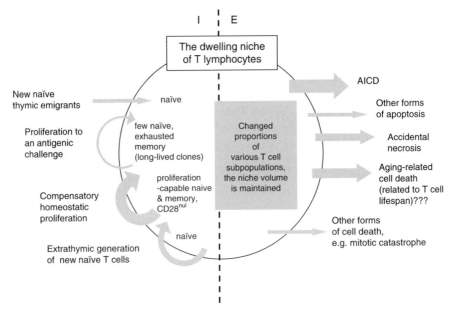

Fig. 3c   The T-cell niche homeostasis in elderly: I ≈ E (proposed model)

Summarizing current knowledge, with aging the production of new cells [both naïve (first of all) and effector as well as memory] seems to be reduced, and the accumulation of post-mitotic, senescent T-cells is increased. On the other hand the AICD and, possibly, other forms of apoptosis and—hypothetically—T-cell death related to the more and more of them attaining cellular old age (senescence) and dying of it, as well as possibly the mitotic catastrophe related to accumulating DNA damage are increased. This would result in the net emptying of the T-cell niche, observed as lower numbers of T-lymphocytes in the circulating blood, reduced volume of the T-cell compartments in the lymphatic tissues etc (Fig. 3b). However, these symptoms do not occur, so some mechanism must maintain the filling of the niche (Fig. 3c).

Why do the T-cells proliferate differently in the aged individuals remains not fully understood. It is well established that various facets of the signal transduction mechanisms leading to the turning on of the DNA replication and cell division are impaired in the T-cells of the elderly [31–33] (see also Tamas Fulop's chapter in this book). The major mechanism governing the progression of the cell cycle when it was already initiated consists of the interplay between the cyclin-dependent kinases (the cdks, in the lymphocytes mostly cdk 2, 4 and 6) that are supposed to phosphorylate specific proteins at specific times during the process, the cyclins (A through G, forming regulatory parts of the active phosphorylating complexes, but must be tightly controlled and timely eliminated or the cell may become neoplastic) and the cyclin-kinase complex inhibitors including the p21cip/waf, p16ink4 etc. The latter are already known to accumulate in many cell types of old individuals including the lymphocytes [36]; ultimately their amount is supposedly that high that the cell cannot perform any cdk-dependent phosphorylation and stops dividing completely, reaching proliferative senescence. On the other hand, the levels of cyclins and the cdks are posing more difficulties for interpretation. It was shown that the levels of cyclins A, G and D (2 and 3) are lowered in the T-cells of old individuals. These observations are related to their increased destruction by the ubiquitin-dependent proteolytic machinery [68–70] and possibly also due to decreased activity of relevant genes [4, 25, 36, 73]. Similarly T-cells of the elderly are containing less cdk kinases, which disrupts the phosphorylation processes needed for cell cycle progression [4, 25, 36, 73]. However, the data available so far do not consider the remodelling of the T-cell pool, including the increase in the proportion of senescent cells. Thus, it is theoretically possible that those T-cells that are still capable to proliferate in the elderly may have these mechanisms even more active than the young ones! In fact this is precisely what we see: using the DCT cytometric technique we had demonstrated more divisions made in vitro by fewer CD4$^+$ cells of the elderly people, associated with increased levels of D1 cyclin (governing the length of the G1 phase of the cycle), both total and cdk-bound in an active complex [93].

This brings us to the whole huge question of possible changes in the cell cycle length and productivity related to aging.

When we consider the actual cell cycle length (or the time between the two consecutive mitoses) we have to bear in mind the serious consequences of shortening or elongation of the cycle by relatively minor span of time per cycle. Using simple enough arithmetic one can show that the cells, for which the cell cycle is shorter, will make more divisions at the same time compared to other with longer cycle. As the average length of the human T-cell cycle is somewhere between 12 and 20 hours [93] and stimulated T-cells are able to perform up to 15 or more division in vitro without artificial support (like feeder cells or IL-2 and other growth factor supplementation), one can easily calculate that after the time the cells with longer cycle spent on x division, those with shorter cycle would make x + 1/cell cycle length * number of cycles until time of observation; eventually, after a precisely calculable time faster cells would make one division more than the slower ones, i.e, at the end of that time, there should be up to twice as many faster cells than slower ones! This may be of physiological importance, for example as a reason for elimination of less active clones by more active ones and changed TCR diversity in the elderly. Thus, it seems important to know if the cell cycle length changes with advancing age.

In fact such studies were performed already a few times for murine and human T-cells from donors of different ages. The methodology applied was mostly staining the cellular DNA after a designed time of stimulation and detecting the proportions of the cells in G0/G1, S, and G2/M stages of the mitotic cycle which, with appropriate analytical tools, allows for approximate estimation of the length of each stage. This technique yielded some intuitively expected results—namely, T-cells from old individuals tended (on average) to have their cell cycle longer than cells from young individuals [4, 25, 73]. While looking at the various stages of the T-cell cycle, various authors reported: no change or elongation of G1 (the latter related to the accumulation of the inhibitor of cyclin D/cdk4/6 kinase complex, the p21 cip/waf (by

BrdUrd/Hoechst staining; [6]) and an elongated S phase (here the example is the Werner's syndrome S phase length [71], but one can easily, intuitively understand that the T-cells (and other cycling cells) of the elderly individuals may have more DNA damage accumulated, and less effective mechanisms of its detection (including the p53 [51]) and repair [3, 39, 77], thus may be prone to slowing down the cycle to allow more time for repairs). Also, and for the same reasons, elongated G2 phase was reported [66, 67]. According to these reports, age-related G2 elongation can be reversed by caffeine which, in turn, is reversed by adenosine (which provokes the—currently unanswered yet—question on the role of changed availability of energy and/or cAMP in the observed process).

Thus, in a model of the T-cell cycle changes related to aging, that arises from the abovementioned observations (Fig. 4a), with aging all or at least some of the cycle phases are elongated, leading to the elongation of the whole cycle. Accordingly, compared to the young, the T-cells of elderly would make fewer divisions in the same time from stimulation and, assuming other factors influencing the progeny number would not change (which is not entirely true, as the level of AICD changes with aging, as do probably other means a T-cell might die) we would see fewer daughter cells at the end of any observation period. This is in agreement with old data on ³H-TdR incorporation in the DNA of mitogen-stimulated T-cells of young and elderly. However, assuming the above as the whole truth we would expect not only the immune response involving the T-cell proliferation to be much less effective (due to not enough effector cells produced on time), but also the numbers of T-cells in the elderly to dwindle quite rapidly, both during activation (AICD and the mitotic catastrophe on the rise) and during the rest period, where the homeostatic mechanisms to fill the niche would also fail. Yet, we do not see a significant change in the volume of lymph nodes, spleen and the MALT when we age, even if their internal histology may change with age [84, 85, 90, 91].

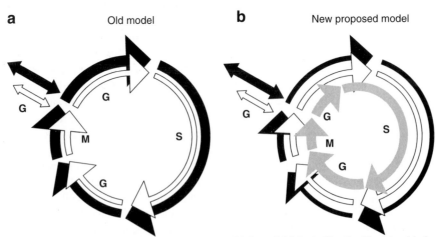

Fig. 4 Changes of the length of cell cycle phases (G0 through M) in the T-cells of healthy elderly. Relative lengths of cell cycle phases of T-cells of young (□), and elderlyindividuals(■—presenescent, ■—homeostatically proliferating). Smaller radius indicates shorter cell cycle

One common mistake in such studies is that the researchers assume some special value for the length of any specific cell cycle stage. For instance, according to Kypreou et al, at 72 hours stimulation (in vitro) the lymphocytes are in the S phase [42]. In fact even if we assume the initial synchronization of these cells' entry in the activation process (by the token of almost immediate contact of all tested cells with the stimulus upon its admixture), we do not know the actual timing of stages preceding the S phase, including first of all the G0→G1 transition as well as the G1 phase itself, which is the most variable and prone to change in length. Thus, any *a priori* assumption of the length of any phase of the cell cycle skews our understanding of possible changes, by not allowing the researcher to assume that any of them might actually be changing with age! As we had demonstrated confirming earlier suggestions, the G0→G1 phase is significantly elongated (in some cases to more than 50 hours!) for the CD4$^+$ cells of healthy elderly and this elongation depends on the availability of CD28 as a source of costimulatory signal [93].

On the other hand, when we applied the abovementioned DCT flow cytometric technique to tag and enumerate dividing human T-cells obtained from people of various age, and the not-so-complicated mathematics for calculations, we have found that, in fact, on average the cell cycle of the CD4$^+$ lymphocytes of the healthy elderly is shorter than that of the same cell type from young people [93]. In detail, the CD4$^+$ population that we studied that way was more diversified: apart from the cells that divided fast (making more divisions per a dividing cell) there were many (more that among the lymphocytes of the young people) those that did not divide at all (senescent?). Also, the shortening of the cell cycle was true for those CD4$^+$ cells that were still expressing some (but FACS-detectable) CD28 on their surface, while the CD4$^+$CD28^{nul} cells of the elderly divided with the speed not different from the same population dwelling in the young. This observation—in our opinion—is indicating that the cell cycle behavior does NOT undergo any COMMON type of changes in aging, even within such a seemingly uniform class of cells like the T-cells; rather, different subpopulations of the T-cells, including those differing in the expression of CD28, but possibly also the broadly different CD4$^+$ and CD8$^+$, naïve and memory cells etc. would follow their separate patterns of cell cycle change, requiring separate studies. In our opinion this once again describes the CD28^{nul} population as an end product of the process of aging. At the end, of course, all of them would fit into the common pattern of remodeled T-cell niche observed in the healthy elderly.

Thus, we propose another model (which according to our experiments is true at least for the CD4$^+$ lymphocytes) where those T-cells of the healthy elderly that still had not reached proliferative senescence would actually divide faster (their cell cycle would be significantly shorter), while these approaching it, but not yet senescent—slower (Fig. 4b). That way in the same time fewer cells than in the young would make more divisions than the dividing lymphocytes of young individuals and the number of their progeny would remain reasonably similar to that seen in the healthy young people. In our opinion, this model fits well in the aged immune system remodeling theory [27, 30], adding a changing functional component to its—already known—changing phenotypic characteristics. The mixed cell population that fills the T-cell niche in the aged organism would therefore consist of increased numbers of the progeny of those clones that can still divide relatively vigorously, steadily reduced numbers of those which still divide slowly (presenescent), and relatively constant or slowly rising numbers of senescent (postproliferative) T-cells clogging the niche (resulting *inter alia* in the observed TCR repertoire contraction)—Fig. 3c. Interestingly, homeostatic proliferation—one that plays a role if filling supposedly empty space in the T-cell niche after the demise of exhausted clones—is reported for both the naïve and memory T-cells of the elderly [60].

The model we propose might gain another aspect, related to the concept of inflamm-aging (readiness of the immune system of elderly to initiate the inflammatory reaction or even permanent state of such mild, subclinical inflammation [17, 29, 75]). It was shown earlier that dexamethasone (a synthetic antiinflammatory glucocorticoid) extends the G1 phase of stimulated human lymphocytes and it is suggested that natural glucocorticoids do the same [7, 8]. The levels of glucocorticoids in the sera of elderly people are variably reported as lowered, unchanged or (quite frequently) increased as compared with these observed in young people; the latter are associated with inter alia worsening of the hypothalamic functions (including memory) [49, 50, 81]. However, these data concern mostly the total levels of the hormone and not the levels of its free, active form. Yet, in our opinion, the inflamm-aging state should be associated with lowered levels of **free** glucocorticoids observed in the elderly. Thus, shorter G1 that we suggest as the reason for overall cell cycle shortening of elderly CD4$^+$ cells might be related not only to high D1 cyclin in these cells that we have reported [93], but also to less free glucocorticoids. Our recent work shows very much decreased amount and activity of cellular β-glucuronidase being the product of Klotho gene in the CD4$^+$ lymphocytes of healthy elderly people [94]. Klotho, recently dubbed the aging hormone, is deeply related to the process of aging, mostly due its involvement in the regulation of calcium and phosphate balances [38, 83, 86]. However, the enzymatic activity of Klotho β-glucuronidase is directed *inter alia* towards the steroid glucuronides (a major water soluble conjugate of steroids manufactured in the liver as means of eliminating the hormones with urine and thus regulating their concentration and activity) and thus, when active, it is keeping the free steroid levels up [35]. In the elderly, decreased Klotho expression and activity would not prevent glucuronidation and elimination of glucocorticoids which then exert less antiinflammatory activity (hence inflamm-aging) and less G1 phase elongating activity (hence shorter G1 phase in the 'Klotho-depleted' T-cells of old people). Accordingly, T-cells of old people seem to be less sensitive to antiproliferative activity of cortisol [45]. Interestingly, very recently Klotho has been described as a direct antagonist of the Wnt gene product, at least in certain stem cells [10, 44]. The role of Wnt—related pathways in the development, differentiation and function of human B- and T-lymphocytes is recognized (for the review, see [72, 80]), and its relation to cellular aging on one hand and to the pathogenesis of rheumatoid arthritis on the other at least strongly suggested [37, 57, 79]. Negative association between Klotho and Wnt opens a new, interesting avenue for aging research.

Concluding, despite already broad and constantly increasing knowledge on the aging-related changes in the dynamics of human T-cell proliferation, this knowledge is so far (end 2007) by no means complete and requires much further study.

References

1. Adibzadeh M, Mariani E, Bartoloni C, Beckman I, Ligthart G, Remarque E, Shall S, Solana R, Taylor GM, Barnett Y, Pawelec G (1996) Lifespans of T-lymphocytes. Mech Ageing Dev 91:145–154

2. Alberti S, Cevenini E, Ostan R, Capri M, Salvioli S, Bucci L, Ginaldi L, De MM, Franceschi C, Monti D (2006) Age-dependent modifications of type 1 and type 2 cytokines within virgin and memory CD4+ T cells in humans. Mech Ageing Dev 127:560–566

3. Annett K, Duggan O, Freeburn R, Hyland P, Pawelec G, Barnett Y (2005) An investigation of DNA mismatch repair capacity under normal culture conditions and under conditions of supra-physiological challenge in human CD4+T cell clones from donors of different ages. Exp Gerontol 40:976–981

4. Arbogast A, Boutet S, Phelouzat MA, Plastre O, Quadri R, Proust JJ (1999) Failure of T lymphocytes from elderly humans to enter the cell cycle is associated with low Cdk6 activity and impaired phosphorylation of Rb protein. Cell Immunol 197:46–54

5. Asquith B, Debacq C, Macallan DC, Willems L, Bangham CR (2002) Lymphocyte kinetics: the interpretation of labeling data. Trends Immunol 23:596–601

6. Bae I, Fan S, Bhatia K, Kohn KW, Fornace A J Jr, O'Connor P M (1995) Relationships between G1 arrest and stability of the p53 and p21Cip1/Waf1 proteins following gamma-irradiation of human lymphoma cells. Cancer Res 55:2387–2393

7. Baghdassarian N, Catallo R, Mahly MA, Ffrench P, Chizat F, Bryon PA, Ffrench M (1998) Glucocorticoids induce G1 as well as S-phase lengthening in normal human stimulated lymphocytes: differential effects on cell cycle regulatory proteins. Exp Cell Res 240:263–273

8. Baghdassarian N, Peiretti A, Devaux E, Bryon PA, Ffrench M (1999) Involvement of p27Kip1 in the G1- and S/G2-phase lengthening mediated by glucocorticoids in normal human lymphocytes. Cell Growth Differ 10:405–412

9. Boucher N, Dufeu-Duchesne T, Vicaut E, Farge D, Effros RB, Schachter F (1998) CD28 expression in T-cell aging and human longevity. Exp Gerontol 33:267–282

10. Brack A S, Conboy MJ, Roy S, Lee M, Kuo CJ, Keller C, Rando T A (2007) Increased Wnt signaling during aging alters muscle stem cell fate and increases fibrosis. Science 317:807–810

11. Bryl E, Vallejo AN, Matteson EL, Witkowski JM, Weyand CM, Goronzy JJ (2005) Modulation of CD28 expression with anti-tumor necrosis factor alpha therapy in rheumatoid arthritis. Arthritis Rheum 52:2996–3003

12. Bryl E, Witkowski JM (2004) Decreased proliferative capability of CD4(+) cells of elderly people is associated with faster loss of activation-related antigens and accumulation of regulatory T cells. Exp Gerontol 39:587–595

13. Brzezinska A, Magalska A, Sikora E (2003) Proliferation of CD8+ in culture of human T cells derived from peripheral blood of adult donors and cord blood of newborns. Mech Ageing Dev 124:379–387

14. Brzezinska A, Magalska A, Szybinska A, Sikora E (2004) Proliferation and apoptosis of human CD8(+)CD28(+) and CD8(+)CD28(-) lymphocytes during aging. Exp Gerontol 39:539–544

15. Consolini R, Legitimo A, Calleri A, Milani M (2000) Distribution of age-related thymulin titres in normal subjects through the course of life. Clin Exp Immunol 121:444–447

16. Davenport MP, Fazou C, McMichael AJ, Callan MF (2002) Clonal selection, clonal senescence, and clonal succession: the evolution of the T-cell response to infection with a persistent virus. J Immunol 168:3309–3317

17. De MM, Franceschi C, Monti D, Ginaldi L (2005) Inflamm-ageing and lifelong antigenic load as major determinants of ageing rate and longevity. FEBS Lett 579:2035–2039

18. Dennett NS, Barcia RN, McLeod JD (2002) Age associated decline in CD25 and CD28 expression correlate with an increased susceptibility to CD95 mediated apoptosis in T cells. Exp Gerontol 37:271–283

19. Douziech N, Seres I, Larbi A, Szikszay E, Roy PM, Arcand M, Dupuis G, Fulop T, Jr (2002) Modulation of human lymphocyte proliferative response with aging. Exp Gerontol 37:369–387

20. Douziech N, Seres I, Larbi A, Szikszay E, Roy PM, Arcand M, Dupuis G, Fulop T Jr (2002) Modulation of human lymphocyte proliferative response with aging. Exp Gerontol 37:369–387

21. Effros RB (1997) Loss of CD28 expression on T-lymphocytes: a marker of replicative senescence. Dev Comp Immunol 21:471–478

22. Effros RB (2000) Costimulatory mechanisms in the elderly. Vaccine 18:1661–1665

23. Effros RB, Allsopp R, Chiu CP, Hausner MA, Hirji K, Wang L, Harley CB, Villeponteau B, West MD, Giorgi JV (1996) Shortened telomeres in the expanded CD28-CD8+ cell subset in HIV disease implicate replicative senescence in HIV pathogenesis. AIDS 10:F17–F22

24. Effros RB, Boucher N, Porter V, Zhu X, Spaulding C, Walford RL, Kronenberg M, Cohen D, Schachter F (1994) Decline in CD28+ T cells in centenarians and in long-term T-cell cultures: a possible cause for both in vivo and in vitro immunosenescence. Exp Gerontol 29:601–609

25. Erickson S, Sangfelt O, Heyman M, Castro J, Einhorn S, Grander D (1998) Involvement of the Ink4 proteins p16 and p15 in T-lymphocyte senescence. Oncogene 17:595–602

26. Fasth AE, Cao D, van VR, Trollmo C, Malmstrom V (2004) CD28nullCD4+ T cells–characterization of an effector memory T-cell population in patients with rheumatoid arthritis. Scand J Immunol 60:199–208

27. Franceschi C (2003) Continuous remodeling as a key to aging and survival: an interview with Claudio Franceschi. Interview by Suresh I S Rattan. Biogerontology 4:329–334

28. Franceschi C, Bonafe M (2003) Centenarians as a model for healthy aging. Biochem Soc Trans 31:457–461

29. Franceschi C, Capri M, Monti D, Giunta S, Olivieri F, Sevini F, Panourgia MP, Invidia L, Celani L, Scurti M, Cevenini E, Castellani G C, Salvioli S (2007) Inflammaging and anti-inflammaging: a systemic perspective on aging and longevity emerged from studies in humans. Mech Ageing Dev 128:92–105

30. Franceschi C, Valensin S, Bonafe M, Paolisso G, Yashin AI, Monti D, De Benedictis G (2000) The network and the remodeling theories of aging: historical background and new perspectives. Exp Gerontol 35:879–896

31. Fulop T, Larbi A, Douziech N, Levesque I, Varin A, Herbein G (2006) Cytokine receptor signaling and aging. Mech Ageing Dev 127:526–537

32. Fulop T Jr, Larbi A, Dupuis G, Pawelec G (2003) Ageing, autoimmunity and arthritis: perturbations of TCR signal transduction pathways with ageing—a biochemical paradigm for the ageing immune system. Arthritis Res Ther 5:290–302

33. Fulop T, Larbi A, Wikby A, Mocchegiani E, Hirokawa K, Pawelec G (2005) Dysregulation of T-cell function in the elderly : scientific basis and clinical implications. Drugs Aging 22:589–603

34. Goronzy JJ, Fujii H, Weyand CM (2006) Telomeres, immune aging and autoimmunity. Exp Gerontol 41:246–251

35. Hayashi Y, Okino N, Kakuta Y, Shiknai T, Tani M, Narimatsu H, Ito M (2007) Klotho-related protein is a novel cytosolic neutral beta-glycosylceramidase. J Biol Chem 282:30889–900

36. Hyland P, Barnett C, Pawelec G (2001) Age-related accumulation of oxidative DNA damage and alterations in levels of p16(INK4a/CDKN2a), p21(WAF1/CIP1/SDI1) and p27(KIP1) in human CD4+ T-cell clones in vitro. Mech Ageing Dev 122:1151–1167

37. Imai K, Morikawa M, D'Armiento J, Matsumoto H, Komiya K, Okada Y (2006) Differential expression of WNTs and FRPs in the synovium of rheumatoid arthritis and osteoarthritis. Biochem Biophys Res Commun 345:1615–1620

38. Imura A, Tsuji Y, Murata M, Maeda R, Kubota K, Iwano A, Obuse C, Togashi K, Tominaga M, Kita N, Tomiyama K, Iijima J, Nabeshima Y, Fujioka M, Asato R, Tanaka S, Kojima K, Ito J, Nozaki K, Hashimoto N, Ito T, Nishio T, Uchiyama T, Fujimori T, Nabeshima Y (2007) Alpha-Klotho as a regulator of calcium homeostasis. Science 316:1615–1618

39. Ju YJ, Lee KH, Park JE, Yi YS, Yun MY, Ham YH, Kim TJ, Choi HM, Han GJ, Lee JH, Lee J, Han JS, Lee KM, Park GH (2006) Decreased expression of DNA repair proteins Ku70 and Mre11 is associated with aging and may contribute to the cellular senescence. Exp Mol Med 38:686–693

40. Kusunoki Y, Akiyama M, Kyoizumi S, Bloom ET, Makinodan T (1988) Age-related alteration in the composition of immunocompetent blood cells in atomic bomb survivors. Int J Radiat Biol Relat Stud Phys Chem Med 53:189–198

41. Kyoizumi S, Umeki S, Akiyama M, Hirai Y, Kusunoki Y, Nakamura N, Endoh K, Konishi J, Sasaki MS, Mori T,(1992) Frequency of mutant T-lymphocytes defective in the expression of the T-cell antigen receptor gene among radiation-exposed people. Mutat Res 265:173–180

42. Kypreou KP, Sourlingas TG, Sekeri-Pataryas KE (2004) Age-dependent response of lymphocytes in the induction of the linker histone variant, H1 degrees and histone H4 acetylation after treatment with the histone deacetylase inhibitor, trichostatin A. Exp Gerontol 39:469–479

43. Li QS, Tanaka S, Kisenge RR, Toyoda H, Azuma E, Komada Y (2000) Activation-induced T-cell death occurs at G1A phase of the cell cycle. Eur J Immunol 30:3329–3337

44. Liu H, Fergusson MM, Castilho RM, Liu J, Cao L, Chen J, Malide D, Rovira II, Schimel D, Kuo CJ, Gutkind JS, Hwang PM, Finkel T (2007) Augmented Wnt signaling in a mammalian model of accelerated aging. Science 317:803–806

45. Luz C, Collaziol D, Preissler T, da C I, Glock L, Bauer ME (2006) Healthy aging is associated with unaltered production of immunoreactive growth hormone but impaired neuroimmunomodulation. Neuroimmunomodulation 13:160–169

46. Lyons AB, Hasbold J, Hodgkin PD (2001) Flow cytometric analysis of cell division history using dilution of carboxyfluorescein diacetate succinimidyl ester, a stably integrated fluorescent probe. Methods Cell Biol 63:375–398

47. Macallan DC, Asquith B, Irvine AJ, Wallace DL, Worth A, Ghattas H, Zhang Y, Griffin G E, Tough D F, Beverley P C (2003) Measurement and modeling of human T-cell kinetics. Eur J Immunol 33:2316–2326

48. Macallan DC, Fullerton CA, Neese RA, Haddock K, Park SS, Hellerstein MK (1998) Measurement of cell proliferation by labeling of DNA with stable isotope-labeled glucose: studies in vitro, in animals, and in humans. Proc Natl Acad Sci U S A 95:708–713

49. Makinodan T, Hirayama R (1985) Age-related changes in immunologic and hormonal activities. IARC Sci Publ 55–70

50. Masoro EJ (1995) Glucocorticoids and aging. Aging (Milano) 7:407–413

51. Matheu A, Maraver A, Klatt P, Flores I, Garcia-Cao I, Borras C, Flores JM, Vina J, Blasco M A, Serrano M (2007) Delayed ageing through damage protection by the Arf/p53 pathway. Nature 448:375–379

52. Mauri D, Wyss-Coray T, Gallati H, Pichler W J (1995) Antigen-presenting T cells induce the development of cytotoxic CD4+ T cells. I. Involvement of the CD80–CD28 adhesion molecules. J Immunol 155:118–127

53. Mclean AR, Michie CA (1995) In vivo estimates of division and death rates of human T-lymphocytes. Proc Natl Acad Sci U S A 92:3707–3711

54. Michie CA, McLean A (1993) Lymphocyte lifespan, immunological memory and retroviral infections. Immunol Today 14:235

55. Michie CA, McLean A, Alcock C, Beverley PC (1992) Lifespan of human lymphocyte subsets defined by CD45 isoforms. Nature%19 360:264–265

56. Nakajima T, Schulte S, Warrington KJ, Kopecky SL, Frye RL, Goronzy JJ, Weyand CM (2002) T-cell-mediated lysis of endothelial cells in acute coronary syndromes. Circulation 105:570–575

57. Nakamura Y, Nawata M, Wakitani S (2005) Expression profiles and functional analyses of Wnt-related genes in human joint disorders. Am J Pathol 167:97–105

58. Namekawa T, Snyder MR, Yen JH, Goehring BE, Leibson PJ, Weyand CM, Goronzy JJ (2000) Killer cell activating receptors function as costimulatory molecules on CD4+CD28null T cells clonally expanded in rheumatoid arthritis. J Immunol 165:1138–1145

59. Nasi M, Troiano L, Lugli E, Pinti M, Ferraresi R, Monterastelli E, Mussi C, Salvioli G, Franceschi C, Cossarizza A (2006) Thymic output and functionality of the IL-7/IL-7 receptor system in centenarians: implications for the neolymphogenesis at the limit of human life. Aging Cell 5:167–175

60. Naylor K, Li G, Vallejo AN, Lee WW, Koetz K, Bryl E, Witkowski J, Fulbright J, Weyand C M, Goronzy J J (2005) The influence of age on T-cell generation and TCR diversity. J Immunol 174:7446–7452

61. Pawelec G (2006) Immunity and ageing in man. Exp Gerontol 41:1239–1242

62. Pawelec G, Barnett Y, Mariani E, Solana R (2002) Human CD4+ T-cell clone longevity in tissue culture: lack of influence of donor age or cell origin. Exp Gerontol 37:265–269

63. Pawelec G, Mariani E, Bradley B, Solana R (2000) Longevity in vitro of human CD4+ T-helper cell clones derived from young donors and elderly donors, or from progenitor cells: age-associated differences in cell surface molecule expression and cytokine secretion. Biogerontology 1:247–254

64. Pfister G, Herndler-Brandstetter D, Grubeck-Loebenstein B (2006) [Results from biomedical aging research. Trends and current examples from immunology]. *Bundesgesundheitsblatt. Gesundheitsforschung. Gesundheitsschutz* 49:506–512

65. Pfister G, Weiskopf D, Lazuardi L, Kovaiou R D, Cioca DP, Keller M, Lorbeg B, Parson W, Grubeck-Loebenstein B (2006) Naive T cells in the elderly: are they still there? Ann N Y Acad Sci 1067:152–157

66. Pincheira J, Bravo M, Santos MJ (1998) G2 repair in Nijmegen breakage syndrome: G2 duration and effect of caffeine and cycloheximide in control and X-ray irradiated lymphocytes. Clin Genet 53:262–267

67. Pincheira J, Gallo C, Bravo M, Navarrete MH, Lopez-Saez JF (1993) G2 repair and aging: influence of donor age on chromosomal aberrations in human lymphocytes. Mutat Res 295:55–62

68. Ponnappan S, Ovaa H, Ponnappan U (2007) Lower expression of catalytic and structural subunits of the proteasome contributes to decreased proteolysis in peripheral blood T-lymphocytes during aging. Int J Biochem Cell Biol 39:799–809

69. Ponnappan U (2002) Ubiquitin-proteasome pathway is compromised in CD45RO+ and CD45RA+ T lymphocyte subsets during aging. Exp Gerontol 37:359–367

70. Ponnappan U, Zhong M, Trebilcock GU (1999) Decreased proteasome-mediated degradation in T cells from the elderly: a role in immune senescence. Cell Immunol 192:167–174

71. Poot M, Hoehn H, Runger TM, Martin GM (1992) Impaired S-phase transit of Werner syndrome cells expressed in lymphoblastoid cell lines. Exp Cell Res 202:267–273

72. Qiang YW, Rudikoff S (2004) Wnt signaling in B- and T-lymphocytes. Front Biosci 9:1000–1010

73. Quadri RA, Arbogast A, Phelouzat MA, Boutet S, Plastre O, Proust JJ (1998) Age-associated decline in cdk1 activity delays cell cycle progression of human T-lymphocytes. J Immunol 161:5203–5209

74. Sabbagh L, Snell LM, Watts TH (2007) TNF family ligands define niches for T-cell memory. Trends Immunol 28:333–339

75. Salvioli S, Capri M, Valensin S, Tieri P, Monti D, Ottaviani E, Franceschi C (2006) Inflammaging, cytokines and aging: state of the art, new hypotheses on the role of mitochondria and new perspectives from systems biology. Curr Pharm Des 12:3161–3171

76. Saurwein-Teissl M, Lung TL, Marx F, Gschosser C, Asch E, Blasko I, Parson W, Bock G, Schonitzer D, Trannoy E, Grubeck-Loebenstein B (2002) Lack of antibody production following immunization in old age: association with CD8(+)CD28(-) T-cell clonal expansions and an imbalance in the production of Th1 and Th2 cytokines. J Immunol 168:5893–5899

77. Scarpaci S, Frasca D, Barattini P, Guidi L, Doria G (2003) DNA damage recognition and repair capacities in human naive and memory T cells from peripheral blood of young and elderly subjects. Mech Ageing Dev 124:517–524

78. Schmidt D, Martens PB, Weyand CM, Goronzy JJ (1996) The repertoire of CD4+ CD28- T cells in rheumatoid arthritis. Mol Med 2:608–618

79. Sen M (2005) Wnt signalling in rheumatoid arthritis. Rheumatology (Oxford). 44:708–713

80. Staal FJ, Meeldijk J, Moerer P, Jay P, van de Weerdt B C, Vainio S, Nolan G P, Clevers H (2001) Wnt signaling is required for thymocyte development and activates Tcf-1 mediated transcription. Eur J Immunol 31:285–293

81. Stein-Behrens BA and Sapolsky RM (1992) Stress, glucocorticoids, and aging. Aging (Milano) 4:197–210

82. Stevens JB, Liu G, Bremer SW, Ye KJ, Xu W, Xu J, Sun Y, Wu GS, Savasan S, Krawetz S A, Ye CJ, Heng HH (2007) Mitotic cell death by chromosome fragmentation. Cancer Res 67:7686–7694

83. Strewler G J (2007) Untangling Klotho's Role in Calcium Homeostasis. Cell Metab 6:93–95

84. Taniguchi I, Murakami G, Sato A, Fujiwara D, Ichikawa H, Yajima T, Kohama G (2003) Lymph node hyalinization in elderly Japanese. Histol Histopathol 18:1169–1180

85. Taniguchi I, Sakurada A, Murakami G, Suzuki D, Sato M, Kohama G I (2004) Comparative histology of lymph nodes from aged animals and humans with special reference to the proportional areas of the nodal cortex and sinus. *Ann Anat* 186:337–347

86. Torres PU, Prie D, Molina-Bletry V, Beck L, Silve C, Friedlander G (2007) Klotho: an antiaging protein involved in mineral and vitamin D metabolism. Kidney Int 71:730–737

87. Umeki S, Kusunoki Y, Cologne JB, Iwamoto KS, Hirai Y, Seyama T, Ohama K., Kyoizumi S (1998) Lifespan of human memory T-cells in the absence of T-cell receptor expression. Immunol Lett 62:99–104

88. Vallejo AN, Nestel AR, Schirmer M, Weyand CM, Goronzy JJ (1998) Aging-related deficiency of CD28 expression in CD4+ T cells is associated with the loss of gene-specific nuclear factor binding activity. J Biol Chem 273:8119–8129

89. Wagner U, Pierer M, Kaltenhauser S, Wilke B, Seidel W, Arnold S, Hantzschel H (2003) Clonally expanded CD4+CD28null T cells in rheumatoid arthritis use distinct combinations of T cell receptor BV and BJ elements. Eur J Immunol 33:79–84

90. Weksler ME (1980) The immune system and the aging process in man. Proc Soc Exp Biol Med 165:200–205

91. Weksler M E (1981) The senescence of the immune system. Hosp Pract *(Off Ed)* 16:53–64

92. Weyand CM, Brandes JC, Schmidt D, Fulbright JW, Goronzy JJ (1998) Functional properties of CD4+ CD28- T cells in the aging immune system. Mech Ageing Dev 102:131–147

93. Witkowski JM, Bryl E (2004) Paradoxical age-related cell cycle quickening of human CD4(+) lymphocytes: a role for cyclin D1 and calpain. Exp Gerontol 39:577–585

94. Witkwski JM, Soroczyńska-Cybula M, Bryl E, Smoleńska Ż, Jóźwik A (2007) Klotho - a common link in physiological and rheumatoid arthritis-related aging of human CD4+ lymphocytes. J Immunol 178:771–777

Mismatch Repair System and Aging: Microsatellite Instability in Peripheral Blood Cells of the Elderly and in the T-cell Clone Longitudinal Model

Simona Neri and Erminia Mariani

Contents

Abbreviations

ACE	angiotensin converting enzyme
AID	activation-induced cytidine deaminase
APOB	apolipoprotein B
APOC	apolipoprotein C
APOE	apolipoprotein E
CD34	cluster of differentiation 34
CD4	cluster of differentiation 4
CD8	cluster of differentiation 8
ExoI	exonuclease I
FES	felin sarcoma oncogene
HLA	human leukocyte antigen
HNPCC	hereditary nonpolyposis colorectal cancer
HRAS	Harvey rat sarcoma oncogene
MLH1	MutL homologue 1
MMR	Mismatch repair
MSH2	MutS homologue 2
MSH3	MutS homologue 3

E. Mariani (✉)
Laboratorio di Immunologia e Genetica
Istituto di Ricerca Codivilla-Putti, IOR
Via di Barbiano 1/10, 40136, Bologna, Italy
Tel.: 0039 051 6366803; Fax: 0039 051 6366807
E-mail: marianie@alma.unibo.it

T. Fulop et al. (eds.), *Handbook on Immunosenescence*,
DOI 10.1007/ 978-1-4020-9062-2_14, © Springer Science+Business Media B.V. 2009

MSH6	MutS homologue 6
MSI	microsatellite instability
MtDNA	mitochondrial DNA
p53	polypeptide 53
PBMC	peripheral blood mononuclear cells
PCNA	proliferating cell nuclear antigen
PCR	polymerase chain reaction
PD	population doublings
PMS1	PostMeiotic Segregation 1
PMS2	PostMeiotic Segregation 2
RER	replication error
RFC	replication factor C
RPA	replication protein A
SNPs	single nucleotide polymorphisms
TCC	T-cell clones
TH	thyrosin hydroxylase
TPOX	thyroid peroxidase
VNTR	variable number of tandem repeats
VWA31	von Willebrand A31

Abstract: Age-related accumulation of DNA damage in human T-cells has been well documented and could be associated with T-cell malfunctions. Therefore, an age-related reduction in DNA repair capacity of human lymphocytes may contribute to this phenomenon and play a key role in the modification of the immune response observed in the elderly. Because the Mismatch Repair system is the main post-replicative pathway for the correction of replication errors and few data suggest a possible alteration with age of this repair pathway, it is conceivable that, also in the immune system, age-related alterations of mismatch repair could contribute to the accumulation of genetic damage. This is particularly true for adaptive immune response, whose function depends on the ability of T-cells to undergo repetitive replications after antigenic challenge. The present chapter will focus on the role of the Mismatch Repair System that is recently emerging as a possible additional mechanism contributing to the accumulation of genetic instability during aging in peripheral blood cells. In vivo data at present available in the literature and results from studies on cloned human T lymphocytes cultured for different periods in vitro, as a model of immunosenescence, will be reviewed.

Keywords: Aging • Microsatellite instability • Mismatch repair system • T-cell clones

1 Introduction

The understanding and prevention of age-related diseases rely on the study of the molecular mechanisms underlying the physiological aging process and different theories have been proposed. According to the "soma theory", the aging process is caused by a life-long accumulation of random damages in somatic cells and tissues (Kirkwood, Kowald 1997) compromising the functional activity of cells and ultimately leading to cell death. This indicates a central role for the different mechanisms of cell care and stress response cooperating in the regulation of life span, allowing a definition of the so-called "network theory of aging" that includes the effects of defective mitochondria, aberrant proteins, free radicals and DNA mutations (Kirkwood, Kowald 1997) as contributors to the overall process of senescence.

2   Aging and DNA Damage

DNA damage might contribute to the aging process by interfering with DNA replication and transcription impairing the functional ability of cells and thus leading to a senescent phenotype, loss of cellular function, cell death or tumours (Walter et al. 1997).

A wide range of damages to the native structure of DNA (single and double strand breaks, apurinic and apyrimidinic sites, base alterations, methylation, inter and intra-chromosomal cross links, bulky and smaller adducts and distortion of helix by intercalation) can occur through spontaneous damages arising from byproducts of the cellular metabolism or by exogenous chemical, radioactive, viral and mutagenic agents (Reddy, Vasquez 2005). However, the steady state level of spontaneous DNA lesions is very low and therefore difficult to evaluate, under normal conditions. Experimental results do not show directly that decreased genomic integrity causes senescence of somatic cells, but many studies have demonstrated direct correlations: base adduct levels in nuclear and mitochondrial genomes shorten life span and are related to decreased functions of aging. In addition, chromosome aberrations in human peripheral blood lymphocytes do increase with age (Prieur et al. 1988), as well as mutation frequencies at the level of specific genes (as HPRT locus) (Vijg 2000). In any case, the critical load of cellular mutation able to induce physiological consequences is still undetermined.

3   Aging and DNA Repair

Genetic stability is controlled by a number of cellular functions including DNA replication, repair and recombination complexes. Mutations in DNA repair genes frequently lead to genome destabilization and consequent increases in the frequency of mutations. Since systems regulating genome stability are considered to be major safety systems for longevity, it is likely that the inactivation of one or more of such pathways accelerates both age-related deterioration/death and mutation accumulation, at the same time. Indeed, several studies have addressed relationships between DNA damage, its repair and aging, and have suggested an age-dependent accumulation of DNA damage as partially responsible for the impairment of cellular functions and an increased rate of diseases, such as cancer, in the elderly. The accumulation of DNA damage with age (Walter et al. 1997; Barnett, Barnett 1998; Vijg 2000; Doria, Frasca 2001) seems to affect various tissues at different rates, as observed in transgenic mice harbouring the LacZ gene (Ono et al. 2000). In addition, a positive correlation between DNA repair capacity and life-span has been demonstrated (Hart, Setlow 1974). The impact of a malfunctioning DNA repair system on genomic integrity is also evidenced by progeroid syndromes in which mutations in DNA repair genes induce a premature aging phenotype characterised by immune defects and increased susceptibility to cancer development (Bohr 2002).

3.1 DNA Repair Pathways

Mammalian DNA repair processes depend on a number of complex pathways to cope with lesions in DNA structure. At least four main pathways have been described so far:

a) the Direct Reversal Repair pathway catalyses a direct reversal only involving single enzymes (e.g., alkyltransferase, removing the methyl group from O6-methylguanine) and DNA ligase (rejoining single-strand breaks) (Harris et al. 1983);

b) the Excision Repair pathway is the predominant mechanism for the maintenance of genomic integrity. This pathway repairs different DNA lesions, ranging from simple base methylations to interstrand adduct formation resulting in major distortion of the DNA structure. Two distinct systems belong to it:

- Nucleotide Excision Repair, which corrects a broad spectrum of structurally unrelated lesions such as UV-induced photoproducts, chemical adducts, intra strand crosslinks and some form of oxidative damage. It can repair any part of the genome, however, damage recognition and repair of trascriptionally active genes (Wood et al. 2001) is performed preferentially by an alternative pathway, termed transcription-coupled repair (Hanawalt 1994);

- Base Excision Repair, which is, perhaps, the most fundamental and ubiquitous DNA repair mechanism in all higher organisms that depend on oxygen for living (Wilson, Bohr 2007). It has evolved to handle the numerous minor alterations (such as spontaneous modification, oxidation, deamination and loss of bases) that can occur in the structure of DNA as a result of cell metabolic activity. This kind of repair is important in post-mitotic tissues, where simple base modifications are likely more prone to occur than major damages;

c) the Recombination Repair pathway that corrects DNA double strand breaks frequently arising from the stalling of the replication fork and from the attack of exogenous agents (such as ionising radiation or chemicals), inducing interstrand or intra-strand cross links and preventing the use of one of the strands as a template for the repair process (Thompson, Schild 2002). Two types of Recombination Repair are described:

- Homologous Recombination, a complex and poorly understood process that entails an intact homologous DNA strand as a template to repair DSB (Sonoda et al. 2006);

– Nonhomologous End Joining that, by contrast, entails relegation of the broken ends without respecting homology and is consequently relatively error prone. Nevertheless, it is a major pathway for double strand break repair in mammalian cells and is thought to be of vital importance in post mitotic tissues (Sonoda et al. 2006).

d) the Mismatch Repair pathway that corrects mispaired bases occurring most frequently during replication (Kolodner, Marsischky 1999).

Finally, the discovery of a number of novel DNA polymerases with the ability to carry out DNA synthesis across a damaged or altered base added new possibilities for understanding DNA repair mechanisms in mammalian cells. These polymerases have different substrate specificities, enabling them to deal with many different types of damaged bases, a process known as translesional synthesis (Rattray, Strathern 2003; Lehmann 2006).

3.2   The Mismatch Repair Pathway (MMR)

The Mismatch Repair system is the main post-replicative pathway for the repair of mismatched DNA (base-base mismatches and insertion/deletion loops occurring during replication, homologous recombination and DNA damage) (Kolodner, Marsischky 1999) and it is essential for maintaining the stability of the genome during repeated duplications. Essential components of the MMR system were identified in *Escherichia coli* and their main activities are reported in the Table 1.

All eukaryotic organisms have MutS (MSH2, MSH3 and MSH6 genes) and MutL (MLH1, PMS1 and PMS2—PostMeiotic Segregation 1 and 2 genes) homologues (Wood et al. 2001; Modrich, Lahue 1996), acting in form of heterodimers, in contrast to bacteria in which MutS and MutL function as homodimers.

In humans, DNA mismatch repair confers to the genome a 100–1,000 fold protection against replication-induced mutations (Loeb 1994). The initial recognition of mismatches is carried out by MutSα and MutSβ, functional heterodimers of Msh2 bound to either Msh6 or Msh3, respectively. They display some functional overlap, with MutSα playing the major role in mismatch correction and being prevalently expressed in the cell. In the following step, MutLα or MutLβ (heterodimers of Mlh1

Table 1   Principal components and functions of the bacterial Mismatch repair system

MutS	Detects mismatches in DNA duplex and initiate the MMR machinery
MutL	Makes a connection between the recognition of a mismatch and its excision from the strand within which it is contained
MutH	Cleaves hemimethylated GATC sites for excision of mismatch-containing strand and formation of nick
Uvr/Helicase	Enters into the nick generated by MutH together with single-stranded DNA-binding proteins

bound to either Pms2 or Pms1, respectively) mediate the recruitment of additional proteins for the completion of the repair process, giving rise to the excision of the mutated strand in either direction to the mismatch and to the resynthesis of the correct sequence (Kolodner, Marsischky 1999). Efficient DNA mismatch repair requires the combined functions of MutS and MutL. The other proteins involved in the repair are: PCNA (Proliferating Cell Nuclear Antigen), whose activity increases the binding of MutSα to mismatched DNA suggesting a role of this protein in the recognition stage (Flores-Rozas et al. 2000; Lau, Kolodner 2003); ExoI (exonuclease I); RPA (replication protein A) and RFC (replication factor C). Once the mutated strand is excised beyond the mismatch, polymerase δ resinthesizes DNA and the nick is sealed by DNA ligases not yet identified (Jun et al. 2006) (Fig. 1).

In addition to a role during replication, MMR proteins have been reported to have other important functions, such as: antirecombination activity between divergent

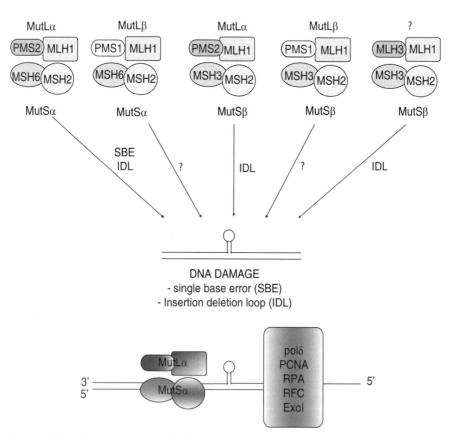

Fig. 1 Schematic representation of the Human DNA Mismatch Repair System. MutS heterodimers (MSH2-MSH6 or MSH2-MSH3) combined with heterodimers of MLH1 with PMS2, PMS1 or MLH3 have different specificities for DNA mismatches or loops (upper panel). Correction is targeted to the primer strand possibly through the interaction with PCNA and additional factors are required to complete the process (lower panel). polδ = polymerase δ; PCNA = proliferating cell nuclear antigen; RPA = replication protein A; RFC = replication factor C; Exo I = exonuclease I

sequences, promotion of meiotic crossover, DNA damage surveillance and diversification of imunoglobulins (Jun et al. 2006). The involvement of MMR in DNA damage response is evidenced by the fact that MMR-defective cells are resistant to alkylating and other DNA damaging agents (Fink et al. 1998). In fact, DNA damage triggers MMR-dependent G2/M arrest, followed by the induction of MMR-dependent apoptosis p53- or p73-mediated. The hypothesis for how MMR is involved in somatic hypermutation and class switch recombination is that, after generation of mutations by AID (activation-induced cytidine deaminase), MMR proteins are recruited to the mismatched DNA and resynthesise the DNA strand with the help of an error-prone polymerase such as polymerase η (Wilson et al. 2005).

Defects in MMR correction pathways are associated with a substantial destabilization of microsatellites, highly polymorphic, tandemly repeated sequences (from one to six bp) interspersed in the genome and particularly prone to slippage during replication. Slippages determine changes of allele length either for insertion or deletion of repeated units. The experimental evidence of this phenomenon is called microsatellite instability (MSI), that is the appearance of additional bands of different lengths or modification of the expected ones. Mutations are observed in repeated sequences, but can also occur randomly in all the genome; therefore, MSI indicates a higher susceptibility to mutations.

Mutator phenotypes due to inactivation of MMR were initially described in HNPCC (hereditary nonpolyposis colorectal cancer) caused by germ line mutations in several members of MMR genes (MLH1 and MSH2 in about 90% of cases), inducing accelerated mutations in microsatellite sequences compared to normal DNA, the so-called replication error (RER) phenotype (Aaltonen et al. 1993; De la Chapelle 1995). Subsequently, it was also described in cancer cell lines and in sporadic cancers of the colon, cervix, endometrium, pancreas, lung, prostate and stomach (Eshleman et al. 1995; Modrich 1996; Kane et al. 1997), due to somatic mutations in MMR genes or, more frequently, to epigenetic mutations, in particular hypermethylation-mediated gene inactivation (Liu et al. 1995; Liu et al. 1996; Moslein et al. 1996; Kane et al. 1997; Herman et al. 1998; Kolodner, Marsischky 1999; Suzuki et al. 1999).

4   Genetic Damage and Immune System

The immune system develops an enormous number of genetically different cells generated by breaking and rejoining DNA sequences coding for antigen receptors, by adapting the DNA repair mechanisms normally used to maintain genome stability. Small populations of naïve and memory T-cells, in order to ensure a correct immune response, have to expand clonally upon antigen stimulation. The ability to expand may depend on the amount of accumulated genetic damage and processes limiting T-cell proliferative capacity might impair the overall immune response. The overlap between DNA repair and immune system efficiency is evidenced by the fact that individuals with defective DNA repair pathways frequently show immunodeficiency.

In addition, immune system efficiency is affected by aging, particularly the T-cell compartment. The impact of age-related immune alterations on lifespan and diseases is in accordance with results from studies in centenarians showing that healthy individuals who have reached the extreme limit of human life in good clinical conditions are equipped with well preserved and efficient immune defence mechanisms (Franceschi et al. 1995).

An age-related accumulation of DNA damage and mutations in human T-cells has been well documented and could be associated with T-cell dysfunctions; it follows that a reduction in DNA repair capacity of human lymphocytes may contribute to this accumulation of DNA damage with age and may play a prominent role in the deterioration of the immune response observed in the elderly and to the development of age-associated immune malfunctions possibly affecting lifespan.

5   MMR System and Aging

MMR deficiency inducing high levels of mutations may only increase the rate of cancer, but not aging. Since cancer is one of the most important causes of mortality in the elderly, it is possible that alterations of the MMR system occurring with age predispose to cancer. Indeed, some emerging evidence indicates that MMR efficiency might be impaired in normal somatic cells with progressive aging.

Msh-2 deficient mice die within one year of cancer with lymphomas (also a common cause of death in aged mice) (Reitmar et al. 1996), while in the first year of life no difference was observed between wild type and Msh2 heterozygotes. MSH2- and PMS2-deficient mice crossbred with transgenic mutation reporter mice generate animals with elevated spontaneous point mutation frequencies in several organs and tissues (Andrew et al. 1997; Narayanan et al. 1997). However, at present nothing is known about mutations accumulated at later ages, since complete lifespan studies on these mice have not yet been performed.

Toyota et al. (1999) found an age-related methylation of CpG islands in normal colon cells affecting different DNA promoter regions, including MLH1 promoter. A large number of CpG in the human genome are progressively methylated during the aging process and, for many genes, this methylation process correlates with reduced expression. The phenomenon appears to be physiologically induced because it is very frequent, it affects large numbers of cells, and it is present in colon tissue from healthy donors and in residual normal colon tissue from cancer patients. The age-related methylation of MLH1 promoter in cancer cells suggests therefore a decreased activity of the MMR system predisposing the elderly to malignant transformation in the colon. In agreement, a spread of methylation in the MLH1 promoter in the normal colonic mucosa closely associated with age and with the development of sporadic MSI in colorectal cancers was found (Nakagawa et al. 2001). The hypermethylation of the MLH1 gene promoter occurring with age correlates with inhibition of its expression and the appearance of MSI.

The frequency of MSI in the pathologic tissue of patients suffering from gastric lymphoma showed a tendency to increase with age, as did microsatellite variability (Starostik et al. 2000).

5.1   Analysis on Peripheral Blood Cells

The immune system, whose impairment is documented with age, is also a possible target of the MMR deficiency, in particular the adaptive immune response that depends on the ability of T-cells to undergo consecutive replications after antigenic challenge. This prominent proliferative stress presumably renders T-cells more prone to possible inefficiencies of DNA repair systems and replicative senescence. In recent years, some data are emerging on age-dependent alterations of the MMR pathway in peripheral blood cells.

A preliminary study demonstrated an age-associated MSI by analysing eight different microsatellite loci on DNA from peripheral blood cell samples from young and old healthy subjects obtained at a ten-year interval (Ben Yehuda et al. 2000). A significantly higher rate of MSI after ten years (in 40% of the loci tested and in 45% of the subjects) was found in older individuals, whereas no difference between paired samples of any of the young subjects was observed. An overall genomic instability in the elderly was subsequently confirmed with an additional panel of microsatellites, together with the lack of an association between MSI and methylation of MLH1 or MSH2 promoters (Krichevsky et al. 2004).

The possible involvement of the MMR system in the accumulation of genetic damage with age was also studied in peripheral blood cell DNA from a wide survey of differently aged subjects (Neri et al. 2005). Five polymorphic microsatellite loci (CD4, p53, VWA31, TPOX and FES), in accordance with the international criteria for the study of MSI in cancer (Boland et al. 1998), were analyzed to find possible age-related instabilities or modifications in allele frequencies. Indications of instability were supplied by both altered allele frequencies in different groups of age and the appearance of trizygosis (three alleles at one locus instead of one or two). Excluding the appearance of plurizygosity, that represents a direct indication of instability, but whose frequency is expected to be low in healthy subjects without germline mutations in MMR genes, in this study it was not possible to compare the allelic pattern with a control (as between normal and tumour DNA from the same patient). For this reason, shifts in allele length, evaluated in terms of age-related modifications of allele frequencies, gave only an indirect indication of genetic instability, possibly due to defective mechanisms of genomic conservation, such as MMR pathway, with progressive aging.

The VWA31 microsatellite showed a significant shortening with increasing age. VWA31 and FES microsatellite alleles presented peculiar distributions in differently aged groups, further suggesting modifications in microsatellite stability as shown by shifts in patterns of allelic frequencies from young (considered as basal condition) to old populations. Only the FES locus, (the most unstable among the five analyzed), resulted trizygotic in five samples among the more than two hundred analyzed. All samples that were trizygotic belonged to the old and the centenarian groups, while no young subjects ever showed this pattern (Fig. 2). In addition, the majority of trizygotic centenarians displayed, among the three, a rare allele, never observed in homo- or heterozygosis (Neri et al. 2005).

These data show both an increased instability in very advanced age and an age-dependent genetic damage affecting repeated sequences (whose stability is predominantly guaranteed by the MMR system), or a weaker ability to balance the increased rate of genetic damage due to advancing age. Cells repeatedly undergoing proliferation were more exposed to the repair activity of the MMR pathway and possibly, due to its inefficiency, accumulated a greater genetic damage than naive cells. A basic characteristic of immunosenescence is the decline of naive T-cells as well as the accumulation of specific T-lymphocyte clones, mostly of memory and effector T-cells, due to persistent exposure to different antigenic challenges (Franceschi et al. 2000; Globerson, Effros 2000) (Epstein-Barr virus and cytomegalovirus, being the most frequent) (Wedderbrun et al. 2001; Ouyang et al. 2004). It is conceivable that these clonal cells, repeatedly expanded in vivo, may have progressively incorporated a genetic damage not evident in young subjects that, conversely, present a prevalent naïve phenotype. The presence of such populations, frequently dramatically expanded, (Ouyang et al. 2004) could justify the finding of additional allele bands (trizygosis) in DNA from heterogeneous populations of circulating peripheral blood cells. In fact, to be detectable, mutated alleles should be present in an adequate amount of cells, since the appearance of new alleles might be undetectable in poorly represented cells (less than 5–10%) among a mixed population, because of the overloading amount of normal alleles, therefore inducing an underestimation of MSI.

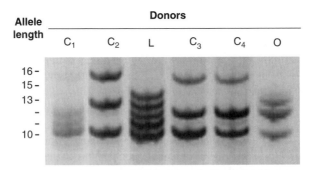

Fig. 2 Trizygosity observed at the FES locus in DNA from peripheral blood lymphocytes of four centenarian (C1-C4) and one old (O) donors. The presence of three alleles at one locus indicates heterogeneity among the analyzed cells, presumably acquired during in vitro replication and giving a different genotype to a portion of cells. Total DNA was amplified by PCR with primers specific for FES microsatellite sequence, then products were electrophoresed on polyacrylamide gel and silver stained. Allele length is indicated on the left and refers to the number of repeats. L= allelic ladder. (from Neri et al. 2005)

As far as the higher instability at the FES locus is concerned, a different sensitivity of this region to the assumed inefficiency of the MMR system is suggested by the evidence that not all sequences are susceptible to, or show the same rate, of MSI. In agreement, a specific FES somatic instability was described in sporadic gastric cancer (Silva et al. 1997) and in lymphocyte clones after in vitro aging (Neri et al. 2004). It is also possible that some alleles undergoing an age-related selection, tend to disappear in the most advanced ages due to a relationship with the FES microsatellite sequence, or with other sequences in linkage disequilibrium with the FES one. The analyzed FES microsatellite lies at intron five of the coding region of FES proto-oncogene that encodes for a nonreceptor protein-tyrosine-kinase whose activation can mediate cellular transformation. Several growth factors, cytokines, immunoglobulin/receptor pairs trigger the activation of cellular FES, shown to play important roles in the regulation of inflammation and immune response (Greer 2002; Yates, Gasson 1996), particularly for survival and terminal differentiation of hematopoietic myeloid lineage (Manfredini et al. 1997). Taking into account the involvement of this factor in the homeostasis of the immune system and modifications of FES-associated microsatellite allele distributions with age, a possible relationship between allelic variants and aging cannot be excluded. Since FES microsatellite alleles are nonexpressed, modifications in allele frequencies might depend on coding sequences in linkage disequilibrium with the analyzed ones, but also on the correlation between the number of repeats and the aging process, thus influencing for example the expression of the gene they are located on, as proposed for VNTR sequences (Bennet et al. 1995). Accordingly, polymorphic alleles of inflammatory cytokines play an important role in age-related chronic inflammatory response diseases, by determining changes in cytokine production (Lio et al. 2002). In addition, it cannot be excluded that polymorphic variations at multiple loci might have produced genotype characteristics contributing to longevity; indeed, a strong familial component of longevity was observed in centenarians (Perls et al. 1998). Different frequencies of variant alleles would indicate a potential functional advantage of those alleles that are more frequent in the disease-free long-lived individuals, as suggested by associations between longevity and allelic variants for polymorphic markers at specific loci such as HLA (Takata et al. 1987), ACE (Schachter et al. 1994), APOB (Kervinen et al. 1994), APOC (Louhija et al. 1994), APOE (Kervinen et al. 1994; Louhija et al. 1994; Schachter et al. 1994), TH and APOB-VNTR (De Benedictis et al. 1998), HRAS1-3'VNTR (Bonafé et al. 2002), as well as mtDNA haplogroups (De Benedictis et al. 1999). Recently, an association between MLH1 gene and longevity was found in centenarians (Kim et al. 2006). In particular, polymorphisms of MLH1 seemed to influence genomic stability and thereby lifespan. By analyzing three SNPs (single nucleotide polymorphisms) leading to amino acid substitutions, a significantly more represented haplotype was found in centenarians than in controls. On the contrary, CD4 (Neri et al. 2005) and p53 (Bonafé et al. 2002; Neri et al. 2005) microsatellites appeared to be stable in different studies, allowing the exclusion of a role of variants of these genes in age-related mortality to such an extent as to alter gene frequency in old people and centenarians.

5.2   The T-cell Clonal Model

To overcome the possible bias of underestimating instability in poorly represented cells, because of the overloading amount of normal alleles, Parsons et al. (1995) performed the analysis on highly diluted peripheral blood lymphocytes in order to amplify the DNA corresponding to maximum three genome equivalents. By analogy, Coolbaugh-Murphy et al. (2005) developed "small pool" PCR for sensitive and quantitative analysis of MSI in somatic tissues by diluting DNA and subsequently amplifying by PCR so that each small pool contained less than a single genome equivalent. Rare mutant fragments contained in one or more small pools would not be overwhelmed by progenitor fragments and could be readily amplified and identified. By using this technique, significant differences in MSI frequencies in DNA from differently aged groups and a positive correlation between age and MSI phenotype were found (Coolbaugh-Murphy et al. 2005). In addition, the frequency of mutant fragments linearly increased with age in peripheral blood lymphocytes from normal individuals, indicating an age-dependent alteration of MMR efficiency.

Long-term CD8+ cell cultures from aged donors undergoing repeated duplications develop MSI as in vitro cell senescence progress, while no MSI develops in young-derived CD8+ T-cells (Krichevsky et al. 2004).

Other studies overcame the problem of heterogeneous cell population analysis by using CD4+ T-cell clones (TCC) (Krickevsky et al. 2004; Neri et al. 2004; Neri et al. 2007). This model allows the longitudinal follow-up of a homogeneous cell population and the functional analysis of a single cell type that, spending its finite lifespan in vitro, provides both important knowledge related to T-cell immunosenescence in vivo and a system to study ways of modulating the aging process (Pawelec et al. 1998; Pawelec et al. 2002). The advantage offered by the analysis of a homogeneous cell population, allowing to join microsatellite instability to increasing duplications in culture, increases the likelihood of detecting new alleles in usually underrepresented cell populations. Indeed, consecutive antigenic stimulation in vitro imposes a marked replicational stress on T-cells, mirroring the antigenic challenge in vivo, as well as, the culture over the entire clonal replicative lifespan mimics the chronic stress thought to really contribute to the possible clonal exhaustion (Hadrup et al. 2006).

Available data indicate that MSI develop with increasing in vitro culture senescence in CD4+ T-cell clones (Krickevsky et al. 2004; Neri et al. 2004), involving different microsatellite sequences, suggesting that a progressive impairment of the MMR system may contribute to the acquisition of genetic damage during chronic antigenic stress in vitro, a phenomenon thought to be of great importance for immune response physiology (Pawelec et al. 2005; Hadrup et al. 2006).

In addition, by a modification of the alkaline comet assay, a reduced ability to repair acridine ICR-191-induced DNA mismatches was observed with aging in culture, indicating that MMR capacity may become deficient in clonal T-cells when they are challenged with supra-physiological levels of DNA damage (Annet et al. 2005).

Moreover, no MSI was observed at increasing population doublings in TCC from young donors, even almost at the end of their finite lifespan in culture (Neri et al. 2004), suggesting an additional relationship between MSI and donor age, in agreement with in vivo data (Ben Yehuda et al. 2000; Krickevsky et al. 2004; Coolbaugh-Murphy et al. 2005; Neri et al. 2005).

Furthermore, microsatellite instability was particularly evident in clones obtained by CD34+ progenitor cells, after undergoing repeated duplication in culture, indicating also the influence of the cell type in addition to in vitro proliferation and aging (Fig. 3).

This may suggest that the efficiency of the MMR system is already optimal in mature T-cells, but that it is less efficient in CD34+ progenitors due to their maturation stage and requirement for differentiation to T-cells in vitro and not in the normal in vivo environment (Pawelec et al. 1998); indeed, early progenitors are

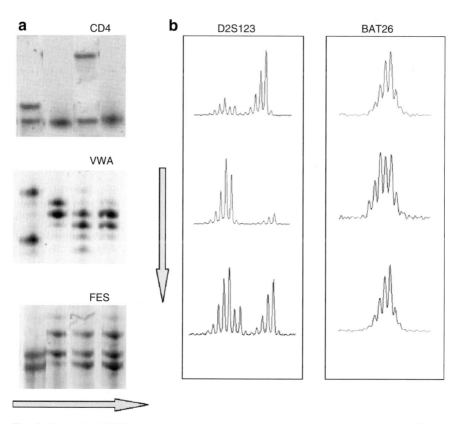

Fig. 3 Example of MSI evidenced during in vitro culture of one clone obtained from CD34+ precursors. CD4, VWA, FES, D2S123 and BAT26 allelic patterns, determined after different population doublings (PD) in culture, are shown. Genotyping was done: a: by PCR followed by analysis on standard acrilamyde gels for CD4, VWA and FES microsatellites; b: by analysis on an automated DNA sequencer for D2S123 and BAT26 microsatellites. Modifications of band length or peak position appear at increasing PD (grey arrows) (Neri et al. 2007)

highly proliferative and, during this period, most susceptible to DNA damage (Park, Gerson 2005). Maturation-dependent alterations in DNA repair function have been demonstrated for the lymphohematopoietic system in association with shifts in DNA repair gene expression profiles (Bracker et al. 2006). In addition, CD34+ cells might have lower levels of genetic integrity control, because they perform T-cell receptor rearrangement in culture. On the other hand, a role of the MMR system in general recombinational processes, VDJ hypermutation and class-switch recombination is well documented (Cascalho et al. 1998; Bellacosa 2001; Larson et al. 2005). Finally, it cannot be excluded that the in vitro system is unable to remove cells that acquired genetic alterations as in vivo occurs by apoptosis. The high instability found during in vitro culture of CD34+ cell-derived clones may suggest the need for particular care for the clinical use of these cells, such as in stem cell transplantation.

The observed MSI did not depend on modifications in the methylation status of MLH1 and MSH2 promoters, as assessed by methylation-specific PCR following bisulfite treatment of clone DNA and no association among methylation status, MMR gene expression, advanced population doublings or presence of MSI was found (Krichevski et al. 2004; Neri et al. 2007).

Semi-quantitative real time RT-PCR showed that transcript levels of the six MMR genes were similar to those observed in total RNA from normal PBMC. MSH6 RNA showed a progressive increase until about 50–60 PD, followed by a slow decrease, while MSH3 mRNA exponentially increased until the more advanced PD, thus suggesting a possible shift from MutSα to MutSβ heterodimer at advanced culture passages. MLH1 RNA did not change significantly during PD, while PMS2 and PMS1 RNA levels increased exponentially (Neri et al. 2007). During aging in culture, unstable clones often presented unstable or decreasing levels of expression, while stable ones constantly increased their expression levels, consistent with a relationship between MMR gene expression, PD and MSI (Neri et al. 2007). In agreement, multivariate regression analysis identified advanced PD as one of the predicting variables for FES MSI, trizygosis and intra-donor changes among clones. MSI and MMR gene expression at the mRNA level were found to correlate, mostly due to a reduced expression of the components of MutL heterodimers, pointing to a role of MMR in the acquisition of DNA damage with in vitro aging: the MutS components MSH6 and MSH3 appeared to be slightly increased in unstable clones; in contrast, the MutL components PMS2 and PMS1 showed decreased transcript levels in unstable compared to stable clones (Neri et al. 2007). This might suggest that unstable TCC maintain the ability to interact with mismatched DNA via MutS, but have a reduced capacity to recruit the enzymes necessary to complete the repair via MutL complexes. Therefore, the upregulation of MutS components in unstable clones, possibly in order to correct DNA mismatches occurring during in vitro proliferation, seems to be not accompanied by an upregulation of MutL components leading to MSI for a reduced expression of PMS2 and PMS1. However, additional posttranscriptional regulation of these genes cannot be definitely excluded. Only limited information is available thus far on the genetic regulation of the MMR system. In MMR proficient cell lines, the regulation seems primarily at the transcriptional level, but mutational inactivation of the components of the system leads to posttranslational down-regulation of heterodimerizing partners. MMR activity appears to be strictly regulated and modulated by changes in gene expression as demonstrated by MSI induction for loss of MLH1 expression secondary to promoter-hypermethylation (Herman et al. 1998) or by overexpression of MLH1 and MSH3 genes (Marra et al. 1998; Shcherbakova, Kunkel 1999). Therefore, it cannot be excluded that the upregulation of RNA for the MutS components is induced by a defect in the corresponding proteins.

Concerning a possible effect of donor age on MSI, clones from centenarians (an example of successful aging and of preserved immune function) presented a level of instability very similar to young-derived clones, despite the presence of significantly higher levels of MMR transcripts. In contrast, clones from old subjects presented a higher instability compared to young ones, but similar levels of MMR gene expression (Fig. 4). This might reflect the importance of up regulating MMR genes in order to maintain genomic stability and to correct DNA errors accumulating with age, thus suggesting a protective effect of higher MMR transcript levels on genomic integrity.

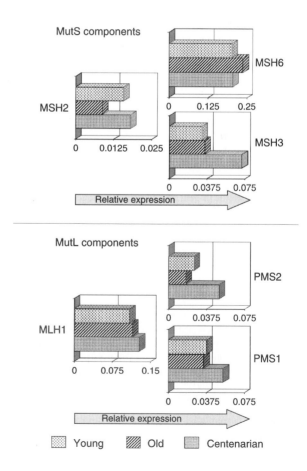

Fig. 4 MMR gene expression at mRNA level (medians) during culture aging of TCC from young, old and centenarian donors (from Neri et al. 2007)

The evidence of differences in allelic patterns among different clones from the same donor suggests the acquisition of new alleles in previous not analyzed culture passages or even before cloning, further supporting the accumulation of MSI even in vivo, as suggested by studies on peripheral blood cells (Ben-Yehuda et al. 2000; Coolbaugh-Murphy et al. 2005; Neri et al. 2005).

In conclusion, it appears that in vitro aging leads to an accumulation of genetic instability manifesting as MSI, possibly to a different extent, depending on cell type, and/or that repeated replication could lead to an accumulation of genetic alterations not counteracted by the MMR system. The correlation between MMR gene expression levels and MSI appeared mostly due to a reduced expression of the components of MutL heterodimers. However, the involvement of other repair pathways (Guo, Loeb 2003) or a possible alteration in polymerase functional activity (Srivastava, Busbee 2003) cannot be excluded. Senescence-associated MMR alterations might also be induced by defects of nuclear localization, assembly and activity of the proteins of this pathway, therefore studies on MMR gene protein levels and functional activity of the MMR system could help in the understanding of these alterations associated to senescence, likely critical for appropriate adaptive immune response.

Acknowledgments This work was partially supported by grants from Bologna University RFO (60% fund), Ricerca Corrente IOR, Italian Health Ministry fund and was performed under the aegis of EU ZINCAGE project (FOOD-CT-2003-506850) and T-CIA (QLK6-CT-2002-02283). The authors thank Mr. Keith Smith for editing.

References

Aaltonen LA, Peltomaki P, Leach F, Sistonen P, Pylkkanen SM, Mecklin J-P, Jarvinen H, Powell S, Jen J, Hamilton SR, Petersen GM, Kinzler KW, Vogelstein B, de la Chapelle A (1993)Clues to the pathogenesis of familial colorectal cancer. Science 260:812–816

Andrew SE, Reitmair AH, Fox J, Hsiao L, Francis A, McKinnon M, Mak TW, Jirik FR (1997) Base transitions dominate the mutational spectrum of a transgenic reporter gene in MSH2 deficient mice. Oncogene 15:123–129

Annett K, Duggan O, Freeburn R, Hyland P, Pawelec G, Barnett Y (2005) An investigation of DNA mismatch repair capacity under normal culture conditions and under conditions of supra-physiological challenge in human CD4+T cell clones from donors of different ages. Exp Gerontol 40:976–981

Atamna H, Cheung I, Ames BN (2000) A method for detecting abasic sites in living cells: age-dependent changes in base excision repair. Proc Natl Acad Sci USA 97:686–691

Barnett YA, Barnett CR (1998) DNA damage and mutation: contributors to the age-related alterations in T cell-mediated immune responses? Mech Aging Dev 102:165–175

Bellacosa A (2001) Functional interactions and signaling properties of mammalian DNA mismatch repair proteins. Cell Death Differ 8:1076–1092

Bennett ST, Lucassen AM, Gough SC, Powell EE, Undlien DE, Pritchard LE, Merriman ME, Kawaguchi Y, Dronsfield MJ, Pociot F, et al (1995) Susceptibility to human type 1 diabetes at IDDM2 is determined by tandem repeat variation at the insulin gene minisatellite locus. Nat Genet 9:284–292

Ben Yehuda A, Globerson A, Krichevsky S, Bar On H, Kidron M, Friedlander Y, Friedman G, Ben Yehuda D (2000) Aging and the mismatch repair system. Mech Aging Dev 121:173–179

Bohr VA (2002) Human premature aging syndromes and genomic instability. Mech Aging Dev 123:987–993

Boland CR, Thibodeau SN, Hamilton SR, Sidransky D, Eshleman JR, Burt RW, Meltzer SJ, Rodriguez-Bigas MA, Fodde R, Ranzani GN, Srivastava S (1998) A National Cancer Institute workshop on microsatellite instability for cancer detection and familial predisposition: development of international criteria for the determination of microsatellite instability in colorectal cancer. Cancer Res 58:5248–5257

Bonafè M, Barbi C, Olivieri F, Yashin A, Andeev KF, Vaupel JW, De Benedictis G, Rose G, Carrieri G, Jazwinski SM, Franceschi C (2002) An allele of HRAS1 3'variable number of tandem repeats is a frailty allele: implication for an evolutionarily-conserved pathway involved in longevity. Gene 286:121–126

Bonafè M, Barbi C, Storci G, Salvioli S, Capri M, Olivieri F, Valensin S, Monti D, Gonos ES, De Benedictis G, Franceschi C (2002) What studies on human longevity tell us about the risk for cancer in the oldest old: data and hypotheses on the genetics and immunology of centenarians. Exp Gerontol 37:1263–1271

Bracker TU, Giebel B, Spanholtz J, Sorg UR, Klein-Hitpass L, Moritz T, Thomale J (2006) Stringent regulation of DNA repair during human hematopoietic differentiation: a gene expression and functional analysis. Stem Cells 24:722–730

Cascalho M, Wong J, Steinberg C, Wabl M (1998) Mismatch repair co-opted by hypermutation. Science 279:1207–1210

Coolbaugh-Murphy MI, Xu J, Ramagli LS, Brown BW, Siciliano MJ (2005) Microsatellite instability (MSI) increases with age in normal somatic cells. Mech Aging Dev 126:1051–1059

De Benedictis G, Carotenuto L, Carrieri G, De Luca M, Falcone E, Rose G, Cavalcanti S, Corsonello F, Feraco E, Baggio G, Bertolini S, Mari D, Mattace R, Yashin AI, Bonafé M, Franceschi C (1998) Gene/longevity association studies at four autosomal loci (REN, THO, PARP, SOD2). Eur J Hum Gen 6:534–541

De Benedictis G, Carotenuto L, Carrieri G, De Luca M, Falcone E, Rose G, Yashin AI, Bonafé M, Franceschi C (1998) Age-related changes of the 3'APOB-VNTR genotype pool in aging cohorts. Ann Hum Genet 62:115–122

De Benedictis G, Rose G, Carrieri G, De Luca M, Falcone E, Passarino G, Bonafé M, Monti D, Baggio G, Bertolini S, Mari D, Mattace R, Franceschi C (1999) Mitochondrial DNA inherited variants are associated with successful aging and longevity in humans. FASEB J 13:1532–1536

De la Chapelle A, Peltomaki P (1995) Genetics of hereditary colon cancer. Annu Rev Genet 29:329–348

Demple B, Harrison L (1994) Repair of oxidative damage to DNA: enzimology and biology. Annu Rev Biochem 63:915–948

Doria G, Frasca D (2001) Age-related changes of DNA damage recognition and repair capacity in cells of the immune system. Mech Aging Dev 122:985–998

Eshleman JR, Markowitz SD (1995) Microsatellite instability in inherited and sporadic neoplasms. Curr. Opin. Oncol. 7:83–89

Fink D, Aebi S, Howell SB (1998) The role of DNA mismatch repair in drug resistance. Clin Cancer Res 4:1–6

Flores-Rozas H, Clark D, Kolodner RD (2000) Proliferating cell nuclear antigen and Msh2p-Msh6p interact to form an active mispair recognition complex. Nat Genet 26:375–378

Franceschi C, Valensin S, Bonafè M, Paolisso G, Yashin AI, Monti D, De Benedictis G (2000) The network and the remodeling theories of aging: historical background and new perspectives. Exp Gerontol 35:879–896

Franceschi C, Monti D, Sansoni P, Cossarizza A (1995) The immunology of exceptional individuals: the lesson of centenarians. Immunol Today 16:12–16

Frasca D, Barattini P, Tirindelli D, Guidi L, Bartoloni C, Errani A, Costanzo M, Tricerri A, Pierelli L, Doria G (1999) Effect of age on DNA binding of the ku protein in irradiated human peripheral blood mononuclear cells (PBMC). Exp Gerontol 34:645–658

Globerson A, Effros RB (2000) Aging of lymphocytes and lymphocytes in the aged. Immunol Today 21:515–521

Goukassian D, Gad F, Yaar M, Eller MS, Nehal US, Gilchrest BA (2000) Mechanisms and implications of the age-associated decrease in DNA repair capacity. FASEB J 14:1325–1334

Greer P (2002) Closing in on the biological functions of Fps/FES and Fer. Nat Rev Mol Cell Biol 3:278–289

Guo HH, Loeb LA (2003) Tumbling down a different pathway to genetic instability. J Clin Invest 112:1793–1795

Hadrup SR, Strindhall J, Kollgaard T, Seremet T, Johansson B, Pawelec G, thor Straten P, Wikby A (2006) Longitudinal studies of clonally expanded CD8 T cells reveal a repertoire shrinkage predicting mortality and an increased number of dysfunctional cytomegalovirus-specific T cells in the very elderly. J Immunol 176:2645–2653

Hanawalt PC (1994) Transcription-coupled repair and human disease. Science 266:1957–1958

Harris AL, Karran P, Lindhal T (1983) O6-Methylguanine-DNA methyltransferase of human lymphoid cells: structural and kinetic properties and absence in repair deficient cells. Cancer Res 43:3247–3252

Hart RW, Setlow RB (1974) Correlation between deoxyribonucleic acid excision-repair and life-span in a number of mammalian species. Proc Natl Acad Sci USA 71:2169–2173

Herman JG, Umar A, Polyak K, Graff JR, Ahuja N, Issa JP, Markowitz S, Willson JK, Hamilton SR, Kinzler KW, Kane MF, Kolodner RD, Vogelstein B, Kunkel TA, Baylin SB (2006) Incidence and functional consequences of hMLH1 promoter hypermethylation in colorectal carcinoma. Proc Natl Acad Sci U S A 95:6870–6875

Jun SH, Kim TG, Ban C (2006) DNA mismatch repair system. Classical and fresh roles. FEBS J 273:1609–1619

Kane MF, Loda M, Gaida GM, Lipman J, Mishra R, Goldman H, Jessup JM, Kolodner R (1997) Methylation of the hMLH1 promoter correlates with lack of expression of hMLH1 in sporadic colon tumors and mismatch repair-defective human tumor cell lines. Cancer Res 57:808–811

Kervinen K, Savolainen MJ, Salokannel J, Hynninen A, Heikkinen J, Ehnholm C, Koistinen MJ, Kesaniemi YA (1994) Apolipoprotein E and B polymorphisms-longevity factors assessed in nonagenarians. Atherosclerosis 105:89–95

Kim DJ, Yi SM, Lee SY, Kang HS, Choi YH, Song YW, Park SC (2006) Association between the MLH1 gene and longevity. Hum Genet 119:353–354

Kirkwood TB, Kowald A (1997) Network theory of aging. Exp Gerontol 32:395–399

Kolodner RD, Marsischky GT (1999) Eukaryotic DNA mismatch repair. Curr Opin Genet Dev 9:89–96

Krichevsky S, Pawelec G, Gural A, Effros RB, Globerson A, Yehuda DB, Yehuda AB (2004) Age related microsatellite instability in T cells from healthy individuals. Exp Gerontol 39:507–515

Larson ED, Duquette ML, Cummings WJ, Streiff RJ, Maizels N (2005) MutS> binds and promotes synapsis of transcriptionally activated immunoglobulin switch regions. Curr Biol 15:470–474

Lau PJ, Kolodner RD (2003) Transfer of the MSH2-MSH6 complex from proliferating cell nuclear antigen to mispaired bases in DNA. J Biol Chem 278:14–17

Lehmann AR Translesion synthesis in mammalian cells. Exp Cell Res 312:2673–2676

Lio D, Scola L, Crivello A, Bonafé M, Franceschi C, Olivieri F, Colonna-Romano G, Candore G, Caruso C (2002) Allele frequencies of +874T-->A single nucleotide polymorphism at the first intron of interferon-gamma gene in a group of Italian centenarians. Exp Gerontol 37:315–319

Liu B, Nicolaides NC, Markowitz S, Willson JK, Parsons RE, Jen J, Papadopolous N, Peltomaki P, de la Chapelle A, Hamilton SR, Kinzler KW, Vogelstein B (1995) Mismatch repair gene defects in sporadic colorectal cancers with microsatellite instability. Nat Genet 9:48–55

Liu B, Parsons R, Papadopoulos N, Nicolaides NC, Lynch HT, Watson P, Jass JR, Dunlop M, Wyllie A, Peltomaki P, de la Chapelle A, Hamilton SR, Vogelstein B, Kinzler KW (1996) Analysis of mismatch repair genes in hereditary non-polyposis colorectal cancer patients. Nat Med 2:169–174

Loeb LA (1994) Microsatellite instability: marker of a mutator phenotype. Cancer Res 54:5059–5063

Louhija J, Miettinen HE, Kontoula K, Miettinen TA, Tilvis RS (1994) Aging and genetic variation of plasma apolipoproteins. Relative loss of the apolipoprotein E4 phenotype in centenarians. Arterioscler Thromb 14:1084–1089

Manfredini R, Balestri R, Tagliafico E, Trevisan F, Pizzanelli M, Grande A, Barbieri D, Zucchini P, Citro G, Franceschi C, Ferrari S (1997) Antisense inhibition of c-FES proto-oncogene blocks PMA-induced macrophage differentiation in HL60 and in FDC-P1/MAC-11 cells. Blood 89:135–145

Marra G, Iaccarino I, Lettieri T, Roscilli G, Delmastro P, Jiricny J (1998) Mismatch repair deficiency associated with overexpression of the MSH3 gene. Proc Natl Acad Sci USA 95:8568–8573

Modrich P, Lahue R (1996) Mismatch repair in replication fidelity, genetic recombination and cancer biology. Annu Rev Biochem 65:101–133

Moslein G, Tester DJ, Lindor NM, Honchel R, Cunningham JM, French AJ, Halling KC, Schwab M, Goretzki P, Thibodeau SN (1996) Microsatellite instability and mutation analysis of hMSH2 and hMLH1 in patients with sporadic, familial and hereditary colorectal cancer. Hum Mol Genet 5:1245–1252

Nakagawa H, Nuovo GJ, Zervos EE, Martin EW Jr, Salovaara R, Aaltonen LA, de la Chapelle A (2001) Age-related hypermethylation of the 5' region of MLH1 in normal colonic mucosa is associated with microsatellite-unstable colorectal cancer development. Cancer Res 61:6991–6995

Narayanan L, Fritzell JA, Baker SM, Liskay RM, Glazer, PM (1997) Elevated levels of mutation in multiple tissues of mice deficient in the DNA mismatch repair gene Pms2. Proc Natl Acad Sci USA 94:3122–3127

Neri S, Cattini L, Facchini A, Pawelec G, Mariani E (2004) Microsatellite instability in in vitro aging of T lymphocyte clones. Exp Gerontol 39:499–505

Neri S, Gardini A, Facchini A, Olivieri F, Franceschi C, Ravaglia G, Mariani E (2005) Mismatch repair system and aging: microsatellite instability in peripheral blood cells from differently aged participants. J Gerontol A Biol Sci Med Sci 60:285–292

Neri S, Pawelec G, Facchini A, Mariani E (2008) Microsatellite instability and compromised Mismatch Repair gene expression during in vitro passaging of monoclonal human T lymphocytes. Rej Res 11:565–572

Ono T, Ikehata H, Nakamura S, Saito Y, Hosoi Y, Takai Y, Yamada S, Onodera J, Yamamoto K (2000) Age-associated increase of spontaneous mutant frequency and molecular nature of mutation in newborn and old lacZ-transgenic mouse. Mutat Res 447:165–177

Ouyang Q, Wagner WM, Zheng W, Wikby A, Remarque EJ, Pawelec G (2004) Dysfunctional CMV-specific CD8(+) T cells accumulate in the elderly. Exp Gerontol 39:607–613

Park Y, Gerson SL (2005) DNA repair defects in stem cell function and aging. Annu Rev Med 56:495–508

Parsons R, Li GM, Longley M, Modrich P, Liu B, Berk T, Hamilton SR, Kinzler KW, Vogelstein B (1995) Mismatch repair deficiency in phenotipically normal human cells. Science 268:738–740

Pawelec G, Muller R, Rehbein A, Hahnel K, Ziegler B (1998) Extrathymic T cell differentiation in vitro from human CD34+ stem cells. J Leukocyte Biol 64:733–739

Pawelec G, Barnett Y, Mariani E, Solana R (2002) Human CD4+ T cell clone longevity in tissue culture: lack of influence of donor age or cell origin. Exp Gerontol 37:265–269

Pawelec G, Akbar A, Caruso C, Solana R, Grubeck-Loebenstein B, Wikby A (2005) Human immunosenescence: is it infectious? Immunol Rev 205:257–268

Perls TT, Bubrick E, Wager CG, Vijg J, Kruglyak L (1998) Siblings of centenarians live longer. Lancet 351:1560

Prieur M, Al Achkar W, Aurias A, Couturier J, Dutrillaux AM, Dutrillaux B, Flury-Herard A, Gerbault-Seureau M, Hoffschir F, Lamoliatte E, Lefrancois D, Lombard M, Muleris M, Ricoul M, Sabatier L, Viegas-Pequignot E (1988) Acquired chromosome rearrangements in human lymphocytes: effect of aging. Hum Genet 79:147–150

Rattray AJ, Strathern JN (2003) Error-prone DNA polymerases: when making a mistake is the only way to get ahead. Annu Rev Genet 37:31–66

Reddy MC, Vasquez KM (2005) Repair of genome destabilizing lesions. Radiat Res 164:345–356

Reitmair AH, Redston M, Cai JC, Chuang TC, Bjerknes M, Cheng H, Hay K, Gallinger S, Bapat B, Mak TW (1996) Spontaneous intestinal carcinomas and skin neoplasms in MSH2-deficient mice. Cancer Res 56:3842–3849

Schachter F, Faure-Delanef L, Guenot F, Rouger H, Froguel P, Lesueur-Ginot L, Cohen D (1994) Genetic associations with human longevity at the APOE and ACE loci. Nat Genet 6:29–32

Silva F, Gusmao L, Alves C, Seruca R, David L, Amorim A (1997) Tetra- and pentanucleotide short tandem repeat instability in gastric cancer. Electrophoresis 18:1633–1636

Shcherbakova PV, Kunkel TA (1999) Mutator phenotypes conferred by MLH1 overexpression and by heterozygosity for mlh1 mutations. Mol Cell Biol 19:3177–3183

Sonoda E, Hochegger H, Saberi A, Taniguchi Y, Takeda S (2006) Differential usage of non-homologous end-joining and homologous recombination in double strand break repair. DNA Repair 5:1021–1029

Srivastava VK, Busbee DL (2003) Replicative enzymes, DNA polymerase alpha (pol alpha), and in vitro aging. Exp Gerontol 38:1285–1297

Starostik P, Greiner A, Schwarz S, Patzner J, Schultz A, Muller-Hermelink HK (2000) The role of microsatellite instability in gastric low- and high-grade lymphoma development. Am J Pathol 157:1129–1136

Suzuki H, Itoh F, Toyota M, Kikuchi T, Kakiuchi H, Hinoda Y, Imai K (1999) Distinct methylation pattern and microsatellite instability in sporadic gastric cancer. Int J Cancer 83:309–313

Takata H, Suzuki M, Ishii T, Sekiguchi S, Iri H (1987) Influence of major histocompatibility complex region genes on human longevity among Okinawan-Japanese centenarians and nonagenarians. Lancet 2:824–826

Thompson LH, Schild D (2002) Recombinational DNA repair and human disease. Mutat Res 509:49–78

Toyota M, Ahuja N, Ohe-Toyota M, Herman JG, Baylin SB, Issa JP (1999) CpG island methylator phenotype in colorectal cancer. Proc Natl Acad Sci USA 96:8681–8686

Vijg J (2000) Somatic mutations and aging: a re-evaluation. Mutat Res 447:117–135

Walter CA, Grabowski DT, Street KA, Conrad CC, Richardson A (1997) Analysis and modulation of DNA repair in aging. Mech Aging Dev 98:203–222

Wedderbrun LR, Patel A, Varsani H, Woo P (2001) The developing human immune system: T-cell receptor repertoire of children and young adults shows a wide discrepancy in the frequency of persistent oligoclonal T-cell expansions. Immunology 102:301–309

Wilson DM III, Bohr VA (2007) The mechanics of base excision repair, and its relationship to aging and disease. DNA Repair:544–559

Wilson TM, Vaisman A, Martomo SA, Sullivan P, Lan L, Hanaoka F, Yasui A, Woodgate R, Gearhart PJ (2005) MSH2-MSH6 stimulates DNA polymerase η, suggesting a role for A:T mutations in antibody genes. J Exp Med 201:637–645

Wood RD, Mitchell M, Sgouros J, Lindahl T (2001) Human DNA repair genes. Science 291:1284–1289

Yates KE, Gasson JC (1996) Role of c-FES in normal and neoplastic hematopoiesis. Stem Cells 14:117–123

Activation-Induced Cell Death of T-cells in Elderly

Ewa Sikora and Agnieszka Brzezińska

Contents

Abstract: The elimination of expanded T-cells at the end of immune response is crucial to maintain homeostasis and avoid any uncontrolled inflammation. Resting mature T-lymphocytes when activated *via* their antigen-specific receptor (TCR) and CD28 coreceptor start to proliferate and acquire resistance to apoptosis. Reactivation of T-cells induces expression of CD95L which after binding to CD95 surface-expressed death receptor triggers signaling pathway to apoptosis. The process is named Activation-Induced Cell Death-AICD. However, in executing AICD death receptor-dependent apoptotic pathway (extrinsic) can overlap with mitochondrial (intrinsic) signaling to apoptosis. Immunosenescence leads to the shrinkage of T-cell repertoire due to the reduction of naïve cells and accumulation of oligoclonal CD8+ and to a lower extent CD4+ cells, which are mainly CD95-positive and CD28-negative. Also, propensity to undergo apoptosis changes with age. However, data so far collected are inconclusive as they show an increased, unchanged or decreased propensity to AICD in the elderly in comparison with young individuals.

1 Introduction

Precursor T-cells from the bone marrow enter the thymus, where they undergo negative or positive selection to produce CD4+ and CD8+ mature cells with diverse functions in the peripheral immune system [34]. In the periphery, T-cells are resting until they encounter foreign antigens and gain the ability to proliferate, differentiate into effector cells, produce cytokines and eliminate target cells. T-cell activation is induced by signal receive through the TCR (T-Cell Receptor) activated by the antigen

E. Sikora (✉) · A. Brzezińska
Molecular Bases of Aging Laboratory
Nencki Institute of Experimental Biology, Polish Academy of Sciences
Pasteura 3, Warsaw Poland
Tel:+4822 5892436
Fax: +4822 8225342
E-mail: e.sikora@nencki.gov.pl

T. Fulop et al. (eds.), *Handbook on Immunosenescence,*
DOI 10.1007/ 978-1-4020-9062-2_15, © Springer Science+Business Media B.V. 2009

presented by APC (Antigen Presenting Cells) in MHC context, and costimulatory molecules, including CD28, adhesion molecules and cytokines (IL-2, IL-13, IL-15). This clonal expansion phase is followed by the contraction phase in which T-cell numbers decline to maintain homeostasis and avoid any uncontrolled inflammation. The majority of activated T-cells die by apoptosis and only a few T-cells that have been exposed to the antigen remain. These cells develop into apoptosis-resistant memory T-cells. The mechanism of memory T-cells' survival is not fully recognized, but it can be controlled by cytokines [27, 46]. Thus, T-cell activation is highly regulated and requires a switch from an apoptosis-resistant (clonal expansion phase) towards an apoptosis-sensitive state (elimination phase). The process in which expanded cells are eventually eliminated is named Activation-Induced Cell Death (AICD).

The term AICD was proposed by Green's group, when they showed that T-cell hybridomas or thymocytes died by apoptosis following activation through their CD3 molecules [44]. It is now know that AICD of hybridomas and of activated T-cells is driven by so called death receptors, such as CD95 (another name is Fas receptor) or the tumor-necrosis factor receptor (TNFR) which, once engaged, activate downstream pathways that lead to cell death by apoptosis [26].

An alternative pathway to that driven by death receptors is activated T-cell autonomous death (ACAD), which is determined by the ratio of anti and proapoptotic BCL-2 family members with the major role of a proapoptotic BIM protein. This type of cell death is known also as death by cytokine deprivation or by neglect [18]. Namely, the absence of appropriate survival signals induces BIM, which on the mitochondrial membrane can bind and neutralize the antiapoptotic BCL-2 or BCL-X_L (see below).

T-cells, similarly to other cells, can undergo Damage-Induced Cell Death (DICD), which is a cell response to DNA damage induced by both extracellular and intracellular insults, such as reactive oxygen species [13].

All three processes, although differentially regulated culminate in apoptotic cell death named also programmed cell death.

2   Apoptotic Pathways in T-cells

Apoptosis, or programmed cell death, is a fundamental process essential for both development and tissue homeostasis (reviewed in [21]). In the immune system, apoptosis plays a crucial role in selection of T-cell repertoire in the thymus, deletion of self-reactive T- and B-lymphocytes both in the central and peripheral lymphoid compartments, and in the killing of target cells by cytotoxic T-lymphocytes and natural killer cells [33]. Defects in apoptosis have been associated with a number of disease states, including autoimmunity and AIDS [48].

Cells undergoing apoptosis exhibit specific morphological changes, including membrane blebbing, cytoplasmic and chromatin condensation, DNA fragmentation, nuclear breakdown and assembly of membrane-enclosed vesicles termed apoptotic bodies, eventually subjected to phagocytosis [55]. The dying cells express "eat-me" signals, such as phosphatidyl serine, which allow the cells to be removed by phagocytosis.

Two major signaling pathways of apoptosis have been described: the extrinsic pathway induced by ligation of death receptors, and the intrinsic pathway comprised of the mitochondrial and endoplasmic reticulum pathways and induced by DNA damage, cytokine deprivation, gluccocorticoids or stress (Fig. 1). There is some crosstalk between these apoptotic pathways, but they lead to activation of different initiator caspases, which in turn activate common effector caspases 3, 6 and 7 [16, 26]. One of the terminal events of the apoptotic signaling pathways is activation of specific endonucleases cleaving DNA into oligunucleosomal fragments: Endo G and DFF/CAD. The latter is activated by effector caspases which cleave the DFF/CAD inhibitory protein [53]. The effector caspases cleave also a number of other important cellular proteins including actin, lamins, gasoline, plectin and others; their degradation in turn leads to the blebbing and formation of apoptotic bodies and final cell destruction.

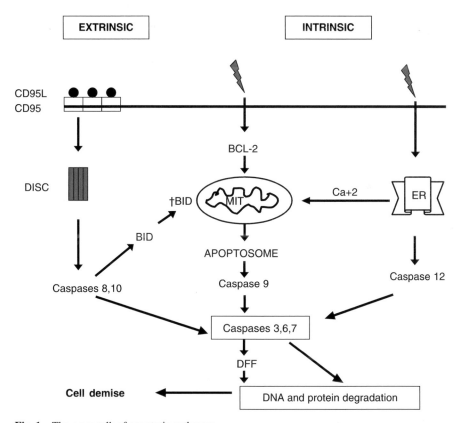

Fig. 1   The cross-talk of apoptotic pathways
The extrinsic pathway is mediated by interaction between death receptor and its ligand and leads to activation of initiator caspases 8, 10. The intrinsic pathway is comprised of the mitochondrial pathway (MIT) and the endoplasmic reticulum (ER) pathway. The mitochondrial pathway leads to activation of initiator caspase 9 and endoplasmic reticulum pathway to activation of initiator caspase 12. All initiator caspases activate effector caspases 3, 6 and 7 which in turn activates specific endonuclease (DFF) and depredate cellular proteins.

The intrinsic apoptotic pathway crucially depends on permeabilization of the outer mitochondrial membrane and mitochondria seem to be integrators of the many apoptotic signals coming from the outside and inside the cell. After receiving an apoptotic signal, mitochondria release a variety of molecules of which cytochrome c seems to be the most important one, which together with cytoplasmic apoptotic-protease-activating factor 1 (APAF1) forms the apoptosome. At the apoptosome initiator caspase 9 is activated. Crucial roles in determining the mitochondrial membrane permeability is controlled primarily by a balance between the antagonistic actions of the proapoptotic and antiapoptotic members of the BCL-2 family. Antiapoptotic members, such as BCL-2 and BCL-X_L possess so named BH1-4 domains. Proapoptotic BCL-2 family proteins comprise two subfamilies: the first including BAX, BAK and BOK, which have BH1-3 domains and the second including BH3-only members, such as BAD, BID, BIM and others. BH3- only proteins, like BIM can bind and neutralize the antiapoptotic BCL-2 or BCL-X_L. This in turn activates proapoptotic BAX or BAK which release cytochrome c from mitochondria.

The extrinsic apoptotic pathway is triggered by signals originating with cell-surface death receptors belonging to the TNF receptor (TNFR) superfamily that are activated by several ligands such as CD95L (also known as FasL), tumor necrosis factor (TNF) or TNF-related apoptosis-inducing ligand (TRAIL). Transduction of the apoptotic signal from the death receptors starts with the formation of a large protein complex at the cell membrane, known as the death inducing signaling complex—DISC. The CD95 DISC consists of trimerized CD95, the adaptor molecule FADD containing so called DD domain, procaspase 8a (also named FLICE), procaspase 8b, procaspase 10 and the cellular FLIP (cFLIP) protein. FLIP protein contains inactive caspase-like domain. Three isoforms of cFLIP are known, but only cFLIPs seem to exert an inhibitory effect on caspase 8 activation. Procaspases 8 and 10 as well as FADD and cFLIP contain DED domain which is required for DISC formation. Thus, formation of the DISC results in the assembly of procaspase 8 and procaspase 10 leading to their autoproteolytic activation. In some cells this signaling pathway suffices to induce executor caspases and eventual cell death (Type I cells). However, the level of CD95 DISC and of active caspase 8 may be too low (Type II cells) and the signal requires on additional amplification loop involving the cleavage of a BH-only BCL-2 family protein, BID, by caspase 8 to form truncated BID (tBID). tBID in turn aggregates BAX or BAK, which leads to mitochondria membrane permebilization and cytochrome c release [26].

3   Mechanism of Activation-Induced Cell Death

AICD is believed to be the major mechanism of elimination of T-cells during the termination phase of immune response. Following pathogen entry, T-cell activation *via* TCR and coreceptors induces their proliferation and clonal expansion. Pathogen killing by effector cells is followed by a severe decrease of T-cell proliferation and the beginning of T-cell elimination by death receptor-dependent apoptosis (Fig. 2)

Fig. 2 Immune response
Following patogen entry,
TCR activation induces T-
cell proliferation and clonal
expansion. Pathogen killing
by effector cells is followed
by cell elimination by death
receptor-driven apoptosis.

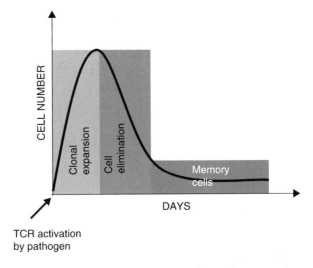

[22]. Upon stimulation of activated T-cells CD95L mRNA and protein expression on the surface of cell are rapidly induced. CD95L binds to the CD95 receptor on the same cell that express CD95L or on neighboring cells and triggers CD95-dependent apoptosis. The first type of CD95/CD95L interaction results in autocrine (suicide) and the second type in paracrine (fratricide) type of death [26].

Studies performed on murine and human T-cells suggested several transcription factors to be involved in activation of CD95L expression, such as Ap-1, NFAT, NFκB, c-Myc, Erg 1 & 3, and others. Cooperation between some of them is necessary for CD95 gene activation. Also, several tyrosine kinases known to be involved, such as PKC, Lck, ZAP-70 and MAPK, among others [14, 19].

An in vitro system of T-cell immune response believed to mimic the shutdown of immune response occurring in vivo has been developed by Krammer's group [24] and now this model is used, with some modifications by many investigators. Originally, freshly isolated primary human T-cells were activated with the non-specific mitogen-PHA for several hours (short–term activated), which respond to CD95 driven apoptosis resistance. However, after in vitro culture lasting for several days (long-term activated), the activated T-cells acquired sensitivity to death receptor-driven cell death, and IL-2 was found to be necessary for this sensitization [27, 43].

CD95 is not expressed on T-cells derived from cord blood or on naïve resting T-cells, but is rapidly up-regulated upon T-cell activation [23]. Although it was shown that long-term activated cells prone to AICD and short-term activated cells resistant to AICD express similar high amounts of CD95 [24]. This observation suggests that the signaling cascade downstream of CD95 must be modulated. Indeed, the cFLIP protein, and particularly its cFLIPs isoform, a potent inhibitor of CD95-mediated apoptosis, was found to be expressed at a high level in short- but not in long-term activated T-cells [2, 20]. Moreover, it was shown that inhibition of IL-2 production or signaling prevented down-regulation of FLIP protein levels and conferred resistance to CD95-mediated apoptosis on TCR-activated cells [2]. It cannot be excluded that expression of antiapoptotic BCL-2 family members, such as BCL-2 and BCL-X$_L$, might provide additional protection against cell death at the level of mitochondria [3].

Overall, AICD regulation is rather complex and involves both extrinsic and intrinsic mechanisms of apoptosis; it is also tightly connected with survival signaling pathways triggered by TCR and cytokines [26] (Fig. 3).

TCR–mediated NFkB signaling is critical for cell survival (death resistance) by inducing prosurvival and antiapoptotic genes [3]. It has been postulated that the hematopoetic progenitor kinase HPK1-C mediates sensitivity towards AICD by suppression of NFκB activity [4].

4 Age-Related Alterations of Activation-Induced Cell Death of Human T-cells

The aging of the immune system, termed immunosenescence involves several components which lead to its decreased functionality contributing to the morbidity and mortality of elderly people. The main aspects of immunosenescence are: (i) the

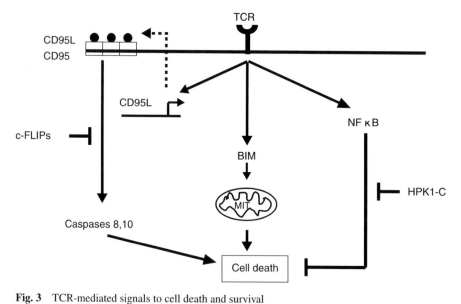

Fig. 3 TCR-mediated signals to cell death and survival
Stimulation of the TCR receptor can lead to CD95L transcription and engagement of CD95, thus activation of the extrinsic apoptotic pathway. TCR stimulation can also cause activation of the intrinsic apoptotic pathway via BH3-only BCL-2 family BIM. The extrinsic death pathway can be connected to the intrinsic pathway by caspase 8-mediated cleavage of the BH3-only BCL-2 family member BID towards truncated BID (tBID). TCR-mediated NFκB signaling is critical for cell survival and can be blocked by HPK1-C. On the other hand, apoptosis can be blocked by c-FLIPs.

involution of the thymus and exhaustion of naïve T-cells; (ii) the diminution of the T-cell repertoire and accumulation of oligoclonal expansions (megaclones) of memory/effector cells; and (iii) a chronic inflammatory state called inflamm-aging [8].

T-cell senescence in humans involves alterations similar to those observed in other cell types, such as changes in functions, cessation of cell proliferation due to shortening of telomeres and a changed propensity to undergo apoptosis. The senescence is seen primarily in the CD8+ T-cell population but it also occurs in CD4+ T-cells [11, 50].

Alterations of apoptosis in T-cells from aged individuals have been reported by many investigators, however, a consensus is still lacking in this matter especially since many studies were only correlative. Some authors show that aging is associated with increased apoptosis of T-cells, whereas others report the opposite (reviewed in [15, 19, 29]). These apparent discrepancies might be due to differences in the stimuli investigated, the phenotype of the cells as well as the general experimental approach. Also, some experiments were performed on lymphocytes undergoing in vitro replicative senescence [45] while others on cells derived from donors of different ages [36]. According to our results, replicative senescence in vitro only partially reflects the in vivo process [5-7].

Moreover, there is profound confusion in the literature concerning the term AICD, partially due to some overlapping of dead receptor-driven and mitochondria-mediated apoptosis in this process. Second, the question is whether the propensity of activated T-cells to undergo apoptosis upon death receptors activation (treatment with CD95L or anti CD95 mAb) can be considered as AICD? Taking into account that AICD is undergoing *via* engagement of death receptors this can help in understanding this process. (Death receptor-driven apoptosis is the subject of another chapter).

However, we must keep in mind that according to classical definition, AICD is induced by religation of TCR on activated cells [25]. Finally, it should be also remembered that AICD is not the only mechanism of T-cell death during shutdown of the immune response [47].

Generally, the literature guides us to three possibilities concerning AICD in the aging process. The first is that **T-cell susceptibility to AICD is increased**.

Despite the induction of CD95L, the main indictor of the cell ability to undergo AICD is the expression of CD95 receptor. While T-cells from cord blood are CD95-negative, the proportion of CD95-positive cells are growing with age [12, 41]. Moreover, Aggarwal and Gupta [1] reported on increased expression of CD95 mRNA in the elderly in comparison with young subjects. Fagnoni et al. [12] postulated the CD95-negative cells disappearing with age are unprimed, naïve cells. We also found a dramatic decrease in percentage of CD95-negative cells with age, from virtually 100% (not shown) in the cord blood to almost undetectable in peripheral blood of centenarians (Fig. 4). However, PBMC cultures from young and old individuals alike show an increase in CD95 expression upon activation, the cells from old individuals reaching even higher CD95 levels than those from young individuals [31, 37, 40]. Therefore, T-cells from the elderly are able to respond to activation with CD95 engagement. Moreover, some studies of T-cells from elderly subjects do appear to show a correlation between the increased CD95 expression and increased activation-induced

Fig. 4 Fraction of CD95-cells in peripheral blood of donors at different ages Young (aged 25–35, N=16), middle (aged 45–55, N=11), old (aged 65, N=37), centenarians (N=32).

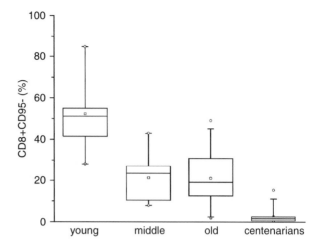

cell death [30, 37, 40]. Lechner et al. [30] observed no differences in the incidence of apoptosis in response to activation between PBMC from young and old subjects. However, under long-term cultivation, namely at replicative senescence in vitro, an increase of AICD was observed and it was more pronounced in T-cell populations from old than from young individuals. Phelouzat et al. [36] reported a greater depletion of T-cells upon stimulation in old than in young PBMC which was shown to be due to apoptosis. Similar results were obtained by Potestio et al. [40]. Schindowski et al. [42] described a slight but statistically significant increase of AICD in elderly in comparison to young individuals. Pawelec et al. [35] reported on increased susceptibility to AICD in a late-passage in comparison to an early-passage CD4+ cultured T-cell clone. Greater CD95-induced apoptosis was found in anti-CD3 stimulated CD4+ than in CD8+ cells derived from healthy donors, and both CD4+ and CD8+ T-cells from the elderly were more sensitive than those from young individuals [1].

The presented so far data indicate that activated T-cells from the elderly are more susceptible to undergoing AICD than cells from younger subjects, moreover, the population of CD4+ cells is more sensitive to cell death then the CD8+ cells.

Based on those studies as well as the results emerging from studies on mice, Ginaldi proposed recently an increased propensity to AICD as a hallmark of aging [13]. However, the literature also shows evidence in favor of other possibilities, namely that **T-cell susceptibility to AICD is unchanged or even decreased with age.** Pinti et al. [38], similarly to others reported on increasing number of CD95-positive cells and an increased level of Fas mRNA with age. Although the reverse trend was observed in the case of FasL in resting cells, the amount of FasL produced by lymphocytes upon activation with anti-CD3 was the same irrespective of the age of donors (young, middle-aged, centenarians). Also AICD level was the same in T-cells from all three groups. This is in agreement with our results showing no differences in AICD levels in T-lymphocytes derived from young in comparison to old donors. Following a slightly modified classical protocol described by Krammer's group [24], PBMC cells were stimulated with PHA for 72 h and then cultured in the presence of IL-2

Fig. 5 AICD of
T-cells derived from
young (aged 25-31, N
= 4) and old (aged 65,
N = 4) donors. PBMC
cells were stimulated
with PHA for 72 h and
then cultured in the
presence of IL-2.

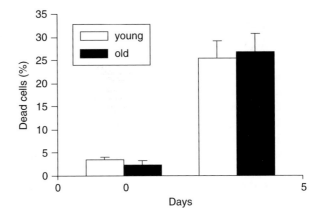

(Fig. 5). However, this protocol does not correctly reflect the situation in vivo, as the production of IL-2 is severely diminished with age. Similar results, namely the same level of AICD in young and old subjects, were obtained by Herndon et al. [17]. However, more recent results from this laboratory indicated for decreased AICD in donors aged 70–85 years in comparison with younger ones (25–65-year old), but also in comparison with nonagenarians. Thus from this results it is difficult to conclude whether AICD is really diminished with the age [19]. Whereas, Donnini et al. clearly showed that the AICD level analyzed in CD4+ cell subsets, namely naïve (CD62L+CD95-) and memory (CD62L-CD95+), did not correlate with the age [10].

Indirect, but convincing arguments of reduced AICD in elderly come from experiments on the role of lipid rafts in immunosenescence. Lipid rafts are involved in many processes, but mainly in signal transduction in T-cells, which is obviously impaired in the elderly [28, 29]. It was shown that disruption of lipid rafts reduced the sensitivity to Fas-mediated apoptosis after TCR restimulation of CD4+ cells. Thus, the redistribution of Fas and other tumor necrosis factor family receptors into and out of lipid rafts may dynamically regulate the efficiency and outcomes of signaling by these receptors [32]. Larbi et al. [29] reported a decreased expression of Fas and FasL in old in comparison with young donors. Expression of Fas was diminished and expression of FasL was completely abolished in stimulated lymphocytes after disruption of lipid rafts. It was shown that activation of lipid rafts was possible only upon ligation of both TCR and CD28, implying that CD28 might be critical in the signal transduction leading to AICD.

5   The Role of CD28 Coreceptor in Age-Dependent AICD of T-cells

Senescence effects numerous changes in the phenotype and the functioning of T-cells. Lifelong and chronic antigenic load may represent the major driving force of immunosenescence due to reducing the number of naïve antigen-nonexperienced cells and their replacement by expanded clones of antigen-experienced effector and memory T-cells with late differentiated phenotype. The thymus releases fewer naïve cells with age and those T-cells remaining, especially the CD8+subset, show increased oligoclonality with age [51].

The recognition of MHC-bound antigen by TCR is a low-affinity interaction unable to sustain activation of T-cells; productive activation requires costimulation with CD28 which serves as an amplifier of the TCR signal [50]. By activating Akt, CD28 acts as a typical transducer of the prosurvival pathway [19].

It is known that T-cell activation leads to CD28 down-regulation. Indeed, various models of T-cell replicative senescence show that subsequent rounds of cell divisions eventually lead to accumulation of CD28-negative cells, which are the progeny of CD28-positive ones [7, 11, 39]. We showed a gradual replacement of CD8+CD28+ cells by CD28- cells in long-term cultures both in the cord blood and in the peripheral blood of donors of different age, including centenarians [7]. It was also shown that purified human CD28+ T-cells progressively lose CD28 during each successive stimulation, with CD8+ T-cells losing CD28 more rapidly than CD4+ cells [50]. Also in vivo the accumulation with age of CD8+CD28- and to lesser extent CD4+CD28- is observed [7, 11, 12, 19, 50, 54]. CD28-negative cells are highly oligoclonal and have very short telomeres [50]. It is believed that they are unable to proliferate, however, we found that this is only true in the case of cells undergoing replicative senescence in vitro, but not for those aging in vivo [7].

As they accumulate progressively through life and large clones persist for years, CD28-negative cells are considered to be resistant to AICD. Indeed, Posnett et al. [39] demonstrated that CD8+CD28- cells activated with a superantigen were less susceptible to apoptosis than their CD8+CD28+ counterparts. Spaulding et al. [45] showed that T-cells reactivated after achieving in vitro the state of replicative senescence acquired resistance do apoptosis induced with different stimuli, including antiCD3 and antiFas.

Many of the CD8+ and CD28- expanded clones seem to result from previous infections by persistent viruses, especially CMV and to lesser extent, EBV and other herpesviruses. These are considered dysfunctional, "anergic" cells possibly at least partly due to apoptosis resistance, however a direct proof of their AICD resistance is lacking [51]. Thus it seems that accumulation with age of long-living CD8+CD28- cells can actually be explained by their relative resistance to AICD. Also CD4+CD28- cells, unlike their CD28+ counterparts, were shown to be protected from AICD due to high expression of cFLIP [49].

On the other hand, the data showing quite opposite correlation between CD28 and AICD can not be neglected. We showed no differences between CD28+ and CD28- in susceptibility to undergo AICD [6], but there are results providing evidences that maintenance of CD28 expression on T-cells may be even crucial for prevention of Fas-mediated apoptosis during the course of antigen engagement. Indeed, it was documented that within a superantigen-activated T-cell population, cells which were sensitive to Fas ligation were characterized by low CD28 expression prior to treatment with Fas [52]. It was also shown that CD28-mediated signaling increases expression of antiapoptotic BCL-X$_L$ and thereby promotes survival implying antiapoptotic activity of CD28. Indeed, Krammer's group reported that activated and cultured in the presence of IL-2 T-cells (undergoing AICD) when co-stimulated by CD28 showed, besides strong up-regulation of BCL-X$_L$, down-regulation of CD95L mRNA and strong up-regulation of cFLIPs [23]. In agreement with these results are data presented by others showing that low CD28 expression predispose to CD95L mediated apoptosis in activated T-cells and CD28 ligation protects from apoptosis [9].

6   Concluding Remarks

Immunosenscence is believed to be driven by thymus involution, continuous pathogen load and common damaging insults. This leads to the shrinkage of T-cell repertoire due to the reduction of naïve cells and accumulation of oligoclonal CD8+ and, to a lesser extent, CD4+ cells, displaying a highly differentiated and senescent phenotype with diminished functioning. Activation-Induced Cell Death plays a crucial role in the proper function of the immune system by elimination of expanded cells at the end of immune response. This logically implies a crucial role of AICD in immunosenescence. Indeed, some data published so far indicates AICD changes in the elderly. Nonetheless, this observations are inconclusive, some showing an increased some a decreased propensity of T-cells to AICD in the elderly. There are also reports of unchanged AICD with age. This apparent controversy probably stems from different experimental approaches and highly fragmentary data, especially concerning human studies. Systematic and comprehensive studies are still needed for a conclusive elucidation of the role of AICD in human aging.

References

1. Aggarwal S, Gupta S (1998) Increased apoptosis of Tcell subsets in aging humans: altered expression of Fas (CD95), Fas ligand, Bcl-2, and Bax. J Immunol 160:1627–1637
2. Algeciras-Schimnich A, Griffith TS, Lynch DH, Paya CV (1999) Cell cycle-dependent regulation of FLIP levels and susceptibility to Fas-mediated apoptosis. J Immunol 162:5205–5211
3. Arnold R, Brenner D, Becker M, Frey CR, Krammer PH (2006) How T lymphocytes switch between life and death. Eur J Immunol 36:1654–1658
4. Brenner D, Golks A, Kiefer F, Krammer PH, Arnold R (2005) Activation or suppression of NFkappaB by HPK1 determines sensitivity to activation-induced cell death. Embo J 24:4279–4290
5. Brzezinska A, Magalska A, Sikora E (2003) Proliferation of CD8+ in culture of human T-cells derived from peripheral blood of adult donors and cord blood of newborns. Mech Ageing Dev 124:379–387
6. Brzezinska A, Magalska A, Szybinska A, Sikora E (2004) Proliferation and apoptosis of human CD8(+)CD28(+) and CD8(+)CD28(−) lymphocytes during aging. Exp Gerontol 39:539–544
7. Brzezinska A (2005) Does in vitro replicative senescence of human CD8+ cells reflect the phenotypic changes observed during in vivo ageing? Acta Biochim Pol 52:931–935

8. Capri M, Monti D, Salvioli S, Lescai F, Pierini M, Altilia S, Sevini F, Valensin S, Ostan R, Bucci L, Franceschi C (2006) Complexity of anti-immunosenescence strategies in humans. Artif Organs 30:730–742

9. Dennett NS, Barcia RN, McLeod JD (2002) Age associated decline in CD25 and CD28 expression correlate with an increased susceptibility to CD95 mediated apoptosis in T-cells. Exp Gerontol 37:271–283

10. Donnini A, Re F, Bollettini M, Moresi R, Tesei S, Bernardini G, Provinciali M (2005) Age-related susceptibility of naive and memory CD4 T-cells to apoptosis induced by IL-2 deprivation or PHA addition. Biogerontology 6:193–204

11. Effros RB, Dagarag M, Spaulding C, Man J (2005) The role of CD8+ T-cell replicative senescence in human aging. Immunol Rev 205:147–157

12. Fagnoni FF, Vescovini R, Passeri G, Bologna G, Pedrazzoni M, Lavagetto G, Casti A, Franceschi C, Passeri M, Sansoni P (2000) Shortage of circulating naive CD8(+) T cells provides new insights on immunodeficiency in aging. Blood 95:2860–2868

13. Ginaldi L, De Martinis M, Monti D, Franceschi C (2004) The immune system in the elderly: activation-induced and damage-induced apoptosis. Immunol Res 30:81–94

14. Green DR, Droin N, Pinkoski M (2003) Activation-induced cell death in T cells. Immunol Rev 193:70–81

15. Gupta S (2005) Molecular mechanisms of apoptosis in the cells of the immune system in human aging. Immunol Rev 205:114–129

16. Gupta S, Gollapudi S (2006) Molecular mechanisms of TNF-alpha-induced apoptosis in naive and memory T cell subsets. Autoimmun Rev 5:264–268

17. Herndon FJ, Hsu HC, Mountz JD (1997) Increased apoptosis of CD45RO- T cells with aging. Mech Ageing Dev 94:123–134

18. Hildeman DA, Zhu Y, Mitchell TC, Kappler J, Marrack P (2002) Molecular mechanisms of activated T cell death in vivo. Curr Opin Immunol 14:354–359

19. Hsu HC, Scott DK, Mountz JD (2005) Impaired apoptosis and immune senescence—cause or effect? Immunol Rev 205:130–146

20. Irmler M, Thome M, Hahne M, Schneider P, Hofmann K, Steiner V, Bodmer JL, Schroter M, Burns K, Mattmann C, Rimoldi D, French LE, Tschopp J (1997) Inhibition of death receptor signals by cellular FLIP. Nature 388:190–195

21. Jacobson MD, Weil M, Raff MC (1997) Programmed cell death in animal development. Cell 88:347–354

22. Kabelitz D, Janssen O (1997) Antigen-induced death of T-lymphocytes. Front Biosci 2: D61–D77

23. Kirchhoff S, Muller WW, Li-Weber M, Krammer PH (2000) Up-regulation of c-FLIPshort and reduction of activation-induced cell death in CD28-costimulated human T cells. Eur J Immunol 30:2765–2774

24. Klas C, Debatin KM, Jonker RR, Krammer PH (1993) Activation interferes with the APO-1 pathway in mature human T cells. Int Immunol 5:625–630

25. Krammer PH (2000) CD95's deadly mission in the immune system. Nature 407:789–795

26. Krammer PH, Arnold R, Lavrik IN (2007) Life and death in peripheral T cells. Nat Rev Immunol 7:532–542

27. Krueger A, Fas SC, Baumann S, Krammer PH (2003) The role of CD95 in the regulation of peripheral T-cell apoptosis. Immunol Rev 193:58–69

28. Larbi A, Dupuis G, Khalil A, Douziech N, Fortin C, Fulop T, Jr. (2006) Differential role of lipid rafts in the functions of CD4+ and CD8+ human T lymphocytes with aging. Cell Signal 18:1017–1030

29. Larbi A, Muti E, Giacconi R, Mocchegiani E, Fulop T (2006) Role of lipid rafts in activation-induced cell death: the fas pathway in aging. Adv Exp Med Biol 584:137–155

30. Lechner H, Amort M, Steger MM, Maczek C, Grubeck-Loebenstein B (1996) Regulation of CD95 (APO-1) expression and the induction of apoptosis in human T cells: changes in old age. Int Arch Allergy Immunol 110:238–243

31. McLeod JD, Walker LS, Patel YI, Boulougouris G, Sansom DM (1998) Activation of human T cells with superantigen (staphylococcal enterotoxin B) and CD28 confers resistance to apoptosis via CD95. J Immunol 160:2072–2079

32. Muppidi JR, Siegel RM (2004) Ligand-independent redistribution of Fas (CD95) into lipid rafts mediates clonotypic T cell death. Nat Immunol 5:182–189

33. Osborne BA (1996) Apoptosis and the maintenance of homoeostasis in the immune system. Curr Opin Immunol 8:245–254

34. Palmer E (2003) Negative selection—clearing out the bad apples from the T-cell repertoire. Nat Rev Immunol 3:383–391

35. Pawelec G, Sansom D, Rehbein A, Adibzadeh M, Beckman I (1996) Decreased proliferative capacity and increased susceptibility to activation-induced cell death in late-passage human CD4+ TCR2 +cultured T cell clones. Exp Gerontol 31:655–668

36. Phelouzat MA, Arbogast A, Laforge T, Quadri RA, Proust JJ (1996) Excessive apoptosis of mature T lymphocytes is a characteristic feature of human immune senescence. Mech Ageing Dev 88:25–38

37. Phelouzat MA, Laforge T, Arbogast A, Quadri RA, Boutet S, Proust JJ (1997) Susceptibility to apoptosis of T lymphocytes from elderly humans is associated with increased in vivo expression of functional Fas receptors. Mech Ageing Dev 96:35–46

38. Pinti M, Troiano L, Nasi M, Bellodi C, Ferraresi R, Mussi C, Salvioli G, Cossarizza A (2004) Balanced regulation of mRNA production for Fas and Fas ligand in lymphocytes from centenarians: how the immune system starts its second century. Circulation 110:3108–3114

39. Posnett DN, Edinger JW, Manavalan JS, Irwin C, Marodon G (1999) Differentiation of human CD8 T cells: implications for in vivo persistence of CD8+ CD28- cytotoxic effector clones. Int Immunol 11:229–241

40. Potestio M, Caruso C, Gervasi F, Scialabba G, D'Anna C, Di Lorenzo G, Balistreri CR, Candore G, Romano GC (1998) Apoptosis and ageing. Mech Ageing Dev 102:221–237

41. Potestio M, Pawelec G, Di Lorenzo G, Candore G, D'Anna C, Gervasi F, Lio D, Tranchida G, Caruso C, Romano GC (1999) Age-related changes in the expression of CD95 (APO1/FAS) on blood lymphocytes. Exp Gerontol 34:659–673

42. Schindowski K, Leutner S, Muller WE, Eckert A (2000) Age-related changes of apoptotic cell death in human lymphocytes. Neurobiol Aging 21:661–670

43. Schmitz I, Krueger A, Baumann S, Schulze-Bergkamen H, Krammer PH, Kirchhoff S (2003) An IL-2-dependent switch between CD95 signaling pathways sensitizes primary human T cells toward CD95-mediated activation-induced cell death. J Immunol 171:2930–2936

44. Shi YF, Sahai BM, Green DR (1989) Cyclosporin A inhibits activation-induced cell death in T-cell hybridomas and thymocytes. Nature 339:625–626

45. Spaulding C, Guo W, Effros RB (1999) Resistance to apoptosis in human CD8+ T cells that reach replicative senescence after multiple rounds of antigen-specific proliferation. Exp Gerontol 34:633–644

46. Sprent J, Tough DF (2001) T cell death and memory. Science 293:245–248

47. Strasser A, Pellegrini M (2004) T-lymphocyte death during shutdown of an immune response. Trends Immunol 25:610–615

48. Thompson CB (1995) Apoptosis in the pathogenesis and treatment of disease. Science 267:1456–1462

49. Vallejo AN, Schirmer M, Weyand CM, Goronzy JJ (2000) Clonality and longevity of CD4+CD28null T cells are associated with defects in apoptotic pathways. J Immunol 165:6301–6307

50. Vallejo AN (2005) CD28 extinction in human T cells: altered functions and the program of T-cell senescence. Immunol Rev 205:158–169

51. Vasto S, Colonna-Romano G, Larbi A, Wikby A, Caruso C, Pawelec G (2007) Role of persistent CMV infection in configuring T cell immunity in the elderly. Immun Ageing 4:2

52. Walker LS, McLeod JD, Boulougouris G, Patel YI, Hall ND, Sansom DM (1998) Downregulation of CD28 via Fas (CD95): influence of CD28 on T-cell apoptosis. Immunology 94:41–47

53. Widlak P, Garrard WT (2005) Discovery, regulation, and action of the major apoptotic nucle-ases DFF40/CAD and endonuclease G. J Cell Biochem 94:1078–1087
54. Wikby A, Ferguson F, Forsey R, Thompson J, Strindhall J, Lofgren S, Nilsson BO, Ernerudh J, Pawelec G, Johansson B (2005) An immune risk phenotype, cognitive impairment, and survival in very late life: impact of allostatic load in Swedish octogenarian and nonagenarian humans. J Gerontol A Biol Sci Med Sci 60:556–565
55. Wyllie AH (1980) Glucocorticoid-induced thymocyte apoptosis is associated with endogenous endonuclease activation. Nature 284:555–556

CD8 Clonal Expansions in Mice: An Age-associated Alteration of CD8 Memory T-cells

Eric T. Clambey, John W. Kappler and Philippa Marrack

Contents

P. Marrack (✉) · E. T. Clambey · J. W. Kappler
Integrated Department of Immunology
Howard Hughes Medical Institute
National Jewish Research & Medical Center
Departments of Medicine, Pharmacology
Biochemistry and Molecular Genetics
University of Colorado Health Sciences Center
Denver, CO 80206, USA
Telephone: +1 303 398 1322
Fax: +1 303 270 2166
E-mail: marrackp@njc.org

T. Fulop et al. (eds), *Handbook on Immunosenescence*,
DOI: 10.1007/978-1-4020-9062-2_16, © Springer Science+Business Media B.V. 2009

Abbreviations

CFSE	5-(and -6) Carboxyfluorescein diacetate succinimidyl ester
EBV	Epstein-Barr virus
HCMV	Human cytomegalovirus
IFN-γ	Interferon gamma
IL	Interleukin
IL-2Rβ	Interleukin-2 receptor, beta chain
IL-7Rα	Interleukin-7 receptor, alpha chain
KLRG1	Killer cell lectin-like receptor G1
LCMV	Lymphocytic choriomeningitis virus
LIP	Lymphopenia-induced proliferation
MHC	Major histocompatibility complex
MP	Memory phenotype
PD-1	Programmed death-1
PMA	Phorbol 12-myristate 13-acetate
SPF	Specific-pathogen free
TCE	T-cell clonal expansion
TCR	T-cell receptor
T_{CM}	Central memory T-cell
T_{EM}	Effector memory T-cell
TRAF	Tumor necrosis factor receptor associated factor
TRAIL	Tumor necrosis factor-related apoptosis-inducing ligand

Abstract: Aging is associated with a variety of perturbations in the immune system. One frequent alteration is a significant skewing of the CD8 T-cell repertoire. This alteration manifests as a clonal expansion of CD8 memory T cells, which in some cases can occupy the majority of the CD8 T-cell pool. CD8 clonal expansions are associated with impaired immunity in the elderly. Although CD8 clonal expansions are commonly found in aging humans and mice, the etiology of this phenomenon is unknown. Here, we describe our current understanding of CD8 clonal expansions as it relates to the current state of knowledge about CD8 T-cell memory. In addition, we discuss the heterogeneity observed between different types of clonal expansions in mice, and how distinct factors may influence both the development and properties of clonal expansions in the aging individual.

Keywords: Ageing • CD8 clonal expansion • CD8 memory T-cell • Homeostasis • TCE

1 T-cells, TCR Diversity and the Phenomenon of CD8 Clonal Expansions

A hallmark of the adaptive immune system is its capacity to respond to a myriad of different challenges. One way that individuals are able to respond to diverse pathogens is through the generation of a highly diverse T-cell repertoire, in which each T-cell expresses a slightly different T-cell receptor (TCR). Each TCR is created through a process of gene rearrangement of TCR gene segments, followed by further diversification methods. Notably, each distinct TCR recognizes a slightly different combination of a short peptide (referred to as antigen) presented in the context of a major histocompatibility complex (MHC) molecule. Once a T-cell (and TCR) encounters its correct antigen and the appropriate stimulatory conditions, the T-cell can undergo a series of steps, including activation, proliferation, and the acquisition of effector functions through which the T-cell mediates its protective effects. CD8+ T-cells recognize antigen in the context of MHC Class I molecules and respond to, and control, a variety of intracellular infections (such as bacteria and viruses).

While young, healthy individuals possess a diverse CD8 T-cell pool, many aged individuals develop significant perturbations in the repertoire of TCR specificities. In these individuals, a single CD8 T-cell achieves a competitive advantage relative to its neighbors and comes to dominate the entire CD8 T-cell pool, a phenomenon referred to as CD8 T-cell clonal expansions (or TCEs). This phenomenon is of significant interest for many reasons. First, it is a common age-associated alteration to the immune system. Second, it results in a significant perturbation to the normally diverse CD8 T-cell repertoire. Third, it has been associated with impaired immunity in the aged. Fourth, it represents a significant breakdown in the normal homeostatic mechanisms that regulate CD8 T-cell survival and proliferation.

This chapter will focus on the biology of CD8 clonal expansions in mice, with only brief discussion of clonal expansions in humans. It should be noted that while there are some differences between clonal expansions in mice and in humans (for further discussion see [24]), CD8 clonal expansions in both species are characterized by the selective outgrowth of a specific subtype of CD8 T-cell, the CD8 memory T-cell. In order to understand the properties of clonal expansions, it is essential to have basic information about CD8 memory T-cells, their development, regulation, and biological properties.

2   CD8 Memory T-cell Differentiation

2.1   Memory T-cell Differentiation Following an Acute Exposure to Antigen

Following TCR stimulation by antigen, a naïve CD8 T-cell initiates a program of activation, proliferation and differentiation (Fig. 1a) [56]. The resulting CD8 T-cell response is characterized by multiple phases: i) proliferation and expansion of antigen-specific CD8 T-cells, during which these cells acquire a variety of effector functions (such as cytokine secretion and the capacity to kill target cells expressing the appropriate antigen), ii) a period of contraction during which 90–95% of the total number of antigen-specific CD8 T-cells undergo apoptosis, and iii) a period of further differentiation during which the remaining 5–10% of antigen-specific CD8 T-cells acquire additional phenotypic changes, to ultimately become a CD8 memory T-cell (Fig. 1a). During the expansion phase, antigen-specific CD8 T-cells can occupy a massive fraction of the CD8 T-cell pool (e.g., during acute lymphocytic choriomeningitis virus (LCMV) infection, at least 80% of the CD8 T-cells in the spleen are specific for LCMV [84]).

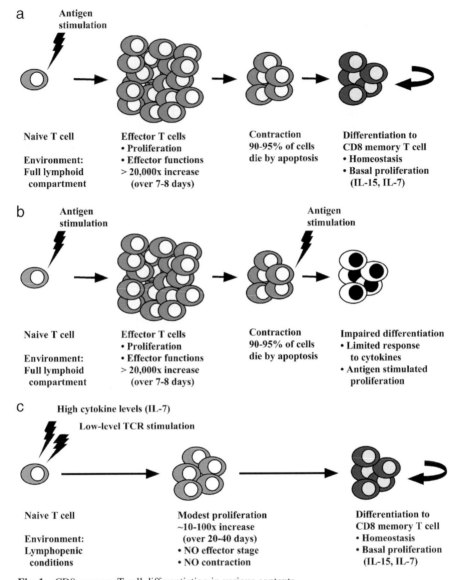

Fig. 1 CD8 memory T-cell differentiation in various contexts

The dynamics of an antigen-specific CD8 T-cell response in individuals possessing a full lymphocyte compartment following either transient, acute antigen exposure (panel a) or prolonged, persistent antigen exposure (panel b). CD8 memory T-cells can also develop when naïve T-cells are placed in a lymphopenic environment, devoid of other lymphocytes (panel c). The different stages of CD8 T-cell differentiation are indicated as follows: naïve (gray cytoplasm, white nucleus), effector cell (red cytoplasm, yellow nucleus), memory cell (deep blue cytoplasm, light blue nucleus). In the case of persistent antigen, there is impaired memory cell differentiation, as indicated by white cytoplasm, black nucleus. Stages of differentiation and factors that influence CD8 T-cell response are discussed further in text. Diagram indicates relative, not absolute abundance of CD8 T-cells at each stage.

CD8 memory T-cells differ from naïve CD8 T-cells in many ways. In contrast to naïve CD8 T-cells, CD8 memory T-cells have an accelerated response to antigen stimulation, are found at many sites in the body and are maintained at very constant levels for months to years following initial antigen exposure (a process facilitated by cytokines). The self-renewing capacity of CD8 memory T-cells can occur in the absence of continued antigen exposure, providing an antigen-independent mechanism of CD8 memory T-cell maintenance. The combination of these characteristics, as well as the increased frequency of antigen-specific CD8 T-cells in antigen-exposed individuals, means that individuals who develop a CD8 memory T-cell response against an antigen will have a rapid, robust response upon antigen reexposure. In many contexts, CD8 memory T-cells provide an important mechanism of immunological protection, or immunity to reinfection [56, 140].

In the context of CD8 clonal expansions, one particularly important property of CD8 memory T-cells is their steady, slow rate of proliferation in the uninfected animal. The long-term proliferation and survival of CD8 memory T-cells is heavily dependent on the cytokines interleukin (IL)-7 and IL-15 [7, 37, 72, 116, 118, 125]. CD8 memory T-cells receive these cytokine cues through expression of the IL-7 receptor alpha chain (IL-7Rα, CD127), the IL-2 receptor beta chain (IL-2Rβ, CD122), and the common gamma chain cytokine receptor. As discussed below, CD8 clonal expansions have alterations in their capacity to respond to these cytokines.

2.2 Memory T-cell Subsets

Though CD8 memory T-cells arise following antigen stimulation, not all CD8 memory T-cells have the same properties. CD8 memory T-cells are most frequently categorized as either central memory (T_{CM}) or effector memory (T_{EM}) cells [113]. While both these subsets of memory cells express cell surface receptors thought to be typical of CD8 memory T-cells (e.g. in the mouse, CD44^{high} CD127^{high} CD122^{high}), these two subsets differ in their expression of L-selectin (CD62L) and the chemokine receptor, CCR7, two proteins that promote trafficking to peripheral lymph nodes. Central memory T-cells are CD62L+ CCR7+, and are found in blood, spleen, and lymph nodes. In contrast, effector memory T-cells do not express CD62L or CCR7, and are found in blood, spleen, and nonlymphoid tissues. T_{EM} cells are generally absent from lymph nodes, except in situations of ongoing inflammation [38, 85].

The precise factors that influence whether a CD8 memory T-cell becomes a central or an effector memory cell remain contentious. One factor that might influence this balance is the magnitude of the initial antigenic stimulus [132]. It should be noted, however, that at this time it is debatable whether the T_{CM} and T_{EM} subdivisions of CD8 memory T-cells represent true independent cell fates, are capable of interconversion, or whether their differences reflect in part the impact of local environments on the phenotype and function of a CD8 memory T-cell (for further discussion see [76]). Regardless of the precise development details of T_{CM} and T_{EM} cells, local tissue environments can significantly influence the phenotype and properties of a CD8 memory T-cell [67, 83, 86].

Following the identification of T_{CM} and T_{EM} subsets of CD8 memory T-cells, further subsets of memory cells have been identified. For example, the IL-7Rα (CD127) was identified as a marker to identify activated CD8 T-cells that gave rise to long-lived memory cells [46, 55]. Subsequent work has shown that the usefulness of this marker varies depending on the experimental system [73], and that IL-7 plays an important but perhaps not instructive role in the development of CD8 memory T-cells [15, 40, 66, 123]. A recent study also identified expression of CD8αα homodimers as a potential marker for CD8 memory T-cell precursors [80], although the significance of this observation remains contentious [21, 135, 143]. Additional subtypes of CD8 memory T-cells, differing by various criteria (e.g., ability to divide in the absence of antigen, tissue distribution, and capacity to respond upon antigen rechallenge) have also been identified [12, 44, 109]. Despite the identification of these various subsets, a major unanswered question is the interrelationship between different types of memory T-cells and the factors that drive these distinct phenotypes and properties.

It is worth noting that in some studies of CD8 memory T-cells, cells have the phenotype of a memory T-cell (in the mouse, typically defined as CD44[high]), but the precise antigen reactivity and origin of this memory cell is poorly defined. These cells are often referred to as CD8 memory phenotype (MP) T-cells. Some CD8 MP T-cells probably result from conditions of lymphopenia (discussed below).

2.3 CD8 Memory T-cell Differentiation in the Context of Chronic Infection

The above discussion of CD8 memory T-cell differentiation focused on this process following an acute, transient infection. It is important to note, however, that CD8 T-cells are highly attuned to external cues, and that the process of CD8 memory T-cell differentiation can be significantly influenced by the nature of the eliciting infection (e.g., [2]). In addition, the phenotypes and properties of a CD8 T-cell can vary between CD8 T-cells responding to different epitopes within the same pathogen [45, 121]. These different outcomes likely reflect differences in the patterns of antigen expression at various stages of infection.

The most dramatic perturbations to CD8 memory T-cell differentiation occur in situations of chronic infection (e.g., certain strains of LCMV) that are characterized by a prolonged, high pathogen burden. In these situations, CD8 T-cells develop an altered state of "memory" in which the resulting CD8 T-cells remain actively dependent on persistent antigen and TCR engagement for their survival (Fig. 1b). These cells express reduced levels of cytokine receptors for IL-7 and IL-15 (IL-7Rα and IL-2Rβ, respectively), and do not achieve antigen-independent survival and proliferation [120, 131]. In addition, these cells can express sustained levels of inhibitory receptors such as programmed death-1 (PD-1), which can actively impair the capacities of a CD8 T-cell [6]. Situations of chronic infection can also result in the continual recruitment of naïve CD8 T-cells into the CD8 memory pool [130].

Based on the above differences, it is worth considering whether the CD8 "memory" T-cells that result during a chronic infection are true CD8 memory T-cells or if they instead exist in an altered state of "quasi-memory". For the purpose of this chapter, we will refer to CD8 memory T-cells that develop in the context of chronic infection as antigen-dependent CD8 memory T-cells (referring to their continued requirement for antigen to survive). This is in contrast to CD8 memory T-cells that arise following an acute infection, which we will refer to as antigen-independent CD8 memory T-cells (referring to their capacity to survive in the absence of antigen).

2.4   An Alternate Way to become a CD8 Memory T-cell: Lymphopenia-induced Proliferation

While CD8 memory T-cells have been traditionally studied in individuals following exposure to a variety of antigens, there is an alternate way for a naïve CD8 T-cell to become a CD8 memory T-cell. This phenomenon occurs in individuals characterized by a state of severely reduced lymphocyte numbers, a condition known as lymphopenia. Lymphopenia is observed in various conditions, including individuals exposed to high dose irradiation or chemotherapy, as well as in neonates [75, 92]. In mice, genetic models of lymphopenia are also available (such as mice completely devoid of T-cells).

The observation that lymphopenia could promote the generation of CD8 memory T-cells was made by multiple groups who transferred naïve, antigen-specific CD8 T-cells into lymphopenic mice (whether irradiated or genetically deficient) (reviewed in [51]). In these studies, naïve CD8 T-cells began to proliferate once placed in the lymphopenic environment, a process referred to as either homeostatic proliferation or lymphopenia-induced proliferation (LIP). In addition to proliferating, however, these CD8 T-cells also acquired many of the characteristics associated with a CD8 memory T-cell [22, 35, 64, 93, 96]. For clarity, these cells will subsequently be referred to lymphopenia-induced proliferation (LIP) CD8 memory T-cells.

At this time, it is unknown whether LIP CD8 memory T-cells and antigen-elicited CD8 memory T-cells are identical. There are clear differences in the generation of these two cell types (compare Fig. 1a and 1c). First, LIP CD8 memory T-cells do not go through a stage of acute activation (e.g., LIP CD8 memory T-cells do not express various early activation markers), in contrast to antigen-elicited CD8 T-cells [22, 93]. In addition, LIP memory cells undergo a much more modest proliferation than antigen-elicited memory T-cells, and have no significant contraction phase [22, 93]. Despite these differences, LIP memory cells do have a transcriptional profile that is similar to that of antigen-elicited CD8 memory T-cells [36], and these cells are capable of mediating a protective response against secondary infection [39].

The observation that a naïve CD8 T-cell can become a memory cell in the absence of strong antigenic stimulation indicates that there is at least one alternate way for a naïve cell to become a memory T-cell (Fig. 1c). While lymphopenia-induced proliferation can be promoted by TCR stimulation by low affinity ligands [30, 34, 64], this phenomenon is also driven by the high levels of unconsumed cytokines (particularly IL-7) present in an environment that is almost devoid of neighboring lymphocytes (reviewed by [51, 124]). At this time, the precise contribution of LIP memory T-cells to the complete CD8 memory T-cell repertoire is unclear. Nonetheless, given some of the factors that influence the development of CD8 clonal expansions (described below), lymphopenia-induced proliferation and memory differentiation may contribute to at least part of this age-associated phenomenon.

3   The Regulation of CD8 Memory T-cell Homeostasis

3.1   The Role of IL-7 and IL-15

As previously alluded to, the regulation of CD8 memory T-cell proliferation and survival is heavily influenced by extracellular factors. The cytokines IL-7 and IL-15 are the best-characterized extracellular proteins that promote the survival and proliferation of CD8 memory T-cells [7, 37, 72, 116, 118, 125, 142]. Both of these cytokines belong to the common gamma chain (γ_c) family of cytokines.

In general, the functions of IL-7 and IL-15 are thought to be compartmentalized, such that IL-7 primarily provides survival signals whereas IL-15 provides proliferative signals (reviewed in [124]). Although excess IL-7 can overcome a deficiency in IL-15 [65], the mechanism by which these two cytokines are perceived differs significantly. IL-7 is present in a secreted, soluble form. In contrast, IL-15 appears to be retained on the cell surface of certain cells, requiring direct cell contact of the CD8 T-cell with an IL-15 presenting cell in order to receive an IL-15 signal [17, 27, 114, 117]. While IL-7 and IL-15 can function alone, their effects can also be influenced by other cytokines. For example, IL-21 can synergize with IL-15 to promote proliferation of CD8 memory T-cells in vitro [141].

Given the central role of IL-7 and IL-15 in promoting CD8 memory T-cell homeostasis, the levels of these cytokines are tightly controlled and for good reasons. Limited cytokine expression appears to be important in limiting excessive proliferation; transgenic mice that express excessive amounts of IL-15 can develop a fatal leukemia [32]. Cytokine signals are also subject to additional regulation. For example, IL-7 can downregulate expression of its own receptor, IL-7Rα [101].

3.2   The Role of Other Cytokines, Cell Surface Receptors and Cells

In addition to IL-7 and IL-15, other cytokines also influence the homeostasis of CD8 memory T-cells. For example, IL-2 appears to be critical for CD8 memory

T-cells to robustly proliferate upon antigen reexposure [136]. In contrast, transforming growth factor beta (TGF-β) appears to limit the rate of proliferation of CD8 memory T-cells, possibly through antagonism of IL-15 signals [79]. High levels of IL-10 can also impair the appropriate formation of CD8 memory T-cells, as revealed by studies of chronic LCMV infection [14, 28].

Various cell surface proteins of the immunoglobulin and tumor necrosis family (TNF) families can also influence the magnitude and homeostasis of CD8 memory T-cells. Mice deficient in the B- and T-lymphocyte attenuator (BTLA), an immunoglobulin superfamily member, have an increased number of CD8 MP T-cells and a higher rate of homeostatic proliferation, indicating that BTLA limits the magnitude of CD8 memory T-cells [69]. In contrast, mice deficient in the TNF receptor ligand 4-1BBL have impaired CD8 memory, suggesting a positive role for 4-1BB signaling in the formation of a robust CD8 memory T-cell response (reviewed in [111]). Similar data indicate a positive role for CD27 and OX40 in promoting CD8 memory T-cell responses [42, 43]. Notably, some of the effects of these proteins may be directly regulated by cytokine cues elicited by IL-15 [107].

While many of the above cues influence the long-term maintenance of CD8 memory T-cells, initial signals received during T-cell activation can also heavily influence the differentiation of a naïve CD8 T-cell to a CD8 memory T-cell. One example of this regulation is the observation that inflammation can prolong the time required for CD8 memory T-cell differentiation [41]. As such, CD8 T-cells activated in a context of minimal inflammation become memory T-cells more rapidly (e.g., following immunization with antigen-pulsed dendritic cells) [5]. At least part of this effect is mediated by the effect of inflammatory cytokines, such as interferon gamma (IFN-γ), on the responding CD8 T-cell [5]. It is worth noting, however, that the effects of IFN-γ on the immune system are pleiotropic, and in some contexts, IFN-γ can promote an optimal CD8 memory T-cell response [133, 134]. IL-12 and type I interferons can also promote optimal CD8 T-cell activation and CD8 memory responses [68, 88].

The properties of CD8 memory T-cells are also heavily influenced by the presence or absence of CD4+ T-cells. Over the past few years, there has been an increasing appreciation that CD8 memory T-cells generated in the absence of CD4 T-cell help can be compromised in various ways (reviewed in [8]). At least part of the defect observed in CD8 memory T-cells that do not receive CD4 T-cell help may be due to tumor-necrosis factor (TNF)-related apoptosis-inducing ligand (TRAIL) induced apoptosis of CD8 memory T-cells upon antigen re-exposure [39, 52]. However, additional mechanisms are also likely involved in CD4 T-cell optimization of CD8 memory T-cell responses [4, 95].

Finally, the properties of CD8 T-cells can be influenced by the frequency of antigen-specific T-cells that participate in a response, as well as subsequent antigenic exposure. Studies analyzing the response of TCR transgenic CD8 T-cells, in which each CD8 T-cell expresses the identical TCR as its neighbors, have revealed that an artificially elevated number of identical antigen-specific T-cells (achieved by adoptive transfer of a high number of TCR transgenic CD8 T-cells) results in CD8 T-cells with distinct properties not observed during an endogenous CD8 T-cell response

[3, 59, 82]. At this time, it is unclear whether this observation reflects an experimental artifact, or whether it reflects some basic physiological regulation observed in certain conditions of CD8 T-cell responses. Although CD8 memory T-cells can be maintained in an antigen-independent manner, subsequent antigen exposures can influence the TCR specificities of CD8 memory T-cells that are maintained [119].

3.3 The Influence of Intracellular Factors

While the properties of CD8 memory T-cells are well defined, the intracellular factors that coordinate these changes remain poorly characterized. CD8 memory T-cells are clearly characterized by a wide variety of transcriptional changes [54], as well as changes in chromatin modifications relative to naïve CD8 T-cells [31, 61, 95]. While there is no identified master regulator for the development of CD8 memory T-cells, there have been an increasing number of transcription factors that either facilitate differentiation to, or the properties of, CD8 memory T-cells. These include Bcl-6 [47], STAT5 [16, 58], eomesodermin and T-bet [49, 103], Bcl-6b/BAZF [81], c-myc [9], MeCP2 [60], and Id2 [19]. At this time, the precise molecular targets of these transcription factors and their contribution to CD8 memory T-cell development remain largely undefined.

Intracellular proteins that influence the proliferation and survival of CD8 T-cells can also impact the development of CD8 memory. The suppressor of cytokine signaling (SOCS) family of proteins is known to inhibit various cytokine signals [1]. In particular, SOCS1 is an important regulator of CD8 T-cell responses to cytokine signals by IL-7 and IL-15, and deficiency of this molecule results in an increased number of CD8 MP T-cells [23, 26, 48].

Regarding proteins that regulate cell survival, the proapoptotic Bcl2-family member, Bim, appears to limit the number of cells entering the CD8 memory T-cell pool [138]. Signal transduction through tumor necrosis factor receptor associated factor (TRAF) 1 is one mechanism that may regulate levels of Bim protein during a CD8 T-cell response [112]. The optimal development of CD8 memory also depends on appropriate protection of CD8 T-cells against internal damage from cytotoxic proteins expressed by CD8 T-cells (e.g. granzymes, cathepsins), something which can be mediated by various serine protease inhibitors expressed in CD8 T-cells [78, 104].

4 The Discovery of CD8 Clonal Expansions

Following the discovery of the T-cell receptor, there was an explosion of reagents to analyze the properties and diversities of the T-cell pool. One technical advance that allowed the discovery of CD8 clonal expansions was the development of monoclonal antibodies that recognized different TCR V alpha (Vα) and V beta (Vβ) gene products. By using these reagents, investigators identified that young, healthy individuals had a relatively consistent number of T-cells expressing each Vα and Vβ gene product [18, 105]. In contrast, aging individuals frequently had significant perturbations in the abundance of T-cells expressing various Vα and Vβ gene products [18, 105]. Significantly, these aged individuals frequently had a massive overrepresentation of a single Vα or Vβ that was at least three standard deviations above the mean Vα and Vβ usage observed in young individuals. The selective outgrowth or accumulation of a single Vα or Vβ gene product within the CD8 T-cell pool suggested that these CD8 T-cells might be clonal expansions. Molecular analysis of the T-cell receptors used by these expanded populations of CD8 T-cells revealed that these overrepresented populations of CD8 T-cells were truly clonal [77, 105]. Notably, these clonal expansions were predominantly found within the CD8 T-cell lineage, and were rarely identified in CD4 T-cells.

Today, CD8 clonal expansions are frequently identified using antibodies against various Vβ gene products (Fig. 2). Based on this method, individuals with CD8 clonal expansions are identified as those with an overabundance of a single Vβ within the CD8 T-cell pool that is increased at least three standard deviations above the mean Vβ usage found for that Vβ in young individuals. The strength of this approach is that it identifies an overabundance of one Vβ within the entire CD8 T-cell pool. CD8 clonal expansions can also be identified by molecular analysis of TCR diversity (e.g. the spectratyping method [97]). When using such molecular methods, however, it is worth noting that these methods can detect reduced diversity within a specific Vβ gene family, despite the fact that that Vβ is not over-represented within the entire CD8 T-cell pool (a phenomenon we have referred to as clonal restriction [24]). Because of this caveat, we consider it preferable to identify the presence of clonal expansions by monoclonal antibodies against the TCR, followed by molecular analysis of TCR diversity. Age-associated clonal expansions are routinely clonal by such analyses.

One important observation about CD8 clonal expansions is that clonal expansions in different individuals express a diverse range of T-cell receptors. Even in genetically identical inbred mice that are housed together, CD8 clonal expansions express a wide variety of TCR Vαs and Vβs. The same is true for humans. Based on these observations, CD8 clonal expansions appear to arise from a diverse set of CD8 T-cells.

5   Properties of Clonal Expansions

5.1   Incidence and Abundance of Clonal Expansions in Humans and Mice

CD8 clonal expansions are a common age-associated alteration within the immune system. In specific-pathogen free (SPF) mice, almost 60% of mice develop clonal

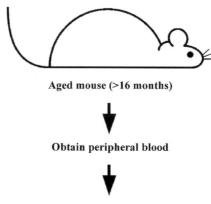

Aged mouse (>16 months)

Obtain peripheral blood

Define TCR Vβ usage in CD8 T cells

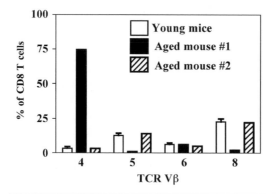

Fig. 2 Methodology to identify CD8 clonal expansions in aged mice
CD8 clonal expansions can be identified based on the percentage of CD8 T-cells expressing various TCR Vβ receptors. While young mice have a highly consistent percentage of CD8 T-cells that
express each Vβ (open bars), certain aged mice (e.g., hypothetical aged mouse #1 in black bars)
have an overabundance of CD8 T-cells expressing one Vβ (in this situation, a Vβ4+ clonal expansion). CD8 clonal expansions are identified in those mice that have an overabundance of one TCR
Vβ, that is increased at least three standard deviations above the mean Vβ usage observed in a
cohort of young mice. Data for young mice indicate mean Vβ usage +/- three standard deviations
of the mean. Young mice are typically between 3–6 months of age. Aged mice develop detectable
clonal expansions by 16 months of age. In this example, aged mouse #2 (hatched bar) does not
have any detectable CD8 clonal expansions.

expansions by 2 years of age [71]. In humans, 33% of adults over the age of 65
have a detectable clonal expansion [108]. CD8 clonal expansions vary widely in
their size within the CD8 T-cell pool. In the most dramatic situations, CD8 clonal

expansions can occupy 50% of the CD8 T-cell pool in humans [33] and 90% of the CD8 T-cell pool in mice (Clambey et al. unpublished data).

Since clonal expansions are found in many, but not all, mice, it is worth noting that studies of T-cell responses in aging mice may be profoundly influenced by whether an individual mouse contains a clonal expansion or does not. Given the idiosyncratic nature of clonal expansions, we strongly recommend that studies of T-cell function in aging mice be carefully controlled to minimize the impact of clonal expansions on the interpretation of the experiment.

5.2 Factors Associated with the Development of Clonal Expansions

While the precise origin of clonal expansions remains unclear, ongoing research has provided clues about potential cues that may facilitate the development of clonal expansions. One of the strongest factors associated with the development of clonal expansions is age. This age-association with clonal expansions is particularly pronounced in the mouse, where CD8 clonal expansions are virtually undetectable until 16 months of age [18]. In humans, increasing age is associated with an increasing prevalence of clonal expansions [108]. In contrast to mice, however, clonal expansions in humans can be found in younger individuals [108]. It is possible that these latter clonal expansions may reflect immune responses to childhood infections, something that would not be observed in SPF mice [50].

Although clonal expansions are particularly observed in aging individuals, it is unknown what factors within the aging environment, if any, contribute to the development of clones. It is worth noting that clonal expansions can be transferred to young individuals and still retain their competitive advantage [70, 91]. This observation indicates that while aging may contribute to the development of clonal expansions, the aging environment is not essential for the maintenance of clonal expansions.

Beyond the correlation of age and the development of clonal expansions, there are two other factors positively associated with the development of clonal expansions.

i) *Humans infected with human cytomegalovirus (HCMV)*. Over the past few years, the use of MHC Class I tetramers has allowed investigators to investigate the TCR specificity of human clonal expansions. Based on these studies, at least some human clonal expansions specifically recognize human cytomegalovirus, a common chronic herpesvirus infection [63, 98]. In the most dramatic case, 27% of CD8 T-cells in one individual were specific against a single HCMV epitope [98]. Although HCMV infection can be controlled in healthy individuals, there is increasing evidence that HCMV infection in the elderly is associated with a variety of negative outcomes [62, 102, 106, 122]. Importantly, while some humans develop clonal expansions against Epstein-Barr virus (EBV), another common chronic Herpes virus infection, these clonal expansions are much smaller in size [62, 97, 129]. Thus, there appear to be certain factors associated with HCMV infection that are capable of eliciting pronounced CD8 clonal expansions in humans. This association may be related in part to the observation that chronic CMV infection can elicit large, and in some cases, highly focused T-cell responses that often increase in size with age, even in individuals without clonal expansions [57, 63, 127].

ii) *Lymphopenia and inflammation in mice.* Additional insights into cues that promote CD8 clonal expansions came from the analysis of CD8 clonal expansions in various mouse models. Significantly, mice characterized by lymphopenia (e.g., mice lacking the IL-7 receptor or mice subjected to adult thymectomy) develop clonal expansions at an earlier age and with a higher prevalence than intact, unmanipulated mice [90]. Although the precise mechanisms behind this outcome remain to be elucidated, one likely explanation for this effect is the increased rate of proliferation of CD8 memory T-cells in lymphopenic conditions [90]. In the same study, it was noted that repeated treatment of mice with adjuvants (compounds known to induce inflammation and to facilitate antigen-specific T- and B-cell responses to coinjected antigen) also modestly increased the incidence of CD8 clonal expansions [90]. It is interesting to note that states of inflammation, such as those of viral infections, have been associated with transient states of lymphopenia (e.g., [87]). Thus, it is possible that adjuvants promote the development of clonal expansions through the temporary generation of lymphopenic conditions. For further discussion of lymphopenia and its effects on the generation of clonal expansions please see chapter by Nikolich-Zugich.

5.3 CD8 Clonal Expansions may Impair Immune Function in the Aged

Given the dominance of CD8 clonal expansions within the aged individual, it is likely that clonal expansions have some impact on the immune function of aged individuals. To date, there are two studies to support this contention. First, in humans, there is a correlation between the presence of clonal expansions and an impaired response to influenza vaccination, a common defect in aged individuals [115]. Second, in mice, there are data that clonal expansions may result in highly focused holes in the T-cell repertoire (particularly in the Vβ subfamily used by the clonal expansion) [89]. These narrow holes may be particularly problematic in individuals responding to infections in which the T-cell response is heavily restricted to use of a single Vβ subfamily. Please see chapter by Nikolich-Zugich for more extensive discussion of the negative impact of clonal expansions on immune function in the aged.

While CD8 clonal expansions can have deleterious effects on immune function, we postulate that perhaps not all clonal expansions are deleterious to health in the elderly. This may be particularly true in the case of clonal expansions specific for HCMV, a chronic virus infection that can cause disease, especially in the immune-suppressed. Although inflated responses to HCMV have often been viewed as a negative indication for health in the elderly (e.g., [102]), this is not to say that these HCMV-specific expansions are not playing some role in containing HCMV infection. Based on this concept, it will be important to test what consequence depletion of CD8 clonal expansions has in animal models of chronic infection (e.g., individuals which develop comparable clonal expansions in response to either mouse or primate cytomegalovirus infection) before further considering the possibility of therapeutic intervention to remove CD8 clonal expansions in the elderly.

One other important consideration when contemplating therapeutic interventions to remove CD8 clonal expansions in the aged is the effect that this depletion might have on subsequent T-cell homeostasis. For example, depletion of a clonal expansion that occupies 50% of the CD8 T-cell pool would likely create a transient state of lymphopenia, which may, in turn, provoke the subsequent development of another clonal expansion.

5.4   CD8 Clonal Expansions are Nonmalignant

Given the growth advantage of CD8 clonal expansions relative to other CD8 T-cells, one curious feature of clonal expansions is that they are nonmalignant. This conclusion is based on the following observations: i) individuals with CD8 clonal expansions do not have an increase in the total number of CD8 T-cells [89] and ii) clonal expansions can exist for an extended period of time without progressing to malignancy (up to 4 years in mice, up to 9 years in humans) (Ku, personal communication) [20]. Given the common occurrence of CD8 clonal expansions, the incidence of human tumors with a CD8 memory phenotype is extremely low [99]. It is important to note that individuals diagnosed with CD8 T-cell lymphomas not only have a clonal expansion of T-cells, but are also characterized by additional abnormalities (including elevated lymphocyte counts and frequent neutropenia) [110, 137]. At this time, there is no known relationship between those individuals with CD8 clonal expansions and those individuals who are diagnosed with T-cell lymphomas.

Despite the similarities of clonal expansions to tumors in terms of their clonality and competitive advantage relative to their neighbors, CD8 clonal expansions are clearly still subject to certain constraints. For example, CD8 clonal expansions do not increase in number above the normal number of CD8 T-cells contained within an individual [89]. Although the precise mechanisms that limit the growth of clonal expansions remain to be elucidated, we propose that a major factor constraining the growth of CD8 clonal expansions is availability for cytokines and other extracellular growth factors.

6   CD8 Clonal Expansions Have an Increased Rate of Proliferation

Many CD8 clonal expansions occupy a sizable fraction of the CD8 T-cell pool. The ability of expansions to out-compete other CD8 T-cells could result from either an increased rate of proliferation or from a decreased rate of attrition (e.g., apoptosis). Currently, there are no published reports rigorously examining the survival properties of CD8 clonal expansions relative to normal CD8 memory T-cells. In contrast, there are clear data regarding the rate of proliferation of CD8 clonal expansions. Initial evidence regarding the rate of proliferation of CD8 clonal expansions came from analysis of the rate of dilution of carboxyfluorescein diacetate succinimidyl ester (CFSE), a fluorescent dye that can be used to track the number of cell divisions of CD8 T-cells. Based on transfer of CD8 clonal expansions into syngeneic, nonirradiated recipients, CD8 clonal expansions had a modest increase in their rate of proliferation (dividing once every 15 days, compared with polyclonal aged CD8 memory T-cells which divided once every 22 days) [70]. Significantly, many CD8 clonal expansions were also capable of growing upon adoptive transfer into mice lacking beta-2 microglobulin and therefore having little to no MHC Class I ligands for the T-cell receptor [70]. This property is consistent with the previous observation that CD8 memory T-cells can achieve long-term antigen-independent proliferation [94]. In sum, these data indicate that clonal expansions have an increased rate of proliferation and that this proliferation is not dependent on active engagement between TCR and MHC.

In this initial study, manipulating cytokine signals also influenced the proliferation of CD8 clonal expansions. Clonal expansions had diminished proliferation when the beta-chain of the IL-2 and IL-15 receptors was blocked by antibody treatment, suggesting that clones were likely growing in response to IL-15 (a common proliferative cue for CD8 memory T-cells) [70]. In contrast, CD8 clonal expansions had accelerated proliferation when mice were treated with IL-2 antibodies [70], a condition now known to create a strong mitogenic signal for CD8 memory T-cells [13].

Since this initial analysis, an additional study examined how CD8 clonal expansions respond to conditions of lymphopenia, a condition known to increase the proliferative rate of CD8 T-cells and to promote the generation of LIP CD8 memory T-cells (discussed above). While these studies showed that CD8 clonal expansions have an increased rate of proliferation in a nonirradiated recipient relative to other CD8 T-cells, they also revealed a surprising finding: CD8 clonal expansions have a relatively constant rate of proliferation that is not accelerated in conditions of lymphopenia [91]. In this study, CD8 clonal expansions were also identified to have a modest increase in the expression of both the IL-7Rα and IL-2Rβ cytokine receptors [91]. Based on these studies, Nikolich-Zugich and colleagues proposed that CD8 clonal expansions have an altered capacity to respond to the homeostatic cues normally perceived by a CD8 T-cell [91]. On one hand, clones do not stop dividing in a full lymphoid compartment. On the other hand, clones do not accelerate their division in a lymphopenic setting. At this time, it is unclear why clonal expansions are capable of accelerating their proliferation in response to strong mitogenic IL-2 signals [70], but do not accelerate their proliferation in lymphopenic settings [91]. One potential explanation for this apparent discrepancy may be that the proliferative cues perceived in a lymphopenic environment are less potent than that received by hyperstimulation with IL-2, IL-2 antibody complexes.

Based on the above data, clonal expansions do not simply have a higher rate of proliferation than other CD8 T-cells, but instead are capable of prolonged, continuous proliferation with little apparent regulation by the normal cues perceived by neighboring CD8 T-cells. One perplexing issue about these observations is that the state of lymphopenia is associated with an increased rate of development of clonal expansions, yet clonal expansions do not seem to have a proliferative advantage in the context of lymphopenia. One possible resolution for this paradox might be that lymphopenia promotes the initiation but not the maintenance of CD8 clonal expansions. For further discussion of this topic, please see chapter by Nikolich-Zugich.

7 The Spectrum of CD8 Clonal Expansions

7.1 Heterogeneous Characteristics of CD8 Clonal Expansions

One of the challenges in understanding CD8 clonal expansions in both mice and humans is the observation that distinct clonal expansions have variable properties. While heterogeneity between clonal expansions might be expected in humans, a genetically diverse population with significant differences in infection history, heterogeneity has also been observed between clonal expansions in genetically identical, inbred mice housed together [18]. To date, heterogeneity between clonal expansions has been best characterized in CD8 clonal expansions in mice [18], as described below.

i) *Stability of clones in vivo:* CD8 clonal expansions have widely discrepant stabilities in vivo. Some CD8 clonal expansions appear to be extremely stable and can continue to grow over a 4-year period, as revealed by serial adoptive transfer studies in mice (Ku, personal communication). In contrast, other CD8 clonal expansions are very unstable and disappear within 2 months of their initial identification [18, 77].

ii) *Response to stimulation in vitro:* CD8 clonal expansions in mice are also variable in their response to stimulation in vitro [18]. For example, some CD8 clonal expansions have a normal proliferative response to polyclonal stimulation in vitro (e.g., following culture with the concanavalin A or phorbol 12-myristate 13-acetate (PMA) and ionomycin). In contrast, other CD8 clonal expansions have an impaired capacity to proliferate and/or survive following similar stimulation conditions, becoming less abundant in bulk cultures following stimulation.

Despite these differences between CD8 clonal expansions, CD8 clonal expansions are uniformly considered to be CD8 memory T-cells, as defined by cell surface markers (in the mouse, CD44^{high} as well as IL-7Rα^{high}IL-2Rβ^{high}) [70, 91]. Many CD8 clonal expansions belong to the T_{CM} subset of CD8 memory T-cells [91]. While our recent data (discussed below) have revealed additional heterogeneity in cell surface phenotypes, to date all clonal expansions are CD44^{high}, consistent with a CD8 memory phenotype in the mouse.

7.2 A New Method to Subclassify CD8 Clonal Expansions in Mice

Given the above heterogeneity between CD8 clonal expansions, we have been interested in identifying methods to subclassify clonal expansions in mice. To do this, we initially focused our efforts on microarray analysis in which we analyzed the transcriptional profile of multiple, independent clonal expansions in mice.

Through this analysis, we identified integrin α4 (also known as very late antigen-4 (VLA-4) or CD49d) as a candidate marker that was differentially expressed in distinct types of clonal expansions. [25] Next, we analyzed the expression of integrin α4 on a large number of age-associated CD8 clonal expansions. This analysis identified that there were two major types of clonal expansions: those expressing high levels of integrin α4 and those expressing low levels of integrin α4.

Based on the differential expression of integrin α4 between different types of clones, we analyzed the properties of integrin α4^{high} and integrin α4^{low} clones. There were clear differences between these two types of clonal expansions [25]. First, these clonal expansions were identified in mice of different ages, with integrin α4^{high} clones identified predominantly in mice 16–20 months of age, while integrin α4^{low} clones were found predominantly in mice 20–36 months of age. Notably, a longitudinal analysis of these two types of clonal expansions revealed that there was no interconversion between these integrin α4 phenotypes. Second, these clones differed in their in vivo growth dynamics, with integrin α4^{high} clones frequently decreasing in size over a 2-month interval, in contrast to integrin α4^{low} clones that rarely decreased in size. Third, integrin α4^{high} clones had an impaired response to in vitro stimulation with PMA and ionomycin, becoming less abundant following stimulation. Integrin α4^{low} clones had no advantage or disadvantage following this same stimulation. Fourth, integrin α4^{high} and integrin α4^{low} clones had differential localization in vivo. Integrin α4^{high} clones were absent from peripheral lymph nodes, while integrin α4^{low} clones were absent from Peyer's patches. Fifth, integrin α4^{high} clones had evidence of chronic TCR stimulation, as revealed by decreased expression of cytokine receptors (both IL-7Rα and IL-2Rβ) and expression of various inhibitory receptors (PD-1 and killer cell lectin-like receptor G1, KLRG1). In sum, integrin α4^{high} clonal expansions had many characteristics of chronic antigen stimulation, whereas integrin α4^{low} clonal expansions appeared similar to an antigen-independent CD8 memory T-cell [25].

The identification of integrin α4-defined clonal expansions in mice is significant for multiple reasons. First, it provides a molecular marker to distinguish between two types of clonal expansions with highly divergent properties. Second, it provides an explanation for the previous dichotomy observed in the properties of clonal expansions [18, 77]. Third, it indicates that these types of clonal expansions may have arisen from very different origins. In particular, we hypothesize that integrin α4^{high} clones may arise due to an inappropriate response against self-antigens, which would result in chronic antigenic stimulation. It is worth noting that while both types of clonal expansions meet the current definition of CD8 clonal expansions, integrin α4^{low} clones appear to be the subtype of expansion that is most capable of long-term growth.

8 Models Regarding the Development and Properties of CD8 Clonal Expansions

8.1 Models to Understand the Development and Properties of Clonal Expansions

Given the heterogeneity between distinct clonal expansions and the apparent differences in clonal expansions between mice and humans (discussed in further detail in [24]), it is challenging to determine whether there are common mechanisms underlying divergent types of CD8 clonal expansions. Here we discuss three conceptual models for the development of CD8 clonal expansions and discuss basic tenants of each model.

Model 1: Clonal expansions arise from natural variation in the rate of proliferation of memory T-cells. Clonal expansions are simply those memory T-cells with the fastest rate of proliferation.

Basic details of this model: This model is based on the principle that there is a range of proliferative rates of memory T-cells present in a normal individual. While the vast majority of cells will proliferate at a very similar rate, there inevitably will be some cells that proliferate slightly faster or slower. At first inspection, this idea is particularly appealing: CD8 clonal expansions only have a modest increase in their rate of proliferation (dividing about once every 15 days compared to CD8 MP T-cells which divide about once every 22 days) [70].

Predictions of this model: CD8 clonal expansions will be identical to CD8 memory T-cells in all parameters, with only a modest acceleration in their rate of proliferation.

Evidence against this model: The major observation that is inconsistent with this model is that CD8 clonal expansions have an altered capacity to respond to proliferative cues typically perceived by lymphocytes in a lymphopenic environment [88]. This property of clones is clearly different than a normal CD8 memory T-cell, and these data indicate that clones are not simply derived from the fastest cell in the

CD8 memory T-cell pool. Despite this, it is worth noting that subtle variations in the expression level of cytokines receptors or inhibitory proteins may still play some role in the basic biology of CD8 clonal expansions.

Model 2: Clonal expansions arise from common alterations to growth regulatory pathways. The variable properties of clonal expansions reflect differences in TCR reactivity and antigen persistence.

Basic details of this model: This model proposes that clonal expansions arise from a discrete set of changes in the expression of growth regulatory proteins (e.g. cell cycle inhibitory proteins or cytokine receptors) (Fig. 3a). These alterations in mRNA or protein expression and/or function may arise to due genetic mutations (i.e., creating mutant gene products) or due to perturbations in epigenetic regulation (e.g., DNA methylation or chromatin alterations that alter transcriptional expression of growth regulatory genes).

Predictions of this model: A basic prediction of this model is that clonal expansions will arise from a common fate, and possess common changes in growth regulatory pathways (e.g., cytokine signaling). Moreover, clonal expansions with divergent biological properties should have similar mRNA and protein expression profiles (discussed further below).

Evidence against this model: Currently, there are two pieces of evidence against this model. The first is that the two major types of clonal expansions in mice (integrin $\alpha 4^{high}$ and integrin $\alpha 4^{low}$) have widely divergent properties, suggesting that they may arise from different age-associated alterations. Integrin $\alpha 4^{high}$ clones have many characteristics consistent with T-cells actively responding against chronic (potentially self) antigen. If these cells are self-reactive, integrin $\alpha 4^{high}$ clones may arise from age-associated alterations in central or peripheral T-cell tolerance. In contrast, integrin $\alpha 4^{low}$ clones do not possess such characteristics, suggesting that they may arise from a distinct mechanism (such as epigenetic inactivation of a growth regulatory gene). The second piece of evidence against this model is microarray analysis, in which integrin $\alpha 4^{high}$ and integrin $\alpha 4^{low}$ clonal expansions appear to have different gene expression profiles (Clambey et al. manuscript in submission). The interpretation of this latter point, however, has caveats (discussed below), and will require analysis of a larger number of integrin $\alpha 4$-defined clonal expansions.

Model 3 : Clonal expansions arise from multiple, distinct age-associated alterations.

Basic details of this model: In contrast to model 2 (above), this model proposes that clonal expansions reflect a common physiological outcome (i.e. selective outgrowth of a single CD8 T-cell), but that these clones arise due to different age-associated alterations (Fig. 3b). As such, different types of clonal expansions have little in common other than their overabundance in the CD8 T-cell pool.

Predictions of this model: In contrast to model 2, a prediction of this model is that different types of CD8 clonal expansions (with different biological properties) will have different gene and protein expression profiles. While different types of clones will have some common expression profiles since they are both CD8 memory T-cells, the underlying molecular changes and growth requirements for these clones will differ. Based on the properties of integrin $\alpha 4^{high}$ and integrin $\alpha 4^{low}$ clones detailed above, integrin $\alpha 4^{high}$ clones would depend on ongoing antigen/

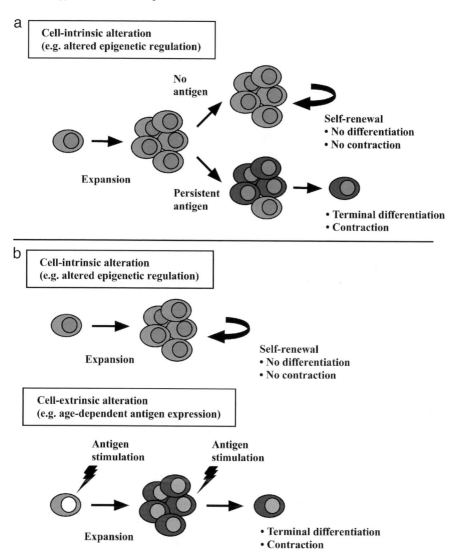

Fig. 3 Models for the development and phenotype of CD8 clonal expansions

In panel a, model 2 (see text for details) proposes that CD8 clonal expansions result from a common set of changes in growth regulatory genes (indicated here by a red nucleus, denoting a common transcriptional alteration). Following their initial expansion, the presence or absence of antigen then significantly influences the properties and dynamics of the clonal expansion. Clones that recognize persistent antigen undergo further differentiation (indicated by a blue cytoplasm). In panel b, model 3 (see text for details) proposes that CD8 clonal expansions result from distinct age-associated changes. While these distinct changes both result in a CD8 clonal expansion, the underlying factors that promote these expansions are completely distinct (indicated by either a red nucleus representing a transcriptional alteration or a blue cytoplasm representing antigen driven stimulation). See text for further discussion of each model.

TCR engagement for their proliferative advantage, whereas integrin $\alpha 4^{low}$ clones would not.

Evidence against this model: Currently there is no direct evidence that contradicts this model.

One important limitation to the above models and predictions is our current inability to distinguish between changes in gene expression profiles that promote the growth of CD8 clonal expansions, compared to changes in gene expression profiles that reflect TCR specificity and the presence or absence of antigen. For example, a clonal expansion responding to a persistent antigen will have major alterations in gene expression (e.g., in the expression of inhibitory receptors such as PD-1). As such, it may be very difficult to discriminate between the influence of TCR and antigen versus the underlying mechanism that creates a clonal expansion. The ability to resolve these issues will only become possible when CD8 clonal expansions can be reliably generated with defined antigen specificities, and such clones can be analyzed in the context of varying conditions of antigen persistence. Future insights into the molecular bases of clonal expansions will be significantly advanced through gain- and loss-of-function studies in both CD8 clonal expansions and CD8 memory T-cells.

8.2   The Probability of Becoming a Clonal Expansion

With regard to models 2 and 3, both models predict that certain stochastic events would change the growth properties of a CD8 memory T-cell. We postulate that this growth-promoting event is a relatively rare event. This statement is based on the observation that not all mice appear to develop CD8 clonal expansions, and mice that do develop clonal expansions frequently only have one clone (Clambey et al.unpublished data). Given that each mouse has more than 1×10^7 CD8 T-cells, the frequency of this growth-promoting event in an aging immune-competent mouse (e.g., C57BL/6J mouse) is probably not more frequent than 1 in 10^7 cells. We predict that the likelihood that a particular CD8 T-cell specificity becomes a clonal expansion would be influenced by the overall abundance of that antigen specificity within the CD8 T-cell pool (further discussed in [24]).

It is interesting to note that lymphopenic mice, which have fewer CD8 T-cells, have an accelerated rate of clonal expansion development, as well as a higher overall incidence of clones [90]. Based on these data, the frequency of the growth-promoting event is increased in conditions of lymphopenia. Since lymphopenic mice are characterized by a higher number of proliferating CD8 T-cells [90], we hypothesize that the probability that a growth-promoting event occurs is directly related to the number of cell divisions that the CD8 T-cell has undergone. Mechanistically, this hypothesis is based on the fact that with each cell division, appropriate epigenetic programming must be perpetuated from the mother to the daughter cells. If there is a certain rate of failure for this event to occur, the more rounds of cell division, the more likely it is that any cell would undergo this growth-promoting event.

8.3 When Do Clonal Expansions Initially Emerge?

In mice, CD8 clonal expansions are not detected until mice are approximately 16 months of age [18]. Although clonal expansions become apparent at this age, it is likely that there is a period during which an emerging clonal expansion remains below the limit of detection within the T-cell repertoire. The events within the early phase of clonal expansions are completely unknown, and at this point, strictly hypothetical. Nonetheless, it is worth considering how long it might take for a clonal expansion to emerge and dominate the CD8 T-cell pool.

CD8 clonal expansions divide once every 15 days, in contrast to polyclonal CD8 MP T-cells that divide once every 22 days [70]. If this was the only advantage that a CD8 clonal expansion had relative to other CD8 T-cells, how long would it take for a clonal expansion to outcompete its neighbors?

In an attempt to approximate the growth history of a clonal expansion, we have used a very simple model to compare the growth dynamics of a clonal expansion relative to a pool of CD8 MP T-cells. In this model, we made the following assumptions:

i) a clonal expansion results from a single CD8 memory T-cell achieving a growth advantage relative to its neighbor
ii) the only advantage that a clonal expansion has relative to other CD8 memory T-cells is its slightly higher rate of proliferation (dividing once every 15 days, instead of once every 22 days)
iii) the relative size of the proliferating, polyclonal CD8 MP T-cell pool contains approximately 10×10^6 cells (Clambey et al. unpublished data) [11, 47, 89] and
iv) both the clonal expansion and the CD8 MP pool have an infinite growth capacity.

While this model is clearly too simplistic (e.g. it does not take into consideration rate of death nor the changing abundance of naïve T-cells with age), it does provide a very useful piece of information (Fig. 4). If a clone only has this subtle growth advantage relative to a large CD8 MP T-cell pool, it would take 855 days (approximately 28.5 months) for the clone to reach just 5% (a small clonal expansion) of the size of the CD8 MP T-cell pool (Fig. 4). However, in mice, larger CD8 clonal expansions are already detectable by 16 months of age (~480 days). Based on this, clonal expansions are likely to have additional factors which promote their dominance within the CD8 T-cell pool.

One condition that could expedite the dominance of a clonal expansion within the CD8 T-cell pool is if there were a higher starting number of cells with a growth advantage. Since clonal expansions are clonal, however, cells with a growth advantage would need to come from a common precursor. One way in which this could happen is if a naïve T-cell achieves a growth-promoting event, and then encounters its antigen. Notably, this growth-promoting event does not need to change the antigen driven proliferation phase or the extent of death following the

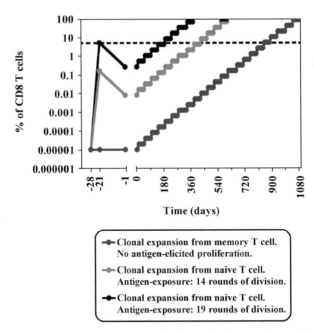

Fig. 4 A simple model to predict how long it takes for a clonal expansion to achieve dominance within the CD8 T-cell pool

Graph indicates the relative abundance of a clonal expansion (dividing once every 15 days) relative to the size of a pool of ten million proliferating CD8 MP T-cells (dividing once every 22 days). This model compares three different growth projections for an emerging clonal expansion: i) in blue, a single CD8 memory T-cell achieves a growth-promoting event that results in an increased rate of proliferation (expansion divides once every 15 days, compared to CD8 MP T-cells that divide once every 22 days) or ii) in black and in red, a single naïve T-cell achieves a growth-promoting event, followed by antigen stimulation. After antigen stimulation, the naïve T-cell goes through a normal phase of expansion and contraction. In contrast to the normal CD8 memory T-cell pool, however, the resulting CD8 memory T-cells all contain a common growth–promoting event that confers an increased rate of proliferation (clonal expansion divides once every 15 days, compared to CD8 MP T-cells that divide once every 22 days). For this latter model, growth projections include two different estimates for the extent of naïve T-cell proliferation following antigen stimulation (either 14 rounds of division indicated in red, or 19 rounds of division indicated in black). Antigen driven proliferation and contraction (95% of cells dying by apoptosis) are indicated from day—28 to day—1. Dashed line indicates 5% of the CD8 T-cell pool, which is a conservative estimate for the detection of a CD8 clonal expansion. Each data point indicates the relative abundance of the clonal expansion relative to the CD8 MP T-cell pool with each round of division (occurring every 15 days). This model presumes that both the clonal expansion and the CD8 MP T-cell pool have an infinite growth capacity, and does not take into consideration rate of death for either population (this parameter is undefined for clonal expansions at this time). See text for further details of model.

peak of the response. Instead, this growth-promoting event simply needs to increase the basal rate of proliferation of the resulting CD8 memory T-cells (so that the resulting cells divide once every 15 days). The end-result of this outcome would be that there would be a higher number of memory cells with a growth advantage. This, in turn, dramatically alters the time required for the clonal expansion to dominate the CD8 T-cell pool. By using a conservative estimate for how many times a naïve T-cell proliferates following an acute antigen exposure (14 rounds of division [3, 10, 84]), a clonal expansion can achieve 5% of the CD8 T-cell pool within 435 days (14.5 months), and occupy more than 30% of the repertoire within 535 days (17.5 months) (Fig. 4, red line). If a naïve T-cell undergoes 19 rounds of division (a recent estimate for naïve T-cell proliferation during acute infection [3]), it would only take 195 days (6.5 months) to achieve 5% of the CD8 T-cell pool, coming to occupy >30% of the repertoire within 285 days (9.5 months).

The bottom line from this overly simplistic model is that although a subtle increase in proliferation may contribute to the development of clonal expansions, there are likely to be other contributing factors. For example, changes in the rate of death could significantly influence the ability of clones to compete with other CD8 T-cells; in addition, if a clone ever goes through a proliferative burst (e.g., following antigen engagement) this could also accelerate the development of clonal expansions. Future reductionist studies will allow a more careful dissection of the time required for a CD8 T-cell to become a clonal expansion.

9 Factors that Influence the Properties of CD8 Clonal Expansions

Regardless of the precise mechanisms that are behind the development of clonal expansions, the phenotype and properties of individual clones are certain to be influenced by multiple factors, most importantly the interaction between the TCR and antigen.

9.1 The Role of Antigen Persistence

It is increasingly clear that the persistence of antigen significantly impacts the phenotype and dynamics of the CD8 T-cell. While CD8 T-cells only require a very brief period of antigen engagement of the T-cell receptor to become activated [53, 128, 139], the duration and context of antigen presentation can significantly influence the capabilities of the resulting CD8 T-cell. The crippling effects of chronic antigen exposure can be best observed in certain models of chronic infection, where CD8 T-cells never differentiate to a state in which they can survive in the absence of antigen [120, 131].

With regard to CD8 clonal expansions, clonal expansions encountering chronic antigen would be predicted to have significantly different cell surface phenotypes (Fig. 3). These changes in cell surface phenotype would likely influence the expression of cytokine receptors for IL-7 and IL-15 (possibly influencing IL-7Rα and IL-2Rβ), as well as result in the upregulation of various inhibitory receptors (such as PD-1 and KLRG1, which are both receptors whose expression is associated with chronically stimulated T-cells [6, 126]). In addition, these clonal expansions would be predicted to disappear if antigen ultimately disappears.

Although chronic antigen exposure would most significantly impact the phenotype and properties of clonal expansions, initial encounter of antigen could also play a more modest effect on the resulting phenotype, for example influencing the fate of the resulting CD8 memory T-cell to become a T_{CM} or a T_{EM} cell.

9.2   The Impact of Initial Conditions of Stimulation

As discussed above, a naïve CD8 T-cell can differentiate into a CD8 memory T-cell by at least two distinct paths: i) engagement of the TCR by its appropriate antigen, resulting in the full activation of the T-cell, followed by subsequent proliferation, contraction and differentiation (referred to as antigen-elicited memory) or ii) lymphopenic conditions in which a naïve CD8 T-cell is capable of undergoing proliferation in the absence of full activation (referred to as LIP memory). While the precise characteristics of these two types of memory cells is a subject of ongoing investigation, it is worth noting that there are surprisingly few differences in the properties of these two types of memory cells. Careful microarray analysis of these two types of memory cells has revealed very similar transcriptional profiles [36], and LIP memory cells can mediate immunological protection, a hallmark of memory T-cells [39]. Although no obvious differences between these two types of memory cells have been identified to date, the very different conditions from which they originate make it highly unlikely that they are absolutely identical.

With regard to CD8 clonal expansions, it appears that CD8 clonal expansions may become CD8 memory T-cells through either an antigen-elicited or LIP mechanism. This conclusion is based on the following data:

i) in mice, conditions of lymphopenia are associated with the accelerated development of clonal expansions indicating that LIP memory cells can become CD8 clonal expansions [90]
ii) mice infected with certain infections such as Sendaivirus, influenza, Herpes simplex virus or LCMV can occasionally develop very large antigen-specific clonal expansions in aged mice ([29, 74], Zajac, personal communication), indicating that antigen-elicited memory cells can become CD8 clonal expansions (see chapters by Woodland and Nikolich-Zugich for further discussion),
iii) humans infected with HCMV can develop HCMV-specific clonal expansions [63, 98].

Given that both LIP and antigen-elicited memory CD8 T-cells can become CD8 clonal expansions, it is worth noting that the relative contribution of these two types of memory cells differs between SPF mice and humans. For example, in SPF mice that are typically used to study clonal expansions in mice, the majority of clonal expansions almost certainly represent LIP memory T-cells given the relative paucity of antigen exposure these animals experience. In contrast, humans have an extremely high rate of antigen exposure, with relatively few memory CD8 T-cells likely to arise from lympho-penia-induced proliferation. Based on this difference, we postulate that the majority of human clonal expansions will recognize a variety of antigens primarily from infectious agents, whereas the majority of clonal expansions in mice will recognize a wide variety of antigens without a bias for infectious agent antigens. Despite this difference, expo-sure of mice to a variety of infections should be capable of recapitulating the diversity of antigen-elicited clonal expansions that we postulate to occur in humans.

10 Major Questions about CD8 Clonal Expansions

CD8 clonal expansions are a common age-associated perturbation in the immune system. The goal in studying this phenomenon is that it will reveal previously unap-preciated effects of the aging environment on CD8 memory T-cell homeostasis, and identify basic cellular and molecular factors that also regulate CD8 memory T-cells in healthy, young individuals. While there is increasing information about this phe-nomenon, there are still many unanswered questions:

1. How does the aging environment influence the development of CD8 clonal expansions?
2. What are the molecular alterations that contribute to increased growth of CD8 clonal expansions?
3. What factors constrain the growth of CD8 clonal expansions?
4. What is the underlying cause for the heterogeneous phenotype of CD8 clonal expansions?
5. Can every subset of CD8 memory T-cell become a clonal expansion?

We anticipate that research in the upcoming years will shed light on many of these questions, providing new insights into how the aging immune system influ-ences the dynamics of CD8 memory T-cell homeostasis.

Acknowledgments   We thank Drs. Linda van Dyk and David Woodland for insightful discus-sion on the underlying forces that drive development of clonal expansions, Dr. Fred Peyerl for discussion on theoretical growth dynamics of clonal expansions, Drs. Megan MacLeod and Linda van Dyk for helpful comments on the manuscript, and Drs. Chia-Chi Ku, David Woodland and Allan Zajac for personal communication of unpublished data. This work was supported by USPHS grants AI-22295 and AI-52225.

References

1. Alexander WS, Hilton DJ (2004) The role of suppressors of cytokine signaling (SOCS) pro-teins in regulation of the immune response. Annu Rev Immunol 22:503–529
2. Appay V, Dunbar PR, Callan M, Klenerman P, Gillespie GM, Papagno L, Ogg GS, King A, Lechner F, Spina CA, Little S, Havlir DV, Richman DD, Gruener N, Pape G, Waters A, Eas terbrook P, Salio M, Cerundolo V, McMichael AJ, Rowland-Jones SL (2002) Memory CD8+ T cells vary in differentiation phenotype in different persistent virus infections. Nat Med 8:379–385

3. Badovinac VP, Haring JS, Harty JT (2007) Initial T cell receptor transgenic cell precursor frequency dictates critical aspects of the CD8(+) T cell response to infection. Immunity 26:827–841

4. Badovinac VP, Messingham KA, Griffith TS, Harty JT (2006) TRAIL deficiency delays, but does not prevent, erosion in the quality of "helpless" memory CD8 T cells. J Immunol 177:999–1006.

5. Badovinac VP, Messingham KA, Jabbari A, Haring JS, Harty JT (2005) Accelerated CD8+ T-cell memory and prime-boost response after dendritic-cell vaccination. Nat Med 11:748–756

6. Barber DL, Wherry EJ, Masopust D, Zhu B, Allison JP, Sharpe AH, Freeman GJ, Ahmed R (2006) Restoring function in exhausted CD8 T cells during chronic viral infection. Nature 439:682–687

7. Becker TC, Wherry EJ, Boone D, Murali-Krishna K, Antia R, Ma A, Ahmed R (2002) Interleukin 15 is required for proliferative renewal of virus-specific memory CD8 T cells. J Exp Med 195:1541–1548

8. Bevan MJ (2004) Helping the CD8(+) T-cell response. Nat Rev Immunol 4:595–602

9. Bianchi T, S Gasser, A Trumpp, HR MacDonald (2006) c-Myc acts downstream of IL-15 in the regulation of memory CD8 T-cell homeostasis. Blood 107:3992–3999

10. Blattman JN, R Antia, DJ Sourdive, X Wang, SM Kaech, K Murali-Krishna, JD Altman, R Ahmed (2002) Estimating the precursor frequency of naive antigen-specific CD8 T cells. J Exp Med 195:657–664

11. Bourgeois C, G Kassiotis, B Stockinger (2005) A major role for memory CD4 T cells in the control of lymphopenia-induced proliferation of naive CD4 T cells. J Immunol 174:5316–5323

12. Boyman O, JH Cho, JT Tan, CD Surh, J Sprent (2006) A major histocompatibility complex class I-dependent subset of memory phenotype CD8+ cells. J Exp Med 203:1817–1825

13. Boyman O, M Kovar, MP Rubinstein, CD Surh, J Sprent (2006) Selective stimulation of T cell subsets with antibody-cytokine immune complexes. Science 311:1924–1927

14. Brooks DG, MJ Trifilo, KH Edelmann, L Teyton, DB McGavern, MB Oldstone (2006) Interleukin-10 determines viral clearance or persistence in vivo. Nat Med 12:1301–1309

15. Buentke E, A Mathiot, M Tolaini, J Di Santo, R Zamoyska, B Seddon (2006) Do CD8 effector cells need IL-7R expression to become resting memory cells? Blood 108:1949–1956

16. Burchill MA, CA Goetz, M Prlic, JJ O'Neil, IR Harmon, SJ Bensinger, LA Turka, P Brennan, SC Jameson, MA Farrar (2003) Distinct effects of STAT5 activation on CD4+ and CD8+ T cell homeostasis: development of CD4+CD25+ regulatory T cells versus CD8+ memory T cells. J Immunol 171:5853–5864

17. Burkett PR, R Koka, M Chien, S Chai, DL Boone, A Ma (2004) Coordinate expression and trans presentation of interleukin (IL)-15Ralpha and IL-15 supports natural killer cell and memory CD8+ T cell homeostasis. J Exp Med 200:825–834

18. Callahan JE, JW Kappler, P Marrack (1993) Unexpected expansions of CD8-bearing cells in old mice. J Immunol 151:6657–6669

19. Cannarile MA, NA Lind, R Rivera, AD Sheridan, KA Camfield, BB Wu, KP Cheung, Z Ding, AW Goldrath (2006) Transcriptional regulator Id2 mediates CD8+ T cell immunity. Nat Immunol 7:1317–1325

20. Chamberlain WD, MT Falta, BL Kotzin (2000) Functional subsets within clonally expanded CD8(+) memory T cells in elderly humans. Clin Immunol 94:160–172

21. Chandele A, SM Kaech (2005) Cutting edge: memory CD8 T cell maturation occurs independently of CD8alphaalpha. J Immunol 175:5619–23.

22. Cho BK, VP Rao, Q Ge, HN Eisen, J Chen (2000) Homeostasis-stimulated proliferation drives naive T cells to differentiate directly into memory T cells. J Exp Med 192:549–556

23. Chong MM, AL Cornish, RDarwiche, EG Stanley, JF Purton, DI Godfrey, DJ Hilton, R Starr, WS Alexander, TW Kay (2003) Suppressor of cytokine signaling-1 is a critical regulator of interleukin-7-dependent CD8+ T cell differentiation. Immunity 18:475–487

24. Clambey ET, LF van Dyk, JW Kappler, P Marrack (2005) Non-malignant clonal expansions of CD8 +memory T cells in aged individuals. Immunol Rev 205:170–189

25. Clambey ET, J White, JW Kappler, P Marrack (2008) Identification of two major types of age-associated CD8 clonal expansions with highly divergent properties. Proc Natl Acad Sci U S A 105:12997–13002

26. Cornish AL, MM Chong, GM Davey, R Darwiche, NA Nicola, DJ Hilton, TW Kay, R Starr, WS Alexander (2003) Suppressor of cytokine signaling-1 regulates signaling in response to interleukin-2 and other gamma c-dependent cytokines in peripheral T cells. J Biol Chem 278:22755–22761

27. Dubois S, J Mariner, TA Waldmann, Y Tagaya (2002) IL-15Ralpha recycles and presents IL-15 In trans to neighboring cells. Immunity 17:537–547

28. Ejrnaes M, CM Filippi, MM Martinic, EM Ling, LM Togher, S Crotty, MG von Herrath (2006) Resolution of a chronic viral infection after interleukin-10 receptor blockade. J Exp Med 203:2461–2472

29. Ely KH, M Ahmed, JE Kohlmeier, AD Roberts, ST Wittmer, MA Blackman, DL Woodland (2007) Antigen-specific CD8+ T cell clonal expansions develop from memory T cell pools established by acute respiratory virus infections. J Immunol 179:3535–3542

30. Ernst B, DS Lee, JM Chang, J Sprent, CD Surh (1999) The peptide ligands mediating positive selection in the thymus control T cell survival and homeostatic proliferation in the periphery. Immunity 11:173–181

31. Fann M, JM Godlove, M Catalfamo, WH Wood, 3rd FJ Chrest, N Chun, L Granger, R Wersto, K Madara, K Becker, PA Henkart, NP Weng (2006) Histone acetylation is associated with differential gene expression in the rapid and robust memory CD8(+) T-cell response. Blood 108:3363–3370

32. Fehniger TA, K Suzuki, A Ponnappan, JB VanDeusen, MA Cooper, SM Florea, AG Freud, M L Robinson, J Durbin, MA Caligiuri (2001) Fatal leukemia in interleukin 15 transgenic mice follows early expansions in natural killer and memory phenotype CD8+ T cells. J Exp Med 193:219–231

33. Fitzgerald JE, NS Ricalton, AC Meyer, SG West, H Kaplan, C Behrendt, BL Kotzin (1995) Analysis of clonal CD8+ T cell expansions in normal individuals and patients with rheumatoid arthritis. J Immunol 154:3538–3547

34. Goldrath AW, MJ Bevan (1999) Low-affinity ligands for the TCR drive proliferation of mature CD8+ T cells in lymphopenic hosts. Immunity 11:183–190

35. Goldrath AW, LY Bogatzki, MJ Bevan (2000) Naive T cells transiently acquire a memory-like phenotype during homeostasis-driven proliferation. J Exp Med 192:557–564

36. Goldrath AW, CJ Luckey, R Park, C Benoist, D Mathis (2004) The molecular program induced in T cells undergoing homeostatic proliferation. Proc Natl Acad Sci U S A 101:16885–16890

37. Goldrath AW, PV Sivakumar, M Glaccum, MK Kennedy, MJ Bevan, C Benoist, D Mathis, E A Butz (2002) Cytokine requirements for acute and Basal homeostatic proliferation of naive and memory CD8+ T cells. J Exp Med 195:1515–1522

38. Guarda G, M Hons, SF Soriano, AY Huang, R Polley, A Martin-Fontecha, JV Stein, RN Germain, A Lanzavecchia, F Sallusto (2007) L-selectin-negative CCR7(-) effector and memory CD8(+) T cells enter reactive lymph nodes and kill dendritic cells. Nat Immunol 8:743–752

39. Hamilton SE, MC Wolkers, SP Schoenberger, SC Jameson (2006) The generation of protective memory-like CD8+ T cells during homeostatic proliferation requires CD4+ T cells. Nat Immunol 7:475–481

40. Hand TW, M Morre, SM Kaech (2007) Expression of IL-7 receptor {alpha} is necessary but not sufficient for the formation of memory CD8 T cells during viral infection. Proc Natl Acad Sci U S A 104:11730–11735

41. Haring JS, VP Badovinac, JT Harty (2006) Inflaming the CD8+ T cell response. Immunity 25:19–29

42. Hendriks J, LA Gravestein, K Tesselaar, RA van Lier, TN Schumacher, J Borst (2000) CD27 is required for generation and long-term maintenance of T cell immunity. Nat Immunol 1:433–440

43. Hendriks J, Y Xiao, JW Rossen, KF Van Der Sluijs, K Sugamura, N Ishii, J Borst (2005) During viral infection of the respiratory tract, CD27, 4-1BB, and OX40 collectively determine formation of CD8+ memory T cells and their capacity for secondary expansion. J Immunol 175:1665–1676

44. Hikono H, JE Kohlmeier, S Takamura, ST Wittmer, AD Roberts, DL Woodland (2007) Activation phenotype, rather than central- or effector-memory phenotype, predicts the recall efficacy of memory CD8+ T cells. J Exp Med 204:1625–1636

45. Hislop AD, NH Gudgeon, MF Callan, C Fazou, H Hasegawa, M Salmon, AB Rickinson (2001) EBV-specific CD8+ T cell memory: relationships between epitope specificity, cell phenotype, and immediate effector function. J Immunol 167:2019–2029

46. Huster KM, V Busch, M Schiemann, K Linkemann, KM Kerksiek, H Wagner, DH Busch (2004) Selective expression of IL-7 receptor on memory T cells identifies early CD40L-dependent generation of distinct CD8+ memory T cell subsets. Proc Natl Acad Sci U S A 101:5610–5615

47. Ichii H, A Sakamoto, M Hatano, S Okada, H Toyama, S Taki, M Arima, Y Kuroda, T Tokuhisa (2002) Role for Bcl-6 in the generation and maintenance of memory CD8+ T cells. Nat Immunol 3:558–563

48. Ilangumaran S, S Ramanathan, J La Rose, P Poussier, R Rottapel (2003) Suppressor of cytokine signaling 1 regulates IL-15 receptor signaling in CD8+CD44high memory T lymphocytes. J Immunol 171:2435–2445

49. Intlekofer AM, N Takemoto, EJ Wherry, SA Longworth, JT Northrup, VR Palanivel, AC Mullen, CR Gasink, SM Kaech, JD Miller, L Gapin, K Ryan, AP Russ, T Lindsten, JS Orange, AW Goldrath, R Ahmed, SL Reiner (2005) Effector and memory CD8+ T cell fate coupled by T-bet and eomesodermin. Nat Immunol 6:1236–1244

50. Jacobsen M, AK Detjen, H Mueller, A Gutschmidt, S Leitner, U Wahn, K Magdorf, SH Kaufmann (2007) Clonal Expansion of CD8+ Effector T Cells in Childhood Tuberculosis. J Immunol 179:1331–1339

51. Jameson SC (2005) T cell homeostasis: keeping useful T cells alive and live T cells useful. Semin Immunol 17:231–237

52. Janssen EM, NM Droin, EE Lemmens, MJ Pinkoski, SJ Bensinger, BD Ehst, TS Griffith, DR Green, SP Schoenberger (2005) CD4+ T-cell help controls CD8+ T-cell memory via TRAIL-mediated activation-induced cell death. Nature 434:88–93

53. Kaech SM, R Ahmed (2001) Memory CD8+ T cell differentiation: initial antigen encounter triggers a developmental program in naive cells. Nat Immunol 2:415–422

54. Kaech SM, S Hemby, E Kersh, R Ahmed (2002) Molecular and functional profiling of memory CD8 T cell differentiation. Cell 111:837–851

55. Kaech SM, JT Tan, EJ Wherry, BT Konieczny, CD Surh, R Ahmed (2003) Selective expression of the interleukin 7 receptor identifies effector CD8 T cells that give rise to long-lived memory cells. Nat Immunol 4:1191–1198

56. Kaech SM, EJ Wherry, R Ahmed (2002) Effector and memory T-cell differentiation: implications for vaccine development. Nat Rev Immunol 2:251–262

57. Karrer U, S Sierro, M Wagner, A Oxenius, H Hengel, UH Koszinowski, RE Phillips, P Klenerman (2003) Memory inflation: continuous accumulation of antiviral CD8+ T cells over time. J Immunol 170:2022–2029

58. Kelly J, R Spolski, K Imada, J Bollenbacher, S Lee, WJ Leonard (2003) A role for Stat5 in CD8+ T cell homeostasis. J Immunol 170:210–217

59. Kemp RA, TJ Powell, DW Dwyer, RW Dutton (2004) Cutting edge: regulation of CD8+ T cell effector population size. J Immunol 173:2923–2927

60. Kersh EN (2006) Impaired memory CD8 T cell development in the absence of methyl-CpG-binding domain protein 2. J Immunol 177:3821–3826

61. Kersh EN, DR Fitzpatrick, K Murali-Krishna, J Shires, SH Speck, JM Boss, R Ahmed (2006) Rapid demethylation of the IFN-gamma gene occurs in memory but not naive CD8 T cells. J Immunol 176:4083–4093

62. Khan N, A Hislop, N Gudgeon, M Cobbold, R Khanna, L Nayak, AB Rickinson, PA Moss (2004) Herpesvirus-specific CD8 T cell immunity in old age: cytomegalovirus impairs the response to a coresident EBV infection. J Immunol 173:7481–489

63. Khan N, N Shariff, M Cobbold, R Bruton, JA Ainsworth, AJ Sinclair, L Nayak, PA Moss (2002) Cytomegalovirus seropositivity drives the CD8 T cell repertoire toward greater clonality in healthy elderly individuals. J Immunol 169:1984–1992

64. Kieper WC, SC Jameson (1999) Homeostatic expansion and phenotypic conversion of naive T cells in response to self peptide/MHC ligands. Proc Natl Acad Sci U S A 96:13306–133011

65. Kieper WC, JT Tan, B Bondi-Boyd, L Gapin, J Sprent, R Ceredig, CD Surh (2002) Overexpression of interleukin (IL)-7 leads to IL-15-independent generation of memory phenotype CD8+ T cells. J Exp Med 195:1533–1539

66. Klonowski KD, KJ Williams, AL Marzo, L Lefrancois (2006) Cutting edge: IL-7-independent regulation of IL-7 receptor alpha expression and memory CD8 T cell development. J Immunol 177:4247–4251

67. Kohlmeier JE, SC Miller, DL Woodland (2007) Cutting edge: Antigen is not required for the activation and maintenance of virus-specific memory CD8+ T cells in the lung airways. J Immunol 178:4721–4725

68. Kolumam GA, S Thomas, LJ Thompson, J Sprent, K Murali-Krishna (2005) Type I interferons act directly on CD8 T cells to allow clonal expansion and memory formation in response to viral infection. J Exp Med 202:637–650

69. Krieg C, O Boyman, YX Fu, J Kaye (2007) B and T lymphocyte attenuator regulates CD8+ T cell-intrinsic homeostasis and memory cell generation. Nat Immunol 8:162–171

70. Ku CC, J Kappler, P Marrack (2001) The growth of the very large CD8+ T cell clones in older mice is controlled by cytokines. J Immunol 166:2186–2193

71. Ku CC, B Kotzin, J Kappler, P Marrack (1997) CD8+ T-cell clones in old mice. Immunol Rev 160:139–144

72. Ku CC, M Murakami, A Sakamoto, J Kappler, P Marrack (2000) Control of homeostasis of CD8+ memory T cells by opposing cytokines. Science 288:675–678

73. Lacombe MH, MP Hardy, J Rooney, N Labrecque (2005) IL-7 receptor expression levels do not identify CD8+ memory T lymphocyte precursors following peptide immunization. J Immunol 175:4400–4407

74. Lang A, JD Brien, I Messaoudi, J Nikolich-Zugich (2008) Age-related dysregulation of CD8+ T cell memory specific for a persistent virus is independent of viral replication. J Immunol 180:4848–4857

75. Le Campion A, C Bourgeois, F Lambolez, B Martin, S Leaument, N Dautigny, C Tanchot, C Penit, B Lucas (2002) Naive T cells proliferate strongly in neonatal mice in response to self-peptide/self-MHC complexes. Proc Natl Acad Sci U S A 99:4538–4543

76. Lefrancois L, AL Marzo (2006) The descent of memory T-cell subsets. Nat Rev Immunol 6:618–623

77. LeMaoult J, I Messaoudi, JS Manavalan, H Potvin, D Nikolich-Zugich, R Dyall, P Szabo, ME Weksler, J Nikolich-Zugich (2000) Age-related dysregulation in CD8 T cell homeostasis: kinetics of a diversity loss. J Immunol 165:2367–2373

78. Liu N, T Phillips, M Zhang, Y Wang, JT Opferman, R Shah, PG Ashton-Rickardt (2004) Serine protease inhibitor 2A is a protective factor for memory T cell development. Nat Immunol 5:919–926

79. Lucas PJ, SJ Kim, CL Mackall, WG Telford, YW Chu, FT Hakim, RE Gress (2006) Dysregulation of IL-15-mediated T-cell homeostasis in TGF-beta dominant-negative receptor transgenic mice. Blood 108:2789–2795

80. Madakamutil LT, U Christen, CJ Lena, Y Wang-Zhu, A Attinger, M Sundarrajan, W Ellmeier, MG von Herrath, P Jensen, DR Littman, H Cheroutre (2004) CD8alphaalpha-mediated survival and differentiation of CD8 memory T cell precursors. Science 304:590–593

81. Manders PM, PJ Hunter, AI Telaranta, JM Carr, JL Marshall, M Carrasco, Y Murakami, M J Palmowski, V Cerundolo, S M Kaech, R Ahmed, DT Fearon (2005) BCL6b mediates the

enhanced magnitude of the secondary response of memory CD8+ T lymphocytes. Proc Natl Acad Sci U S A 102:7418–7425

82. Marzo AL, KD Klonowski, A Le Bon, P Borrow, DF Tough, L Lefrancois (2005) Initial T cell frequency dictates memory CD8+ T cell lineage commitment. Nat Immunol 6:793–799

83. Marzo AL, H Yagita, L Lefrancois (2007) Cutting edge: migration to nonlymphoid tissues results in functional conversion of central to effector memory CD8 T cells. J Immunol 179:36–40

84. Masopust D, K Murali-Krishna, R Ahmed (2007) Quantitating the magnitude of the lymphocytic choriomeningitis virus-specific CD8 T-cell response: it is even bigger than we thought. J Virol 81:2002–2011

85. Masopust D, V Vezys, AL Marzo, L Lefrancois (2001) Preferential localization of effector memory cells in nonlymphoid tissue. Science 291:2413–2417

86. Masopust D, V Vezys, EJ Wherry, DL Barber, R Ahmed (2006) Cutting edge: gut microenvironment promotes differentiation of a unique memory CD8 T cell population. J Immunol 176:2079–2083

87. McNally JM, CC Zarozinski, MY Lin, MA Brehm, HD Chen, RM Welsh (2001) Attrition of bystander CD8 T cells during virus-induced T-cell and interferon responses. J Virol 75:5965–5976

88. Mescher MF, JM Curtsinger, P Agarwal, KA Casey, M Gerner, CD Hammerbeck, F Popescu, Z Xiao (2006) Signals required for programming effector and memory development by CD8 +T cells. Immunol Rev 211:81–92

89. Messaoudi I, J Lemaoult, JA Guevara-Patino, B M Metzner, J Nikolich-Zugich (2004) Age-related CD8 T cell clonal expansions constrict CD8 T cell repertoire and have the potential to impair immune defense. J Exp Med 200:1347–1358

90. Messaoudi I, J Warner, D Nikolich-Zugich, M Fischer, J Nikolich-Zugich (2006) Molecular, cellular, and antigen requirements for development of age-associated T cell clonal expansions in vivo. J Immunol 176:301–308

91. Messaoudi I, J Warner, J Nikolich-Zugich (2006) Age-related CD8+ T cell clonal expansions express elevated levels of CD122 and CD127 and display defects in perceiving homeostatic signals. J Immunol 177:2784–2792

92. Min B, R McHugh, GD Sempowski, C Mackall, G Foucras, WE Paul (2003) Neonates support lymphopenia-induced proliferation. Immunity 18:131–140

93. Murali-Krishna K, R Ahmed (2000) Cutting edge: naive T cells masquerading as memory cells. J Immunol 165:1733–1737

94. Murali-Krishna K, LL Lau, S Sambhara, F Lemonnier, J Altman, R Ahmed (1999) Persistence of memory CD8 T cells in MHC class I-deficient mice. Science 286:1377–1381

95. Northrop JK, RM Thomas, AD Wells, H Shen (2006) Epigenetic remodeling of the IL-2 and IFN-gamma loci in memory CD8 T cells is influenced by CD4 T cells. J Immunol 177:1062–1069

96. Oehen S, K Brduscha-Riem (1999) Naive cytotoxic T lymphocytes spontaneously acquire effector function in lymphocytopenic recipients: A pitfall for T cell memory studies? Eur J Immunol 29:608–614

97. Ouyang Q, WM Wagner, S Walter, CA Muller, A Wikby, G Aubert, T Klatt, S Stevanovic, T Dodi, G Pawelec (2003) An age-related increase in the number of CD8+ T cells carrying receptors for an immunodominant Epstein-Barr virus (EBV) epitope is counteracted by a decreased frequency of their antigen-specific responsiveness. Mech Ageing Dev 124:477–485

98. Ouyang Q, WM Wagner, A Wikby, S Walter, G Aubert, AI Dodi, P Travers, G Pawelec (2003) Large numbers of dysfunctional CD8+ T lymphocytes bearing receptors for a single dominant CMV epitope in the very old. J Clin Immunol 23:247–257

99. Pandolfi F, TP Loughran Jr, G Starkebaum, T Chisesi, T Barbui, WC Chan, JC Brouet, G De Rossi, RW McKenna, F Salsano, et al (1990) Clinical course and prognosis of the lymphoproliferative disease of granular lymphocytes. A multicenter study. Cancer 65:341–348

100. Pannetier C, M Cochet, S Darche, A Casrouge, M Zoller, P Kourilsky (1993) The sizes of the CDR3 hypervariable regions of the murine T-cell receptor beta chains vary as a function of the recombined germ-line segments. Proc Natl Acad Sci U S A 90:4319–4323

101. Park JH, Q Yu, B Erman, JS Appelbaum, D Montoya-Durango, HL Grimes, A Singer (2004) Suppression of IL7Ralpha transcription by IL-7 and other prosurvival cytokines: a novel mechanism for maximizing IL-7-dependent T cell survival. Immunity 21:289–302

102. Pawelec G, A Akbar, C Caruso, R Solana, B Grubeck-Loebenstein, A Wikby (2005) Human immunosenescence: is it infectious? Immunol Rev 205:257–268

103. Pearce EL, AC Mullen, GA Martins, CM Krawczyk, AS Hutchins, VP Zediak, M Banica, CB DiCioccio, DA Gross, CA Mao, H Shen, N Cereb, SY Yang, T Lindsten, J Rossant, CA Hunter, SL Reiner (2003) Control of effector CD8+ T cell function by the transcription factor Eomesodermin. Science 302:1041–1043

104. Phillips T, JT Opferman, R Shah, N Liu, CJ Froelich, PG Ashton-Rickardt (2004) A role for the granzyme B inhibitor serine protease inhibitor 6 in CD8+ memory cell homeostasis. J Immunol 173:38013809

105. Posnett DN, R Sinha, S Kabak, C Russo (1994) Clonal populations of T cells in normal elderly humans: the T cell equivalent to "benign monoclonal gammapathy". J Exp Med 179:609–618

106. Pourgheysari B, N Khan, D Best, R Bruton, L Nayak, PA Moss (2007) The Cytomegalovirus-Specific CD4 +T-Cell Response Expands with Age and Markedly Alters the CD4+ T-Cell Repertoire. J Virol 81:7759–7765

107. Pulle G, M Vidric, TH Watts (2006) IL-15-dependent induction of 4-1BB promotes antigen-independent CD8 memory T cell survival. J Immunol 176:2739–2748

108. Ricalton NS, C Roberton, JM Norris, M Rewers, RF Hamman, BL Kotzin (1998) Prevalence of CD8+ T-cell expansions in relation to age in healthy individuals. J Gerontol A Biol Sci Med Sci 53:B196–B203

109. Romero P, A Zippelius, I Kurth, MJ Pittet, C Touvrey, EM Iancu, P Corthesy, E Devevre, D E Speiser, N Rufer (2007) Four functionally distinct populations of human effector-memory CD8+ T lymphocytes. J Immunol 178:4112–4119

110. Rose MG, N Berliner (2004) T-cell large granular lymphocyte leukemia and related disorders. Oncologist 9:247–258

111. Sabbagh L, LM Snell, TH Watts (2007) TNF family ligands define niches for T cell memory. Trends Immunol 28:333–339

112. Sabbagh L, CC Srokowski, G Pulle, LM Snell, BJ Sedgmen, Y Liu, EN Tsitsikov, TH Watts (2006) A critical role for TNF receptor-associated factor 1 and Bim down-regulation in CD8 memory T cell survival. Proc Natl Acad Sci U S A 103:18703–18708

113. Sallusto F, D Lenig, R Forster, M Lipp, A Lanzavecchia (1999) Two subsets of memory T lymphocytes with distinct homing potentials and effector functions. Nature 401:708–712

114. Sandau MM, KS Schluns, L Lefrancois, SC Jameson (2004) Cutting edge: transpresentation of IL-15 by bone marrow-derived cells necessitates expression of IL-15 and IL-15R alpha by the same cells. J Immunol 173:6537–6541

115. Saurwein-Teissl M, TL Lung, F Marx, C Gschosser, E Asch, I Blasko, W Parson, G Bock, D Schonitzer, E Trannoy, B Grubeck-Loebenstein (2002) Lack of antibody production following immunization in old age: association with CD8(+)CD28(-) T cell clonal expansions and an imbalance in the production of Th1 and Th2 cytokines. J Immunol 168:5893–5899

116. Schluns KS, WC Kieper, SC Jameson, L Lefrancois (2000) Interleukin-7 mediates the homeostasis of naive and memory CD8 T cells in vivo. Nat Immunol 1:426–432

117. Schluns KS, KD Klonowski, L Lefrancois (2004) Transregulation of memory CD8 T-cell proliferation by IL-15Ralpha+ bone marrow-derived cells. Blood 103:988–994

118. Schluns KS, K Williams, A Ma, XX Zheng, L Lefrancois (2002) Cutting edge: requirement for IL-15 in the generation of primary and memory antigen-specific CD8 T cells. J Immunol 168:4827–4831

119. Selin LK, MA Brehm, YN Naumov, M Cornberg, SK Kim, SC Clute, RM Welsh (2006) Memory of mice and men: CD8+ T-cell cross-reactivity and heterologous immunity. Immunol Rev 211:164–181

120. Shin H, SD Blackburn, JN Blattman, EJ Wherry (2007) Viral antigen and extensive division maintain virus-specific CD8 T cells during chronic infection. J Exp Med 204:941–949

121. Sierro S, R Rothkopf, P Klenerman (2005) Evolution of diverse antiviral CD8+ T cell populations after murine cytomegalovirus infection. Eur J Immunol 35:1113–1123

122. Stowe RP, EV Kozlova, DL Yetman, DM Walling, JS Goodwin, R Glaser (2007) Chronic herpesvirus reactivation occurs in aging. Exp Gerontol 42:563–570

123. Sun JC, SM Lehar, MJ Bevan (2006) Augmented IL-7 signaling during viral infection drives greater expansion of effector T cells but does not enhance memory. J Immunol 177:4458–4463

124. Surh CD, O Boyman, JF Purton, J Sprent (2006) Homeostasis of memory T cells. Immunol Rev 211:154–163

125. Tan JT, B Ernst, WC Kieper, E LeRoy, J Sprent, CD Surh (2002) Interleukin (IL)-15 and IL-7 jointly regulate homeostatic proliferation of memory phenotype CD8+ cells but are not required for memory phenotype CD4+ cells. J Exp Med 195:1523–1532

126. Thimme R, V Appay, M Koschella, E Panther, E Roth, AD Hislop, AB Rickinson, SL Rowland-Jones, HE Blum, H Pircher (2005) Increased expression of the NK cell receptor KLRG1 by virus-specific CD8 T cells during persistent antigen stimulation. J Virol 79:12112–12116

127. Trautmann L, M Rimbert, K Echasserieau, X Saulquin, B Neveu, J Dechanet, V Cerundolo, M Bonneville (2005) Selection of T cell clones expressing high-affinity public TCRs within Human cytomegalovirus-specific CD8 T cell responses. J Immunol 175:6123–6132

128. van Stipdonk MJ, EE Lemmens, SP Schoenberger (2001) Naive CTLs require a single brief period of antigenic stimulation for clonal expansion and differentiation. Nat Immunol 2:423–429

129. Vescovini R, A Telera, FF Fagnoni, C Biasini, MC Medici, P Valcavi, P di Pede, G Lucchini, L Zanlari, G Passeri, F Zanni, C Chezzi, C Franceschi, P Sansoni (2004) Different contribution of EBV and CMV infections in very long-term carriers to age-related alterations of CD8+ T cells. Exp Gerontol 39:1233–1243

130. Vezys V, D Masopust, CC Kemball, DL Barber, LA O'Mara, CP Larsen, TC Pearson, R Ahmed, AE Lukacher (2006) Continuous recruitment of naive T cells contributes to heterogeneity of antiviral CD8 T cells during persistent infection. J Exp Med 203:2263–2269

131. Wherry EJ, DL Barber, SM Kaech, JN Blattman, R Ahmed (2004) Antigen-independent memory CD8 T cells do not develop during chronic viral infection. Proc Natl Acad Sci US A 101:16004–16009

132. Wherry EJ, V Teichgraber, TC Becker, D Masopust, SM Kaech, R Antia, UH von Andrian, R Ahmed (2003) Lineage relationship and protective immunity of memory CD8 T cell subsets. Nat Immunol 4:225–234

133. Whitmire JK, B Eam, N Benning, JL Whitton (2007) Direct Interferon-{gamma} Signaling Dramatically Enhances CD4+ and CD8+ T Cell Memory. J Immunol 179:1190–1197

134. Whitmire JK, JT Tan, JL Whitton (2005) Interferon-gamma acts directly on CD8+ T cells to increase their abundance during virus infection. J Exp Med 201:1053–1059

135. Williams MA, MJ Bevan (2005) Cutting edge: a single MHC class Ia is sufficient for CD8 memory T cell differentiation. J Immunol 175:2066–2069

136. Williams MA, AJ Tyznik, MJ Bevan (2006) Interleukin-2 signals during priming are required for secondary expansion of CD8+ memory T cells. Nature 441:890–893

137. Wlodarski MW, AE Schade, JP Maciejewski (2006) T-large granular lymphocyte leukemia: current molecular concepts. Hematology 11:245–256

138. Wojciechowski S, MB Jordan, Y Zhu, J White, AJ Zajac, DA Hildeman (2006) Bim mediates apoptosis of CD127(lo) effector T cells and limits T cell memory. Eur J Immunol 36:1694–1706

139. Wong P, EG Pamer (2001) Cutting edge: antigen-independent CD8 T cell proliferation. J Immunol 166:5864–5868

140. Woodland DL, RJ Hogan, W Zhong (2001) Cellular immunity and memory to respiratory virus infections. Immunol Res 24:53–67
141. Zeng R, R Spolski, SE Finkelstein, S Oh, PE Kovanen, CS Hinrichs, CA Pise-Masison, MF Radonovich, JN Brady, NP Restifo, JA Berzofsky, WJ Leonard (2005) Synergy of IL-21 and IL-15 in regulating CD8+ T cell expansion and function. J Exp Med 201:139–148
142. Zhang X, S Sun, I Hwang, DF Tough, J Sprent (1998) Potent and selective stimulation of memory-phenotype CD8+ T cells in vivo by IL-15. Immunity 8:591–599
143. Zhong W, EL Reinherz (2005) CD8 alpha alpha homodimer expression and role in CD8 T cell memory generation during influenza virus A infection in mice. Eur J Immunol 35:3103–3110

Generation and Gene Expression of CD28⁻ CD8 T-cell in Human

Nan-ping Weng

Contents

Abstract: Increase of CD28⁻CD8 T-cells is one of the hallmarks of aging in the human immune system. Recent studies reveal the mechanism of generation and gene expression features of CD28⁻CD8 T-cells. Here, I summarize the recent progress focusing on the role of interleukin-15 (IL-15) in generation of CD28⁻CD8 T-cells and the identification of unique gene expression in CD28⁻CD8 T-cells by microarray gene expression analysis. These new findings enhance our understanding of the origin and function of the CD28⁻CD8 T-cells and may provide new means for clinical intervention.

1 Overview

CD8 T-cells play an essential role in the control of intracellular pathogens and cancerous growths for the host. The capability of the immune system, particularly CD8 T-cells, to protect the host declines with age [1, 2]. Accumulating evidence suggest that increase of CD28⁻CD8 T-cells in peripheral blood, a consistent age-associated change, account for the decline of CD8 T-cell mediated protection in the elderly [3–6]. However, the mechanisms underlying the age-associated changes in the immune system are complex and have just begun to be understood.

CD28, a membrane glycoprotein serving as a major co-stimulatory receptor for TCR mediated activation, plays multiple roles during T-cell activation from amplification of the TCR signal to induction of key cytokine production such as IL-2 to

N.-p. Weng (✉)
Laboratory of Immunology
National Institute on Aging, National Institutes of Health
251 Bayview Blvd, Suite 100, Baltimore, Maryland 21224
E-mail: wengn@mail.nih.gov

T. Fulop et al. (eds.), *Handbook on Immunosenescence*,
DOI 10.1007/ 978-1-4020-9062-2_17, © Springer Science+Business Media B.V. 2009

ensure a complete activation of T-cells after stimulation with antigen [7, 8]. Loss of CD28 expression has profound impact on the function of T-cells [9]. For example: (1) decreased production of IL-2 and IFN-γ in response to stimulation [10]; (2) resistance to apoptosis [11]; (3) reduced antigen repertoire diversity [5], and (4) associated with the lack of antibody production after immunization [12]. In addition, CD28⁻CD8 T-cells gain expression of some NK cell markers such as KIRs, CD16, CD56, KLRK1 (NKG2D), and retain or increase cytotoxicity with high expression of granzyme B and perforin [3].

Despite recent findings, the key issues related to CD28⁻CD8 T-cells remain to be elucidated. What are the causes of CD28⁻CD8 memory T-cells? How CD28⁻CD8 memory T-cells are maintained in vivo? What are the molecular features of CD28⁻CD8 memory T-cells compared to CD28⁺CD8 memory T-cells? In this chapter, I review the ontogeny of CD28⁻CD8 memory T-cells and summarize the genome-wide analysis of gene expression profiles of CD28⁻CD8 memory T-cells from peripheral blood. I will discuss the features of gene expression of CD28⁻CD8 memory T-cells as compared to their CD28⁺ counterparts.

2   Ontogeny of CD28⁻CD8 T-cells

In newborn human, all T-cells in the peripheral blood express CD28 on the cell surface [3, 13]. As CD28⁻ T-cells appear after birth and gradually increase with age [14], it has been suggested that CD28⁻CD8 T-cells are derived from CD28⁺CD8 T-cells. In the past decades, accumulating evidence support such a notion and the causes of CD28⁻CD8 T-cells are begun to be understood. There is overwhelming evidence indicating that repeated antigenic stimulation, mostly viral challenge, is one major cause of down-regulation of CD28 expression in T-cells [15, 16]. More recently, homeostatic cytokines such as IL-15 are also capable of induce down-regulation of CD28 expression in CD8 T-cells [17, 18].

2.1   *Antigenic Stimulation Induced CD28⁻CD8 T-cells*

An increasing number of publications shows that increase of CD28⁻CD8 T-cells are found in patients with a variety of viral infections including human immuno-deficiency virus (HIV) [19, 20], cytomegalovirus (CMV) [21, 22], Epstein-Barr virus (EBV) [23, 24], and Hepatitis C virus (HCV) [25, 26]. A common feature of these viral infections is relative persistent in the host and their interaction with immune system is often long lasting and results in varing degree of increase of effector T-cells, particularly in the CD8 T-cells. In the CD8 T-cell compartment, most of these responding CD8 T-cells are CD28⁻CD8 T-cells. The notion that these CD28⁻CD8 T-cells are derived from their precursor CD28⁺CD8 T-cells after viral stimulation is supported by several findings. (1) CD28+CD8 T-cells stimulated in vitro loss CD28 expression to become CD28⁻CD8 T-cells [4]. The loss of CD28 expression in these viral antigen primed CD8 T-cells appears stable, which is different from a transient down-regulation of CD28 expression on T-cells occurs after antigenic stimulation [27].

2.2   Cytokine Mediated Loss of CD28 Expression in CD8 T-cells

Recently, down-regulation of CD28 expression in T-cells by cytokines sharing the common γ-chain receptors has been reported [17, 18]. Although Borthwick showed that IL-2, IL-7, and IL-15 were capable of down-regulation of CD28 expression in T-cells after a short term culture, it is unclear if such down-regulation is transient or stable and what mechanisms are responsible for these cytokine-mediated down-regulations of CD28. In addition, TNF-α, a proinflammatory cytokine secreted by various types of cells including T-cells, has also been shown to down-regulate CD28 expression in CD4 T-cells [28]. However, the relationship of cytokines of the common γ-chain family and the TNF family in down-regulation of CD28 expression is not fully understood.

Loss of CD28 expression in memory CD8 T-cells under homeostatic cytokine IL-15 in a longer term of culture has been analyzed in more detail [18]. In general, CD28 expression was relatively stable during the initial few rounds of cell divisions under IL-15 but a significant loss of CD28 expression occurred after the fifth cell division. The average ratio of CD28⁻ to CD28+CD8 memory T-cells is 0.43 for the cells that had undergone fewer than five cell divisions while this CD28⁻ to CD28+CD8 memory T-cell ratio increases to 1.4 in cells undergone five or more cell divisions. Further analysis to determine if loss of CD28 expression was limited to the surface expression or occurred at the transcription level, we found that CD28 mRNA was absent in CD28⁻CD8 memory T-cells, suggesting that the down-regulation of CD28 expression under IL-15 is at transcriptional level. Finally, the loss of CD28 expression in CD8 memory T-cells is quite stable under IL-15-culture and there is no obvious re-gain of CD28 expression in those CD28⁻CD8 T-cells over a month of culture. These findings suggest that IL-15-mediated down-regulation of CD28 expression occurs primarily in actively dividing CD28+CD8 memory T-cells and that IL-15-induced loss of CD28 expression in CD8 memory T-cells is stable under continuous IL-15 stimulation.

How does IL-15 induce down-regulation of CD28 expression in CD8 memory T-cells? We found that IL-15 induced production of TNF-α in CD8 memory T-cells and blocking TNF-α effect with the neutralizing anti-TNF-α antibody reduced CD28⁻CD8 T-cells by approximately 15% ($p=0.002$, $n=12$) after 14-day IL-15 culture [18]. More dramatically, supplement of recombinant TNF-α(200 ng/ml) in IL-15 culture induced significantly more CD28⁻CD8 T-cells than that of the control cultures (IL-15 alone) at day 14 (195% increase, $p= 7.1×10^{-6}$). The loss of CD28 expression in CD8 memory T-cells induced by exogenous TNF-α is time and dosage-dependent. Supplement of recombinant TNF-α at the beginning of culture accelerated CD28 down-regulation in CD8 memory T-cells as early as 7 days of culture. The effect of TNF-α on down-regulation of CD28 expression in IL-15 cultured CD8 memory T-cells is seen as low as 50 ng/ml of TNF-α. Together, these findings indicate that IL-15 induced down-regulation of CD28 expression in CD8 memory T-cells is partially through production of TNF-α.

2.3   Transcriptional Regulation of CD28 Expression in CD8 T-cells

Loss of CD28 expression in CD28⁻CD8 T-cells appears to be regulated at the transcription level [29, 30]. Analysis of the promoter of CD28 reveals that an inoperative transcriptional initiator (INR) consisting of two motifs α and β at the proximal region of CD28 promoter is involved in the regulation of transcription of CD28 [30]. Loss of α and β bound complexes is found in CD28⁻ T-cells and two proteins, nucleolin and heterogeneous nuclear ribonucleoprotein-D0 isoform A (hnRNP-D0A), bind to the α motif of INR [31]. The binding of these proteins to the α motif of INR is required for transcription of CD28 as lack of nucleolin and hnRNP-D0A at the α site INR site appears to be associated with the loss of transcription of CD28 in CD28⁻ T-cell lines [31]. Because these findings were derived from cell lines, it remains to be confirmed if the same regulation works in normal/primary T-cells during chronic infection and replicative senescence. Equally important is to understand how the chronic stimulation and/or replicative senescence lead to the loss of the α/β INR complexes in the promoter of CD28 gene.

3   Gene Expression Analysis of CD28⁻CD8 T-cells

3.1   Experimental Design

Memory phenotype CD8 T-cells that are CD28⁺ and CD28⁻ were isolated from peripheral blood of healthy adults based on the surface markers CD8, CD45RA⁻ and CD28 by cell sorting. The purity of sorted CD28⁺ and CD28⁻ memory phenotype CD8 T-cells was over 95%. Total RNA were extracted immediately from half of the sorted cells or after 5-day culture with human recombinant IL-15 (50 ng/ml, Peprotech, Boston, MA) of the rest of sorted cells. The quality and quantity of total RNA were analyzed by an Agilent Bioanalyzer (Agilent Technologies, Palo Alto, CA) and only the high quality RNA were used in the microarray experiment and in real time quantitative RT-PCR. To minimize the potential differences among individuals, RNA was pooled from 2–3 donors and a total of three RNA pools were generated for microarray experiments and for real time quantitative RT-PCR analysis. A fourth RNA pool was made for additional real time quantitative RT-PCR analysis to ensure the changes identified here were common between CD28$^+$ and CD28⁻CD8 memory T-cells.

The microarray gene chips were purchased from Agilent Technologies (Whole Human Genome Oligo Chip). This Whole Human Genome Oligo Chip consists of the vast majority of the genes and transcripts in human genome (36,866) on a single slide. The targets on the chip were 60-mer oligonucleotides which offer an overall excellent balance between sensitivity and specificity. The two-fluorescent dyes detection system with a standard universal reference RNA was used in the signal detection to allow a uniformed comparison among different chips. As only three biological replications in this experiment, we applied a conservative error model to reduce the false positives. Statistical significance was determined using the false discovery rate (FDR). The FDR was set to 0.05, which corresponds to the average proportion of false positives = 5% in combination with the pair-wise mean comparison of the signal intensity difference was set to be greater than 2 fold. Finally, real time RT-PCR was applied to independently confirm these selected significant genes. Most of them were confirmed by real time RT-PCR, and the agreeable rate was 85%.

3.2 Gene Expression Changes in CD28⁻CD8 Memory T-cells

Overall, CD28⁻ and CD28$^+$CD8 memory T-cells expressed similar number of genes at the comparable levels. A small number of genes (58 out of 36,866 analyzed) displayed significant difference in mRNA level between CD28⁻ and CD28$^+$CD8 memory T-cells. The majority of these differentially expressed genes are known genes (78%, 45 out of 58 genes) and they serve a wide range of functions and are discussed below.

3.2.1 Expression of Co-Stimulatory Receptors in CD28⁻CD8 T-cells

The CD28 co-stimulatory receptor family consists of five known members, CD28, CTLA-4 (CD152), inducible costimulator (ICOS), program death-1 (PD-1), and B and T Lymphocyte Attenuator (BTLA) [8]. The CD28 family transmembrane proteins have a single extracellular IgV domain and a cytoplasmic tail. CD28 is constitutively expressed on the cell surface of most T-cells and plays a primary role in augmenting TCR signals upon activation. The expression of CD28 decreases after activation. CTLA-4 increases expression after activation and serves as an inhibitory receptor [32, 33]. ICOS expression increases after activation and may play a role in sustained stimulation of effector functions of T-cells [34]. PD-1 and BTLA are both expressed on T and B cells and serve as inhibitory receptors [35, 36]. Among the five members of CD28 family, we found that only CD28 expression was significantly diminished in CD28⁻CD8 memory T-cells compared to CD28$^+$ counterparts.

CD40L and CD70 are members of the TNF superfamily and both serve as co-stimulatory receptors during T-cell activation. The expression pattern of CD40L is similar to CTLA4 during CD8 T-cell differentiation. CD70 is a ligand for CD27, a receptor that is member of the tumor necrosis factor receptor (TNFR family). The signal generated from CD27/CD70 interaction is temporally or spatially segregated from CD28 during T-cell activation [37]. The T-cell activation/survival signals generated by different co-stimulators have some functions in common and yet distinct from each other in other aspects to allow effectiveness and longevity of the T-cell response and survival. The levels of CD27 and CD70 are stable from naive to memory (CD28$^+$ to CD28$^-$) cells. Decreased CD27 expression associated with increased CD70 expression are found in the effector memory CD8 T-cells. The significance of this altered balance of CD27/CD70 expression remains to be determined. It is clear, however, that the parallel loss of CD27 and CD28 expression has profound impact on CD8 T-cell function.

Not all co-stimulatory receptors were down-regulated in CD28$^-$CD8 memory T-cells. Two co-stimulatory receptors (4-1BB and SLAMF7) express higher in CD28$^-$ CD8 memory T-cells. 4-1BB (CD137) belongs to the TNFR gene family and plays a key role in activation-induced cell division, survival, and effector function of CD8 T-cells [38, 39]. An increased 4-1BB expression along with a diminished expression of CD154 coexists in CD28$^-$CD8 memory T-cells, suggesting that an elevated 4-1BB could facilitate the growth and survival of CD28$^-$CD8 memory T-cells in vivo. If this is true, 4-1BB might facilitate the age-associated accumulation of CD28$^-$CD8 T-cells. CD2-like receptor activating cytotoxic cells (CRACC, SLAMF7) also belongs to the SLAM gene family and is expressed on cytotoxic T-cells, activated B cells, and mature dendritic cells [40]. Engagement of SLAMF7 activates NK cell-mediated cytotoxicity [40]. The mRNA level of SLAMF7 was highly expressed in ex vivo CD28$^-$CD8 memory T-cells and was stable after IL-15 treatment. Although the mRNA level of SLAMF7 was lower in ex vivo CD28$^+$CD8 memory T-cells, the level of SLAMF7 was similar between CD28$^-$ and CD28$^+$CD8 memory T-cells after IL-15 treatment.

Alteration of co-stimulatory receptors expression in CD28$^-$CD8 memory T-cells appears to be complex. While loss of expression of some receptors (CD28 and CD154) was apparent, elevated expression of other co-stimulatory receptors (4-1BB and SLAMF7) may provide a compensatory measure for the co-stimulatory function. The questions are: How are these different co-stimulatory receptors regulated in CD8 memory T-cells, particularly in CD28$^-$CD8 memory T-cells? Can an elevated expression of 4-1BB and SLAMF7 compensate the loss of CD28 and CD154? Further studies are required to address these issues and to better understand the activation associated defects of CD28$^-$CD8 memory T-cells and the mechanisms of the age-associated decline of immune function.

3.2.2   Expression of NK Cell Receptors in CD28$^-$CD8 T-cells

The NK cell receptors are initially identified on the surface of NK cells and NK T-cells. Based on their structures, NK cell receptors can be divided into (1) the Immunoglobulin-like NK cell receptors including natural cytotoxicity receptors (NCR), killer immunoglobulin-like receptor (KIR), and CD244, and (2) the C-type lectin-like NK cell receptors including the killer cell lectin-like receptor (KLR) [41]. According to their functions, NK cell receptors can be divided into inhibitory and stimulatory receptors. While engagement of the inhibitory receptors prevents NK cells and CD8 T-cells from killing target cells, interaction of stimulatory receptors results in the trigging of NK cell or CD8 T-cell-mediated cytotoxicity. Expression of NK cell receptors on CD28⁻ CD8 T-cells have been reported [42]. Here we discuss the expression of seven NK cell receptors: KIR2DL2, KIR3DL2, NCR1, CD244, KLRD1, KLRF1, and KLRG1 during CD8 T-cell differentiation identified from microarray analysis.

KIR2DL2, KIR3DL2, NCR1, and CD244 belong to the Ig-like NK cell receptor family. KIR2DL2 (NKAT6) and KIR3DL2 (NKAT4) bind to the polymorphic MHC class I molecules and inhibits lymphocyte cytotoxicity. In contrast, NCR1 and CD244 are stimulatory NK receptors that activate NK-mediated cytotoxicity. The engagement of CD244 (2B4) with its ligand (CD48) or with an anti-CD244 antibody results in enhanced production of interferon gamma (IFN-γ) and cytotoxicity in CD8 T-cells and NK cells [43, 44]. Despite their opposite function, the expression patterns of these four NK cell receptors are similar: all of them are expressed in naïve cells, down-regulated in CD28⁺ memory T-cells, increased in CD28⁻ memory T-cells, and elevated in effector memory cells. After IL-15 treatment, all of them are down-regulated in CD28⁻CD8 memory T-cells [45]. As NCR1 is considered to be exclusively expressed in NK cells, the role of its elevated expression in effector memory T-cells remains to be determined. It has been shown that CD244 level is elevated in CMV-specific effector CD8 T-cells while absent in naïve CD8 T-cells [44]. This enhanced expression of CD244 in effector memory cells agrees with the elevated effector function of the CMV specific CD8 T-cells.

KLRD1, KLRF1, and KLRG1 belong to the C-type lectin-like NK cell receptor family. KLRD1 (CD94) forms heterodimers with KLRC3 (NKG2E) or other members. The KLRD1/KLRK1 (CD94/NKG2D) heterodimer is expressed primarily in NK cells and CD8 T-cells. KLRF1 (NKp80) is expressed in all NK cells and CD56⁺ T-cells and cross-linking of KLRF1 results in induction of cytolytic activity. KLRG1 is a newly identified member of the KLR family and is expressed in NK cells and a subset of T-cells. Although all of them are highly expressed in CD28⁻CD8 T-cells, the patterns of their expression differ. A down-regulation of expression from naïve to memory (CD28⁺) is observed for KLRD1 and KLRF1 but not for KLRG1. The identification of elevated expression of different NK cell receptors in CD28⁻CD8 memory T-cells suggests that NK cell receptors may play roles in CD28⁻CD8 T-cell function. The physiological significance of acquiring these NK cell receptors in CD28⁻CD8 T-cells is not clear and will require further study.

3.2.3 Expression of Cytolytic Molecules in CD28⁻CD8 T-cells

The function of cytotoxic CD8 T-cells is inducing rapid apoptosis of intracellular pathogen-infected or transformed cells. This cellular killing is mediated by two distinct pathways: the granule exocytosis pathway that releases perforin and granzymes from the granule cores and the Fas ligand (FasL)/Fas pathway [46]. The granule exocytosis pathway consists of secretory granules that contain perforin and granzymes. Perforin is expressed only in cytotoxic T-cells and form a pore structure on the targeT-cell membrane to facilitate the entry of granzymes [47]. Granzymes are proteinases that consist of five members in humans: A, B, H, K and M. Each member of granzymes has a different substrate specificity [46]. Granzyme A (GZMA) and granzyme B (GZMB) are expressed in CD8 CTL, $\gamma\delta$ T-cells, and NK cells [48, 49], granzyme H (GZMH) and granzyme K (GZMK) appear to be expressed mainly in CD8 CTL [50, 51], and granzyme M (GZMM) is expressed mainly in NK cells [52].

Perforin is detected in freshly isolated CD8 memory T-cells and is up-regulated after in vitro stimulation by TCR crosslinking or by treatment with IL15 [53]. The levels of perforin mRNA was higher in CD28⁻CD8 memory T-cells than their CD28⁺ counterparts [13, 45]. After culture with IL-15, there is no obvious increase of perforin mRNA levels in CD28⁻CD8 memory T-cells but significantly increased perforin in CD28⁺CD8 memory T-cells. The increase of proforin mRNA in IL-15 treated CD28⁺CD8 memory T-cells is compatible to the level of freshly isolated CD28⁻CD8 memory T-cells.

GZMB and GZMH share a high degree of similarity in amino acid sequence [50]. However, the expression patterns of GZMB and GZMH are quite different. The GZMB level is low in freshly isolated T-cells, but increases after activation [54]. The GZMH level is low in both freshly isolated and activated T-cells [55]. In CD28⁻ CD8 memory T-cells, both GZMB and GZMH are highly expressed, resembling a mixed feature of activated T-cells and NK cells. GZMA and GZMK are functionally overlapping as up-regulation of GZMK has been found in GZMA deficient mice [51]. The levels of GZMA mRNA are similar between CD28⁻ and CD28⁺ CD8 memory T-cells, but a low level of GZMK is found in CD28⁻CD8 memory T-cells compared to their CD28⁺ counterparts. The level of GZMM expression was similar between CD28⁻ and CD28⁺CD8 memory T-cells. Following culture with IL-15, the expression of both GZMA and GZMB were increased in both CD8 memory T-cell subsets. Although activation by antigen do not significantly increase the expression of GZMH [55], IL-15 treatment induces up-regulation of GZMH in CD28⁺CD8 memory T-cells. But CD28⁻CD8 memory T-cells still have higher levels of both GZMB and GZMH than CD28⁺CD8 memory T-cells. This indicates that CD28⁻ CD8 memory T-cells possessed more cytolytic granule enzymes than CD28⁺ counterparts before and after IL-15 culture, providing a molecular basis for high levels of cytotoxicity of CD28⁻CD8 memory T-cells.

The Fas ligand (FasL)/Fas pathway provides another means of T-cell cytotoxicity, which applies not only to regular target cells such as intracellular pathogen infected and transformed cells but also to immune cells as a negative feedback regulation to the generation and expansion of CD4 and CD8 T-cells [46, 56]. It has been reported that FasL can block expression of CD28 at the transcriptional level in Jurkat cells [57], suggesting the role of FasL/Fas in the age-related decline of CD28 expression. The level of FasL mRNA appears higher in CD28⁻CD8 memory T-cells than in

CD28⁺ counterparts, and IL-15 treatment did not increase FasL expression in CD28⁻ CD8 memory T-cells but increased in CD28⁺CD8 memory T-cells. Together, the elevated expression of key molecules in both the granule exocytosis pathway and the FasL/Fas pathway indicates an enhancement of cytolytic capability in CD28⁻ CD8 memory T-cells.

3.2.4 Expression of Cytokines, Chemokines and Their Receptors in CD28⁻CD8 T-cells

Cytokines and chemokines are secreted proteins and play essential roles in many aspects of immune functions. In lymphocytes, cytokines or chemokines can promote their survival or death through strict regulation of their expression and their receptor expression during lymphocyte development and differentiation. Activation of lymphocytes induces production of a variety of cytokines and chemokines in turn these cytokines and chemocykes influence the effectiveness or determine the consequence of an immune response. Therefore, alteration of expression of cytokines and chemokines and their receptors could lead to mild or even severe defects of immune function [58].

Changes in cytokine and chemokine production in CD28⁻CD8 T-cells after in vitro stimulation have been previously reported [10, 12, 59]. In freshly isolated CD28⁻CD8 memory T-cells, the mRNA levels of interleukin 12A (IL12A), interleukin 13 (IL13), chemokine (C-C motif) ligand 4 (CCL4, MIP1-β), chemokine (C-X3-C motif) receptor 1 (CX3CR1, CCRL1), and chemokine-like receptor 1 (CMKLR1) are more highly expressed than do CD28⁺CD8 memory T-cells. In contrast, the mRNA levels of interleukin 3 (IL3), interleukin 23A (IL23A), interleukin 7 receptor (IL7R), and interleukin 12 receptor β2 (IL12RB2) were more highly expressed in CD28⁺CD8 memory T-cells compared with the CD28⁻ cells.

IL-12 and IL-23 are cytokines that are composed of two subunits, one common subunit (IL12B, p40), and one unique subunit IL12A (p35) and IL23A (p19) for IL12 and IL23, respectively [60, 61]. Functionally, IL-12 induces the production of IFN-γ in NK and T-cells, facilitates Th1 differentiation, and serves as a bridge between non-specific innate resistance and antigen specific adaptive immunity [60]. In contrast, IL-23 participates in the proliferative signal in memory T-cells [60, 61]. At the mRNA level, IL12A is higher in CD28⁻CD8 memory T-cells ex vivo but down-regulated after IL-15 treatment. In contrast, IL23A is highly expressed in CD28⁺CD8 memory T-cells ex vivo, but was not changed after IL-15 treatment. The increased level of IL12 in CD28⁻CD8 memory T-cells could contribute to the cytotoxicity of these cells while decreased levels of IL23A may affect the proliferative response of CD28⁻CD8 memory T-cells.

IL-13 is produced primarily by Th2 cells and NK cells and promotes survival, differentiation, and proliferation of hematopoietic progenitor cells [62]. It also exerts immunoregulatory functions including anti-inflammatory effects, Th2 cell development, and B cell proliferation and IgE production [63]. By regulating cell-mediated immunity, IL-13 modulates resistance to several intracellular organisms [63]. IL13 mRNA level was higher in CD28⁻ than in CD28⁺CD8 memory T-cells ex vivo. After IL-15 culture, IL13 mRNA level does not increase in CD28⁻CD8 memory T-cells but increases in CD28⁺CD8 memory T-cells. The precise role of IL-13 in CD28⁻CD8 memory T-cells requires further study.

IL-7 is an essential cytokine during T-cell development and also plays a key role in homeostasis of memory CD8 T-cells [64]. IL-7 receptor is a dimmer that consists of IL-7 unique α receptor (IL7R) and the common γ chain. The function of IL7 depends on the expression of IL7R, which appears to be regulated in T-cells by the availability of IL-7 [65]. The mRNA level of IL7R is lower in CD28⁻CD8 memory T-cells than in the CD28⁺CD8 memory T-cells and is further down-regulated in both subsets after IL-15 treatment. These findings suggest that IL-7 may not be a key survival cytokine for CD28⁻CD8 memory T-cells.

The primary function of chemokines is regulating lymphocyte migration but they are also involved in lymphocyte development, differentiation, and effector function. Like cytokines, different expression patterns of chemokines and their receptors were also observed between CD28⁻ and CD28⁺CD8 memory T-cells. CD28⁻CD8 memory T-cells express higher levels of CCL4 (MIP-1β) and CX3CR1 compared to CD28⁺ counterparts. Both are involved in the regulation of adhesion and migration of T-cells and NK cells [66, 67]. In addition, the expression of CX3CR1 is found in CTL and NK cells [68, 69]. Interaction of CX3CR1 with its ligand, CX3CL1 (Fractalkine), induces the adhesion function as well as promotes subsequent migration to the secondary chemokines such as CCL4 or IL-8/CXCL8 [69]. After IL-15 treatment, the mRNA levels of CCL4 and CX3CR1 are increased in both subsets of memory cells. In addition, the mRNA levels of chemokines XCL1 (lymphotactin-α) and XCL2 (lymphotactin-β) are induced to significantly higher levels after IL15 treatment in CD28⁻CD8 memory T-cells compared to their CD28⁺ counterparts. Since they induce both T-cell and NK cell migration [70], elevated expression of XCL1 and XCL2 may facilitate migration of CD28⁻CD8 memory T-cells. Three chemokine receptors, CCR2, CCR6, and CCR7, express more highly expressed in CD28⁺CD8 memory T-cells than in CD28⁻CD8 memory T-cells. After IL-15 culture, the mRNA levels of CCR2 and CCR6 are increased while the level of CCR7 was decreased in both subsets of memory cells.

3.2.5 Differentially Expressed Transcription Factors in CD28⁻CD8 T-cells

The interaction between T-cells and other cells at various lymphoid compartments mediated by different ligands/receptors on the cell surface is an ongoing process throughout the life of T-cells. The consequence of these interactions depends on the specific interaction, the strength of the interaction, and the states of interacting cells, which are essential for the development, differentiation, and function of T-cells. One of the consequences of the surface ligand/receptor interaction is activation of transcription factors. Here, we will discuss four transcription factors that are differentially highly expressed either in CD28⁻ (TBX21, EOMES, and MYC) or in CD28⁺ (CEBPD) CD8 memory T-cells.

T-box 21 (TBX21, T-bet) is a member of T-box containing gene family and is involved in initiating Th1 lineage development from naive precursor cells and regulation of Ig class switching in effector cells [71, 72]. In addition, it is also involved in regulation of the effector function by promoting IFN-γ production and cytotoxicity in CD8 T-cells [73, 74]. The level of TBX21 mRNA is higher in CD28⁻CD8 memory T-cells than in the CD28⁺ counterparts but there is no significant difference in the levels of IFN-γ and other Th1 cytokine genes between CD28⁻ and CD28⁺CD8 memory T-cells. Thus, it is plausible that elevated expression of TBX21 may serve as a regulator behind the elevated cytotoxicity in CD28⁻CD8 memory T-cells.

Eomesodermin (EOMES) is also a member of the T-box containing gene family within the same subfamily of TBX21. EOMES has been shown to induce IFNγ, perforin, and GZMB in CD8 T-cells [75]. The level of EOMES is higher in CD28⁻CD8 memory T-cells than in their CD28⁺ counterparts. After IL-15 treatment, the levels of EOMES are decreased only in CD28⁻CD8 memory T-cells but did in CD28⁺CD8 memory T-cells. As EOMES shares similar function with TBX21 in regulation of effector functions of CD8 T-cells, their elevated expression in CD28⁻CD8 memory T-cells provides a transcriptional basis of enhanced cytotoxicity in CD28⁻CD8 memory T-cells.

MYC and its family transcription factors are key regulators of cell growth and proliferation as well as inhibition of terminal differentiation and induction of apoptosis [76]. Dysregulation of MYC expression leads to unlimited cell growth and ultimately development of tumors [77]. MYC is up-regulated after T-cell activation and is also involved in the induction of apoptosis [78]. The level of MYC mRNA is higher in freshly isolated CD28⁻CD8 memory T-cells than their CD28⁺ counterparts. After IL-15 culture, MYC mRNA levels are highly increased in both CD28⁻ and CD28⁺CD8 memory T-cells. However, the difference of MYC mRNA level remained significantly higher in CD28⁻CD8 memory T-cells compared to their CD28⁺ counterparts. As previously studies showed CD28⁻CD8 memory T-cells are resistant to apoptosis, MYC in CD28⁻CD8 memory T-cells may facilitate cell division and resistant to apoptosis.

CEBPD is a member of the CCAAT/enhancer-binding protein (C/EBP) family that contains a highly conserved of leucine zipper DNA binding motif [79]. Members of the C/EBP family have been shown to regulate the differentiation of myelomonocytic marrow cells [80]. CEBPD is also involved in regulating the expression of IL6 that plays an important role in regulating immune and inflammatory response [81].The level of CEBPD mRNA is higher in CD28⁺CD8 memory T-cells than in CD28⁻CD8 memory T-cells. Although CEBPD expression is tightly regulated in G(0) growth-arrested mouse mammary epithelial cells (MEC) [82], IL-15 induced proliferation does not appear to affect the levels of CEBPD mRNA in either CD28⁻ or CD28⁺CD8 memory T-cells. It remains to be determined the significance of down-regulated expression of CEBPD in CD28⁻CD8 memory T-cells.

4   Conclusion

Studies of the generation of CD28⁻CD8 T-cells indicate that both antigenic stimulation and homeostatic proliferation are causes for loss of CD28 expression in CD28⁺ CD8 T-cells. Thus, it is likely that age-associated accumulation of CD28⁻CD8

T-cells is the combinational consequence of antigenic stimulation and homeostatic expansion of memory T-cells. Genome-wide analysis of gene expression profiles between CD28⁻ and CD28⁺CD8 T-cells reveals the molecular changes in CD28⁻ CD8 memory T-cells. The gain and loss of these specific gene expressions in CD28⁻ CD8 T-cells may reflect an adaptive process of the immune system in which an induced cytotoxicity is replaced by a constant cytotoxicity in CD8 memory T-cells in compensation of the inability of robust proliferation. Further characterization of the regulation and function of those differentially expressed genes in CD28⁻ CD8 T-cells will help us to better understand this age-associated change in T-cell function and may open new avenues of clinical intervention to slow or reverse this aging-associated process.

Acknowledgment   The author want to thank Monchou Fann, Kevin Becker, and William Wood III for conducting and assisting microarray experiments; Karen Chiu and Jason Godlove for the study of IL-15 induced down-regulation of CD28 expression, Robert Wersto, Joe Chrest and Coung Nguyen for cell sorting, Karen Madara and her staff at the NIA Apheresis Unit for processing the blood samples. This research was supported by the Intramural Research Program of the National Institute on Aging, National Institutes of Health (NIH).

References

1. Longo DL (2004) Immunology of aging. In Paul WE (ed) Fundamental immunology, 5th edn. Lippincott Williams & Wilkins pp 1043–1075
2. Weng NP (2006) Aging of the immune system: how much can the adaptive immune system adapt? Immunity 24:495–499
3. Azuma M et al (1993) CD28- T lymphocytes: antigenic and functional properties. J Immunol 150:1147–1159
4. Effros RB et al (1994) Decline in CD28+ T-cells in centenarians and in long-term T-cell cultures: a possible cause for both in vivo and in vitro immunosenescence. Exp Gerontol 29: 601–609
5. Posnett D N et al (1994) Clonal populations of T-cells in normal elderly humans: the T cell equivalent to "benign monoclonal gammapathy". J Exp Med 179:609–618
6. Fagnoni FF et al (1996) Expansion of cytotoxic CD8+CD28- T-cells in healthy ageing people, including centenarians. Immunology 88:501–507
7. Acuto O, Michel F (2003) CD28-mediated co-stimulation: a quantitative support for TCR signalling. Nat Rev Immunol 3:939–951
8. Riley JL, June CH (2005) The CD28 family: a T cell rheostat for therapeutic control of T-cell activation. Blood 105:13–21
9. Effros RB et al (2003) CD8 T-cells and aging. Crit Rev Immunol 23:45–64
10. Nociari MM et al (1999) Postthymic development of CD28-CD8+ T cell subset: age-associated expansion and shift from memory to naive phenotype. J Immunol 162:3327–3335
11. Spaulding C et al (1999) Resistance to apoptosis in human CD8+ T-cells that reach replicative senescence after multiple rounds of antigen-specific proliferation. Exp Gerontol 34:633–644
12. Saurwein-Teissl M et al (2002) Lack of antibody production following immunization in old age: association with CD8(+)CD28(-) T cell clonal expansions and an imbalance in the production of Th1 and Th2 cytokines. J Immunol 168:5893–5899
13. Posnett DN et al (1999) Differentiation of human CD8 T-cells: implications for in vivo persistence of CD8+CD28- cytotoxic effector clones. Int Immunol 11:229–241

14. Boucher N et al (1998) CD28 expression in T cell aging and human longevity. Exp Gerontol 33:267–282
15. Effros RB et al (1996) Shortened telomeres in the expanded CD28-CD8+ cell subset in HIV disease implicate replicative senescence in HIV pathogenesis. AIDS 10:F17–F22
16. Hazzan M et al (1997) Recall response to cytomegalovirus in allograft recipients: mobilization of CD57+, CD28+ cells before expansion of CD57+. Transplantation 63:693–698
17. Borthwick NJ et al (2000) Loss of CD28 expression on CD8(+) T-cells is induced by IL-2 receptor gamma chain signalling cytokines and type I IFN, and increases susceptibility to activation-induced apoptosis. Int Immunol 12:1005–1013
18. Chiu WK et al (2006) Generation and growth of CD28nullCD8+ memory T-cells mediated by IL-15 and its induced cytokines. J Immunol 177:7802–7810
19. Fiorentino S et al (1996) Predominant involvement of CD8+CD28- lymphocytes in human immunodeficiency virus-specific cytotoxic activity. J Virol 70:2022–2026
20. Weekes MP et al (1999) Human CD28-CD8+ T-cells contain greatly expanded functional virus- specific memory CTL clones. J Immunol 162:7569–7577
21. Wills MR et al (1999) Human virus-specific CD8+ CTL clones revert from CD45ROhigh to CD45RAhigh in vivo: CD45RAhighCD8+ T-cells comprise both naive and memory cells. J Immunol 162:7080–7087
22. Ouyang Q et al (2003) Large numbers of dysfunctional CD8+ T lymphocytes bearing receptors for a single dominant CMV epitope in the very old 5. J Clin Immunol 23:247–257
23. Roos MT et al (2000) Changes in the composition of circulating CD8+ T-cell subsets during acute epstein-barr and human immunodeficiency virus infections in humans 6. J Infect Dis 182:451–458
24. Klatt T et al (2005) Expansion of peripheral CD8+CD28- T-cells in response to Epstein-Barr virus in patients with rheumatoid arthritis. J Rheumatol 32:239–251
25. Scognamiglio P et al (1999) Presence of effector CD8 + T-cells in hepatitis C virus-exposed healthy seronegative donors 17. J Immunol 162:6681–6689
26. Appay V et al (2002) Memory CD8+ T-cells vary in differentiation phenotype in different persistent virus infections2. Nat Med 8:379–385
27. Linsley PS et al (1993) CD28 engagement by B7/BB-1 induces transient down-regulation of CD28 synthesis and prolonged unresponsiveness to CD28 signaling. J Immunol 150:3161–3169
28. Bryl E et al (2001) Down-regulation of CD28 expression by TNF-alpha. J Immunol 167:3231–3238
29. Vallejo AN et al (1998) Aging-related deficiency of CD28 expression in CD4+ T-cells is associated with the loss of gene-specific nuclear factor binding activity. J Biol Chem 273:8119–8129
30. Vallejo,A.N. et al (1999) Modulation of CD28 expression: distinct regulatory pathways during activation and replicative senescence. J. Immunol. 162, 6572–6579
31. Vallejo AN et al (2002) Molecular basis for the loss of CD28 expression in senescent T-cells. J Biol Chem 277:46940–46949
32. Sharpe AH, Freeman GJ (2002) The B7-CD28 superfamily. Nat Rev Immunol 2:116–126
33. Wang S, Chen L (2004) Co-signaling molecules of the B7-CD28 family in positive and negative regulation of T lymphocyte responses. Microbes Infect 6:759–766
34. Riley JL et al (2001) ICOS costimulation requires IL-2 and can be prevented by CTLA-4 engagement. J Immunol 166:4943–4948
35. Freeman GJ et al (2000) Engagement of the PD-1 immunoinhibitory receptor by a novel B7 family member leads to negative regulation of lymphocyte activation. J Exp Med 192:1027–1034
36. Watanabe N et al (2003) BTLA is a lymphocyte inhibitory receptor with similarities to CTLA-4 and PD-1. Nat Immunol 4:670–679
37. Watts TH (2005) TNF/TNFR family members in costimulation of T-cell responses. Annu Rev Immunol 23:23–68
38. Cannons JL et al (2001) 4-1BB ligand induces cell division, sustains survival, and enhances effector function of CD4 and CD8 T-cells with similar efficacy. J Immunol 167:1313–1324

39. Cooper D et al (2002) 4-1BB (CD137) controls the clonal expansion and survival of CD8 T-cells in vivo but does not contribute to the development of cytotoxicity. Eur J Immunol 32:521–529
40. Bouchon A et al (2001) Activation of NK cell-mediated cytotoxicity by a SAP-independent receptor of the CD2 family. J Immunol. 167, 5517–5521
41. Biassoni R et al (2003) Human natural killer cell receptors: insights into their molecular function and structure. J Cell Mol Med 7:376–387
42. Phillips JH et al (1995) Superantigen-dependent, cell-mediated cytotoxicity inhibited by MHC class I receptors on T lymphocytes. Science 268:403–405
43. Kubin MZ et al (1999) Molecular cloning and biological characterization of NK cell activation-inducing ligand, a counterstructure for CD48. Eur J Immunol 29:3466–3477
44. Speiser DE et al (2001) The activatory receptor 2B4 is expressed in vivo by human CD8+ effector alpha beta T-cells. J Immunol 167:6165–6170
45. Fann M et al (2005) Gene expression characteristics of CD28null memory phenotype CD8+ T-cells and its implication in T-cell aging. Immunol Rev 205:190–206
46. Henkart PA, Sikovsky MV (2003) Cytotoxic T lymphocytes. In Paul WE (ed) Fundamental immunology, 5th edn. Lippincott Williams & Wilkins, pp 1127–1150
47. Catalfamo M, Henkart PA (2003) Perforin and the granule exocytosis cytotoxicity pathway. Curr Opin Immunol 15:522–527
48. Lieberman J, Fan Z (2003) Nuclear war: the granzyme A-bomb. Curr Opin Immunol 15:553–559
49. Trapani JA, Sutton VR (2003) Granzyme B: pro-apoptotic, antiviral and antitumor functions. Curr Opin Immunol 15:533–543
50. Haddad P et al (1991) Structure and evolutionary origin of the human granzyme H gene. Int Immunol 3:57–66
51. Shresta S et al (1997) Residual cytotoxicity and granzyme K expression in granzyme A-deficient cytotoxic lymphocytes. J Biol Chem 272:20236–20244
52. Sayers TJ et al (2001) The restricted expression of granzyme M in human lymphocytes. J Immunol 166:765–771
53. Liu K et al (2002) IL-15 mimics T-cell receptor crosslinking in the induction of cellular proliferation, gene expression, and cytotoxicity in CD8+ memory T-cells. Proc Natl Acad Sci U S A 99:6192–6197
54. Clement MV et al (1990) Granzyme B-gene expression: a marker of human lymphocytes "activated" in vitro or in renal allografts. Hum Immunol 28:159–166
55. Sedelies KA et al (2004) Discordant regulation of granzyme H and granzyme B expression in human lymphocytes. J Biol Chem 279:26581–26587
56. Ashany D et al (1995) Th1 CD4+ lymphocytes delete activated macrophages through the Fas/APO-1 antigen pathway. Proc Natl Acad Sci U S A 92:11225–11229
57. Ma S et al (2003) FasL-induced downregulation of CD28 expression on jurkat cells in vitro is associated with activation of caspases. Cell Biol Int 27:959–964
58. Noguchi M et al (1993) Interleukin-2 receptor gamma chain mutation results in X-linked severe combined immunodeficiency in humans. Cell 73:147–157
59. Bandres E et al (2000) The increase of IFN-gamma production through aging correlates with the expanded CD8(+high)CD28(-)CD57(+) subpopulation. Clin Immunol 96:230–235
60. Trinchieri G (2003) Interleukin-12 and the regulation of innate resistance and adaptive immunity. Nat Rev Immunol 3:133–146
61. Frucht DM (2002) IL-23: a cytokine that acts on memory T-cells. Sci STKE 2002:E1
62. Shelburne CP, Ryan JJ (2001) The role of Th2 cytokines in mast cell homeostasis. Immunol Rev 179:82–93
63. Wynn TA (2003) IL-13 effector functions. Annu Rev Immunol 21:425–456
64. Schluns KS et al (2000) Interleukin-7 mediates the homeostasis of naive and memory CD8 T-cells in vivo. Nat Immunol 1:426–432

65. Park JH et al (2004) Suppression of IL7Ralpha transcription by IL-7 and other prosurvival cytokines: a novel mechanism for maximizing IL-7-dependent T-cell survival. Immunity 21:289–302

66. Tanaka Y et al (1993) T-cell adhesion induced by proteoglycan-immobilized cytokine MIP-1 beta. Nature 361:79–82

67. Imai T et al (1997) Identification and molecular characterization of fractalkine receptor CX3CR1, which mediates both leukocyte migration and adhesion. Cell 91:521–530

68. Foussat A et al (2000) Fractalkine receptor expression by T lymphocyte subpopulations and in vivo production of fractalkine in human. Eur J Immunol 30:87–97

69. Nishimura M et al (2002) Dual functions of fractalkine/CX3C ligand 1 in trafficking of perforin+/granzyme B+ cytotoxic effector lymphocytes that are defined by CX3CR1 expression. J Immunol 168:6173–6180

70. Kennedy J et al (1995) Molecular cloning and functional characterization of human lymphotactin. J Immunol 155:203–209

71. Szabo SJ et al (2000) A novel transcription factor, T-bet, directs Th1 lineage commitment. Cell 100:655–669

72. Peng SL et al (2002) T-bet regulates IgG class switching and pathogenic autoantibody production. Proc Natl Acad Sci U S A 99:5545–5550

73. Szabo SJ et al (1995) Developmental commitment to the Th2 lineage by extinction of IL-12 signaling. Immunity 2:665–675

74. Sullivan BM et al (2003) Antigen-driven effector CD8 T cell function regulated by T-bet. Proc Natl Acad Sci U S A 100:15818–15823

75. Pearce EL et al (2003) Control of effector CD8+ T-cell function by the transcription factor Eomesodermin. Science 302:1041–1043

76. Secombe J et al (2004) Myc: a weapon of mass destruction. Cell 117:153–156

77. Popescu NC, Zimonjic DB (2002) Chromosome-mediated alterations of the MYC gene in human cancer. J Cell Mol Med 6:151–159

78. Genestier L et al (1999) Transforming growth factor beta1 inhibits Fas ligand expression and subsequent activation-induced cell death in T-cells via downregulation of c-Myc. J Exp Med 189:231–239

79. Landschulz WH et al (1988) The leucine zipper: a hypothetical structure common to a new class of DNA binding proteins. Science 240:1759–1764

80. Scott LM et al (1992) A novel temporal expression pattern of three C/EBP family members in differentiating myelomonocytic cells. Blood 80:1725–1735

81. Kinoshita S et al (1992) A member of the C/EBP family, NF-IL6 beta, forms a heterodimer and transcriptionally synergizes with NF-IL6. Proc Natl Acad Sci U S A 89:1473–1476

82. Sivko GS et al (2004) CCAAT/enhancer binding protein delta (C/EBPdelta) regulation and expression in human mammary epithelial cells: II. Analysis of activating signal transduction pathways, transcriptional, post-transcriptional, and post-translational control. J Cell Biochem 93:844–856

Role of Regulatory Subsets During Aging

Piotr Trzonkowski

Contents

Abstract: Efficient immune response requires both vigorous effector responses and regulation via regulatory subsets. Any disturbances in the balance between these two opposite activities of immune system result in either autoimmunity or excessive immunosuppression. Undoubtedly immunosenescence contributes to this balance as it affects the majority of populations taking part in immune response. This chapter describes activities of regulatory subsets, alterations associated with their ageing and clinical consequences of these changes.

Keywords: CD25+CD4+ Treg cells • Tr1 cells • Th3 cells • Interleukin 10 (IL10) • Transforming growth factor β (TGFβ) • Tolerogenic dendritic cells • CD28-CD8+ T suppressor cells • NKT cells

1 Introduction

Aggressive action of immune system against alien agents has to be strictly controlled in order to prevent destruction of self tissues. There are several subsets within lymphoid system which are responsible for the control of selective targeting of alloanti-

P. Trzonkowski (✉)
Laboratory of Experimental Transplantology
Department of Histology and Immunology
Medical University of Gdańsk
Ul. Dębinki 1, 80-211 Gdańsk, Poland
Tel.: 0048 58 3491430; Fax: 0048 58 3491436
E-mail: ptrzon@amg.gda.pl

T. Fulop et al. (eds.), *Handbook on Immunosenescence*,
DOI 10.1007/ 978-1-4020-9062-2_18, © Springer Science+Business Media B.V. 2009

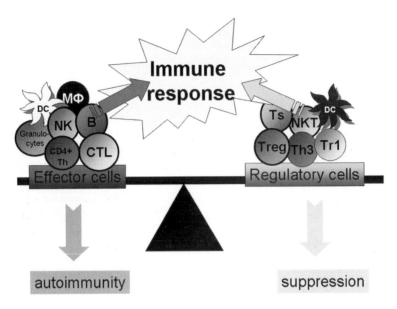

Fig. 1 The balance is required for efficient immune response. Coordinated function of effector and regulatory subsets guarantees efficient immune response. Imbalance in this regulation results is either autoimmune phenomena or exaggerated immunosuppression

gens and, at the same time, keeping the immune system neutral to autoantigens. The awareness of such immunosuppressive subsets started with Owen's notion, who found that the intraplacental transfusion of blood in cattle caused that each dizygote twin tolerated skin transplants from the other (Owen RD 1945). Soon after, Medawar performed a series of excellent Nobel Prize awarded experiments with infusion of alloantigens to newborn mice inducing selective alloantigen tolerance during their adulthood (Billingham RE 1953). The leading role of T-cells in tolerance induction was proved in 70s and 80s (Gershon RK 1970; Fujimoto S 1975; North RJ 1984); however, a detailed phenotype of those cells has been discovered only recently. In 1995, Sakaguchi reported that deficiency of CD4+ T-cells with expression of IL2Rα (CD4+CD25+), so-called T regulatory cells (Treg), in mice was associated with multiple autoimmune diseases (Sakaguchi S 1995). Without any doubt, different subsets of Treg cells have taken a central stage in immunology since that time. Nevertheless, induction of tolerance is much wider than Treg cells as some other subsets, such as CD28-CD8+ T suppressor cells (Ts), NKT cells, and some dendritic cells, were also found to confer it in immune system. Making the story even more complex, recent reports have suggested that efficient regulation of immune response is not limited to immunosuppressive cells, but it is more a balance between suppressive and proinflammatory effector cells. Interestingly, having opposite activities, at least some of those cells have common origin. Thus, keeping adequate proportions between aggressive effector phase of immune response and self-limitation of immune response is probably the best definition of the function of all the above mentioned regulatory subsets.

2   CD25^{high}CD4⁺ T Regulatory Cells (Treg)

2.1   Biology

CD4+ T-cells play the central role in T-cell mediated regulation. There are two main subsets of CD4+ Treg cells in the body: naturally occurring and adaptive ones. As the discovery of Treg cells is relatively fresh, it is very often difficult to distinguish between these lineages due to their common features. Naturally occurring or intrinsic Treg cells (nTreg) in humans can be defined as CD25^{high}FoxP3+CD4+ T-cells. The expression of CD25 receptor is related to their high dependency on IL2, and FoxP3 is a transcription factor that drives intracellular signals which results in suppressive abilities of nTreg cells. Of note, FoxP3 is currently considered as the most characteristic intracellular marker of nTreg cells (Baecher-Allan C 2001; Hori S 2003). nTreg cells originate from the thymus. Maturing nTreg cells are self-reactive with intermediate to low affinity to autoantigens and yet they escape from central deletion. It is distinctive feature of their development in the thymus. Probably, they do not only arise as a result of the presentation of self antigens through TCR-dependent process but also by means of some other not well understood mechanisms. It has been only recently discovered that their intrathymic lineage commitment is maintained by interactions with medullary thymic epithelial cells expressing the autoimmune regulator AIRE (Aschenbrenner 2007). Intracellular mechanisms related to the maturation of Treg lineage are still far from final conclusions. The studies with *Scurfy* mice, that is, mice without active Treg cells due to the knockout of FoxP3 gene, revealed that these animals suffer from severe lymphoproliferative autoimmune disease (Fontenot JD 2003). Similar defect, so-called IPEX (IPEX–Immune dysregulation, Polyendocrinopathy, Enteropathy, X-linked syndrome) was also found to be caused by mutations in FoxP3 gene in men (Bennett CL 2001). Genome-wide profiling revealed that transcription factor FoxP3 can bind to around 700 genes imposing phenotypic features of nTreg cells (Zheng Y 2007). Although FoxP3 takes a part in both differentiation and functioning of these cells, it appears that its action solidifies only pre-established features acquired by developing nTreg cells in the thymus as it has been shown that inactive nTreg may develop in the thymus even in the absence of FoxP3 (Gavin MA 2007; Wan YY 2007). Moreover, early stage of activation may be associated with transient expression of FoxP3 in T effector cells (Kretschmer K 2005). Despite self-specificity, nTreg do not damage own tissues at the periphery as they are highly anergic. The anergy might by explained by high differentiation of nTreg cells. It has been revealed that the expression of many surface markers locate them within memory phenotype, their proliferation is very much limited, they are characterised by short telomeres and easily undergo apoptosis (Taams LS 2001, 2002). The most important function of nTreg cells is the suppression of other immune cells. Autoreactive cells are not the only targets for nTreg cells. They are also highly efficient suppressors of alloresponses. Broad range of responses inhibited by nTreg cells caused that they were initially thought to be non-specific. However, more recent data, mainly from in vitro nTreg expansion experiments, proved that their suppressive effect can be directed against responses driven by specific antigens (Masteller EL 2006). This inconsistency might have come from low affinity of their receptors and the phenomenon of bystander regulation exerted by nTreg cells, *i.e.* nTreg cells specific to particular antigen may impose tolerance to other antigens when activated (Waldmann H 2006). At first, only CD4+ T effector cells were described to be inhibited by nTreg cells (Suri-Payer E 1998). Twelve years after the discovery Treg cells were found to interfere with CD8+ T-cells, NK cells, NKT cells, monocytes, dendritic cells, and granulocytes (Piccirillo CA 2001; Trzonkowski P 2004; Taams LS 2005; Lewkowicz P 2006). Upon stimulation, which usually occurs at the site of inflammation as well as in the local lymphoid tissue, nTreg interact with effectors in a direct cell-to-cell manner suppressing their proliferation and effector activities (Taams LS 2001; Trzonkowski P 2004). Although nTreg cells were found to produce suppressive cytokines, such as IL10 or TGFβ, direct contact with other cells is regarded as the most important way of their action. The most important receptor of Treg cells cooperating in the immune synapse with both CD4+ and CD8+ T effector cells is CTLA-4 molecule (Cytotoxic T lymphocyte antigen 4, CD152). Engagement of this receptor in the presence of TCR ligation triggers suppressive activity of nTreg cells (Takahashi T 2000; Sansom DM 2006). There are several mechanisms of this suppression. Initially, it was postulated that nTreg cells may physically interfere with the interaction of effector T-cells with APCs by competing for the costimulatory molecules on APCs (Takahashi T 2000). It might be possible as, in comparison to the ligands expressed on T effectors, CTLA-4 has higher affinity for B7 family receptors on APC (Linsley PS 1992). In addition, nTreg cells express variety of adhesive molecules, such as ICAM-1 (CD54) and integrins LFA-1 (CD11a/CD18), α4β7 (LPAM-1), αEβ7 (CD103) and α4β1 (CD49d/CD49), that may additionally give Treg cells the advantage of cell-to-cell interaction with APC that is stronger than the interaction of APC with effectors (Takahashi T 2000; Stassen M 2004; Marski M 2005). Another explanation is that the interaction between CTLA-4 on nTreg cells and B7 family receptors on APC, notably in dendritic cells (DC), induces the expression of enzyme indolamine 2,3-dioxygenase (IDO) in the latter (Grohmann U 2003). IDO changes metabolic pathway of tryptophan to kynurenines, which suppresses T-cell responses (Mellor AL 2002). It has been also described that the engagement of CTLA-4 on nTreg induces secretion of TGFβ that subsequently strongly suppresses T effector cells (Chen W 1998). Apart from T-cells, cell-to-cell interactions were also described in the regulation of other immune cells by nTreg cells. Membrane-anchored TGFβ on nTreg cells is crucial for the inhibition of NK cells and TLR receptors expressed on nTreg cells are prerequisite for the regulation of the activity and survival of granulocytes (Ghiringhelli F 2005; Lewkowicz P 2006). The competition between nTreg cells and T effectors is not limited to the binding of surface receptors of APC. nTreg cells are highly dependent on IL2 but devoid of capabilities of its production. Thus, they compete with effector cells for IL2 which decreases the amount of IL2 available at the site of immune reaction and therefore tempers activities of T effectors (Thornton AM 1998). Moreover, despite dependency on IL2, Treg cells suppress production of IL2 by CD4+ T effectors which additionally decreases availability of the cytokine during immune response. The most extreme pathway of the regulation revealed during research upon nTreg cells is their cytotoxicity. Namely, it has been found that these cells upon stimulation kill autologous cells by means of secreted cytotoxic perforin and granzymes (Grossman WJ 2004; Gondek DC 2005).

Peripherally induced or adaptive Treg cells constitute another subset of CD4+ Treg cells. It is a small number of cells generated during each and every immune response from activated naïve CD4+ T-cells at the periphery (Karim M 2004). These cells are antigen-specific as they arise in response to specific antigens and their activation is dependent on expressed TCR receptors. Importantly, it is a source of Treg cells independent of the thymus. Apart from that, basic characteristics of these so-called adaptive Treg cells, including the most important marker FoxP3, are similar to thymic-derived nTreg cells (O'Neill 2004).

There are also some other subsets of adaptive CD4+ Treg cells induced at the periphery. In contrast to nTreg cells, these cells do not suppress in cell-to-cell mode and their action is dependent mainly on secreted suppressive cytokines. Based on secreted cytokines at least two different groups may be distinguished—Tr1 cells, which function relies on secreted IL10 (Groux H 1997), and Th3 cells, which produce mainly TGFβ (Fukaura H 1996). Apart from cytokine-dependent mode of suppression, their basic characteristics are also different from nTreg cells. Tr1 cells are anergic mainly due to autocrine action of IL10. These cells seem to be dependent on IL2 family of cytokines as they constitutively express high levels of IL2 family receptors IL2Rβ (CD122) and IL2Rγ (CD132) and can be expanded in the presence of IL2 and IL15. On the other hand, normal level of IL2Rα (CD25) on Tr1 cells can be achieved only upon TCR-mediated stimulation (Battaglia M 2006). Also the expression of FoxP3 in Tr1 is not constitutive but can be upregulated upon activation (Vieira PL 2004). The most consistent intracellular protein postulated as a marker of Tr1 cells is the repressor of GATA-3 (ROG); however, its expression was also noted in T effectors (Cobbold SP 2003). The most important inducer of IL10-producing Tr1 are immature DC (Levings MK 2005). IL10 secreted during interaction of Tr1 with DC limits the production of IL12 and TNFα by DC and macrophages which subsequently quenches induction of Th1 and Th2 responses (Moore KW 2001). Tr1 cells were found to promote tolerance to both auto- and alloantigens. Their suppressive role was described in allotransplantations of bone marrow and solid organs, down-regulation of immune responses in rheumatoid diseases and other autoimmune pathologies, allergies and, inflammatory bowel diseases. On the other hand, their deficit was found to facilitate chronic course of some infections (Battaglia M 2006). It might be important in ageing that IL10 is secreted not only by Tr1 cells but also by other T-cells, monocytes, macrophages and nonlymphoid cells. IL10 from all those sources is often treated as a counterbalance to proinflammatory cytokines, notably to IL6 (Saurwein-Teissl M 2000; Ye SM 2001; Hacham M 2004).

Like Tr1 cells, TGFβ-producing Th3 cells are distinctive in several aspects. First of all, their function is linked mainly to oral tolerance. This aspect is of great importance as Th3 cells generated with orally administered antigens might exert bystander regulation, which has implications in pathology as well as in potential therapeutic strategies (Ochi H 2006). Unlike other Treg cells, the generation of Th3 cells is dependent on IL4 (Fukaura H 1996; Hafler DA 1997). Also TGFβ on its own, or augmented by IL10, may generate Th3 cells from naïve T-cells (Chen W 2003; Kitani A 2003). Immunosuppressive action of TGFβ secreted by Th3 cells is directed against Th1 responses as it downregulates expression of IL12R and transcription factor T-bet in Th1 cells (Kitani A 2000; Gorelik L 2002). TGFβ may work as soluble cytokine but also as membrane-anchored receptor. The action of the latter form, in relation to TGFβ type 1 on Treg cells, was initially described as an important tool of cell-to-cell regulation of T effectors, B cells (Nakamura K 2001) as well as NK cells (Ghiringhelli F 2005). Membrane-anchored TGFβ seems to work as an executor of several pathways of regulation as its function can be activated by several factors, for example, latency-associated protein (LAP) or thrombospondin (Faria AM 2005). Like the system associated with IL10, TGFβ-dependent regulation appears to be much wider than Th3-mediated effects. The cytokine is fully capable of suppression of T-cells responses when produced by nonlymphoid lineages, such as macrophages or enterocytes (Barnard JA 1993; Galliaerde V 1995).

2.2 Ageing

The regulation of immune responses through Treg cells in ageing appears to have some distinctive features. When compared to younger subjects, the elderly are characterised by higher number of Treg cells but per-cell activity of those cells seems to be altered.

Several laboratories reported increased frequency of Treg cells in aged individuals (Trzonkowski P 2003; Gregg R 2005; Gottenberg JE 2005). The percentage of CD25^{high}CD4+ T-cells in the peripheral blood is surprisingly high at birth reaching in some cases even 9.5% of total CD4+ T-cells in cord blood (Godfrey WR 2005), but then decreases during childhood and remains on a stable level not exceeding 5% of total CD4+ T-cells in young and middle aged subjects (Cao D 2004; Beyer M 2005; Gottenberg JE 2005). In more advanced age the number of Treg cells gradually increases and, in the extreme, it may be even fivefold higher than that noted in earlier phases of ontogeny (Trzonkowski P 2006). There might be several sources which give rise to the increased number of Treg cells with ageing. First of all, longer life means longer time when the cells can be generated. Although thymic involution causes reduced output of naturally occurring Treg cells with age, adaptive Treg cells may be generated continuously at the periphery throughout entire lifespan. To a great extent, this idea was confirmed in animal model. Shimizu's group found that age-associated increase in FoxP3+ T-cells with regulatory properties was mainly attributed to CD25-CD4+ T-cells and not to the classical thymus-derived nTreg cells (Shimizu J 2003). In humans, FoxP3+ Treg cells were shown to arise from rapidly dividing, highly differentiated memory CD4+ T-cells (Vukmanovic-Stejic M 2006). Since both memory and regulatory subsets in particular subjects were revealed to share the same TCR repertoire, the authors of this report concluded that every challenge with specific antigen generates both memory and regulatory cells. This finding, consistent with other reports (Cobbold SP 2006), is of special importance in quantitative studies upon Treg cells in aging as it gives a link between the number of immune responses and potency of regulation in particular subject. It seems to be logic that aged individuals have had higher chance to be challenged with higher number of pathogens than the young, simply because they live longer. Thus, as it comes from Akbar's studies, the elderly are not only characterised by increased number of memory cells but also those regulatory (Vukmanovic-Stejic M 2006). Consistently with this view, when the number of Treg cells was compared between subjects of the same age, the higher number was found in those with the history of more frequent inflammatory events and exposures to higher number of antigenic challenges (Trzonkowski P 2003). Thus, it is not surprising that frail elderly with inflammatory burden (Pawelec G 2005) are characterized by higher number of Treg cells than their healthy counterparts (Trzonkowski P 2006). Preferential accumulation of Treg cells in unhealthy individuals may be recognized as a kind of "vicious circle," when Treg cells arising during particular responses make the patient more susceptible to subsequent infections and these infections induce more Treg cells. It may be especially detrimental in aged subjects as their "vicious circle" lasts for a long time and therefore the number of Treg cells is exceptionally high in frail elderly (Trzonkowski P 2006).

It has to be highlighted that the estimation from peripheral blood might not correlate with total number of Treg cells in the body as Treg cells are capable of efficient trafficking through lymphoid tissues where their level may be substantially higher than that measured in the peripheral blood. For example, Treg cells in mice were found to constitute 40% of CD4+ T-cells in the bone marrow or even more, in terms of absolute numbers, in the spleen (Hoffmann P 2002). Moreover, the trafficking through the tissues seems to be crucial for the function of Treg cells as the expression of receptors allowing them to enter lymphoid tissues, such as CD62L or CCR7, was associated with higher capabilities of immunosuppression (Fu S 2004; Taylor PA 2004; Ermann J 2005). Since the expression of these receptors declines with age on T-cells, it might be the reason that Treg cells in the elderly are not capable of extravasation and their level is increased in the peripheral blood but not in the tissues. These receptors are also markers of naïve cells which implies that Treg cells, like other T-cells, may be on different levels of their differentiation. Indeed, "naïve" CD45RA+FoxP3+CD4+ T-cells, which characteristics are close to other naïve T subsets, was described as a subset of Treg cells in humans. The percentage of these cells was shown to be substantially reduced with age (Valmori D 2005). Initially, no difference in ex vivo suppressive activity was found between CD45+ and CD45RA- Treg cells (Valmori D 2005; Seddiki N 2006). Nevertheless, it might have been dependent on incomplete phenotyping and assessment based on single sampling of the probands. More recent study, in which authors followed phenotype of Treg cells over time during ex vivo expansion, proved superiority of Treg cells derived from CD45RA+ precursors above those CD45RA- (Hoffmann P 2006).

Bearing in mind that the majority of Treg cells in the elderly are highly differentiated and their development, to some extent, is parallel to memory/effector cells, it might be possible that their accumulation might be an attempt of the counteraction to the process of "shrinkage and filling up of the immunological space" hypothesized initially by Franceschi's group (Franceschi C 2003). The theory is based on the observation that lymphoid system in aged individuals is filled with expanded clones of anergic CD8+ T-cells that block proper immune responses to new challenges (Ku CC 1997). Homeostatic proliferation seems to be an important phenomenon responsible for the generation of CD8+ T clones during ageing (Ku CC 2000; Surh CD 2000; Goronzy JJ 2007). The process has not yet been fully understood but it is known that it is regulated by homeostatic cytokines IL15, IL7, CCL19, CCL21, and MHC-signaling which allow T-cells for rapid expansion in the absence of any external stimuli. Interestingly, recent reports have proved that Treg cells are important players in the limitation of homeostatic proliferation of nonregulatory T effector cells (Shen S 2005). Moreover, Treg cells do not undergo homeostatic expansion on their own (Liu W 2006; Seddiki N 2006). In the light of these facts, their accumulation with age might be surprising as the logic indicates that homeostatic proliferation should preferentially give rise to the increased number of CD8+ T clones and, at the same time, keep the number of Treg cells low. The explanation comes from the nature of resistance of Treg cells to the homeostatic mechanism. Namely, Treg cells are devoid of the expression of IL7R (CD127; Liu W 2006; Seddiki N 2006) and therefore, in contrast to other CD4+ T-cells, they do not require IL7 for survival. The level of this homeostatic cytokine declines with age together with the shrinkage of its main producer, the stroma of the thymus and other lymphoid organs (Fry TJ 2001; Aspinall R 2002). Thus, independence from IL7 may be the reason that CD4+ Treg cells, in contrast to non-regulatory CD4+ T-cells, accumulate with age. Making the image complete, CD8+ T clones are able to accumulate in a homeostatic manner even more vigorously than Treg cells because they are not very much dependent on IL7 and utilize IL15 instead (Chiu WK 2006). Importantly, IL2 is prerequisite for Treg cells to inhibit homeostatic proliferation of other T-cells (Murakami M 2002). In this regard, the role of Treg cells in the suppression of homeostatic proliferation might be somewhat ambiguous as, on the one hand, Treg cells require IL2 for the limitation of homeostatic proliferation of other cells but, on the other hand, they inhibit production of this cytokine by CD4+ T effectors (Piccirillo CA 2001). It might be possible that beyond some threshold the accumulation of Treg cells may be the reason of self-limitation of their activity due to deprivation of IL2. Reaching this point, Treg cells no longer prevent from homeostatic proliferation of T effectors. Indeed, frail elderly seem to "cross the threshold" as they are characterized by extremely high number of Treg cells concomitantly with deep deficiency of IL2 (Trzonkowski P 2006). It seems that the regulation of homeostatic proliferation by Treg cells was designed by the evolution for short-living individuals. Long-lasting or repetitive stimulation, such as continuous stimulation with pathogens like CMV described widely during ageing, might be capable of destabilization of this regulatory circuit which subsequently results in detrimental expansion of oligoclonal CD8+ T-cells found preferentially in frail elderly.

It is not a long time since the discovery of Tr1 and Th3 cells was made and therefore the data specifically on these two subsets in ageing are scarce yet. Up to date, many questions related to these two suppressive subsets of CD4+ T-cells remain not addressed. In many cases, it is not possible to split up the function of different regulatory subsets of CD4+ T-cells in a given experimental model. Performed studies very often suggest overlapping between phenotype and function of different subsets. The main suppressive cytokines, TGFβ and IL10, are not only secreted by CD4+ T-cells but also by other lymphocytes and nonlymphoid cells and they do not only exert action on immune system but also on other tissues. IL10, in particular, is associated with regulation in ageing as it is often contrasted with proinflammatory activities of IL6 and other proinflammatory cytokines reported to be overexpressed in the elderly. Polymorphic variant -1082GG of IL10 gene, which is associated with high production of IL10 (Persico M 2006), was found to be preferentially spared in centenarian males (Lio D 2002). Interestingly, animal studies suggest surprisingly well preserved secretion of IL10 in old animals versus young ones in epithelial organs such as intestine and kidney (Hacham M 2004). This finding is consistent with previous reports that IL10, also secreted by Tr1 cells, modulate preferentially mucosal immune responses (Nakagome K 2005; Uhlig HH 2006). The cytokine secreted by Tr1 cells might be also involved in aging of cardiovascular system. High levels of IL10 were found in hearts from old mice during their healthy ageing (Hacham M 2004). Increased expression of IL10 in the wall of aorta after adoptive transfer of Treg cells was found to be an agent slowing down atherosclerosis in apolipoprotein E-knockout mice (Mor A 2007). Involvement of IL10 in the circulatory system was also described in humans where low levels of IL10 were associated with complicated recovery after coronary artery bypass grafting (Wei M 2003). Some other studies did not find age-related differences in the levels of IL10 but pointed at increased levels of soluble form of TGFβ in plasma of the elderly (Forsey RJ 2003). Increased secretion of TGFβ type 1 was revealed in response to elevated levels of IL6, being a counterbalance to proinflammatory activity of the latter (Villiger PM 1993). Both TGFβ type 1 and 2 were found to interfere with IL7 in thymopoiesis which might contribute to faster involution of the thymus (Chantry D 1989). At the periphery, TGFβ was described to suppress many different cells. It seems that apart from inhibitory action on T-cells (Letterio JJ 2000), TGFβ is involved in the inhibition of macrophages, which might be of great importance in the prevention of inflammageing (Erwig LP 1998). High levels of TGFβ in aged individuals appear to be consistent with increased expression of CTLA-4 on T-cells reported in this age group (Wakikawa A 1997; Leng Q 2002). Reciprocal interrelation between TGFβ and CTLA-4 may have some functional implications. Cross-linking of CTLA-4 results in the secretion of TGFβ by CD4+ T-cells (Chen W 1998). On the other hand, TGFβ accelerates the expression of CTLA-4 on T precursors which facilitates transformation of CD4+CTLA-4+ T precursors to adaptive Treg cells (Zheng SG 2006). As mentioned above, TGFβ secreted by regulatory cells must be separated from other sources as, for example, locally decreased production of this factor by fibroblasts was linked to impaired wound healing in the elderly (Kudravi SA 2000). Moreover, soluble form of the cytokine is significantly less functional than that membrane-bound and the level of the latter was found to drop down quite early in life in animal model (Gregg RK 2004). Nevertheless, we still lack the knowledge about age-related differences in the expression of membrane-bound TGFβ in humans.

Despite many efforts, there is no certainty that the accumulation of Treg subsets with age results in oversuppression of the immune system in the elderly. For example, inflammageing, one of the most commonly accepted theories of ageing, contradicts exaggerated immunosuppression in the elderly. Indeed, some reports suggest that the activity of Treg cells declines with age (Tsaknaridis L 2003). Importantly, these studies compare suppressive ability of equal numbers of highly purified Treg cells sorted from either elderly or young subjects in various in vitro suppression assays. In fact, lower responsiveness of Treg cells from the elderly, as compared to the young, in these tests may simply illustrate an impairment of aged Treg cells on a per-cell basis. If the quality of single Treg cell taken from aged subject is not as good as that from the young, it is not surprising that the same number of Treg cells taken from the elderly and the young does not reveal similar suppressive abilities in the assay. The suggestion that per-cell Treg activity from older subject is lower than that from the young is of great importance in the light of reports that local rather than systemic level of Treg cells is associated with clinical outcomes (Liu W 2006). As such, small proportion Treg cells trafficking to the place of local inflammation, might be effective enough in the young but insufficient in the elderly. Bearing in mind this quality issue, the accumulation of Treg cells reported in the elderly may be not necessarily associated with high suppressive abilities but rather recognized as a compensation for their per-cell impaired functioning. Indeed, altered phenotype of Treg cells with age, manifested as low proportion of CD45RA+ naïve Treg cells, seems to prove this hypothesis. Another example of impaired "molecular hardware" of aged Treg cells is their inability to undergo apoptosis. It was described mainly in frail elderly and was recognized as a reason of Treg cell accumulation with age (Trzonkowski P 2006). Of note, although the level of Treg cells was revealed to be extremely high in frail elderly, they were unable of efficient action as those patients were the most affected by detrimental effects of inflammageing (Trzonkowski P 2003). It clearly indicates that aged Treg cells are somehow defective. It is possible that prolonged exposure to environmental factors throughout the lifespan might be responsible for defects of Treg cells. Such environmental influence in the elderly was already described as a cause of damage of naïve CD4+ T-cells (Haynes L 2002).

Although accumulation of Treg cells was not found to be faster in any gender, some specific physiological milestones of human life were linked with sudden increase or decrease in the suppressive activity of Treg cells, notably per-cell Treg cell activity. The best described effects are associated with pregnancy when Treg mediated suppression increases in order to tolerate foetal tissues (Aluvihare VR 2004; Somerset DA 2004). However, slightly increased suppressive activity can be also detected during each and every luteal phase of menstrual cycle being interpreted as an action facilitating implantation of the embryo (Mysliwska J 2000; Trzonkowski P 2001). It is very likely that protolerant action of Treg cells towards embryonic tissues is the most pronounced locally. For example, primary idiopathic infertility is associated with low density of Treg cells in endometrium (Jasper MJ

2006). Obviously, the activity of Treg cells in these phenomena is driven by sex hormones, notably oestradiol (Prieto GA 2006). No surprise, fading hormonal activity around menopause is associated with loss of per-cell Treg activity that tips the effector/suppressor balance in favor of the former (Rachon D 2002; Arruvito L 2007). For example, a peak of some Th1-dependent autoimmune diseases associated with menopause in women, such as rheumatoid arthritis, might be triggered by decreased per-cell activity of Treg cells (Ehrenstein MR 2004). Somehow similar effects, but less clear, were also described for androgens (Page ST 2006). Importantly, also other steroid hormones, both endogenous and administered as drugs, are known to keep proper physiological activity of Treg cells (Fattorossi A 2005).

In general, the discussion about suppression in immune system should take into account effector/suppressor balance rather than suppressors only. It might be of special interest in the elderly, where the activation of immune system is prolonged and elevated. Namely, it was found in animal model that Treg cells generated throughout life regulate weak to moderate immune responses mediated by T effector cells. On the other hand, strong stimulation of T effector cells could not be stopped by endogenous Treg cells and only adoptive transfer of relatively high number of Treg cells specific to the stimulus was able to limit the response (Billiard F 2006). Are these conditions adaptable in humans? Would it be possible that we are able to control our immune responses to some level and when the input of activatory signals is too high or too long, like in the case of inflammageing and CMV, endogenous Treg cells are no longer capable of control over T effectors? Some experimental data answers in the affirmative. Some factors associated with inflammation may turn the effector/suppressor balance in favor of exaggerated effector responses. Proinflammatory cytokines, such as TNFα and IL6 were described as strong inhibitors of Treg cell function (Valencia X 2006; Wan S 2007). Bearing in mind that inflammageing is associated with extremely high production of TNFα and IL6, it is not surprising that above some threshold Treg cells in the elderly are no longer able to counteract inflammation. Moreover, recently discovered strong proinflammatory subset of CD4+ T-cells, Th17 cells, were found to have common ties with Treg cells on a very early stage of development. Th17 cells exert their actions mainly through secreted members of IL17 family cytokines, which are very strong stimulators of inflammatory responses (Veldhoen M 2006). In the extreme, as it comes from animal models, they may be involved in the development of chronic inflammation and autoimmune diseases (Romagnani S 2006). Pathways leading to transition of precursor cells to either Treg cells or Th17 cells were proved to have some common features. Like in the case of adaptive Treg cells, the generation of Th17 cells requires TGFβ (Bettelli E 2006; Veldhoen M 2006). However, the transition to Th17 cells needs also the addition of IL6. The secretion of IL6 by DC stimulated with lipopolysaccharide, in the presence of TGFβ, was necessary to generate Th17 cells. Interestingly Treg cells could be a source of TGFβ in this process and secretion of TGFβ by Treg cells in the presence of IL6 results inevitably in the generation of Th17 cells and not Treg cells. Other inflammatory stimuli, TNFα and IL1, were not necessary but strongly enhanced this process (Veldhoen M 2006). Moreover, activated Treg cells could themselves differentiate into Th17 cells in the presence of IL6 (Xu L

2007). This mechanism of regulation is of special importance in the elderly, where inflammageing phenomena may easily add inflammatory stimuli to those secreted by Treg cells and generate Th17 cells and disturb effector/suppressor balance. Ironically, accumulation of Treg cells in frail elderly would not prevent from inflammageing but rather gave more signals necessary to generate Th17 cells.

2.3   Infectious Diseases

The accumulation of Treg cells with age is an attractive explanation of commonly known susceptibility to infections and high incidence of some tumours among the elderly. However, regulation mediated by suppressive mechanisms should not be always treated as a "pure evil." Effective regulation seems to be inevitable to focus immune response on the pathogen clearance and not on unnecessary exaggerated inflammation leading to destruction of self tissues. For example, lack of IL10-dependent regulatory circuit, as shown in IL10-deficient mice, was responsible for high sensitivity to lysteriosis (Deckert M 2001), gram-negative peritonitis (Sewnath ME 2001) or chronic active *Helicobacter pylori* gastritis (Chen W 2001). TLR4-defective mice were also found to be highly susceptible to infection with *Bordetella pertussis* due to low production of IL10 (Higgins SC 2003). In all those models immune response was fulminant and led to a damage of self tissues and not to elimination of invading pathogen.

Of note, TLR-dependent activity is the example of yet another way of regulation of antipathogen responses by Treg cells. It has been only recently found that Treg cells are able to directly sense pathogens through expressed TLR receptors (TLR4, TLR5, TLR8 in humans; Caramalho I 2003). Signals received by Treg cells through at least some of those receptors (TLR2 in mice and TLR8 in humans) were found to decrease suppressive abilities of those cells at the time of acute infection which allowed for effective immune response. However, the same signals promoted proliferation of Treg cells. Thus, it is hypothesized that TLR-dependent regulation makes the activity of Treg cells low during pathogen clearance and, at the same time, promotes the generation of expanded clones of Treg cells that attenuate potentially harmful responses of residual T effectors left when the infection is gone (Peng G 2005; Sutmuller RP 2006). The delay in TLR-stimulated activity of Treg cells, as compared to other subsets regulated by TLR stimulation, comes from the fact that Treg cells need much stronger signals (more microbial products) than other immune cells to be activated via TLR receptors (Raghavan S 2005). In the light of this mechanism, repetitive infections may explain accumulation of suppressive Treg cells with age. It might be relevant in the clinic as some authors tempt to speculate that the protection from atopic diseases in adults might be linked to increased frequency of regulatory cells generated during frequent infections with some pathogens during childhood (Braun-Fahrlander C 2002; Yazdanbakhsh M 2002). It is possible that it is yet another example of "short-sightedness of evolution," when the mechanism good for young individuals might be disastrous in the elderly. At some point, accumulation of Treg cells may become detrimental as it leads to insufficient responses to new infectious challenges, which results in chronic nature of infections in the elderly or, in the worst case, can prove fatal.

As already mentioned, Treg cells are capable of inhibition of the variety of immune cells. The suppression of effector cells, when affects somehow deteriorated T-cells in the elderly, might be a reason of too weak effector responses. Looking into the spectrum of cells suppressed by Treg cells it is not surprising that Th1 responses are the most depressed. Treg cells suppress efficiently cells with abilities to exert cytotoxic effect, such as CTL, NK and macrophages. Thus, infections that are cleared by cellular type of immunity, where cytotoxic activity is crucial, are more difficult to control in patients with increased activity of Treg cells. It is very much important in the elderly. Treg cells, mainly nTreg cells, make infections chronic by decreasing cytotoxic abilities of effectors as revealed in persistent infections caused by *Hepatitis C virus, Herpes simplex virus* and CMV (Boettler T 2005; Vahlenkamp TW 2005). Involvement of those cells was also described in some other infections known to be associated with deteriorated immunity in ageing, such as candidiasis (Netea MG 2004), tuberculosis (Chen X 2007) or pneumocystis pneumonia (McKinley L 2006).

2.4 Tumors

Increased frequency of tumors is recognized as another consequence of increased frequency of Treg cells in the elderly (Sharma S 2006). The presence of Treg cells associated with tumors might be extremely dangerous in aged individuals as a high proportion of those cells recognize self-antigens. As such, these cells mediate tolerance also to aplastic self tissue of growing tumors, which additionally hampers immune response compromised already by ageing. Accumulation of Treg cells was revealed in a wide variety of tumors of different origin (Betts GJ 2006). Some of the studies managed even to correlate increasing level of Treg cells with disease progression and patient survival (Curiel TJ 2004; Wolf D 2005). Importantly, high number of the studies reported increased number of Treg cells in cancer, predominant type of tumors in the elderly (De Pinho RA 2000). The most convincing link between Treg cells and tumor immunity comes from the studies on NK cells. NK cells are one of the most important elements of immune surveillance against tumors. It is remarkable that aged individuals characterized by low activity of NK cells are at higher risk of cancer onset when compared to those with high NK activity (Imai K 2000). It has been described that Treg cells, mainly nTreg cells, are strong inhibitors of NK cells (Trzonkowski P 2004). Utilizing membrane-bound TGFβ, Treg cells inhibit cytotoxic activity of NK cells in the site of tumor as well as in local lymph nodes and peripheral blood. Importantly, the effect appeared to be quite universal as it was found against gastrointestinal stroma tumors (GIST), melanoma, different types of cancer and, leukaemia cells in both humans and animals (Wolf AM 2003; Ghiringhelli F 2005; Smyth MJ 2006). Apart from NK cells, also CD8+ T-cells were found to be directly inhibited by Treg cells within the tumor mass (Curiel TJ 2004).

It might be also possible that tumor environment on its own is able to induce regulatory cells from naïve precursors. For example, it is widely known that many tumors secrete TGFβ necessary to transform naïve T-cells to Treg cells. Consistent with this finding, tumor-infiltrating Treg cells are mainly Tr1 and Th3 cells which suppress effector cells via secreted cytokines (Chacrabarty NG 1999; Liyanage UK 2002). Moreover, some tumor cells and tumor-infiltrating inflammatory cells secrete chemokines, such as CCL22, attracting Treg cells to the site of tumor (Curiel TJ 2004).

Some anti-tumor drugs were confirmed to have an impact on Treg cells. Small dose of cyclophosphamide was confirmed to induce selective apoptosis of Treg cells in humans and animals (Ghiringhelli F 2004; Lutsiak ME 2005). Similar effect was also described after administration of another oncological drug, fludarabine (Beyer M 2005). There are also attempts of more specific immunotherapy targeting Treg cells. For example, depletion of those cells resulted in a better immune response to tumors or when performed prior to the administration of ant-itumor vaccines, enhanced effects of anti-tumor vaccines against cancer cells in animals (Dannull J 2005; Nair S 2007). It is of special importance in the elderly as the effectiveness of anti-tumor vaccines in preclinical models was revealed to be low at this age and there are suggestions that age-associated accumulation of adaptive Treg cells might have been responsible for this effect (Gravekamp C 2007).

2.5 Autoimmunity

The role of Treg cells in the elderly is intriguing when autoimmunity is taken into account. It is surprising that there is an accumulation of Treg cells and, at the same time, the incidence of autoimmune phenomena during ageing is higher than during earlier ontogeny (Stacy S 2002). Nevertheless, there are few characteristic features of autoimmunity in aged individuals, which may explain this apparent paradox. First important feature is the hormonal introduction to senescence. Menopause, and less evident andropause, are associated with a peak of incidence of some autoimmune diseases, mainly those Th1-dependent like rheumatoid arthritis or Hashimoto's thyroiditis. As already mentioned, lack of hormonal protection starting with menopause (and to a lesser extent with andropause) might be associated with a decrease in regulatory function of Treg cells which facilitates the onset of such disorders (Arruvito L 2007). Later phases of senescence are more associated with Th2-dependent autoimmunity. Shrunk naïve compartment and cytokine balance skewed towards Th2 cytokines makes B memory cells the leading cause of autoimmune phenomena in the elderly. Of note, the control provided by Treg cells over B cells, notably over B memory cells, is very much limited. It is rather indirect suppression as Treg cells regulate mainly CD4+ T helper cells cooperating with B cells (Guay HM 2007). Moreover, as B memory cells are less dependent on signals from CD4+ T helper cells than their naïve precursors, therefore B memory cells are the least affected by Treg cells. Hence, a wide variety of autoantibodies can be found in the elderly (Stacy S 2002). Streaking feature of these autoantibodies is that the vast majority of them is not linked to any autoimmune disease and seem to be not interfering with the health status (Xavier RM 1995; Nilsson BO 2006). It might be possible that, like during earlier life, crucial immunodominant self antigens are still protected from autoaggression in the elderly. Obviously, accumulation of Treg cells is relevant for this regulation but it is not the only event contributing to this phenomenon (Specht C 2003). Increased proportion of CD5+ B1 cells and elevated level of antiidiotypic antibodies together with low affinity and avidity of autoantibodies in aged individuals is probably more important in this regulation (Doria G 1978; Arreaza EE 1993; Zhao KS 1995).

Although high incidence of autoimmune diseases is noted in the elderly, many of these diseases have started earlier in life and their presence in aged individuals simply reflects the fact that nowadays medicine allows affected individuals reaching the age ≥ 65 years. It has to be stressed that the characteristics of late-onset autoimmune diseases, *i.e.* diseases starting mainly in the elderly, differs from those starting earlier. For example, pernicious anaemia, Sjögren syndrome, myasthenia gravis are relatively slowly progressing as compared to a dramatic course of, occurring mainly in children, diabetes mellitus type I. Taking into account that the pressure of autoimmune phenomena in the elderly is thought to be much higher than that in the young, it seems that immunoregulatory mechanisms in aged individuals might be surprisingly well-preserved. Is it due to the accumulation of Treg cells? Obviously, Treg cells are only a small piece of the puzzle.

2.6   Interventions—Vaccinations

Prophylaxis with vaccines in the elderly is one of the most important medical interventions protecting from exacerbation of symptoms of various medical conditions which very often complicate infections at this age. The most advised for the elderly are anti-influenza and pneumococcal vaccines. As a leading goal of this form of therapy is to transform naïve lymphocytes into specific memory/effector cells, immune alterations associated with immunosenescence make it more difficult than in the young. The accumulation of Treg cells should be considered as a one of such harmful alterations. Treg cells were found to limit postimmunization effector and memory cell numbers (Toka FN 2004; Belkaid Y 2005). Consequently, depletion of Treg cells in animal model resulted in improved immune responses to variety of vaccines (Moore AC 2005). It is clinically relevant in geriatrics as Treg cells accumulate the most in frail elderly, that is, patients at the highest risk of complications, if the vaccination did not protect them from infection (Trzonkowski P 2006). Both serological and cellular protection achieved after anti-influenza vaccination was found to be the lowest in such individuals (Trzonkowski P 2003). The association, at least in case of cellular response, was not a co-incidence but proved interrelation as in vitro studies revealed that the addition of Treg cells to the cultures of CTL or NK cells resulted in the suppression of responses to the vaccine antigens. Cell-to-cell interactions were revealed as the leading mechanism of this suppression (Trzonkowski P 2004). However, in some experimental types of vaccinations, IL10 secreted by Treg cells was the master regulator of immunization efficiency (Stober CB 2005). It has to be mentioned at this point that surprisingly low efficiency of vaccines against some pathogens, mainly parasites, is highly attributed to the effect of immune evasion that involves Treg cells. Namely, parasites protects themselves utilizing host Treg cells that suppress the action of the host effector mechanisms. Such situation during immunization against parasites results in low clinical effectiveness of anti-parasite vaccines (Belkaid Y 2005). Some indirect effects might be also very much relevant to the final outcome of the vaccination. For example, Treg cells may limit production of specific antibodies via suppression of CD4+ T helper cells cooperating with B cells during antigen encounter. As a result, the titer of specific protective antibodies after vaccination is low in patients characterized by high number of Treg cells, that is, mainly frail elderly (Trzonkowski P 2003). Also the fact, that Treg cells are consumers of IL2 might additionally decrease effectiveness of the immunization as this cytokine is necessary to generate protective post-immunization immune memory (Effros RB 1983; Provinciali M 1994). Again, Treg cells make the deficit of IL2 more severe in the group of patients characterized already by the lowest levels of this cytokine, *i.e.* in frail elderly (Trzonkowski P 2003). High number of Treg cells prior to the vaccination is not the only obstacle for efficient responses. It has been shown that immunization on its own, due to the challenge with administered vaccine peptides, generates vaccine-specific Treg cells which may additionally decrease immunization efficiency (Bauer T 2007). Specificity of Treg cells seems to be a key point in obtaining good post-immunization responses. For example, low response of CTL after immunization with immunodominant peptide of *Herpes simplex virus* was attributed to antigen-specific Treg cells. Namely, Treg cells isolated from mice chronically infected with *Herpes simplex virus* were much more potent in the suppression of *anti-herpes* CTL responses than Treg cells obtained from healthy mice (Suvas S 2003). In contrary, there are experimental data from mice which proves that very potent graft-specific Treg cells that keep operational tolerance to transplanted organs in recipient animals are not the obstacle in efficient cytotoxic responses to the challenge with influenza virus antigens as these antigens are different from those expressed by the graft (Bushell A 2005).

Interestingly, in some models Treg cells were required to receive efficient postimmunization responses. For example, depletion of Treg cells was associated with poor antibody responses to the vaccination and subsequent challenge with *Borrelia burgdorferi* (Nardelli DT 2006). Another interesting mode of regulation, in which regulatory T-cells are necessary to maintain post-immunization immune memory, is provided by the hypothesis of anti-idiotypic T-cells. This theory states that after a challenge with a given peptide, CD4+ T-cells create a network of idiotypic /anti-idiotypic T-cells (to some extent it is similar to Jerne's idiotypic network of antibodies; Nayak R 2001). According to this theory, antiidiotypic T-cells were in fact antigen-specific Treg cells, which presence was necessary to maintain long-term immune memory within both B and T subsets (Nayak R 2001; Lal G 2006). Some dysfunctionalities in this complex network over years of life might have been responsible for insufficient responses to vaccines in the elderly.

2.7   Interventions—Transplantation

Modern medicine has reached the point when the barrier of age is less important and even high-level invasive medical procedures are considered to be applied in the elderly. It is the most obvious in transplantation, which significance in geriatrics increases parallel with increasing number of elderly patients that received transplanted cells or organs. It is not a long time since modern drugs harnessed the major problem in transplantation, that is, incidence of acute rejections. Yet, their action is associated with many severe adverse effects which limit their use. It is of special importance in the elderly, in whom their administration may additionally deteriorate existing medical conditions or, in some cases, it is precluded due to insufficiency of organs taking part in their metabolism. Thus, dose reduction, application of novel less toxic drugs or tolerance induction strategies are one of the primary goals of nowadays transplantation. Fortunately, immunity compromised with age can be considered as an ally in these strategies. There are number of organs which have been reported to be better tolerated in the elderly as compared to the young after transplantation. Lower incidence of acute rejections in the elderly was reported in kidney, liver, heart, lung and corneal transplantations (Renlund DG 1987; Snell GI 1993; Vail A 1997; Zetterman RK 1998; Bradley BA 2000). While the majority of these studies are based on limited number of patients, renal transplantations can be analyzed with great statistical accurateness due to the widespread of this procedure. The analysis of around 80, 000 cases from the United Network of Organ Sharing (transplant registry in the US) fully confirmed that the level of acute rejections is lower in the elderly and the dose of immunosuppressive drugs in the elderly might be reduced (Bradley BA 2001, 2002). The need for reduced immunosuppression protocols in the elderly is urgent as the majority of posttransplant deaths at this age is associated with exacerbated circulatory diseases, tumors and infections, which are clear adverse effects of overimmunosuppression (Bradley BA 2001; Dębska-Ślizień A 2007). No doubt, accumulation of Treg cells with age may contribute to the deterioration of immunity and better transplantation outcomes in the elderly. Importantly, the action and number of Treg cells is modified with the use of particular immunosuppressive drugs which might have implications in establishing of immunosuppression protocols. For example glicocorticosteroids and mTOR inhibitors have been found to increase the number and function of Treg cells (Fattorossi A 2005; Game DS 2005), while calcineurin inhibitors depressed the activity of those cells (Zeiser R 2006). Of note, mTOR inhibitors are superior above other immunosuppressants as they have less adverse effects. This feature can make mTOR inhibitors a "drug-of-choice" in the elderly (Halloran PF 2004). Also the dose of strong and toxic calcineurin inhibitors can be reduced in the elderly as it was found that aged T-cells activated with alloantigens are less resistant to these drugs than T-cells from young recipients (Bradley BA 2001b). Surprisingly, the incidence of chronic rejections, currently known as chronic allograft nephropathy (CAN), is higher in the elderly than in the young. The most widely described cause of CAN is oversecretion of TGFβ (Suthanthiran M 1997). As already mentioned, the level of this cytokine is increased in the elderly but, apart from lymphocytes, it is secreted by a variety

Table 1 Regulatory subsets in humans

Subset	Phenotype	Mechanism	Origin
Naturally occurring CD4+ T regulatory cells	CD3+CD4+CD25^{high}FoxP3+ CD127-*	Cell-to-cell contact	Thymus
Adaptive CD4+ T regulatory cells	CD3+CD4+FoxP3+	Cell-to-cell contact	Conversion from nonregulatory CD4+ T-cells at the periphery
CD4+ Tr1 cells	CD3+CD4+IL10+ROG+	via IL10	Conversion from non-regulatory (usually naïve) CD4+ T-cells at the periphery
CD4+ Th3 cells	CD3+CD4+TGFβ+	via TGFβ and sometimes IL10	Conversion from non-regulatory (usually naïve) CD4+ T-cells at the periphery
CD28-CD8+ type 1 T suppressor cells	CD3+CD28-CD8+	Cell-to-cell contact, DC-dependent	Terminally differentiated CD8+ T-cells (generated in vitro by multiple rounds of stimulation with APC)
CD28-CD8+ type 2 T suppressor cells	CD3+CD28-CD8+IL6+IFNγ+	via soluble factors, IL6 and IFNγ required	Terminally differentiated CD8+ T-cells (generated in vitro in 1-week coculture with monocytes, GM-CSF and, IL2)
CD28-CD8+ type 3 T suppressor cells	CD3+CD28-CD8+IL10+	via IL10	Conversion of naïve CD8+ T-cells by IL10-producing plasmacytoid DC
NKT cells	'Classical' NKT: CD56+ CD3+TCRαβ(Vα24i)+ 'Nonclassical' NKT: CD56+CD3+TCRγd(Vγ9/Vd2)+	via IL10, IL13	Thymus
Immature dendritic cells	Lin^{neg}HLA-DR+CD80^{low} CD86^{low} CD83^{low}	Cell-to-cell contact, IL10 and tryptophan deprivation (IDO)	From myeloid and lymphoid precursors
Plasmacytoid dendritic Cells	Lin^{neg}HLA-DR+CD11c^{low}CD123^{high}	Cell-to-cell contact, IL10 and tryptophan deprivation (IDO)	From lymphoid precursors
Cytokine-modulated mature dendritic cells	Lin^{neg}HLA-DR+CD80^{high} CD86^{high}CD83^{high}	IL10, TGFβ, TNFα, GM-CSF, G-CSF, M-CSF, VIP, IL21, thymic stromal lymphopoietin	From immature DC

* Other markers suggested but also expressed on other subsets: GITR+, CTLA-4+, neuropilin1+, CD45RB-, CD103+, CD62L+, CD54+, CD122+, CD134+, CD137+

of nonimmune cells. In transplanted kidney affected by CAN, TGFβ secreted by fibroblasts is suspected to be responsible for fibrosis, medial hyperplasia and therefore vessel narrowing. It is very much possible that proinflammatory activity in the elderly may contribute to CAN as proinflammatory cytokines directly stimulate production of TGFβ and activate mononuclear cells facilitating their trafficking and infiltration of the graft (Bradley BA 2002). Not to mention, that synergistic action of TGFβ and proinflammatory cytokines results in the generation of highly inflammatory Th17 cells. However, it has to be highlighted that pathogenesis of CAN is complex and consists of plenty, also non-immune, factors.

2.8 Interventions—Perspectives

Adoptive transfer or depletion of Treg cells is recognized as a manoeuvre suppressing or improving immune response, respectively. Bearing in mind that one of the major features of immune risk phenotype is a low level of dysfunctional CD4+ T-cells, intervention affecting CD4+ T-cells might be of interest in geriatrics. In theory, depletion of Treg cells can be specifically obtained using anti-CD25 antibody, the drug commonly used during allogeneic transplantations in humans. Although initially confirmed, the depletion was subsequently denied by other reports (Kreijveld E 2007). It was reported in some oncological studies that the administration of the antibody improved anti-tumor responses but did not kill but rather blocked the activity of Treg cells (Fecci PE 2006). On the other hand, the use of other antibodies in humans, such as anti-CD3, anti-CD52, anti-lymphocyte globulin preparations, was reported to induce different subsets of Treg cells (Belghith M 2003; Ciancio G 2005; Lopez M 2006). Currently, a lot of effort has been put into attempts of ex vivo large-scale generation of Treg cells which might be subsequently used as immunosuppressive medication (Tang Q 2006). Apparently, in the light of the fact that Treg cells accumulate in aged subjects, these attempts seem to be irrelevant for the elderly. Nevertheless, aged population is a substantial consumer of various immunosuppressive drugs and therapy with Treg cells is thought to be substantially less toxic alternative to those drugs.

3 Other Regulatory Subsets

3.1 Dendritic Cells

Although CD4+ T-cells are robust in their regulatory abilities, it is not the only subset having such potential. It is not surprising that DC are also considered as they are often the first sensors of pathogen pattern. Their action directs all subsequent responses of the immune system. While mature DC trigger mainly robust effector responses, immature DC have the capability of immunosuppression in order to protect self tissue against uncontrolled effector activity of immune system. DC might be of importance as they seem to be relatively slightly affected by age (Agrawal A 2007). Some known age-dependent alterations in DC functioning, such as low expression of MHC receptors and costimulatory molecules (Shurin MR 2007), make the phenotype of aged DC close to immature tolerogenic DC. Namely, it is widely known that immature DC, that is, DC with low expression of MHC and costimulatory molecules, are capable of induction of anergy in effector T-cells and transition of naïve T-cells to adaptive subsets of Treg cells (Steinbrink K 1997; Steinbrink K 1999; Jonuleit H 2000; Vigoroux S 2004). Immature DC are so effective in this process as they have become a laboratory tool in expansion of Treg cells for therapeutic purposes (Yamazaki S 2006). The mechanism of action of tolerogenic DC is associated with release of IL10 (by DC and adaptive Treg cells stimulated by DC) and expression of indoleamine 2,3-dioxygenase (IDO; Steinbrink K 1999; Munn DH 2002). The latter mechanism is very intriguing as increased expression of this enzyme in immune cells of aged individuals was described as predictive for mortality (Pertovaara M 2006). As lymphocytes require tryptophan for their proper functioning, its deprivation triggered by IDO is recognized as ``immunosuppression by starvation of immune system'' (Mellor AL 1999). In addition, IDO in DC metabolises tryptophan to kynurenines and these products suppress T-cells. To a great extent, anergy of T-cells in such environment is dependent on upregulation of GCN2 kinase in T-cells and induction of adaptive Treg cells (Munn DH 2002; Mellor AL 2003). The activity of the enzyme was found to be increased in late-onset autoimmune diseases and chronic infections (Mellor AL 1999; Pertovaara M 2005). Interestingly, the activity of IDO, including the isoform expressed in immune cells, is associated with serotonin deficit in depression (Cubala WJ 2006). There are assumptions that the enzyme might be an important link between chronic stress, inflammation and neurohormonal alterations in this disease (Muller N 2007). As depression is one of the most important medical conditions in the elderly and serotonin deficit is the target for a very potent group of antidepressive drugs (SSRI), the research upon IDO will for sure find its continuation in the elderly. Recently, a growing attention in the field of immune regulation has been given specifically to immature plasmacytoid DC (PDC or DC2) which were found to be extremely powerful regulators of immune responses. Utilizing IDO-related mechanisms, immature PDC significantly reduce antigen presentation, which leads to immunosuppression (Munn DH 2004). Induction of anergy of CD4+ T-cells by immature PDC occurs in direct cell-to-cell interaction between MHC and TCR receptor which prevents from upregulation of CD40L, and possibly other costimulatory molecules, on T-cells (Kuwana M 2001). Particular relevance of these cells for the clinic comes from the fact that the presence of immature PDC promotes vigorous progression of tumor growth and significantly decreases efficiency of anti-tumor vaccines (Munn DH 2004; Shurin MR 2007). While there is single study that reported no difference in the activity of PDC between young and adult mice (Dakic A 2004), there is still no convincing data on the activity of PDC in aged humans (Shurin MR 2007). It has to be mentioned that mature DC, in some specific conditions, are also capable of immunosuppression. It is mainly due to the action of various cytokines, such as

IL10, TGFβ, TNFα, GM-CSF, G-CSF, M-CSF, VIP, IL21 and, thymic stromal lymphopoietin, that modulate activity of mature DC (Rutella S 2006).

3.2   CD28– CD8+ T-Cells

CD28-CD8+ T-cells, described elsewhere in this book as a substantial burden for immunity in ageing, have some regulatory abilities when cooperate with other immune subsets. Because of that they are often described as T suppressor cells (Ts). Thus, anergy of these cells should be also evaluated in the context of regulation of particular immune responses. First of all, CD28-CD8+ Ts cells are heterogeneous with at least three subsets distinguished already (Filaci G 2002). Ts type 1 cells trigger anergy of CD4+ T effector cells through interaction with DC presenting specific antigens to these effectors (Liu Z 1998). As such, the inhibition is MHC-restricted. Anergy occurs due to the inhibition of expression of CD40 receptor on the surface of DC, which further prevents from upregulation of B7 molecules on DC. Ts type 1 cells also upregulate expression of the immunoglobulin-like transcripts ILT3 and ILT4 on DC (Chang CC 2002). The expression of these transcripts upon stimulation with Ts type 1 cells not only is responsible for anergy of CD4+ T effector cells but also for promotion of adaptive Treg cells (Suciu-Foca N 2005). Ts type 2 cells were generated from CD8+ T-cells in vitro in the presence of monocytes, exogenous IL2 and GM-CSF (Balashov KE 1995). These cells are capable of suppression of cytotoxic cells via secreted cytokines in MHC unrestricted way (Filaci G 2002). Interestingly, IL6 and IFNγ secreted by Ts type 2 cells were indispensable in this mode of suppression (Filaci G 2001). Finally, Ts type 3 cells can be generated by the stimulation of naïve CD8+ T-cells with IL10-producing PDC. Ts type 3 cells acquires then the ability to secrete IL10 on their own and suppress other naïve, but not effector, CD8+ T-cells. IL10 secretion, rather than downregulation of CD28 receptor, is the characteristic feature of Ts type 3 cells. Despite IL10-dependent mode of action, the inhibitory effects appear to be antigen-specific and limited to the antigens presented initially by PDC to Ts type 3 cells (Gilliet M 2002).

   Like in the case of many other elements of immune response, generation of CD28-CD8+ T-cells might be considered profitable during particular infections as these cells control effector cells and prevent from damage of self tissues. On the other hand, frequent infections, accumulation of infectious episodes throughout life or chronic form of infections may result in continuous generation of CD28-CD8+ T-cells which skews effector/ suppression balance during aging towards suppression (Pawelec G 2005). Important way of escape from this age-dependent dysregulation, a kind of "rescue circuit of regulation," might be acquired expression of KIR receptors on CD28-CD8+ T-cells (Abedin S 2005). Unlike the level of intrinsic NKT cells, the level of NK-like T-cells expressing KIR receptors is increased in aged individuals (Tarazona R 2000; Peralbo E 2007). The expression of KIR receptors is not a constant feature of CD28-CD8+ T-cells and becomes evident at late phase of their differentiation (Arlettaz L 2004). Diversity and function of KIR receptors implies that the expression of some of them make CD28-CD8+ T-cells tolerant towards self antigens, while the others are capable of triggering their cytotoxic response. Thus, it is probable that the expression of different sets of KIR receptors might be responsible for fine tuning of the function of CD28-CD8+ T-cells (Abedin S 2005).

3.3 NKT-Cells

Intrinsic NKT-cells are another subset with regulatory abilities. NKT-cells merge the characteristics of T-cells and NK-cells but the facts that the repertoire of their TCR is restricted (invariant Vα and limited diversity of Vβ) and they recognize very limited range of glycolipids, via CD1d on APC cells classically, place them on the border between acquired and innate immunity (Biron CA 2001; Kinjo Y 2005). Their proportion in peripheral blood is small and reaches not more than 2–3% of T-cells. In peripheral tissues they preferentially migrate to the bone marrow and liver, where they constitute 10–20% and 30–40% of T-cells, respectively (Emoto M 2003). The most classically, NKT cells are generated in the thymus and traffic mainly to the liver (Abo T 2000). The number of NKT-cells was found to be increased in aged mice but diminished in the general population of the elderly humans with exception of very old subjects. It might be important for aged immune system that the liver can serve as a site of extrathymic development of NKT-cells which results in increased number of those cells in centenarians (Watanabe H 1996; Miyaji C 2000). Regardless of number discrepancies, it is altered function of NKT-cells that influences substantially the activity of immune system (DelaRosa O 2002; Faunce DE 2005; Peralbo E 2007). On the one hand, NKT-cells were found to control autoimmune diseases, such as diabetes mellitus type I, rheumatoid arthritis, inflammatory bowel disease, systemic sclerosis (Sumida T 1995; Hong S 2001; Lee PT 2002; van Kaer L 2005) and promote tolerance to transplanted organs (Jiang X 2005, 2007), but on the other hand, they significantly improve anti-tumor responses and potentialize efficiency of vaccines (Cui J 1997). These ambiguous results might be explained by the mechanisms of their action, which suggest their regulatory activity (Kronenberg M 2005). When stimulated, they produce both Th1 and Th2 cytokines. Production of Th1 cytokines, mainly IFNγ, is responsible for augmented anti-tumor and viral responses via stimulated NK cells (Cui J 1997), while Th2 cytokines, mainly IL4 and IL10, are responsible for NKT-mediated suppression (Kronenberg M 2005). Ageing is associated with decreased secretion of IFNγ by NKT cells, which is recognized as an important reason of deficits in antiviral and antitumor responses in the elderly (Miyaji C 2000; Mocchegiani E 2004). On the other hand, the secretion of Th2 cytokines, like IL10, remains unchanged or even increases with age (Faunce DE 2005). It seems to be a powerful regulatory mechanism as the secretion of IL10 by NKT cells was found to be a major inducer of tolerance to many allotransplants (Oh K 2005; Jiang X 2007). Moreover, increased suppressive activity of NKT cells stimulate secretion of IL10 by CD4+ and CD8+ T-cells and DC (Jiang X 2007;

Wahl C 2007). NKT cells were also found to suppress CD8+ T-cells via secreted IL13 (Terabe M 2000). However, the most convincing proof of the regulatory activity of NKT cells comes from the fact of reciprocal influence of NKT cells and Treg cells. Some NKT cells were found to secrete IL2 stimulating proliferation of Treg cells (Jiang S 2005). In several models, NKT cells were found to promote oral tolerance via induction of adaptive Treg cells which secreted IL10 and TGFβ (Roelofs-Haarhuis K 2004; Kim HJ 2006). Also the shift towards Th2 cytokines produced by gut-associated NKT cells was revealed to be associated with local increase in the number of Treg cells (Ronet C 2005). In contrary, Treg cells were found to suppress activity of NKT cells in cell-to-cell manner (Azuma T 2003). It is probably relevant in the clinic as the interference of Treg cells with NKT cells was proved to promote enhancement of some tumors (Nishikawa H 2003).

References

Abedin S, Michel JJ, Lemster B, Vallejo AN (2005) "Diversity of NKR expression in aging T cells and in T cells of the aged: the new frontier into the exploration of protective immunity in the elderly." Exp Gerontol 40(7):537–548

Abo T, Kawamura T, Watanabe H (2000) "Physiological responses of extrathymic T cells in the liver." Immunol Rev 174:135–149

Agrawal A, Agrawal S, Gupta S,(2007) "Dendritic cells in human aging." Exp Gerontol 42(5):421–426

Aluvihare VR, Kallikourdis M, Betz AG (2004) "Regulatory T cells mediate maternal tolerance to the fetus." Nat Immunol 5(3):266–271

Arlettaz L, Degermann S, De Rham C, Roosnek E, Huard B (2004) "Expression of inhibitory KIR is confined to CD8+ effector T cells and limits their proliferative capacity." Eur J Immunol 34(12):3413–3422

Arreaza EE, Gibbons JJ, Siskind GW, Weksler ME (1993) "Lower antibody response to tetanus toxoid associated with higher auto-anti-idiotypic antibody in old compared with young humans." Clin Exp Immunol 92(1):169–173

Arruvito L, Sanz M, Banham AH, Fainboim L (2007) "Expansion of CD4+CD25+and FOXP3+ regulatory T cells during the follicular phase of the menstrual cycle: implications for human reproduction." J Immunol 178(4):2572–2578

Aschenbrenner K, D'Cruz LM et al. (2007) "Selection of Foxp3 +regulatory T cells specific for self antigen expressed and presented by Aire+ medullary thymic epithelial cells." Nat Immunol 8(4):351–358

Aspinall R, Andrew D, Pido-Lopez J (2002) "Age-associated changes in thymopoiesis." Springer Semin Immunopathol 24:87–101

Azuma T, Takahashi T, Kunisato A, Kitamura T, Hirai H (2003) "Human CD4+ CD25+ regulatory T cells suppress NKT cell functions." Cancer Res 63(15):4516-4520

Baecher-Allan C, Brown JA, Freeman GJ, Hafler DA. (2001) "CD4+CD25high regulatory cells in human peripheral blood." J Immunol 167:1245–1253

Balashov KE, Khoury SJ, Hafler DA, Weiner HL (1995) "Inhibition of T cell responses by activated human CD8+ T cells is mediated by interferon-gamma and is defective in chronic progressive multiple sclerosis." J Clin Invest 95(6):2711–2719

Barnard JA, Warwick GJ, Gold LI (1993) "Localization of transforming growth factor beta isoforms in the normal murine small intestine and colon." Gastroenterology 105(1):67–73

Battaglia M, Gregori S, Bacchetta R, Roncarolo MG (2006) "Tr1 cells: from discovery to their clinical application." Semin Immunol 18(2):120–127

Bauer T, Günther M, Bienzle U, Neuhaus R, Jilg W (2007) "Vaccination against hepatitis B in liver transplant recipients: pilot analysis of cellular immune response shows evidence of HBsAg-specific regulatory T cells." Liver Transpl 13(3):434–442

Belghith M, Bluestone JA, Barriot S, Megret J, Bach JF, Chatenoud L (2003) "TGF-beta-dependent mechanisms mediate restoration of self-tolerance induced by antibodies to CD3 in overt autoimmune diabetes." Nat Med 9(9):1202–1208

Belkaid Y, Rouse BT (2005) "Natural regulatory T cells in infectious disease." Nat Immunol 6(4):353–360

Bennett CL, Christie J, Ramsdell F, Brunkow ME, Ferguson PJ, Whitesell L, Kelly TE, Saulsbury FT, Chance PF, Ochs HD (2001) "The immune dysregulation, polyendocrinopathy, enteropathy, X-linked syndrome (IPEX) is caused by mutations of FOXP3." Nat Genet 27(1):20–21

Bettelli E, Carrier Y, Gao W et al (2006) "Reciprocal developmental pathways for the generation of pathogenic effector TH17 and regulatory T cells." Nature 441:235–238

Betts GJ, Clarke SL, Richards HE, Godkin AJ, Gallimore AM (2006) "Regulation the immune response to tumours." Adv Drug Deliv Rev 58:948–961

Beyer M, Kochanek M, Darabi K, Popov A, Jensen M, Endl E, Knolle PA, Thomas RK, von Bergwelt-Baildon M, Debey S, Hallek M, Schultze JL (2005) "Reduced frequencies and suppressive function of CD4+CD25hi regulatory T cells in patients with chronic lymphocytic leukemia after therapy with fludarabine." Blood 106(6):2018–2025

Billiard F, Litvinova E, Saadoun D, Djelti F, Klatzmann D, Cohen JL, Marodon G, Salomon BL (2006) "Regulatory and effector T cell activation levels are prime determinants of in vivo immune regulation." J Immunol 177(4):2167–2174

Billingham RE, Brent L, Medawar PB (1953) "Activity acquired tolerance of foreign cells." Nature 172:603–606

Biron CA, Brossay L (2001) "NK cells and NKT cells in innate defense against viral infections." Curr Opin Immunol 13(4):458–464

Boettler T, Spangenberg HC, Neumann-Haefelin C, Panther E, Urbani S, Ferrari C, Blum HE, von Weizsacker F, Thimme R (2005) "T cells with a CD4+CD25+ regulatory phenotype suppress in vitro proliferation of virus-specific CD8+ T cells during chronic hepatitis C virus infection." J Virol 79(12):7860–7867

Bradley BA (2000) "Acute rejection: the impact of recipient age. In: Pawelec G EUCAMBIS: Immunology and ageing in Europe, pp. 77–79. Amsterdam, IOS Press

Bradley BA (2002) "Rejection and recipient age." Transplant Immunol 10:125–132

Bradley BA, Gausul Haque KM, Truman C et al (2001b) "Loss of cyclosporin-resistant allospecific T cells with age." Transplant Proc 33(1–2):1056

Bradley BA, Takemoto S, Gjertson D, Reed E, Cecka M (2001) "Elderly transplant recipients may require less immunosuppression." Transplant Proc 33(1–2):1115–1116

Braun-Fahrlander C et al (2002) "Environmental exposure to endotoxin and its relation to asthma in school-age children." N Engl J Med 347:869–877

Bushell A, Jones E, Gallimore A, Wood K (2005) "The generation of CD25+ CD4+ regulatory T cells that prevent allograft rejection does not compromise immunity to a viral pathogen." J Immunol 174(6):3290–3297

Cao D van Vollenhoven R, Klareskog L, Trollmo C, Malmström V (2004) "CD25brightCD4+ regulatory T cells are enriched in inflamed joints of patients with chronic rheumatic disease." Arthritis Res Ther 6(4):R335–R346

Caramalho I, Lopes-Carvalho T, Ostler D, Zelenay S, Haury M, Demengeot J (2003) "Regulatory T cells selectively express toll-like receptors and are activated by lipopolysaccharide." J Exp Med 197(4):403–411

Chacrabarty NG, Li L, Sporn JR, Kurtzman SH, Ergin MT, Mukherji B (1999) "Emergence of regulatory CD4+ T cell response to repetitive stimulation with antigen-presenting cells in vitro: implications in designing antigen-presenting cell-based tumour vaccines." J Immunol 162:5576–5583

Chang CC, Ciubotariu R, Manavalan JS, Yuan J, Colovai AI, Piazza F, Lederman S, Colonna M, Cortesini R, Dalla-Favera R, Suciu-Foca N (2002) "Tolerization of dendritic cells by T(S) cells: the crucial role of inhibitory receptors ILT3 and ILT4." Nat Immunol 3(3):237–243

Chantry D, Turner M, Feldmann M (1989) "Interleukin 7 (murine pre-B cell growth factor/lymphopoietin 1) stimulates thymocyte growth: regulation by transforming growth factor beta." Eur J Immunol 19(4):783–786

Chen W, Jin W, Hardegen N et al (2003) "Conversion of peripheral CD4+CD25- naive T cells to regulatory T cells by TGFbeta induction of transcription factor FoxP3." J Exp Med 198:1875–1886

Chen W, Jin W, Wahl SM (1998) "Engagement of cytotoxic T lymphocyte-associated antigen 4 (CTLA-4) induces transforming growth factor beta (TGF-beta) production by murine CD4(+) T cells." J Exp Med 188(10):1849–1857

Chen W, Shu D, Chadwick VS (2001) "Helicobacter pylori infection: mechanism of colonization and functional dyspepsia. Reduced colonization of gastric mucosa by Helicobacter pylori in mice deficient in IL10." J Gastroenterol Hepatol 16:377–383

Chen X, Zhou B, Li M, Deng Q, Wu X, Le X, Wu C, Larmonier N, Zhang W, Zhang H, Wang H, Katsanis E (2007) "CD4(+)CD25(+)FoxP3(+) regulatory T cells suppress Mycobacterium tuberculosis immunity in patients with active disease." Clin Immunol 123(1):50–59

Chiu WK, Fann M, Weng NP (2006) "Generation and growth of CD28nullCD8+ memory T cells mediated by IL-15 and its induced cytokines." J Immunol 177(11):7802–7810

Ciancio G, Burke GW, Gaynor JJ, Carreno MR, Cirocco RE, Mathew JM, Mattiazzi A, Cordovilla T, Roth D, Kupin W, Rosen A, Esquenazi V, Tzakis AG, Miller J (2005) "A randomized trial of three renal transplant induction antibodies: early comparison of tacrolimus, mycophenolate mofetil, and steroid dosing, and newer immune-monitoring." Transplantation 80(4):457–465

Cobbold SP (2006) "The hidden truth about gene expression in Tregs: is it what you don't see that counts?" Eur J Immunol 36(6):1360–1363

Cobbold SP, Nolan KF, Graca L, Castejon R, Le Moine A, Frewin M, Humm S, Adams E, Thompson S, Zelenika D, Paterson A, Yates S, Fairchild PJ, Waldmann H (2003) "Regulatory T cells and dendritic cells in transplantation tolerance: molecular markers and mechanisms." Immunol Rev 196:109–124

Cubala WJ, Godlewska B, Trzonkowski P, Landowski J (2006) "Indicators of the persistent proinflammatory activation of the immune system in depression." Psychiatr Pol 40(3): 431–444.

Cui J Shin T, Kawano T, Sato H, Kondo E, Toura I, Kaneko Y, Koseki H, Kanno M, Taniguchi M (1997) "Requirement for Valpha14 NKT cells in IL-12-mediated rejection of tumors." Science 278(5343):1623–1626

Curiel TJ, Coukos G, Zou L, Alvarez X, Cheng P, Mottram P, Evdernon-Hogan M, Conejo-Garcia JR, Zhang L, Burow M, Zhu Y, Wei S, Kryczek I, Daniel B, Gordon L, Myers L, Lackner A, Disis ML, Knutson KL, Chen L, Zou W (2004) "Specific recruitment of regulatory T cells in ovarian carcinoma fosters immune privilege and predicts reduced survival." Nat Med 10:942–949

Dakic A, Shao QX, D'Amico A, O'Keeffe M, Chen WF, Shortman K, Wu L (2004) "Development of the dendritic cell system during mouse ontogeny." J Immunol 172(2):1018–1027

Dannull J, Su Z, Rizzieri D, Yang BK, Coleman D, Yancey D, Zhang A, Dahm P, Chao N, Gillboa E et al (2005) "Enhancement of vaccine-mediated anti-tumour immunity in cancer patients after depletion of regulatory T cells." J Clin Invest 115:3623–3633

De Pinho RA (2000) "The age of cancer." Nature 408:248–254

Deckert M et al (2001) "Endogenous IL10 is required for prevention of a hyperinflammatory intracerebral immune response to Lysteria mnocytogenes meningocephalitis." Infect Immun 69:4561–4571

DelaRosa O, Tarazona R, Casado JG, Alonso C, Ostos B, Pena J, Solana R (2002) "Valpha24+ NKT cells are decreased in elderly humans." Exp Gerontol 37(2–3):213–217

Dębska-Ślizień A, Jankowska MM, Wołyniec W, Ziętkiewicz M, Gortowska M, Moszkowska G, Chamienia A, Zadrożny D, Śledziński Z, Rutkowski B (2007) "A single centre experience of renal transplantation in elderly patients: a paired-kidney analysis." Transplantation 83:1188–1192

Doria G, D'Agostaro G, Poretti A (1978) "Age-dependent variations of antibody avidity." Immunology 35(4):601–611

Effros RB, Waldford RL (1983) "The immune response of aged mice to influenza: diminished T-cell proliferation, IL2 production and cytotoxicity." Cell Immunol 81:298–305

Ehrenstein MR, Evans JG, Singh A, Moore S, Warnes G, Isenberg DA, Mauri C (2004) "Compromised function of regulatory T cells in rheumatoid arthritis and reversal by anti-TNFalpha therapy." J Exp Med 200(3):277–285

Emoto M, Kaufmann SH (2003) "Liver NKT cells: an account of heterogeneity." Trends Immunol 24(7):364–369

Ermann J, Hoffmann P, Edinger M, Dutt S, Blankenberg FG, Higgins JP, Negrin RS, Fathman CG, Strober S (2005) "Only the CD62L+ subpopulation of CD4+CD25+ regulatory T cells protects from lethal acute GVHD." Blood 105(5):2220–2226

Erwig LP, Kluth DC, Walsh GM, Rees AJ (1998) "Initial cytokine exposure determines function of macrophages and renders them unresponsive to other cytokines." J Immunol 161(4):1983–1988

Faria AM, Weiner HL (2005) "Oral tolerance." Immunol Rev 206:232–259

Fattorossi A, Battaglia A, Buzzonetti A, Ciaraffa F, Scambia G, Evoli A (2005) "Circulating and thymic CD4 CD25 T regulatory cells in myasthenia gravis: effect of immunosuppressive treatment." Immunology 116(1):134–141

Faunce DE, Palmer JL, Paskowicz KK, Witte PL, Kovacs EJ (2005) "CD1d-restricted NKT cells contribute to the age-associated decline of T cell immunity." J Immunol 175(5):3102–3109

Fecci PE, Sweeney AE, Grossi PM, Nair SK, Learn CA, Mitchell DA, Cui X, Cummings TJ, Bigner DD, Gilboa E, Sampson JH (2006) "Systemic anti-CD25 monoclonal antibody administration safely enhances immunity in murine glioma without eliminating regulatory T cells." Clin Cancer Res 12(14 Pt 1):4294–4305

Filaci G, Bacilieri S, Fravega M, Monetti M, Contini P, Ghio M, Setti M, Puppo F, Indiveri F (2001) " Impairment of CD8+ T suppressor cell function in patients with active systemic lupus erythematosus." J Immunol 166(10):6452–6457

Filaci G, Suciu-Foca N (2002) "CD8+ T suppressor cells are back to the game: are they players in autoimmunity?" Autoimmun Rev 1(5):279–283

Fontenot JD, Gavin MA, Rudensky AY (2003) "Foxp3 programs the development and function of CD4+CD25+ regulatory T cells." Nat Immunol 4(4):330–336

Forsey RJ, Thompson JM, Ernerudh J, Hurst TL, Strindhall J, Johansson B, Nilsson BO, Wikby A (2003) "Plasma cytokine profiles in elderly humans." Mech Ageing Dev 124(4):487–493

Franceschi C, Bonafe M (2003) "Centenarians as a model for healthy aging." Biochem Soc Trans 31(2):457–461

Fry TJ, Mackall CL (2001) "IL7: Master regulator of T cell homeostasis?" Trends Immunol 22:564–571

Fu S, Yopp AC, Mao X, Chen D, Zhang N, Chen D, Mao M, Ding Y, Bromberg JS (2004) "CD4+ CD25+ CD62+ T-regulatory cell subset has optimal suppressive and proliferative potential." Am J Transplant 4(1):65–78

Fujimoto S, Greene M, Sehon AH (1975) "Immunosuppressor T cells in tumour bearing host." Immunol Commun 4: 201–217

Fukaura H, Kent SC, Pietrusewicz MJ, Khoury SJ, Weiner HL, Hafler DA (1996) "Induction of circulating myelin basic protein and proteolipid protein-specific transforming growth factor-beta1-secreting Th3 T cells by oral administration of myelin in multiple sclerosis patients." J Clin Invest 98(1):70–77

Galliaerde V, Desvignes C, Peyron E, Kaiserlian D (1995) "Oral tolerance to haptens: intestinal epithelial cells from 2,4-dinitrochlorobenzene-fed mice inhibit hapten-specific T cell activation in vitro." Eur J Immunol 25(5):1385–1390

Game DS, Hernandez-Fuentes MP, Lechler RI (2005) "Everolimus and basiliximab permit suppression by human CD4+CD25+ cells in vitro." Am J Transplant 5:454

Gavin MA, Rasmussen JP, Fontenot JD, Vasta V, Manganiello VC, Beavo JA, Rudensky AY (2007) "Foxp3-dependent programme of regulatory T-cell differentiation." Nature 445(7129):771–775

Gershon RK, Kondo SK (1970) "Cell interactions in the induction of tolerance:the role of thymic lymphocytes." Immunology 18:723–737

Ghiringhelli F, Larmonier N, Schmitt E, Parcellier A, Cathelin D, Garrido C, Chauffert B, Solary E, Bonnotte B, Martin F (2004) "CD4+CD25+ regulatory T cells suppress tumor immunity but are sensitive to cyclophosphamide which allows immunotherapy of established tumors to be curative." Eur J Immunol 34(2):336–344

Ghiringhelli F, Ménard C, Terme M, Flament C, Taieb J, Chaput N, Puig PE, Novault S, Escudier B, Vivier E, Lecesne A, Robert C, Blay JY, Bernard J, Caillat-Zucman S, Freitas A, Tursz T, Wagner-Ballon O, Capron C, Vainchencker W, Martin F, Zitvogel L (2005) "CD4+CD25+ regulatory T cells inhibit natural killer cell functions in a transforming growth factor-beta-dependent manner." J Exp Med 202(8):1075–1085

Gilliet M, Liu YJ (2002) "Generation of human CD8 T regulatory cells by CD40 ligand-activated plasmacytoid dendritic cells." J Exp Med 195(6):695–704

Godfrey WR, Spoden DJ, Ge YG, Baker SR, Liu B, Levine BL, June CH, Blazar BR, Porter SB (2005) "Cord blood CD4(+)CD25(+)-derived T regulatory cell lines express FoxP3 protein and manifest potent suppressor function." Blood 105(2):750–758

Gondek DC, Lu LF, Quezada SA, Sakaguchi S, Noelle RJ (2005) "Cutting edge: contact-mediated suppression by CD4+CD25+ regulatory cells involves a granzyme B-dependent, perforin-independent mechanism." J Immunol 174(4):1783–1786

Gorelik L, Constant S, Flavell RA (2002) "Mechanism of TGFbeta-induced inhibition of T helper type 1 differentiation." J Exp Med 195:1499–1505

Goronzy JJ, Lee WW, Weyand CM (2007) " Aging and T-cell diversity." Exp Gerontol 42(5):400–406

Gottenberg JE, Lavie F, Abbed K, Gasnault J, Le Nevot E, Delfraissy JF, Taoufik Y, Mariette X (2005) "CD4 CD25high regulatory T cells are not impaired in patients with primary Sjögren's syndrome." J Autoimmun 24(3):235–242

Gravekamp C (2007) "Cancer vaccines in old age." Exp Gerontol 42(5):441–450

Gregg R, Smith CM, Clark FJ, Dunnion D, Khan N, Chakraverty R, Nayak L, Moss PA (2005) "The number of human peripheral blood CD4+ CD25high regulatory T cells increases with age." Clin Exp Immunol 140(3):540–546

Gregg RK, Jain R, Schoenleber SJ, Divekar R, Bell JJ, Lee HH, Yu P, Zaghouani H (2004) "A sudden decline in active membrane-bound TGF-beta impairs both T regulatory cell function and protection against autoimmune diabetes." J Immunol 173(12):7308–7316

Grohmann U, Puccetti P (2003) "CTLA-4, T helper lymphocytes and dendritic cells: an internal perspective of T-cell homeostasis." Trends Mol Med 9(4):133–135

Grossman WJ, Verbsky JW, Barchet W, Colonna M, Atkinson JP, Ley TJ (2004) "Human T regulatory cells can use the perforin pathway to cause autologous target cell death." Immunity 21(4):589–601

Groux H, O'Garra A, Bigler M, Rouleau M, Antonenko S, de Vries JE, Roncarolo MG (1997) "A CD4+ T-cell subset inhibits antigen-specific T-cell responses and prevents colitis." Nature 389(6652):737–742

Guay HM, Larkin J, Picca CC, Panarey L, Caton AJ (2007) "Spontaneous autoreactive memory B cell formation driven by a high frequency of autoreactive CD4+ T cells." J Immunol 178(8):4793–4802

Hacham M, White RM, Argov S, Segal S, Apte RN (2004) "Interleukin-6 and interleukin-10 are expressed in organs of normal young and old mice." Eur Cytokine Netw 15(1):37–46

Hafler DA, Kent SC, Pietrusewicz MJ, Khoury SJ, Weiner HL, Fukaura H (1997) "Oral administration of myelin induces antigen-specific TGF-beta 1 secreting T cells in patients with multiple sclerosis." Ann N Y Acad Sci 835:120–131

Halloran PF (2004) "Immunosuppressive drugs for kidney transplantation." N Engl J Med 351:2715

Haynes L, Eaton SM, Swain SL (2002) "Effect of age on naive CD4 responses: impact on effector generation and memory development." Springer Sem Immunopathol 24:53–60

Higgins SC et al (2003) "TLR4-mediated innate IL10 activates antigen-specific regulatory T cells and confers resistance to Bordetella pertussis by inhibiting inflammatory pathology." J Immunol 171:3119–3127

Hoffmann P, Eder R, Boeld TJ, Doser K, Piseshka B, Andreesen R, Edinger M (2006) "Only the CD45RA+ subpopulation of CD4+CD25high T cells gives rise to homogeneous regulatory T-cell lines upon in vitro expansion." Blood 108(13):4260-4267

Hoffmann P, Ermann J, Edinger M, Fathman CG, Strober S (2002) "Donor-type CD4(+)CD25(+) regulatory T cells suppress lethal acute graft-versus-host disease after allogeneic bone marrow transplantation." J Exp Med 196(3):389–399

Hong S, Wilson MT, Serizawa I, Wu L, Singh N, Naidenko OV, Miura T, Haba T, Scherer DC, Wei J, Kronenberg M, Koezuka Y, Van Kaer L (2001) "The natural killer T-cell ligand alpha-galactosylceramide prevents autoimmune diabetes in nonobese diabetic mice." Nat Med 7(9):1052–1056

Hori S, Nomura T, Sakaguchi S (2003) "Control of regulatory T cell development by the transcription factor Foxp3." Science 299(5609):1057–1061

Imai K, Matsuyama S, Miyake S, Suga K, Nakachi K (2000) "Natural cytotoxic activity of peripheral blood lymphocytes and cancer incidence: an 11-year follow-up study of a general population." Lancet 356:1795–1799

Jasper MJ, Tremellen KP, Robertson SA (2006) "Primary unexplained infertility is associated with reduced expression of the T-regulatory cell transcription factor Foxp3 in endometrial tissue." Mol Hum Reprod 12(5):301–308

Jiang S, Game DS, Davies D, Lombardi G, Lechler RI (2005) "Activated CD1d-restricted natural killer T cells secrete IL-2: innate help for CD4+CD25+ regulatory T cells?" Eur J Immunol 35(4):1193–1200

Jiang X, Kojo S, Harada M, Ohkohchi N, Taniguchi M, Seino KI (2007) "Mechanism of NKT cell-mediated transplant tolerance." Am J Transplant 7(6):1482–1490

Jiang X, Shimaoka T, Kojo S, Harada M, Watarai H, Wakao H, Ohkohchi N, Yonehara S, Taniguchi M, Seino K (2005) "Cutting edge: critical role of CXCL16/CXCR6 in NKT cell trafficking in allograft tolerance." J Immunol 175(4):2051–2055

Jonuleit H, Schmitt E, Schuler G, Knop J, Enk AH (2000) "Induction of IL10-producing, nonproliferating CD4+ T cells with regulatory properties by repetitive stimulation with allogeneic immature human dendritic cells." J Exp Med 192:183–191

Karim M, Kingsley CI, Bushell AR, Sawitzki BS, Wood KJ (2004) "Alloantigen-induced CD25+CD4+ regulatory T cells can develop in vivo from CD25-CD4+ precursors in a thymus-independent process." J Immunol 172(2):923–928

Kim HJ, Hwang SJ, Kim BK, Jung KC, Chung DH (2006) "NKT cells play critical roles in the induction of oral tolerance by inducing regulatory T cells producing IL-10 and transforming growth factor beta, and by clonally deleting antigen-specific T cells." Immunology 118(1):101–111

Kinjo Y, Wu D, Kim G, Xing GW, Poles MA, Ho DD, Tsuji M, Kawahara K, Wong CH, Kronenberg M (2005) "Recognition of bacterial glycosphingolipids by natural killer T cells." Nature 434(7032):520–525

Kitani A, Chua K, Nakamura K, Strober W (2000) "Activated self-MHC-reactive T cells have the cytokine phenotype of TH3/T regulatory cell 1 T cells." J Immunol 165:691–702

Kitani A, Fuss I, Nakamura K, Kumaki F, Usui T, Strober W (2003) "Transforming growth factor (TGF)-beta1-producing regulatory T cells induce Smad-mediated interleukin 10 secretion that facilitates coordinated immunoregulatory activity and amelioration of TGF-beta1-mediated fibrosis." J Exp Med 198(8):1179–1188

Kreijveld E, Koenen HJ, Klasen IS, Hilbrands LB, Joosten I (2007) "Following anti-CD25 treatment, a functional CD4+CD25+ regulatory T-cell pool is present in renal transplant recipients." Am J Transplant 7(1):249–255

Kretschmer K, Apostolou I, Hawiger D, Khazaie K, Nussenzweig MC, von Boehmer H (2005) "Inducing and expanding regulatory T cell populations by foreign antigen." Nat Immunol 6(12):1219–1227

Kronenberg M (2005) "Toward an understanding of NKT cell biology: progress and paradoxes." Annu Rev Immunol 23:877–900

Ku CC, Kappler J, Marrack P (1997) "Characteristics and maintenance of CD8+ T-cell clones found in old mice." Mech Ageing Dev 94(1–3): 41–53

Ku CC, Murakami M, Sakamoto A, Kappler J, Marrack P (2000) "Control of homeostasis of CD8+ memory T cells by opposing cytokines." Science 288(5466):675–678

Kudravi SA, Reed MJ (2000) "Aging, cancer, and wound healing." In Vivo 14(1):83–92.

Kuwana M Kaburaki J, Wright TM, Kawakami Y, Ikeda Y. (2001). "Induction of antigen-specific human CD4(+) T cell anergy by peripheral blood DC2 precursors." Eur J Immunol 31(9):2547–2557

Lal G, Shaila MS, Nayak R (2006) "Booster immunization of antigen primed mice with anti-idiotypic T cells generates antigen-specific memory T cell response." Vaccine 24(8):1149–1158

Lee PT, Putnam A, Benlagha K, Teyton L, Gottlieb PA, Bendelac A (2002) "Testing the NKT cell hypothesis of human IDDM pathogenesis." J Clin Invest 110(6):793–800

Leng Q, Bentwich Z, Borkow G (2002) "CTLA-4 upregulation during aging." Mech Ageing Dev 123(10):1419–1421

Letterio JJ (2000) "Murine models define the role of TGF-beta as a master regulator of immune cell function." Cytokine Growth Factor Rev 11(1–2):81–87

Levings MK, Gregori S, Tresoldi E, Cazzaniga S, Bonini C, Roncarolo MG (2005) "Differentiation of Tr1 cells by immature dendritic cells requires IL-10 but not CD25+CD4+ Tr cells." Blood 105(3):1162–1169

Lewkowicz P, Lewkowicz N, Sasiak A, Tchorzewski H (2006) "Lipopolysaccharide-activated CD4+CD25+ T regulatory cells inhibit neutrophil function and promote their apoptosis and death." J Immunol177(10):7155–7163

Linsley PS, Brady W, Urnes M, Grosmaire LS, Damle NK, Ledbetter JA (1992) "Coexpression and functional cooperation of CTLA-4 and CD28 on activated T lymphocytes." J Exp Med 176:1595–1599

Lio D, Scola L, Crivello A, Colonna-Romano G, Candore G, Bonafe M, Cavallone L, Franceschi C, Caruso C (2002) "Gender-specific association between -1082 IL-10 promoter polymorphism and longevity." Genes Immun 3(1):30–33

Liu W, Putnam AL, Xu-Yu Z, Szot GL, Lee MR, Zhu S, Gottlieb PA, Kapranov P, Gingeras TR, Fazekas de St Groth B, Clayberger C, Soper DM, Ziegler SF, Bluestone JA (2006) "CD127 expression inversely correlates with FoxP3 and suppressive function of human CD4+ T reg cells." J Exp Med 203(7):1701–1711

Liu Z, Tugulea S, Cortesini R, Suciu-Foca N (1998) "Specific suppression of T helper alloreactivity by allo-MHC class I-restricted CD8+CD28- T cells." Int Immunol 10(6):775–783

Liyanage UK, Moore TT, Joo HG, Tanaka Y, Herrmann V, Doherty G, Drebin JA, Strassberg SM, Eberlein TJ, Goedegebuure PS et al (2002) "Prevalence of regulatory T cells is increased in peripheral blood and tumor microenvironment of patients with pancreas or breast adenocarcinoma." J Immunol 169:2756–2761

Lopez M, Clarkson MR, Albin M, Sayegh MH, Najafian N (2006) "A novel mechanism of action for anti-thymocyte globulin: induction of CD4+CD25+Foxp3 +regulatory T cells." J Am Soc Nephrol 17(10):2844–2853

Lutsiak ME, Semnani RT, De Pascalis R, Kashmiri SV, Schlom J, Sabzevari H (2005) "Inhibition of CD4(+)25+ T regulatory cell function implicated in enhanced immune response by low-dose cyclophosphamide." Blood 105(7):2862–2868

Marski M, Kandula S, Turner JR, Abraham C (2005) "CD18 is required for optimal development and function of CD4+CD25+ T regulatory cells." J Immunol 175(12):7889–7897

Masteller EL, Tang Q, Bluestone JA (2006) "Antigen-specific regulatory T cells—ex vivo expansion and therapeutic potential." Semin Immunol 18(2):103–110

McKinley L, Logar AJ, McAllister F, Zheng M, Steele C, Kolls JK (2006) "Regulatory T cells dampen pulmonary inflammation and lung injury in an animal model of pneumocystis pneumonia." J Immunol 177(9):6215–6226

Mellor AL, Baban B, Chandler P, Marshall B, Jhaver K, Hansen A, Koni PA, Iwashima M, Munn DH (2003) "Induced indoleamine 2,3 dioxygenase expression in dendritic cell subsets suppresses T cell clonal expansion." J Immunol 171(4):1652–1655

Mellor AL, Keskin DB, Johnson T, Chandler P, Munn DH (2002) "Cells expressing indoleamine 2,3-dioxygenase inhibit T cell responses." J Immunol 168(8):3771–3776

Mellor AL, Munn DH (1999) "Tryptophan catabolism and T-cell tolerance: immunosuppression by starvation?" Immunol Today 20:469–473

Miyaji C, Watanabe H, Toma H, Akisaka M, Tomiyama K, Sato Y, Abo T (2000) "Functional alteration of granulocytes, NK cells, and natural killer T cells in centenarians." Hum Immunol 61(9):908–916

Mocchegiani E, Giacconi R, Cipriano C, Gasparini N, Bernardini G, Malavolta M, Menegazzi M, Cavalieri E, Muzzioli M, Ciampa AR, Suzuki H (2004) "The variations during the circadian cycle of liver CD1d-unrestricted NK1.1+TCR gamma/delta+ cells lead to successful ageing. Role of metallothionein/IL-6/gp130/PARP-1 interplay in very old mice." Exp Gerontol 39(5):775–788

Moore AC, Gallimore A, Draper SJ, Watkins KR, Gilbert SC, Hill AV (2005) "Anti-CD25 antibody enhancement of vaccine-induced immunogenicity: increased durable cellular immunity with reduced immunodominance." J Immunol 175(11):7264–7273

Moore KW, de Waal Malefyt R, Coffman RL, O'Garra A (2001) "Interleukin 10 and the interleukin 10 receptor." Annu Rev Immunol 19:683–765

Mor A, Planer D, Luboshits G, Afek A, Metzger S, Chajek-Shaul T, Keren G, George J (2007) "Role of naturally occurring CD4+ CD25+ regulatory T cells in experimental atherosclerosis." Arterioscler Thromb Vasc Biol 27(4):893–900

Muller N, Schwarz MJ (2007) "The immune-mediated alteration of serotonin and glutamate: towards an integrated view of depression." Mol Psychiatry (in press)

Munn DH, Sharma MD, Hou D, Baban B, Lee JR, Antonia SJ, Messina JL, Chandler P, Koni PA, Mellor AL (2004) "Expression of indoleamine 2,3-dioxygenase by plasmacytoid dendritic cells in tumor-draining lymph nodes." J Clin Invest 114(2):280–290

Munn DH, Sharma MD, Lee JR, Jhaver KG, Johnson TS, Keskin DB, Marshall B, Chandler P, Antonia SJ, Burgess R, Slingluff CL Jr, Mellor AL (2002) "Potential regulatory function of human dendritic cells expressing indoleamine 2,3-dioxygenase." Science 297(5588):1867–1870

Murakami M, Sakamoto A, Bender J, Kappler J, Marrack P (2002) "CD25+CD4+ T cells contribute to the control of memory CD8+ T cells." Proc Natl Acad Sci 99(13):8832–8837

Mysliwska J, Trzonkowski P, Bryl E, Lukaszuk K, Mysliwski A (2000) " Lower interleukin-2 and higher serum tumor necrosis factor-a levels are associated with perimenstrual, recurrent, facial Herpes simplex infection in young women." Eur Cytokine Netw 11(3):397–406

Nair S, Boczkowski D, Fassnacht M, Pisetsky D, Gilboa E (2007) "Vaccination against the forkhead family transcription factor Foxp3 enhances tumor immunity." Cancer Res 67(1):371–380

Nakagome K, Dohi M, Okunishi K, Komagata Y, Nagatani K, Tanaka R, Miyazaki J, Yamamoto K (2005) "In vivo IL-10 gene delivery suppresses airway eosinophilia and hyperreactivity by down-regulating apc functions and migration without impairing the antigen-specific systemic immune response in a mouse model of allergic airway inflammation " J Immunol 174:6955–6966

Nakamura K, Kitani A, Strober W (2001) "Cell contact-dependent immunosuppression by CD4(+)CD25(+) regulatory T cells is mediated by cell surface-bound transforming growth factor beta." J Exp Med1 94(5):629–644

Nardelli DT, Warner TF, Callister SM, Schell RF (2006) "Anti-CD25 antibody treatment of mice vaccinated and challenged with Borrelia spp. does not exacerbate arthritis but inhibits borreliacidal antibody production." Clin Vaccine Immunol 13(8):884–891

Nayak R, Mitra-Kaushik S, Shaila MS (2001) "Perpetuation of immunological memory: a relay hypothesis." Immunology 102(4):387–395

Netea MG, Sutmuller R, Hermann C, Van Der Graaf CA, Van Der Meer JW, van Krieken JH, Hartung T, Adema G, Kullberg BJ (2004) "Toll-like receptor 2 suppresses immunity against Candida albicans through induction of IL-10 and regulatory T cells." J Immunol 172(6):3712–3718

Nilsson BO, Skogh T, Ernerudh J, Johansson B, Löfgren S, Wikby A, Dahle C (2006) "Antinuclear antibodies in the oldest-old women and men." J Autoimmun 27(4):281–288

Nishikawa H, Kato T, Tanida K, Hiasa A, Tawara I, Ikeda H, Ikarashi Y, Wakasugi H, Kronenberg M, Nakayama T, Taniguchi M, Kuribayashi K, Old LJ, Shiku H (2003) "CD4+ CD25+ T cells responding to serologically defined autoantigens suppress antitumor immune responses." Proc Natl Acad Sci 100(19):10902–10906

North RJ, Bursuker I (1984) "Generation and decay of the immune response to a progressive fibrosarcoma.I.Ly-1 + 2 – suppressor T cells downregulate the generation of Ly-1 –2 + effector T cells." J Exp Med 159:1295–1311

O'Neill EJ et al (2004) "Natural and induced regulatory T cells." Ann N Y Acad Sci 1029:180–192

Ochi H, Abraham M, Ishikawa H, Frenkel D, Yang K, Basso AS, Wu H, Chen ML, Gandhi R, Miller A, Maron R, Weiner HL (2006) "Oral CD3-specific antibody suppresses autoimmune encephalomyelitis by inducing CD4+ CD25- LAP+ T cells." Nat Med 12(6):627–635

Oh K, Kim S, Park SH, Gu H, Roopenian D, Chung DH, Kim YS, Lee DS (2005) "Direct regulatory role of NKT cells in allogeneic graft survival is dependent on the quantitative strength of antigenicity." J Immunol 174(4):2030–2036

Owen RD (1945) "Immunogenetic consequences of vascular anastomoses between bovine twins." Science 102:400–401

Page ST, Plymate SR, Bremner WJ, Matsumoto AM, Hess DL, Lin DW, Amory JK, Nelson PS, Wu JD (2006) "Effect of medical castration on CD4 +CD25+ T cells, CD8+ T cell IFN-gamma expression, and NK cells: a physiological role for testosterone and/or its metabolites." Am J Physiol Endocrinol Metab 290(5):E856–E863

Pawelec G, Akbar A, Caruso C, Solana R, Grubeck-Loebenstein B, Wikby A (2005) "Human immunosenescence: is it infectious?" Immunol Rev 205:257–268

Peng G, Guo Z, Kiniwa Y, Voo KS, Peng W, Fu T, Wang DY, Li Y, Wang HY, Wang RF (2005) "Toll-like receptor 8-mediated reversal of CD4+ regulatory T cell function." Science 309(5739):1380–1384

Peralbo E, Alonso C, Solana R (2007) "Invariant NKT and NKT-like lymphocytes: Two different T cell subsets that are differentially affected by ageing." Exp Gerontol (in press)

Persico M, Capasso M, Persico E, Masarone M, Renzo A, Spano D, Bruno S, Iolascon A (2006) "Interleukin-10 - 1082 GG polymorphism influences the occurrence and the clinical characteristics of hepatitis C virus infection." J Hepatol 45(6):779–785

Pertovaara M, Raitala A, Lehtimäki T, Karhunen PJ, Oja SS, Jylhä M, Hervonen A, Hurme M (2006) "Indoleamine 2,3-dioxygenase activity in nonagenarians is markedly increased and predicts mortality." Mech Ageing Dev 127(5):497–499

Pertovaara M, Raitala A, Uusitalo H, Pukander J, Helin H, Oja SS, Hurme M (2005) "Mechanisms dependent on tryptophan catabolism regulate immune responses in primary Sjögren's syndrome." Clin Exp Immunol 142(1):155–161

Piccirillo CA, Shevach EM (2001) "Control of CD8+ T cell activation by CD4+CD25+ immunoregulatory cells." J Immunol 167:1137–1140

Prieto GA, Rosenstein Y (2006) "Oestradiol potentiates the suppressive function of human CD4 CD25 regulatory T cells by promoting their proliferation" Immunology 118(1):58–65

Provinciali M, Di Stefano G, Colombo M, Della Croce F, Gandolfi MC, Daghetta L, Anichini M, Della Bitta R, Fabris NM (1994) "Adjuvant effect of low-dose interleukin2 on antibody response to influenza virus vaccination in healthy elderly subjects." Mech Ageing Dev 77:75–82

Rachon D, Mysliwska J, Suchecka-Rachon K, Wieckiewicz J, Mysliwski A (2002) "Effects of oestrogen deprivation on interleukin-6 production by peripheral blood mononuclear cells of postmenopausal women." J Endocrinol 172(2):387–395

Raghavan S, Holmgren J (2005) "CD4+CD25+ suppressor T cells regulate pathogen induced inflammation and disease." FEMS Immunol Med Microbiol 44(2):121–127

Renlund DG, Gilbert EM, O'Connell JB et al (1987) "Age-associated decline in cardiac allograft rejection." Am J Med 83(3):391–398

Roelofs-Haarhuis K, Wu X, Gleichmann E (2004) "Oral tolerance to nickel requires CD4+ invariant NKT cells for the infectious spread of tolerance and the induction of specific regulatory T cells." J Immunol 173(2):1043–50

Romagnani S (2006) "Regulation of the t cell response." Clin and Exp Allergy 36:1357–1366

Ronet C, Darche S, Leite de Moraes M, Miyake S, Yamamura T, Louis JA, Kasper LH, Buzoni-Gatel D (2005) "NKT cells are critical for the initiation of an inflammatory bowel response against Toxoplasma gondii." J Immunol 175(2):899–908

Rutella S, Danese S, Leone G (2006) "Tolerogenic dendritic cells: cytokine modulation comes of age." Blood 108(5):1435–1440

Sakaguchi S, Sakaguchi N, Asano M, Itoh M, Toda M (1995) " Immunologic self-tolerance maintained by activated T cells expressing IL-2 receptor alpha-chains (CD25). Breakdown of a single mechanism of self-tolerance causes various autoimmune diseases." J Immunol 155(3):1151–1164

Sansom DM, Walker LS (2006) "The role of CD28 and cytotoxic T-lymphocyte antigen-4 (CTLA-4) in regulatory T-cell biology." Immunol Rev 212:131–148

Saurwein-Teissl M, Blasko I, Zisterer K, Neuman B, Lang B, Grubeck-Loebenstein B (2000) "An imbalance between pro- and anti-inflammatory cytokines, a characteristic feature of old age." Cytokine 12(7):1160–1161

Seddiki N, Santner-Nanan B, Martinson J, Zaunders J, Sasson S, Landay A, Solomon M, Selby W, Alexander SI, Nanan R, Kelleher A, Fazekas de St Groth B (2006) "Expression of interleukin (IL)-2 and IL-7 receptors discriminates between human regulatory and activated T cells." J Exp Med 203(7):1693–1700

Seddiki N, Santner-Nanan B, Tangye SG, Alexander SI, Solomon M, Lee S, Nanan R, Fazekas de Saint Groth B (2006) " Persistence of naive CD45RA +regulatory T cells in adult life." Blood 107(7):2830–2838

Sewnath ME et al (2001) "IL10-deficient mice demonstrate multiple organ failure and increased mortality during Escherichia coli peritonitis despite an accelerated bacterial clearance." J Immunol 166:6323–6331

Sharma S, Dominguez AL, Lustgarten J (2006) "High accumulation of T regulatory cells prevents the activation of immune responses in aged animals." J Immunol 177(12):8348–8355

Shen S, Ding Y, Tadokoro CE, Olivares-Villagomez D, Camps-Ramirez M, Curotto de Lafaille MA, Lafaille JJ (2005) "Control of homeostatic proliferation by regulatory T cells." J Clin Invest 115(12):3517–3526

Shimizu J, Moriizumi E (2003) "CD4+CD25- T cells in aged mice are hyporesponsive and exhibit suppressive activity." J Immunol 170(4):1675–1682

Shurin MR, Shurin GV, Chatta GS (2007) "Aging and the dendritic cell system: Implications for cancer." Crit Rev Oncol Hematol (in press)

Smyth MJ, Teng MW, Swann J, Kyparissoudis K, Godfrey DI, Hayakawa Y (2006) "CD4+CD25+ T regulatory cells suppress NK cell-mediated immunotherapy of cancer." J Immunol 176(3):1582–1587

Snell GI, De Hoyos A, Winton T, Maurer JR (1993) "Lung transplantation in patients over the age of 50." Transplantation 55(3): 562–566

Somerset DA, Zheng Y, Kilby MD, Sansom DM, Drayson MT (2004) "Normal human pregnancy is associated with an elevation in the immune suppressive CD25+ CD4+ regulatory T-cell subset." Immunology 112(1):38–43

Specht C, Schluter B, Rolfing M, Bruning K, Pauels HG, Kolsch E (2003) "Idiotype-specific CD4+CD25 +T suppressor cells prevent, by limiting antibody diversity, the occurrence of anti-dextran antibodies crossreacting with histone H3." Eur J Immunol 33(5):1242–1249

Stacy S, Krolick KA, Infante AJ, Kraig E (2002) " Immunological memory and late onset autoimmunity." Mech Ageing Dev 123(8):975–985

Stassen M, Fondel S, Bopp T, Richter C, Muller C, Kubach J, Becker C, Knop J, Enk AH, Schmitt S, Schmitt E, Jonuleit H (2004) " Human CD25+ regulatory T cells: two subsets defined by the integrins alpha 4 beta 7 or alpha 4 beta 1 confer distinct suppressive properties upon CD4 +T helper cells." Eur J Immunol 34(5):1303–1311

Steinbrink K, Jonuleit H, Muller G, Schuler G, Knop J, Enk AH (1999) "IL10-treated human dendritic cells induce a melanoma-antigen-specific anergy in CD8+ T cells resulting in a failure to lyse tumor cells." Blood 93:1634–1645

Steinbrink K, Wolfl M, Jonuleit H, Knop J, Enk AH (1997) "Induction of tolerance by IL10-treated dendritic cells." J Immunol 159:4772–4782

Stober CB, Lange UG, Roberts MT, Alcami A, Blackwell JM (2005) "IL-10 from regulatory T cells determines vaccine efficacy in murine Leishmania major infection." J Immunol 175(4):2517–2524

Suciu-Foca N, Manavalan JS, Scotto L, Kim-Schulze S, Galluzzo S, Naiyer AJ, Fan J, Vlad G, Cortesini R (2005) "Molecular characterization of allospecific T suppressor and tolerogenic dendritic cells: review." Int Immunopharmacol 5(1):7–11

Sumida T, Sakamoto A, Murata H, Makino Y, Takahashi H, Yoshida S, Nishioka K, Iwamoto I, Taniguchi M (1995) "Selective reduction of T cells bearing invariant V alpha 24J alpha Q antigen receptor in patients with systemic sclerosis." J Exp Med 182(4):1163–1168

Surh CD, Sprent J (2000) " Homeostatic T cell proliferation: how far can T cells be activated to self-ligands?" J Exp Med 192(4):F9–F14

Suri-Payer E, Amar AZ, Thornton AM, Shevach EM (1998) "CD4+CD25+ T cells inhibit both the induction and effector function of autoreactive T cells and represent a unique lineage of immunoregulatory cells." J Immunol 160(3):1212–1218

Suthanthiran M (1997) "Clinical application of molecular biology: a study of allograft rejection with polymerase chain reaction." Am J Med Sci 313(5):264–267

Sutmuller RP, den Brok MH, Kramer M, Bennink EJ, Toonen LW, Kullberg BJ, Joosten LA, Akira S, Netea MG, Adema GJ (2006) "Toll-like receptor 2 controls expansion and function of regulatory T cells." J Clin Invest 116(2):485–494

Suvas S, Kumaraguru U, Pack CD, Lee S, Rouse BT (2003) "CD4+CD25+ T cells regulate virus-specific primary and memory CD8+ T cell responses." J Exp Med 198(6):889–901

Taams LS, Smith J, Rustin MH, Salmon M, Poulter LW, Akbar AN (2001) "Human anergic/suppressive CD4(+)CD25(+) T cells: a highly differentiated and apoptosis-prone population." Eur J Immunol 31(4):1122–1131

Taams LS, van Amelsfort JM, Tiemessen MM, Jacobs KM, de Jong EC, Akbar AN, Bijlsma JW, Lafeber FP (2005) "Modulation of monocyte/macrophage function by human CD4+CD25+ regulatory T cells." Hum Immunol 66(3):222–230

Taams LS, Vukmanovic-Stejic M, Smith J, Dunne PJ, Fletcher JM, Plunkett FJ, Ebeling SB, Lombardi G, Rustin MH, Bijlsma JW, Lafeber FP, Salmon M, Akbar AN (2002) "Antigen-specific T cell suppression by human CD4+CD25+ regulatory T cells." Eur J Immunol 32(6):1621–1630

Takahashi T, Tagami T, Yamazaki S, Uede T, Shimizu J, Sakaguchi N, Mak TW, Sakaguchi S (2000) "Immunologic self-tolerance maintained by CD25(+)CD4(+) regulatory T cells constitutively expressing cytotoxic T lymphocyte-associated antigen 4." J Exp Med 192(2):303–10

Tang Q, Bluestone JA (2006) "Regulatory T-cell physiology and application to treat autoimmunity." Immunol Rev 212:217–237

Tarazona R, DelaRosa O, Alonso C, Ostos B, Espejo J, Pena J, Solana R (2000) "Increased expression of NK cell markers on T lymphocytes in aging and chronic activation of the immune system reflects the accumulation of effector/senescent T cells." Mech Ageing Dev 121(1–3):77–88

Taylor PA, Panoskaltsis-Mortari A, Swedin JM, Lucas PJ, Gress RE, Levine BL, June CH, Serody JS, Blazar BR (2004) "L-Selectin(hi) but not the L-selectin(lo) CD4+25+ T-regulatory cells are potent inhibitors of GVHD and BM graft rejection." Blood 104(12):3804–3812

Terabe M, Matsui S, Noben-Trauth N, Chen H, Watson C, Donaldson DD, Carbone DP, Paul WE, Berzofsky JA (2000) "NKT cell-mediated repression of tumor immunosurveillance by IL-13 and the IL-4R-STAT6 pathway." Nat Immunol 1(6):515–520

Thornton AM, Shevach EM (1998) "CD4+CD25+ immunoregulatory T cells suppress polyclonal T cell activation in vitro by inhibiting interleukin 2 production." J Exp Med 188(2):287–296

Toka FN, Suvas S, Rouse BT (2004) "CD4+ CD25+ T cells regulate vaccine-generated primary and memory CD8+ T-cell responses against herpes simplex virus type 1." J Virol 78(23):13082–13089

Trzonkowski P, Mysliwska J, Lukaszuk K, Szmit E, Bryl E, Mysliwski A (2001) "Luteal phase of the menstrual cycle in young healthy women is associated with decline in interleukin 2 levels." Horm Metab Res 33(6):348–353

Trzonkowski P, Myśliwski A (2003) "Vaccination against influenza in the elderly (in Polish]." Medical University of Gdańsk Press

Trzonkowski P, Szmit E, Mysliwska J, Dobyszuk A, Mysliwski A (2004) "CD4+CD25+ T regulatory cells inhibit cytotoxic activity of T CD8+ and NK lymphocytes in the direct cell-to-cell interaction." Clin Immunol 112(3):258–267

Trzonkowski P, Szmit E, Mysliwska J, Mysliwski A (2006) "CD4+CD25+ T regulatory cells inhibit cytotoxic activity of CTL and NK cells in humans-impact of immunosenescence." Clin Immunol 119(3):307–316

Tsaknaridis L, Spencer L, Culbertson N, Hicks K, LaTocha D, Chou YK, Whitham RH, Bakke A, Jones RE, Offner H, Bourdette DN, Vandenbark AA (2003) "Functional assay for human CD4+CD25+ Treg cells reveals an age-dependent loss of suppressive activity." J Neurosci Res 74(2): 296–308

Uhlig HH, Coombes J, Mottet C, Izcue A, Thompson C, Fanger A, Tannapfel A, Fontenot JD, Ramsdell F, Powrie F (2006) "Characterization of Foxp3+CD4+CD25 +and IL-10-secreting CD4+CD25+ T cells during cure of colitis." J Immunol 177(9):5852–5860

Vahlenkamp TW, Tompkins MB, Tompkins WA (2005) "The role of CD4+CD25+ regulatory T cells in viral infections." Vet Immunol Immunopathol 108(1–2):219–225

Vail A, Gore SM, Bradley BA, Easty DL, Rogers CA, Armitage WJ (1997) "Conclusions of the corneal follow-up study. Collaborating Surgeons." Br J Ophthalmol 81(8):631–636

Valencia X, Stephens G, Goldbach-Mansky R, Wilson M, Shevach EM, Lipsky PE (2006) "TNF downmodulates the function of human CD4+CD25hi T-regulatory cells." Blood 108(1): 253–261

Valmori D, Merlo A, Souleimanian NE, Hesdorffer CS, Ayyoub M (2005) "A peripheral circulating compartment of natural naive CD4 Tregs." J Clin Invest 115(7):1953–1962

van Kaer L (2005) "Alpha-galactosylceramide therapy for autoimmune diseases: prospects and obstacles." Nat Rev Immunol 5:31–42

Veldhoen M, Hockinger RJ, Atkins CJ, Locksley RM, Stockinger B (2006) "TGFbeta in the context of an inflammatory cytokine millieu supports de novo differentiation of IL17-producing T cells." Immunity 24:179–189

Veldhoen M, Stockinger B (2006) "TGFbeta1, a 'Jack of all trades': the link with pro-inflammatory IL17-producing T cells." Trends Immunol 27(8):358–361

Vieira PL, Christensen JR, Minaee S, O'Neill EJ, Barrat FJ, Boonstra A, Barthlott T, Stockinger B, Wraith DC, O'Garra A (2004) "IL-10-secreting regulatory T cells do not express Foxp3 but have comparable regulatory function to naturally occurring CD4+CD25+ regulatory T cells." J Immunol 172(10):5986–5993

Vigoroux S, Yvon E, Biagi E, Brenner MK (2004) "Antigen-induced regulatory T cells." Blood 104: 26–33

Villiger PM, Kusari AB, ten Dijke P, Lotz M (1993) "IL-1 beta and IL-6 selectively induce transforming growth factor-beta isoforms in human articular chondrocytes." J Immunol 151(6): 3337–3344

Vukmanovic-Stejic M, Zhang Y, Cook JE, Fletcher JM, McQuaid A, Masters JE, Rustin MH, Taams LS, Beverley PC, Macallan DC, Akbar AN (2006) " Human CD4+ CD25hi Foxp3+ regulatory T cells are derived by rapid turnover of memory populations in vivo." J Clin Invest 116(9):2423–2433

Wahl C, Bochtler P, Schirmbeck R, Reimann J (2007) "Type I IFN-producing CD4 Valpha14i NKT cells facilitate priming of IL-10-producing CD8 T cells by hepatocytes." J Immunol 178(4): 2083–2093

Wakikawa A, Utsuyama M, Hirokawa K (1997) "Altered expression of various receptors on T cells in young and old mice after mitogenic stimulation: a flow cytometric analysis." Mech Ageing Dev94(1–3):113–122

Waldmann H, Chen TC, Graca L, Adams E, Daley S, Cobbold S, Fairchild PJ (2006) "Regulatory T cells in transplantation." Semin Immunol 18(2):111–119

Wan S, Xia C, Morel L (2007) "IL-6 Produced by dendritic cells from Lupus-Prone mice inhibits CD4+CD25+ T cell regulatory functions." J Immunol 178:271–279

Wan YY, Flavell RA (2007) "Regulatory T-cell functions are subverted and converted owing to attenuated Foxp3 expression." Nature 445(7129): 766–770

Watanabe H, Miyaji C, Seki S, Abo T (1996) "c-kit+ stem cells and thymocyte precursors in the livers of adult mice." J Exp Med 184(2):687–693

Wei M, Kuukasjärvi P, Laurikka J, Pehkonen E, Kaukinen S, Laine S, Tarkka M (2003) "Imbalance of pro- and anti-inflammatory cytokine responses in elderly patients after coronary artery bypass grafting." Aging Clin Exp Res 15(6):469–474

Wolf AM, Wolf D, Steurer M, Gastl G, Gunsilius E, Grubeck-Loebenstein B (2003) "Increase of regulatory T cells in peripheral blood of cancer patients." Clin cancer Res 9:606–612

Wolf D, Wolf AM, Rumpold H, Fiegl H, Zeimet AG, Muller-Holzner E, Deibl M, Gastl G, Gunsilius E, Marth C (2005) "The expression of the regulatory T cell specific forkhead box transcription factor FoxP3 is associated with poor prognosis in ovarian cancer." Clin Cancer Res 11:8326–8331

Xavier RM, Yamauchi Y, Nakamura M, Tanigawa Y, Ishikura H, Tsunematsu T, Kobayashi S (1995) "Antinuclear antibodies in healthy aging people: a prospective study." Mech Ageing Dev 78(2):145–154

Xu L, Kitani A, Fuss I, Strober W (2007) "Regulatory T cells induce CD4+CD25-Foxp3- T cells or are self-induced to become Th17 cells in the absence of exogenous TGF-beta." J Immunol 178:6725–6729

Yamazaki S, Inaba K, Tarbell KV, Steinman RM (2006) "Dendritic cells expand antigen-specific Foxp3+ CD25+ CD4+ regulatory T cells including suppressors of alloreactivity." Immunol Rev 212:314–329

Yazdanbakhsh M, Kremsner PG, van Ree R (2002) "Allergy, parasites, and the hygiene hypothesis." Science 296:490–494

Ye SM, Johnson RW (2001) "An age-related decline in interleukin-10 may contribute to the increased expression of interleukin-6 in brain of aged mice." Neuroimmunomodulation 9(4):183–192

Zeiser R, Nguyen VH, Beilhack A, Buess M, Schulz S, Baker J, Contag CH, Negrin RS (2006) "Inhibition of CD4+CD25+ regulatory T-cell function by calcineurin-dependent interleukin-2 production." Blood 108(1):390–399

Zetterman RK, Belle SH, Hoofnagle JH et al (1998) "Age and liver transplantation: A report of the Liver Transplantation Database." Transplantation 66(4):500–506

Zhao KS, Wang YF, Guéret R, Weksler ME (1995) "Dysregulation of the humoral immune response in old mice." Int Immunol 7(6):929–934

Zheng SG, Wang JH, Stohl W, Kim KS, Gray JD, Horwitz DA (2006) "TGF-beta requires CTLA-4 early after T cell activation to induce FoxP3 and generate adaptive CD4+CD25+ regulatory cells." J Immunol 176(6):3321–3329

Zheng Y, Josefowicz SZ, Kas A, Chu TT, Gavin MA, Rudensky AY (2007) "Genome-wide analysis of Foxp3 target genes in developing and mature regulatory T cells." Nature 445(7130):936–940

Cellular Immunosenescence - B Cells

Transcription Factors in Mature B-Cells During Aging

Daniela Frasca, Richard L. Riley and Bonnie B. Blomberg

Contents

Abbreviations

AID	activation-induced cytidine deaminase
ARE	adenylate/uridylate-rich elements
BAFF	B-cell-activating factor
BCMA	B-cell maturation antigen
bHLH	basic helix loop helix
BSAP	B-cell lineage-specific activator protein
CSR	class switch recombination
EMSA	electrophoretic mobility shift assay
HEB	E-box binding protein
Ig	Immunoglobulin
MZ	marginal zone
NF-κB	nuclear factor-κB
RAG	recombination activating enzyme
RT-PCR	reverse transcription-polymerase chain reaction
SL	surrogate light (chain)
TACI	transmembrane activator and CAML interactor
TdT	deoxynucleotidyl transferase
TD	thymus-dependent
TI	thymus-independent
TTP	tristetraprolin
UTR	untranslated region

D. Frasca (✉) · R. L. Riley · B. B. Blomberg
Department of Microbiology and Immunology
University of Miami Miller School of Medicine
P.O. Box 016960 (R-138)
Miami, FL 33101, USA
Tel.: 305-243 6225
Fax: 305-243 4623
E-mail: dfrasca@med.miami.edu

D. Frasca
Graduate School of Cell Biology and Development
University of Rome La Sapienza
Rome, Italy

T. Fulop et al. (eds.), *Handbook on Immunosenescence*,
DOI 10.1007/978-1-4020-9062-2_19, © Springer Science+Business Media B.V. 2009

Abstract: The purpose of this chapter is to give an overview of the age-related changes in the expression and function of the major transcription factors regulating mature B-cells. We also summarize our recent work and show that the age-related defects in Ig class switch are directly related to the decrease in the transcription factor E47 which controls the expression of AID, needed for CSR. The age-associated effects on the expression and function of the transcription factors NF-κ B and Pax-5 are also described. Blimp-1 seems not to be modified by aging. For other transcription factors relevant for mature B-cell functions, such and IRF4 and Notch2, no effects of aging have been reported so far. The defects presented herein for aged B-cells should allow the discovery of mechanisms to improve humoral immune responses in both humans and mice in the near future.

1   E Proteins

Class I basic helix loop helix (bHLH) proteins, also known as E proteins, were first identified based on their ability to bind with relatively high affinity to the palindromic DNA sequence CANNTG, referred to as an E-box site (Ephrussi et al. 1985; Henthorn et al. 1990; Quong et al. 2002), found in the promoter and enhancer regions of many B lineage-specific genes, such as the enhancers in the immunoglobulin (Ig) loci and the promoters of mb-1, λ5 and RAG-1 (Quong et al. 2002). The E protein family includes E12, E47, HeLa E-box binding protein (HEB), and E2-2, in vertebrates, and the Drosophila gene product, daughterless (Massari and Murre 2000). E12 and E47, arising through differential splicing of the exon encoding for the HLH domain of the *E2A* gene (Murre et al. 1989), regulate a plethora of processes involved in B-cell commitment and differentiation. In particular, they initiate Ig rearrangements; and regulate the expression of the surrogate light (SL) chain, the recombination activating enzymes RAG-1 and RAG-2, the enzyme terminal deoxynucleotidyl transferase (TdT), the IL-7Rα chain, which together with the common γ chain (γc) comprises the high affinity IL-7 receptor (IL-7R), and the genes encoding the signal transduction molecules Igα (mb-1) and Igβ (B29; Schlissel et al. 1991; Sigvardsson et al. 1997; Massari and Murre 2000; Kee et al. 2002). E2A also induces the expression of EBF, which acts in synergy with E2A to promote SL chain transcription.

In B lymphocytes, the active DNA-binding complex consists of E47 homodimer, as opposed to E12/E12 or E12/E47 complexes, whereas in the bone marrow pro-B/early pre-B cells the predominant form is E12/E47 (Frasca et al. 2003). The formation and the function of the homodimer or heterodimer depend on the balance between the *E2A*-encoded proteins, other class I bHLH proteins (HEB and E2-2) and the E protein inhibitory proteins, Id 1-4, which lack the DNA-binding domain and function as dominant negative inhibitors of E proteins (Rivera and Murre 2001). The paradigm of HLH function is that an ubiquitously expressed class I bHLH protein dimerizes with a tissue-specific class II factor, such as MyoD (skeletal muscle) or NeuroD (neurons), to regulate cell-specific gene transcription. E2A-deficient mice display a complete block in B lineage development at a very early stage prior to the onset of IgH DJ rearrangement, whereas myeloid development is normal. Transgenic introduction of either E47 or E12 restores B lymphopoiesis in E2A-deficient mice, although E47 promotes pre-B cell differentiation more effectively, likely because it has a higher DNA-binding affinity than does E12 (Shen and Kadesch 1995). Mice expressing a transgene for Id proteins, the inhibitors of E protein activity, have a phenotype similar to the E2A$^{-/-}$ mice (Quong et al. 2002). These mice display the same block in B-cell development, and its severity is dependent on the level of expression of the transgene.

E2A activity is necessary for class switch recombination (CSR; Quong et al. 1999; Sugai et al. 2003), as the E47 transcription factor has been shown to be important in transcriptional regulation of *Aicda*, the gene encoding the activation-induced cytidine deaminase (AID; Sayegh et al. 2003), the enzyme responsible for breaking the DNA in the switch regions, the first step in the CSR process. Briefly, it has been shown that ectopic expression of Id3 in splenic activated B-cells inhibits CSR (Quong et al. 1999) because of reduced AID transcription and overexpression of E47 can directly induce *Aicda* gene expression both in a B-cell line and in splenic B-cells activated in vitro (Sayegh et al. 2003). A cis-regulatory element (E-box) in the *Aicda* locus has been identified and shown to be activated by E-proteins. Ectopic expression of AID in splenic activated B-cells retrovirally transduced with Id3 only partially rescues the ability of these cells to undergo CSR. The Authors concluded that the efficient induction of *Aicda* expression is dependent on E-proteins, but also suggest that E-proteins have roles in CSR in addition to their induction of *Aicda* expression. However, the level of restoration of AID was not complete in these experiments and therefore an alternative interpretation of these results would be that optimal E47, which would induce optimal AID, would itself completely restore CSR. Our data showing no decrease in germline μ transcripts in old or in E2A$^{+/-}$ B-cells support this hypothesis (Frasca et al. 2004a).

In senescent mice, we have previously shown that in vitro stimulated splenic B-cells are deficient in production of multiple class switch isotypes (IgG1, G2a, G3, and E), and CSR (Frasca et al. 2004a, b). This occurs concomitant with decreased induction of E47 and AID. The reduced CSR observed in old splenic activated B-cells is not the consequence of defective B-cell proliferation, as B-cells from old mice can be effectively activated in vitro, but their capacity to undergo CSR is impaired. Our results are in line with the findings that expression of the receptors for CD40, and IL-4 are unaffected by aging in mice and humans, as already reported (Whisler et al. 1991; Song et al. 1997; Zheng et al. 1997; Bergler et al. 1999). Although it is known that there are defects in T as well as B-cells during aging, our studies indicate that an intrinsic B-cell defect may not be able to be rescued by modifying/enhancing T-cell activity alone by itself in aged individuals. Both DNA-binding (EMSA) and expression (Western blot) of E47 are decreased in stimulated splenic B-cells from old mice. We have previously shown (Frasca et al. 2003) that the endogenous E47 DNA-binding is low, and importantly, twofold lower than that in unstimulated young spleen cells in the majority of aged mice individually tested (65%). Activation of B-cells up-regulates E47 DNA binding in young and to a significantly lower extent in old mice. Therefore, both basal and activated levels of E47 are decreased in splenic B-cells in aged mice. These findings suggest that the down-regulation of this transcriptional regulator may help explain not only decreased CSR in activated splenic B-cells from old mice, but also age-related changes in affinity maturation and SHM affecting the quality of the Ab response. Other results from our laboratory showing that CSR is perturbed in E2A[+/-] mice further support the important role of this transcription factor in the generation of Abs with different isotypes (Frasca et al. 2004a).

In order to determine a mechanism for the age-related decrease in the amounts of E47 protein in nuclear extracts, we found that E47 mRNA levels were decreased in stimulated splenic B-cells from old as compared with young mice. RNA stability assays showed that the rate of E47 mRNA decay was accelerated in stimulated splenic B-cells from old mice, but E47 protein degradation rates were comparable in young versus aged B-cells, indicating that the regulation of E47 expression in activated splenic B-cells occurs primarily by mRNA stability (Frasca et al. 2005b, 2007b). In contrast with splenic activated B-cells, E47 mRNA expression is comparable in bone marrow-derived IL-7-expanded pro-B/early pre-B cells from young and old mice (Van der Put et al. 2004). Thus, the reduced expression and DNA-binding of the E12/E47 transcription factor in aged B-cell precursors is not transcriptionally regulated, but is due to reduced protein stability (Van der Put et al. 2004; King et al. 2007) mediated presumably via the ubiquitin–proteasome pathway (Kho et al. 1997; Huggins et al. 1999). This instability is largely due to PEST (proline, glutamic acid, serine, threonine) residues common to degradation domains (Huang et al. 1998).

The stability of labile mRNA may be controlled by signal transduction cascades, where the final product of the cascade phosphorylates a protein which interacts with adenylate/uridylate-rich elements (ARE) in the 3′ untranslated region (UTR) of mRNA and modifies its stability (Chen et al. 1995; Bevilacqua et al. 2003). ARE sequences have been found in the 3′-untranslated region (UTR) of many mRNAs, including those for transcription factors. ARE motifs have been previously classified into at least three categories based in part upon the distribution of AUUUA pentamers. Class I AREs, found in early response gene mRNAs like c-fos and c-myc, contain multiple isolated AUUUA motifs; class II AREs, found exclusively in cytokine mRNAs, contain two or more overlapping copies of the AUUUA motif; class III AREs contain no AUUUA motifs but generally contain U-rich or AU-rich regions and possibly other unknown features for their destabilizing function. The E47 mRNA is a class I/III mRNA, because it has one AUUUA sequence and multiple AU/U-rich regions. At least part of the decreased stability of E47 mRNA seen in aged B-cells is mediated by proteins. We have found that tristetraprolin (TTP), a physiological regulator of mRNA expression and stability, is involved in the degradation of the E47 mRNA. Because many studies have shown TTP expression and function in macrophages, monocytes, mast cells and T-cells, but little is known about the expression and function of TTP in primary B-cells, we have investigated TTP mRNA and protein expression in splenic B-cells from young and old mice. Our recently published results (Frasca et al. 2007b) show that TTP mRNA and protein levels are higher in stimulated splenic B-cells from old as compared with young mice. TTP has been described to be directly phosphorylated by p38 MAPK in macrophages (Carballo et al. 2001; Chrestensen et al. 2004; Cao et al. 2006). We show that inhibition of the p38 MAPK signaling pathway significantly reduces TTP protein expression in B-cells. Old B-cells in response to LPS make less phospho-p38 MAPK (Frasca et al. 2007b) and there-fore, as would be expected, make less phospho-TTP. This leads to an increase in the amount of TTP bound to the 3′-UTRs, and therefore decrease mRNA stability (of E47) in old B-cells. Our studies demonstrate for the first time that TTP is regu-lated in activated B-cells during aging, that TTP is involved in the degradation of the E47 mRNA, and show the molecular mechanism for the decreased expression of E47, AID and CSR in aged B-cells.

2 NF-κB

The transcription factor, nuclear factor-κ B (NF-κB), has also been shown to be impor-tant for Ig class switch (Snapper et al. 1996). NF-κB has been shown to be strongly activated by anti-CD40/IL-4, but not by anti-CD40 or IL-4 stimulation alone in splenic B-cells and to be involved in CSR to IgG1/IgE in both humans (Jeppson et al. 1998) and mice (Tinnell et al. 1998; Pioli et al. 1999; Kaku et al. 2002). It has also been shown to be the key transcription factor in mouse or human B-cells undergoing CSR in response to BAFF, the B-cell-activating factor, also called BLyS, TALL-1, THANK, ZTNF4 or TNF13B (Litinskiy et al. 2002; Castigli et al. 2005; Yamada et al. 2005).

We have recently investigated the ability of BAFF/IL-4, as compared to anti-CD40/IL-4, to induce CSR to γ_1 in splenic B-cells from young and old mice (Frasca et al. 2007a). We found that anti-CD40/IL-4 is a better CSR stimulus than BAFF/IL-4 in young B-cells, as measured by RT-PCR of postswitch transcripts and flow cytometry. CSR is reduced in old B-cells with both stimuli, but the suboptimal CSR seen in young mice to BAFF/IL-4 shows less reduction in the old B-cells. AID and γ_1PSTs are significantly reduced in old B-cells stimulated with anti-CD40/IL-4, and less reduced with BAFF/IL-4 stimulus. BAFF receptor mRNA expression (BAFF-R, TACI, and BCMA) is not affected by aging. The age-related decrease in CSR induced by anti-CD40/IL-4 is primarily associated with a decrease in E47, whereas the less affected response to BAFF/IL-4 is associated with decreases in both E47 and NF-κB. Therefore, NF-κB is not involved in the decreased response of old B-cells to anti-CD40/IL-4. These differences in B-cell responses to CD40/IL-4 and BAFF/IL-4 may help to explain at least a partial maintenance of TI (more BAFF/IL-4-depend-ent) versus TD responses in senescent mice (Smith 1976; Weksler et al. 1978).

The mechanisms by which NF-κB controls CSR are known only in part. Recent results show that signals delivered via CD40 that activate NF-κB synergize with signals delivered via the IL-4 receptor that activate Stat-6 to induce optimal AID gene expression (Dedeoglu et al. 2004). The importance of Stat-6 and NF-κB in induction of AID expression by IL-4 and CD40 was demonstrated in studies of Stat-6$^{-/-}$ and p50$^{-/-}$ mice. However, in this study (Dedeoglu et al. 2004) the ability of

CD40 ligation to induce AID expression and to synergize with IL-4 in AID induction in B-cells was only partially impaired in p50$^{-/-}$ mice, suggesting that NF-κB is only one of the transcription factors involved in inducing AID expression and CSR in B-cells. Our studies show that the defect in aging seen in CSR is due primarily to E47 and not to NF-κB (Frasca et al. 2007a).

3 Pax-5 (BSAP)

Pax-5, also called B-cell lineage-specific activator protein (BSAP), is critical for B-cell lineage commitment, B-cell development and CSR in GC B-cells, but it is not expressed in terminally differentiated B-cells (Max et al. 1995; Nutt et al. 1998, 1999; Linn et al. 2002; Gonda et al. 2003). B-cell-specific target genes for Pax-5 are λ5, CD19, mb-1, blk, RAG-2, J-chain, and IgH genes (Kozmick et al. 1992; Neurath et al. 1994; Zwollo et al. 1994; Michaelson et al. 1996; Lauring and Schlissel 1999). Binding sites for Pax-5 have been identified in the promoters of multiple genes as well as at multiple sites within the IgH locus (Neurath et al. 1994; Michaelson et al. 1996). Pax-5-dependent repression of X box binding protein-1 (XBP-1) is probably critical for inhibiting plasmacytic differentiation in the GC (Shaffer 2002). It has recently been demonstrated that a putative regulatory region in the *Aicda* gene contains both E2A- and Pax-5-binding sites, and the latter site is indispensable for AID gene expression (Gonda et al. 2003). Id proteins have been shown to interact with Pax-5, and inhibit its DNA-binding (Roberts et al. 2001; Gonda et al. 2003). E2A proteins have been described to regulate Pax-5 not directly but through its regulation of EBF (Kee and Murre 1998). Consistent with these observations is the finding that the Pax-5 promoter contains functional EBF binding sites (O'Riordan and Grosschedl 1999).

Pax-5 DNA-binding activity (for the active Pax-5a isoform) has been shown to be strongly reduced in resting splenic B-cells from aged mice, whereas protein levels did not change significantly (Anspach et al. 2001). Decreased Pax-5 binding activity is not the result of decreased levels of Pax-5 RNA transcripts or overall protein levels, as shown by RNase protection and Western blot analyses, suggesting a posttranslational mechanism affecting Pax-5 activity in aged B-cells, possibly involving its oxidation status (the oxidative form does not bind to DNA; Tell et al. 1998). Unlike E2A, Pax-5 is regulated posttranscriptionally in splenic B-cells. Preliminary results from our laboratory have shown that in splenic activated B-cells Pax-5 may also be regulated by mRNA stability (Landin, Frasca and Blomberg, work in progress).

4 Blimp-1

Blimp-1, encoded by the *prdm1* gene (Lin et al. 2003), is a transcriptional repressor which represses proliferation and induces maturation of B-cells into antibody-secreting plasma cells. It blocks the alternative GC B-cell fate by inhibiting Bcl-6,

Pax-5, BCR signaling, E2A, EBF, CSR, activation and homing to follicles (Lin et al. 2002; Shaffer et al. 2002; Johnson and Calame 2003, Calame et al. 2003). Blimp-1 has been detected in plasma cells, but not in early bone marrow B-cells, splenic memory B-cells in spleen, and GC B-cells (Tunyaplin et al. 2004).

As demonstrated by Han et al. (2003), there is a substantially higher number of antibody-secreting cells in the spleens of old mice than in the spleens of young mice. Therefore, we measured Blimp-1 mRNA expression in cultures of splenic B-cells from young and old mice activated for different times with LPS. We also determined the percentages of plasma cells (CD138$^+$B220^{low}) in cultures of LPS-stimulated B-cells from young and old mice. The expression of mRNA for Blimp-1 is induced by LPS and suppressed by IL-4 (Knodel et al. 2001). Our results (Frasca et al. 2004b) showed that Blimp-1 mRNA was undetectable in unstimulated B-cells, increased at days 2 and 3, reached the optimum levels at day 4 and then decreased at day 7 in both young and old mice. Blimp-1 mRNA expression was comparable in young and old splenic B-cells. These results again point to the main defect in aged stimulated B-cells being at the level of CSR, and not due to differentiation to antibody-secreting (plasma) cells.

5 IRF4

IRF4, also called Pip, LSIRF, ICSAT or MUM1 (Iida et al. 1997) is a member of the interferon-regulatory factor family of transcription factors characterized by a specific DNA-binding domain and by the ability to bind to regulatory elements in promoters of interferon-inducible genes. In the B lineage, IRF4 is expressed in immature B-cells in the bone marrow, is absent from proliferating centroblasts and then is re-expressed in plasma cells (Lu et al. 2003; Klein et al. 2006). IRF4, together with Blimp-1, is required for the generation of plasma cells, both transcription factors acting upstream of the transcription factor XBP-1 (Klein et al. 2006). No aging effects have been reported so far for IRF4.

6 Notch2

The Notch family of receptors plays an important role in the development of hematopoietic cells (Maillard et al. 2005). Notch1 regulates T-cell development, whereas Notch2 is preferentially expressed in mature B-cells (Saito et al. 2003). Conditionally targeted deletion of Notch2 results in a defect in marginal zone (MZ) B-cells and their precursors (Kuroda et al. 2003). Among Notch target genes, the expression level of Deltex1 is prominent in MZ cells and strictly dependent on that of Notch2, suggesting that Deltex1 may play a role in MZ cell differentiation. No aging effects have been reported so far for Notch2.

7   Conclusions

In conclusion, particular transcription factors have been shown to be decreased with age in activated murine B-cells, *e.g.* E47, or in resting B-cells, *e.g.* Pax-5. The stage of differentiation as well as activation of the cell types studied appears to be important as our data on E2A in murine bone marrow versus the spleen has shown decreases with age but using different molecular mechanisms (Frasca et al. 2005a; Riley 2005). Further studies should help to better determine the molecular mechanisms for these suboptimal expression of transcription factors, their molecular consequences, and provide avenues for correction of the immune deficiencies created by them.

References

Anspach J, Poulsen G, Kaattari I, Pollock R, Zwollo P (2001) Reduction in DNA binding activity of the transcription factor Pax-5a in B lymphocytes of aged mice. J Immunol 166:2617–2626

Bergler W, Adam S, Gross HJ, Hormann K, Schwartz-Albiez R (1999) Age-dependent altered proportions in subpopulations of tonsillar lymphocytes. Clin Exp Immunol 116:9–18

Bevilacqua A, Ceriani MC, Capaccioli S, Nicolin A (2003) Post-transcriptional regulation of gene expression by degradation of messenger RNAs. J Cell Physiol 195:356–372

Calame KL, Lin KI, Tunyaplin C (2003) Regulatory mechanisms that determine the development and function of plasma cells. Ann Rev Immunol 21:205–230

Cao H, Deterding LJ, Venable JD, Kennington EA, Yates JR 3rd, Tomer KB, Blackshear PJ (2006) Identification of the anti-inflammatory protein tristetraprolin as a hyperphosphorylated protein by mass spectrometry and site-directed mutagenesis. Biochem J 394:285–297

Carballo E, Cao H, Lai WS, Kennington EA, Campbell D, Blackshear PJ (2001) Decreased sensitivity of tristetraprolin-deficient cells to p38 inhibitors suggests the involvement of tristetraprolin in the p38 signaling pathway. J Biol Chem 276: 42580–42587

Castigli E, Wilson SA, Scott S, Dedeoglu F, Xu S, Lam KP, Bram RJ, Jabara H, Geha RS (2005) TACI and BAFF-R mediate isotype switching in B cells. J Exp Med 201:35–39

Chen CY, Shyu AB (1995) AU-rich elements: characterization and importance in mRNA degradation. Trends Biochem Sci 20:465–470

Chrestensen CA, Schroeder MJ, Shabanowitz J, Hunt DF, Pelo JW, Worthington MT, Sturgill TW (2004) MAPKAP kinase 2 phosphorylates tristetraprolin on in vivo sites including Ser178, a site required for 14-3-3 binding. J Biol Chem 279:10176–10184

Dedeoglu F, Horwitz B, Chaudhuri J, Alt FW, Geha RS (2004) Induction of activation-induced cytidine deaminase gene expression by IL-4 and CD40 ligation is dependent on STAT6 and NFkappaB. Int Immunol 16:395–404

Ephrussi A, Church GM, Tonegawa S, Gilbert W (1985) B lineage—specific interactions of an immunoglobulin enhancer with cellular factors in vivo. Science 227:134–140

Frasca D, Nguyen D, Riley RL, Blomberg BB (2003) Decreased E12 and/or E47 transcription factor activity in the bone marrow as well as in the spleen of aged mice. J Immunol 170:719–726

Frasca D, Van Der Put E, Riley RL, Blomberg BB (2004a) Reduced Ig class switch in aged mice correlates with decreased E47 and activation-induced cytidine deaminase. J Immunol 172: 2155–2162

Frasca D, Riley RL, Blomberg BB (2004b) Effect of age on the immunoglobulin class switch. Crit Rev Immunol 24:297–320

Frasca D, Riley RL, Blomberg BB (2005a) Humoral immune response and B-cell functions including immunoglobulin class switch are downregulated in aged mice and humans. Semin Immunol 17:378–384

Frasca D, Van Der Put E, Landin AM, Gong D, Riley RL, Blomberg BB (2005b) RNA stability of the E2A-encoded transcription factor E47 is lower in splenic activated B cells from aged mice. J Immunol 175:6633–6644

Frasca D, Riley RL, Blomberg BB (2007a) Aging murine B cells have decreased class switch induced by anti-CD40 or BAFF. Exp Gerontol 42:192–203

Frasca D, Landin AM, Alvarez JP, Blackshear PJ, Riley RL, Blomberg BB (2007b) Tristetraprolin, a negative regulator of mRNA stability, is increased in old B cells and is involved in the degradation of e47 mRNA. J Immunol 179:918–927

Gonda H, Sugai M, Nambu Y, Katakai T, Agata Y, Mori KJ, Yokota Y, Shimizu A (2003) The balance between Pax5 and Id2 activities is the key to AID gene expression. J Exp Med 198: 1427–1437

Han S, Yang K, Ozen Z, Peng W, Marinova E, Kelsoe G, Zheng B (2003) Enhanced differentiation of splenic plasma cells but diminished long-lived high-affinity bone marrow plasma cells in aged mice. J Immunol 170:1267–1273

Henthorn P, Kiledjian M, Kadesch T (1990) Two distinct transcription factors that bind the immunoglobulin enhancer microE5/kappa 2 motif. Science 247:467–470

Huang LE Gu J, Schau M, Bunn HF (1998) Regulation of hypoxia-inducible factor 1alpha is mediated by an O2-dependent degradation domain via the ubiquitin-proteasome pathway. Proc Natl Acad Sci U S A 95:7987–7992

Huggins GS, Chin MT, Sibinga NE, Lee SL, Haber E, Lee ME (1999) Characterization of the mUBC9-binding sites required for E2A protein degradation. J Biol Chem 274:28690–28696

Iida S, Rao PH, Butler M, Corradini P, Boccadoro M, Klein B, Chaganti RS, Dalla-Favera R (1997) Deregulation of MUM1/IRF4 by chromosomal translocation in multiple myeloma. Nat Genet 17:226–230

Jeppson JD, Patel HR, Sakata N, Domenico J, Terada N, Gelfand EW (1998) Requirement for dual signals by anti-CD40 and IL-4 for the induction of nuclear factor-kappa B, IL-6, and IgE in human B lymphocytes. J Immunol 161:1738–1742

Johnson K, Calame K (2003) Transcription factors controlling the beginning and end of B-cell differentiation. Curr Opin Genet Dev 13:522–528

Kaku H, Horikawa K, Obata Y, Kato I, Okamoto H, Sakaguchi N, Gerondakis S, Takatsu K (2002) NF-kappaB is required for CD38-mediated induction of C(gamma)1 germline transcripts in murine B lymphocytes. Int Immunol 14:1055–1064

Kee BL, Bain G, Murre C (2002) IL-7Ralpha and E47: independent pathways required for development of multipotent lymphoid progenitors. EMBO J 21:103–113

Kee BL, Murre C (1998) Induction of early B cell factor (EBF) and multiple B lineage genes by the basic helix-loop-helix transcription factor E12. J Exp Med 188:699–713

Kho CJ, Huggins GS, Endege WO, Hsieh CM, Lee ME, Haber E (1997) Degradation of E2A proteins through a ubiquitin-conjugating enzyme, UbcE2A. J Biol Chem 272:3845–3851

King AM, Van Der Put E, Blomberg BB, Riley RL (2007) Accelerated Notch-dependent degradation of E47 proteins in aged B cell precursors is associated with increased ERK MAPK activation. J Immunol 178:3521–3529

Klein U, Casola S, Cattoretti G, Shen Q, Lia M, Mo T, Ludwig T, Rajewsky K, Dalla-Favera R (2006) Transcription factor IRF4 controls plasma cell differentiation and class-switch recombination. Nat Immunol 7:773–782

Knodel M, Kuss AW, Berberich I, Schimpl A (2001) Blimp-1 over-expression abrogates IL-4- and CD40-mediated suppression of terminal B cell differentiation but arrests isotype switching. Eur J Immunol 31:1972–1980

Kozmik Z, Wang S, Dorfler P, Adams B, Busslinger M (1992) The promoter of the CD19 gene is a target for the B-cell-specific transcription factor BSAP. Mol Cell Biol 12:2662–2672

Kuroda K, Han H, Tani S, Tanigaki K, Tun T, Furukawa T, Taniguchi Y, Kurooka H, Hamada Y, Toyokuni S, Honjo T (2003) Regulation of marginal zone B cell development by MINT, a suppressor of Notch/RBP-J signaling pathway. Immunity 18:301–312

Lauring J, Schlissel MS (1999) Distinct factors regulate the murine RAG-2 promoter in B- and T-cell lines. Mol Cell Biol 19:2601–2612

Lin KI, Angelin-Duclos C, Kuo TC, Calame K (2002) Blimp-1-dependent repression of Pax-5 is required for differentiation of B cells to immunoglobulin M-secreting plasma cells. Mol Cell Biol 22:4771–4780

Lin KI, Tunyaplin C, Calame, K (2003) Transcriptional regulatory cascades controlling plasma cell differentiation. Immunol Rev 194:19–28

Litinskiy MB, Nardelli B, Hilbert DM, He B, Schaffer A, Casali P, Cerutti A (2002) DCs induce CD40-independent immunoglobulin class switching through BLyS and APRIL. Nat Immunol 3:822–829

Lu R, Medina KL, Lancki DW, Singh H (2003) IRF-4,8 orchestrate the pre-B-to-B transition in lymphocyte development. Genes Dev 17:1703–1708

Maillard I, Fang T, Pear WS (2005) Regulation of lymphoid development, differentiation, and function by the Notch pathway. Annu Rev Immunol 23:945–974

Massari ME, Murre C (2000) Helix-loop-helix proteins: regulators of transcription in eucaryotic organisms. Mol Cell Biol 20:429–440

Max EE, Wakatsuki Y, Neurath MF, Strober W (1995) The role of BSAP in immunoglobulin isotype switching and B-cell proliferation. Curr Top Microbiol Immunol 194:449–458

Michaelson JS, Singh M, Birshtein BK (1996) B cell lineage-specific activator protein (BSAP). A player at multiple stages of B cell development. J Immunol 156:2349–2351

Murre C, McCaw PS, Baltimore D (1989) A new DNA binding and dimerization motif in immunoglobulin enhancer binding, daughterless, MyoD, and myc proteins. Cell 56:777–783

Neurath MF, Strober W, Wakatsuki Y (1994) The murine Ig 3' alpha enhancer is a target site with repressor function for the B cell lineage-specific transcription factor BSAP (NF-HB, S alpha-BP). J Immunol 153:730–742

Nutt SL, Morrison AM, Dorfler P, Rolink A, Busslinger M (1998) Identification of BSAP (Pax-5) target genes in early B-cell development by loss- and gain-of-function experiments. EMBO J 17:2319–2333

Nutt SL, Heavey B, Rolink AG, Busslinger M (1999) Commitment to the B-lymphoid lineage depends on the transcription factor Pax5. Nature 401:556–562

O'Riordan M, Grosschedl R (1999) Coordinate regulation of B cell differentiation by the transcription factors EBF and E2A. Immunity 11:21–31

Pioli C, Gatta L, Ubaldi V, Doria G (2000) Inhibition of IgG1 and IgE production by stimulation of the B cell CTLA-4 receptor. J Immunol 165:5530–5536

Quong MW, Harris DP, Swain SL, Murre C (1999) E2A activity is induced during B-cell activation to promote immunoglobulin class switch recombination. EMBO J 18:6307–6318

Quong MW, Romanow WJ, Murre C (2002) E protein function in lymphocyte development. Annu Rev Immunol 20:301–322

Riley RL, Van Der Put E, King AM, Frasca D, Blomberg, BB (2005) Deficient B lymphopoiesis in murine senescence: potential roles for dysregulation of E2A, Pax-5, and STAT5. Semin Immunol 17:330–336

Rivera R, Murre C (2001) The regulation and function of the Id proteins in lymphocyte development. Oncogene 20:8308–8316

Roberts EC, Deed RW, Inoue T, Norton JD, Sharrocks AD (2001) Id helix-loop-helix proteins antagonize pax transcription factor activity by inhibiting DNA binding. Mol Cell Biol 21:524–533

Saito T, Chiba S, Ichikawa M, Kunisato A, Asai T, Shimizu K, Yamaguchi T, Yamamoto G, Seo S, Kumano K, Nakagami-Yamaguchi E, Hamada Y, Aizawa S, Hirai H (2003) Notch2 is preferentially expressed in mature B cells and indispensable for marginal zone B lineage development. Immunity 18:675–685

Sayegh CE, Quong MW, Agata Y, Murre C (2003) E-proteins directly regulate expression of activation-induced deaminase in mature B cells. Nat Immunol 4:586–593

Schlissel M, Voronova A, Baltimore D (1991) Helix-loop-helix transcription factor E47 activates germ-line immunoglobulin heavy-chain gene transcription and rearrangement in a pre-T-cell line. Genes Dev 5:1367–1376

Shaffer AL, Lin KI, Kuo TC, Yu X, Hurt EM, Rosenwald A, Giltnane JM, Yang L, Zhao H, Calame K, Staudt LM (2002) Blimp-1 orchestrates plasma cell differentiation by extinguishing the mature B cell gene expression program. Immunity 17:51–62

Shen C-P, Kadesch T (1995) B-cell-specific DNA binding by an E47 homodimer. Mol Cell Biol 15:4518–4524

Sigvardsson M, O'Riordan M, Grosschedl R (1997) EBF and E47 collaborate to induce expression of the endogenous immunoglobulin surrogate light chain genes. Immunity 7:25–36

Smith AM (1976) The effects of age on the immune response to type III pneumococcal polysaccharide (SIII) and bacterial lipopolysaccharide (LPS) in BALB/c, SJL/J, and C3H mice. J Immunol 116:469–474

Snapper CM, Zelazowski P, Rosas FR, Kehry MR, Tian M, Baltimore D, Sha, WC (1996) B cells from p50/NF-kappa B knockout mice have selective defects in proliferation, differentiation, germ-line CH transcription, and Ig class switching. J Immunol 156:183-191

Song H, Price PW, Cerny J (1997) Age-related changes in antibody repertoire: contribution from T cells. Immunol Rev 160:55–62

Sugai M, Gonda H, Kusunoki T, Katakai T, Yokota Y, Shimizu A (2003) Essential role of Id2 in negative regulation of IgE class switching. Nat Immunol 4:25–30

Tell G, Scaloni A, Pellizzari L, Formisano S, Pucillo C, Damante G (1998) Redox potential controls the structure and DNA binding activity of the paired domain. J Biol Chem 273:25062–25072

Tinnell SB, Jacobs-Helber SM, Sterneck E, Sawyer ST, Conrad DH (1998) STAT6, NF-kappaB and C/EBP in CD23 expression and IgE production. Int Immunol 10:1529–1538

Tunyaplin C, Shaffer AL, Angelin-Duclos CD, Yu X, Staudt LM, Calame KL (2004) Direct repression of prdm1 by Bcl-6 inhibits plasmacytic differentiation. J Immunol 173:1158–1165

Van Der Put E, Frasca D, King AM, Blomberg BB, Riley RL (2004) Decreased E47 in senescent B cell precursors is stage specific and regulated posttranslationally by protein turnover. J Immunol 173:818–827

Weksler MC, Innes JD, Goldstein G (1978) Immunological studies of aging. IV. The contribution of thymic involution to the immune deficiencies of aging mice and reversal with thymopoietin32-36. J Exp Med 148:996–1006

Whisler RL, Williams JW, Jr, Newhouse YG (1991) Human B cell proliferative responses during aging. Reduced RNA synthesis and DNA replication after signal transduction by surface immunoglobulins compared to B cell antigenic determinants CD20 and CD40. Mech Ageing Dev 61:209–222

Yamada T, Zhang K, Yamada A, Zhu D, Saxon A (2005) B lymphocyte stimulator activates p38 mitogen-activated protein kinase in human Ig class switch recombination. Am J Respir Cell Mol Biol 32:388–394

Zheng B, Han S, Takahashi Y, Kelsoe G (1997) Immunosenescence and germinal center reaction. Immunol Rev 160:63–77

Zwollo P, Desiderio S (1994) Specific recognition of the blk promoter by the B-lymphoid transcription factor B-cell-specific activator protein. J Biol Chem 269:15310–15317

B-Cell Repertoire Changes in Mouse Models of Aging

Jean L. Scholz, William J. Quinn III and Michael P. Cancro

Contents

Abstract: Changes in the antibody repertoire are a well-established feature of immunosenescence. These reflect an aggregate of age-associated alterations in the generation, numbers, and proportions of B-cell subsets; as well as the homeostatic and selective processes governing them. A basic understanding of these relationships, coupled with integrated assessments of how they change with age, should reveal mechanisms underlying the immunosenescent phenotype. Mouse models provide powerful tools for these analyses, allowing controlled manipulation of key genetic, cellular, and microenvironmental factors. Here we summarize current understanding of how primary and antigen-experienced murine B-cell repertoires are established, as well as how they shift with age.

M. P. Cancro (✉)
Department of Pathology and Laboratory Medicine
University of Pennsylvania School of Medicine
36th and Hamilton Walk
Philadelphia, PA 19104-6082, USA
Tel.: 215 898 8067; Fax: 215 573 2350
E-mail: cancro@mail.med.upenn.edu

T. Fulop et al. (eds.), *Handbook on Immunosenescence*,
DOI 10.1007/ 978-1-4020-9062-2_20, © Springer Science+Business Media B.V. 2009

1   Introduction

Immunosenescence, the progressive dysregulation of immune function with age, reflects a mosaic of genetic, epigenetic, and microenvironmental changes [10, 11, 34, 42, 44, 77, 101, 102, 125–127, 158]. This complexity confounds minimal explanations of the overall phenomenon, and underscores the need to exploit systems whereby defined factors can be deliberately manipulated. Accordingly, mouse model systems, which have been refined as immunologic experimental tools, should yield insights into the underlying mechanistic relationships.

Altered clonotype repertoires are a consistent feature of immunosenescence. This is anecdotally evident from the shifts in immune responsiveness, increased autoimmunity, and clonal expansions that accompany age; and is corroborated through empirical evidence in human and animal models. For example, both the frequency and clonotypic composition of hapten- and virus-specific primary B-cells change with age [76, 112–114, 136, 182, 184, 185]; and nearly all laboratory mouse strains display an age-associated appearance of autoantibodies [29, 30]. Most observations addressing these age-associated repertoire shifts are based on assessments at single time points. While these can *identify* repertoire changes, the underlying mechanisms resist interrogation via such static sampling approaches, because lymphocytes comprise multiple, dynamic populations under stringent selective and homeostatic controls.

Lymphocyte dynamics involve the continuous generation and corresponding loss of cells, such that relatively constant numbers are maintained. Thus, the stability of lymphocyte numbers disguises underlying and ongoing cellular and molecular processes. For example, commitment rates to the B lineage per se, as well as the entrance rates and lifespan of B-cells in different functional subsets, can vary. Further, these compartments not only play differing immunological roles, but also can interact with and impact one another's behavior. Finally, selective events based on B-cell receptor (BCR) specificity, innate ligand responsiveness, and homeostatic factors are superimposed on this dynamically changing landscape. Accordingly, effective interrogation of repertoire changes—including those associated with advancing age—requires simultaneous, longitudinal assessments of lymphocyte generation, homeostasis, and selection.

Indeed, the size, proportions, and dynamics of nearly all progenitor and mature B lineage subsets shift with age in the mouse, so overall changes in clonotype frequency and composition likely reflect the aggregate of these shifts. Understanding age-associated repertoire changes therefore requires an appreciation of the molecular and cellular mechanisms governing primary and antigen-experienced repertoires. Herein we review currently accepted notions about the identity and relationships of B lineage subsets and their progenitors, emphasizing the selective and homeostatic processes impacting repertoire composition. With this as background, age-associated changes in these parameters and their potential relationship to repertoire shifts in primary and antigen-experienced B-cell subsets are discussed. A schematic summary of these overall changes is provided in Fig. 1.

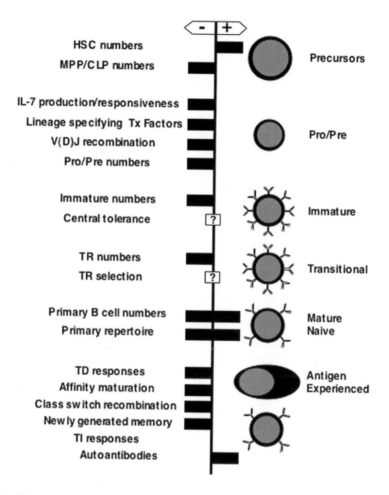

Fig. 1 Changes in B-cell traits with age. Major B-cell subsets are shown at right with character-istic traits and/or processes at left. Bars indicate changes in aged mice compared to young adults. Bars left-of-center denote age-associated reductions, while bars right-of-center indicate age-asso-ciated increases, of a characteristic. Disparate or mixed results are indicated as bi-directional bars, and currently unexplored issues are signified by a central question mark.

2 Primary Repertoire Development

2.1 Lineage Commitment and Developing Bone Marrow B-Cell Subsets

In adults, B-cells are generated in the bone marrow (BM), where pluripotent hematopoietic stem cells (HSCs) give rise to multipotent progenitor (MPPs) that initiate lymphoid-restricted gene expression. This yields common lymphoid progenitors (CLPs) [65], a population enriched for B lineage specified precursors that subsequently become committed to the B lineage [2]. Several transcription factors and cytokine receptors comprise a regulatory network for B lineage specification and commitment [16, 66, 90, 106, 117, 151] (also see Frasca et al., this volume). For example, Ikaros is expressed in all hematopoietic lineages and controls the emergence of lymphoid progenitors [68, 111]; the proto-oncogene PU.1 is critical for both myeloid and lymphoid differentiation [149]; and the transcriptional repressor Bcl11A is essential for normal B- and T-cell development [72]. The E protein family members E2A and EBF coordinately activate the expression of B-cell specific genes, especially those governing pre-BCR production and function [64, 66, 119, 150] and also regulate Pax-5 [140], a key mediator that activates B lineage-specific genes and represses genes associated with other lineages [16, 17]. IL-7/IL-7R is a key cytokine axis for early B lineage development, promoting both survival and differentiation [2]. Complex interplay between cell intrinsic and extrinsic signals characterizes the regulation of these transcriptional systems [26, 90, 150].

Although these transcriptional and signaling events occur prior to antigen receptor gene rearrangement, they can nonetheless influence repertoire composition in several ways. First, they dictate the rate of lineage commitment, thus impacting B-cell production rates and shifting downstream homeostatic demands. Second, they influence the rate and specificity of key intracellular events, thus coloring the likelihood and nature of heavy and light chain gene rearrangements.

Subsequent to lineage commitment, B-cell differentiative stages are characterized according to surface markers and Ig gene rearrangement status [46–48, 94, 121, 122, 138]. In the pro-B stage, cells rearrange their Ig heavy chain genes [40, 180]. This is followed by surface Ig heavy chain expression with surrogate light chain and BCR signaling molecules, delineating onset of the pre-B-cell stage. Surface pre-BCR expression and signaling are required for transit from the pro- to pre-B-cell stage [61, 92, 93, 123, 133, 134, 164, 165], and result in a proliferative burst characteristic of the large pre-B-cell compartment. Light chain gene rearrangement during the late pre-B-cell stage leads to the expression of a complete BCR, defining the immature (IMM) BM B-cell. Once in the IMM subset, cells either die or exit the BM to complete maturation [6, 7].

2.2 Peripheral Maturation and Primary B-Cell Subsets

Recent marrow émigrés have been dubbed transitional (TR) B-cells [73], and can be further divided into subsets termed T1, T2, and T3 [1]. While historically viewed as a linear progression from the IMM marrow stage through the successive TR compartments, it now appears that branched, asynchronous models for transit into and through these subsets are more likely [5, 91, 145, 153]. Cells that successfully complete TR differentiation enter the mature peripheral B-cell pools.

Mature follicular (FO) B-cells, also termed B2 or "conventional" B-cells, encompass the majority (>80%) of peripheral B-lymphocytes, and are the progenitors of both primary antibody forming cells and memory B-cells. Additional subsets of mature B-cells include marginal zone (MZ) B-cells, which are phenotypically, functionally, and anatomically distinct from FO B-cells and play a major role in responses to T-cell independent (TI) antigens. In peritoneal and pleural cavities the B1 subset predominates (reviewed in [52]). B1 B-cells appear first in ontogeny and are maintained by self-renewal [48, 49, 53]. The MZ and B1 subsets share several functional attributes, particularly participation in TI immune responses [63, 74, 75, 83]. The derivation of B1 B-cells, though distinct from the other B-cell subsets, is not yet entirely clear [1, 14, 52, 54, 74, 104, 176]. However, in the context of age-associated repertoire shifts, it is noteworthy that while production from BM B2 progenitors predominates in young adults, this wanes in aged mice. Therefore, if B1 progenitors are stable and distinct from B2 progenitors, the B1 lineage may wax with advancing age; thus altering the combined B-cell repertoire [104, 105].

2.3 Selection and Homeostasis Among Emerging and Primary B-Cells

Although they occur before complete BCR expression and perforce cannot be specificity-driven, heavy and light chain gene rearrangement processes, as well as heavy chain selection at the pre-BCR stage, will influence the incipient B-cell repertoire. For example, only heavy chains with structural characteristics affording surrogate light chain pairing are selected for further differentiation [81, 95]. In addition, heavy and light chain gene rearrangement processes rely on multiple factors, including the expression of appropriate enzyme and targeting complexes, accessibility and marking of heavy and light chain loci, and the activity of DNA damage resistance and repair systems (for reviews see [32, 59, 62, 107, 108, 139, 142–144]).

The interaction of homeostasis and selection powerfully impacts all B-cell subsets downstream of BCR expression, directly determining repertoire composition. A critical notion emerging from appreciation of this interplay is that events acting upstream of mature B-lymphocyte pools can impact downstream populations. Since advancing age is accompanied by substantial shifts in both B-cell generation and the success rate of IMM and TR differentiation, distinguishing primary lesions from homeostatic compensation is critical to a mechanistic understanding of age-related changes [19, 99, 131].

Stringent specificity-based selection occurs at the IMM stage, where high avidity interactions yield secondary Ig gene rearrangements or death [21, 22, 41, 109, 110, 115, 116, 128–130, 162]. These central tolerance mechanisms result in the loss of ~90% of all IMM cells formed [7, 120]. While it is possible that the IMM pool is governed by homeostatic mechanisms to preserve its size, this remains speculative and does not seem tied to BCR-mediated negative selection. Instead, BCR signal strength is the major, if not sole, determinant of survival at the IMM stage.

Specificity-based selection continues to act on newly formed cells that exit the marrow to join TR pools. Whereas high avidity BCR interactions lead to cell death, a lack of minimal BCR signaling precludes maturation and entrance to mature peripheral pools [20, 23, 33, 51, 82, 169]. While BM negative selection depends on BCR signal strength (and is therefore cell-intrinsic), the likelihood that a given cell completes TR differentiation to join a mature B-cell subset is based on both BCR signal strength and the availability of B-lymphocyte stimulator (BLyS, also termed BAFF). BLyS is the limiting resource for which TR, FO, and MZ B-cells compete (reviewed in [18] and [100]). Through this competitive mechanism, steady state numbers of mature B-cells are governed by ambient BLyS levels that vary the proportion of TR cells completing maturation, as well as the lifespan of FO and MZ B-cells [50, 57]. This connection between BCR specificity and fitness for interclonal competition indicates that BLyS availability, within the context of the emerging clonotypic cohort, will determine thresholds for TR selection. This relationship has recently been confirmed in several transgenic systems [56, 70, 161].

The relationship between BLyS availability, antigen receptor specificity, and TR selective stringency makes several implications relevant to age-associated changes in the primary repertoire. First it implies that BCR- and BLyS-mediated signals must be integrated, possibly via cross-talk between intracellular signaling systems [154]. Although the molecular details remain the subject of intense research, age associated perturbations of any of these systems may influence primary repertoire diversity. Moreover, decreased B-cell generation rates in BM—a feature of the aging immune system—might permit a broader array of clonotypes, including autoreactive cells, to enter peripheral pools as competition wanes [100].

3   Antigen-Experienced Pools

3.1   Establishing and Maintaining Antigen-Experienced Subsets

Antigen-experienced subsets contain the descendants of primary B-cells recruited into immune responses, and thus include activated cells themselves, as well as the resulting effector and memory pools. Humoral immune responses are generally characterized as T-dependent (TD) or T-independent (TI), depending on their requirement for cognate T help. In general, protein antigens engender TD responses, reflecting the requisite for MHC class II restricted presentation that affords delivery of costimulation. These responses primarily involve FO B-cells, and typically lead to long-term humoral immunity. A key characteristic of TD responses is the formation of germinal centers (GCs), where proliferating B-cells undergo class switch recombination, as well as the somatic hypermutation (SHM) and affinity-based selection processes that culminate in cells producing high-affinity antibody [86]. In contrast, TI responses do not require cognate help, although T-cell derived cytokines may promote limited isotype switching [15]. TI responses elicit little if any memory, lack substantial hypermutation or affinity maturation, and consist predominantly of IgM. Two classes of TI antigens exist: TI-1 responses are induced via pattern recognition receptors [148]; whereas TI-2 responses are generated by antigens with densely repeating epitopes. Both TI-1 and TI-2 responses preferentially arise from

B1 and MZ B-cells. Whether this reflects intrinsic bias in the pre-immune repertoires of these cells or more extensive expression of pattern recognition receptors [58, 84]—both of which are empirically observed—remains debated.

Antigen activation yields a series of short-lived cells, which are detectable for only days or weeks following antigen challenge; as well as several subsets of long-lived cells, which persist for months or years [80, 141, 163]. During TD responses, antigen activated B-cells become either GC B-cells, or short-lived plasma cells (PC), in a differentiation decision dictated by BCR affinity [124]. Short-lived PC arise in the first few days of an immune response, congregating at the T/B-cell interface and extrafollicular regions of secondary lymphoid organs [86]. The critical relationship between BCR repertoire and recruitment into long-lived pools has been revealed using transgenic systems [24, 25]. For example, B-cells with low initial affinity for antigen can participate in GC reactions when higher affinity competition is eliminated, suggesting that initial repertoire can shape the pool of antigen-reactive B-cells that ultimately succeed and contribute to immune responses. Long-lived antigen-experienced populations include a group of long-lived PC, as well as a separate group termed memory B-cells [79, 87]. The delineation of these groups based on surface markers is debated; however, a clear functional difference is that long-lived PC secrete antibody, while memory cells do not [9, 28, 78, 85, 87–89]. The lineal relationships between various antigen-experienced subsets are unclear. For example, whether long-lived populations are generated from cells within the generally short-lived populations, or instead differentiate from distinct progenitors through a separate selective mechanism, is debated.

3.2   Homeostasis in Antigen Experienced Subsets

The concept of a biological niche for naïve B-cells is well established, with the BLyS/BR3 ligand/receptor axis playing a central role. In contrast, knowledge of factors governing the size and composition of antigen-experienced B-cell subsets is more limited. As with naïve pools, interplay between homeostasis and selection seems likely in the establishment and maintenance of antigen-experienced subsets. Multiple steps in the generation of effector and memory B-cells rely on selective decisions. These include the relationship between BCR affinity and recruitment into the extrafollicular PC pool versus the GC [124]; affinity maturation per se; as well as commitment to long-lived PC versus memory B-cells [8, 31].

Homeostatic controls, while evident in antigen-experienced pools, also remain poorly understood. While neither short-term effectors or long lived antigen experienced populations compete with primary B-cells for survival, the trophic factors and relationships are only now being explored. Recent evidence suggests that additional BLyS family receptors or ligands, such as TACI, BCMA and APRIL likely play a role. In support of this idea, TACI is associated with activated B-cells and regulates some TI immune responses [163, 168], whereas BCMA is required for survival of long-lived PC in BM [118]. Further, ongoing immune responses appear to create temporary homeostatic niches for short-lived populations, while leading to little change in long-term protective memory pools [132]. Finally, long-lived BM PC survival is competitive [78–80], possibly involving cell extrinsic stromal factors, as well as Fc-gammaRIIb expression [177].

4 Age-Associated Changes in Progenitor and Primary Pools

An extensive literature suggests the primary repertoire shifts with age. For example, the phosphorylcholine-specific repertoire shifts from one predominated by the T15 clonotype to a more diverse pool [113, 114, 136, 185]. On the other hand, overall diversity in the primary pool is not altered extensively, as assessed by fine specificity analyses [113, 183]. Nonetheless, clonal expansions in both the B and T-cell pools suggest that some specificities can be inordinately expanded. Understanding the basis for these changes requires considering all events likely to impact repertoire generation, selection, and maintenance. These include changes in the size and behavior of generative pools, as well as changes in the primary pools themselves.

4.1 B-Cell Generative Rates and Subsets Change with Age

Age-associated changes in B lineage development include reductions in precursor frequencies, lowered expression of critical regulatory genes, diminished pro- and pre B-cell numbers, and damped responsiveness to differentiation cues [35, 39, 60, 69, 97, 136, 146, 156, 157, 166]. Together, these observations indicate overall diminution of B-cell generation and throughput.

The impact of aging is first manifested in HSCs and CLPs. Somewhat paradoxically, while HSC numbers are maintained and possibly expanded in aged mice [179], the MPP/ELP and CLP pools are reduced [3, 97, 98]. Although the basis for this remains unclear, correlations with age-associated reductions in stromal IL-7 production [156]; as well as reduced expression of E2A and EBF and genes they control, suggest these may contribute [35, 39, 147, 166, 167]. As might be expected from these changes in upstream pools, pro-B-cell numbers are reduced, with an even greater proportional reduction in pre-B-cell numbers [4, 131, 135]. This decline in part reflects reduced IL-7-mediated proliferation at the pro- to pre-B transition [103, 155]. Hormonal changes may be another important extrinsic factor, since pregnancies delay the age-associated reduction in BM B-cell production [12].

The dynamics of developing B-cells also change with age. In vivo BrdU labeling studies [60, 67, 69] showed reductions in successful pro- to pre B-cell transit, yielding a fourfold drop in pre-B-cell numbers, and a corresponding decrease in the IMM B-cell generation rate. However, the throughput of pre-B-cells increased, so a twofold greater proportion of pre-B-cells enter the IMM pool. In addition, residency within the IMM pool is longer. Together, these apparent compensatory features result in an IMM pool that is only about twofold smaller than in young adults.

4.2 Dynamics and Proportions of Peripheral Subsets Change with Age

Reflecting the upstream reductions in IMM B-cell numbers, TR pools are reduced in throughput and size; however, because residency time is extended, TR cell numbers are not significantly reduced. Similarly, the FO pool's turnover rate is reduced in aged mice [60, 67, 131], so FO pool size is maintained in the face of reduced marrow production. Despite this fairly stable overall size, B-cell clonal expansions are more prevalent in aged mice [13, 171, 172]. In contrast, the MZ and B1 pools are unaffected or even enlarged in aged mice, but this may vary by strain [4, 131, 171].

Whether the homeostatic mechanisms controlling primary B-cell numbers change with age has not been extensively interrogated. However, several recent observations suggest this is likely. For example, in young adults, emerging cells expressing high levels of the BLyS receptor, TACI, are selected during TR differentiation. This process is dampened in aged mice, allowing cells with lower TACI levels to join the mature FO pool [131]. In addition, FO B-cells from aged mice more effectively capture BLyS-mediated survival signals in vitro, although the underlying mechanism is unclear. These observations suggest a model whereby selection at the marrow-periphery interface is relaxed in aged mice; yet competition among mature B-cells may be more severe, reflecting lifelong selection for optimally fit clonotypes [131].

4.3 Developing and Primary Repertoires Change with Age

Alterations in the BM pre-selection repertoire might be expected, given the numerous age-associated changes in cytokine and transcription factors, many of which are involved in Ig gene rearrangement [39, 69, 146, 147, 156]. There is a correlation between the age-associated reduction of pre-B-cell numbers and reduced RAG gene expression, V(D)J recombinase activity, and V to (D)J rearrangement [69, 159, 160]. Evidence for age-associated, intrinsic shifts in V gene segment use are suggested by studies showing an increased frequency of phosphorylcholine-responsive cells arising from sIg⁻ BM cells in aged BALB/c mice [185]. These increases included clonotypes bearing VhS107 (T15) as well as other Vh segments.

The interplay of intrinsic and microenvironmental changes in aged BM could affect the pre-selection repertoire in several ways. Shifts in heavy chain allele choice at the pre-BCR stage or in light chain choice at the pre-B stage could alter repertoire composition. Decreased pre-B-cell production may mean that fewer B-cells of different clonotypes are generated. However, this effect may be at least partially offset if extended residency time in the IMM stage affords greater opportunity for receptor editing or Vh gene replacement. Finally, the existence of multiple B differentiation lineages whose Vh gene preferences differ and whose dominance varies with age might underlie some of these observations.

There is ample evidence for age-associated shifts in the primary repertoire, but whether these act to generally expand or contract diversity is uncertain. The phosphorylcholine-specific response in young BALB/c and B6 mice is dominated by VhS107/Vk22 gene segments, whereas aged mice use a broader range of Vh and Vk segments [112, 113]. Moreover, phosphorylcholine-binding monoclonal antibodies generated from aged mice show greater polyreactivity. In contrast, while the frequency of NP-responsive cells is about twofold lower in aged mice, there is no accompanying change in repertoire diversity or clonotype distrubution [184]; and repertoire diversity to influenza hemagglutinin is similar in aged and young mice [183]. Finally, the autoreconstituting repertoire that emerges after irraditaion- or drug-induced lymphopenia is truncated in aged mice, when assessed by CDR3 length heterogeneity [71].

5 Immune Responses and Antigen-Experienced Pools Change With Age

Some age-related changes in immune responses may be related to shifts in the pre-selection or primary repertoires, while others may be the result of alterations that are observed as or after responding cells have encountered antigen. Immune responses in aged mice sometimes—but not always—involve reduced antibody production and/or antibody of lower affinity in comparison to young mice; however, overall diversity of the responding repertoire is retained or enhanced. Short-lived PC responses and pools are normal to increased in aged individuals, whereas long-lived PC and memory cell numbers are reduced. All of this suggests that the antigen-experienced repertoire is different in quality and possibly quantity in aged mice.

Extensive age-associated changes have been reported in TD immune responses. These include impaired GC formation and kinetics, defective cellular interactions, and deficiencies in SHM and affinity maturation (reviewed in [187]). The antibody response to NP-CGG in aged B6 mice is impaired in terms of primary response kinetics and the amount of antibody produced; moreover, the average affinity of NP-binding antibodies is sixfold lower than in young mice [96]. Although GCs form in aged mice, their number and size are significantly reduced, their kinetics are delayed, and there is no detectable SHM. In apparent contrast, some experimental systems suggest that SHM yields increased diversity of serum Igs in aged mice [175]. These different results are not necessarily contradictory, as SHM may occur even when B-cells are activated outside of GCs [173, 174]. Microenvironment may play an important role: Peyer's patch GC B-cells from aged B6D2F1 mice were similar in frequency and activation phenotype to those observed in young mice, yet showed higher somatic mutation frequencies [137].

Cellular interactions are also altered with age [43, 152, 178]. T-cell intrinsic changes may account for some of this; for example, a decrease in IL-2 production with age leads to reduced CD40L expression as well as a general CD4+T-cell population shift away from a naive phenotype and towards either a memory or a regulatory phenotype [55]. The proportion of antigen-responsive B-cells to DNP-specific stimulation is decreased in aged mice, and T-cells from aged mice can down-regulate B-cell responsiveness [181, 182]. In an Igh^b scid chimera system with donor lymphocytes from young or aged mice, where the primary response to NP is highly restricted to use of Vh186.2/lambda-1 gene segments, aged donor helper T-cells—but not aged B-cells—are less effective at inducing GC formation, and shift Vh gene segment use away from Vh186.2 to include higher proportions of others, particularly C1H4 [178]. In addition, SHM in GC B-cells was reduced in frequency with aged donor T- or B cells. Thus, both germline repertoire use and SHM are likely altered in aged mice; and immunosenescence likley results from changes in both B- and T cell compartments.

Class-switch recombination also appears impaired in aged mice [36–38]. B-cells from old BALB/c mice stimulated in vitro with optimal levels of CD40L and IL-4 display a reduced ability to isotype switch [38]. Defects in isotype switching as well as SHM are associated with an age-related downregulation of E47, which leads to reduced expression of the activation-induced cytidine deaminase (AID) [37].

Mirroring the spectrum of observations in primary repertoire analyses, whether age impacts the magnitude or diversity of antibody responses depends on the model antigen employed, as well as the strain of mice studied. For example, the magnitude of the antibody response to S. pneumoniae vaccine and TNP-BA differ in B6 and BALB/c mice, indicating a role for genetic factors in the immune response [113]. However, the clonotypic diversity of the response to both antigens and to phosphorylcholine is greater in aged mice of both strains [112, 113]. In contrast, both primary and secondary responses to DNP-BGG are reduced in aged mice [43, 170]. A study of the IgM component of the primary response to TNP-KLH shows that the peak IgM response is delayed in aged mice but the spectrum and affinity of antibodies are similar to those seen in young animals [186].

Several studies have shown decreased affinity or avidity of antibodies produced by aged mice in TD responses, in some cases along with evidence for a role for altered T-cell responses [27, 43, 114, 170, 186]. When mixtures of phosphorylcholine-specific antibodies from young or aged donor mice are injected into recipients that subsequently receive a lethal dose of S. pneumoniae, only antibodies from young donors allowed survival [114]. Moreover, the average affinity of antibodies from aged donors is lower than that of young donors for free PC hapten [114]. Thus the efficacy of antibodies produced by aged mice may be quite different from those produced by young mice. In accord with this overall picture, aged mice challenged with NP-CGG show a higher antigen-forming cell (AFC) response than young mice, but smaller and fewer GCs [45]. Most of the AFC in old mice were low-affinity IgM producers, and the number of high-affinity AFC was half that of young controls. There were significantly fewer AFC in BM of aged mice following immunization, and reconstitution experiments demonstrated that aged BM was defective in supporting AFC. Thus, the spleen may prove the primary source of the antibody response in aged mice, in contrast to BM in young mice. This shift in AFC location could reflect several potential age related defects in the B-cell response including potential BM homing problems, an altered antigen specific precursor frequency, reduced capacity for AFCs in the BM environment, or a combination of these and other factors. Due to the unclear relationship between naïve B-cells and long-lived PC generation, it is difficult to determine whether impaired humoral immunity in the aged is due to a failure to generate cells capable of seeding the BM and becoming PC memory, or if the defect is downstream. It has been proposed that long-lived PC occupy a highly specialized, tightly regulated niche, and it is possible that this niche is unable to support the entrance of newly formed long-lived PC in old mice, due to intensive competition for survival factors [132].

Only a few studies have addressed TI responses in aged mice. Zharhary [186] made a direct comparison of the IgM response following immunization with TD versus TI forms of the TNP hapten. While the peak IgM response was delayed in aged mice for the TD antigen, there was no delay for the TI antigen. Similarly, Weksler [170] reports that TI responses are generally less impaired than TD responses in aged mice.

It is tempting to speculate that because TI responses are largely B-cell-intrinsic, they will be less severely impacted by age-related changes in T-cell function. Moreover, TI responses may be further preserved by the age-associated persistence of MZ and B1 cells [131], which are largely responsible for antibody production to TI antigens. Thus, the comparative resilience of TI responses may increasingly impact repertoire composition with advancing age.

6   Summary and Perspective

Assessing the nature and basis for repertoire changes is a first-order consideration in our understanding of immunosenescence. Multiple processes appear to act in concert to alter repertoire with age. These include reduced B-cell generation, shifts in V gene choice, and altered subset dynamics and selection overlaid with compensatory homeostatic mechanisms. Murine model systems are attractive routes to interrogate the underlying mechanisms, not only because of their substantial similarities to age associated shifts in human immune responsiveness, but also because they provide an opportunity to approach basic questions experimentally. Some important questions include why and how BM B-cell generation decreases with age, and how this impacts repertoire; whether the stringency of central or TR tolerance change with age; and how B-cell repertoire shifts and impaired immune responses in aged individuals are linked.

References

1. Allman D, Lindsley RC, DeMuth W, Rudd K, Shinton SA, Hardy RR (2001) Resolution of three nonproliferative immature splenic B cell subsets reveals multiple selection points during peripheral B cell maturation. J Immunol 167(12):6834–6840

2. Allman D, Miller JP (2003) Common lymphoid progenitors, early B-lineage precursors, and IL-7: characterizing the trophic and instructive signals underlying early B cell development. Immunol Res 27(2–3):131–140

3. Allman D, Miller JP (2005) The aging of early B-cell precursors. Immunol Rev 205:18–29

4. Allman D, Miller JP (2005) B cell development and receptor diversity during aging. Curr Opin Immunol 17(5):463–467

5. Allman D, Srivastava B, Lindsley RC (2004) Alternative routes to maturity: branch points and pathways for generating follicular and marginal zone B cells. Immunol Rev 197:147–160

6. Allman DM, Ferguson SE, Cancro MP (1992) Peripheral B cell maturation. I. Immature peripheral B cells in adults are heat-stable antigenhi and exhibit unique signaling characteristics. J Immunol 149(8):2533–2540

7. Allman DM, Ferguson SE, Lentz VM, Cancro MP (1993) Peripheral B cell maturation. II. Heat-stable antigen(hi) splenic B cells are an immature developmental intermediate in the production of long-lived marrow-derived B cells. J Immunol 151(9):4431–4444

8. Angelin-Duclos C, Cattoretti G, Lin KI, Calame K (2000) Commitment of B lymphocytes to a plasma cell fate is associated with Blimp-1 expression in vivo. J Immunol 165(10):5462–5471

9. Arce S, Luger E, Muehlinghaus G, Cassese G, Hauser A, Horst A, Lehnert K, Odendahl M, Honemann D, Heller KD et al (2004) CD38 low IgG-secreting cells are precursors of various CD38 high-expressing plasma cell populations. J Leukoc Biol 75(6):1022–1028

10. Aspinall R, Andrew D (2000) Immunosenescence: potential causes and strategies for reversal. Biochem Soc Trans 28(2):250–254

11. Aw D, Silva AB, Palmer DB (2007) Immunosenescence: emerging challenges for an ageing population. Immunology 120(4):435–446

12. Barrat FS, Lesourd BM, Louise AS, Boulouis H, Thibault DJ, Neway T, Pilet CA (1999) Pregnancies modulate B lymphopoiesis and myelopoiesis during murine ageing. Immunology 98(4):604–611

13. Ben-Yehuda A, Szabo P, LeMaoult J, Manavalan JS, Weksler ME (1998) Increased VH 11 and VH Q52 gene use by splenic B cells in old mice associated with oligoclonal expansions of CD5 + B cells. Mech Ageing Dev 103(2):111–121

14. Berland R, Wortis HH (2002) Origins and functions of B-1 cells with notes on the role of CD5. Annu Rev Immunol 20:253–300

15. Borisova TK (2006) Role of cytokines in immune response to T-independent antigens, type 2. Zh Mikrobiol Epidemiol Immunobiol (1):44–47

16. Busslinger M (2004) Transcriptional control of early B cell development. Annu Rev Immunol 22:55–79

17. Busslinger M, Urbanek P (1995) The role of BSAP (Pax-5) in B-cell development. Curr Opin Genet Dev 5(5):595–601

18. Cancro MP (2004) The BLyS family of ligands and receptors: an archetype for niche-specific homeostatic regulation. Immunol Rev 202:237–249

19. Cancro MP (2005) B cells and aging: gauging the interplay of generative, selective, and homeostatic events. Immunol Rev 205:48–59

20. Cancro MP, Kearney JF (2004) B cell positive selection: road map to the primary repertoire? J Immunol 173(1):15–19

21. Casellas R, Shih TA, Kleinewietfeld M, Rakonjac J, Nemazee D, Rajewsky K, Nussenzweig MC (2001) Contribution of receptor editing to the antibody repertoire. Science 291(5508):1541–1544

22. Chen C, Nagy Z, Prak EL, Weigert M (1995) Immunoglobulin heavy chain gene replacement: a mechanism of receptor editing. Immunity 3(6):747–755

23. Clarke SH, McCray SK (1993) VH CDR3-dependent positive selection of murine VH12-expressing B cells in the neonate. European J Immunol 23:3327–3334

24. Dal Porto JM, Haberman AM, Kelsoe G, Shlomchik MJ (2002) Very low affinity B cells form germinal centers, become memory B cells, and participate in secondary immune responses when higher affinity competition is reduced. J Exp Med 195(9):1215–1221

25. Dal Porto JM, Haberman AM, Shlomchik MJ, Kelsoe G (1998) Antigen drives very low affinity B cells to become plasmacytes and enter germinal centers. J Immunol 161(10):5373–5381

26. DeKoter RP, Lee HJ, Singh H (2002) PU.1 regulates expression of the interleukin-7 receptor in lymphoid progenitors. Immunity 16(2):297–309

27. Doria G, D'Agostaro G, Poretti A (1978) Age-dependent variations of antibody avidity. Immunology 35(4):601–611

28. Driver DJ, McHeyzer-Williams LJ, Cool M, Stetson DB, McHeyzer-Williams MG (2001) Development and maintenance of a B220- memory B cell compartment. J Immunol 167(3):1393–1405

29. Eaton-Bassiri AS, Mandik-Nayak L, Seo SJ, Madaio MP, Cancro MP, Erikson J (2000) Alterations in splenic architecture and the localization of anti-double-stranded DNA B cells in aged mice. Int Immunol 12(6):915–926

30. Erikson J, Mandik L, Bui A, Eaton A, Noorchashm H, Nguyen KA, Roark JH (1998) Self-reactive B cells in nonautoimmune and autoimmune mice. Immunol Res 17(1–2):49–61

31. Fairfax KA, Corcoran LM, Pridans C, Huntington ND, Kallies A, Nutt SL, Tarlinton DM (2007) Different kinetics of blimp-1 induction in B cell subsets revealed by reporter gene. J Immunol 178(7):4104–4111

32. Feeney AJ, Goebel P, Espinoza CR (2004) Many levels of control of V gene rearrangement frequency. Immunol Rev 200:44–56

33. Forsdyke DR (2005) "Altered-self" or "near-self" in the positive selection of lymphocyte repertoires? Immunol Lett 100(2):103–106

34. Franceschi C, Passeri M, De Benedictis G, Motta L (1998) Immunosenescence. Aging (Milano) 10(2):153–154

35. Frasca D, Nguyen D, Van Der Put E, Riley RL, Blomberg BB (2003) The age-related decrease in E47 DNA-binding does not depend on increased Id inhibitory proteins in bone marrow-derived B cell precursors. Front Biosci 8:a110–a116

36. Frasca D, Riley RL, Blomberg BB (2004) Effect of age on the immunoglobulin class switch. Crit Rev Immunol 24(5):297–320

37. Frasca D, Riley RL, Blomberg BB (2005) Humoral immune response and B-cell functions including immunoglobulin class switch are downregulated in aged mice and humans. Semin Immunol 17(5):378–384

38. Frasca D, Riley RL, Blomberg BB (2007) Aging murine B cells have decreased class switch induced by anti-CD40 or BAFF. Exp Gerontol 42(3):192–203

39. Frasca D, Van Der Put E, Riley RL, Blomberg BB (2004) Age-related differences in the E2A-encoded transcription factor E47 in bone marrow-derived B cell precursors and in splenic B cells. Exp Gerontol 39(4):481–489

40. Fuxa M, Skok J, Souabni A, Salvagiotto G, Roldan E, Busslinger M (2004) Pax5 induces V-to-DJ rearrangements and locus contraction of the immunoglobulin heavy-chain gene. Genes Dev 18(4):411–422

41. Gay D, Saunders T, Camper S, Weigert M (1993) Receptor editing: an approach by autoreactive B cells to escape tolerance. J Exp Med 177(4):999–1008

42. Ginaldi L, Loreto MF, Corsi MP, Modesti M, De Martinis M (2001) Immunosenescence and infectious diseases. Microbes Infect 3(10):851–857

43. Goidl EA, Innes JB, Weksler ME (1976) Immunological studies of aging. II. Loss of IgG and high avidity plaque-forming cells and increased suppressor cell activity in aging mice. J Exp Med 144(4):1037–1048

44. Gruver AL, Hudson LL, Sempowski GD (2007) Immunosenescence of ageing. J Pathol 211(2):144–156

45. Han S, Yang K, Ozen Z, Peng W, Marinova E, Kelsoe G, Zheng B (2003) Enhanced differentiation of splenic plasma cells but diminished long-lived high-affinity bone marrow plasma cells in aged mice. J Immunol 170(3):1267–1273

46. Hardy RR CC, Shinton SA, Kemp JD, Hayakawa K (1991) Resolution and characterization of pro-B and pre-pro-B cell stages in normal mouse bone marrow. J Exp Med 173(5):1213–1225

47. Hardy RR, Hayakawa K (1991) A developmental switch in B lymphopoiesis. Proc Natl Acad Sci U S A 88(24):11550–11554

48. Hardy RR, Hayakawa K (2001) B cell development pathways. Annu Rev Immunol 19:595–621

49. Hardy RR, Hayakawa K, Parks DR, Herzenberg LA, Herzenberg LA (1984) Murine B cell differentiation lineages. J Expt Med 159:1169–1178

50. Harless SM, Lentz VM, Sah AP, Hsu BL, Clise-Dwyer K, Hilbert DM, Hayes CE, Cancro MP (2001) Competition for BLyS-mediated signaling through Bcmd/BR3 regulates peripheral B lymphocyte numbers. Curr Biol 11(24):1986–1989

51. Hayakawa K, Asano M, Shinton SA, Gui M, Allman D, Stewart CL, Silver J, Hardy RR (1999) Positive selection of natural autoreactive B cells. Science 285(5424):113–116

52. Hayakawa K, Hardy RR (2000) Development and function of B-1 cells. Curr Opin Immunol 12(3):346–353

53. Hayakawa K, Li YS, Wasserman R, Sauder S, Shinton S, Hardy RR (1997) B lymphocyte developmental lineages. Ann N Y Acad Sci 815:15–29

54. Hayakawa K, Shinton SA, Asano M, Hardy RR (2000) B-1 cell definition. Curr Top Microbiol Immunol 252:15–22

55. Haynes L, Eaton SM, Swain SL (2002) Effect of age on naive CD4 responses: impact on effector generation and memory development. Springer Semin Immunopathol 24(1):53–60

56. Hondowicz BD, Alexander ST, Quinn WJ 3rd, Pagan AJ, Metzgar MH, Cancro MP, Erikson J (2007) The role of BLyS/BLyS receptors in anti-chromatin B cell regulation. Int Immunol 19(4):465–475

57. Hsu BL, Harless SM, Lindsley RC, Hilbert DM, Cancro MP (2002) Cutting edge: BLyS enables survival of transitional and mature B cells through distinct mediators. J Immunol 168(12):5993–5996

58. Hsu MC, Toellner KM, Vinuesa CG, Maclennan IC (2006) B cell clones that sustain long-term plasmablast growth in T-independent extrafollicular antibody responses. Proc Natl Acad Sci U S A 103(15):5905–5910

59. Johnson K, Angelin-Duclos C, Park S, Calame KL (2003) Changes in histone acetylation are associated with differences in accessibility of V(H) gene segments to V-DJ recombination during B-cell ontogeny and development. Mol Cell Biol 23(7):2438–2450

60. Johnson KM, Owen K, Witte PL (2002) Aging and developmental transitions in the B cell lineage. Int Immunol 14(11):1313–1323

61. Jumaa H, Wollscheid B, Mitterer M, Wienands J, Reth M, Nielsen PJ (1999). Abnormal development and function of B lymphocytes in mice deficient for the signaling adaptor protein SLP-65. Immunity 11(5):547–554

62. Jung D, Giallourakis C, Mostoslavsky R, Alt FW (2006) Mechanism and control of V(D)J recombination at the immunoglobulin heavy chain locus. Annu Rev Immunol 24:541–570

63. Kearney JF (2005) Innate-like B cells. Springer Semin Immunopathol 26(4):377–383

64. Kee BL, Murre C (1998) Induction of early B cell factor (EBF) and multiple B lineage genes by the basic helix-loop-helix transcription factor E12. J Exp Med 188(4):699–713

65. Kee BL, Paige CJ (1995) Murine B cell development: commitment and progression from multipotential progenitors to mature B lymphocytes. Int Rev Cytol 157:129–179

66. Kee BL, Quong MW, Murre C (2000) E2A proteins: essential regulators at multiple stages of B-cell development. Immunol Rev 175:138–149

67. Kline GH, Hayden TA, Klinman NR (1999) B cell maintenance in aged mice reflects both increased B cell longevity and decreased B cell generation. J Immunol 162(6):3342–3349

68. Koipally J, Kim J, Jones B, Jackson A, Avitahl N, Winandy S, Trevisan M, Nichogiannopoulou A, Kelley C, Georgopoulos K (1999) Ikaros chromatin remodeling complexes in the control of differentiation of the hemo-lymphoid system. Cold Spring Harb Symp Quant Biol 64:79–86

69. Labrie JE 3rd, Sah AP, Allman DM, Cancro MP, Gerstein RM (2004) Bone marrow microenvironmental changes underlie reduced RAG-mediated recombination and B cell generation in aged mice. J Exp Med 200(4):411–423

70. Lesley R, Xu Y, Kalled SL, Hess DM, Schwab SR, Shu HB, Cyster JG (2004) Reduced competitiveness of autoantigen-engaged B cells due to increased dependence on BAFF. Immunity 20(4):441–453

71. Jin F, Freitas A, Szabo P, Weksler ME (2001) Impaired regeneration of the peripheral B cell repertoire from bone marrow following lymphopenia in old mice. Eur J Immunol 31(2):500–505

72. Liu P, Keller JR, Ortiz M, Tessarollo L, Rachel RA, Nakamura T, Jenkins NA, Copeland NG (2003) Bcl11a is essential for normal lymphoid development. Nat Immunol 4(6):525–532

73. Loder F, Mutschler B, Ray RJ, Paige CJ, Sideras P, Torres R, Lamers MC, Carsetti R (1999) B cell development in the spleen takes place in discrete steps and is determined by the quality of B cell receptor-derived signals. J Exp Med 190(1):75–89

74. Lopes-Carvalho T, Foote J, Kearney JF (2005) Marginal zone B cells in lymphocyte activation and regulation. Curr Opin Immunol 17(3):244–250

75. Lopes-Carvalho T, Kearney JF (2004) Development and selection of marginal zone B cells. Immunol Rev 197:192–205

76. YF, Cerny J (2002) Repertoire of antibody response in bone marrow and the memory response are differentially affected in aging mice. J Immunol 169(9):4920–4927

77. Malaguarnera L, Ferlito L, Imbesi RM, Gulizia GS, Di Mauro S, Maugeri D, Malaguarnera M, Messina A (2001) Immunosenescence: a review. Arch Gerontol Geriatr 32(1):1–14

78. Manz RA, Arce S, Cassese G, Hauser AE, Hiepe F, Radbruch A (2002) Humoral immunity and long-lived plasma cells. Curr Opin Immunol 14(4):517–521

79. Manz RA, Radbruch A (2002) Plasma cells for a lifetime? Eur J Immunol 32(4):923–927

80. Manz RA, Thiel A, Radbruch A (1997) Lifetime of plasma cells in the bone marrow. Nature 388(6638):133–134

81. Martin DA, Bradl H, Collins TJ, Roth E, Jack HM, Wu GE (2003) Selection of Ig mu heavy chains by complementarity-determining region 3 length and amino acid composition. J Immunol 171(9):4663–4671

82. Martin F, Kearney JF (2000) Positive selection from newly formed to marginal zone B cells depends on the rate of clonal production, CD19, and btk. Immunity 12(1):39–49

83. Martin F, Kearney JF (2002) Marginal-zone B cells. Nat Rev Immunol 2(5):323–335

84. Martin F, Oliver AM, Kearney JF (2001) Marginal zone and B1 B cells unite in the early response against T-independent blood-borne particulate antigens. Immunity 14(5):617–629

85. McHeyzer-Williams LJ, Cool M, McHeyzer-Williams MG (2000) Antigen-specific B cell memory: expression and replenishment of a novel b220(-) memory B cell compartment. J Exp Med 191(7):1149–1166

86. McHeyzer-Williams LJ, Driver DJ, McHeyzer-Williams MG (2001) Germinal center reaction. Curr Opin Hematol 8(1):52–59

87. McHeyzer-Williams LJ, McHeyzer-Williams MG (2005) Antigen-specific memory B cell development. Annu Rev Immunol 23:487–513

88. McHeyzer-Williams MG, McLean MJ, Lalor PA, Nossal GJ (1993) Antigen-driven B cell differentiation in vivo. J Exp Med 178(1):295–307

89. McHeyzer-Williams MG, Nossal GJ, Lalor PA (1991) Molecular characterization of single memory B cells. Nature 350(6318):502–505

90. Medina KL, Singh H (2005) Gene regulatory networks orchestrating B cell fate specification, commitment, and differentiation. Curr Top Microbiol Immunol 290:1–14
91. Mehr R, Shahaf G, Sah A, Cancro M (2003) Asynchronous differentiation models explain bone marrow labeling kinetics and predict reflux between the pre- and immature B cell pools. Int Immunol 15(3):301–312
92. Melchers F (1997) Control of the sizes and contents of precursor B cell repertoires in bone marrow. Ciba Found Symp 204:172–182; discussion 182–176
93. Melchers F, Haasner D, Grawunder U, Kalberer C, Karasuyama H, Winkler T, Rolink A (1994) Roles of IgH and L chains and of surrogate H and L chains in the development of cells of the B lymphocyte lineage. Ann Rev Immunol 12:209–225
94. Melchers F, Strasser A, Bauer SR, Kudo A, Thalmann P, Rolink A (1989) Cellular stages and molecular steps of murine B cell development. Cold Spring Harb Symp Quant Biol LIV:183–189
95. Melchers F, ten Boekel E, Seidl T, Kong XC, Yamagami T, Onishi K, Shimizu T, Rolink AG, Andersson J (2000) Repertoire selection by pre-B-cell receptors and B-cell receptors, and genetic control of B-cell development from immature to mature B cells. Immunol Rev 175:33–46
96. Miller C, Kelsoe G (1995) Ig VH hypermutation is absent in the germinal centers of aged mice. J Immunol 155(7):3377–3384
97. Miller JP, Allman D (2003) The decline in B lymphopoiesis in aged mice reflects loss of very early B-lineage precursors. J Immunol 171(5):2326–2330
98. Miller JP, Allman D (2005) Linking age-related defects in B lymphopoiesis to the aging of hematopoietic stem cells. Semin Immunol 17(5):321–329
99. Miller JP, Cancro MP (2007) B cells and aging: balancing the homeostatic equation. Exp Gerontol 42(5):396–399
100. Miller JP, Stadanlick JE, Cancro MP (2006) Space, selection, and surveillance: setting boundaries with BLyS. J Immunol 176(11):6405–6410
101. Mishto M, Santoro A, Bellavista E, Bonafe M, Monti D, Franceschi C (2003) Immunoproteasomes and immunosenescence. Ageing Res Rev 2(4):419–432
102. Mocchegiani E, Malavolta M (2004) NK and NKT cell functions in immunosenescence. Aging Cell 3(4):177–184
103. Monroe JG, Allman D (2004) Keeping track of pro-B cells: a new model for the effects of IL-7 during B cell development. Eur J Immunol 34(10):2642–2646
104. Montecino-Rodriguez E, Dorshkind K (2006) New perspectives in B-1 B cell development and function. Trends Immunol 27(9):428–433
105. Montecino-Rodriguez E, Leathers H, Dorshkind K (2006) Identification of a B-1 B cell-specified progenitor. Nat Immunol 7(3):293–301
106. Morrison AM, Nutt SL, Thevenin C, Rolink A, Busslinger M (1998) Loss- and gain-of-function mutations reveal an important role of BSAP (Pax-5) at the start and end of B cell differentiation. Semin Immunol 10(2):133–142
107. Mostoslavsky R, Alt FW, Bassing CH (2003) Chromatin dynamics and locus accessibility in the immune system. Nat Immunol 4(7):603–606
108. Murre C (2005) Helix-loop-helix proteins and lymphocyte development. Nat Immunol 6(11):1079–1086
109. Nemazee D, Russell D, Arnold B, Haemmerling G, Allison J, Miller JFAP, Morahan G, Buerki K (1991) Clonal deletion of autospecific B lymphocytes. Immunol Rev 122:117–132
110. Nemazee D, Weigert M (2000) Revising B cell receptors. J Exp Med 191(11):1813–1817
111. Ng SY, Yoshida T, Georgopoulos K (2007) Ikaros and chromatin regulation in early hematopoiesis. Curr Opin Immunol 19(2):116–122
112. Nicoletti C, Borghesi-Nicoletti C, Yang XH, Schulze DH, Cerny J (1991) Repertoire diversity of antibody response to bacterial antigens in aged mice. II. Phosphorylcholine-antibody in young and aged mice differ in both VH/VL gene repertoire and in specificity. J Immunol 147(8):2750–2755

113. Nicoletti C, Cerny J (1991) The repertoire diversity and magnitude of antibody responses to bacterial antigens in aged mice: I. Age-associated changes in antibody responses differ according to the mouse strain. Cell Immunol 133(1):72–83

114. Nicoletti C, Yang X, Cerny J (1993) Repertoire diversity of antibody response to bacterial antigens in aged mice. III. Phosphorylcholine antibody from young and aged mice differ in structure and protective activity against infection with Streptococcus pneumoniae. J Immunol 150(2):543–549

115. Nossal G, Pike B (1975) Evidence for the clonal abortion theory of B-lymphocyte tolerance. J Exp Med 141:904–917

116. Nossal GJV. 1983. Cellular mechanisms of immunologic tolerance. Ann Rev Immunol 1:33–62

117. Nutt SL, Rolink AG, Busslinger M (1999) The molecular basis of B-cell lineage commitment. Cold Spring Harb Symp Quant Biol 64:51–59

118. O'Connor BP, Raman VS, Erickson LD, Cook WJ, Weaver LK, Ahonen C, Lin LL, Mantchev GT, Bram RJ, Noelle RJ (2004) BCMA is essential for the survival of long-lived bone marrow plasma cells. J Exp Med 199(1):91–98

119. O'Riordan M, Grosschedl R (1999) Coordinate regulation of B cell differentiation by the transcription factors EBF and E2A. Immunity 11(1):21–31

120. Osmond D (1991) Proliferation kinetics and the lifespan of B cells in central and peripheral lymphoid organs. Curr Opin Immunol 3:179–185

121. Osmond DG (1990) B cell development in the bone marrow. Seminars in Immunology 2:173

122. Osmond DG, Park Y-H (1987) B lymphocyte progenitors in mouse bone marrow. Int Rev Immunol 2:241–261

123. Osmond DG, Rolink A, Melchers F (1998) Murine B lymphopoiesis: towards a unified model. Immunol Today 19(2):65–68

124. Paus D, Phan TG, Chan TD, Gardam S, Basten A, Brink R (2006) Antigen recognition strength regulates the choice between extrafollicular plasma cell and germinal center B cell differentiation. J Exp Med 203(4):1081–1091

125. Pawelec G (2003) Immunosenescence and human longevity. Biogerontology 4(3):167–170

126. Pawelec G, Koch S, Griesemann H, Rehbein A, Hahnel K, Gouttefangeas C (2006) Immunosenescence, suppression and tumour progression. Cancer Immunol Immunother 55(8):981–986

127. Pawelec G, Wagner W, Adibzadeh M, Engel A (1999) T cell immunosenescence in vitro and in vivo. Exp Gerontol 34(3):419–429

128. Pelanda R, Schwers S, Sonoda E, Torres RM, Nemazee D, Rajewsky K (1997) Receptor editing in a transgenic mouse model: site, efficiency, and role in B cell tolerance and antibody diversification. Immunity 7(6):765–775

129. Prak EL, Trounstine M, Huszar D, Weigert M (1994) Light chain editing in kappa-deficient animals: a potential mechanism of B cell tolerance. J Exp Med 180(5):1805–1815

130. Prak EL, Weigert M (1995) Light chain replacement: a new model for antibody gene rearrangement. J Exp Med 182(2):541–548

131. Quinn WJ 3rd, Scholz JL, Cancro MP (2005) Dwindling competition with constant demand: can homeostatic adjustments explain age-associated changes in peripheral B cell selection? Semin Immunol 17(5):362–369

132. Radbruch A, Muehlinghaus G, Luger EO, Inamine A, Smith KG, Dorner T, Hiepe F (2006) Competence and competition: the challenge of becoming a long-lived plasma cell. Nat Rev Immunol 6(10):741–750

133. Reth M (1991) Regulation of B-cell development by pre-B-cell receptors. Curr Biol 1(3):198–199

134. Reth M, Petrac E, Wiese P, Lobel L, Alt FW (1987) Activation of V kappa gene rearrangement in pre-B cells follows the expression of membrane-bound immunoglobulin heavy chains. EMBO J 6(11):3299–3305

135. Riley RL, Kruger MG, Elia J (1991) B cell precursors are decreased in senescent BALB/c mice, but retain normal mitotic activity in vivo and in vitro. Clin Immunol Immunopathol 59(2):301–313

136. Riley SC, Froscher BG, Linton PJ, Zharhary D, Marcu K, Klinman NR (1989) Altered VH gene segment utilization in the response to phosphorylcholine by aged mice. J Immunol 143(11):3798–3805

137. Rogerson BJ, Harris DP, Swain SL, Burgess DO (2003) Germinal center B cells in Peyer's patches of aged mice exhibit a normal activation phenotype and highly mutated IgM genes. Mech Ageing Dev 124(2):155–165

138. Rolnik A, Melchers F (1991) Molecular and cellular orgins of B lymphocyte diversity. Cell 66:1081–1094

139. Schatz DG, Oettinger MA, Schlissel MS (1992) V(D)J recombination: molecular biology and regulation. Annu Rev Immunol 10:359–383

140. Schebesta M, Heavey B, Busslinger M (2002) Transcriptional control of B-cell development. Curr Opin Immunol 14(2):216–223

141. Schittek B, Rajewsky K (1990) Maintenance of B-cell memory by long-lived cells generated from proliferating precursors. Nature 346(6286):749–751

142. Schlissel MS (2003) Regulating antigen-receptor gene assembly. Nat Rev Immunol 3(11):890–899

143. Schlissel MS (2004) Regulation of activation and recombination of the murine Igkappa locus. Immunol Rev 200:215–223

144. Schlissel MS, Stanhope-Baker P (1997) Accessibility and the developmental regulation of V(D)J recombination. Semin Immunol 9(3):161–170

145. Shahaf G, Allman D, Cancro MP, Mehr R (2004) Screening of alternative models for transitional B cell maturation. Int Immunol 16(8):1081–1090

146. Sherwood EM, Blomberg BB, Xu W, Warner CA, Riley RL (1998) Senescent BALB/c mice exhibit decreased expression of lambda5 surrogate light chains and reduced development within the pre-B cell compartment. J Immunol 161(9):4472–4475

147. Sherwood EM, Xu W, King AM, Blomberg BB, Riley RL (2000) The reduced expression of surrogate light chains in B cell precursors from senescent BALB/c mice is associated with decreased E2A proteins. Mech Ageing Dev 118(1–2):45–59

148. Shih TA, Roederer M, Nussenzweig MC (2002) Role of antigen receptor affinity in T cell-independent antibody responses in vivo. Nat Immunol 3(4):399–406

149. Singh H, DeKoter RP, Walsh JC (1999) PU.1, a shared transcriptional regulator of lymphoid and myeloid cell fates. Cold Spring Harb Symp Quant Biol 64:13–20

150. Singh H, Medina KL, Pongubala JM (2005) Contingent gene regulatory networks and B cell fate specification. Proc Natl Acad Sci U S A 102(14):4949–4953

151. Singh H, Pongubala JM (2006) Gene regulatory networks and the determination of lymphoid cell fates. Curr Opin Immunol 18(2):116–120

152. Song H, Price PW, Cerny J (1997) Age-related changes in antibody repertoire: contribution from T cells. Immunol Rev 160:55–62

153. Srivastava B, Lindsley RC, Nikbakht N, Allman D (2005) Models for peripheral B cell development and homeostasis. Semin Immunol 17(3):175–182

154. Stadanlick JE, Cancro MP (2006) Unraveling the warp and weft of B cell fate. Immunity 25(3):395–396

155. Stephan RP, Lill-Elghanian DA, Witte PL (1997) Development of B cells in aged mice: decline in the ability of pro-B cells to respond to IL-7 but not to other growth factors. J Immunol 158(4):1598–1609

156. Stephan RP, Reilly CR, Witte PL (1998) Impaired ability of bone marrow stromal cells to support B-lymphopoiesis with age. Blood 91(1):75–88

157. Stephan RP, Sanders VM, Witte PL (1996) Stage-specific alterations in murine B lymphopoiesis with age. Int Immunol 8(4):509–518

158. Stout RD, Suttles J (2005) Immunosenescence and macrophage functional plasticity: dysregulation of macrophage function by age-associated microenvironmental changes. Immunol Rev 205:60–71
159. Szabo P, Shen S, Telford W, Weksler ME (2003) Impaired rearrangement of IgH V to DJ segments in bone marrow Pro-B cells from old mice. Cell Immunol 222(1):78–87
160. Szabo P, Shen S, Weksler ME (1999). Age-associated defects in B lymphocyte development. Exp Gerontol 34(3):431–434
161. Thien M, Phan TG, Gardam S, Amesbury M, Basten A, Mackay F, Brink R (2004) Excess BAFF rescues self-reactive B cells from peripheral deletion and allows them to enter forbidden follicular and marginal zone niches. Immunity 20(6):785–798
162. Tiegs SL, Russell DM, Nemazee D (1993) Receptor editing in self-reactive bone marrow B cells. J Exp Med 177(4):1009–1020
163. Treml LS, Crowley JE, Cancro MP (2006) BLyS receptor signatures resolve homeostatically independent compartments among naive and antigen-experienced B cells. Semin Immunol 18(5):297–304
164. Tsubata T, Reth M (1990) The products of pre-B cell-specific genes (lambda 5 and VpreB) and the immunoglobulin mu chain form a complex that is transported onto the cell surface. J Exp Med 172(3):973–976
165. Tsubata T, Tsubata R, Reth M (1992) Crosslinking of the cell surface immunoglobulin (mu-surrogate light chains complex) on pre-B cells induces activation of V gene rearrangements at the immunoglobulin kappa locus. Int Immunol 4(6):637–641
166. Van Der Put E, Frasca D, King AM, Blomberg BB, Riley RL (2004) Decreased E47 in senescent B cell precursors is stage specific and regulated posttranslationally by protein turnover. J Immunol 173(2):818–827
167. Van Der Put E, Sherwood EM, Blomberg BB, Riley RL (2003) Aged mice exhibit distinct B cell precursor phenotypes differing in activation, proliferation and apoptosis. Exp Gerontol 38(10):1137–1147
168. von Bulow GU, van Deursen JM, Bram RJ (2001) Regulation of the T-independent humoral response by TACI. Immunity 14(5):573–582
169. Wang H, Clarke SH (2004) Positive selection focuses the VH12 B-cell repertoire towards a single B1 specificity with survival function. Immunol Rev 197:51–59
170. Weksler MC, Innes JD, Goldstein G (1978) Immunological studies of aging. IV. The contribution of thymic involution to the immune deficiencies of aging mice and reversal with thymopoietin 32–36. J Exp Med 148(4):996–1006
171. Weksler ME (2000) Changes in the B-cell repertoire with age. Vaccine 18(16):1624–1628
172. Weksler ME, Szabo P (2000) The effect of age on the B-cell repertoire. J Clin Immunol 20(4):240–249
173. Weller S, Braun MC, Tan BK, Rosenwald A, Cordier C, Conley ME, Plebani A, Kumararatne DS, Bonnet D, Tournilhac O et al (2004) Human blood IgM "memory" B cells are circulating splenic marginal zone B cells harboring a prediversified immunoglobulin repertoire. Blood 104(12):3647–3654
174. William J, Euler C, Christensen S, Shlomchik MJ (2002) Evolution of autoantibody responses via somatic hypermutation outside of germinal centers. Science 297(5589):2066–2070
175. Williams GT, Jolly CJ, Kohler J, Neuberger MS (2000) The contribution of somatic hypermutation to the diversity of serum immunoglobulin: dramatic increase with age. Immunity 13(3):409–417
176. Wortis HH, Berland R (2001) Cutting edge commentary: origins of B-1 cells. J Immunol 166(4):2163–2166
177. Xiang Z, Cutler AJ, Brownlie RJ, Fairfax K, Lawlor KE, Severinson E, Walker EU, Manz RA, Tarlinton DM, Smith KG (2007) FcgammaRIIb controls bone marrow plasma cell persistence and apoptosis. Nat Immunol 8(4):419–429
178. Yang X, Stedra J, Cerny J (1996) Relative contribution of T and B cells to hypermutation and selection of the antibody repertoire in germinal centers of aged mice. J Exp Med 183(3):959–970

179. Zediak VP, Maillard I, Bhandoola A (2007) Multiple prethymic defects underlie age-related loss of T progenitor competence. Blood 110(4):1161–1167

180. Zhang Z, Espinoza CR, Yu Z, Stephan R, He T, Williams GS, Burrows PD, Hagman J, Feeney AJ, Cooper MD (2006) Transcription factor Pax5 (BSAP) transactivates the RAG-mediated V(H)-to-DJ(H) rearrangement of immunoglobulin genes. Nat Immunol 7(6):616–624

181. Zharhary D (1986) T cell involvement in the decrease of antigen-responsive B cells in aged mice. Eur J Immunol 16(9):1175–1178

182. Zharhary D, Klinman NR (1983) Antigen responsiveness of the mature and generative B cell populations of aged mice. J Exp Med 157(4):1300–1308

183. Zharhary D, Klinman NR (1984) B cell repertoire diversity to PR8 influenza virus does not decrease with age. J Immunol 133(5):2285–2287

184. Zharhary D, Klinman NR (1986) The frequency and fine specificity of B cells responsive to (4-hydroxy-3-nitrophenyl)acetyl in aged mice. Cell Immunol 100(2):452–461

185. Zharhary D, Klinman NR (1986) A selective increase in the generation of phosphorylcho-line-specific B cells associated with aging. J Immunol 136(2):368–370

186. Zharhary D, Segev Y, Gershon H (1977) The affinity and spectrum of cross reactivity of anti-body production in senescent mice: the IgM response. Mech Ageing Dev 6(5):385–392

187. Zheng B, Han S, Takahashi Y, Kelsoe G (1997) Immunosenescence and germinal center reaction. Immunol Rev 160:63–77

B-Cells and Antibodies in Old Humans

Kate L. Gibson and Deborah K. Dunn-Walters

Contents

1 Role of B-Cells in Age-Associated Susceptibility to Infection

It has been well established that the efficiency of the immune system declines with increasing age. Immunosenescence causes increased susceptibility to infectious diseases, and infection is, in fact, the third leading cause of mortality in people aged 65 and over [1]. As is clearly apparent from the other chapters of this book, there are many components of the immune system that can change with age, and are crucial to maintaining an effective immune system. The humoral immune system interacts with the other components, both as part of its own development and via its effector mechanisms. The most important function of B-cells is to produce antibodies, the indispensable soluble effectors of many functions. There are a number of different stages of development for B-cells and their antibodies (Fig. 1).

In the primary B-cell response antibodies that recognize pathogen, although not necessarily with high affinity, are rapidly produced. They may include the so-called "polyspecific" antibodies, which have the ability to recognize multiple antigens [2]. The first antibodies are of the IgM isotype and are crucial for opsonizing pathogens, inducing phagocytosis and activating the complement cascade. These

D.K. Dunn-Walters (✉) · K. L. Gibson
Department of Immunobiology
2nd Floor, Borough Wing Guy's
King's and St. Thomas School of Medicine
King's College London
Guy's Hospital, Great Maze Pond
London SE1 9RT
E-Mail: Deborah.Dunn-Walters@kcl.ac.uk

T. Fulop et al. (eds.), *Handbook on Immunosenescence,*
DOI 10.1007/ 978-1-4020-9062-2_21, © Springer Science+Business Media B.V. 2009

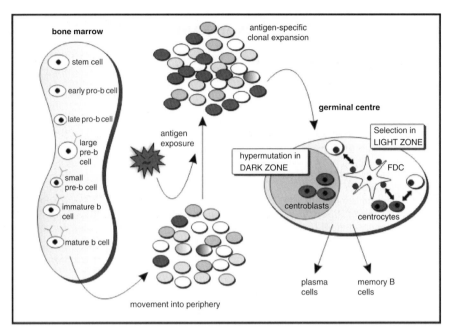

Fig. 1 B-cell development. The humoral immune response is mediated by antibodies produced from plasma cells. These plasma cells are the end point in B-cell development, which is characterized by (a) generation of a huge diversity of different B-cells, each carrying a different antibody gene in the bone marrow and (b) selection processes using the affinity of the membrane-bound form of the antibody (the B-cell receptor) for it's antigen as the selection criteria. Diversity is generated by a process of gene rearrangement early on in the development of the cell, in the bone marrow prior to antigen encounter. The selection processes are twofold. Firstly B-cells are selected for survival, or not, on the basis of their antibody recognition—to eliminate inappropriate self-reactivity and encourage reactivity with foreign pathogens. Secondly there is a mutation step in development, and the resultant B-cells carrying improved antibodies are selected—this occurs in the germinal centre of secondary tissues, after encounter with antigen, and serves to increase the affinity of the antibody for the relevant antigen. Both generation of diversity and selection of antibody are complex processes that are crucial for an effective humoral immune system. A clear understanding of these processes, and how they are affected with age, is needed in order to comprehend the etiology of age-related inflammatory and infectious disease

antibody functions, and the rapidity of this primary response, have been shown to play a vital role in protection from extracellular bacterial pathogens [3]. Antibodies afford protection against viral infection by neutralizing the virus particles; binding and blocking key molecules involved in cellular infection. Similarly they can also neutralize toxins. Later maturation of the B-cells in the immune response is slower but results in the generation of more highly specific antibodies, which may be of a different isotype, following a process known as affinity maturation. In addition to the neutralizing and opsonizing functions of antibody, B-cells are also important as modulators of inflammation [4, 5], regulators of the immune response [6] and as antigen presenting cells and activators of T-cells [7–10].

The elderly are susceptible to infections by a wide variety of pathogens, all of which involve B-cells and antibodies in the normal course of the immune response (Table 1). The lungs are, in common with other mucosal surfaces of the gastrointestinal and genito-urinary tracts, particularly vulnerable to infection by virtue of their exposure to the environment. As is illustrated in Table 1, pulmonary infections are common in older people. The elderly are usually the first to be affected by annual epidemics of respiratory infections, and frequently suffer the worst clinically. Mortality figures attributable to influenza and pneumonia are confused by the fact that influenza is very often followed by a secondary infection—most notably by *Streptococcus pneumoniae*. Some would argue that this confounding factor results in a two to threefold underestimate of influenza mortality [23]. It is also argued that mortality due to influenza is negligible and it is the secondary bacterial infection that causes almost all deaths [24, 25]. Whichever way round, it is generally agreed that older people are the worst affected by these diseases. It has been reported that 90% of all pneumonia and influenza deaths and 88% of respiratory syncytial virus-associated deaths occur in those aged over 65 years [26]. In the oldest old (85 years and over) there was a 32-fold increased chance of mortality from influenza or influenza-associated pneumonia compared with those aged 65–69 years [26]. According to the Department of Health, in the UK there are more than 18,000 hospitalizations resulting from pneumococcal pneumonia each year in those aged 65 years and over [27]. There is also an increased incidence of pneumococcal septicemia in old people associated with *S. pneumoniae* infection [28].

Table 1 Pathogens found frequently in elderly subjects with respiratory or urinary tract infections. (adapted from [1])

Organ system	Pathogen found frequently	B-cell role in immune response to pathogen
Respiratory tract (upper and lower)	Bacteria *Streptococcus pneumoniae* *Hemophilus influenza*	B-cells are crucial to the TI-II response [11] Mucosal IgA has a protective role independent of serum antibody levels [12]
	Legionella pneumophila *Chlamydia pneumoniae* Viruses	B-cells are required for opsonization [13] Neutralization by antibody [14]
	Rhinoviruses *Coronaviruses* *Influenza* *Respiratory syncytial*	Antibody-mediated neutralization [15,16]
Urinary tract	Bacteria *Escherichia coli*	IgA secretion and antigen-specific Ig inhibits attachment of bacteria [17,18]
	Proteus *Klebsiella*	An increase in IgM and IgA aids protection [19,20]
	Pseudomonas aeruginosa *Enterococci*	Opsonization [21] Antibody alone not hugely effective, but effective in the presence of complement [22]

It is known that specific antibodies, generated during a T-dependent B-cell response, are crucial for protection against influenza. Ineffective influenza-specific antibody, as assessed by the Haemagglutination inhibition (HI) test, is associated with lowered protection from the disease [29]. Studies have shown that 25% or more of the elderly fail to develop HI titres of a protective level following vaccination [30, 31]. In vivo studies in mice have shown that higher levels of B-cells and IgG2a antibody confer increased levels of protection [32]. It has been said that an age-related decrease in influenza protection can be solely accounted for by the reduced T-cell help available in the diminished elderly T-cell repertoire. However, this does not take into account the fact that the CD4+ T-cells themselves may rely on fully functioning B-cells for their activation [7, 10].

In other areas of humoral immunity the B-cells are even less reliant on T-cells for help. Pneumonia is a bacterial infection, caused by a number of different organisms (e.g. *Streptococcus pneumoniae* [33], *Staphylococcus aureus* [34], *Streptococcus pyogenes* [35]) although *S. pneumoniae* is the major cause [33]. Immunity against *S. pneumoniae* is particularly reliant on a healthy B-cell population. This is because the antigenic portion of *S. pneumoniae* is a capsular polysaccharide and a T-independent type II (TI-II) antigen. Unlike a T-dependent B-cell response, where the maturation of the B-cell antibody relies on T-cell help and therefore any failure to respond could be attributed to a failure of T-cells, the TI-II response is independent of direct T-cell help. Therefore a failure to protect against *S. pneumoniae* is more likely to be a failure ascribable to deficits in the B-cells themselves.

In children a reduced pneumococcal response can be explained by a lack of marginal zone B-cells in the spleen, where the main TI-II responding B-cells are thought to reside. However, older people appear to have a fully functioning splenic marginal zone [36] so the lack of effective pneumococcal protection in the elderly still remains a mystery. One good candidate for further study is the IgM response. It has been shown, in mice, that the classical complement pathway, partially mediated by binding of natural IgM to bacteria, is vital for innate immunity to S. pneumoniae [3]. Human studies have also shown that antibody of the IgM isotype is vital in providing efficient protection against S. pneumoniae [37], although this has been mainly attributed to "IgM memory," with mutated IgM genes. The exact roles and relationships between natural antibody, IgM memory and class switched memory in the pneumococcal response remain to be determined.

The immune response of the elderly to RSV is less well studied than that against other pulmonary infections. Recent data shows that the senescence accelerated mouse has a severely compromised cellular immune system and produces less virus-specific local IgA in response to RSV infection [38].

Although pulmonary infections of the elderly are the most notable, by virtue of the fact that they cause the most mortality, there are also significant increases in morbidity and mortality from other infections. Bacterial infections of the skin, urinary tract, soft tissue, and gastrointestinal tract are all increased with age [1]. The exact role of the humoral response in this declined protection has yet to be elucidated.

2 Vaccination in the Elderly

Vaccines are an extremely important tool in preventing deaths from infection, and since they are routinely administered as part of a normal health care routine they are the main source of data on immune responses in man. It has been consistently shown that the effectiveness of vaccines is severely diminished in older people. The most commonly studied vaccine is that against influenza. The cellular response, i.e. T-cells and release of cytokines, macrophages and natural killer cells, is decreased with age [39]. In terms of the humoral response the antibody titre, in the form of IgG, is significantly lower [39–41]. While vaccination of the elderly against influenza is widely accepted as a valid health strategy to reduce disease incidence, and studies support this, [42–44] other studies suggest that influenza vaccination does not significantly decrease influenza-related mortality in older people [45, 46]. The age-related reduction in specific antibody production also occurs in response to other vaccines, such as against hepatitis B [47], tetanus and tick-borne encephalitis (TBE) [48]. Data on some of the less common vaccines is more scarce, but gradually becoming available with the advent of an older population which travels more widely. Some travel vaccines, such as hepatitis A, also show a reduced specific antibody response [49], while others such as yellow fever seem to show an undiminished antibody response but have an increased risk of adverse events in the elderly [50].

A possible explanation for a decrease in specific antibody is that the process of affinity maturation is defective. During one study on influenza vaccine it was discovered that an age-related decrease in specific antibody was accompanied by an increase in antibodies against double stranded DNA—indicative of self reactive/polyclonal B-cells [51]. Polyclonal B-cells are often associated with naive B-cells that have not been through the affinity maturation process and are reacting in either a low-affinity manner to specific antigen, or in a non-specific manner by virtue of their innate pattern recognition responses. It was this finding that led to the idea that perhaps humoral immunity in the older person was better represented by the T-independent response. However, as mentioned above, there is a large T-independent component to immune protection against *S. pneumoniae* and general protection is decreased with age. Cross-reactive antibodies certainly appear to be increased in older people treated with the polysaccharide pneumococcal vaccine [52], although the failure of the vaccine to adequately protect against pneumonia [53–57] implies that they are not adequate compensation for the reduction in specific antibody that is also seen [52].

3 Autoantibodies and Age

There is a well-documented shift towards self-reactive antibody production with age. One of the most common autoantibody types, frequently associated with disease, is antinuclear antibodies (ANAs). These have consistently been found to be increased in the old (over 65) in the absence of disease; a prospective study showed persistence of these raised levels throughout older life [58]. The significance of this increase has not yet been determined, and attempts to relate these antibodies with general levels of disease and frailty have shown no associations. The Swedish longitudinal NONA immune study [59] showed significantly higher ANA levels in the oldest old (86–95 years) but found there to be no association nor any correlation to other immune risk factors (e.g. CD4/CD8 T-cell ratio, CMV seropositivity). These findings are echoed by a Finnish study, where ANA positivity at the age of 90 did not show any correlation with survival, or with the levels of serum markers of inflammation [60]. It has even been suggested that an increase in ANA antibodies may have beneficial effects by virtue of a possible anti-tumor activity [61].

ANAs are not the only auto-antibodies to increase with age. The study by Xavier et al. [58] also noted an increase in the frequency of anti-ssDNA antibodies, as have other studies [62, 63]. Increases in antibodies against many other auto-antigens have been reported, for example against cardiolipin, dsDNA and rheumatoid factor, [62–65] although, again, there were no associations found with mortality [62]. The Danish study by Andersen-Ranberg et al. [65] did find a correlation between autoantibodies and comorbidity and disability, although this was only for the organ-specific antibodies, indicating that these were more likely a result of age-associated disease.

Although the aetiology of Rheumatoid arthritis (RA) is not yet fully elucidated, it is an age-related inflammatory autoimmune disorder. Coincidentally, as reported above, there is also an increased incidence of rheumatoid factor (RF) with age— regardless of whether the subject has RA or not [62–65]. There has been a decline in incidence of the disease that has been observed over the last 40 years [66] which has been attributed to environmental factors. One possible contributor to this is the gradual decrease in the number of smokers. Recent evidence has shown that the presence of another auto-antibody, anti-cyclic citrullinated peptide (anti-CCP) is associated with smoking and a higher risk of RA [67]. The successful use of therapies such as Rituximab, which utilize an anti-CD20 monoclonal antibody to ablate peripheral B-cells, is ample evidence that B-cells play an important part in the disease process of RA [68]. In addition to the obvious mechanism of depleting auto-antibody producing cells, there is increasing evidence for a role of B-cells in RA as antigen-presenting cells, activating T-cells, and producing and responding to cytokines [69]. A further complication in understanding the role of B-cells is the fact that B-cells have recently been shown to be capable of immunosuppression—including in animals models of arthritis [70, 71].

4 Immunodysregulation of B-cells in Aging

The above observations are all evidence that the humoral immune system is dysregulated in older people. At first glance it would appear that there is no easily identifiable quantitative defect in the humoral immune system with age. However, although the range of B-cell numbers, as a percentage of peripheral blood lymphocytes, varies greatly between individuals, it has been reported that there is a slight decline in the number of CD19+ B-cells in old age [72–75]. It has also been reported that having a higher number of CD19+ B-cells is associated with better survival [76, 77]. When CD20 is used as a marker for B-cells no age-related change could be found [78]. The number of antibody molecules circulating in the periphery of older adults remains relatively stable [79, 80]. Similarly, studies have been conducted on the ratio of different Ig isotypes in the elderly and most show no significant change during later life [75, 81, 82]; although it has been reported that an increase of the mucosal IgA antibody in the serum can be a predictor of mortality [83]. In general the picture is one of a qualitative change in the antibody repertoire rather than a quantitative one [84].

4.1 Generation of High Affinity Antibodies

Since the lack of high affinity antibodies is a key feature of the older immune system, and our expertise is in the study of Ig genes, we initially investigated the affinity maturation process. Affinity maturation occurs in the germinal centre (GC) and involves the expansion of antigen-specific B-cells, mutation of their Ig genes (resulting in altered antibody function), followed by selection of the B-cells producing the best antibody [85–87]. Contained within the dynamic microenvironment of the GC are B-cells, T-cells, and follicular dendritic cells (FDCs) all in close proximity to allow the exchange of costimulatory molecules and cytokine signaling.

Following antigenic stimulation, selected B-cells migrate and converge on the GC FDCs, making contact with their long processes [88] and differentiating into centroblasts. The FDCs are the stromal cells of the GC and play a key role in regulating the humoral immune respone [89]. Unlike antigen presenting cells (APCs), FDCs present intact antigen–antibody complexes on their cell surface [88], in the form of immune complexes which are highly immunogenic, and assist GC B-cell proliferation [90–92]. Proliferating GC B-cells are known as centroblasts. During centroblast proliferation, in the dark zone of the GC, hypermutation of the immunoglobulin (Ig) genes encoding antibody occurs. The B-cells move into the light zone, as centrocytes, and will die through apoptosis unless they receive rescue signals conditional on efficient recognition of the antigen by the newly formed B-cell receptor. Rescue signals are provided by FDCs and T-cells [93]. The helper T-cells in the GC are a particular subset of CD4+ T-cells, expressing CD57. These cells have unique characteristics that have yet to be fully elucidated [94]. Since FDC and T-cell help is limiting there is competition between B-cells and therefore selection of those B-cells with the highest affinity for antigen occurs. The resulting B-cells can switch the class of their antibody, from IgM to IgG/IgA/IgE, and this also requires T-cell help. B-cells with high affinity antibody differentiate into either memory B-cells, to provide for an efficient recall response, or plasma cells to secrete antibody. We have addressed the possible age-related changes in the GC reaction in three main areas: proliferation of B-cells, hypermutation of the Ig genes, and selection of high-affinity, antigen-specific, antibodies.

4.2 Proliferation

A defect in B-cell proliferation would have severe consequences for the GC reaction, since the loss of cells due to deleterious mutations acquired by hypermutation is extremely large and the pool of B-cells required to counter this is therefore also large. For some cell types proliferating cells can reach replicative senescence— where the telomeres at the ends of the chromosomes erode at each division and therefore there is a limit to the amount of proliferation one cell line can undergo set by the length of the telomere [95]. It has been shown that telomere length decreases with age in T-cells, and to a lesser extent in B-cells [96, 97]. However, we do not believe that the proliferative capacity of B-cells in the GC is impaired in this way as a result of old age. Telomerase, the enzyme that elongates telomeres, is upregulated in the GC, being high in centroblasts and higher still in centrocytes. This results in B-cells leaving the GC for the periphery with substantially longer telomeres than when they first entered, up to 4 kb longer as determined by Southern blotting [98]. Further to this, memory B-cells have telomeres on average 2 bp longer than naïve B-cells [97].

There has been much debate as to whether the overall size and number of GCs decrease with age. Several studies have pointed to this though they have all been conducted in rodent models [99–101]. Immunohistochemical studies measuring the size and overall number of B-cell follicles in human spleen, Peyer's patches [36] and lymph nodes [78] have not shown any age-related difference. However, there have been two studies of human tonsil, performed by flow cytometry rather than measuring individual GC sizes, which have both reported a decrease in GC B-cells with age [99, 102]. Tissue specific differences may account for these discrepancies and further work would be needed to clarify the issue.

4.3 Hypermutation of B-Cells

As outlined above, somatic hypermutation occurs following activation of the B-cells by antigen and entry into the GC reaction. The mutations introduced are generally point mutations, though some insertions and deletions may occur, and tend to be in areas containing hotspot motifs [103–105].

There is conflicting opinion regarding whether there is a quantitative change in hypermutation in the ageing individual. Reports have indicated no change [106–108], a decrease [109, 110] or increase [99, 111, 112] in mutation with increasing age. The fact that these studies do not agree is hardly surprising as they do not take into account patient health history i.e. prior immune responses. The tissue origin of samples can also make a significant difference to the number of mutations observed, for example we have shown consistently that B-cells of mucosal origin have a higher level of mutations than those from, say, spleen or blood [113].

We addressed these issues by attempting to quantitate the frequency of hypermutation in individual B-cell GC expansions. We microdissected histologically-defined areas of GC from the spleen and Peyer's patch follicles of young and old humans so that only the mutations in that particular GC reaction were counted [114, 115]. Individual B-cell expansions were identified by their Ig gene characteristics; by identifying Ig gene sequences that have the same CDR3 region we can identify related B-cell clones (Fig. 2, *see* later for a more detailed explanation of Ig gene rearrangement). Furthermore, we can draw a lineage tree of individual B-cell clonal expansions (Fig. 3) by analyzing the order of accumulation of mutations in the hypermutation process [114, 115]. In this way we look at the number of mutations that occurred within that particular clonal expansion, and can compare lineage trees from subjects of different ages. We have shown that there was no difference in the frequency of mutation occurring in human GC reactions in the spleen and Peyer's patch with age.

4.4 Selection of High Affinity B-Cells and Class Switching

Lineage tree construction can furnish information on the affinity maturation dynamics by measurement of lineage tree shape parameters. The shape of the lineage tree can help indicate the degree of selection that has taken place. For instance, a 'pruned' tree (few branches) indicates high selection pressure whereas a 'bushy' tree (many branches), indicates less selection (Fig. 3). Since a failure of adequate selection

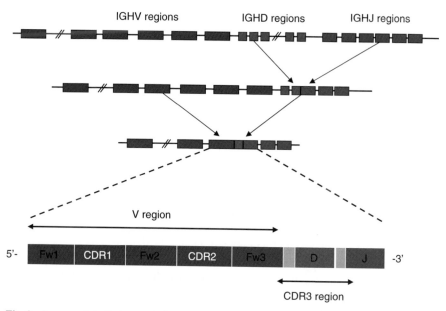

Fig. 2 Immunoglobulin heavy chain gene structure and the complementarity determining region (CDR) 3 region. The rearranged immunoglobulin gene contains 3 CDR regions (that form the antigen binding site) and 3 framework (Fw) regions (that provide structural integrity). During germline Ig gene rearrangement, a variable (V) region is joined to a diversity (D) region and a joining (J) region. During the rearrangement process, random N-nucleotides (N) are inserted into the junctions to form a unique CDR3 sequence

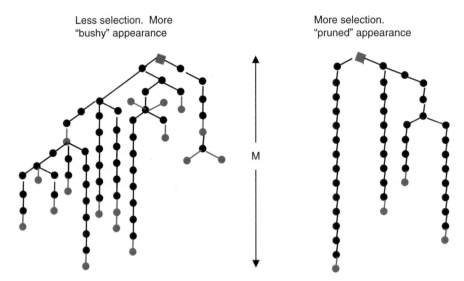

Fig. 3 Representations of lineage trees from clonal expansions of B-cells in the germinal centre reaction. Each node (round) represents one mutation away from the germline sequence (square). The shape of the lineage tree reflects the degree of selection acting on the clonal expansion as shown. The relative frequency of mutation in each lineage tree is compared by comparing the distances between the top and bottom of the lineage trees (M)

could result in the production of a population of cells with low affinity, such as is seen in the elderly, we investigated lineage trees from GC reactions in samples from patients of different ages for selection differences. We found a significant decrease in the degree of selection pressure acting on GC B-cells in the Peyer's patch of the gut (but not the spleen). These data were confirmed by further analysis of the distribution of mutations within the Ig gene. A high level of replacement mutations in the complementarity-determining areas of the gene (relative to the more conserved Framework areas, Fig. 2) is expected in a selected Ig gene, and is indeed seen in the younger Peyer's patch GC samples but not the old [114, 115].

An explanation for these apparent changes in selection is still elusive, but several factors could contribute. It may be solely a failure of the quality of B-cells in terms of specificity or signaling function. However, since FDCs and T-cells are important in the selection process they are also good candidates to investigate for the failure of selection pressure.

There is a well-documented age-related decline in thymus size and a reduced T-cell output. Homeostatic regulation in the face of reduced levels of naïve T-cells causes skewing of the T-cell repertoire which may reduce the availability of appropriate T-cell help for B-cells. Immunohistochemically stained human tissue sections have illustrated changes in T-cell populations in B-cell follicles [36,102]. The CD8+ T-cell numbers decline with age resulting in an increased CD4+/CD8+ ratio. Since it is CD4+ cells that are important in the affinity maturation process the significance of these findings is not known. There is, as yet, no information on whether the GC-specific T helper cells (CD4+ CD57+) are changed with age. CD40 ligand on GC

T-cells interacts with CD40 expressed on B-cells and this relationship is critical to T-cell dependent activation of B-cell proliferation, memory formation and class-switch recombination in the GC. Aged CD4 T-cells in mice have shown reduced CD40L expression [116] and in these animals there is a decrease in IgG levels reminiscent of the decreased IgG production in response to influenza vaccination in humans [40,41].

It has been suggested that the function of FDCs declines with increasing age [101, 117, 118]. Defects may be intrinsic to the FDCs themselves, or may be a failure of the FDC-B-cell interactions. FDCs have Fc receptors (FcR) and complement receptors 1 and 2 (CR1 and CR2) on their surface which retain antigen as immune complexes [119], and these interactions are crucial for the signaling and activation of antigen-specific B-cells. The immune complexes coat the FDCs to form bodies known as iccosomes. Aged FDCs have been reported to produce few to none of these iccosomes [117]. This may be due to the apparent down-regulation of FDC-FcγRII expression by FDC-bound immune complexes demonstrated in the GCs of old mice [120]. The resulting decrease in immune complex retention and presentation to B-cells would lead to lowered B-cell activation in the GC.

Although there is clearly a role for accessory cell failure in the age-related changes in GC responses, changes intrinsic to the B-cell itself are also responsible. The key enzyme in affinity maturation of B-cells is Activation Induced Cytidine Deaminase (AID) which is directly responsible for both hypermutation of Ig genes and class switching. Class switch recombination, from IgM to either IgG, IgA or IgE isotypes, creates antibodies with the same antigen specificity but different effector functions (e.g. complement fixing, secretory, opsonizing). AID expression is regulated by the E2A-encoded transcription factor E47. It has been shown, in mice, that E47 and AID expression is reduced in old B-cells [121], and that this reduction is due to a failure in the CD40 signaling pathway (indicative of T-dependent interactions) and the BAFF signaling pathway (indicative of T-independent reactions) [122]. Preliminary results also suggested that there was a similar decrease of E47 and AID in human peripheral blood B-cells [121].

4.5   Diversity of the B-Cell Repertoire

Evidence from our lineage tree studies on individual GCs indicated that in some instances the founder B-cells of a GC may have already been mutated. This occurred more often in the older samples and led us to postulate that B-cells which have previously been through the affinity maturation process might be being re-used in subsequent immune responses. If the starting population of B-cells has already been modified in response to a different antigen, then its ability to effectively change to accommodate a new antigen may be compromised. This could partially explain the compromized selection noted above. Naive B-cells are characterized by their IgD expression, and memory B-cells are characterized by having mutated Ig genes and expressing CD27 on their surface. It has been shown in mice that the older B-cell population is made up of a greater number of B-cells carrying mutated Ig genes—i.e. memory B-cells [123]. Observations of an increased number of CD27+ B-cells in humans concur with this [124,125]. A change in serum IgD, which may also reflect an increase in the proportion of IgD-, memory, B-cells, has also been noted [84]. It is now well established, in mice, that naïve B-cell output into the periphery decreases with age [see p. 395 Scholz et al.]. There is, as yet, no evidence that human bone marrow B-cell output decreases with age, although it is known that children reconstitute B-cell function after bone marrow transplants more rapidly than adults do [126]. Therefore, if the overall number of B-cells is not drastically reduced, and there are less naive cells being produced, an increased proportion of memory B-cells is a logical conclusion [127]. Since B-cell memory appears to be maintained by proliferation [125] it is possible that proliferating memory B-cell clones make up for any shortfall in immunological space caused by lower naive B-cell input. However, a decrease in the number of memory B-cells with age has also been reported [128], so it would seem that this issue is still not completely resolved.

Our postulation, that GC reactions in the older samples were using "second hand" B-cells, lead us to further investigate B-cell diversity. A diverse and functional repertoire of antibodies is essential to produce an effective humoral immune response. If the repertoire of B and plasma cells is reduced, then the ability to recognize foreign antigen is severely compromised. B-cell diversity and antibody specificity are defined during the early stages of B lymphocyte differentiation, where the Ig genes are formed. The remarkable way in which gene segment rearrangement forms a complete Ig gene from different segments (Fig. 2) results in millions of different B-cells, each with a unique Ig sequence capable of producing antibody with distinctive specificity. Briefly, the Ig molecule consists of both heavy and light chains. There are three types of gene segments, variable (V), diversity (D, heavy chain only) and joining (J). The segments are randomly recombined to generate a V(D)J for the heavy chain (Fig. 2) or VJ for the light chain. Thus a germline repertoire of just 165 different V,D or J genes can result in a possible 8,116 different gene rearrangements. Combination of the heavy and light chains results in a possible 2,643,840 combinations. The region where the junctions join together is further diversified by an incomplete joining process. Addition and deletion of nucleotides by terminal deoxynucleotidy transferase (TdT) activity at these joints leads to junctional diversity. The VDJ joining region of the heavy chain, the CDR3 region, is so highly variable that it can be considered to be a fingerprint for that particular gene and the B-cell (and its progeny) that carries it.

There have been a number of studies which have looked for an age-related change in diversity by investigating the gene segment usage in Ig genes. The studies vary in design (looking at specific gene families only, or at specific isotypes, or only in response to a particular challenge) which may account for some of the discrepancies between them. The earliest report is probably the most comprehensive in terms of VH repertoire, although limited in the number of different subjects used (five old and one young) [106]. They showed an increase in usage of certain IGHV genes, in particular of the IGHV4 family [106]. However, this has since been contradicted. In another sequencing-based study of the IGHV4 repertoire in elderly human tonsil

Kolar et al. did not find any change [99]. The IGHV repertoire has also been analyzed, in a small group of individuals, using a family-specific PCR-based approach. This showed consistency in the IGHV repertoire between samples of the same individual at time points 10 years apart [107]. IGHV family specific studies alone may not pick up functionally significant differences in the repertoire. Although the IGHV3 family usage in response to pneumococcal polysaccharide vaccination showed no overall difference between the elderly and young adults, there was a significant loss of focus in the elderly response as evidenced by a loss of oligoclonality [52]. Furthermore, in the same experiments, a difference in Ig light chain usage was observed [129].

Other studies of B-cell diversity have concentrated on the CDR3 region. This, being the most variable region of the gene and having importance in antigen binding, has traditionally been an area used to define monoclonality and oligoclonality in pathology [130]. However, due to the cumbersome nature of sequencing and identifying V-D-J regions, the numbers of patients studied have generally been low, or limited to particular subsets of genes. For example, one study by Xue et al. [131] looked at D and J

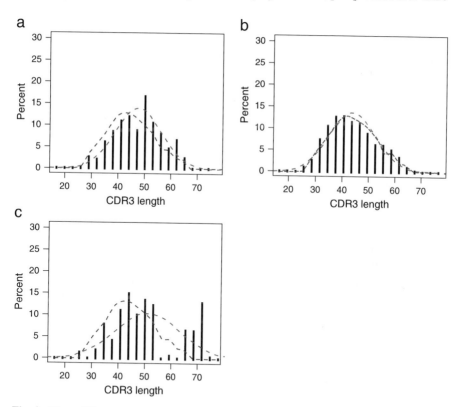

Fig. 4 Three different spectratype profiles. All are from old individuals (>88 years). Black bars represent the percentage of cdr3 regions of each different length. The red line represents the mean distribution for the young controls. The blue line shows the best fit for the individual sample data shown. A shows some B-cell repertoire restriction, B shows normally distributed cdr3 lengths, C shows an individual with very restricted B-cell repertoire. Approximately one-third of the old blood samples analyzed show restricted IgH repertoire along the lines of the spectratype in C

region usage as determined by sequencing and found no difference between younger and older samples. However, they had only seven young and seven old samples and only studied the CDR3 regions of IGHV5 family IgM genes. A more tractable method of looking at CDR3 diversity was also employed by them, using PCR to amplify all CDR3 regions and look at the spread of different sized fragments. This method of spectratyping has also been used in the analysis of T-cell repertoires [132–134] and enables the study of a much greater number of samples. We performed B-cell spectratyping on samples from peripheral blood of 33 old and 24 young subjects. The old samples are from the Swedish NONA Immune Longitudinal Study [135], from patients over 86 years of age. Preliminary data has shown that the B-cell repertoire is indeed restricted in a subgroup (approximately one third) of older people (Fig. 4).

4.6 Association of Monoclonal B-Cell Expansions With Age

Skewed B-cell spectratypes of the kind we have observed may have a number of aetiologies. It may indeed be true that a decreasing naïve B-cell output in the face of homeostatic mechanisms to keep the total number of B-cells the same has resulted in the repertoire being increasingly made up of antigen-experienced expansions of cells. Alternatively there may be pathological monoclonal expansions of B-cells, such as are seen in leukemia or lymphoma. Usually, these are diagnosed conditions, and individuals with this sort of medical history are excluded from studies on B-cell diversity. However, it might be possible that a pre-clinical condition exists in some people. An increase in monoclonal expansions of B-cells, both of CD5+ and CD5- phenotype, has previously been reported in older people [136]. Monoclonal gammopathy of undetermined significance (MGUS) is a predominant plasma-cell disorder [137] and has been shown to increase with age in both humans [137,138] and mouse [139]. It is characterized by an increase in presence of serum monoclonal Ig. MGUS is not found in young subjects, is prevalent in around 2% of over 50s and has been reported to vary in the elderly from 11% to 38% [138,140]. There is an association between MGUS and onset of multiple myeloma or related malignant condition with average risk assessed at about 1% per year [141]. Questions still remain as to what significance these populations have in the aging human. Obviously there is the possibility that MGUS accounts for some of the observed repertoire restriction with increasing age. However, our data does not suggest a high prevalence of such monoclonal expansions, and the restricted repertoires often have a more oligoclonal appearance.

5 Summary

We have outlined the different factors that are involved in making and maintaining an effective humoral immune response and how these may be affected by increasing age. It is clear that the ability to produce high affinity antibody with age is diminished but there are many possible explanations as to why this might be. We have identified the most likely areas as being a decrease in the ability to select B-cells producing high affinity antibodies, and a decrease in the available repertoire in the first instance.

Many of the studies on B-cells in old age are carried out in mice and the data in humans is sadly lacking. Hopefully this situation will change in the future and maybe the advent of the use of B-cell depletion therapies for the treatment of autoimmune disease can help provide more human data on B-cell dynamics in individuals of different ages.

References

1. Albright JF, Albright JW (2003) Aging, immunity, and infection. Humana Press, New Jersey
2. Wing MG (1995) The molecular basis for a polyspecific antibody. Clin Exp Immunol 99:313–315
3. Brown JS, Hussell T, Gilliland SM et al (2002) The classical pathway is the dominant complement pathway required for innate immunity to Streptococcus pneumoniae infection in mice. Proc Natl Acad Sci 99(26):16969–16974
4. Arnaboldi PM, Behr MJ, Metzger DW (2005) Mucosal B cell deficiency in IgA-/- mice abrogates the development of allergic lung inflammation. J Immunol 175(2):1276–1285
5. Maglione PJ, Xu J, Chan J (2007) B cells moderate inflammatory progression and enhance bacterial containment upon pulmonary challengewith Mycobacterium tuberculosis. J Immunol 178(11):7222–7234
6. Fillatreau S, Sweenie CH, McGeachy MJ et al (2002) B cells regulate autoimmunity by provision of IL-10. Nat Immunol 3(10):944–950
7. Crawford A, Macleod M, Schumacher T et al (2006) Primary T cell expansion and differentiation in vivo requires antigen presentation by B cells. J Immunol 176(6):3498–3506
8. Lund FE, Hollifield M, Schuer K et al (2006) B cells are required for generation of protective effector and memory CD4 cells in response to Pneumocystis lung infection. J Immunol 176(10):6147–6154
9. Linton PJ, Harbertson J, Bradley LM (2000) A critcal role for B cells in the development of memory CD4 cells. J Immunol 165(10):5558–5565
10. Rivera A, Chen CC, Ron N et al (2001) Role of B cells as antigen-presenting cells in vivo revisited: antigen-specific B cells are essential for T cell expansion in lymph nodes and for systemic T cell responses to low antigen concentrations. Int Immunol 13(12):1583–1593
11. Barrett DJ, Ayoub EM (1986) IgG2 subclass restriction of antibody to pneumococcal polysaccharides. Clin Exp Immunol 63:127–134
12. Pichichero ME, Hall CB, Insel RA (1981) A mucosal antibody response following systemic Haemophilus influenzae type B infection in children. J Clin Invest 67:1482–1489
13. Brieland JK, Heath LA, Huffnagle GB et al (1996) Humoral immunity and regulation of intrapulmonary growth of Legionella pneumophila in the immunocompetent host. J Immunol 157(11):5002–5008
14. Peterson EM, de la Maza LM, Brade L et al (1998) Characterization of a neutralizing monoclonal antibody directed at the lipopolysaccharide of Chlamydia pneumoniae. Infect Immun 66(8):3848–3855
15. Smith TJ, Chase ES, Schmidt TJ, et al (1996) Neutralizing antibody to human rhinovirus 14 penetrates the receptor-binding canyon. Nature 383(6598):350–354
16. Zhong X, Yang H, Guo ZF, et al (2005) B-cell responses in patients who have recovered from severe acute respiratory syndrome target a dominant site in the S2 domain of the surface glycoprotein. J Virol 79(6):3401–3408

17. Trinchieri A, Braceschi L, Tiranti D, et al (1990) Secretory immunoglobulin A and inhibitory activity of bacterial adherence to epithelial cells in urine from patients with urinary tract infections. Urol Res 18(5):305–308
18. Kantele A, Mottonen T, Ala-Kaila K et al (2003) P fimbria-specific B cell responses in patients with urinary tract infection. J Infect Dis 188(12):1885–1891
19. Lepper PM, Moricke A, Held TK, et al (2003) K-antigen-specific, but not O-antigen-specific natural human serium antibodies promote phagocytosis of Klebsiella pneumoniae. FEMS Immunol Med Microbiol 35(2):93–98
20. Deo SS, Vaidva AK (2004) Elevated levels of secretory immunoglobulin a (sIgA) in urinary tract infections. Indian J Pediatr 71(1):37–40
21. Mueller-Ortiz SL, Drouin SM, Wetsel RA (2004) The alternative activation pathway and complement component CS are critical for a protective immune reponse against Pseudomonas aeruginosa in a murine model of pneumonia. Infect Immun 72(5):2899–2906
22. Harvey BS, Baker CJ, Edwards MS (1992) Contributions of complement and immunoglobulin to neutrophil=mediated killing of enterococci. Infect Immun 60(9):3635–3640
23. Brinkhof MWG, Spoerr A, Birrer A et al (2006) Influenza-attributable mortality among the elderly in Switzerland. Swiss Med Wkly 136:302–309
24. Van Der Sluijs KF, van Elden LJ, Nijhuis M, et al. (2004) IL-10 is an important mediator of the enhanced susceptibility to pneumococcal pneumonia after influenza infection. J Immunol 172(12):7603–7609
25. Seki M, Yanagihara K, Higashiyama Y, et al (2004) Immunokinetics in severe pneumonia due to influenza virus and bacteria coinfection in mice. Eur Respir J 24(1):143–149
26. Thompson WW, Shay DK, Weintraub E et al (2003) Mortality associated with influenza and respiratory syncytial virus in the United States. JAMA 289(2):179–186
27. http://www.dhsspsni.gov.uk/publichealth-pnemofactsheet03.pdf
28. McIntosh EDG, Conway P, Willingham J, et al (2005) Pneumococcal pneumonia in the UK—how herd immunity affects the cost-effectiveness of 7-valent penumococcal conjugate vaccine (PCV). Vaccine 23:1739–1745
29. Goodeve A, Potter CW, Clark A, et al (1983) A graded-dose study of inactivated, surface antigen influenza B vaccine in volunteers: reactogenicity, antibody response and protection to challenge virus infection. J Hyg (Lond) 90(1):107–115
30. Keren G, Segev S, Morag A, et al (1988) Failure of influenza vaccination in the aged. J Med Virol 25(1):85–89
31. Beyer WE, Palache AM, Baljet M, et al (1989) Antibody induction by influenza vaccines in the elderly: a review of the literature. Vaccine 7(5):385–394
32. Jayasekera JP, Vinuesa CG, Karupiah G et al (2006) Enhanced anti-viral antibody secretion and attenuated immunopathology during influenza virus infection in nitric oxide synthase-2-deficient mice. J Gen Virol 87(11):3361–3371
33. AlonsodeVelasco E, Verheul AFM, Verhoef J, et al (1995) Streptococcus pneumoniae: virulence factors, pathogenesis, and vaccines. Microbiol Rev 59(4):591–603
34. Hageman JC, Uyeki TM, Francis JS, et al (2006) Severe community-acquired pneumonia due to Staphylococcus aureus, 2003-04 influenza season. Emerg Infect Dis 12(6):894–899
35. Birch C, Gowardman J (2000) Streptococcus pyogenes: a forgotten cause of severe community-acquired pneumonia. Anaesth Intensive Care 28(1):87–90
36. Banerjee M, Sanderson JD, Spencer J et al (2000) Immunohistochemical analysis of ageing human B and T cell populations reveals an age-related decline of CDb T cells in spleen but not gut-associated lymphoid tissue (GALT). Mech Ageing Dis 115(1–2):85–99
37. Kruetzmann S, Rosado MM, Weber H et al (2003) Human immunoglobulin M memory B cells controlling Streptococcus pneumoniae infections are generated in the spleen. J Exp Med 197(7):939–945
38. Liu B, Kimura Y (2007) Local immune response to respiratory syncytial virus infection is diminished in senescence-accelerated mice. J Gen Virol 88(9):2552–2558
39. Bernstein ED, Gardner EM, Abrutyn E et al (1998) Cytokine production after influenza vaccination in a healthy elderly population. Vaccine 16(18):1722–1731

40. Gardner EM, Bernstein ED, Dran S et al () Characterization of antibody responses to annual influenza vaccination over four years in a healthy elderly population. Vaccine 19:4610–4617

41. Murasko DM, Bernstein ED, Gardner EM et al (2002) Role of humoral and cell-mediated immunity in protection from influenza disease after immunization of healthy elderly. Exp Gerontol 37:427–439

42. Keitel WA, Atmar RL, Cate TR et al (2006) Safety of high doses of influenza vaccine and effect on antibody responses in elderly persons. Arch Intern Med 166(10):1121–1127

43. Maciosek MV, Solberg LI, Coffield AB, et al (2006) Influenza vaccination health impact and cost effectiveness among adults aged 50 to 64 and 65 and older. Am J Prev Med 31(1):72–79

44. Odelin MF, Momplot C, Bourlet T, et al (2003) Temporal surveillance of the humoral immunity against influenza vaccine in the elderly over 9 consecutive years. Gerontology 49(4):233–239

45. Simonsen L, Reichart TA, Viboud C, et al (2005) Impact of influenza vaccination on seasonal mortality in the US elderly population. Arch Intern Med 165(3):265–272

46. Rizzo C, Viboud C, Montomoli E et al (2006) Influenza-related mortality in the Italian elderly: No decline associated with increasing vaccination coverage. Vaccine. 24:6468–6475

47. Cook JM, Gualde N, Hessel L, et al (1987) Alterations in the human immune response to the hepatitis B vaccine among the elderly. Cell Immunol 109(1):89–96

48. Hainz U, Jenewein B, Asch E et al (2005) Insufficient protection for healthy elderly adults by tetanus and TBE vaccines. Vaccine 23:3232–3235

49. Genton B, D'Acremont V, Furrer HJ, et al (2006) Hepatitis A vaccines and the elderly. Travel Med Infect Dis 4(6):303–312

50. Monath TP, Cetron MS, McCarthy K, et al (2005) Yellow fever 17D vaccine safety and immunogenicity in the elderly. Hum Vaccine 1(5):207–214

51. Huang YP, Gauthey L, Michel M, et al (1992) The relationship between influenza vaccine-induced specific antibody responses and vaccine-induced non-specific autoantibody responses in healthy older women. J Gerontol 47:50–55

52. Kolibab K, Smithson SL, Rabquer B et al (2005) Immune response to pneumococcal polysaccharides 4 and 14 in elderly and young adults:analysis of the variable heavy chain repertoire. Inf Imm 73(11):7465–7476

53. Rubins JB, Janoff EN (2001) Pneumococcal disease in the elderly: what is preventing vaccine efficacy? Drugs Aging 18(5):305–311

54. Ortqvist A, Hedlund J, Burman LA et al (1998) Randomised trial of 23-valent pneumococcal capsular polysaccharide vaccine in prevention of pneumonia in middle-aged and elderly people. Swedish Pneumococcal Vaccination Study Group. Lancet 351(9100):399–403

55. Ortqvist A, Henckaerts I, Hedlund J, Poolman J (2007) Non-response to specific serotypes likely cause for failure to 23-valent pneumococcal polysaccharide vaccine in the elderly. Vaccine 25(13):2445–2450

56. Koivula I, Stén M, Leinonen M, Mäkelä PH (1997) Clinical efficacy of pneumococcal vaccine in the elderly: a randomized, single-blind population-based trial. Am J Med 103(4):281–90

57. Simberkoff MS, Cross AP, Al-Ibrahim M, et al (1986) Efficacy of pneumococcal vaccine in high-risk patients. Results of a Veterans Administration Cooperative Study. N Engl J Med 315(21):1318–1327

58. Xavier RM, Yamauchi Y, Nakamura M et al (1995) Antinuclear antibodies in healthy aging people: a prospective study. MAD 78:145–154

59. Nilsson B-O, Skogh T, Ernerudh J et al (2006) Antinuclear antibodies in the oldest-old women and men. J AutoImm 27:281–288

60. Hurme M, Korkki S, Lehtimaki T, et al (2007) Autoimmunity and longevity: presence of antinuclear antibodies is not associated with the rate of inflammation or mortality in nonagenarians. Mech Ageing Dev 128(5–6):407–408

61. Torchilin VP, Iakoubov LZ, Estrov Z (2001) Antinuclear autoantibodies as potential antine-oplastic agents. Trends Immunol 22(8):424–427
62. Ioannidis JP, Katsifis GE, Stavropoulos ED et al (2003) Evaluation of the association of autoantibodies with mortality in the very elderly: a cohort study. Rheumatology (Oxford) 42(2):357–361
63. Manoussakis MN, Tzioufas AG, Silis MP, et al () High prevalence of anti-cardiolipin and other autoantibodies in a healthy elderly population. Clin Exp Immunol 69(3):557–565
64. Njemini R, Meyers I, Demanet C, et al (2002) The prevalence of autoantibodies in an eld-erly sub-Saharan African population. Clin Exp Immunol 127(1):99–106
65. Andersen-Ranberg K, Hoier-Madsen M, Wiik A et al (2004) High prevalence of autoanti-bodies among Danish centenarians. Clin Exp Immunol 138:158–163
66. Doran MF, Pond GR, Crowson CS et al (2002) Trends in incidence and mortality in rheumatoid arthritis in Rochester, Minnesota, over a forty-year period. Arthritis Rheum 46(3):625–631
67. Michou L, Teixeira VH, Pierlot C et al (2007) Associations between genetic factors, tobacco smoking and autoantibodies in familial and sporadic rheumatoid arthritis. Ann Rheum Dis (in press)
68. Edwards JCW, Szczepanski L, Szechinski J et al (2004) Efficacy of B-cell targeted therapy with Rituximab in patients with Rheumatoid Arthritis. N Engl J Med 350(25):2572–2581
69. Bugatti S, Codullo V, Caporali R et al (2007) B cells in rheumatoid arthritis. Arthritis Rheum 6:482–487
70. Mauri C, Gray D, Mushtaq N, et al (2003) Prevention of arthritis by interleukin 10-produc-ing B cells. J Exp Med 197(4):489–501
71. Evans JG, Chavez-Rueda KA, Eddaoudi A et al (2007) Novel suppressive function of tran-sitional 2 B cells in experimental arthritis. J Immunol 178(12):7868–7878
72. Huppert FA, Solomou W, O'Connor S, et al (1998) Aging and lymphocyte subpopulations: whole-blood analysis of immune markers in a large population sample of healthy elderly individuals. Exp Gerontol 33(6):593–600
73. Ginaldi L, De Martinis M, D'Ostilio A, et al (2001) Changes in the expression of surface receptors on lymphocyte subsets in the elderly: quantitative flow cytometric analysis. Am J Hematol 67(2):63–72
74. Colonna-Romano G, Bulati M, Aquino A et al (2003) B cells in the aged: CD27, CD5, and CD40 expression. Mech Aging Dis 124:389–393
75. Chong Y, Ikematsu H, Yamaji K et al (2005) CD27+ (memory) B cell decrease and apop-tosis-resistant CD271485; (naïve) B cell increase in aged humans: implications for age-related peripheral B cell developmental disturbances. Int Immunol 17(4):383–390
76. Huppert FA, Pinto EM, Morgan K et al (2003) Survival in a population sample if predicted by proportions of lymphocyte subsets. Mech Aging Dev 124:449–451
77. Ferguson FG, Wikby A, Maxson P et al (1995) Immune parameters in a longitudinal study of a very old population of Swedish people: a comparison between survivors and nonsurvi-vors. J Gerontol A Biol Sci Med Sci 50(6):B378–B382
78. Lazuardi L, Jenewein B, Wolf AM et al (2005) Age-related loss of naïve T cells and dys-regulation of T-cell/B-cell interactions in human lymph nodes. Immunol 14(1):37–43
79. Potter KN, Orchard J, Critchley E et al (2003) Features of the overexpressed V1-69 genes in the unmutated subset of chronic lymphocytic leukaemia are distinct from those in the healthy elderly repertoire. Blood 101:3082–3084
80. Veneri D, Franchini M, Vella A et al (2007) Changes of human B and B-1a peripheral blood lymphocytes with age. Heamatol 12(4):337–341
81. Butterworth M, McClellan B, Allansmith M (1967) Influence of sex in immunoglobulin levels. Nature 214(5094):1224–1225
82. Buckley CE, Dorsey FC (1970) The effect of aging on human serum immunoglobulin con-centrations. J Immunol 105(4):964–972
83. Hurme M, Paavilainen PM, Pertovaara M et al (2005) IgA levels are predictors of mortality in Finnish nonagenarians. Mech Aging Dis 126:829–831

84. Listi FLOR, Candore GIUS, Modica MA et al (2006) A study of serum immunoglobulin levels in elderly persons that provides new insights into B cell immunosenescence. Ann N Y Acad Sci 1089(1):487–495

85. Jacob J, Kelsoe G, Rajewsky K et al (1991) Intraclonal generation of antibody mutants in germinal centres. Nature 354(6352):389–392

86. MacLennan IC (1994) Germinal centers. Annu Rev Immunol 12:117–139

87. Han S, Zheng B, Takahashi Y et al (1997) Distinctive characteristics of germinal center B cells. Sem Immunol 9:255–260

88. Park C–S, Choi YS (2005) How do follicular dendritic cells interact intimately with B cells in the germinal centre? Immunol 114(1):2–10

89. Tew JG, Wu J, Qin D et al (1997) Follicular dendritic cells and presentation and antigen and costimulatory signals to B cells. Immunol rev 156(1):39–52

90. Qin D, Wu J, Vora KH et al () Fc1543;RIIB on follicular dendritic cells regulates the B cell recall response. J Immunol 164(12):6268–6275

91. Choe J, Kim HS, Zhang X et al (1996) Cellular and molecular factors that regulate the differentiation and apoptosis of germinal center B cells. Anti–Ig down-regulates Fas expression of CD40 ligand-stimulated germinal center B cells and inhibits Fas-mediated apoptosis. J Immunol 157(3):1006–1016

92. Li L, Zhang X, Kovacic S et al (2000) Identification of a human follicular dendritic cell molecule that stimulates germinal center B cell growth. J Exp Med 191(6):1077–1084

93. Zhang X, Li L, Jung J et al (2001) The distinct roles of T cell-derived cytokines and a novel follicular dendritic cell-signaling molecule 8D6 in germinal center-B cell differentiation. J Immunol 167(1):49–56

94. Marinova E, Hans S, Zheng B (2007) Germinal center helper T cells are dual functional regulatory cells with suppressive activity to conventional CD4+ T cells. J Immunol 178(8):5010–5017

95. Goronzy JJ, Fujii H, Weyand CM (2006) Telomeres, immune aging and autoimmunity. Exp Gerontol 41:246–251

96. Son NH, Murray S, Yanovski J et al (2000) Lineage-specific telomere shortening and unaltered capacity for telomerase expression in human T and B lymphocytes with age. J Immunol 165:1191–1196

97. Martens UM, Brass V, Sedlacek L et al (2002) Telomere maintenance in human B lymphocytes. Br J Haematol 119(3):810–818

98. Norrback KF, Hultdin M, Dahlenborg K et al (2001) Telomerase regulation and telomere dynamics in germinal centers. Eur J Haematol 67(5–6):309–317

99. Kolar GR, Mehta D, Wilson PC et al (2006) Diversity of the Ig repertoire is maintained with age in spite of reduced germinal centre cells in human tonsil lymphoid tissue. Scand J Immunol 64(3):314–324

100. Gonzalez-Fernandez A, Gilmore D, Milstein C (1994) Age-related decrease in the proportion of germinal center B cells from mouse Peyer's patches is accompanied by an accumulation of somatic mutations in their immunoglobulin genes. Eur J Immunol 24(11):2918–2921

101. Aydar Y, Balogh P, Tew JG et al (2004) Follicular dendritic cells in aging, a "bottle-neck" in the humoral immune response. Ageing Res Rev 3(1):15–29

102. Mattila PS, Tarkkanen J (1997) Age-associated changes in the cellular composition of the human adenoid. Scand J Immunol 45(4):423–427

103. Rogozin IB, Kolchanov NA (1992) Somatic hypermutagenesis in immunoglobulin genes. II. Influence of neighbouring base sequences on mutagenesis. Biochim Biophys Acta 1171(1):11–8

104. Spencer J, Dunn M, Dunn-Walters DK (1999) Characteristics of sequences around individual nucleotide substitutions in IgVH genes suggest different GC and AT mutators. J Immunol 162(11):6596–6601

105. Rogozin IB, Diaz M (2004) Cutting edge: DGYW/WRCH is a better predictor of mutability at G:C bases in Ig hypermutation than the widely accepted RGYW/WRCY motif and prob-

ably reflects a two-step activation-induced cytidine deaminase-triggered process. J Immunol 172(6):3382–3384

106. Wang X, Stollar BD (1999) Immunoglobulin VH gene expression in human aging. Clin Immunol 93(2):132–142

107. Van Dijk-Hard I, Soderstrom I, Feld S et al (1997) Age-related impaired affinity maturation and differential D-JH gene usage in human VH6-expressing B lymphocytes from healthy individuals. Eur J Immunol 27(6):1381–1386

108. Boursier L, Dunn-Walters DK, Spencer J (1999) Characteristics of IgVH genes used by human intestinal plasma cells from childhood. Immunol 97(4):558–564

109. Troutaud D, Drouet M, Decourt C et al (1999) Age-related alterations of somatic hypermutation and CDR3 lengths in human Vkappa4-expressing B lymphocytes. Immunol 97(2):197–203

110. Rosner K, Winter DB, Kasmer C et al (2001) Impact of age on hypermutation of immunoglobulin variable genes in humans. J Clin Immunol 21(2):102–115

111. Chong Y, Ikematsu H, Yamaji K et al (2003) Age-related accumulation of Ig VH gene somatic mutations in peripheral B cells from aged humans. Clin Exp Immunol 133(1):59–66

112. Dunn-Walters DK, Boursier L, Spencer J. Hypermutation, diversity and dissemination of human intestinal lamina propria plasma cells. Eur J Immunol 1997;27(11):2959–2964

113. Dunn-Walters D, Hackett M, Boursier L et al (2000) Charcteristics of human IgA and IgM genes used by plasma cells in the salivary gland resemble those used in duodenum but not those used in the spleen. J Immunol 164:1595–1601

114. Banerjee M, Mehr R, Belelovsky A et al (2002) Age- and tissue-specific differences in human germinal center B cell selection revealed by analysis of IgVH gene hypermutation and lineage trees. Eur J Immunol 32:1947–1957

115. Dunn-Walters DK, Banerjee M & Mehr R (2003) Effects of age on antibody affinity maturation. Biochem Soc Trans 31(2):447–448

116. Eaton SM, Burns EM, Kusser K et al (2004) Age-related defects in CD4 T cell cognate helper function lead to reduction in humoral responses. J Exp Med 200(12):1613–1622

117. Szakal AK, Kosco MH, Tew JG (1988a) A novel in vivo follicular dendritic cell-dependent iccosome-mediated mechanism for delivery of antigen to antigen-processing cells. J Immunol 140(2):341–353

118. Szakal AK, Taylor JK, Smith JP et al (1988b) Morphometry and kinetics antigen transport and developing antigen retaining reticulum of follicular dendritic cells in lymph nodes of aging immune mice. Aging: Immunol Infect Dis 1:7–22

119. Yoshida K, Van Den Berg TK, Dijkstra CD (1993) Two functionally different follicular dendritic cells in secondary lymphoid follicles of mouse spleen, as revealed by CR1/2 and Fc1543;RII-mediated immune-complex trapping. Immunol 80:34–39

120. Aydar Y, Balogh P, Tew JG et al (2003) Altered regulation of FcgRII on aged follicular dendritic cells correlates with immunoreceptor tyrosine-based inhibition motif signaling in B cells and reduced germinal center formation. J Immunol 171(11):5975–5987

121. Frasca D, Riley RL & Blomberg BB (2005) Humoral immune response and B-cell functions including immunoglobulin class switch are downregulated in aged mice and humans. Sem Immunol 17(5):378–384

122. Frasca D, Riley RL, Blomber BB (2007) Aging murine B cells have secreased class switch induced by anti-CD40 or BAFF. Exp Gerontol 42(3):192–203

123. Williams GT, Jolly CJ, Kohler J et al (2000) The contribution of somatic hypermutation to the diversity of serum immunoglobulin: dramatic increase with age. Immunity 13(3):409–417

124. Colonna-Romano G, Aquino A, Bulati M et al (2006) Memory B cell subpopulations in the aged. Rejuv Res 9(1):149–152

125. Macallan DC, Wallace DL, Zhang Y et al (2005) B-cell kinetics in humans: rapid turnover of peripheral blood memory cells. Blood 105(9):3633–3640

126. Savage WJ, Bleesing JJ, Douek D et al (2001) Lymphocyte reconstitution following non-myeloblative hematopoietic stem cell transplantation follows two patterns depending on age and donor/recipient chimerism. Bone Marrow Transplant 28(5):463–471

127. Johnson SA, Cambier JC (2004) Ageing, autoimmunity and arthritis: senescence of the B cell compartment – implications for humoral immunity. Arthritis Res Ther 6(4):131–139

128. Breitbart E, Wang X, Leka LS et al (2002) Altered memory B-cell homeostasis in human aging. J Gerontol A Biol Sci Med Sci 57(8):B304–B311

129. Smithson SL, Kolibab K, Shriner AK et al (2005) Immune response to pneumococcal polysaccharides 4 and 14 in elderly and young adults: analysis of the variable light chain repertoire. Infect Immun 73(11):7477–7484

130. Bakkus MH (1999) Ig gene sequences in the study of clonality. Pathol Biol (Paris) 47(2):128–147

131. Xue W, Luo S, Adler WH et al (1997) Immunoglobulin heavy chain junctional diversity in young and aged humans. Human Immunol 57:80–92

132. Pannetier C, Cochet M, Darche S et al (1993) The sizes of the CDR3 hypervariable regions of the murine T-cell receptor beta chains vary as a function of the recombined germ-line segments. Proc Natl Acad Sci 90(9):4319–4323

133. Gorski J, Yassai M, Zhu X et al (1994) Circulating T cell repertoire complexity in normal individuals and bone marrow recipients analyzed by CDR3 size spectratyping. J Immunol 152:5109–5119

134. Liu D, Callahan JP, Dau PC (1995) Interfamily fragment analysis of the T cell receptor beta chain CDR3 region. J Immunol Methods 187(1):139–150

135. Wikby A, Johansson B, Olsson J et al (2002) Expansions of peripheral blood CD8 T-lymphocyte subpopulations and an association with cytomegalovirus seropositivity in the elderly: the Swedish NONA immune study. Exp Gerontol 37:445–453

136. Ghia P, Prato G, Scielzo C et al (2004) Monoclonal CD5+ and CD51485; B-lymphocyte expansions are frequent in the peripheral blood of the elderly. Blood 103:2337–2342

137. Kyle RA, Therneau TM, Rajkumar SV et al (2006) Prevalence of monoclonal gammopathy of undetermined significance. N Engl J Med 354:1362–1369

138. Ligthart GJ, Radl J, Corberand JX et al (1990) Monoclonal gammopathies in human aging: increased occurrence with age and correlation with health status. MAD 52(2–3):235–243

139. Radl J (1990) Age-related monoclonal gammopathies: clinical lessons from the aging C57BL mouse. Immunol Today 11(7):234–236

140. Kyle RA, Therneau TM, Rajkumar SV et al (2002) A long-term study of prognosis in monoclonal gammopathy of undetermined significance. NEJ Med 346(8):564–569

141. Kyle RA, Rajkumar SV (2003) Monoclonal gammopathies of undetermined significance: a review. Imm rev 194:112–139

Cellular Immunosenescence - Neutrophils

Neutrophil Granulocyte Functions in the Elderly

Peter Uciechowski and Lothar Rink

Contents

Abstract: The immune response weakens during aging. Especially, the altered functions of the lymphocytes of the adaptive immune system have been extensively studied. Aged persons > 65 years display a predisposition to inflammation and infection combined with an increase in morbidity and mortality than younger individuals. In the past few years it has been discovered that certain functions of the innate immune system, which build the first line of defense against pathogenic microorganisms, are altered with aging. Among the cells of the innate immune system, neutrophilic granulocytes (polymorphonuclear leukocytes, PMN, neutrophils) eliminate invaded bacteria and fungi and play an accepted important role in regulation of the immune response. In vitro studies demonstrate that neutrophilic functions such as phagocytosis, generation of reactive oxygen species (ROS), intracellular killing, degranulation, and possibly chemotaxis are changed in elderly persons whereas the number of circulating neutrophils are unaltered compared to young persons. However, the reported data of different investigators regarding the above-mentioned functions are sometimes controversial. This may result from the use of different isolation methods of neutrophils, the degree of contaminating cells and preactivation of neutrophils during isolation. It could be shown that most of the adhesion surface molecules and receptors of neutrophils are not impaired in function and expression with age. But there is increasing evidence that age-related changes affect receptor-dependent signal transduction and membrane content and fluidity, which in turn lead to a decline in function and in inhibition of apoptosis. Further research

L. Rink (✉) · P. Uciechowski
Institute of Immunology
RWTH Aachen University Hospital
Pauwelsstr. 30
52074 Aachen, Germany
Tel.: +49 241 80 80208
Fax: +49 241 80 82613
E-mail: lrink@ukaachen.de

T. Fulop et al. (eds.), *Handbook on Immunosenescence,*
DOI 10.1007/978-1-4020-9062-2_22, © Springer Science+Business Media B.V. 2009

has to be done to identify the molecular mechanisms that are responsible for the age-related modulations in human neutrophils.

Keywords: Adhesion • Polymorphonuclear leukocytes • Neutrophils • Phagocytosis • Chemotaxis • Degranulation • Intracellular killing • Inflammation • Apoptosis • G-CSF • GM-CSF • fMLP • IL-1RA • IL-1β • IL-3 • IL-8 • TNF-α • Toll-like receptor • MAPK • MyD88 • IRAK • p38 • ERK1/2 • Membrane fluidity • CD62L

1 Introduction

Elderly persons are more susceptible to microbial infections with an increase in morbidity and mortality due to declining immune status, termed immune senescence. In general, age-related changes include a decreased response to vaccination, increased incidence of inflammatory and autoimmune diseases and cancer. There are many efforts to clear up the molecular and cellular changes surrounding immune system dysfunctions. However, other factors such as nutrition, fitness, social components and diseases influence immunity of elderly persons making it difficult to detect single, age-dependent changes. To exclude those factors, the SENIEUR protocol was created to clearly separate age-related from nonage-related alterations of the immune system [1, 2]. This protocol sets the criteria in order for a healthy elderly person to participate in immunogerontological studies. The effects of aging are well-documented for the adaptive immune system, e.g. the alterations in T-cell count, phenotype, and function as well as reduced ability of B-cells to synthesize high affinity antibodies. But in the meantime, the importance of the innate immune system in fighting invading microorganisms and the cooperation with the adaptive immune system to ensure optimal immune response has become more widely accepted. Neutrophils display alterations of function, surface molecule expression, apoptosis and signal transduction with aging. These changes and their effect on the attenuation of neutrophil functions will be summarized and discussed by reviewing the literature.

2 Neutrophils

Polymorphonuclear leukocytes (PMN or neutrophils) are key effector cells of the innate immune system. They are the first cells to migrate rapidly to sites of infection and recognize and engulf microorganisms by phagocytosis. Neutrophils destroy and degrade invaded pathogenic bacteria and fungi via the release of reactive oxygen species and antimicrobial and proteolytic granule proteins, which are delivered to the phagosomes and to the extracellular environment. Additionally, neutrophils produce chemokines and cytokines that recruit and regulate the inflammatory response of macrophages, T-cells and neutrophils themselves. Finally, activated neutrophils initiate an apoptotic programme where they are digested by macrophages without causing tissue damage and necrosis and therefore support the resolution of the inflammatory response [3].

Neutrophils are short-lived cells and die by apoptosis spontaneously within 12–24 h of their release from the bone marrow. The adult bone marrow has to produce 1–2×10^{11} neutrophils per day to sustain a sufficient cell number to efficiently fight infections [4]. This continuous production is controlled by granulocyte colony-stimulating factor (G-CSF), granulocyte/macrophage colony-stimulating factor (GM-CSF) and interleukin-3 (IL-3). To maintain the function of neutrophils summoned to infected tissue, "survival" factors such as lipopolysaccharide (LPS), hypoxic environment, complement and pro-inflammatory cytokines counteract apoptotic programs in neutrophils (Fig. 1) [5–8]. To fulfill their tasks in the defense against bacterial and fungal infections specific functions are regulated by specific receptors. These receptors are formyl-methionyl-leucyl peptide (fMLP), GM-CSF, complement, IgG Fc and interleukin-8 (IL-8) receptors [9]. Additionally, pattern recognition receptors, e.g. toll-like receptors (TLR), binding conserved molecular structures of most microorganisms, participate in the inflammatory response of PMN and other cells of the innate and adaptive immune system [10].

Historically, the role of neutrophils and their immune response has been underestimated and their function has been reduced to being only phagocytic active cells. In the past few years the views on the ability of neutrophils to bridge and regulate innate and adaptive immune responses have been shifted [11]. Using an isolation method to acquire highly purified human neutrophils without preactivation it was shown that neutrophils synthesize only a limited pattern of cytokines released, mainly IL-8, after stimulation [12, 13]. In addition, neutrophils produce large amounts of the antiinflammatory interleukin-1 receptor antagonist (IL-1RA) after stimulation or after high accumulation of neutrophils [14, 15]. Interestingly, neutrophils do not synthesize proinflammatory cytokines such as interleukin-1ß (IL-1ß), tumor necrosis factor-α (TNF- α) and interleukin-6 (IL-6) as described by others [16], which may be explained as a result of monocyte contaminations in the PMN isolates. Therefore, neutrophils not only recruit other immune cells to sites of infection but are also able to create an antiinflammatory environment that helps resolve inflammation.

3 Neutrophils and Aging

It is well-known that aging results in a predisposition to inflammation as well as to infections, which is associated with higher rates of mortality and morbidity [17, 18].

One might assume that impaired defense against invading pathogens such as fungi and bacteria is accompanied by a reduced amount of neutrophils as seen within the T- and B-cell system of elderly persons. But there are no alterations in the number of precursor cells in the bone marrow or of circulating neutrophils [19, 20]. Moreover, neutrophils have been described to be significantly increased in the aged [21]. Neutrophil precursor cells show a reduced proliferative response to G-CSF only (Fig. 1),

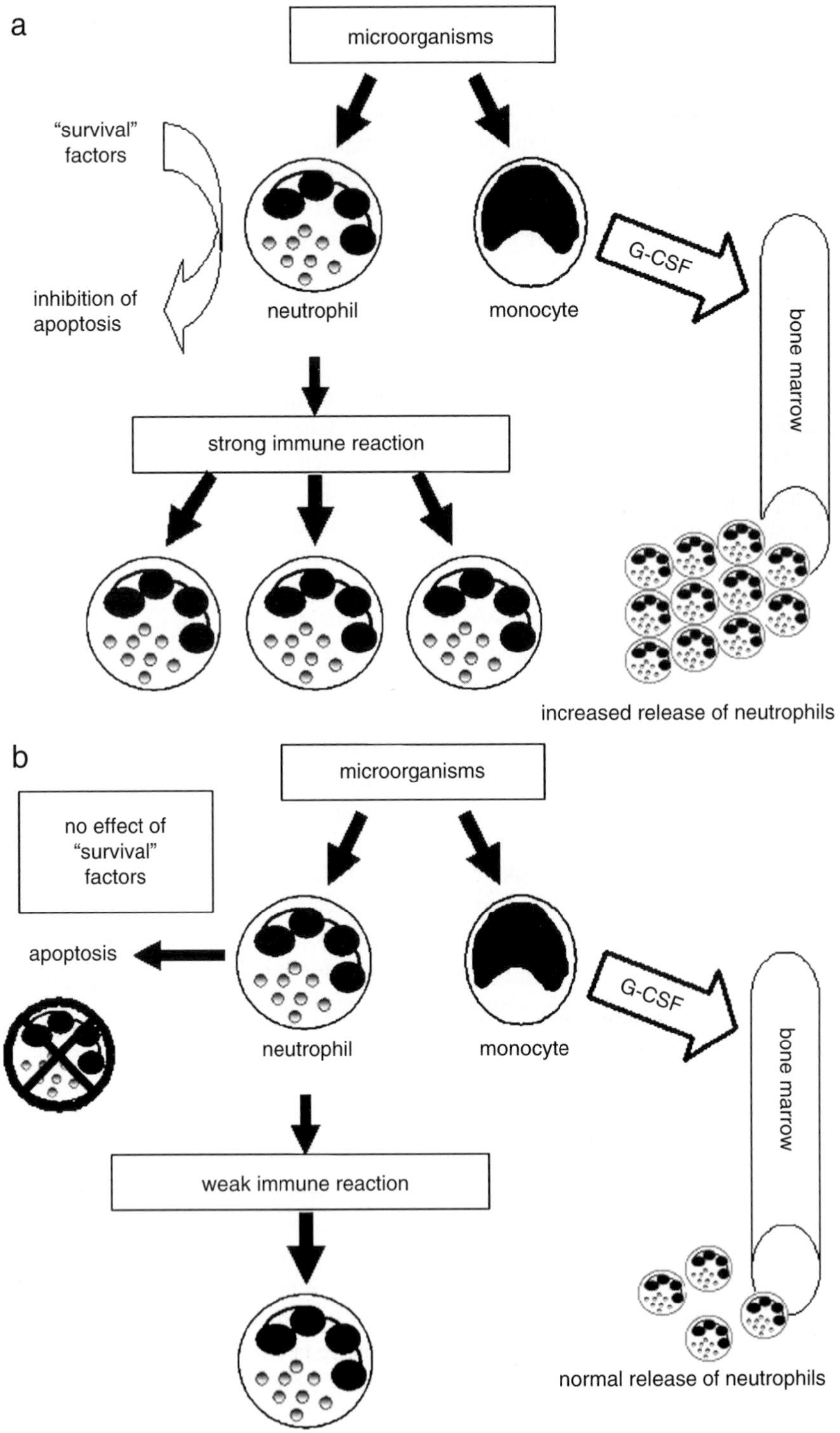

a

microorganisms

"survival" factors

inhibition of apoptosis

neutrophil

monocyte

G-CSF

bone marrow

strong immune reaction

increased release of neutrophils

b

microorganisms

no effect of "survival" factors

apoptosis

neutrophil

monocyte

G-CSF

bone marrow

weak immune reaction

normal release of neutrophils

whereas responses to GM-CSF and IL-3 are not affected [19]. Elderly persons also display a normal neutrophilia during infection [22], indicating that GM-CSF and IL-3 mediate sufficient neutrophil production. However, loss of apoptotic rescue and a normal recruitment of neutrophils by G-CSF during infection might promote an impaired immune response with age (Fig. 1). In the case of severe chronic infection, neutropenia can be observed in the elderly, suggesting that persistent infection in the elderly impairs neutrophil recruitment [20].

4 Function

Although neutrophil count is elevated and adherence to endothelia is unchanged in elderly persons, impaired neutrophilic functions can be seen including a decline in phagocytic capacity in healthy elderly individuals accompanied by reduced intracellular killing [22–24]. This decline in function may contribute to increased susceptibility to bacterial infections in the elderly population. In contrast, aged persons fulfilling the SENIEUR criteria who also exhibit elevated numbers of granulocytes are functionally normal [25–28].

Studies that analyze phagocytosis of opsonized bacteria or yeast and opsonized zymosan by neutrophils have all demonstrated a significant impairment in phagocytic function in the elderly [29–33]. Additionally, the antibody-dependent phagocytosis mediated by Fc-receptors is also decreased [33]. Interestingly, the functions of these receptors are not changed, immunoglobulin and complement levels are normal and serum from elderly donors opsonize bacteria normally so that phagocytosis itself is impaired [32–34]. Butcher et al. [33] have shown that one of the receptors involved in recognizing antibodies on the surface of bacteria, CD16 (FcγRIII), is significantly reduced with age and may contribute to the observed decline in neutrophil phagocytic function with age [33].

After phagocytosis of pathogenic microorganisms, the phagosomes fuse with lysosomes containing bactericidal substances and build the phagolysosome. Therein the pathogen will be intracellularly killed. Besides other destructive components contained within the phagolysosome, intracellular killing is dependent on the generation of ROS, termed respiratory burst. This respiratory burst causes production of superoxide, hydrogen peroxide, and hypochloric acid, which are all toxic to microbes. Contradictory findings describing the respiratory burst after fMLP stimulation in neutrophils of the elderly have been reported. Some groups determined decreased respiratory burst activity after either fMLP [35–38], GM-CSF, or LPS stimulation [39, 40]. Wenisch et al. [32] showed a significant reduction in generation of ROS after stimulation with

Fig. 1 Recruitment and apoptosis of neutrophils during infection
a) After phagocytosis of invading microorganisms the apoptosis of neutrophils in young individuals is blocked via the release of survival factors. Additionally, G-CSF induces the release of a large number of neutrophils from the bone marrow leading to physiological neutrophil leukocytosis.
b) In elderly persons the inhibition of apoptosis of neutrophils is impaired and the recruitment of neutrophils from the bone marrow is not enhanced. This might result in an exhaustion of neutrophils and consequently lead to a reduced immune response with age.

Staphylococcus aureus (*S. aureus*) in contrast to no reduction after stimulation with *Escherichia coli*. These results are in concordance with the reported reduced ability of elderly to fight infections caused by gram-positive bacteria [41], since *S. aureus* frequently causes postoperative sepsis in the elderly.

Others studies using SENIEUR selected persons could not detect a difference in respiratory burst compared to younger persons even after stimulation with fMLP [22, 23]. The application of different stimuli led to various results, based on the assumption that distinct pathways of neutrophilic activation are involved. An early report by Tortorella et al. [42] showed that signal pathways may be impaired. Neutrophils obtained from elderly humans and stimulated with GM-CSF displayed a significant reduction in phosphorylated ERK1/2 levels and an even larger decrease in ERK1/2 activation. No changes in GM-CSF-induced p38 MAPK phosphorylation were observed [42]. This coincides with Larbi and colleagues reporting that p38 signaling is not involved in GM-CSF delayed apoptosis in any age-groups [43]. There are few reports about intracellular killing of fungi and bacteria in elderly people. They described that the capability of stimulated and unstimulated neutrophils to destroy *Candida albicans* is reduced by 10–50% in the elderly, and *E. coli* killing is 44% lower than that of young persons [39, 44]. The reason for impaired intracellular killing in neutrophils of the elderly is not clear yet. Although Piazzolla postulated that cytoskeleton affecting compounds are responsible for the alteration of fMLP stimulated superoxide generation [45], this does not illuminate the selective discrimination of one stimulant against the other. It is possible that triggering various signal transduction pathways after recognition of the pathogen and consequent activation of the neutrophil are responsible for an impaired defense towards one pathogen whereas the response to another remains unaltered in the elderly.

Neutrophils respond to various chemotactic products released either by the host or by the invading organism [46, 47]. Chemotaxis results from the initial contact and adhesion of PMN to endothelial cells through cell adhesion molecules, followed by migration through the endothelium following a chemotactic gradient to inflamed sites. Some investigators reported that chemotaxis remains largely unaltered in the elderly [34] or at least display a normal reaction after stimulation with fMLP [22, 23]. Other research groups found impaired chemotaxis when using other chemotactic substances and complement [32, 48, 49]. The consequence of the latter is that a fast recruitment to sites of infection is functionally restricted. That might explain the occurrence of severe wound infections by elderly persons since small numbers of pathogens cannot be efficiently eliminated. Corberand et al. [50] reported significantly decreased chemotaxis in people over the age of 80 years, and no significant difference in 60- to 70-year-old compared with young persons. Curiously, Niwa et al. [49] presented contrary results. They found a correlation between 60- and 70 year-old volunteers with diminished PMN chemotaxis and respiratory burst and mortality 7 years after the initial study. No difference between people older than 80 years old and the young could be seen. The explanation they offer was that there was no difference between the over-80-year-old persons and the younger ones because individuals with the more suitable neutrophils survived into the oldest age group [49, 50]. Similar data have been obtained for degranulation and superoxide production in response to stimulants such as fMLP [31, 38].

5 Apoptosis

Apoptosis is involved not only in differentiation, development of tissue and home-ostasis, but also in neurogenerative and immune diseases and cancer. Neutrophils display a fast apoptotic rate in vitro as well as in vivo. Apoptosis has to be well-balanced to ensure their survival and production; if the balance is shifted, the risk of chronic inflammatory diseases is enhanced.

The regulation of apoptosis of neutrophils is important to maintain longer survival in inflamed tissue or the resolution of inflammation. Without stimulation, the susceptibility of neutrophils to apoptosis is either slightly increased in the elderly or unaffected by aging [51–53].

It has been shown that the functions and the rescue from apoptosis by survival factors G-CSF, GM-CSF, IL-2 and LPS of PMN diminish with aging. In comparison to younger persons only GM-CSF alters apoptotic neutrophils slightly in the elderly [53]. Increased apoptotic rates of neutrophils at the site of infection might cause decreased bactericidal function (Fig. 1). DiLorenzo and coworkers reported a significant age-related decrease of formation of O^{2-} and chemotaxis whereas no significant correlation between age and the expression of the death receptor CD95 (APO1, Fas) on the granulocyte membrane could be detected. The authors suggest that an increase of CD95-mediated apoptosis of neutrophils might play a minor role in the impairment of neutrophilic function [54]. Fulop et al. [55, 56] investigated the role of antiapoptotic Mcl1 and pro-apoptotic Bax in decreased apoptosis inhibition in PMN of the elderly. The authors found that the expression of Bax was unchanged in elderly and young persons; also treatment with GM-CSF could not modulate the Bax expression. Similar results were obtained by examining Mcl1, which was upregulated after GM-CSF stimulation in young persons, whereas in the elderly no difference was found between stimulation and spontaneous apoptosis. By comparing the Bax/Mcl1 ratio after GM-CSF stimulation in younger and aged persons there was only a slight difference in the Bax/Mcl1 ratio in the elderly, whereas Mcl1 expression was increased relative to Bax in neutrophils from younger individuals. These findings indicate an important role of Bax and Mcl1 in the survival of neutrophils mediated by GM-CSF. The Janus tyrosine kinase (Jak)2-signal transducer and activator of transcription (Stat)5 signal transduction pathway is also modulated in elderly persons [44, 56]. Since Jak2 is related to the expression of antiapoptotic Bcl-2 there might be a possible link between Jak2 and Mcl1 being involved in the decreased rescue of neutrophils from apoptosis (Fig. 2) [56]. Larbi et al. [43] presented evidence that a modulation in the p42/p44 (ERK1/2) mitogen activated protein kinase (MAPK) activation occurs in PMN of elderly subjects under GM-CSF stimulation and is in part responsible for the decreased apoptotic decline of PMN in the elderly. This might be the reason why GM-CSF was not able to down-regu-

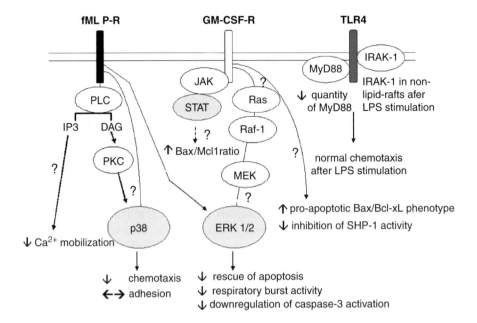

Fig. 2 Signaling in neutrophils of the elderly
Age-related impairment in intracellular signaling after binding of the appropriate ligands to their
receptors leading to altered functions of neutrophils. Question marks display defects in different
signal pathways associated with age (modified and adapted from Fulop et al. [56]). PLC, phospholipase C; DAG, diacylglycerol; IP3, inositol triphosphate; MEK, MAPK (mitogen-activated
protein kinase)/ERK kinase; PKC, protein kinase C.

late caspase-3 activation in neutrophils of elderly persons. Interestingly, the authors
observed that GM-CSF changed the proapoptotic phenotype to an antiapoptotic
phenotype by alteration of the bcl-2 family members Bax and Bcl-xL in young
neutrophils in an MAPK independent way whereas this could not be seen in aged
neutrophils [43]. Taken together, these modulations might be responsible for the
creation of a proapoptotic environment and could explain the increased incidence of
infections in the elderly (Figs. 1, 2).

6 Signal Transduction

Activation of the fMLP receptor via phospholipase C (PLC) leads to the production of diacylglycerol (DAG) and inositolphosphate 3 (IP3), the latter initiates the
enhancement of intracellular Ca^{2+}. DAG induces the membrane translocation of protein kinase C (PKC) and phosphorylation of MAPK family members. Intracellular
Ca^{2+} is decreased in stimulated neutrophils from elderly persons (Fig. 2), suggesting
that there is an impairment in Ca^{2+} flux during cell signaling [53, 56–59]. Interestingly, resting neutrophils of elderly subjects show an enhanced level of intracel-

lular Ca^{2+} [32, 57, 60]. Preactivation, modulation of the aged plasma membrane followed by altered receptor and adapter protein linkage and defects in the early phase of signal transduction might lead to the impairment of Ca^{2+} mobilization of aged neutrophils after fMLP stimulation. By investigating the impaired Ca^{2+} mobilization in aged neutrophils, Klut et al. [61] found heterogeneity of the examined neutrophils concerning time and magnitude of the response. A reduced number of neutrophils in the elderly were able to generate an effective reaction, hinting at a possible subpopulation [61].

After fMLP stimulation, PKC might also activate the p38 signal pathway, which is involved in regulating gene transcription, chemotaxis and adhesion. The ERK1/2 signal pathway is also triggered after fMLP stimulation playing a role in adhesion and respiratory burst activity. Defects in the signal cascades of both pathways and the decrease in activation and phosphorylation levels of p38 and ERK1/2 MAPKs are suggested to affect impaired neutrophilic functions in the elderly (Fig. 2) [56].

GM-CSF is able to activate the JAK/STAT pathway, the Ras-Raf-1-MEK-ERK1/2 pathway and phosphatidyl-inositol 3 kinase (PI-3K) triggered signaling [56]. Investigating the role of protein tyrosine phosphatases (PTP), especially Src homology domain-containing protein tyrosine phosphatase-1 (SHP-1), Fortin et al. [62] suggested a differential effect of GM-CSF on phosphatase activity in modulating neutrophil functions with aging. SHP-1 is a negative regulator of signal transduction and can negatively regulate Src kinases, such as the Jak or Lyn kinase, elicited by GM-CSF in PMN. When recruited to the plasma membrane and activated, SHP-1 dephosphorylates proteins activated by receptors, and inhibits cell activation. The authors could show that SHP-1 phosphatase activity cannot be down-regulated after short stimulation with GM-CSF in the neutrophils of the elderly persons in contrast to neutrophils of young. In lipid rafts from neutrophils of elderly, SHP-1 is continuously present, whereas in the neutrophils of young donors, SHP-1 is rapidly dissociated after stimulation by GM-CSF and is recruited back during a longer period of stimulation. In contrast to younger persons, SHP-1 is constantly recruited to Lyn, which cannot be relieved by GM-CSF. These modulations together with the above-mentioned changes in the Jak2-Stat5 and ERK1/2 signal pathways might contribute to the decreased GM-CSF effects on neutrophils [62]. Fig. 2 summarizes the effects of aging in signal transduction.

7   Adhesion, Surface Molecules and Receptors

After receiving a chemotactic signal, the rolling neutrophil adheres via integin molecules to endothelial cells and migrates through the endothelium (diapedesis) towards the site of infection. Adhesion appears not to be impaired in the elderly. After stimulation with fMLP, zymosan, phorbol myristate acetate (PMA), or calcium ionophores, human neutrophils from young and elderly persons displayed no difference in adhesion to plastic, gelatin, and bovine aortic endothelium [37, 44].

Additionally, a normal or enhanced adherence of neutrophils to endothelia or thrombocytes has been described, but it is not clear whether this has an effect on increased tissue migration in vivo. One might argue that increased adherence is caused by slightly enhanced expression of CD15 (Lewis X) and CD11b (Mac-1, complement receptor 3) on neutrophils [31]. In contrary, no increase of CD11b and CD15 but a decrease of CD62L (L-selectin) was observed by others [33, 63]. Interestingly, the expression of the other two integrins, CD11a (leukocyte function antigen, LFA-1) and CD11c (p150, 95) involved in cell adhesion, is not affected [22, 23, 31, 33].

De Martinis et al. [64] compared the expression of CD50 (ICAM-3; a ligand for CD11a/CD18) and CD62L adhesion molecules in peripheral blood granulo-cytes and monocytes between healthy elderly and young persons. They found a decrease in the percentage of granulocytes and monocytes expressing CD62L in the elderly but no alteration in the density expression on both cell types sug-gesting a preactivation which might contribute to the proinflammatory status in aging. The authors described a downregulation of the density expression of CD50 at a per cell level on granulocytes and a decrease of CD50 density expression on monocytes but an expansion of CD50 positive cells in elderly persons. This indi-cates that the loss of CD62L on granulocytes leads to impairment in cell adhesion and likely contributes to the enhanced susceptibility to acute infections in elderly persons.

Noble et al. [65] observed a significantly lower recruitment of early activa-tion marker CD69 from the vesicles to the plasma membrane after stimulation with PMA in elderly people (fulfilling the SENIEUR criteria) than in younger persons. fMLP in contrast had no influence in different expression of CD69 in young and elderly persons, suggesting again the impairment of distinct pathways within aging. Interestingly, also the CD69 expression in natural killer (NK) cells is decreased [66].

There is growing evidence that aging is accompanied by changes in receptor signaling pathways and membrane fluidity [22, 24, 37, 43, 56, 62]. In contrast to other cells the fluidity of the PMN membrane increases with age, caused by altera-tions in the cholesterol/phospholipid content of the membrane [56, 67, 68]. These modulations result in changed function of lipid rafts, which directly influence TLRs and GM-CSF signaling. Additionally actin, which may play a role in cell-surface receptor movement and expression, has been indicated to contribute to the changed ROS production [69]. In summary, these alterations in signaling may impair the effector functions of neutrophils in aging.

After stimulation, the fMLP receptor which is coupled to a Pertussis toxin-sen-sitive G protein induces the production of superoxide anion, hydrogen peroxide, nitrite oxide (NO) and an increase in intracellular free calcium. The influence of aging on the release of free radicals has been investigated by different laboratories for a long period of time (reviewed by Ref. 24). Some investigators reported a decreased synthesis of free radicals by neutrophils of elderly persons, but found no change in the expression of fMLP receptor number, [37, 38, 56] whereas others could not confirm those data [22]. A recent study by Fulop et al. [56] examining neutrophils isolated from young and aged persons who met criteria defined by the SENIEUR protocol, showed a significantly lower production of superoxide anion under fMLP stimulation and/or GM-CSF priming in PMN from elderly persons compared with younger ones. Fulop et al. [56] postulate the existence of a subpopulation of neutrophils in aged persons, which seems to be responsible for a significantly higher superoxide anion production after 48 h when compared with younger PMN, although they found a reduced superoxide anion production after 24 h stimulation with fMLP and GM-CSF in elderly persons. The authors suggest that PMN from elderly persons might act heterogeneously to down-regulate responses to stimulation than PMN from younger persons, which react more efficiently.

Toll-like receptors belong to the family of pattern recognition receptors and have a specificity to bind substances consisting of conserved motifs of bacteria, fungi and virus. To date, ten different human TLR have been identified, including three intracellularly located types. After ligand binding, the central adapter molecule, myeloid differentiation primary response protein 88 (MyD88), transduces signals into the cell by recruiting a cascade of serine–threonine kinases and IL-1 receptor-associated protein kinases (IRAKs), leading to nuclear factor kappa B (NF-kB)-dependent transcription of proinflammatory genes. Although there is a MyD88 independent way, stimulation via TLR leads to the release of pro-inflammatory cytokines such as interleukin-1, IL-6 or TNF-α. The additional production of chemokines and upregulation of surface molecules through TLR signaling build a bridge between innate and adaptive immune responses. Few reports about the influence of age on TLR exist at present. Renshaw et al. [70] described that LPS (ligand for TLR4, gram- bacteria)-stimulated macrophages from aged mice synthesize less IL-6 and TNF-α than younger ones. This study was confirmed by Boehmer [71]. Additionally, a lower TLR4 mRNA level compared with those of younger macrophages was found in aged macrophages by Renshaw et al. [70, 71], whereas others did not observe a variation in TLR4 surface expression with age. These results are not compatible with the situation in elderly human beings where elevated levels of circulating proinflammatory cytokines are generally observed; especially since elderly monocytes after LPS stimulation produce significantly higher amounts of IL-6 and TNF-α [24, 72, 73].

By studying the expression of TLR2 (ligand: components of gram+ bacteria) and TLR4, Fulop et al. [56] did not observe any changes in the proportion of neutrophils expressing TLR2/4 nor in the expression of both receptors on the surface of neutrophils. They also observed no differences of fMLP and GM-CSF receptor expression with aging [56]. What they found was an increase of TLR4 expression in unstimulated raft and nonraft fractions and no redistribution after LPS stimulation in elderly persons in contrast to younger individuals.

Although the TLR2 and TLR4 expression remains unchanged, one key component of the TLR signaling, IRAK-1, was not found to be associated with lipid-rafts after stimulation with LPS. Additionally, the main adapter protein of the TLR signal pathway, MyD88, was significantly reduced in the plasma membrane of elderly persons (Fig. 2). These observations confirm the thesis that age-related

Fig. 3 Overview of impaired neutrophilic functions with aging

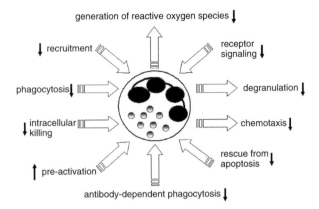

alterations influence receptor-driven signal transduction but do not explain normal LPS mediated chemotaxis of neutrophils of elderly persons. One might speculate that other signal pathways are involved or a nonreceptor-driven function of LPS might exist [56, 72].

The views regarding the importance of neutrophils in immune responses have been changed over the past few years. In immunogerontological studies, contradictory data may result from different isolation techniques of neutrophils, distinct amounts of contaminating cells, preactivation of neutrophils during isolation, and selection criteria of aged persons.

Taken together, the neutrophils are also affected through aging. The changes are found in decreased chemotactic functions which may be associated with the loss of CD62L. Therefore, CD62L-mediated migration might be hampered and this might lead to increased infection. The shedding of CD62L from the cell surface of neutrophils is also a sign of preactivation as postulated by other groups [17, 18] and conforms well to the observation of enhanced Ca^{2+} flux in elderly persons. Yet, one has to be cautious with regards to the purification process of neutrophils since some substances may cause a decrease in CD62L expression [12, 13, 24]. With the exception of CD62L, CD50 and CD16 other surface molecules such as CD11a, b, c/CD18 were not found to be modulated in aged persons when compared to younger individuals. Recent publications indicate a decline in signal transduction as being responsible for receptor-mediated responses and apoptotic rescue mechanisms. Additionally, altered plasma membrane content and fluidity of neutrophils in the elderly appear to influence signal transduction. It should be pointed out that different PMN isolation techniques and monocyte contaminations cannot be excluded as a possible explanation for the controversial results published by distinct groups of investigators [24]. The importance of purity and preactivation of PMN preparations in defining and differentiating PMN signals from those by others could be demonstrated recently [13, 14]. By investigating cytokine production of neutrophils in the elderly, one must also take into account that aged monocytes produce significantly more proinflammatory cytokines after stimulation than those of younger persons [72, 74].

Table 1 Age-related changes of neutrophils

Parameter/function	Stimulants/targets	Reported effect
Number of circulating neutrophils		←→19, 20 ↑21
Number of precursors in bone marrow		←→19
Proliferation of neutrophilic precursors in response to	G-CSF	↓19
	IL-3	←→19
	GM-CSF	←→19
Phagocytosis	Opsonized bacteria, yeast	↓29–33
	Antibody-dependent CD16-mediated	↓33
Respiratory burst	fMLP	↓ 35–38←→ 22, 23
	GM-CSF, LPS	↓39, 40
	Gram positive bacteria	↓32, 48
	Gram negative bacteria	←→32
Degranulation	fMLP	↓31, 38
Chemotaxis	fMLP, GM-CSF, LPS	↓32, 48–50←→22, 23, 34
Intracellular killing	Gram negative bacteria, fungi	↓39, 44
Adhesion	Endothelia, thrombocytes	←→37↗31
	CD11a-c/CD18	←→33, 63, 65↗31 (CD11b)
	CD15	←→63↗31
	CD50	↘64
	CD62L	↓64
Apoptosis		←→51, 52↗53
rescue by	IL-2, LPS, G-CSF, GM-CSF	↓51, 53
CD95 induced apoptosis; expression of CD95		←→54
down-regulation of caspase-3 activity	GM-CSF	↓43
Bax/Mcl1	GM-CSF	↑55, 56
Antiapoptotic phenotype	GM-CSF	↓43
inhibition SHP-1 activity	GM-CSF	↓62
Jak2-Stat5 pathway	GM-CSF	↓56
Signal transduction		↗42, 56
intracellular Ca^{2+} level		↑32, 57, 60
intracellular Ca^{2+} mobilization	fMLP	↓57–59
ERK1/2 MAPK pathway	GM-CSF	↓42
p38 MAPK pathway	GM-CSF	←→42, 43
plasma membrane fluidity	Receptor signaling in relation with lipid rafts	↓56, 67, 68
Expression of surface molecules		
	CD69	↓65
	fMLP-R	←→ 37, 38, 53↘22
	GM-CSF-R	←→ 56
	TLR2, 4	←→ 56

↓, decreased; ↘, slightly decreased; ↑, increased; ↗, slightly increased; ←→, unchanged

8 Conclusions

Although neutrophilic counts are normal or slightly increased in aged persons compared to young individuals aging influences the functional properties of neutrophils. The changes affect phagocytosis in neutrophils from elderly subjects where significant reduction along with decreased antibody-dependent phagocytosis was observed. Also, the other toxic mechanisms to destroy pathogenic microorganisms such as ROS generation, degranulation and intracellular killing, are impaired by age. Studies of chemotaxis have shown contrary results, so it has to be clarified if migratory responses of neutrophils from healthy, elderly persons are in fact altered. The decline in functionality, impaired Ca^{2+} mobilization and delayed rescue from apoptosis during aging appear to arise from defects of several signaling pathways, altered plasma membrane components and modulated protein tyrosine phosphatase activity. The molecular mechanisms responsible for those alterations in signal transduction and why distinctive stimuli cause different effects are still poorly understood. Fig. 3 and Table 1 summarize the age-related changes in neutrophils.

Further research is required since neutrophils display more features than formerly assumed, it would spread light on the deficiencies that occur during the aging process and could be beneficial to the elderly in the future.

Acknowledgment   We would like to thank Romney Haylett for critical reading of the manuscript.

References

1. Ligthart GJ, Corberand JX, Fournier C et al (1984) Admission criteria for immunogerontological studies in man: the SENIEUR protocol. Mech Ageing Dev 28:47–55
2. Ligthart GJ, Corberand JX, Geertzen HGM et al (1994) Necessity of the assessment of health status in human immunogerontological studies: evaluation of the SENIEUR protocol. Mech Ageing Dev 55:89–105
3. Theilgaard-Mönch K, Porse BT, Borregaard N (2006) Systems biology of neutrophil differentiation and immune response. Curr Opin Immunol 18:54–60
4. Hellewell PG, Williams TJ (1994) The neutrophil. In: Hellewell PG, Williams TJ, (eds) Immunopharmacology of neutrophils. London, Academic Press, pp 1–4
5. Lee A, Whyte MK, Haslett C (1993) Inhibition of apoptosis and prolongation of neutrophil functional longevity by inflammatory mediators. J Leukoc Biol 54:283–288
6. Hannah S, Mecklenburgh K, Rahman I et al (1995) Hypoxia prolongs neutrophil survival in vitro. FEBS Lett 372:233–237
7. Moulding DA, Quayle JA, Hart CA et al (1998) Mcl-1 expression in human neutrophils: regulation by cytokines and correlation with cell survival. Blood 92:2495–2502
8. Chilvers ER, Cadwallader KA, Reed BJ et al (2000) The function and fate of neutrophils at the inflamed site: prospects for therapeutic intervention. J R Coll Physicians Lond 34:68–74
9. Fulop T Jr (1994) Signal transduction changes in granulocytes and lymphocytes with ageing. Immunol Lett 40:259–268
10. O'Neill L (2006) How Toll–like receptors signal: what we know and what we don't know. Curr Opin Immunol 18:3–9

11. Nathan C (2006) Neutrophils and immunity: challenges and opportunities. Nat Rev Immunol 6:173–182
12. Altstaedt J, Kirchner H, Rink L (1996) Cytokine production of neutrophils is limited to interleukin-8. Immunology 89:563–568
13. Schröder AK, von der Ohe M, Kolling U et al (2006) Polymorphonuclear leucocytes selectively produce anti-inflammatory interleukin-1 receptor antagonist and chemokines, but fail to produce pro-inflammatory mediators. Immunology (Epub Jul 25)
14. Schröder AK, von der Ohe M, Fleischer D et al (2005) Differential synthesis of two interleukin-1 receptor antagonist variants and interleukin-8 by peripheral blood neutrophils. Cytokine 32:246–253
15. Kolling UK, Hansen F, Braun J et al (2001) Leucocyte response and anti-inflammatory cytokines in community acquired pneumonia. Thorax 56:121–125
16. Lloyd AR, Oppenheim JJ (1992) Poly's lament: the neglected role of the polymorphonuclear neutrophil in the afferent limb of the immune response. Immunol Today 13:169–172
17. Meyer KC, Rosenthal NS, Soergel P et al (1998) Neutrophils and low grade inflammation in the seemingly normal aging human lung. Mech Ageing Dev 104;169–181
18. Franceschi C, Bonafe M, Valensin S et al (2000) Inflamm-aging. An evolutionary perspective on immunosenescence. Ann N Y Acad Sci 908:244–254
19. Chatta GS, Andrews RG, Rodger E et al (1993) Hematopoietic progenitors and aging: alterations in granulocytic precursors and responsiveness to recombinant human G-CSF, GM-CSF, and IL-3. J Gerontol 48:M207–M212
20. Born J, Uthgenannt D, Dodt C et al (1995) Cytokine production and lymphocyte subpopulations in aged humans. An assessment during nocturnal sleep. Mech Ageing Dev 84:113–126
21. Cakman I, Kirchner H, Rink L (1997) Zinc supplementation reconstitutes the production of interferon-alpha by leukocytes from elderly persons. J.Interferon Cytokine Res 17:469–472
22. Lord JM, Butcher S, Killampali V et al (2001) Neutrophil ageing and immunesenescence. Mech Ageing Dev 122:1521–1535
23. Butcher S, Chahel H, Lord JM (2000) Ageing and the neutrophil: no appetite for killing? Immunology 100:411–416
24. Schröder AK, Rink L (2003) Neutrophil immunity of the elderly. Mech Ageing Dev 124:419–425
25. Rabatic S, Sabioncello A, Dekaris D et al (1988) Age-related changes in functions of peripheral blood phagocytes. Mech Ageing Dev 45:223–229
26. Ginaldi L, De Martinis M, D'Ostilio A et al (1999) The Immune system in the elderly I. Specific humoral immunity. Immunol Res 20:101–108
27. Ginaldi L, De Martinis M, D'Ostilio A et al (1999) The Immune system in the elderly II. Specific cellular immunity. Immunol Res 20:109–115
28. Ginaldi L, De Martinis M, D'Ostilio A et al (1999) The immune system in the elderly: III. Innate immunity. Immunol Res 20:117–126
29. Emmanuelli, G, Lanzio, M, Anfossi, T et al (1986) Influence of age on polymorphonuclear leukocytes in vitro: phagocytic activity in healthy human subjects. Gerontology 32:308–316
30. Mege, JL, Capo, C, Michel, B et al (1988) Phagocytic cell function in aged subjects. Neurobiol Aging 9: 217–220
31. Esparza B, Sanchez H, Ruiz M et al (1996) Neutrophil function in elderly persons assessed by flow cytometry. Immunol Invest 25:185–190
32. Wenisch C, Patruta S, Daxbock F et al (2000) Effect of age on human neutrophil function. J Leukoc Biol 67:40–45
33. Butcher SK, Chahel H, Nayak L et al (2001) Senescence in innate immune responses: reduced neutrophil phagocytic capacity and CD16 expression in elderly humans. J Leukoc Biol 70:881–886
34. MacGregor RR, Shalit M (1990) Neutrophil function in healthy elderly subjects. J Gerontol 45:M55–M60
35. Braga PC, Sala MT, Dal Sasso M et al (1998) Age-associated differences in neutrophil oxidative burst (chemiluminescence). Exp Gerontol 33:477–484

36. Braga PC, Sala MT, Dal Sasso M et al (1998) Influence of age on oxidative bursts (chemilumi-nescence) of polymorphonuclear neutrophil leukocytes. Gerontology 44:192–197
37. Biasi D, Carletto A, Dell'Agnola C et al (1996) Neutrophil migration, oxidative metabolism, and adhesion in elderly and young subjects. Inflammation 20:673–681
38. Tortorella C, Piazzolla G, Spaccavento F et al (2000) Regulatory role of extracellular matrix proteins in neutrophil respiratory burst during aging. Mech Ageing Dev 119:69–82
39. Seres I, Csongor J, Mohacsi A et al (1993) Age-dependent alterations of human recombinant GM-CSF effects on human granulocytes. Mech Ageing Dev 71:143–154
40. Tortorella, C, Polignano, A, Piazzolla, G et al (1996) Lipopolysaccharide-, granulocyte-monocyte colony stimulating factor- and pentoxifylline-mediated effects on formyl-methio-nyl- leucine-phenylalanine-stimuated neutrophil respiratory burst in the elderly. Microbios 85:189–198
41. Whitelaw DA, Rayner BL, Willcox PA (1992) Community-acquired bacteremia in the elderly: a prospective study of 121 cases. J Am Geriatr Soc 40:996–1000
42. Tortorella C, Stella I, Piazzolla G et al (2004) Role of defective ERK phosphorylation in the impaired GM-CSF-induced oxidative response of neutrophils in elderly humans. Mech Age-ing Dev 8:539–546
43. Larbi A, Dupuis G, Douziech N et al (2004) Low-grade inflammation with aging has conse-quences for T-lymphocyte signaling. Ann N Y Acad Sci 1030:125–133
44. Plackett TP, Boehmer ED, Faunce DE et al (2004) Aging and innate immune cells. J Leukoc 76:291–299
45. Piazzolla G, Tortorella C, Serrone M et al (1998) Modulation of cytoskeleton assembly capacity and oxidative response in aged neutrophils. Immunopharmacol Immunotoxicol 20:251–266
46. Babior BM (1992) Neutrophil function as related to neutrophil–endothelial interactions. Nouv Rev Fr Hematol 34 (Suppl.):829–835
47. Rossi AG, Hellewell PG (1994) Mechanisms of neutrophil accumulation in tissues. In: Hellewell PG, Williams TJ, (eds) Immunopharmacology of neutrophils. London, Academic Press, pp 223–243
48. McLaughlin B, O'Malley K, Cotter TG (1986) Age-related differences in granulocytochemo-taxis and degranulation. Clin Sci 70:59–62
49. Niwa Y, Kasama T, Miyachi Y et al (1989) Neutrophil chemotaxis, phagocytosis and param-eters of reactive oxygen species in human aging: cross-sectional and longitudinal studies. Life Sci 44:1655–1664
50. Corberand J, Ngyen F, Laharrague P et al (1981) Polymorphonuclear functions and aging in humans. J Am Geriatr Soc 29;391–397
51. Tortorella C, Piazzolla G, Spaccavento F, Pece S, Jirillo E, Antonaci S (1998) Spontaneous and Fas-induced apoptotic cell death in aged neutrophils. J Clin Immunol 18:321–329
52. Tortorella C, Piazzolla G, Spaccavento F et al (1999) Age related effects of oxidative metabo-lism and cyclic AMP signaling on neutrophil apoptosis. Mech Ageing Dev 110;195–205
53. Fulop Jr T, Fouquet C, Allaire P et al (1997) Changes in apoptosis of human polymorphonu-clear granulocytes with aging. Mech Ageing Dev 96:15–34
54. Di Lorenzo G, Balistreri CR, Candore G et al (1999) Granulocyte and natural killer activity in the elderly. Mech Ageing Dev 108:25–38
55. Fulop Jr T, Larbi A, Linteau A et al (2002) Role of Mcl-1 and Bax expression alterations in the decreased rescue of human neutrophils from apoptosis by GM-CSF with aging. Ann N Y Acad Sci 973: 305–308
56. Fulop T, Larbi A, Douziech N et al (2004) Signal transduction and functional changes in neu-trophils with aging. Aging Cell 3:217–226
57. Varga Z, Kovacs EM, Paragh G et al (1988) Effect of elastin peptides and N-formyl-methionyl-leucyl phenylalanine on cytosolic free calcium in polymorphonuclear leukocytes of healthy middle-aged and elderly subjects. Clin Biochem 21:127–130
58. Fulop Jr T, Varga Z, Csongor J et al (1989) Age related impairment in phosphatidylinositol breakdown of polymorphonuclear granulocytes. FEBS Lett 245:249–252

59. Lipschitz DA, Udupa KB, Indelicato SR et al (1991) Effect of age on second messenger generation in neutrophils. Blood 78:1347–1354

60. Mohacsi A, Fulop Jr T, Kozlovszky B et al (1992) Superoxide anion production and intracellular free calcium levels in resting and stimulated polymorphonuclear leukocytes obtained from healthy and arteriosclerotic subjects of various ages. Clin Biochem 25:285–288

61. Klut ME, Ruehlmann DO, Li L et al (2002) Age-related changes in the calcium homeostasis of adherent neutrophils. Exp Gerontol 37:533–541

62. Fortin CF, Larbi A, Lesur O et al (2006) Impairment of SHP-1 down-regulation in the lipid rafts of human neutrophils under GM-CSF stimulation contributes to their age-related, altered functions. J Leukoc Biol 79:1061–1072

63. Walrand S, Guillet C, Boirie Y et al (2006) Insulin differentially regulates monocyte and polymorphonuclear neutrophil functions in healthy young and elderly humans. J Clin Endocrinol Metab 91:2738–2748

64. De Martinis M, Modesti M, Ginaldi L (2004) Phenotypic and functional changes of circulating monocytes and polymorphonuclear leucocytes from elderly persons. Immunol Cell Biol 82:415–420

65. Noble JM, Ford GA, Thomas TH (1999) Effect of aging on CD11b and CD69 surface expression by vesicular insertion in human polymorphonuclear leukocytes. Clin Sci 97:323–329

66. Solana R, Alonso MC, Pena J (1999) Natural killer cells in healthy aging. Exp Gerontol 34:435–443

67. Yuli I, Tamonga A, Snyderman R (1982) Chemoattractant receptor functions in human polymorphonuclear leukocytes are divergently altered by membrane fluidizers. Proc Natl Acad Sci U S A 79:5906–5910

68. Alvarez E, Ruiz-Guttierrez V, Sobrino F et al (2001) Age-related changes in membrane lipid composition, fluidity and respiratory burst in rat peripheral neutrophils. Clin Exp Immunol 124;95–102

69. Rao KMK, Currie MS, Padmadabhan J et al (1992) Age-related alterations in actin cytoskeleton and receptor expression in human leukocytes. J Gerontol 47:B37–B44

70. Renshaw M, Rockwell J, Engleman C et al (2002) Cutting edge: impaired Toll-like receptor expression and function in aging. J Immunol 169:4697–4701

71. Boehmer ED, Goral J, Faunce DE et al (2004) Age dependent decrease in Toll-like receptor 4-mediated proinflammatory cytokines by production and mitogen-activated protein kinase expression. J Leukoc Biol 75:342–349

72. Gabriel P, Cakman I, Rink L (2002) Overproduction of monokines by leukocytes after stimulation with lipopolysaccharide in the elderly. Exp Gerontol 37:235–247

73. Ibs KH, Rink L (2001) The immune system in aging. Z Gerontol Geriatr 34:480–485

74. Fagiolo U, Cossarizza A, Scala E et al (1993) Increased cytokine production in mononuclear cells of healthy elderly people. Eur J Immunol 23:2375–2378

Signal Transduction Changes in fMLP, TLRs, TREM-1 and GM-CSF Receptors in PMN with Aging

Carl F. Fortin, Anis Larbi, Gilles Dupuis and Tamas Fulop

Abstract: It is well known that the immune response is decreased with aging leading to a higher susceptibility to infections, cancers and autoimmune disorders. The most widely studied alterations are relative to the adaptive immune response. Recently, the role of the innate immune response as first line of defence

T. Fulop (✉)
Research Center on Aging
Department of Medicine
Immunology Graduate Programme
Faculty of Medicine University of Sherbrooke
Sherbrooke, Quebec, Canada

C. F. Fortin
Clinical Research Center
Immunology Graduate Programme
Faculty of Medicine
University of Sherbrooke
Sherbrooke, Quebec, Canada

A. Larbi
Center for Medical Research
Section for Transplant-Immunology and Immuno-Hematology
Tuebingen Aging and Tumor Immunology Group
University of Tuebingen
Tuebingen, Germany

G. Dupuis
Clinical Research Center
Department of Biochemistry
Immunology Graduate Programme, Faculty of Medicine
University of Sherbrooke
Sherbrooke, Quebec, Canada

T. Fulop et al. (eds.), *Handbook on Immunosenescence*,
DOI 10.1007/ 978-1-4020-9062-2_23, © Springer Science+Business Media B.V. 2009

against bacterial invasion and modulator of the adaptive immune response has been widely recognized. One of the most important cell components of the innate response is neutrophils. It is now accepted that neutrophil functions are changed with age however the degree of these changes is still debated. With aging there is an alteration of the receptor driven functions of human neutrophils, such as superoxide anion production, chemotaxis and apoptosis. One of the alterations underlying these functional changes is the decrease of the receptor signalling elicited by specific receptors. Alterations were also found in the neutrophil membrane lipid rafts. These alterations in neutrophils functions and signal transduction occurring with aging might contribute to the increased infections with aging.

1 Introduction

Neutrophils, also known as polymorphonuclear leukocytes (PMN), are the first cells to arrive at the site of an aggression (Medzhitov and Janeway, 2000). Their role is to eliminate the aggression in a non specific way to prevent ongoing tissue damage and in the mean time regulate and determine the adaptive immune response. They are very efficacious to combat the bacterial and fungal infections (Lehrer et al. 1988). The neutrophils are very short lived cells except if they receive a proinflammatory signal. These signals may prolong the survival of neutrophils to be more effective in eliminating pathogens. Neutrophil functions with aging are changing, mainly those of chemotaxis, free radical production and adherence. Most of these functions are mediated through the engagement of a receptor including formyl methionyl leucine peptide (fMLP), granulocyte macrophage colony stimulating factor (GM-CSF), interleukin-8 (IL-8) receptors (Fulop and Seres, 1994). Recently, novel class of receptors emerged and, they have profound impact on the functions of human PMN. Among them, the pattern recognition receptors (PRRs), including at least 10 toll like receptors (TLRs) which recognize conserved molecular structures, related mostly to pathogens, were described and extensively studied (Medzhitov 2001; Krishnana et al. 2007). Furthermore, the triggering receptor expressed on myeloid cells-1 (TREM-1) is a recent addition to the growing members of activating receptors that are members of the Ig superfamily and, is up-regulated at the surface of PMN and monocytes in infection and LPS-induced sepsis in mice (Bouchon et al. 2000; Bleharski et al. 2003; Gibot 2006). Over the past few years, it has been demonstrated that PMN-specific receptor-driven effector functions are altered with aging (Fulop et al. 1997; Varga et al. 1997; Fulop et al. 2004). One of the causes of these decreased functions could be the alteration of signalling with aging via various receptors of neutrophils (Fulop et al. 1985a,b; Vlahos and Matter, 1992; Wenisch et al. 2000; Lord et al. 2001; Schröder and Rink, 2003; Fulop et al. 2001; Biasi et al. 1996; Seres et al. 1993). This chapter will describe our present knowledge concerning the signal transduction pathways in neutrophils with aging elicited by fMLP, GM-CSF, TLR and TREM-1 ligands.

2 Neutrophil Function Changes with Aging

PMN are short-lived cells that play important roles in both host defence and acute inflammation. They represent the first line of defence against an assault. They are committed to die in circulation within 18 hours unless activated (Akgul et al. 2001). This activation results in the initiation of an inflammatory response leading to chemotaxis via adhesion to endothelial cells, migration and the development of effector functions such as free radical production (Babior 2000). The adhesion (Butcher et al. 2001) and migration (Biasi et al. 1996) functions of PMN were found unchanged with aging. Recent data on chemotaxis indicate a decrease during aging towards fMLP and GM-CSF as chemoattractants (Fulop et al. 2004). The inability of GM-CSF to prime PMN of elderly for superoxide anion production was also described (Seres et al. 1993). It is of note that the number of receptors involved in PMN chemotaxis has not been found to change with aging. We have demonstrated some time ago that the production of free radicals by PMN of elderly subjects was decreased under fMLP stimulation while the number of fMLP receptors did not change (Fulop et al. 1985a, 1989) and, this was also found by many laboratories (Braga et al. 1998; Biasi et al. 1996), while others found no changes (Lord et al. 2001). It is of note that the variations in PMN superoxide production with aging were dependent on the stimuli indicating different pathways of neutrophil activation. It was shown that gram positive pathogens induce a decreased production, while gram-negative ones induce no reduction (Wenisch et al. 2000). Insofar, these pathogens modulate PMN functions through different TLRs (Hayashi et al. 2003).Certain proinflammatory cytokines, or other molecules, were shown to prolong the life span and the functional survival of PMN (Whyte et al. 1999). Among these molecules are GM-CSF, LPS and IL-6. Other bacterial products such as fMLP, LPS, lipoteichoic acid modulate the effector functions of neutrophils. We and others have found that the PMN of elderly subjects can not be rescued from apoptosis by various agents known to be very effective for PMN of young subjects (Fulop et al. 1997; Tortorella et al. 1998, 2001).

Thus, we can hypothesize that alterations of the signal transduction pathways of the various receptors are involved in the altered neutrophil functions with aging (Fulop and Seres 1994; Fulop et al. 2001). This altered signal transduction can be related to changes in the physico-chemical properties of the PMN membrane with ageing determining its fluidity. It has been shown that changes in membrane fluidity affect PMN functions, such as chemotaxis, superoxide anion production (Yuli 1982; Alvarez et 2001). An age-dependent decrease in plasma membrane fluidity has been shown in various cell types (Rivnay et al. 1980; Shinitzki 1987) including T-lymphocytes (Larbi 2004a,b), whereas in neutrophils an increase was observed in the membrane fluidity (Fulop et al. 2004). These data suggest that either of these changes in membrane fluidity with aging could be deleterious for cellular functions. It should be remembered that PMN are very short lived cells in contrast to all the others studied, explaining the differential changes of membrane fluidity with aging. Very recently, the presence of lipid rafts in PMN cell membrane has been described and an important role in PMN signal transduction has been suggested for them (Kandzelskii et al. 2004; Sitrin 2004; Fortin 2007b, c). Changes in membrane fluidity will affect the function of lipid rafts (Simons and Ehehalt 2002; Simons and Ilkonen 1997), which are special membrane microdomains for signalling that are playing an important role in cellular functions, including chemotaxis (Ibanez 2004). Thus, age-related changes in the cell membrane affect the membrane properties, which in turn determine the signal transduction leading to altered effector functions, such as chemotaxis, superoxide anion production and apoptosis. This might influence the sequence of all the other effector functions of PMN with aging. We will review herein some specific receptor signalling changes with aging.

3 Signal Transduction Changes and Lipid Rafts in Neutrophils in Relation to fMLP, GM-CSF and Toll-like Receptors with Ageing

There are rather few data concerning the signal transduction in PMN with aging as compared to those in T-lymphocytes (Larbi et al. 2004a). Nevertheless, accumulating data suggest that aging cause alterations of specific receptor signalling pathways in PMN (Fulop and Seres 1994; Fulop et al. 2004; Lord et al. 2001; Schröder and Rink 2003; Tortorella et al. 2007). The recent description of lipid rafts in PMN membrane will also rapidly improve our understanding on PMN signalling pathways and permit their extension to a better investigation of the PMN signal transduction with aging.

3.1 fMLP Receptor

Formyl peptides engage receptors that belong to the seven transmembrane G protein-coupled receptor (GPCR) family and trigger neutrophil responses, i.e., chemotaxis, up-regulation of surface receptors, release of proteolytic enzymes from granules and, ROS production (Varga et al. 1988; Mcleish et al. 1989; Varga et al. 1989; Rabiet et al. 2007). These responses are largely inhibited by Bordetella pertussis toxin, indicating that signal transduction is dependent on a heterotrimeric G protein of the Gi type. We will review current knowledge about the peptide-induced activation of chemoattractant receptors and their regulation, with special emphasis on the human formyl peptide receptor family (FPR, FPRL1, and FPRL2). Upon chemoattractant binding, receptors undergo a conformational change that enables them to interact with the Gi2 protein thereby triggering both the exchange of GDP to GTP in the G protein α subunit and, the dissociation of the βγ complex from the α subunit (Gierschik et al. 1989). Following its dissociation from the α subunit, the G protein βγ subunits activate the phospholipase Cβ2 (PLCβ2) (Camps et al. 1992) and the phosphoinositide 3-kinase γ (PI3Kγ) (Stoyanov et al. 1995). PI3Kγ

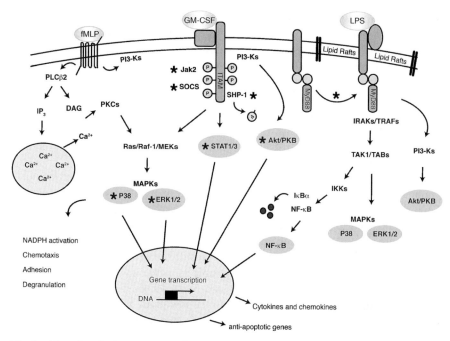

Fig. 1 Alterations in the receptor-mediated signal transduction in human neutrophils with aging. In neutrophils, fMLPR engagement leads to activation of PI3-K and PLCγ2, this in turn leads to the production of DAG and the influx of Ca^{2+} to the cytosol where they activate the PKCs. The PKCs activate the downstream MAPKs P38 and ERK1/2 through Ras. The ligand of GM-CSFR, for its part, induces the phosphorylation of residues in the ITAM of the common β-chain These events will induce the recruitment of various signalling molecules to the GM-CSFR, and will lead to the activation of the MAPKs P38 and ERK1/2, the Jak2-STAT1/3 and the PI3-K-Akt/PKB signalling pathway. The down-regulation of the GM-CSFR is mediated by phosphatases, like SHP-1, that removes phospho-groups on the ITAM, or the SOCS family of protein, which bind Jak2 and other activating upstream kinases thereby impeding the recruitment of signalling molecules on the receptor. Upon engagement, TLR4 is recruited into lipid rafts and, with the accessory molecule MyD88, leads to the activation of the MAPKs P38 and ERK1/2 and the transcription factor NF-κB through the IRAK/TRAFs and TAK1/TABs complexes. It also activates the PI3-K-Akt/PKB pathway through largely unknown mechanisms. The downstream kinases and the transcription factors elicited by these receptors mediate, in the cytosol and in the nucleus, the functional responses of human neutrophils such as respiratory burst, chemotaxis, degranulation and production of cytokines and chemokines. The asterisks indicate impairment that have been found in the signalling pathways of these receptor with aging in human neutrophils. One can appreciate the work that remains to be done as the absence of asterisk indicates that potential alterations were not studied in the elderly for these signalling molecules

converts the membrane phosphatidylinositol-4,5-bisphosphate (PIP$_2$) into phosphatidylinositol-3,4,5-trisphosphate (PIP$_3$) which is required for both the directed migration of neutrophils in a gradient of fMLP and the generation of superoxide mediated by the stimulation of chemoattractant receptors. The activation of PLCβ2, which induces the production of IP$_3$, leads to an increase of intracellular free calcium and of DAG, which result in the translocation of PKC to the membrane and, leading to the phosphorylation of members of the MAPK family (Chang and Wang 1999). Neutrophils express the classical PKC isoforms (α, βI, and βII), the novel PKC isoforms δ and the atypical PKC isoforms ζ. The activation of PKC isoforms play a role in the regulation of NADPH oxidase activity. The extracellular signal-regulated kinases (ERK1/2) and the stress-activated p38 MAP kinase are activated by chemoattractants in neutrophils. These two signalling pathways are thought to participate at different degrees in adherence, chemotaxis and superoxide production. PLA$_2$-α is phosphorylated by MAP kinases and is translocated to the plasma membrane in a calcium-dependent manner where it produces free fatty acids and lysophospholipids.

Stimulation of the cells by fMLP induces, via the production of IP$_3$ and the opening of calcium channels in the membrane, an increase in intracellular free calcium. This increase is normally very rapid and returns to the prestimulation level relatively quickly. There is a slight difference between young and elderly subjects in the intracellular free calcium kinetics stimulated by fMLP in PMN (Biasi et al. 1996). The amount of the intracellular free calcium inside the cells is higher under fMLP stimulation in PMN of young than elderly subjects, while it was higher in the PMN of elderly at unstimulated status (Fulop and Seres 1994). This indicates a slight activation status of PMN with aging due to the low grade inflammation occurring with physiological aging (Franceschi et al. 2000; Meyer et al. 1998). The return of the intracellular free calcium must be tightly regulated, because if it remains high this could lead to cell death via the activation of certain intracellular proteases such as calpains or endonucleases. These data indicate that aging is associated with a decrease in the early phase of signal transduction in PMN.

The induction of PKC via the ras pathway in turn induces the activation of MAPK family members when the PMN are stimulated by fMLP (Zu et al. 1998). MAPKs are a family of serine/threonine kinases that are activated by a cascade of protein kinase reactions (Kyriakis and Avrach 1996), which are not completely elucidated in human neutrophils, even after fMLP stimulation. In rat neutrophils the activation of Lyn is associated with binding to the Shc adaptor protein and allows the G protein-coupled receptors to modulate the activity of the Ras/ERK cascade (Chang and Wang 1999). Nevertheless, investigations of human neutrophils have suggested that p38 MAPK is involved in an intracellular cascade that regulates stress-activated signal transduction. The p38 MAPK can phosphorylate transcription factors, thereby regulating gene expression and, can also phosphorylate other proteins to stimulate NADPH oxidase activity, adhesion and chemotaxis (Kyriakis and Avreach 1996; Zu et al. 1998; Heuertz et al. 1999; Yagisawa et al. 1999; Chang and Wang 2000). fMLP has been shown to induce the activities of ERK1 and ERK2, thus playing a role in neutrophil adherence and respiratory burst activity as well as inducing p38 and contributing to chemotaxis and superoxide anion production (Zu et al. 1998). Recent data obtained in our laboratory (Larbi et al. 2005) indicate that aging is associated with a decrease of ERK and p38 tyrosine phosphorylation in PMN under fMLP stimulation, suggesting a decreased activity of these MAPKs. These alterations could explain the decrease found in effector functions of PMN with aging such as superoxide anion production, as well as chemotaxis. Altogether we assist to an alteration of the human fMLP receptor signalling with aging.

3.2   GM-CSF Receptor

GM-CSF is a powerful modulator of granulopoiesis and the priming of mature PMN to a second stimulation such as fMLP. GM-CSF is able to rescue PMN from apoptosis by interacting with its specific receptor on the PMN plasma membrane. The receptor for GM-CSF is a member of the superfamily of cytokine receptors (Miyajima et al. 1992). Its structure consists of a receptor-specific α subunit and a β subunit (βc) that is shared by the receptors for IL-3 and IL-5 (Miyajima et al. 1993). Although the GM-CSF receptor is not endowed with intrinsic protein kinase activity, its occupation triggers the phosphorylation of its βc subunit on tyrosine residues, most probably by Jak2 (Quelle et al. 1994) and, the phosphorylation of a host of cytoplasmic proteins on tyrosine residues, the expression of early response genes and the proliferation of hematopoietic cells. GM-CSF has been shown to activate three distinct pathways in various cells: 1. the JAK/STAT pathway, 2. the Ras-Raf-1-MEK-MAP kinase pathway and, 3. the PI3-kinase intracellular signalling events (Sato et al. 1993; Watanabe et al. 1997). Recently, the MAPK and PI3K pathways were suggested to be involved with the GM-CSF antiapoptotic effect in PMN (Klein et al. 2000). These signalling pathways modulate the executioner phase of apoptosis, mediated by a family of cysteine proteases, the caspases, as well as members of the bcl-2 family, which are key players in the regulation of apoptosis.

Our recent studies suggest that aging is accompanied by a decrease in GM-CSF-signal transduction (Fortin et al. 2007a). PMN functions were shown to decrease with aging, as well as the antiapoptotic effect of GM-CSF (Fulop et al. 2004). Thus, we also investigated whether the Jak/STAT pathway in PMN under GM-CSF stimulation could be altered with aging. We have demonstrated that activation of the Jak/STAT pathway is altered in PMN of elderly subjects under GM-CSF stimulation. Neither short, nor sustained phosphorylation of Jak2 could be demonstrated and this inability of GM-CSF to induce Jak2 activation was translated in the decreased activation of STAT3 and STAT5. Moreover, the density of GM-CSF receptor β subunit did not change with age. The unchanged βc-subunit expression would assure an equal possibility of signalling in PMN of young and elderly subjects. This is supported by the fact that the physical association between the GM-CSF receptor β subunit and Jak2 did not change neither with aging, nor with GM-CSF stimulation. One other explanation could be an alteration in the membrane composition rendering difficult the mobility of the receptors to facilitate the phosphorylation of Jak2 (Fulop et al. 2004). Recently, the presence of lipid rafts in the cell membrane of PMN was demonstrated (Sitrin et al. 2004; Kindzelskii et al. 2004). These lipid rafts are privileged microdomains in the membrane enriched in cholesterol, sphyngolipids and various proteins, such as signalling proteins (Simons and Ikonen 1997). We found with aging a significant alteration in the composition and properties of lipid rafts of T-cells (Larbi et al. 2004a). In PMN, our group showed in a recent paper an over activation of the protein tyrosine phosphatase SHP-1, a negative regulator of signal transduction, in the lipid rafts with aging. This over activation caused the defects in the activation of the Src Kinase Lyn and contributed to the impaired functions of PMN with aging (Fortin et al. 2006). Moreover, an over activation or a deregulated termination of Jak2 negative regulators, including SOCS, with aging cannot be ruled out and is currently under investigation by, among others, the group of Tortorella (2007). They demonstrated that both SOCS1 and SOCS3 levels were significantly higher in unstimulated neutrophils from elderly individuals than in their younger counterparts and, unlike the neutrophils of young subjects, they did not further increase following GM-CSF stimulation. As a result, a more effective SOCS1 and SOCS3 binding to either the GM-CSF receptor or Jak2, which would largely account for the GM-CSF dependent defect of PI3-K/Akt/ERK activation, might occur in senescent neutrophils. This finding is in line with recent demonstration of elevated SOCS3 levels in resting lymphocytes from elderly donors. Therefore, the increase in this class of inhibitory molecules may be considered as a general phenomenon associated with aging (Tortorella et al. 2007).

We also investigated whether this alteration in the activation of the Jak/STAT signalling pathway could be linked to the decreased antiapoptotic effect of GM-CSF in PMN of elderly subjects. We found that GM-CSF was unable to modulate the Caspase-3 activity in the elderly subjects (Fortin et al. 2007a). Moreover, our results show that AG490 could not modulate the already decreased anti-apoptotic effect of GM-CSF. It is difficult to determine what the exact contribution of the Jak/STAT pathway is, but these results indicate that it plays an important role in the GM-CSF failure to rescue PMN of elderly subjects from apoptosis. Thus, PMN of elderly subjects seem to be in a dominant negative status leading to a decreased response to GM-CSF. This also precludes that if the Jak2 activation is decreased, other downstream signalling pathways could be also altered, such as the PI3-kinase pathway (our unpublished results and Tortorella et al. 2007). Thus, Jak2 might play an upstream and essential role in the signalling cascade to provide survival signal to STATs and other signalling pathways.

PI3-K and the downstream serine/threonine kinase Akt/protein kinase B (Akt/PKB) have a central role in modulating neutrophil respiratory burst activation, chemotaxis and apoptosis. Tortorella et al. (2007) studied the functional activity of the neutrophil PI3-K/Akt pathway in the elderly and found, similarly to the ERK1/2, higher baseline levels of phosphorylated Akt forms and lower GM-CSF-induced phosphorylation of Akt with respect to younger subjects. The link once more between these signalling alterations and the age-related inability of GM-CSF to prolong neutrophil survival emerged from observations using various pharmacological inhibitors such as PD98059, LY294002 or wortmannin. These alterations in the PI3-K/Akt pathways could explain the alterations in the MAPK ERK1/2 activation, as they seem to be activated in succession. In fact, others and we have showed significant alterations in the GM-CSF induced ERK1 and ERK2 tyrosine phosphorylation and, even a higher decrease in ERK1/2 activation with respect to baseline in PMN from elderly subjects compared to young subjects (Larbi et al. 2005). The p38 MAPK pathway was also found altered in PMN from elderly under GM-CSF activation (Larbi et al. 2005).

It is of note that bypassing the GM-CSF receptor by direct inhibition of Caspase-3 was able to rescue PMN from apoptosis in both groups of age (Fortin et al. 2007a). This further indicates that the GM-CSF inability to rescue PMN of elderly from apoptosis is linked, in part, to the alteration of the signalling pathway that leads from GM-CSFR to Caspase-3. However, it is not the sole factor as there is a significant fraction of residual procaspase-3 in the PMN of the elderly donors after 18h of culture. Moreover, after 18h of culture with GM-CSF there is even a larger fraction of inactive procaspase-3 in the elderly. These results would be surprising if the inhibition of Jak2 by AG490 did resulted in a complete cleavage of procaspase-3 in the elderly as it did in the young donors. We can only hypothesize that the inability of GM-CSF to rescue PMN of elderly from apoptosis is not mediated by the cleavage of procaspase-3 but rather by other mechanisms, especially as the Caspase-3 enzymatic activity has been found to be higher in this paper (Fortin et al. 2007a). Others mechanisms include an altered ratio of antiapoptotic vs. proapoptotic members of the Bcl-2 protein family, such as Bax, BclXL, Bad and A1 (Fulop et al. 2002; Fulop et al. 2004) and, deregulation of the activity of negative regulators of GM-CSF signal transduction like SHP-1 (Fortin et al. 2006). Supporting this notion, GM-CSF has been shown to up-regulate the expression of the antiapoptotic Mcl-1 (Moulding et al. 1998) while interferon-α/γ had similar surviving effects by increasing the expression of the cIAP2 protein (Sakamoto et al. 2005). Moreover, the failure of GM-CSF to sustain STAT3 phosphorylation in the elderly may promote PMN apoptosis by not counteracting the proapoptotic effects of activated STAT1, as it is the case for Mel80 cells. Moreover, these observations in elderly subjects bear a resemblance to the phenomenon observed in T-cells. The T-cell receptor (TCR) signalling is altered leading to deficient proliferation with aging, while bypassing the TCR by PMA and Ca2+ ionophore stimulation restore their proliferative capacity. This could be of importance when we consider the increase of infections with aging and the modulation of PMN function might go through a nonspecific manner.

The Jak/STAT, PI3-K/Akt and MAPK pathways were found to be altered with aging in PMN upon GM-CSF receptor stimulation (Fortin et al. 2007a; Larbi et al. 2005; Tortorella et al. 2007). However, there is no decrease in the GM-CSFR number with aging. The primary alteration could be the Jak/STAT pathway as it seems to regulate all the others. Not only the positive signalling events but also the negative signalling events are altered under GM-CSF stimulation in PMN with aging. This leads to an altered functioning of the PMN with aging concerning apoptosis, chemotaxis and free radical productions.

3.3   Toll-like Receptors

Toll-like receptors (TLRs) are pattern recognition receptors that recognize conserved molecular patterns on microbes and link innate and adaptive immune systems. There exists actually of 10 different TLRs. Ligands for the TLR2 are gram-positive bacteria, while gram-negative bacterial product, LPS, is a ligand for TLR4 and, both of them are found on neutrophils (Remer et al. 2003; Kurt-Jones et al. 2002). The signalling pathways activated by TLRs are broadly classified into MyD88-dependent and independent pathways (Takeda and Akira 2005) as MyD88 is the universal adapter protein recruited by all TLRs, except TLR3. The MyD88-independent pathway of TLR4 signalling is not used in human PMN (Tamassia et al. 2007). The major pathways activated by TLR engagement are using IκB kinase (IKK), MAPK and phosphatidylinositol 3-kinase (PI3-K)/Akt pathways. These pathways regulate the balance between cell viability and inflammation. There are currently four cytosolic adaptor proteins that are thought to play a crucial role in specificity of individual TLR-mediated signalling pathways. Amongst them, TLR4 signalling involves all four adapter proteins, MyD88 (myeloid differentiation primary response gene 88), MyD88 adapter like [MAL; also known as TIRAP (TIR domain-containing adapter protein)], TIR domain-containing adapter protein inducing IFN-β [TRIF; also known as TICAM1 (TIR domain-containing adapter molecule 1)], and TRIF-related adapter molecule [TRAM; also known as TICAM2 (TIR domain-containing adapter molecule 2)] (McGettrick and O'Neill, 2004). The differential recruitment of these adapter proteins by different TLRs form the basis for the specificity in the signalling process activated by them. However, the signal transduction pathway initiated by these interactions is mediated initially by an adaptor molecule, MyD88, recruiting various serine-threonine kinases, IRAKs and finally leading to NF-κB translocation (Kobayashi and Flavell 2004). Among IRAK family proteins IRAK-4 and IRAK-1 play major roles in signal transduction under LPS stimulation. This interaction ultimately results in the secretion of pro-inflammatory cytokines (Cloutier et al. 2007) that recruit the cells of adaptive immune response. That is why the function of TLRs is very important not only for an adequate innate, but also for the adaptive immune response. Moreover, there exists a synergy between TLR2 and GM-CSF receptors (Hayashi et al. 2003).

There exists almost no data concerning the TLRs receptor number and signal transduction in PMN in relation to aging. Renshaw et al. (2002) reported impaired TLR expression and function with aging in mice macrophages. A recent comprehensive evaluation of TLR function in monocytes from older adults was conducted using a multivariable mixed statistical model to account for covariates (van Duin and Shaw 2007). It found that cytokine production after TLR1/2 engagement, which is essential for the recognition of triacylated lipopeptides found in a variety of bacteria, is substantially lower in monocytes from older adults. The up-regulation of costimulatory proteins such as CD80, essential for optimal activation of T-cells, on monocytes from older adults was less for all TLR ligands tested than for cells from young individuals and, the extent of CD80 up-regulation predicted subsequent antibody response to influenza immunization. These and other consequences of aging on human TLR function may impair activation of the immune response and contribute to poorer vaccine responses and greater morbidity and mortality from infectious diseases in older adults. That is why we investigated the TLR4 and TLR2 receptor numbers on PMN of young and elderly subjects by flow cytometry. We found that there is no change in the percentage of PMN expressing TLR4 and TLR2 with aging. Similar results were obtained when we measured, by comparing the Mean Fluorescence Intensity (MFI), the amount of TLR4 or TLR2 receptors expressed by PMN in each age groups (Fulop et al. 2004). These results show that there is no change with aging in the expression of TLR2 and TLR4 receptors on PMN.

One other element, as mentioned above, which recently changed our comprehension of the signalling mechanism through the membrane is the existence of specific signalling microdomains in the membrane, called lipid rafts (Simon and Ilkonen 1997). These were demonstrated in numerous cells and recently in PMN too (Shao et al. 2003). These microdomains, enriched in sphyngolipids, cholesterol and signalling molecules either are parts of, or are recruited to the signalling complexes of the cell membrane. Presently, a few data exist in relation to aging on the existence of these lipid rafts in PMN membranes and how these lipid rafts could be structured and functioning (Fortin et al. 2006, 2007b, 2007c). Therefore, we also studied, whether the unchanged number of TLRs found by FACScan is reinforced by the study of the expression of TLR2 and TLR4 in the PMN membrane lipid rafts. We showed for the first time that LPS not only increases the expression of TLR4 in PMN of young subjects, but increases also its recruitment in the rafts and nonrafts fractions. In contrast, the expression of TLR4 in rafts and nonraft fractions were increased with aging already at the basal status compared to that of PMN of young subjects while no-redistribution occurred after LPS stimulation. It is of note that the apparent increase at basal status of TLR4 expression in the membrane of PMN of elderly could be in accordance with the slight stimulated status of PMN with aging, as already demonstrated (Fulop and Seres 1994). This is also in accordance with the low-grade inflammation present with aging as stated by the inflamm-aging theory of Franceschi et al. (2000). It is of note that no significant changes in TLR2 recruitment occurred in rafts and nonrafts fractions of PMN under LPS stimulation in either young subjects or elderly subjects. These results indicate that even if the number of receptors seems not to change with aging the differential recruitment between raft and nonraft fractions could induce an altered signalling of the receptors, mainly in case of TLR4 under LPS stimulation with aging.

We also studied the early signal transduction events elicited by LPS through the TLR4. The signal transduction of TLR4 under LPS stimulation is mediated at the early phases by MyD88 and IRAKs (Kobayashi and Flavell 2004). We studied the expression of MyD88 and IRAK-1 under LPS stimulation in membrane rafts and nonrafts fractions of PMN. MyD88 was evenly distributed before and after LPS stimulation in the rafts and nonrafts fractions of the membranes in young and elderly subjects. Thus, no differences in the MyD88 distribution could be found with aging, however the quantity of MyD88 in the membrane of PMN of elderly subjects was significantly decreased after stimulation (Fulop et al. 2004). MyD88 is an adaptor protein found very close to the membrane, which could explain that no change in its physical distribution can be observed under stimulation. In contrast, there is a recruitment of IRAK-1 molecules from nonrafts fractions to lipid rafts in PMN of young subjects under LPS stimulation while this recruitment is totally absent in PMN of elderly subjects. It is of note that IRAK-1 was already in the rafts fraction at basal status, in accordance with the slightly activated status of PMN with aging. All these results suggest an alteration in the signal transduction of TLR4 under LPS stimulation with aging either in the redistribution of IRAK-1 signalling protein among rafts and nonrafts fractions, or in the quantity of the MyD88 molecule between rafts and nonrafts fractions. These results provide evidence for a lipid rafts dependant activation of neutrophils via the Toll-like receptor pathway. However, they cannot explain why the LPS was efficient for chemotaxis of PMN with aging. We can only speculate that either this function is mediated through different signalling pathway(s) or this is a nonreceptor dependent function of LPS, playing the role of a nonspecific chemoattractant.

Altogether, the studies on signal transduction pathways elicited by the stimulation of various PMN receptors suggest that there exists an altered signal transduction in PMN with aging. These alterations does not seem to arise from a change in the receptor number, but most probably from an alteration related to the cell membrane physico-chemical status with aging. We and others have found that the fluidity of PMN with aging, in contrast to other cells, is increasing due to the alteration in the membrane cholesterol/phospholipid composition (Yuli et al. 1982; Alvarez et al. 2001). The cholesterol content does not change while the phospholipid content is increasing. These changes affect the functionality of lipid rafts which are important microdomains for the receptor signalling, as was shown in the case of TLRs and GM-CSF receptors. A dysfunction of the signalling due to age-related changes in actin cytoskeleton function (Rao et al. 1992) has been also suggested to be a contributing factor. Ultimately these changes in signalling decrease the effectors functions of PMN with aging.

3.4   TREM-1

This receptor is a recent addition to the growing members of activating receptors that are members of the Ig superfamily and, is up-regulated at the surface of PMN and macrophages in infection and LPS-induced sepsis in mice (Bouchon et al. 2000). This family mediate their signal transduction with an adapter molecule, for TREM-1 the adapter is DAP12, to elicit a number of common signalling molecules (Bouchon et al. 2000; Klesney-Tait et al. 2006; Tessarz and Cerwenka 2007). Its ligand is still unknown, but the functional responses elicited by the engagement of TREM-1 on monocytes/macrophages and PMN is well known. TREM-1 triggers the release of cytokines and chemokines, ROS production, degranulation and phagocytosis (Bouchon et al. 2000; Bleharski et al. 2003; Radsak et al. 2004; Fortin et al. 2007b). Of note, stimulation of PMN with both TREM-1 and TLR ligands resulted in a synergistic effect on functional responses (Bleharski et al. 2003; Radsak et al. 2004; Fortin et al. 2007b) hence amplifying the inflammatory response and, suggesting potentially aggravating consequences in infections with aging. Inasmuch, our group recently found that TREM-1 and TLR4 colocalized in human PMN upon stimulation with LPS (Fortin et al. 2007b) and, silencing of TREM-1 in macrophages with siRNA resulted in down-regulation of key signalling molecules of the TLR4 pathway (Ornatowska et al. 2007). Thus, emerging data are showing an unsuspected link between the TLR4 and TREM-1 and, it is possible that multimeric complexes are responsible for the recognition of noncytokines mediators of inflammation such as the ligands of TREM-1 (Klesney-Tait and Colonna 2007). We have already evoke the possibilty of an innateosome, which would be responsible for the recognition of LPS and TREM-1 ligands in human PMN, when we showed that stimulation of either receptors lead to the phosphorylation of IRAK1 and the colocalization at the membrane of TRL4 and TREM-1 (Fortin et al. 2007b). Furthermore, the importance of soluble TREM-1, the shedding of TREM-1 occurs in sepsis or with LPS stimulation of macrophages, in a clinical context it is established that this is a relevant marker for human sepsis and, the use of decoy TREM-1 with blocking ability favored a positive outcome of the resolution of sepsis (Gibot 2006).

So far, only our group studied the impact of aging on the TREM-1-induced functions on cells of the immune system. PMN from elderly donors were found to have impaired response following TREM-1 engagement (Fortin et al. 2007c). Notably, TREM-1 could not prime the production of ROS in the elderly as it did in the young donors and, altered signal transduction of downstream TREM-1-elicited molecules (Akt and PLCγ) was found. Of particular interest, TREM-1 engagement could not reverse PMN survival following incubation with LPS or GM-CSF in the elderly whereas it did in the young. This particular alteration in TREM-1 response could possibly be a contributing factor in the higher incidence of sepsis-related deaths in the elderly population as resolution of inflammation requires clearance of effectors cells. Finally, TREM-1 engagement could not drive the recruitment of TREM-1 in the lipid-rafts of the elderly explaining in part the altered response. Although data exist in human relative to the amount of soluble TREM-1 found in the plasma of patient with or without sepsis, the study was carried only for one age group (mean age 60 ± 15) (Gibot et al. 2004). In keeping with the contributions of TREM-1 in inflammation and the aforementioned alterations in the TEM-1-induced functions in the PMN of the elderly, it would be extremely interesting to have data on lethal outcome of sepsis vs. age of hospitalized patients.

4   Conclusion

PMN are very important part of the immune response towards invading organisms. They are the first line defence being part of the innate immune response and, are essential modulators of the adaptive immune response. It is well known that the incidence of infections is increasing with age. Decrease in specific receptor mediated functions including free radical production, chemotaxis and apoptosis/survival of PMN with aging resulting from an alteration of the positive and negative events in the signalling pathways have been recently demonstrated. These alterations might contribute to the increased incidence of infections with aging. However, these changes in neutrophil functions remain controversial with aging. Elucidation with more rigorous and sophisticated methods of PMN function alterations with aging is needed as these changes could have a great impact on the adaptive immune response. The recent demonstration of lipid rafts in PMN, as being fundamental platforms for signal transduction, will help to better understand the mechanism of age-related signalling changes. These changes should be also taken into account when tentative is made to increase the immune response of the elderly by immunomodulating agents for improving the quality of life of elderly persons.

Acknowledgments This work was supported by a grant-in-aid from the National Science and Engenineering Research Council of Canada (No 249549), Research Center on Aging of Sherbrooke, the Clinical Researh Center and the Canadian Institute of Health Research (No 63149).

References

Akgul C, Moulding DA, Edwards SW (2001) Molecular control of neutrophil apoptosis. FEBS Lett 487:318–322

Alvarez E, Ruiz-Guttierrez V, Sobrino F, Santa-Maria C (2001) Age-related changes in membrane lipid composition, fluidity and respiratoty burst in rat peripheral neutrophils. Clin Exp Immunol 124:95–102

Babior BM (2000) Phagocytes and oxidative stress. Am J Med 109: 33–44

Biasi D, Carletto A, Dellagnola C, Caramaschi P, Montesanti F, Zavateri G, Zeminian S, Bellavite P, Bambara LM (1996) Neutrophil migration, oxidative metabolism, and adhesion in elderly and young subjects. Inflammation 20:673–681

Bleharski JR, Kiessler V, Buonsanti C, Sieling PA, Stenger S, Colonna M, Modlin RL (2003) A role for triggering receptor expressed on myeloid cells-1 in host defense during the early-induced and adaptive phases of the immune response. J Immunol 170:3812–3818

Bouchon A, Dietrich J, Colonna M (2000) Cutting edge: inflammatory responses can be triggered by TREM-1, a novel receptor expressed on neutrophils and monocytes. J Immunol 164:4991–4995

Braga PC, Sala MT, Dal Sasso M, Mancini L, Sandrini MC, Annoni G (1998) Age-associated differences in neutrophil oxidative burst (chmiluminsescence). Exp Gerontol 33:477–484

Butcher SK, Chahal H, Nayak L, Sinclair A, Henriquez NV, Sapet E, O'Mahony D, Lord JM (2001) Senescence in innate immune responses: reduced neutrophil phagocytic capacity and and CD16 expression in elderly humans. J Leukocyte Biol 70: 881–886

Camps M, Carozzi A, Schnabel P, Scheer A, Parker PJ, Gierschik P (1992) Isozyme-selective stimulation of phospholipase C-b2 by G protein bgsubunits. Nature 360:684–689

Chang LC, Wang JP (1999) Examination of the signal transduction pathways leading to activation of extracellular signal-regulated kinase by formyl-methionyl-leucyl-phenylalanine in rat neutrophils. FEBS Lett 454:165–168

Chang LC, Wang JP (2000) Activation of p38 mitogen-activated protein kinase by formyl-methionyl-leucyl-phenylalanine in rat neutrophils. Eur J Pharmacol 390: 61–66

Cloutier A, Ear T, Blais-Charron E, Dubois CM, McDonald PP (2007) Differential involvement of NF-kappaB and MAP kinase pathways in the generation of inflammatory cytokines by human neutrophils. J Leukocyte Biol 81: 567–577

Fortin CF, Larbi A, Lesur O, Douziech N, Fulop T (2006) Impairment of SHP-1 down-regulation in the lipid rafts of human neutrophils under GM-CSF stimulation contributes to their age-related, altered functions. J Leukocyte Biol 79:1061–1072

Fortin CF, Larbi A, Dupuis G, Lesur O, Fulop T (2007a) GM-CSF activates the Jak/STAT pathway to rescue polymorphonuclear neutrophils from spontaneous apoptosis in young but not elderly individuals. Biogerontology 8:173–187

Fortin CF, Lesur O, Fulop T (2007b) Effects of TREM-1 activation in human neutrophils: activation of signaling pathways, recruitment into lipid rafts and association with TLR4. Int Immunol 19:41–50

Fortin CF, Lesur O, Fulop T (2007c) Effects of aging on triggering receptor expressed on myeloid cells (TREM)-1-induced PMN functions. FEBS Lett 581:1173–1178

Franceschi C, Bonafe M, Valensin S, Olivieri F, De Luca M, Ottaviani E, De Benedictis G (2000) Inflamm-ageing. An evolutionary perspective on immunosenescence. Ann N Y Acad Sci 908:244–254

Fulop T Jr, Foris G, Worum I, Paragh G, Leovey A (1985a). Age-related variations of some PMNL functions. Mech Age Dev 29:1–8

Fulop T Jr, Foris G, Worum I, Leovey A (1985b) Age-dependent alterations of Fc receptor mediated effector functions of human polymorphonuclear leukocytes. Clin Exp Immunol 61:425–432

Fulop T Jr, Varga Zs, Csongor J, Foris G, Leovey A (1989) Age-related impairment of phosphatidylinositol breakdown of polymorphonuclear granulocytes. FEBS Lett 245:249–252

Fulop T Jr, Seres I (1994) Signal transduction changes in granulocytes and lymphocytes with ageing. Immunol Lett 40:259–268

Fülöp T Jr, Fouquet C, Allaire P, Perrin N, Lacombe G, Stankova J, Rola-Pleszczinsky M, Wagner, JR, Khalil A, Dupuis G (1997) Changes in apoptosis of human polumorphonuclear granulocytes with ageing. Mech Ageing Dev 96:15–31

Fulop T Jr, Douziech N, Jacob MP, Hauck M, Wallach J, Robert L (2001) Age-related alterations in the signal transduction pathways of the elastin-laminin receptor. Pathol Biol 49:339–348

Fulop T Jr, Larbi, A, Linteau A, Desgeorges S, Douziech N (2002) Role of Mcl-1 and Bax expression alterations in the decreased rescue of human neutrophils from apoptosis by GM-CSF with ageing. Ann NY Acad Sci 973:305–308

Fulop T, Larbi A, Douziech N, Fortin CF, Guerard KP, Lesur O, Khalil A, Dupuis G, Fulop T (2004) Signal transduction and functional changes in neutrophils with aging. Aging Cell 3:217–226

Gibot S (2006) The therapeutic potential of TREM-1 modulation in the treatment of sepsis and beyond. Curr Opin Investig Drugs 7:438–442

Gibot S, Kolopp-Sarda MN, Bene MC, Cravoisy A, Levy B, Faure GC, Bollaert PE (2004) Plasma level of a triggering receptor expressed on myeloid cells-1: its diagnostic accuracy in patients with suspected sepsis. Ann Intern Med 141:9–15

Gierschik P, Sidoropoulos D, Jakobs KH (1989) Two distinct Gi-proteins mediate formyl peptide receptor signal transduction in human leukemia (HL-60) cells. J Biol Chem 264:21470–21473

Harman D (1956) Aging: a theory based on free radical and radiation chemistry. J Gerontol 11:298–300

Hayashi F, Means TK, Luster AD (2003) Toll-like receptors stimulate human neutrophil functions. Blood 102:2660–2669

Heuertz RM, Tricomi SM, Ezekiel UR, Webster RO (1999) C-reactive protein inhibits chemotactic peptide-induced p38 mitogen-activated protein kinase activity and human neutrophil movement. J Biol Chem 274:17968–17974

Ibanez CF (2004) Lipid rafts as organizing platforms for cell chemotaxis and axon guidance. Neuron 42:3–5

Kindzelskii AL, Sitrin RG, Petty HR (2004) Cutting edge: optical microspectrophotometry supports the existence of gel phase lipid rafts at the lamellipodium of neutrophils: apparent role in calcium signalling. J Immunol 172:4681–4685

Klein JB, Rane MJ, Scherzer JA, Coxon PY, Kettritz R, Methiesen JM, Buridi A, McLeish KR (2000) Granulocyte-macrophage colony stimulating factor delays neutrophil constitutive apoptosis through phosphoinisitide 3-kinase and extracellular signal regulated kinase pathways. J Immunol 164:4286–4291

Klesney-Tait J and Colonna M (2007) Uncovering the TREM-1-TLR connection. Am J Physiol Lung Cell Mol Physiol 293:L1374–L1376

Klesney-Tait J, Turnbull IR, Colonna M (2006) The TREM receptor family and signal integration. Nat Immunol 7:1266–1273

Kobayashi KS, Flavell RA (2004) Shielding the double-edged sword: negative regulation of the innate immune response. J Leukocyte Biol 75:428–433

Krishnan J, Selvarajoo K, Tsuchiya M, Lee G, Choi S (2007) Toll-like receptor signal transduction. Exp Mol Med 39:421–438

Kurt-Jones EA, Mandell L, Whitney C et al (2002) Role of toll-like receptor-2 (TLR2) in neutrophil activation: GM-CSF enhances TLR2 expression and TLR2-mediated interleukin responses in neutrophils. Blood 100:1860–1868

Kyriakis JM, Avrach J (1996) Sounding the alarm: protein kinase cascades activated by stress and inflammation. J Biol Chem 271:24313–24316

Larbi A, Douziech N, Dupuis G, Khalil A, Pelletier H, Guérard KP, Fülöp T Jr (2004a) Age-associated Alterations in the Recruitment of Signal Transduction Proteins to Lipid Rafts in Human T lymphocytes J Leukocyte Biol 75:373–381

Larbi A, Douziech N, Khalil A, Dupuis G, Gheraïri S, Guérard P, Fülöp T Jr (2004b) Effects of Methyl-β-cyclodextrin on T lymphocytes lipid rafts with ageing. Exp Gerontol 39:551–558

Larbi A, Douziech N, Fortin CF, Linteau A, Dupuis G, Fulop T (2005) The role of the MAPK pathway alterations in GM-CSF modulated human neutrophil apoptosis with aging. Immun Ageing 2:6

Larbi A, Dupuis G, Khalil A, Douziech N, Fortin CF, Fulop T (2006) Differential role of lipid rafts in the functions of CD4+ and CD8+ human T lymphocytes with aging. Cell Signal 18:1017–1030

Lehrer HI, Ganz T, Selsted ME, Babior BM, Curnutte JT (1988) Neutrophils and host defence. Ann Int Med 109:127–142

Lord JM, Butcher S, Killampali V, Lascelles D, Salmon M (2001) Neutrophil ageing and immunesenescence. Mech Ageing Dev 122:1521–1535

Makinodan T, Kay MMB (1980) Age influence on the immune system. Adv Immunol 29:287–300

McGettrick AF, O'Neill LA. (2004) The expanding family of MyD88-like adaptors in Toll-like receptor signal transduction. Mol Immunol 41:577–582

Mcleish KR, Gierschik P, Schepers T, Sidiropoulos D, Jakobs KH (1989) Evidence that activation of a common G-protein by receptors for leukotriene B4 and N-formylmethionyl-leucyl-phenylalanine in HL-60 cells occurs by different mechanisms. Biochemical J 260:427–434

Medzhitov R, Janeway C (2000) Innate immunity. N Engl J Med 343:338–344

Medzhitov R (2001) Toll-like receptors and innate immunity. Nat Rev Immunol 1:135–145

Meyer KC, Rosenthal NS, Soergel P, Peterson K (1998) Neutrophils and low grade inflammation in the seemingly normal ageing human lung. Mech Age Dev 104:169-181

Miyajima A, Kitamura T, Harada N, Yokota T and Arai K (1992) Cytokine receptors and signal transduction. Annu Rev Immunol 10:295–331

Miyajima A, Mui AL, Ogorochi T and Sakamaki K (1993) Receptors for granulocytemacrophage colony-stimulating factor, interleukin-3, and interleukin-5. Blood 82:1960–1974

Moulding DA, Quayle JA, Hart CA, Edwards SW. (1998) Mcl-1 expression in human neutrophils: regulation by cytokines and correlation with cell survival. Blood 92:2495–2502

Ornatowska M, Azim AC, Wang X, Christman JW, Xiao L, Joo M, Sadikot RT (2007) Functional genomics of silencing TREM-1 on TLR4 signaling in macrophages. Am J Physiol Lung Cell Mol Physiol 293:L1377–L1384

Quelle FW, Sato N, Witthuhn BA, Inhorn RC, Eder M, Miyajima A, Griffin JD and Ihle JN (1994) JAK2 associates with the beta c chain of the receptor for granulocytemacrophage colony-stimulating factor, and its activation requires the membrane proximal region. Mol Cell Biol 14:4335–4341

Rabiet MJ, Huet E, Boulay F (2007) The N-formyl peptide receptors and the anaphylatoxin C5a receptors: An overview. Biochimie 89:1089–1106

Radsak MP, Salih HR, Rammensee HG, Schild H (2004) Triggering receptor expressed on myeloid cells-1 in neutrophil inflammatory responses: differential regulation of activation and survival. J Immunol 172:4956–4963

Rao KMK, Currie MS, Padmadabhan J, Cohen HJ (1992) Age-related alterations in aktin cytoskeleton and receptor expression in human leukocytes. J Gerontol 47:B37–B44

Remer KA, Brcic M, Jungi TW (2003) Toll-like receptor-4 is invovlved in eliciting an LPS-induced oxidative burst in neutrophils. Immunol Lett 85:75–80

Renshaw M, Rockwell J, Engleman C, Gewirtz A, Katz J, Sambhara S. (2002) Cutting edge: impaired Toll-like receptor expression and function in aging. J Immunol 169;4697–4701

Rivnay B, Bergman S, Shinitzky M, Globerson A (1980) Correlations between membrane viscosity, serum cholesterol, lymphocytes activation and ageing in man. Mech Age Dev 12:119–126

Sakamoto E, Hato F, Kato T, Sakamoto C, Akahori M, Hino M, Kitagawa S. (2005) Type I and Type II interferons delay human neutrophil apoptosis via activation of STAT3 and up-regulation of cellular inhibitor of apoptosis 2. J Leukocyte Biol 78: 301–309

Sato N, Sakamaki K, Terada N, Arai K, Miyajima A (1993) Signal transduction by the high-affinity GM-CSF receptor: two distinct cytoplasmic regions of the common beta subunit responsible for different signalling. EMBO J 12:4181–4189

Schröder KA, Rink L (2003) Neutrophil immunity of the elderly. Mech Age Dev 124:419–425

Seres I, Csongor J, Mohacsi A, Leovey A, Fulop T Jr (1993) Age-dependent alterations of human recombinant GM-CSF effects on human granulocytes. Mech Ageing Dev 71:143–154

Shao D, Segal AW, Dekker LV (2003) Lipid rafts determine efficiency of NADPH oxidase activation in neuitrophils. FEBS Lett 550:101–106

Shinitzky M (1987) Patterns of lipid changes in membranes of the aged brain. Gerontology 33:149–154

Simons K, Ehehalt, R (2002) Cholesterol, lipid rafts, and disease. J Clin Invest 110:597–603

Simons K, Ikonen E (1997) Functional rafts in cell membranes. Nature 387:569–572

Sitrin RG, Johnson DR, Pan PM, Harsh DM, Huang J, Petty HR, Blackwood RA (2004) Lipid rafts compartmentalization of urokinase receptor signalling in human neutrophils Am J Respir Cell Mol Biol 30:233–241

Stoyanov B, Volinia S, Hanck T, Rubio I, Loubtchenkov M, Malek D, Stoyanova S, Vanhaesebroeck B, Dhand R, Nurnberg B, Gierschik P, Seedorf K, Hsuan JJ, Waterfield MD,Takeda K, Akira S. (2005) Toll-like receptors in innate immunity. Int Immunol 17:1–14

Tamassia N, Le Moigne V, Calzetti F, Donini M, Gasperini S, Ear T, Cloutier A, Martinez FO, Fabbri M, Locati M, Mantovani A, McDonald PP, Cassatella M (2007) The MyD88-independent pathway is not mobilized in human neutrophils stimulated via TLR4. J Immunol 178:7344–7356

Tessarz AS and Cerwenka A (2007). The TREM-1/DAP12 pathway. Immunol Lett doi:10.1016/j.imlet.2007.11.021

Tortorella C, Piazzolla G, Spaccavento F, Pece S, Jirillo E, Antonaci S (1998) Spontaneous and Fas induced apoptotic cell death in aged neutrophils. J Clin Immunol 18:321–329

Tortorella C, Piazzolla G, Napopi N, Antonaci S (2001) Neutrophil apoptotic cell death: does it contribute to the increased infectious rsik in ageing? Microbios 106:129–136

Tortorella C, Simone O, Piazzolla G, Stella I, Antonaci S. (2007) Sge-related impairment of GM=CSF-induced signalling in neutrophils: role of SHP-1 and SOCS proteins. Ageing Res Rev 2:81–93

van Duin D, Shaw AC (2007) Toll-Like Receptors in Older Adults Journal Am Geriatr Soci 55:1438–1444

Varga ZS, Kovacs EM, Paragh G, Jacob MP, Robert L, Fulop T Jr (1988) Effects of Kappa elastin and fMLP on polymorphonuclear leukocytes of healthy middle-aged and elderly. K-elastin induced changes in intracellular free calcium. Clin Biochem 21:127–130

Varga ZS, Jacob MP, Robert L, Fulop T Jr,(1989) Identification and signal transduction mechanism of elastin peptide receptor in human leukocytes. FEBS Lett 258:5–8

Varga ZS, Jacob MP, Robert L, Fulop T Jr (1997) Studies on effector functions of soluble elastin receptors of phagocytic cells at various ages. Exp Gerontol 32:653–662

Vlahos CJ, Matter WF (1992) Signal transduction in neutrophil activation. Phosphatidylinositol 3-kinase is stimulated without tyrosine phosphorylation. FEBS Lett 309:242–248

Watanabe S, Itoh T, Arai K (1997) Roles of JAK kinase in human GM-CSF receptor signals. Leukemia 11 (Suppl 3):76–78

Wenisch, C, Patruta S, Daxbock F, Krause R, Horl W (2000) Effect of age on human neutrophil function. J Leukocyte Biol 67:40–5

Whyte M, Renshaw S, Lawson R, Bingle C (1999) Apoptosis and the regulation of neutrophil lifespan. Biochem Soc Trans 27:802–807

Yagisawa M, Saeki K, Okuma E, Kitamura T, Kitagawa S, Hirai H, Yazaki Y, Takaku F, Yuo A (1999) Signal transduction pathways in normal human monocytes stimulated by cytokines and mediators: comparative study with normal human neutrophils or transformed cells and the putative roles in functionality and cell biology. Exp Hematol 27:1063–1076

Yuli I, Tamonga A, Snyderman R (1982) Chemoattractant receptor functions in human polymor-phonuclear leukocytes are divergently altered by membrane fluidizers. Proc Natl Acad Sci USA 79:5906–5910

Zu YL, Qi J, Gilchrist A, Fernandez GA, Vazquez-Abad D, Kreutze DL, Huang CK, Sha'afi RI (1998) p38 mitogen-activated protein kinase activation is required for human neutrophil func-tion triggered by TNF-alpha or fMLP stimulation. J Immunol 160:1982–1989

Synergistic Effects of Ageing and Stress on Neutrophil Function

Janet M. Lord, Anna C. Phillips and Wiebke Arlt

Contents

Abstract: Although ageing is a complex process, we now know much of what happens with age at the cellular and tissue level. In contrast, our understanding of how the various age-related changes interact to result in frailty and pathology is incomplete. For example, ageing is accompanied by a loss of immune function (Immunesenescence), an increase in the level of circulating proinflammatory cytokines (Inflammaging), a decline in adrenal androgen production (Adrenopause) whilst concurrently peripheral glucocorticoid availability increases. In this article we propose that these changes in combination increase the susceptibility of older adults to the adverse effects of physical and emotional stress, exacerbating the age-related decline in immune competence and exposing the older individual to increased risk of infections. We have focused upon the effects of stress and ageing

J. M. Lord (✉)
MRC Centre for Immune Regulation
Division of Immunity and Infection
Birmingham University Medical School
Birmingham B15 2TT, United Kingdom
Tel: +44 121 414 4399
Fax: +44 414 3599
E-mail: J.M.Lord@bham.ac.uk

A. C. Phillips
School of Sport and Exercise Science
University of Birmingham
Birmingham B15 2TT, United Kingdom

W. Arlt
Division of Medical Sciences
University of Birmingham
Birmingham B15 2TT
United Kingdom

T. Fulop et al. (eds.), *Handbook on Immunosenescence*,
DOI 10.1007/978-1-4020-9062-2_24, © Springer Science+Business Media B.V. 2009

on neutrophil function, an element of the immune system that has received less attention from immunogerontologists, despite the primary role of neutrophils in fighting bacterial infections and the major contribution of such infections to age-related morbidity and mortality. We propose that physical and emotional stressors elicit an exaggerated response in older adults that synergises with the age-related loss of neutrophil function, to compromise antibacterial mechanisms. Moreover, the molecular basis of this effect may lie with the significant changes in tissue concentrations of cortisol and dehydroepiandrosterone in peripheral target cells including the immune compartment.

1   Ageing, Stress and Infection

It is now well established that the efficiency of the immune system declines with age and this is highlighted most obviously at the functional level by the increased risk of morbidity and mortality from infection in older adults [1–3]. The three major causes of death in the UK in those aged over 65 are cardiovascular diseases, cancer and respiratory disease (Fig. 1). Approximately 1 in 6 older adults will die as a result of the latter, the majority succumbing to respiratory infections. Older adults show a threefold greater incidence of bacterial dysentery than younger subjects, 50% higher mortality from gram-negative bacterial sepsis, and deaths from gastrointestinal infections, pneumonia and influenza are largely confined to patients over 65 years of age [4, 5]. Age-related reactivation of latent infections previously held in check by the immune system is a further indicator of the age-related decline in immune function (immunesenescence). Thus the incidence of tuberculosis is raised in the elderly, indicating reduced functioning of macrophages [6] and reduced T-lymphocyte function is reflected by reactivation of latent Herpes viruses such as Varicella Zoster (shingles) in older age [7]. Older adults are also at increased risk of postsurgical complications such as infections, which include infections at the wound site; but are dominated by bacterial chest and urinary tract infections [8]. Furthermore, delayed wound healing with age has particular relevance in the context of surgery and has underlying contributions from senescent fibroblasts as well as senescent immune

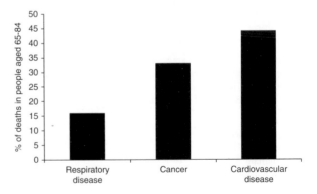

Fig. 1 The figure shows the major causes of death in adults aged 65-84 in the UK, (adapted from data presented in the House of Lords Science and Technology Committee 1st report on Ageing: Scientific Aspects, 2005, Figure 4, page 42)

cells which are key players in the wound healing response (9). The increased risk of infection following surgery may therefore reflect compromised immune and wound healing responses and underline the significant effect of physical stress upon immunity.

It is now well accepted that prolonged exposure to stress, whether psychosocial or physical, has detrimental effects upon immunity. Immune suppression associated with chronic stress has significant clinical consequences, including increased risk of illness and death from infectious disease [10, 11]. In the area of psychosocial stress there is now a solid literature showing reduced immunity, suboptimal responses to infectious agents and vaccines and increased susceptibility to infection in adults following bereavement [12–14] extended care-giving [15, 16], or low social support [10, 17–20]. In an elegant study by Cohen et al. [21] the effect of psychosocial stress on resistance to infection was clearly demonstrated. In this study almost 400 volunteers were exposed to five different respiratory viruses and incidence and severity of infection for each virus was found to be positively correlated with their scores on a psychological stress index. The reader is referred to a recent comprehensive review of this area by Kiecolt-Glaser and Glaser [22].

Moderate physical trauma is also a potent mediator of immune suppression, with 1 in 3 trauma patients succumbing to one or more infections [23]. An extensive retrospective analysis of infections in over 10,000 trauma patients revealed that 32% of patients developed respiratory tract infections and 17% had urinary tract infections [24]. In older adults the most frequent trauma results from falls leading to hip-fractures. Falls are the leading cause of admission into care homes and a frequent cause of death in the elderly population. Again, one of the major health risks associated with falls and hip-fracture is infection, such as osteomyelitis, respiratory infections and infections at the surgical wound site [24–26].

2   Ageing and Neutrophil Function

The high incidence of bacterial infections in older adults is particularly suggestive of a suboptimal neutrophil response, as these leucocytes form the primary response to bacterial, fungal and yeast infections. The preponderance of urinary tract infections in older adults would also support this conclusion. As the effect of ageing on neutrophil function is covered in detail elsewhere in this volume, this topic will be covered only briefly here to allow discussion of the combined effect of age and stress on neutrophil function.

Neutrophils are the dominant leucocyte in the circulation, making up 60% of the white cell count. They are also the shortest lived blood cell, dying by apoptosis approximately 24h after leaving the bone marrow [27, 28]. Their function can be enhanced by proinflammatory cytokines, such as GM-CSF, TNFα and Type 1 interferon, which not only amplify their basic bactericidal functions, such as generation of reactive oxygen species, but also extend their lifespan at sites of infection by inhibiting apoptosis [29, 30]. Neutrophils are recruited to sites of infection via chemotactic signals, such as the chemokine CXCL8 (also known as IL8). Once in contact with the pathogen they uptake the microbe by phagocytosis mediated via opsonic receptors (CD11b/CD18, CD16, CD32, CD64) that detect complement proteins C3b and C3Bi or antibody coating the microbe. Once inside the neutrophil, pathogens are killed as a result of the generation of reactive oxygen and nitrogen species and the release of a range of proteolytic enzymes from cytoplasmic granules. Phagocytosis and generation of superoxide trigger the death of the neutrophil, which is then removed by macrophages leading to the resolution of inflammation [27].

Comparison of neutrophils from peripheral blood of healthy young and old adults has shown in a majority of studies that chemotaxis is not significantly affected by ageing, with adherence of neutrophils to endothelium [31, 32] and expression of adhesion molecules [31, 33] both unaltered with ageing. In contrast, bactericidal (superoxide generation and degranulation) and phagocytic function is dramatically reduced in neutrophils from older adults [34–37]. For superoxide generation, responses to the bacterial peptide fMLP and to gram-negative bacteria appear to be unaltered by ageing [31, 34, 38], whereas superoxide generation in response to a gram-positive stimulus such as *Staphylococcus aureus,* was significantly reduced in neutrophils from older donors [37]. The latter is of clinical importance bearing in mind the reduced ability of older adults to resolve infections with gram-positive bacteria [39]. The cause of reduced superoxide generation with age is not fully understood, though reduced signaling via calcium in activated neutrophils has been suggested [36] and reduced responsiveness to proinflammatory cytokines such as GM-CSF has also been shown [40, 41]. This is an important finding as cytokines such as GM-CSF prime neutrophil function leading to improved bactericidal responses to bacterial components such as fMLP. In addition, as stated above GM-CSF is also a potent neutrophil survival factor and reduced responsiveness to this cytokine would limit neutrophil lifespan extension at sites of inflammation.

Loss of phagocytic capacity has been investigated reasonably thoroughly. Neutrophils from older subjects retain their ability to phagocytose opsonized bacterial pathogens *per se*, but their phagocytic capacity (phagoctyic index, the number of microbes ingested per cell) is significantly compromised [34, 35, 42–44]. The level of expression of opsonic receptors is known to be a determinant of phagocytic capacity and our data showed a significant reduction in one of the cell surface opsonin receptors (CD16) that binds to antibody coating bacterial pathogens. Taken together these data indicate that neutrophils should be able to respond to chemotactic signals from a site of infection, but will then be severely compromised in their bactericidal function and also their ability to respond to local survival factors such as GM-CSF.

In addition to the obvious consequences of reduced neutrophil function for ability to combat bacterial infections, neutrophils also play a key role in wound healing. In response to tissue injury cytokines are released, including CXCL8, which attract neutrophils to the site. Neutrophils then aid resolution of the damage by removing microbial pathogens and restoring sterility, thus removing the inflammatory stimulus. Whether neutrophils play a positive role in wound healing beyond clearance of pathogens is still a hotly debated topic. Neutrophils release cytokines important for revascularization and tissue repair, such as CXCL8 and VEGF [45], but this has to be balanced with their ability to produce tissue-damaging agents if they persist at a sterile wound site. Reduced phagocytosis of microbes will lead to persistence of inflammation and prevention of wound healing by the presence of high levels of inflammatory cytokines. Although this aspect of innate immunesenescence has received less attention, it is potentially a significant factor in the development and persistence of ulcerated wounds in the elderly.

3   Stress and Neutrophil Function

Stress, whether physical or psychological, is broadly sensed by 2 endocrine regulatory systems, the Hypothalamic-Pituitary-Adrenal (HPA) axis and the sympathetic-adrenal-medullary (SAM) system. Stress induces the release of catecholamines (adrenalin and noradrenalin) from the adrenal medulla and the sympathetic nervous system and, mediated via an increased pituitary ACTH secretion, results in an acute increase in cortisol and dehydroepiandrosterone (DHEA) release from the adrenal cortex. Catecholamines and cortisol are both immune suppressive [46,47], whereas DHEA is a precursor to sex hormones and is generally thought to be immune enhancing [48–52], though evidence for the latter is less substantial due to lack of data generated in humans and human cell-based systems. In particular, all DHEA replacement studies in humans have been carried out in healthy older subjects only [53–55] and not under conditions of stress in which this hormone may play its vital role in counteracting the negative effects of cortisol (discussed below).

As the effects of stress on adaptive immune functions are dealt with separately in this volume, the focus here will be upon neutrophil function in response to stress.

3.1   Acute Stress

The impact of acute psychological stress on neutrophils has received little attention within the immune literature. In animals, acute psychological stress can be applied in a variety of ways including inescapable intermittent electric shock, overcrowding, or restraint in an enclosed space. Acute psychological stressors in humans usually involve brief laboratory-based tasks such as public speaking or mental arithmetic in front of an audience and/or under time pressure, or the cold-pressor test (submersion of the hand in ice-cold water), although some studies have used examination stress as a short-term stressor. Overall, the literature suggests that periods of acute stress have beneficial effects on neutrophil function. Mice that had received 2.5 hours of restraint stress showed increased infiltration of neutrophils into a surgically implanted sponge in comparison to unstressed control mice [57]. In addition, an increase in neutrophil adhesion and aggregation has also been shown to be induced by short periods of inescapable foot shock in rats [58], an acute anticipatory stressor in healthy young adults [59, 60], and stroop and mirror tracing tasks in men aged 30–59 [61].

Acute stress has also been shown to modulate phagocytosis: periods of social conflict stress between mice for less than one day resulted in increased phagocytosis by neutrophils and other phagocytic cells in comparison to nonstressed mice [62]. When neutrophils are activated, they undergo a respiratory burst and produce toxic superoxides that kill the pathogens they have phagocytosed. In humans, a 15 minute time pressured stress task (Raven's Advanced Progressive Matrices) induced an immediate significant increase in the number of activated neutrophils relative to resting baseline and in comparison to a nonstressed control group. This increase in activation state had returned to baseline 10 minutes following the end of the stress task. A comparison of neutrophil function in students between final examination week and nonexamination weeks showed that the short-term stress of examinations was associated with an increase in neutrophil superoxide production [63, 64], and this increase was maintained at 2–3 weeks post examinations [63]. In rats, superoxide production was increased in response to 1 hour of open field stress [65]; and superoxide production at the site of inflammation following experimental *E.coli* injection was observed to be higher in rats previously exposed to inescapable tail shock in restraint tubes for two hours in comparison to non-stressed rats. In the latter study, stressed rats also showed a complete resolution of the inflammatory response to the infection two weeks faster than control nonstressed rats, potentially indicating a stress-induced elevation in neutrophil response resulting in more effective bactericidal activity [66]. This increase in neutrophil function parallels other acute stress induced changes in nonspecific immunity such as the increased production of secretory immunoglobulin A [67].

In summary, acute stress appears to have an overall positive impact upon neutrophil function, particularly when acute stress is applied in the context of an inflammatory challenge, although the mechanisms of such effects are unclear at present.

3.2 Chronic Stress

In contrast to acute stress, the effects of chronic exposure to stress are detrimental to immune function. A meta-analysis of thirty years literature on the effect of stress on the immune system concluded that chronic stress such as bereavement or physical trauma resulted in suppression of cellular and humoral immunity and increased susceptibility to infection [68]. As with acute stress there is very little information relating to neutrophil function and the research emphasis has been placed upon adaptive immune responses. However, chronic stress and depression in cancer patients is associated with neutrophilia, but also with decreased neutrophil phagocytic ability and raised cortisol levels [69]. Intense or long duration exercise is also associated with raised circulating cortisol and adrenalin, together with reduced neutrophil bactericidal responses namely degranulation and superoxide generation [70]. Our own studies of the effect of physical stress (limb or hip-fracture) on neutrophil function confirmed a profound neutrophilia in response to stress, but also a significant suppression of superoxide generation in response to a bacterial peptide challenge which correlated with raised cortisol levels [71].

Glucocortoids are likely to be major mediators of the negative effects of chronic stress upon neutrophil biology and function [72]. For example, studies of the effects of cortisol infusions in humans have shown a profound neutrophilia, which is achieved in part by the inhibition of neutrophil apoptosis thus extending neutrophil lifespan in the circulation [73, 74]. Cortisol can also enhance G-CSF mediated stimulation of granulopoiesis in the bone marrow [75], further contributing to raised neutrophil numbers in response to cortisol. Unfortunately the potential benefit of an increased level of circulating neutrophils with raised cortisol is not realized, as cortisol also inhibits neutrophil chemotaxis and extravasation [76]. The clinical significance of this observation is seen in studies that reported reduced neutrophil chemotaxis in trauma patients and a strong correlation with increased incidence of infection [77, 78]. In vitro studies also suggest that the suppression of neutrophil superoxide generation after trauma is mediated by cortisol. We and others have shown that superoxide generation by cytokine-primed neutrophils in vitro was suppressed by cortisol [71, 79], though we found no effect of cortisol on phagocytic function (S.K. Butcher, unpublished data). Taken together these data indicate that raised cortisol levels will impact negatively upon neutrophil function, which could in turn increase susceptibility to bacterial infections.

The meta-analysis carried out by Segerstrom and Miller [68] also revealed that the loss of immunity in response to stress was much greater in older adults, which in turn concurs with reports of excess infection-related morbidity and mortality in older trauma patients [80–82]. Our own studies have compared responses to stress in young and old trauma patients and revealed that the detrimental effect of physical stress was most marked in older adults [71, 83], supporting an influence of age upon stress mediated suppression of neutrophil responses. That neutrophil function was affected by chronic stress in patients with cancer, an age-related disease, adds further weight to this proposal. Synergy between the effects of stress and immunesenescence on immune function, has also been proposed in relation to psychosocial stress and the immune system [22, 84] and there is now a real need to compare the differential effects of stress on a broad range of immune responses in young and old subjects.

4 Ageing and Stress Hormones

While cortisol secretion by the adrenocortical zona fasciculata appears to remain largely unchanged throughout life [85], adrenal dehydroepiandrosterone (DHEA) secretion from the adrenal zona reticularis exhibits a characteristic, age-associated pattern. Intraindividual maximum levels of DHEA and its sulphate ester DHEAS are reached during early adulthood, followed by a steady decline throughout adult life, eventually decreasing to 10–20% of previous maximum levels by 70–80 years of age [86, 87]. This age-associated decline in DHEA synthesis has been termed "adreno-pause", which is somewhat imprecise given that adrenocortical glucocorticoid and mineralocorticoid secretion is maintained without change across the lifespan. Inter-estingly, an age-associated secretion pattern of DHEA is only observed in humans and higher nonhuman primates [88, 89] and it is important to recognize that rodent adrenals are not capable of DHEA secretion, yielding only very low circulating DHEA concentrations of primarily gonadal origin, thereby limiting the suitabil-ity of rodents for studies on the significance of DHEA for human physiology and disease. Adrenopause is independent of menopause, and it occurs in both sexes; it shows high interindividual variability and has been suggested to be associated with a macroscopically visible decrease in size of the adrenal zona reticularis [90]. There is also a suggestion of an age related increase in senescent and apoptotic cells within the zona reticularis, though whether this contributes to loss of cells in this region of the adrenal cortex, or might influence functional activity of the zona reticularis cells, has not been established [91].

DHEA secretion exhibits a diurnal rhythm similar to that of cortisol and ongo-ing age has been shown to be associated with an attenuation of the diurnal rhythm and the pulse amplitude of DHEA secretion [92]. Furthermore, the adrenal stress response seems to be partially impaired with ageing, with a significant reduction of acute DHEA release following an acute exogenous ACTH challenge whilst the cortisol response remains intact [93]. In young healthy subjects it has been shown that an acute psychosocial stressor such as an arithmetic challenge or public speak-ing test results in an acute rise in cortisol [94], but neither the impact of this on DHEA release nor its modification in the aged has been investigated to date. We have recently shown that acute sepsis leads to an up-regulation of both cortisol and DHEA [95], however, comprehensive data on chronic exposure to physical or psy-chological stress are lacking.

Whilst cortisol mediates its action via the cytosolic glucocorticoid receptor that, once activated, translocates to the nucleus and initiates the transcription of gluco-corticoid effector genes, the exact mechanisms underlying the actions of DHEA and its sulphate ester DHEAS still remain controversial. High affinity binding sites for DHEA have been described in murine and human T-lymphocytes [96, 97] and human vascular endothelial cells [98, 99], but their specificity as opposed to active androgens is still debated. DHEA has also been shown to have neurosteroidal prop-erties and exerts stimulatory effects on NMDA receptors and inhibitory effects on $GABA_A$ receptors in the brain [87]. However, the current view is that the majority of its actions are mediated indirectly, via downstream conversion to sex steroids and other steroids of potentially distinct activity including the putatively immune modu-latory steroids androstenediol, androstenetriol and 7α-OH-DHEA [100] (Fig. 2).

DHEA represents a paradigm for prereceptor metabolism as its action will mainly depend on the expression of enzymes responsible for its conversion to other ster-oids in the specific target cell of interest. Lymphocytes and macrophages have been shown previously to express steroidogenic enzymes involved in the downstream

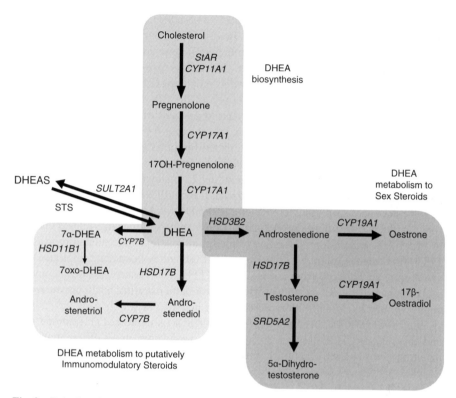

Fig. 2 Dehydroepiandrosterone (DHEA) biosynthesis from cholesterol via StAR (steroidogenic acute regulatory protein), CYP11A1 (side chain-cleavage enzyme) and CYP17A1 (17α-hydroxy-lase/17, 20 lyase) as well as its downstream metabolism to sex steroids and potentially immune-modulatory steroids via HSD3B (3β-hydroxysteroid dehydrogenase Type 1 and 2), HSD17B (17β-hydroxysteroid dehydrogenases), SRD5A1 (5a-reductase Type 1 and 2), CYP19A1 (Aromatase), CYP7B (7α-hydroxylase) and HSD11B1 (11β-hydroxysteroid dehydrogenase Type 1). Lipophilic DHEA can be converted to its hydrophilic sulphate ester DHEAS by SULT2A1 (DHEA sulphotransferase) and back by STS (steroid sulfatase)

metabolism of DHEA [101–103], but their presence in neutrophils has not been determined. We have recently shown that the expression level of these enzymes changes with ageing and demonstrated enhanced conversion of DHEA to andros-tenediol as well as increased androgen activation by 5α-reductase in lymphocytes from older men as compared to young men [104]. Concurrently circulating levels of DHEAS and testosterone were significantly lower in the older men, suggesting that the up-regulation of steroidogenic enzymes in the lymphocyte compartment may be a counter-regulatory event aiming to maintain intracellular availability of androstenediol and dihydrotestosterone.

Although circulating cortisol levels do not change significantly with aging, intracellular availability of active glucocorticoids within the peripheral target cells including immune cells may well be altered with age. The major regula-tory switch controlling tissue-specific activation of glucocorticoids is the enzyme

11β-hydroxysteroid dehydrogenase Type 1 (11β-HSD1), which converts inactive cortisone to active cortisol [105] (Fig. 3). 11β-HSD1 has two activities; in vivo it mainly acts as an oxoreductase, activating cortisone to cortisol, whereas in vitro it mostly exhibits dehydrogenase activity, converting cortisol to inactive cortisone. 11β-HSD1 is anchored in the endoplasmic reticulum (ER) membrane and has its catalytic domain directed towards the lumen of the ER. Only recently it has been elucidated that its oxoreductase activity is dependent on NADPH generation by the endoplasmic reticulum luminal enzyme hexose-6-phosphate dehydrogenase (H6PDH) [106, 107] (Fig. 3). It is well established that expression and functional activity of 11β-HSD1 can be up-regulated by inflammatory cytokines, e.g., in adipose tissue and bone [108, 109]. As ageing leads to a cytokine profile that is more proinflammatory, with raised levels of IL-1β, IL-6 and TNFα [110], it can be readily hypothesized that increased activity of 11β-HSD1 would lead to increased tissue-specific glucocorticoid availability and action. A precedent for age related changes in 11β-HSD1 expression may relate to the brain, where an age related increase in 11β-HSD1 might explain why cerebrospinal fluid cortisol concentrations rise with age despite unchanged serum cortisol levels [111]. This concept has been convincingly supported by recent human in vivo data demonstrating an improvement in cognitive function by inhibition of 11β-HSD1 activity [112].

Interestingly, it has been shown that 11β-HSD1 is expressed in immune cells and that 11β-HSD1 expression is induced in monocytes upon differentiation to macrophages [113]. By contrast, intracellular glucocorticoid activation by 11β-

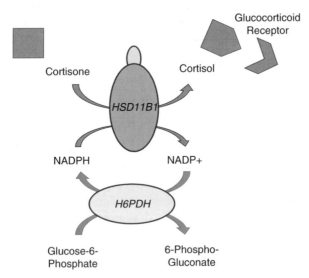

Fig. 3 The oxoreductase activity of 11β-hydroxysteroid dehydrogenase (HSD11B1) converts inactive cortisone to active cortisol that binds and activates the glucocorticoid receptor (GR). HSD11B1 is predominantly an oxoreductase *in vivo*, however *in vitro*, following disruption of the endoplasmic reticulum integrity, mainly acts as a dehydrogenase, inactivating cortisol to cortisone. HSD11B1 is anchored in the ER membrane with its catalytic domain towards the ER lumen and its oxoreductase activity is dependent on NADPH delivery by the intraluminal enzyme hexose-6-phosphate dehydrogenase (H6PD)

HSD1 oxoreductase activity sharply declines during the maturation of monocyte-derived dendritic cells [114]. Whether macrophage and dendritic cell function are differentially modulated by cortisol remains an interesting possibility. The loss of DHEA with age, accompanied by increased 11β-HSD1 in immune cells and tissues induced by inflammaging, may thus result in increased glucocorticoid activity in inflamed tissues, further dampening the immune response in older adults. In addition, inhibition of 11β-HSD1 decreases cortisol half-life [115] and the observed increase in cortisol half-life in the elderly (by as much as 40%) may be a reflection of enhanced 11β-HSD1 activity [116]. Thus we postulate that ageing represents a state of tissue specific cortisol excess in the context of normal circulating levels and that this will impair the peripheral immune response in tissues throughout the body.

5   Stress Hormones and Neutrophil Function

The vast majority of literature on this topic is focused upon the immune suppressive activity of cortisol, with little attention paid to DHEA or its downstream metabolites. Moreover, very few studies of stress hormone effects on immune cells have considered neutrophils. The active glucocorticoid cortisol exhibits a variety of immune suppressing effects [117], which appear to be counteracted by DHEA. For example, it has been suggested that DHEA and glucocorticoids have opposing effects on T-helper cell 1 (Th1)/Th2 balance [118] with evidence for protection of a Th1 cytokine profile by DHEA [119]. In rodents, DHEA antagonizes dexamethasone-induced suppression of lymphocyte proliferation and prevents glucocorticoid-induced thymic and splenic atrophy [120]. DHEA and dexamethasone may have opposing effects on dendritic cell differentiation [121]. DHEA and the glucocorticoid receptor antagonist RU486 equally reverse the suppressive effects of glucocorticoids on immune function [49]. In vitro studies utilizing human immune cells have demonstrated an increase in IL-2 secretion [52] and natural killer cell cytotoxicity [122] following exposure to DHEA. Conversely, DHEA has been shown to inhibit IL-6 release and circulating DHEAS levels have been shown to negatively correlate with serum IL-6 [123, 124]. Thus DHEA appears to counteract the changes in cytokine secretion characteristically observed with ageing, i.e. decreased IL-2 and increased IL-6 levels. DHEA replacement in patients with adrenal insufficiency and thus pronounced DHEA deficiency has been shown to increase the number of circulating regulatory T-cells [125], but this study did not provide details on functional activity.

In relation to neutrophil function, as described above cortisol is a potent suppressor of neutrophil bactericidal responses inhibiting neutrophil superoxide generation [79]. Our own work has confirmed these reports and shown that DHEAS was able to enhance neutrophil superoxide generation in vitro and to overcome the suppressive effects of cortisol on primed neutrophil superoxide generation [71]. Indirect support for the ability of DHEA to counteract the immune suppressive effects of cortisol in vivo, comes from animal studies of DHEA supplementation. For example, dietary

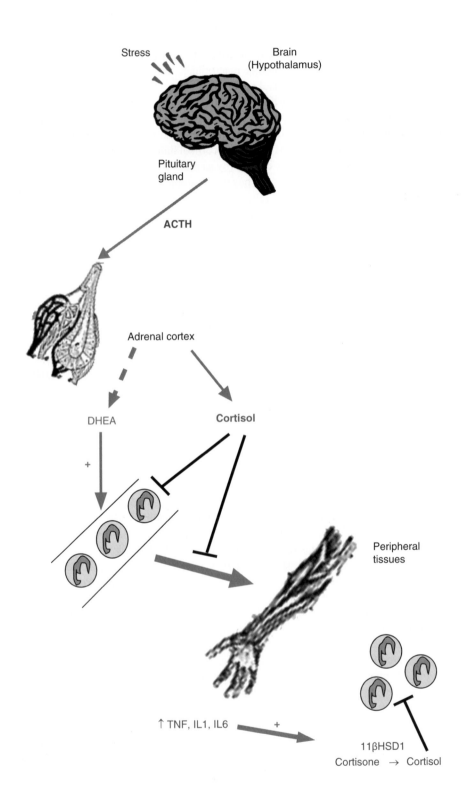

DHEA supplementation of rodents exposed to physical trauma resulted in reduced mortality from the trauma induced sepsis [126]. The latter may be due not only to improved neutrophil function in the presence of DHEA, but also to moderation of the shock response which can produce excessive neutrophil accumulation in tissues leading to nonspecific tissue damage. In this respect DHEA has been reported to down-regulate induction of adhesion molecule expression by LPS [127]. It is thus clear that both cortisol and DHEA appear to modulate neutrophil function, but much more research is necessary to determine the extent of these effects and their mechanisms, i.e. whether the effects of DHEA are direct or via downstream metabolites.

Peripheral actions of glucocorticoids may also be modified by DHEA. DHEA reverses glucocorticoid-associated immune changes after trauma/haemorrhage in mice, concurrently leading to normalisation of elevated corticosterone levels [128], which may suggest an effect upon the prereceptor modulation of glucocorticoids, specifically on 11β-HSD1. Down-regulation of 11β-HSD1 expression and activity by DHEA was recently demonstrated in rat hepatocytes [129], in murine adipocytes [130] and in human skeletal muscle [131]. Thus in the situation of ageing we predict an increase in glucocorticoid action in immune cells due to enhanced tissue-specific activation by 11β-HSD1 whilst the potentially counteracting DHEA pool diminishes due to the age-associated decline in adrenal DHEA production.

In summary, there is still a paucity of data generated in human based systems that informs about DHEA-induced immune effects, in particular there are few studies investigating the effect of DHEA or DHEAS on neutrophil function. The data available to date do however suggest that DHEA can counteract the immune suppressive effects of corticosteroids, including suppression of neutrophil function [132].

6   Ageing, Stress and Neutrophil Function

We propose that the age-related immune and endocrine changes outlined above have specific implications for resilience to stress in older adults. We hypothesize that the combination of adrenopause, leading to a relative preponderance of cortisol over DHEA, with increased tissue levels of 11β-HSD1 resulting in raised peripheral cortisol availability and an already reduced immune defence against infection, leave this population particularly susceptible to the negative effects of stress on immunity. For example, relative to age-matched controls, older adults exposed to the chronic stress of being the primary caregiver for a partner with dementia have

Fig. 4 Stress is sensed by the hypothalamus which secretes corticotrophin releasing hormone, stimulating the pituitary gland to produce adrenocorticotropic hormone (ACTH). ACTH acts upon the adrenal gland causing release of glucocorticoids (cortisol) and DHEA into the circulation. Cortisol suppresses neutrophil function, including extravasation, whereas DHEA counteracts the effects of cortisol and promotes neutrophil function. With age the ability to produce DHEA is reduced (indicated by the dashed line) giving a relative excess of cortisol. Raised levels of inflammatory cytokines induce 11β-HSD1 expression in peripheral tissues increasing conversion of inactive cortisone to active cortisol. The overall effect of age and stress is to diminish the antibacterial actions of neutrophils, thus increasing susceptibly to these infections in older adults

shown a variety of immunological decrements. These include a reduced response to pneumococcal pneumonia vaccination and poorer *in vitro* NK-cell cytotoxicity [133, 134]. More recently, *in vivo* assessments of immune function, such as healing rates of experimentally administered wounds and antibody response to vaccination, have been used to provide clinically relevant outcome measures of the effects of stress on immunity. These studies have supported the previous work suggesting that psychosocial stress is associated with reduced immune functioning in older populations. For example, older adults providing long-term care-giving have shown delayed wound healing in the mouth [135]. Further, experimentally induced punch biopsy wounds took significantly longer to heal in chronically stressed older caregivers and immune cells from the caregivers produced significantly less of the cytokine IL-1β in response to stimulation *in vitro* than the cells of women who were not caregivers [135]. Although an interaction between stress and ageing has not, to our knowledge, been tested directly in the context of psychological stress, there is evidence that younger care-givers of multiple sclerosis patients do not demonstrate reduced antibody responses to vaccination compared to controls [136]. In addition, influenza vaccination responses were reduced in chronically stressed older adults to a much greater extent than young adults [137].

Physical bodily trauma, such as hip-fracture, can also be considered as a chronic stressor, and is associated with decrements in immune function. For example, the experience of hip-fracture in adults aged over 65 years was associated with diminished neutrophil function (generation of superoxide) and a significant incidence (43%) of bacterial infection [83]. Interestingly, this effect of trauma on neutrophil function and infection rates was not observed in younger adults with limb fractures, suggesting that this immune impact of stress is worsened by the presence of immunesenescence. This finding supports the hypothesis that nonacute stress, whether physical [132] or psychosocial [84] exacerbates the negative influence of ageing on the immune system.

7   Conclusions and Future Directions

Ageing has been defined classically as the increasing frailty of an organism with time that reduces its ability to deal with stress, resulting in increased probability of disease and death. The age-related loss of innate immune function, including reduced neutrophil bactericidal function, contributes to such frailty by increasing susceptibility of older adults to bacterial, fungal and yeast infections. Chronic stress is also detrimental to immune function and although the literature regarding neutrophils is sparse, the negative effects of cortisol are well documented. We propose that the age-related increase in proinflammatory cytokines will increase tissue levels of cortisol via induction of 11β-HSD1, contributing to peripheral immune suppression in old age. Furthermore, the negative effects of cortisol appear to be modified by the counter stress hormone DHEA and we suggest that the loss of this hormone with age mediates a synergistic down regulation of innate immune function by chronic stress and immunesenescence.

There is currently a paucity of experimental data concerning differential responses to stress with age and in particular the effects of stress on neutrophil function in older adults. Future intervention strategies to improve neutrophil function at times of stress may therefore usefully target the altered HPA axis, either by elevating circulating DHEA levels or by functional antagonism of cortisol at the cellular level.

References

1. Bonomo RA (2002) Resistant pathogens in respiratory tract infections in older people. J Am Geriatr Soc 50:S236–S241
2. Fein AM (1999) Pneumonia in the elderly: Overview of diagnostic and therapeutic approaches. Clin Infect Dis 28:726–729
3. Gavazzi G, Krause KH (2002) Ageing and infection. Lancet Infect Dis 2:659–666
4. Martin GS, Mannino DM, Moss M (2006) The effect of age on the development and outcome of adult sepsis. Crit Care Med 34:15–21
5. Liang SY, Mackowiak PA (2007) Infections in the elderly. Clin Geriatr Med 23:441–456
6. Rajagopalan S, Yoshikawa TT (2000) Tuberculosis in long-term-care facilities. Infect Control Hosp Epidemiol 21:611–615
7. Laube S (2004) Skin infections and ageing. Ageing Res Rev 3:69–89
8. Butcher SK, Killampalli V, Chahal H, Kaya AE, Lord JM (2003) Effect of age on susceptibility to post-traumatic infection in the elderly. Biochem Soc Trans 31:449–451
9. Pittman J (2007) Effect of aging on wound healing—Current concepts. J Wound Ostomy Continence Nurs 34:412–415
10. Cohen F, Kemeny ME, Kearney KA, Zegans LS, Neuhaus JM, Conant MA (1999) Persistent stress as a predictor of genital herpes recurrence. Arch Intern Med 159:2430–2436
11. Lien L, Haavet OR, Thoresen M, Heyerdahl S, Bjertness E (2007) Mental health problems, negative life events, perceived pressure and the frequency of acute infections among adolescents— Results from a cross-sectional, multicultural, population-based study. Acta Paediatr 96:301–306
12. Keynes WM (1994) Medical response to mental stress. J Royal Soc Med 87:536–539
13. Leserman J (2003) The effects of stressful life events, coping, and cortisol on HIV infection. CNS Spectr 8:25–30
14. Phillips AC, Carroll D, Bums VE, Ring C, Macleod J, Drayson M (2006) Bereavement and marriage are associated with antibody response to influenza vaccination in the elderly. Brain Behav Immun 20:279–289
15. Glaser R, Kiecolt-Glaser JK (1997) Chronic stress modulates the virus-specific immune response to latent herpes simplex virus type 1. Ann Behav Med 19:78–82
16. Kiecolt-Glaser JK, Glaser R, Gravenstein S, Malarkey WB, Sheridan J (1996) Chronic stress alters the immune response to influenza virus vaccine in older adults. Proc Natl Acad Sci USA 93:3043–3047
17. Clausing P, Bocker T, Diekgerdes J, Gartner K, Guttner J, Haemisch A, Veckenstedt A, Weimer A (1994) Social isolation modifies the response of mice to experimental mengo virus infection. J Exp Anim Sci 36:37–54
18. Radek KA, Elias P, Gallo RL (2007) Psychological and physiological stress increases susceptibility to skin infection by Group A Streptococcus due to glucocorticoid-mediated changes in innate immune function. J Invest Dermatol 127:S72

19. Pressman SD, Cohen S, Miller GE, Barkin A, Rabin BS (2005) Loneliness, social network size, and immune response to influenza vaccination in college freshmen. J Health Psychol 24:297–306

20. Phillips AC, Burns VE, Carroll D, Ring C, Drayson M (2005) The association between life events, social support, and antibody status following thymus-dependent and thymus-independent vaccinations in healthy young adults. Brain Behav Immun 19:325–333

21. Cohen S (2005) The Pittsburgh common cold studies: Psychosocial predictors of susceptibility to respiratory infectious illness. Int J Behav Med 12:123–131

22. Glaser R, Kiecolt-Glaser JK (2005) Science and society—Stress-induced immune dysfunction: implications for health. Nat Rev Immunol 5:243–251

23. Papia G, McLellan BA, El Helou P, Loiue M, Rachlis A, Szalai JP, Simor AE (1999) Infection in hospitalized trauma patients: incidence, risk factors and complications. J Trauma 47:923–927

24. Caplan ES, Hoyt NJ (1985) Identification and treatment of infections in multiply traumatised patients. Am J Med 79:68–76

25. Bhattacharrya T, Iorio R, Healy WL (2002) Rate of and risk factors for acute inpatient mortality after othropaedic surgery. J Bone Joint Surg Am 84:562–572

26. Nichols RL, Smith JW, Klein DB, Trunkey DD, Cooper RH, Adinolfi MF, Mills J (1984). Risk of infection after penetrating abdominal trauma. N Engl J Med 311:1065–1070

27. Savill JS, Wyllie AH, Henson JE, Walport MJ, Henson PM, Haslett C (1989) Macrophage phagocytosis of aging neutrophils in inflammation. Programmed cell death in the neutrophil leads to its recognition by macrophages. J Clin Invest 83:865–875

28. Scheel-Toellner D, Wang KQ, Webb PR, Wong SH, Craddock R, Assi LK, Salmon M, Lord JM (2004) Early events in spontaneous neutrophil apoptosis. Biochem Soc Trans 32:461–464

29. Brach MA, deVos S, Gruss H-J, Herrmann F (1992) Prolongation of survival of human polymorphonuclear neutrophils by granulocyte-macropahge colony stimulating factor is caused by inhibition of programmed cell death. Blood 80:2920–2924

30. Scheel-Toellner D, Pilling D, Akbar AN, Hardie D, Lombardi G, Salmon M, Lord JM (1999) Inhibition of T cell apoptosis by IFN-beta rapidly reverses nuclear translocation of protein kinase C-delta. Eur J Immunol 29:2603–2612

31. Esparza B, Sanchez H, Ruiz M, Barranquero M, Sabino E, Merino F (1996) Neutrophil function in elderly persons assessed by flow cytometry. Immunol Invest 25:185–190

32. MacGregor RR, Shalit M (1990) Neutrophil function in healthy elderly subjects. J Gerontol 45:M55–M60

33. Rao KMK (1996) Age-related decline in ligand-induced actin polymerisation in human leukocytes and platelets. J Gerontol 41:561–566

34. Butcher SK, Chahal H, Nayak L, Sinclair A, Henriquez NV, Sapey E, O'Mahony D, Lord JM (2001) Senescence in innate immune responses: reduced neutrophil phagocytic capacity and CD16 expression in elderly humans. J. Leukocyte Biol 70:881–886

35. Fulop T, Komaromi I, Foris G Worum I, Leovey A (1986) Age-dependent variations of intralysosomal enzyme release from human PMN leukocytes under various stimuli. Immunobiology 171:302–310

36. Lipschitz DA, Udupa KB, Milton KY, Thompson CO (1984) Effect of age on hematopoieisis in man. Blood 63:502–509

37. Wenisch C, Patruta S, Daxbock F, Krause R, Horl W (2000) Effect of age on human neutrophil function. J Leukocyte Biol 67:40–45

38. Corberand J, Ngyen F, Laharrague P, Fontanilles AM, Gleyzes B, Gyrard E, Senegas C (1981) Polymorphonuclear functions and aging in humans. J Am Geriatr Soc 29:391–397

39. Whitelaw DA, Rayner BL, Wilcox PA (1992) Community acquired bacteremia in the elderly—a prospective study of 121 cases. J Am Geriatr Soc 40:996–1004

40. Fulop T, Larbi A, Douziech N, Fortin C, Guerard K-L, Lesur O, Khalil A, Dupuis G (2004) Signal transduction and functional changes in neutrophils with aging. Aging Cell 3:217–226

41. Fortin CF, Larbi A, Lesur O, Douziech N, Fulop T. Jr (2006) Impairment of SHP-1 down-regulation in the lipid rafts of human neutrophils under GM-CSF stimulation contributes to their age-related, altered functions. J Leukocyte Biol 79:1061–1072
42. Emanuelli G, Lanzio M, Anfossi T, Romano S, Anfossi G, Calcamuggi G (1986) Influence of age on polymorphonuclear leukocytes in vitro: phagocytic activity in healthy human subjects. Gerontology 32:308–316
43. Fulop T, Foris G, Worum I, Leovey A (1985) Age-dependent alterations of Fc gamma receptor-mediated effector functions of human polymorphonuclear leucocytes, editors. Clin Exp Immunol 61:425–432
44. Mege JL, Capo C, Michel B, Gastaut JL, Bongrand P (1988) Phagocytic cell function in aged subjects. Neurobiol Aging 9:217–220
45. McCourt M, Wang JH, Sookhai S, Redmond HP (1999) Proinflammatory mediators stimulate neutrophil-directed angiogenesis. Arch Surg 134:1325–1331
46. Irwin M (1993) Stress-Induced Immune Suppression Role of the Autonomic Nervous System. Ann N Y Acad Sci 697:203–218
47. Parrillo JE, Fauci AS (1979) Mechanisms of glucocorticoid action on immune processes. Annu Rev Pharmacol Toxicol 19:179–201
48. Arlt W, Hewison M (2004) Hormones and immune function: implications of aging. Aging Cell 3:209–216
49. Araneo B, Daynes R (1995) Dehydroepiandrosterone functions as more than an antiglucocorticoid in preserving immunocompetence after thermal injury. Endocrinology 136:393–401
50. Daynes RA Dudley DJ Araneo BA (1990) Regulation of murine lymphokine production in vivo. II. Dehydroepiandrosterone is a natural enhancer of interleukin 2 synthesis by helper T cells. Eur J Immunol 20:793–802
51. Padgett DA, MacCallum RC, Loria RM, Sheridan JF (2000) Androstenediol-induced restoration of responsiveness to influenza vaccination in mice. J Gerontol A Biol Sci Med Sci 55: B418–B424
52. Suzuki T, Suzuki N, Daynes RA, Engleman EG (1991) Dehydroepiandrosterone enhances IL2 production and cytotoxic effector function of human T cells. Clin Immunol Immunop 61:202–211
53. Baulieu EE, Thomas G, Legrain S, Lahlou N, Roger M, Debuire B, Faucounau V, Girard L, Hervy MP, Latour F, Leaud MC, Mokrane A, Pitti-Ferrandi H, Trivalle C, de Lacharriere O, Nouveau S, Rakoto-Arison B, Souberbielle JC, Raison J, Le Bouc Y, Raynaud A, Girerd X, Forette F (2000) Dehydroepiandrosterone (DHEA), DHEA sulfate, and aging: Contribution of the DHEAge Study to a sociobiomedical issue. Proc Natl Acad Sci USA 97:4279–4284
54. Arlt W, Callies F, Koehler I, van Vlijmen JC, Fassnacht M, Strasburger CJ, Seibel MJ, Huebler D, Ernst M, Oettel M, Reincke M, Schulte HM, Allolio B (2001) Dehydroepiandrosterone supplementation in healthy men with an age-related decline of dehydroepiandrosterone secretion. J Clin Endocrinol Metab 86:4686–4692
55. Percheron G, Hogrel JY, Denot-Ledunois S, Fayet G, Forette F, Baulieu EE, Fardeau M, Marini JF (2003) Effect of 1-year oral administration of dehydroepiandrosterone to 60-to 80-year-old individuals on muscle function and cross-sectional area—A double-blind placebo-controlled trial. Arch Intern Med 163:720–727
56. Nair KS, Smith G (2007) DHEA and testosterone in the elderly—reply. N Engl J Med Med 356:637
57. Viswanathan K, Dhabar FS (2005) Stress-induced enhancement of leukocyte trafficking into sites of surgery or immune activation. Proc Natl Acad Sci USA 102:5808–5813
58. Harmsen AG, Turney TH (1985) Inhibition of in vivo neutrophil accumulation by stress. Inflammation 9:9–20
59. Arber N, Berliner S, Arber L, Lipshitz A, Sinai Y, Zajicek G, Eilat Y, Pinkhas J, Aronson M (1992) The state of leukocyte adhesiveness-aggregation in the peripheral blood is more sensitive than the white blood cell count for the detection of acute mental stress. J Psychosom Res 36:37–46

60. Arber N, Berliner S, Tamir A, Liberman E, Segal G, Pinkhas J, Aronson M (1991) The state of leukocyte adhesiveness-aggregation in the peripheral blood – a new and independnet marker of mental. Stress Medicine 7:75–78

61. Steptoe A, Magid K, Edwards S, Brydon L, Hong Y, Erusalimsky J (2003) The influence of psychological stress and socioeconomic status on platelet activation in men. Atherosclerosis 168:57–63

62. Lyte M, Baissa B, Nelson S (1991) Neuroendocrine examination of the social-conflict stress-induced enhancement of phagocytosis in mice. Faseb J. 5:A1386

63. Kang DH, Coe CL, McCarthy DO (1996) Academic examinations significantly impact immune responses, but not lung function, in healthy and well-managed asthmatic adolescents. Brain Behav Immun 10:164–181

64. Kang DH, Coe CL, Karaszewski J, McCarthy DO (1998) Relationship of social support to stress responses and immune function in healthy and asthmatic adolescents. Res Nurs Health 21:117–128

65. Kang DH, McCarthy DO (1994) The effect of psychosocial stress on neutrophil superoxide release. Res Nurs Health 17:363–370

66. Campisi J, Leem TH, Fleshner M (2002) Acute stress decreases inflammation at the site of infection: A role for nitric oxide. Physiol Behav 77:291–299

67. Ring C, Carroll D, Willemsen G, Cooke J, Ferraro A, Drayson M (1999) Secretory immunoglobulin A and cardiovascular activity during mental arithmetic and paced breathing. Psychophysiology 36:602–609

68. Segerstrom SC, Miller GE (2004) Psychological stress and the human immune system: A meta-analytic study of 30 years of inquiry. Psychol Bull 130:601–630

69. Reiche EMV, Morimoto HK, Nunes SOV (2006) Stress and depression-induced immune dysfunction: Implications for the development and progression of cancer. Int Rev Psychiatry 17:515–527

70. Peake JM (2002) Exercise-induced alterations in neutrophil degranulation and respiratory burst activity: possible mechanisms of action. Exerc Immunol Rev 8:49–100

71. Butcher SK Killampalli V, Lascelles D, Wang K, Alpar E, Lord JM (2005) Raised cortisol: DHEAS ratios in the elderly after injury: Potential impact upon neutrophil function and immunity. Aging Cell 4:319–324

72. Padgett DA, Glaser R (2003) How stress influences the immune response. Trends Immunol 24:444–448

73. Weyts FAA, Flik G, Verburg-van Kemenade BML (1998) Cortisol inhibits apoptosis in carp neutrophilic granulocytes. Dev Comp Immunol 22:563–572

74. Zhang XH, Moilanen E, Kankaanranta H (2001) Beclomethasone, budesonide and fluticasone propionate inhibit human neutrophil apoptosis. Eur J Pharmacol 431:365–371

75. Dror Y, Ward AC, Touw IP, Freedman MH (2000) Combined corticosteroid/granulocyte colony-stimulating factor (G-CSF) therapy in the treatment of severe congenital neutropenia unresponsive to G-CSF: Activated glucocorticoid receptors synergize with G-CSF signals. Exp Hematol 28:1381–1389

76. Davis KA, Fabian TC, Ragsdale DN, Trenthem LL, Croce NA, Proctor KG (2001) Combination therapy that targets secondary pulmonary changes after abdominal trauma. Shock 15:479–484

77. Egger G, Aigner R, Glasner A, Hofer HP, Mitterhammer H, Zelzer S (2004) Blood polymorphonuclear leukocyte migration as a predictive marker for infections in severe trauma: comparison with various inflammation parameters. Intensive Care Med 30:331–334

78. Egger G, Burda A, Mitterhammer H, Baumann G, Bratschitsch G, Glasner A (2003) Impaired blood polymorphonuclear leukocyte migration and infection risk in severe trauma. J Infect 47:148–154

79. Bekesi G Kakucs R, Varbiro S, Racz K, Sprintz D, Feher J, Szekacs B (2000) In vitro effects of different steroid hormones on superoxide anion production of human neutrophil granulocytes. Steroids 65:889–894

80. Wood DJ, Ions GK, Quinby JM, Gale DW, Stevens J (1992) Factors which influence mortality after subcapital hip fracture. J Bone Joint Surg 74:199–202

81. Dai YT, Wu SC, Weng R (2002) Unplanned hospital readmission and its predictors in patients with chronic conditions. J Formos Med Assoc 101:779–785

82. Khasraghi FA, Lee EJ, Christmas C, Wenz JF (2003) The economic impact of medical complications in geriatric patients with hip fracture. Orthopedics 26:49–53

83. Butcher SK, Killampalli V, Chahal H, Alpar EK, Lord JM (2003) Effect of age on susceptibility to post-traumatic infection in the elderly. Biochem Soc Trans 31:449–451

84. Graham JE, Christian LM, Kiecolt-Glaser JK (2006) Stress, age, and immune function: Toward a lifespan approach. J Behav Med 29:389–400

85. Laughlin GA, Barrett-Connor E (2000) Sexual dimorphism in the influence of advanced aging on adrenal hormone levels: The Rancho Bernardo Study. J J Clin Endocrinol Metab 85:3561–3568

86. Orentreich N, Brind JL, Vogelman JH, Andres R, Baldwin H (1992) Long-term longitudinal measurements of plasma dehydroepiandosterone sulfate in normal men. J Clin Endocrinol Metab 75:1002–1004

87. Arlt W (2004) Dehydroepiandrosterone and ageing. Best Practice Res. J Clin Endocrinol Metab 18:363–380

88. Arlt W, Martens JWM, Song MS, Wang JT, Auchus RJ, Miller WL (2002) Molecular evolution of adrenarche: Structural and functional analysis of P450c17 from four primate species. Endocrinology 143:4665–4672

89. Smail PJ, Faiman C, Hobson WC, Fuller GB, Winter JSD (1982) Further studies on adrenarche in non-human primates. Endocrinology 111:844–848

90. Parker CR, Mixon RL, Brissie RM, Grizzle WE (1997) Aging alters zonation in the adrenal cortex of men. J Clin Endocrinol Metab 82:3898–3901

91. Hornsby PJ (2002) Aging of the human adrenal cortex. Ageing Res Rev 1:229–242

92. Liu CH, Laughlin GA, Fischer UG, Yen SSC (1990) Marked attenuation of ultradian and circadian rhythms of dehydroepiandrosterone in post-menopausal women—evidence for a reduced 17,20-Desmolase enzymatic activity. J Clin Endocrinol Metab 71:900–906

93. Parker CR, Slayden SM, Azziz R, Crabbe SL, Hines GA, Boots LR, Bae S (2000) Effects of aging on adrenal function in the human: responsiveness and sensitivity of adrenal androgens and cortisol to adrenocorticotropin in premenopausal and postmenopausal women. J Clin Endocrinol Metab 85:48–54

94. Kudielka BM, Hellhammer J, Hellhammer DH, Wolf OT, Pirke KM, Varadi E, Pilz J, Kirschbaum C (1998) Sex differences in endocrine and psychological responses to psychosocial stress in healthy elderly subjects and the impact of a 2-week dehydroepiandrosterone treatment. J Clin Endocrinol Metab 83:1756–1761

95. Arlt W, Hammer F, Sanning P, Butcher SK, Lord JM, Allolio B, Annane D, Stewart PM (2006) Dissociation of serum dehydroepiandrosterone and dehydroepiandrosterone sulfate in septic shock. J Clin Endocrinol Metab 91:2548–2554

96. Meikle AW, Dorchuck RW, Araneo BA, Stringham JD, Evans TG, Spruance SL, Daynes RA (1992) The presence of dehydroepiandrosterone-specific receptor binding complex in murine T-cells. J Steroid Biochem Mol Biol 42:293–304

97. Okabe T, Haji M, Takayanagi R, Adachi M, Imasaki K, Kurimoto F, Watanabe T, Nawata H (1995) Up-regulation of high affinity dehydroepiandrosterone binding activity by dehydroepiandrosterone in activated human T lymphocytes. J Clin Endocrinol Metab 80:2993–2996

98. Liu DM, Dillon JS (2002) Dehydroepiandrosterone activates endothelial cell nitric-oxide synthase by a specific plasma membrane receptor coupled to G alpha(i2,3). J Biol Chem 277:21379–21388

99. Liu DM, Si HW, Reynolds KA, Zhen W, Jia ZQ, Dillon JS (2007) Dehydroepiandrosterone protects vascular endothelial cells against apoptosis through a G alpha(i) protein-dependent activation of phosphatidylinositol 3-kinase/Akt and regulation of antiapoptotic Bcl-2 expression. Endocrinology 148:3068–3076

100. Loria RM, Padgett DA, Huynh PN (1996) Regulation of the immune response by dehydroepiandrosterone and its metabolites. J Endocrinol 150:S209–S220

101. Zhou ZF, Speiser PW (1999) Regulation of HSD17B1 and SRD5A1 in lymphocytes. Mol Genet Metab 68:410–417

102. Zhou ZF, Shackleton CHL, Pahwa S, White PC, Speiser PW (1998) Prominent sex steroid metabolism in human lymphocytes. Mol Cell Endocrinol 138:61–69
103. Schmidt M, Kreutz M, Loffler G, Scholmerich J, Straub RH (2000) Conversion of dehydroepiandrosterone to downstream steroid hormones in macrophages. J Endocrinol 164:161–169
104. Hammer F, Drescher DG, Schneider SB, Quinkler M, Stewart PM, Allolio B, Arlt W (2005) Sex steroid metabolism in human peripheral blood mononuclear cells changes with aging. J Clin Endocrinol Metab 90:6283–6289
105. Tomlinson JW, Walker EA, Bujalska IJ, Draper N, Lavery GG, Cooper MS, Hewison M, Stewart PM (2004) 11 beta-hydroxysteroid dehydrogenase type 1: A tissue-specific regulator of glucocorticoid response. Endocr Rev 25:831–866
106. Draper N, Walker EA, Bujalska IJ, Tomlinson JW, Chalder SM, Arlt W, Lavery GG, Bedendo O, Ray DW, Laing I, Malunowicz E, White PC, Hewison M, Mason PJ, Connell JM, Shackleton CHL, Stewart PM (2003) Mutations in the genes encoding 11 beta-hydroxysteroid dehydrogenase type 1 and hexose-6-phosphate dehydrogenase interact to cause cortisone reductase deficiency. Nat Genet 34:434–439
107. Lavery GG, Walker EA, Draper N, Jeyasuria P, Marcos J, Shackleton CHL, Parker KL, White PC, Stewart PM (2006) Hexose-6-phosphate dehydrogenase knock-out mice lack 11 beta-hydroxysteroid dehydrogenase type 1-mediated glucocorticoid generation. J Biol Chem 281:6546–6551
108. Cooper MS, Bujalska I, Rabbitt E, Walker EA, Bland R, SHEPPARD MC, Hewison M, Stewart PM (2001) Modulation of 11 beta-hydroxysteroid dehydrogenase isozymes by proinflammatory cytokines in osteoblasts: An autocrine switch from glucocorticoid inactivation to activation. J Bone Miner Res 16:1037–1044
109. Tomlinson JW, Moore J, Cooper MS, Bujalska I, Shahmanesh M, Burt C, Strain A, Hewison M, Stewart PM (2001) Regulation of expression of 11 beta-hydroxysteroid dehydrogenase type 1 in adipose tissue: tissue-specific induction by cytokines. Endocrinology 142:1982–1989
110. Franceschi C, Capri M, Monti D, Giunta S, Olivieri F, Sevini F, Panouraia MP, Invidia L, Celani L, Scurti M, Cevenini E, Castellani GC, Salvioli S (2007) Inflammaging and anti-inflammaging: A systemic perspective on aging and longevity emerged from studies in humans. Mech Ageing Dev 128:92–105
111. Murakami K, Nakagawa T, Shozu M, Uchide K, Koike K, Inoue M (1999) Changes with aging of steroidal levels in the cerebrospinal fluid of women. Maturitas 33:71–80
112. Sandeep TC, Yau JLW, MacLullich AMJ, Noble J, Deary IJ, Walker BR, Seckl JR (2004) 11 beta-Hydroxysteroid dehydrogenase inhibition improves cognitive function in healthy elderly men and type 2 diabetics. Proc Natl Acad Sci USA 101:6734–6739
113. Thieringer R, Le Grand CB, Carbin L, Cai TQ, Wong BM, Wright SD, Hermanowski-Vosatka A (2001) 11 beta-hydroxysteroid dehydrogenase type 1 is induced in human monocytes upon differentiation to macrophages. J Immunol 167:30–35
114. Freeman L, Hewison M, Hughes SV, Evans KN, Hardie D, Means TK, Chakraverty R (2005) Expression of 11 beta-hydroxysteroid dehydrogenase type 1 permits regulation of glucocorticoid bioavailability by human dendritic cells. Blood 106:2042–2049
115. Kasuya Y, Yokokawa A, Takashima S, Shibasaki H, Furuta T (2005) Use of 11 alpha-deuterium labeled cortisol as a tracer for assessing reduced 11 beta-HSD2 activity in vivo following glycyrrhetinic acid ingestion in a human subject. Steroids 70:117–125
116. Tornatore KM, Logue G, Venuto RC, Davis PJ (1994) Pharmacokinetics of methylprednisolone in elderly and young healthy males. J Am Geriatr Soc 42:1118–1122
117. Asadullah K, Schacke H, Cato AC (2002) Dichotomy of glucocorticoid action in the immune system. Trends Immunol 23:120–122
118. Rook GAW, Hernandez-Pando R, Lightman SL (1994) Hormones, peripherally activated hormones and regulation of the TH1/TH2 balance. Immunol Today 15:301–303
119. Hernandez-Pando R, Streber MDL, Orozco H, Arriaga K, Pavon L, Al Nakhli SA, Rook GAW (1998) The effects of androstenediol and dehydroepiandrosterone on the course and cytokine profile of tuberculosis in BALB/c mice. Immunology 95:234–241

120. Blauer KL, Poth M, Rogers WM, Bernton EW (1991) Dehydroepiandrosterone antagonizes the suppressive effects of dexamethasone in lymphocyte proliferation. Endocrinology 129:3174–3179

121. Canning MO, Grotenhuis K, de Wit HJ, Drexhage HA (2000) Opposing effects of dehydroepiandrosterone and dexamethasone on the generation of monocyte-derived dendritic cells. Eur J Endocrinol 143:687–695

122. Solerte SB, Fioravanti M, Vignati G, Giustina A, Cravello L, Ferrari E (1999) Dehydroepiandrosterone sulfate enhances natural killer cell cytotoxicity in humans via locally generated immunoreactive insulin-like growth factor I. J Clin Endocrinol Metab 84:3260–3267

123. Straub RH, Konecna L, Hrach S, Rothe G, Kreutz M, Scholmerich J, Falk W, Lang B (1998) Serum dehydroepiandrosterone (DIEA) and DHEA sulfate are negatively correlated with serum interleukin-6 (IL-6), and DHEA inhibits IL-6 secretion from mononuclear cells in man in vitro: Possible link between endocrinosenescence and immunosenescence. J Clin Endocrinol Metab 83:2012–2017

124. Gordon CM, LeBoff MS, Glowacki J (2001) Adrenal and gonadal steroids inhibit IL-6 secretion by human marrow cells. Cytokine 16:178–186

125. Coles AJ, Thompson S, Cox AL, Curran S, Gurnell EM, Chatterjee VK (2005) Dehydroepiandrosterone replacement in patients with Addison's disease has a bimodal effect on regulatory (CD4(+)CD25(hi) and CD4(+)FoxP3(+)) T cells. Eur J Immunol 35:3694–3703

126. Angele MK, Catania RA, Ayala A, Cioffi WG, Bland KI, Chaudry IH (1998) Dehydroepiandrosterone—An inexpensive steroid hormone that decreases the mortality due to sepsis following trauma-induced hemorrhage. Arch Surg 133:1281–1287

127. Barkhausen T, Westphal BM, Puetz C, Krettek C, van Griensven M (2006) Dehydroepiandrosterone administration modulates endothelial and neutrophil adhesion molecule expression in vitro. Crit Care 10:R109–R119

128. Catania RA, Angele MK, Ayala A, Cioffi WG, Bland KI, Chaudry IH (1999) Dehydroepiandrosterone restores immune function following trauma-haemorrhage by a direct effect on T lymphocytes. Cytokine 11:443–450

129. Gu S, Ripp SL, Prough RA, Geoghegan TE (2003) Dehydroepiandrosterone affects the expression of multiple genes in rat liver including 11 beta-hydroxysteroid dehydrogenase type 1: A cDNA array analysis. Mol Pharmacol 63:722–731

130. Apostolova G, Schweizer RAS, Balazs Z, Kostadinova RM, Odermatt A (2005) Dehydroepiandrosterone inhibits the amplification of glucocorticoid action in adipose tissue. Am J Physiol Endocrinol Metab 288:E957–E964

131. Whorwood CB, Donovan SJ, Wood PJ, Phillips DIW (2001) Regulation of glucocorticoid receptor alpha and beta isoforms and type I 11 beta-hydroxysteroid dehydrogenase expression in human skeletal muscle cells: A key role in the pathogenesis of insulin resistance? J Clin Endocrinol Metab 86:2296–2308

132. Butcher SK, Lord JM (2004) Stress responses and innate immunity: aging as a contributory factor. Aging Cell 3:151–160

133. Esterling BA, KiecoltGlaser JK, Glaser R (1996) Psychosocial modulation of cytokine-induced natural killer cell activity in older adults. Psychosomatic Med 58:264–272

134. Glaser R, Sheridan J, Malarkey WB, MacCallum RC, Kiecolt-Glaser JK (2000) Chronic stress modulates the immune response to a pneumococcal pneumonia vaccine. Psychosom Med 62:804–807

135. Kiecolt-Glaser JK, Marucha PT, Malarkey WB, Mercado AM, Glaser R (1995) Slowing of wound healing by psychological stress. Lancet 346:1194–1196

136. Vedhara K, McDermott MP, Evans TG, Treanor JJ, Plummer S, Tallon D, Cruttenden KA, Schifitto G (2002) Chronic stress in nonelderly caregivers - Psychological, endocrine and immune implications. J Psychosom Res 53:1153–1161

137. Kiecolt-Glaser JK, Glaser R, Gravenstein S, Malarkey WB, Sheridan J (1996) Chronic stress alters the immune response to influenza virus vaccine in older adults. Proc Natl Acad Sci USA 93:3043–3047

Cellular Immunosenescence - Antigen Presenting Cells

Role of Dendritic Cells in Aging

Anshu Agrawal, Sudhanshu Agrawal and Sudhir Gupta

Contents

Abstract: Immunesenescence is characterized by a decline in immune functions which is responsible for majority of morbidity and mortality associated with aging. The possible consequences of this progressive aging of the immune system are an increase in autoimmune phenomena, incidence of malignancies and predisposition to infections. Innate immune system is the primary defense against invading pathogens. Moreover, it also initiates and modulates the functions of adaptive immune system. This review focuses on the age-associated changes in the functions of dendritic cells, the major antigen presenting cells of the innate immune system.

1 Introduction

The immune system is composed of two major defenses—1) innate immune or nonspecific defense mechanisms consisting of cells such as granulocytes, macrophages and dendritic cells (DCs) and proteins such as cytokines which allows an extremely rapid response to pathogens. 2) The adaptive immune or specific immune defense mechanisms consist mainly of cells such as T- and B-lymphocytes and follow the innate immune response. This response is exquisitely tailored and specific

S. Gupta (✉)
Medical Sciences I, C-240, University of California, Irvine
CA 92697, USA
Tel: (949) 824-5818
Fax: (949) 824-4362w
E-mail: sgupta@uci.edu

A. Agrawal · S. Agrawal
Division of Basic and Clinical Immunology, University of California
Irvine, CA 92697

T. Fulop et al. (eds.), *Handbook on Immunosenescence,*
DOI 10.1007/ 978-1-4020-9062-2_25, © Springer Science+Business Media B.V. 2009

to the particular pathogen and is responsible for generating long-term memory against subsequent challenges. These two defense mechanisms are interlinked together and the nature of innate immune response dictates the nature or quality of adaptive immune response. The proper function of both systems is thus essential for generating effective immunity. Adaptive immune functions are known to be severely compromised with increasing age and believed to be the majo r cause for immunosenescence [18, 23, 26, 27, 35, 36, 42, 44, 60]. The knowledge regarding the contribution of innate immune cells such as DCs in immunosenescence is still in its infancy. This review summarizes the findings on DC functions in aging.

2   Dendritic Cells

Dendritic cells (DCs) are the most potent of antig en-presenting cells [6, 58] of the immune system present at various portals of entry of pathogens like skin, airways etc., sensing pathogens, ready to initiate and amplify the immune response. DCs serve as critical mediators of both immunity and tolerance [6, 57, 58] by virtue of their ability to ascertain that inflammatory immune responses against commensals of the physiologic skin microflora, ingested food antigens, or inhaled airborne microorganisms are prevented while potent immune responses against harmful pathogens are sustained.

DCs can be activated by various stimuli including microbes, dying cells, and inflammatory cytokines. An array of Toll-like receptors (TLRs), C-type lectin receptors (CLRs) and intracytoplasmic NOD-like receptors (NLRs) in DCs aid them in sensing pathogens [5, 28, 50]. The sensing and capture of antigen by DCs initiates their differentiation and maturation. During maturation they lose their antigen capturing capacity and upregulate the expression of MHC and costimulatory molecules, thus becoming the efficient antigen presenting cells [6, 57, 58]. Maturation of DCs also results in the upregulation of CCR-7 which allows them migrate to T-cell areas in the lymphoid organs where antigens are presented to the T-cells, initiating an adaptive immune response. In addition to an up-regulation of various markers, activation of DCs initiates an inflammatory response through secretion of a broad array of cytokines and other inflammatory mediators which allows them to communicate between themselves and other cells of the immune system, exerting a broad influence on the immune system [6, 50]. For example, DCs can dictate the type of T-cell responses by virtue of the cytokines they secrete in response to a stimulus. IL-12 or IL-23 secretion by DCs [1, 13, 34] primes TH1/TH17 responses while IL-10 gives rise to TH2 or T-regulatory type of responses [2, 3].

Maintenance of tolerance is another key function of DCs [57, 58]. Under steady state conditions DCs continuously sample self-antigens from dying cells. However, no immune response is initiated since these do not activate DCs. These immature DCs interact with T-cells in the absence of costimulation leading to T-cell anergy or the development of T-regulatory cells. The presence of danger signals such as proinflammatory cytokines can cause DCs to mature resulting in break of tolerance. The proinflammatory cytokines and other inflammatory mediators that are increased during aging can modulate functions of dendritic cells affecting the magnitude and quality of both innate and adaptive immune responses [10, 19, 30, 45].

3 Dendritic Cell Subsets

In humans, two major subsets of DCs [6] have been identified that function differently in both the innate and adaptive immune responses: myeloid DCs (mDCs), – interstitial DCs and Langerhans cells are found in peripheral tissue, secondary lymphoid organs and blood, and plasmacytoid DCs (pDCs) are present in the blood and secondary lymphoid organs. mDCs are professional APCs with a strong capacity to prime naive T-cells and to induce and regulate T-cell responses through secretion of IL-12. pDCs on the other hand are characterized by their plasma cell-like morphology, low phagocytic capacity and production of large amounts of Type I interferons in response to viral, bacterial and parasitic infections [38]. The two subsets of DCs differ in their expression of highly conserved microbial pattern recognition receptors (PRRs), known as Toll-like receptors (TLR). Circulating pDCs express TLR1, 6, 7, 9 and 10, but not TLR4 [29, 51], while blood mDCs express TLR1, 2, 3, 4, 5, 6, 7, 8 and 10, but not TLR9 [51].

4 DCs in Aging

Aging is associated with multiple changes in the cytokine microenvironment that could have either inhibitory or stimulatory effect on the activation and/or maturation of DCs [9, 10, 19, 30, 45, 49]. The increased TNF-α and prostaglandins would result in premature DC activation altering their antigen uptake capacity [30]. Similarly elevated IL-10 and glucocorticoid levels in aging may result in the suppression of activation of DCs [10, 45]. A change in the microenvironment such as age-associated increase in proinflammatory cytokines like TNF-α, may act as a trigger for maturation of DCs, and in combination with apoptotic cells may lead to immune activation and associated inflammation.

Studies on DCs in aging in humans have been focused primarily on the function of myeloid DC subset because it was believed to be the major DC subset involved in T-cell priming.

5 DC Numbers and Phenotype

Most studies in humans have reported no change in numbers or phenotype of DCs in aging [39, 56, 61]. In our study we found normal numbers and phenotype of circulating and monocyte-derived DCs (MDDCs) in aged humans [4]. However,

Della-bella et al. [15] reported progressive decline in the number of circulating mDCs with age while there was no change in pDC numbers. They also found that DCs from aged individuals have a more mature phenotype with an increased proportions of cells expressing CD86 and CD83 as compared to young individuals. Recent mouse studies by Grolleau–Julius et al. [22] and Tesar et al. [59] also did not report any–significant difference in the numbers and phenotype of blood or lymphoid DCs. However, HLA-DR expression on peripheral blood DCs and DCs from a strain of senescence-accelerated mouse (SAMP-1) was found to be reduced [24]. A few earlier studies in mice document a decrease in the number Langerhan cells in the skin [11, 14, 55].

6   DC Pathogen Sensing and Cytokine Secretion

H. Influenzae and *Streptococcus pneumoniae* infections account for substantial mortality [31, 41] in aged individuals resulting in increased susceptibility to infections with age. Alterations in PRR functions in aging may impair activation of the immune response and contribute to poorer vaccine responses and greater morbidity and mortality from infectious diseases. Proinflammatory cytokines are increased during aging. A greater understanding of PRR functions in aging is extremely relevant in view of the interest in TLR agonists as therapeutic agents not only for infections, but also for allergic, autoimmune, and malignant diseases.

Amongst the PRRs, TLRs are most studied in aging because of their important role in clearing viral and bacterial pathogens. Numerous studies have investigated the expression of these receptors on the innate immune cells of both humans and mice. Alterations in TLR expression pattern in aging seem to be cell specific with monocytes showing decreased expression of certain TLRs while dendritic cells appear to express similar level of TLRs as the young.

Some earlier studies [8, 48, 54, 61, 62] had reported decreased expression and function of TLRs in macrophages from aged mice; however, recent studies by Tesar et al. [59] found that TLR expression and function (in vivo) is intact in myeloid DCs and macrophages from aged mice. They found that both circulating mDCs and bone-marrow derived DCs from aged and young mice expressed comparable levels of maturation markers following activation with various TLR ligands. The levels of cytokine secretion between the groups were also comparable. In contrast, Grolleau-Julius et al. [22] reported decreased secretion of TNF-α and IL-6 and increased IL-10 secretion from bone-marrow derived DCs from aged mice. The reason for this discrepancy is presently unclear. Previous studies [39, 56] have reported comparable levels of activation and cytokine secretion by MDDCs from the aged and young subjects following TLR stimulation. Our studies [4] found no differences in TLR expression in MDDCs from aged and young subjects at the gene level (Affymatrix analyses) and protein level (TLR4). There was no difference in the expression of CD40, CD80, CD83, CD86 and HLA-DR on MDDCs before and after activation with TLR-4 ligand, LPS between aged and young subjects. However, we observed an increased secretion of TNF-α and IL-6 from MDDCs from aged compared to young subjects, when stimulated with TLR-4 or TLR8 ligand. The levels of IL-10, IL-12p40 and IL-12p70 were comparable between the two groups. Della bella et al. [15] report decreased IL-12 secretion from LPS-stimulated circulating mDCs in humans. Unpublished data from our laboratory indicates that circulating mDCs in the aged subjects also secrete higher levels of TNF-α and IL-6 upon TLR stimulation. In summary, TLR expression and function in DCs during aging appears to be intact except an increased secretion of proinflammatory cytokines TNF-α and IL-6. High IL-6 and TNF-α levels are poor prognostic factors for a number of age-associated diseases. For example, higher IL-6 levels lead to the production of C-reactive protein which is identified as a major risk factor for myocardial infarction. Increased serum IL-6 and C-reactive protein play a major role in Type-2 diabetes; rheumatoid arthritis and osteoporosis, all diseases which show increased incidence with age [12, 16, 43]. Likewise there is positive correlation between IL-6 levels and congestive heart failure. Increase in another proinflammatory cytokine TNF-α has been found to be associated with higher incidence of arteriosclerosis in older men [47]. Thus overactivation of the dendritic cells in response to TLR may be contributing to age-associated inflammation.

7   Antigen Capture

Phagocytosis is the major mechanism used by DCs to remove pathogens and cell debris and therefore is important for maintaining both immunity and tolerance [57,58]. Our studies [4] have shown that both, the phagocytosis of dextran beads and pinocytosis of Lucifer Yellow dye was found to be impaired in MDDCs from aged subjects when compared to young. This suggested that MDDCs from aged displayed reduced capacity to capture antigen via both receptor-dependent and independent mechanisms. In addition to foreign antigens, DCs also capture and present self-antigens in the periphery [25,57,58]. In fact the uptake of apoptotic cells by DCs in the periphery and presentation to T-cells in the absence of costimulation, is considered to be the major mechanism of maintenance of peripheral self-tolerance. Our investigations indicated that DCs from aged individuals were also impaired in their capacity to phagocytose apoptotic cells [4]. Impaired clearance of apoptotic cells in aging would lead to accumulation of apoptotic cells which will become necrotic and lyse to release auto-antigens such as nucleic acids, heat shock proteins, HMGB1, ATP and uric acid along with other cell debris. In contrast to apoptotic cells which are known to inhibit maturation of DCs, necrotic cells lead to activation of DCs and secretion of proinflammatory cytokines. Thus these auto-antigens can be taken up by DCs and presented to T-cells leading to inflammation and autoimmunity associated with age. Therefore, a reduction in the phagocytic capacity of DCs with age would not only result in reduced clearance of infections but would contribute to age-associated loss of peripheral self-tolerance, autoimmunity and chronic inflammation.

8   Migration of DCs

Following activation, DCs migrate to T- and B-cell areas after activation in order
to induce effective cellular immune responses. Stimulation of immature DCs with
TLR ligands results in the down-regulation of CCR6 and up-regulation of CCR7,
which enhances their ability to migrate from the peripheral tissues to the draining
lymph node. CCL21 and CCL19 both bind to the CCR7 receptor and are potent
chemoattractants for mature DCs [32]. Mice deficient in CCR7 are unable to mount
effective T-cell immunity [20]. Relatively few studies have addressed the question of migration of DCs in aging. We determined the migration of DCs from aged
and young human subjects using a transwell system where the DCs in the upper
chamber migrate through a transwell of defined pore size to the lower chamber
in response to a chemokine gradient [4]. We observed that DCs from aged subjects were impaired in their capacity to migrate in response to CCL19 and SDF-1
compared to DCs from young. This was not a consequence of reduced CCR7 or
CXCR4 expression. Neither did we observe a significant difference in the secretion
of basal level of the chemokines from DCs between aged and young individuals.
Bhushan et al. [7] observed significantly impaired migration of LCs in response to
TNF-α in elderly subjects. The same group also found decreased TNF-α induced
LC migration in aged animals. Choi and Sauder [11] reported decreased LCs mobilization and the subsequent accumulation of DCs in the regional lymph nodes in
aged mice in response to topical challenge with a chemical agent; however, contact
hypersensitivity responses were not compromised. Linton et al. [37] have reported
in vivo impaired migration of DCs from aged mice to the draining lymph nodes, in
a TCR transgenic mice model. They suggest it to be due to both intrinsic defect of
DCs and aged microenvironment. Contrary to above studies, Pietschmann et al. [46]
observed normal trans-endothelial migration of peripheral blood myeloid-enriched
lymphocyte-depleted cells in elderly subjects. This could be due to the difference
in the model system. Impaired migration of DCs has also been observed in mice
[14, 17]. Since the migration of DCs to lymph nodes is pivotal to the establishment of the immune response, reduced migration may contribute to age-associated
immune dysfunction.

9   Dendritic Cells and Adaptive Immunity

DCs play a key role in sensing and processing microbial information and directing the differentiation of naïve lymphocytes to effector cells suitable against particular types of infection. They have the unique capacity to prime naïve T-cells
among the antigen presenting cells of the body, therefore they are critical for
mounting immune responses against new antigens. The engagement of TLRs on
DCs leads to an increased expression of MHC–peptide complexes and costim-

ulatory molecules, as well as the production of immunomodulatory cytokines, all of which have a profound effect on T-cell priming and differentiation. The up-regulation of costimulatory molecules on DCs dictates the decision between tolerance and immunity. Antigen presentation by DCs in the absence of costimulation results in the generation of anergic and/ or regulatory T-cells [25]. DCs also dictate the nature of TH (TH1, TH2, Treg, TH17) response generated through the type of cytokine secreted by them. For example, IL-12 from DCs induces T-cells to secrete IFN-γ [2] while IL-23 will induce IL-17 from T-cells [13, 34]. Secretion of IL-10 by DCs on the other hand induces either a TH2 or a T-regulatory type of response [2, 3]. It is thus clear that any alteration in the function of DCs with age, would affect T-cell responses.

There is some controversy regarding capacity of DCs in old age to stimulate T-cells. Earlier studies in aged mice demonstrated decrease in antigen presentation and T-cell priming capacity of DCs in the lymph nodes [17, 33, 55]. However, the two recent studies in mice are contradictory. Study by Tesar et al. [59] suggests the intrinsic defect in T-cells during age is responsible for the age-associated reduced T-cell function. Grollaeu-julius [22] on the other hand found old bone-marrow derived DCs less effective than young DCs in stimulating syngeneic ova–specific CD4 T-cell proliferation. They also reported a decrease in tumor regression in mice treated with the ovalbumin peptide-pulsed aged DCs than with ovalbumin peptide-pulsed young DCs.

Similar to the findings of Tesar et al. in mice [59], MDDCs from elderly subjects were not impaired in their capacity to induce T-cell responses. Steger et al. [56] and Grewe et al. [21] reported that DCs from young and aged subjects have similar stimulatory capacity to induce proliferation of T-cell lines developed in long-term cultures. Our preliminary studies with MDDCs show reduced proliferation of young T-cells when cultured with aged DCs. The reason for this discrepancy is not clear.

10 Plasmacytoid DCs and Aging

Studies described above are all focused on the mDC subset from either the blood or in vitro monocyte-derived DCs. Except for a report by Schodell et al. [53] documenting a decrease in the number and IFN-α secretion by pDCs in aging, virtually nothing is known about the functions of the pDC subset in aging. pDCs are key players in the elimination of infections and upon activation produce extremely high amounts of Type I IFNs. Type I IFN production by pDCs regulates the cytotoxic potential of NK and CD8 T-cells [38]. It also induces differentiation of B-cells to plasma cells. The NK and CD8 cytotoxicity are reduced with age along with a reduction in specific antibody responses. Studies of pDC functions with age may help in identification of mechanisms responsible for the reduced B and T-cell functions and the associated increased susceptibility to infections.

11   Conclusion

Though the numbers and phenotype of DCs are relatively unchanged during aging dendritic cell functions are altered with age resulting in an enhanced secretion of proinflammatory cytokines. This increased in proinflammatory cytokines may be due decreased sensitivity of the cells to these cytokines, a phenomenon similar to what is observed with insulin resistance. Reduced phagocytosis and migration on the other hand increases the susceptibility of the elderly to infections. Therefore, it appears that dysfunction of DCs may contribute to T-and B-cell immunosenescence and chronic inflammation associated with aging.

Acknowledgment   Work cited here was in part supported by grant AG 27512 from NIH and partly by new scholar grant from the Ellison Medical Foundation.

References

1. Aggarwal S, Ghilardi N, Xie MH, de Sauvage FJ Gurney AL (2003) Interleukin 23 promotes a distinct CD4 +T cell activation state characterized by the production of IL-17. J Biol Chem 278:1910–1914
2. Agrawal S, Agrawal A, Doughty B, Gerwitz A, Blenis J,Van Dyke T, Pulendran B (2003) Cutting edge: different toll-like receptor agonists instruct dendritic cells to induce distinct Th responses via differential modulation of extracellular signal-regulated kinase-mitogen-acti- vated protein kinase and c-Fos. J Immunol 171:4984–4989
3. Agrawal A, Kaushal P, Agrawal S, Gollapudi S, Gupta S (2007) Thimerosal affects human dendritic cell functions promoting a TH2 response. J Leukocyte Biology 81:474–483
4. Agrawal A, Agrawal S, Cao JN, Su H, Osann K, Gupta S (2007) Altered innate immune func- tioning of dendritic cells in aging humans: Role of PI3Kinase signaling pathway. J Immunol 178:6912–6922
5. Akira S, Uematsu S, Takeuchi O (2006) Pathogen recognition and innate immunity. Cell. 124:783–801
6. Banchereau J, Briere F, Caux C, Davoust J, Lebecque S, Liu YJ, et al (2000) Immunobiology of dendritic cells. Annu Rev Immunol 18:767–811
7. Bhushan M, Cumberbatch M, Dearman RJ, Andrew SM, Kimber I and Griffiths CE (2002) Tumor necrosis factor-alpha-induced migration of human Langerhans cells: the influence of ageing. Br J Dermatol 146:32–40
8. Boehmer ED, Meehan MJ, Cutro BT, Kovacs EJ (2005) Aging negatively skews macrophage TLR2- and TLR4-mediated proinflammatory responses without affecting the IL-2-stimulated pathway. Mech Ageing Dev 126:1305–1313
9. Bruunsgaard H, Pedersen M, Pedersen BK (2001) Aging and proinflammatory cytokines. Curr Opin Hematol 8:131–136
10. Caux C, et al (1994) Interleukin 10 inhibits T cell alloreaction induced by human dendritic cells. Int Immunol. 8:1177–1185
11. Choi KL, Sauder DN (1987) Epidermal Langerhans cell density and contact sensitivity in young and aged BALB/c mice. Mech Age Dev 39:69–79
12. Cohen HJ, Pieper CF, Harris T, Rao KM, Currie MS (1997) The association of plasma IL-6 levels with functional disability in community-dwelling elderly. J Gerontol A Biol Sci Med Sci 52: M201–M208
13. Cua DJ, Sherlock J, Chen Y, Murphy CA, Joyce B, Seymour B, Lucian L, To W, Kwan S, Chura- kova T, Zurawski S, Wiekowski M, Lira SA, Gorman D, Kastelein RA, Sedgwick JD (2003)

Interleukin-23 rather than interleukin-12 is the critical cytokine for autoimmune inflammation of the brain. Nature 421:744–748

14. Cumberbatch M, Dearman RJ, Kimber I (2000) Influence of ageing on Langerhans cell migration in mice: identification of a putative deficiency of epidermal interleukin-1beta. Immunology 105:466–477

15. Della Bella S, Bierti L, Presicce P, Arienti R, Valenti M, Saresella M, Vergani C, Villa ML (2007) Peripheral blood dendritic cells and monocytes are differently regulated in the elderly. 2007. Clin Immunol. 122:220-228

16. Dobbs RJ, Charlett A, Purkiss AG, Dobbs SM, Weller C, Peterson, DW (1999) Association of circulating TNF-alpha and IL-6 with ageing and parkinsonism. Acta Neurol Scand 100:34–41

17. Donnini A, Argentati K, Mancini R, et al (2002) Phenotype, antigen-presenting capacity, and migration of antigen-presenting cells in young and old age. Exp Gerontol 37:1097–1112

18. Dunn-Walters D K, Banerjee M, Mehr R (2003) Effects of age on antibody affinity maturation. Biochem Soc Trans 31:447–448

19. Fagiola U, Cossarizza A, Scala E, Fanales-Belasio E, Ortolani C, Cozzi E, Monti D, Franceschi C, Paganelli R (1993) Increased cytokine production in mononuclear cells of healthy elderly people. Eur J Immunol 23:2375–2378

20. Forster R, Schubel A, Brietfeld D, Kremmer E, Renner-Muller I, Wolf E, Lipp M (1999) CCR-7 coordinates primary immune response by establishing functional microenvironments in secondary lymphoid organs. Cell 99:23–33

21. Grewe M (2001) Chronological ageing and photoageing of dendritic cells. Clin Exp Dermatol 26:608–612

22. Grolleau-Julius A, Garg MR, Mo R, Stoolman LL, Yung RL (2006) Effect of aging on bone marrow-derived murine CD11c+CD4-CD8alpha—dendritic cell function. J Gerontol A Biol Sci Med Sci 61:1039–1047

23. Gupta S, Bi R, Su K, Yel L, Chiplunkar S, Gollapudi S (2004) Characterization of naive, memory and effector CD8+ T cells: effect of age. Exp Gerontol 39:545–550

24. Haruna H, Inaba M, Inaba K, Taketani S, Sugiura K, Fukuba Y, Doi H, Toki J, Tokunaga R, Ikehara S (1995) Abnormalities of B cells and dendritic cells in SAMP1 mice. Eur J Immunol 25:1319–1325

25. Hawiger D, Inaba K, Dorsett Y, Guo M, Mahnke K, Rivera M, Ravetch JV, Steinman RM, Nussenzweig MC (2001) Dendritic cells induce peripheral T cell unresponsiveness under steady state conditions in vivo. J Exp Med 194:769–779

26. Haynes L, Eaton SM, Burns EM, Randall TD, Swain SL (2003) CD4 T cell memory derived from young naïve cells functions well into old age, while memory generated from Elderly naïve cells functions poorly. Proc Natl Acad Sci USA 100:15053–15058

27. Hirokawa K (1999) Age-related changes of signal transduction in T cells. Exp Gerontol 34:7–18

28. Iwasaki A, Medzhitov R (2004) Toll-like receptor control of the adaptive immune responses. Nat Immunol 5:987–995

29. Jarrossay D, Napolitani G, Colonna M, Sallusto F, Lanzavecchia A (2001) Specialization and complementarity in microbial molecule recognition by human myeloid and plasmacytoid dendritic cells Eur J Immunol 31:3388–3393

30. Jonuleit H, Kuhn U, Muller G, Steinbrink K, Paragnik L, Schmitt E, Knop J, Enk AH (1997) Proinflammatory cytokines and prostaglandins induce maturation of potent immunostimulatory dendritic cells under fetal calf serum-free conditions. Eur J Immunol 27(12):3135–3142

31. Katz JM, Plowden J, Renshaw-Hoelscher M, Lu X, Tumpey TM, Sambhara S (2004) Immunity to influenza: the challenges of protecting an aging population. Immunol Res 29:113–124

32. Kellermann SA, Hudak S, Oldham ER, Liu YJ, McEvoy LM (1999) TheCCchemokine receptor-7 ligands 6Ckine and macrophage inflammatory protein 3 are potent chemoattractants for in vitro- and in vivo-derived dendritic cells. J Immunol 162:3859–3864

33. Komatsubara S, Cinader B, Muramatsu S (1986) Functional competence of dendritic cells of ageing C57BL/6 mice. Scand J Immunol 24:517–525

34. Langrish CL, Chen Y, Blumenschein WM, Mattson JD, Chen T, Smith K, Basham B, McClana-han T, Kastelein RA, Cua DJ (2005) IL-23-drives a pathogenic T cell population that induces autoimmune inflammation. J Exp Med 201:233–240

35. Linton PJ, Haynes L, Klinman NR, Swain SL (1996) Antigen-independent changes in naive CD4 T cells with aging. J Exp Med 184:1891–1900

36. Linton PJ, Dorshkind, K (2004) Age-related changes in lymphocyte development and func-tion. Nat Immunol 5:133–139

37. Linton PJ, Li SP, Zhang Y, Bautista B, Huynh Q, Trinh T (2005) Intrinsic versus environmental influences on T-cell responses in aging. Immunol Rev 205:207–219

38. Liu YJ (2005) IPC: professional type 1 interferon-producing cells and plasmacytoid dendritic cell precursors. Annu Rev Immunol 23:275–306

39. Lung TL, Saurwein-Teissl M, Parson W, Schonitzer D, Grubeck-Loebenstein B (2000) Unim-paired dendritic cells can be derived from monocytes in old age and can mobilize residual function in senescent T cells. Vaccine 18:1606–1612

40. McGeer PL, McGeer, EG (2004) Inflammation and the degenerative diseases of aging. Ann N Y Acad Sci (2004) 1035:104–116

41. McBean AM, Hebert PL (2004) New estimates of influenza-related pneumonia and influenza hospitalizations among the elderly. Int J Infect Dis 8:227–235

42. Miller RA, Garcia G, Kirk CJ, Witkowski, JM (1997) Early activation defects in T lym-phocytes from Elderly mice. Immunol Rev 160:79–90

43. Paolisso G, Rizzo MR, Mazziotti G, Tagliamonte MR, Gambardella A, Rotondi M (1998) Advancing age and insulin resistance: role of plasma tumor necrosis factor-alpha. Am J Phys-iol 275:E294–E299

44. Pawalec G, Remarque E, Barnett Y, Solana R (1998) T cells and aging. Front Biosci 3: D59–D99

45. Piemonti L, Monti P, Allavena P, Sironi M, Soldini L, Leone BE, Socci C (1999) Glucocorticoids affect human dendritic cell differentiation and maturation. J Immunol 162(11):6473–6481

46. Pietschmann P, Hahn P, Kudlacek S, Thomas R, Peterlik M (20 Surface markers and transen-dothelial migration of dendritic cells from elderly subjects. Exp Gerontol 35:213–222

47. Rees D, Miles EA, Banerjee T (2006) Dose-related effects of eicosapentaenoic acid on innate immune function in healthy humans: a comparison of young and older men. Am J Clin Nutr 83:331–342

48. Renshaw M, Rockwell J, Engleman C, Gewirtz A, Katz J, Sambhara S (2002) Cutting edge: impaired Toll-like receptor expression and function in aging. J Immunol 169:4697–4701

49. Rink I, Kirchner H (1998) Altered cytokine production in the elderly. Mech Ageing Dev 102:199–209

50. Schnare M, Barton GM, Holt AC, Takeda K, Akira S, Medzhitov, R (2001) Toll-like receptors control activation of adaptive immune responses. Nat Immunol 2:947–650

51. Seeds RE, Gordon S, Miller JL (2006) Receptors and ligands involved in viral induction of type I interferon production by plasmacytoid dendritic cells. Immunobiology 211(6–8):525–535

52. Sharma S, Dominguez AL, Lustgarten J (2006) Aging affect the anti-tumor potential of den-dritic cell vaccination, but it can be overcome by co-stimulation with anti-OX40 or anti-4-1BB, Exp Gerontol 41:78–84

53. Shodell M, Siegal FP (2002) Circulating, interferon-producing plasmacytoid dendritic cells decline during human ageing. Scand J Immunol 56(5):518–521

54. Solana R, Pawelec G, Tarazona R (2006) Aging and innate immunity. Immunity 24:491–494

55. Sprecher E, Becker Y, Kraal G, Hall E, Harrison D, Shultz LD (1990) Effect of aging on epi-dermal dendritic cell populations in C57BL/6J mice. J Invest Dermatol 94:247–253

56. Steger MM, Maczek C, Grubeck-Loebenstein B (1996) Morphologically and functionally intact dendritic cells can be derived from the peripheral blood of aged individuals. Clin Exp Immunol 105:544–550

57. Steinman RM, Turley S, Mellman I, Inaba K (2000) The induction of tolerance by dendritic cells that have captured apoptotic cells. J Exp Med 191:411–416

58. Steinman RM, Hawiger D, Nussenzweig MC (2003) Tolerogenic dendritic cells [review]. Annu Rev Immunol 21:685–711
59. Tesar BM, Walker WE, Unternaehrer J, Joshi NS, Chandele A, Haynes L, Kaech S, Goldstein DR (2006) Murine [corrected] myeloid dendritic cell-dependent toll-like receptor immunity is preserved with aging. Aging Cell 5:473–486
60. Utsuyama M, Hirokawa K, Kurashima C, Fukayama M, Inamatsu T, Suzuki K, Hashimoto W, Sato K (1992) Differential age-change in the numbers of CD4+CD45RA+ and CD4+CD29+ T cell subsets in human peripheral blood. Mech Ageing Dev 63:57–68
61. Uyemura K, Castle SC, Makinodan T (2002) The frail elderly: role of dendritic cells in the susceptibility of infection. Mech Ageing Dev 123(8):955–962
62. Van Duin D, Mohanty S, Thomas V, Ginter S, Montgomery RR, Fikrig E, Allore HG, Medzhitov R, Shaw AC (2007) Age-associated defect in human TLR-1/2 function. J Immunol 178:970–975

Phenotypic and Functional Changes of Circulating Monocytes in Elderly

Lia Ginaldi and Massimo De Martinis

Contents

Abstract: Immunosenescence has been envisaged as a situation in which the specific immune system deteriorates with age, while the innate immunity is negligibly affected and, in some cases, almost upregulated. Ageing represents a state of paradox where chronic inflammation is associated with declining immune responses. This peculiar finding, known as inflammageing, is mainly sustained by cells of the innate immunity. One of the key constituents of the innate immune system are monocytes. Therefore, although the age-related changes in the specific immunity are commonly considered the hallmarks of immunosenescence, the central role of the complex remodelling of first line defence cells, such as monocytes, is gradually emerging. For example, chemotaxis and phagocytosis, as well as antigen processing and presentation, are depressed, whereas cell activation and the secretion of inflammatory cytokines, such as IL-1, IL-6, TNF, are markedly increased. Changes in the expression of functionally important cellular receptors on monocyte surface can also contribute to the modification of immune function characteristic of the elderly.

1 Monocyte Biology and Function

One of the key constituents of the immune system are monocyte–macrophages. Monocytes originate in the bone marrow and migrate through blood to body tissues as macrophages. Monocytes therefore represent the immature macrophages when in transit from bone marrow to tissues. These cells, also known as mononuclear phagocytes, share a common precursor with neutrophils. Through the expression

Prof. L. Ginaldi (✉) · M. De Martinis
Department of Internal Medicine and Public Health
University of L'Aquila
Coppito-67100 L'Aquila, Italy
Tel.: +39 0861 211395
Fax: +39 0861 211395
E-mail: liaginaldi@alice.it

T. Fulop et al. (eds.), *Handbook on Immunosenescence*,
DOI 10.1007/978-1-4020-9062-2_26, © Springer Science+Business Media B.V. 2009

of a series of transcription factors differentiation takes place [67]. Human bone marrow produces approximately 5×10^9 monocytes per day. Under the influence of cytokines, a small number of macrophages in tissues differentiate and, depending on the anatomical sites, may become osteoclasts (bone), Kupffer cells (liver), microglia (brain), etc., all of which exhibit unusual morphological features and functional capacities. Monocytes proliferate in the presence of growth factors, such as monocyte colony-stimulating factor (M-CSF), granulocyte-macrophage colony-stimulating factor (GM-CSF) or IL-3. When these cells are needed at the inflammatory loci, in order to become activated and fully functional, they must interact with interferon-γ (IFN-γ), a cytokine released by activated T-lymphocytes that interacts with the specific receptor [52, 71].

B- and T lymphocytes have specific recognition systems (immunoglobulins and the T-cell receptor, respectively), that interact with specific antigens. This mechanism allows the survival of just the small number of lymphocytes that are needed to recognize and remove foreign material. However, monocytes are members of innate immunity and thus present nonspecific systems on their cell surface to recognize and discriminate self from nonself.

Monocyte–macrophages play a crucial role in immune response and act through several mechanisms: (a) directly, by destroying bacteria, parasites, viruses and tumor cells; (b) indirectly, by releasing mediators, such as interleukin-1 (IL-1), tumor necrosis factor-α (TNF-α), etc., which can activate other cells; (c) by processing antigens and presenting digested peptides to T lymphocytes; and (d) by repairing tissue damage [70].

Monocyte–macrophages can produce an impressive array of cytokines, chemokines, enzymes, arachidonic acid metabolites, and reactive radicals upon activation. Many of these functions appear to antagonize or counter each other. These cells can clearly enhance or suppress adaptive immune responses. Macrophages display both proinflammatory and antiinflammatory functions, produce metalloproteinases and inhibitors of these metalloproteinases, and produce toxic radicals that contribute to tissue cell destruction as well as cytokines that promote tissue regeneration and wound healing. All of these functions are not expressed simultaneously but are thought to be regulated such that macrophages display a balanced, harmonious pattern of functions [79].

In the classic acute inflammatory response, blood monocytes enter the damaged tissue shortly after neutrophils. Encounter with bacteria, their products, and damaged tissue results in the activation of pro-inflammatory activities, such as the production of TNF-α, IL-1, and IL-6 and the secretion of metalloproteinases [102].

In addition to the inflammatory, clearance and tissue regenerative activities, macrophages also play a critical liaison role in the communication between the innate and adaptive immune systems. Macrophages can display antigen presenting activity and phenotype [46, 95] and the inflammatory milieu created by monocyte–macrophages can significantly impact the maturation of myeloid dendritic cells and thus influence the nature of the adaptive immune response that will be elicited [47, 117]. A function-polarizing synergy can develop between T-cells and macrophages wherein the functional pattern displayed by the macrophages influences the nature of the adaptive immune response and the nature of the adaptive immune response (TH 1 vs. TH2) influences the functional pattern displayed by the macrophages. Th 1 cytokines, such as IFN-γ and TNF-α, promote inflammatory and cytotoxic activities of macrophages. In contrast, Th2 cytokines, such as IL-4 and IL-10, promote anti-inflammatory and/or tissue regenerative activities. Ligation of surface receptors such as CD40, TNF-αR, or Toll-like receptors (TLR) on macrophages initiates signal cascades that provide a strong activating stimulus for macrophage function. IFN-γ selectively upregulates LPS-induced inflammatory cytokine production and NOS and oxidase expression while down-regulating other functions, such as arginase and PGE2 and LTC4 production [75, 103, 104].

2 The Impact of Ageing on Monocyte Function

The immune system is affected by ageing, causing an increased susceptibility to infections and mortality, as well as a major incidence of immune diseases and cancer in the elderly. Because mononuclear phagocytes are an essential component of both innate and adaptive immunity, altered function of these cells with aging may play a key role in immunosenescence [98, 50].

Human immunosenescence has been envisaged as a situation in which the specific immune system deteriorates with age, while the innate immunity is negligibly affected and, in some cases, almost upregulated [46]. Aging represents a state of paradox where chronic inflammation is associated with declining immune responses [1, 107].

Inflammageing is considered the common and most important driving force of age-related pathologies, such as neurodegeneration, atherosclerosis, diabetes and sarcopenia, among others, all of which share an inflammatory pathogenesis [36]. The cell types more involved in the inflammatory processes and therefore in the inflammageing are cells of the innate immunity, such as monocytes/macrophages. For example, adhesion of monocytes to the arterial wall, via specific cell surface adhesion molecules, is an important early event in the development of atherosclerotic lesions [112]. Similarly, the increased incidence of tumours in the elderly has been related to a modified antitumour innate defence [63]. In addition, the interface between innate and adaptive immunity, implicates that many of the changes of monocytes influence the initiation of specific immune responses. Impaired ability of antigen presenting cells (APCs) to stimulate T-cells in elderly has been shown [13, 29]. Therefore, although the age-related changes in the specific immunity are commonly considered the hallmarks of immunosenescence, the central role of the complex remodeling of first line defence cells, such as monocytes, is gradually emerging. Some functions of the innate immunity are depressed in the elderly, while many other functions are upregulated, exerting a global and peculiar reshaping. For example, while chemotaxis and phagocytosis, as well as antigen processing and presentation, are depressed, cell activation and the secretion of inflammatory cytokines, such as IL-1, IL-6, TNF, or mononuclear phagocytic cell specific enzymes, are markedly increased [24, 43, 46, 66].

Healthy elderly subjects and centenarians show a decreased susceptibility of monocytes to oxidative stress-induced apoptosis [77]. The respiratory burst of monocytes during ageing decreases between 45% and 70%. Scavenger receptor activity and the expression of apolipoprotein E are reduced in healthy elderly men [37] as is the inflammatory wound healing response, which may be related to poor expression of cell adhesion molecule-1 [6].

Reports on the impact of advanced age on the recruitment of monocytes into excisional wound sites vary from observations of no significant effect to observatians of long delays in attainment of peak monocyte numbers [25].

Chemotactic activity decreases with advanced age [82, 106]. Phagocytosis and clearance of infectious organisms is also reduced with advanced age [2, 4, 12, 73]. Expression of class II MHC and antigen presentation by macrophages have been reported to be reduced in aged rodents and humans [39, 69, 118]. The production of fibroblast growth factor (FGF-2), vascular endothelial growth factor (VEGF), platelet derived growth factor (PDGF), epithelial growth factor (EGF), and transforming growth factor-beta (TGF-β) are reduced and/or delayed, as is the expression of their corresponding receptors [136]. The result is a delay and/or deficiency in reepithelialization, collagen deposition, and angiogenesis in excisional wounds of the elderly.

Haematopoietic stem cells age and have a limited functional lifespan [40]. This may explain the hypocellularìty observed in the bone marrow of elderly people [81]. Of particular interest is the decrease with age of CD68 positive cells, which are markers of macrophage population [70].

Cell lifespan may be regulated by multiple factors. Recently, telomeres and telomerase have been implicated in the regulation of replicative lifespan [56]. Several studies using peripheral blood mononuclear cells consisting of 10–15% monocytes and 60–70% lymphocytes have shown that these structures shorten with age at a rate comparable with that of purified lymphocytes. Mature monocytes do not undergo further cell division after activation. Thus, the variations in telomere length in monocytes with aging may reflect the changes in telomere length in hematopoietic progenitor cells. While mature monocytes do not express telomerase, myeloid progenitor cells do [111].

There are several potential molecular mechanisms that may affect monocyte ageing. An important and universal mechanism that leads to a wide spectrum of intracellular damage during aging are the reactive oxygen species (ROS), which are natural by-products of cellular metabolism. Exposure to ROS may lead to structural changes in macromolecules that impair their function, such as cross-linking of intracellular and intramitochondrial structural and functional proteins, carbohydrates and the oxidation of fats and lipids in membranes. A likely cause of monocyte ageing is the acquisition of defects in genomic DNA. This may occur through a reduced ability to repair even small amounts of DNA damage or very stringent requirements on DNA repair machinery for the maintenance of DNA fidelity, or both. In addition, an increased number of spontaneous mutations may occur, thereby producing DNA damage [105].

3 The Interface Between Innate and Adaptive Immunity

The complex process of immune activation is dependent on the close participation of T-cells and APCs. APCs are responsible for uptake, processing, and presentation of antigen to T-cells. Impaired ability of APCs to stimulate T-cells in elderly has been shown. Expression of costimulatory molecules that assist in the efficiency of cell to cell communication may be altered in old subjects and thus alter cytokine production by APCs, which regulates downstream T-cell effector functions [46, 48, 86]. However, some studies have shown enhanced antigen presentation by APCs from healthy elderly, associated with increased levels of IL-10 and IL-12. It is hypothesized that this upregulation in IL-12 production by APCs may be compensatory to an inherent age-related decline in T-cell function to maintain immunocompetence [46].

Antigenic presentation is a very complex phenomenon involving the formation of the immunological synapse via the activation of the T-cell receptor (TCR) and coreceptors. This interaction determines whether the interacting T-cell becomes tolerant or proliferates and differentiates into a functional effector T-cell. The capacity for immune synapse formation between APC and T-lymphocyte is altered with age. This may be partly due to an alteration in the membrane properties and costimulatory molecules of the cells of the innate immune system with ageing. The innate immune system also influences the adaptive immune response through the timing, type and strength of cytokines produced. Ageing is associated even in healthy persons with a non specific increase in the production of proinflammatory cytokines originating from monocyte to macrophages [50].

Dendritic cells (DCs) are the major APCs responsible for initiating an immune response. Agrawal et al. [1] compared the innate immune functions of monocyte-derived myeloid DCs from elderly subjects with DCs from young individuals. They showed that, although phenotypically comparable, DCs from the aging are functionally different from DCs from the young. In contrast to DCs from the young, DCs from elderly individuals display (1) significantly reduced capacity to phagocytose antigens via macropinocytosis and endocytosis as determined by flow cytometry (2) impaired capacity to migrate in vitro in response to the chemokines MIP-3β and stromal cell-derived factor-1 and (3) significantly increased LPS and ssRNA-induced secretion of TNF-α and IL-6, as determined by ELISA. Investigations of intracellular signalling revealed reduced phosphorylation of AKT in DCs from the ageing, indirectly suggesting decreased activation of the PI3K pathway. Because the PI3K-signaling pathway plays a positive regulatory role in phagocytosis and migration, and also functions as a negative regulator of (TLR) signaling by inducing activation of p38MAPK, this may explain the aberrant innate immune functioning of DCs from elderly subjects. Results from real-time PCR and protein expression by flow cytometry demonstrated an increased expression of phosphatase and tensin homolog, a negative regulator of the PI3K-signaling pathway, in DCs from the aging. Increased phosphatase and tensin homolog may thus be responsible for the defect in AKT phosphorylation and, therefore, the altered innate immune response of DCs from elderly humans [57, 58, 83, 116].

Della Bella et al. [21] analyzed the number, phenotype and function of peripheral blood DCs from elderly subjects by using flow cytometric methods that allow cell characterization directly in whole blood samples. They demonstrated that the number of myeloid DCs progressively declines with age. This finding was accompanied by a decrease of CD34+ precursors and increase of circulating monocytes, suggesting that the entire differentiation process of APCs is partially dysregulated in the elderly. DCs from aged individuals also appeares to have a more mature phenotype and impaired ability to produce IL-12 upon stimulation [85].

The frequency of CD34+ cells progressively declines with age, suggesting that in aged subjects a reduced availability of these cells may contribute to reduce the frequency of DCs [99]. On the other hand the frequency of monocytes, that not only may differentiate into DCs but also represent another main population of professional APCs, shows a progressive increase with ageing. Therefore, the entire differentiation process of APCs is partially dysregulated in the elderly. The analysis of the plasmatic levels of factors known to affect the differentiation of monocytes and DCs from their precursors demonstrates in the elderly increased levels of TGF-β, which does promote the maturation and differentiation of monocytic cells [33]; and increased levels of VEGF, which does impair the differentiation of CD34+ cells into mature DCs [63]. The percentage of peripheral blood dendritic cells (PBDCs) expressing the costimulatory molecule CD86 and the maturation marker CD83 are slightly increased in the aged individuals. The easier explanation for this finding is that this partial activation and maturation of PBDCs may be sustained by the increased inflammatory activity that accompanies ageing [65]. The finding of higher plasma levels of TNF-α in the aged subjects seems to corroborate this hypothesis.

4 Age-Related Phenotypic Changes of Monocytes

The phenotype of monocytes in the elderly is consistently remodelled [43]. Changes in the expression of functionally important cellular receptors can contribute to the modification of immune function characteristic of the elderly [42, 45].

Our previous studies [23, 24, 44] demonstrated important cell adhesion receptor modifications on lymphocyte subsets in the elderly, related to peculiar lymphocyte dysfunctions. A significant expansion of CD14dim CD16bright subpopulation of circulating monocytes in elderly subjects, that may indicate a state of in vivo activation, has been demonstrated [96]. Cell adhesion molecules (CAMs) are surface receptors mediating cell-cell and cell-matrix interactions [102]. CAMs are essential molecules involved in chemotaxis, phagocytosis and killing of microbes and neoplastic cells. The increased susceptibility of elderly people to cancer and infections could be partly explained as a failure in such basic immune defence functions [24].

Since leukocyte adhesion molecules play important roles in mediating a wide variety of leukocyte functions, age-related changes in their expression on monocyte surface could be partially responsible for immune dysfunctions during senescence. Chiricolo et al. [17] documented a decrease in monocyte subpopulations bearing the adhesion molecule CD11a/CD18 and an increase in CD44 antigen density on monocytes in the elderly. These changes might be an event in the mechanism leading to the decreased lymphocyte proliferative response in vitro and to other immunological dysfunctions reported in old subjects.

Considering the central role of the innate immunity in the process of immunosenescence and the involvement of CAMs in the great majority of leukocyte functions, we studied the expression of CD50 and CD62L adhesion molecules in peripheral blood monocytes in the elderly. Such adhesion receptors mediate important cellular functions. CD50 (ICAM-3) is an Ig-related molecule which functions both in cell adhesion and activation processes [20]. Moreover, ICAM-3 is important in the initial scanning of the APC surface by T-cells and, therefore, in generating the specific immune response [78]. CD62L (L-selectin) is an important leucocyte homing receptor which is required to initiate leukocyte capture, rolling and adhesive interactions. In response to inflammatory stimulation, the endothelium expresses a distinct ligand for L-selectin that is sufficient for capture of leukocytes. CD62L is up regulated on circulating leucocytes early after injury and L-selectin mediated signalling may directly initiate or amplify neutrophil activation and localization selectively at sites of inflammation. The percentages of monocytes expressing CD62L is decreased in the elderly, whereas its density expression is unchanged. CD50 expression on monocytes from old subjects show a peculiar attitude: its density expression decreases whereas the number of positive cells is expanded. CD50 is associated with tyrosine kinase activity and functions as a ligand for LFA-1 [24].

CD50 on the surface of APCs plays an important role in the initiation of the immune. Its lower expression on monocytes could therefore contribute to the impaired antigen presentation in the elderly. On the other hand, the increased number of CD50 positive monocytes in the elderly, despite its decreased density expression at a per cell level, could be interpreted as a tentative to counteract the inability to mount strong immune responses [76].

Under some conditions, engagement of surface adhesion molecules induces activation of intracellular signaling cascades (outside-in signaling) that causes altered cellular function and responses. CD50 stimulation on monocytes potently induces secretion and spreading of chemokines (MIP-1alpha, IL-8, and MCP-1 by monocytes and IL-8 by neutrophils) [62]. The increased production of chemokines in the elderly is a well known phenomenon [89]. Therefore CD50 downregulation, as the consequence of its engagement by specific ligand and consequent activation, is the first cellular step in chemokine production.

CD50 and CD62L are released to the medium upon cell stimulation. The increased proportion of granulocytes and monocytes lacking CD62L and the downregulation of CD50 intensity expression may suggest a state of in vivo activation. The presence of soluble CAMs in plasma might serve as a physiological adhesion regulatory system to prevent undesirable leukocyte cell–cell interaction or the attachment of leucocytes to endothelium [22]. Serum levels of solubile cell adhesion receptors are increased in patients with several pathologic states, as well as in the elderly. Therefore CD50 and CD62L shedding from the cell surface of activated monocytes could be interpreted as a tentative to counteract the dangerous effects of an excessive chronic inflammation in the elderly. However, the increased proportion of CD62L negative monocytes in the elderly leads to an impairment in cell adhesion which is the first line of response to acute inflammatory stimuli. This phenomenon likely contributes to the increased susceptibility to acute infections of elderly people.

5   Hormone Modulation and the Stress Response in Senescent Monocytes

Several hormones, differentially modulated during ageing, can regulate immune cell function. For example, ageing is associated with various degrees of insulin resistance together with reduced immune cell activity. Since monocytes express insulin receptors, the perturbation of insulin pathway has been proposed as possible pathogenetic mechanism in the immune derangement in the elderly. Walrand et al. [110] measured circulating monocyte receptor expression and density using flow cytometric detection. The density of monocyte insulin receptors was not affected by age. Therefore, notwithstanding the presence of insulin receptors on monocytes, insulin dysfunction pathway has a limited action on monocyte function during ageing.

Alterations in retinoid metabolism and thyroid dysfunction occur with senescence. Vitamin A and retinoid acid have a wide variety of profound effects on growth, epithelial tissue differentiation and homeostasis, and are involved in maintaining an efficient immune system [74]. An age-related hypo-activation of the retinoid and thyroid nuclear pathways has also been demonstrated on monocytes and lymphocytes [31].

Monocytes play early roles in triggering an acute inflammatory response to many stressful conditions. The expression of leucocyte L-selectin increases during acute stress events such as injury and is temporally related to an early neuroendocrine response. Adrenaline up-regulates whereas TNF-α down-regulates the surface expression of L-selectin on monocytes [90]. The stress response in the elderly is impaired as well as the secretion of stress response hormons (cortisol, catecolamines) thus contributing to the decreased CD62L expression on both monocytes and granulocytes with consequent inhability to trigger acute inflammatory reactions. The downregulation of CD62L on the cell surface could also be the consequence of the increase of proinflammatory cytokines, such as TNF-α, which characterizes immunosenescence [24].

The effect of age in the production of heat shock proteins (Hsp) is very controversial. Hsp are highly conserved proteins and their synthesis is ubiquitous. Constitutive and stress-inducible Hsp play diverse roles in cellular function. Under normal physiological conditions constitutively synthesised Hsp act as molecular chaperones modulating protein folding, assembly, intracellular localisation, secretion, and degradation. When cells endure stress such as high temperature, exercise, oxidative stress, osmotic stress, and inflammation, the expression of inducible

Hsp is increased and these proteins participate in protein refolding and protection, in dissolving aggregated proteins, and in targeting them for degradation. Hsp27 is able to induce an increase in cellular glutathione levels, which works together with ascorbic acid and coenzyme Q as a redox buffer for cellular protection. With ageing there is a general decline in the capacity of cells to respond to stressors and oxidative insult [80].

Some investigators have reported an increase in the basal levels of Hsp with age, which is indicative of an adaptive response to cumulative intracellular stress during ageing and may be associated with increased oxidative stress. On the other hand, a decrease or no effect of age on Hsp basal levels have also been reported [30].

Njemini R et al. [80] investigated the effect of age and inflammation on the induction of Hsp27 in human peripheral blood monocytes, using flow cytometry. There is an age-related decrease in the level of Hsp27, which disappeares in the presence of inflammation. A relationship between the circulating levels of C reactive protein (CRP), IL-6 and TNF-α with Hsp27 levels exists, indicating that cytokines are able to influence the production of Hsp27. The basal level of Hsp27, measured as mean fluorescence intensity (MFI) or as percentage of Hsp27 producing cells, is inversely related to age, for both lymphocytes and monocytes. The expression of Hsp27 as well as Hsp70 is high in monocytes compared to other leukocyte subsets. Because Hsp27 is up-regulated following oxidative stress a likely explanation for this phenomenon is the higher capacity of monocytes to induce ROS and thus to promote oxidative stress. Since Hsp27 production increases with inflammation, it is possible that it exerts some antiinflammatory or immune modulatory effects on leukocytes. Inflammation results in the neutralisation of the age induced Hsp27 repression. Acute phase factors, which mediate the regulation of Hsp genes by interacting with several signaling pathways are most likely involved in this process. TNF-α might be one such factor, since there is a correlation with the percentages of monocytes producing Hsp27. This observation is compatible with the known proinflammatory tendency that is observed during ageing, and might explain the lower values for Hsp27 in the elderly compared to the younger subjects.

6 Monocyte–Macrophage Subset and Cytokine Dysregulation

Monocyte–macrophage heterogeneity has been recognized recently, and an imbalance in subsets could be a reason for the difference between the young adult versus the aged. Mononuclear phagocytes have been subdivided into M-1 and M-2 phenotypes depending on their ability to produce NO and proinfíammatory cytokines (M-1 type) or antiinflammatory agents such as IL-1RA and arginase (M-2 type), suggesting a possibility that one of these types of macrophages accumulates in the spleens of the aged [41, 75]. NOS-2 and arginase, respectively, unique to M-1 and M-2 macrophages, are reduced in macrophages from the aged. It has also been shown that macrophages can be activated by IL-4, leading to suppression of proinflammatory cytokines and enhanced expression of major histocompatibility complex class II (MHC II) genes as well as IL-1RA [47]. As the aged have been shown to have an increased incidence of TH2 T-cells [55], it is conceivable that the macrophages in the aged have markers of IL-4 activation. Mosser and colleagues [3] identified a uniquely hyporesponsive macrophages in spleens from the aged, which has profound influences on immune responses to polysaccharide antigens and may affect the overall ability of the aged to generate an inflammatory response necessary to contain infections. Several studies have examined the capacity of phagocytic mononuclear cells to produce cytokines or chemokines [4, 79]. There are reports of increases, decreases or no effects of age on cytokine release by monocytes, either spontaneously or after LPS stimulation [80, 81]. The decreased response of monocytes from aged persons to LPS in relation to the production of IL-6 and TNF-α has been associated with deficiencies in the activation of protein kinase C (PKC), mitogen-activated protein kinase (MAPK) and deficient expression of c-Fos and c-Jun [57, 59, 91].

Ageing is associated with progressive muscle wasting and low-grade systemic increases in cytokines such as IL-6 and TNF-α. Higher systemic cytokine levels are associated with functional decline and often cachectic disease [7, 93, 109]. Monocytes are involved in skeletal muscle repair through proinflammatory and alternative functions [49, 51]. Przybyla B et al. [88] quantified the total number of macrophages and their pro- and antiinflammatory subpopulations, as well as related cytokine expression, in muscle from young and elderly subjects before and after exercise and found that the number of macrophages within skeletal muscle from the elderly is decreased and their functional properties show defects both at rest and in response to resistance exercise, which could contribute mechanistically to age-related muscle loss [72].

The macrophage lineage displays extreme functional and phenotypic heterogeneity which appears to due in large part to the ability of macrophages to functionally adapt to changes in their tissue microenvironment. This functional plasticity plays a critical role in their ability to respond to tissue damage and/or infection and to contribute to clearance of damaged tissues and invading microorganisms, to contribute to recruitment of the adaptive immune system, and to contribute to resolution of the wound and of the immune response. Ageing alters the proportion and abundance of monocuclear phagocyte subsets. Immune cell functions, including monocyte–macrophage functional plasticity, are known to decrease with age [105].

Evidence has accumulated that environmental influences, such as stromal function and imbalances in hormones and cytokines, contribute significantly to the dysfunction of the adaptive as well as innate immune system in the elderly. A current hypothesis is that the age-associated dysfunction of monocyte–macrophages is the result of their functional adaptation to the age-associated changes in tissue environments. The resultant loss of orchestration of the functional capabilities of these cells would undermine the efficacy of both the innate and adaptive immune systems. Both the T-lymphocyte and B-lymphocyte compartments of the adaptive immune system deteriorate progressively with advancing age [34, 35, 64, 84, 108]. The implications of this hypothesis are that mononuclear phagocyte function may change with age in a tissue specific manner, that changes in macrophage function may contribute significantly to decreased clearance of microorganisms and decreased responsiveness of the adaptive immune system.

DCs and monocytes are progressively affected during ageing. A numerical reduction of PBDCs concomitant with increase of monocytes and an impaired ability of both populations to produce IL-12 have been documented during senescence. The ability of PBDCs to produce IL-12 upon lipopolysaccharide (LPS) stimulation progressively declines with age, while their ability to produce IL-10 remains unaffected. Monocytes show the same selective impairment. Given the central role of IL-12 in the induction of protective immunity, this finding appears relevant to the increased incidence of morbidity and mortality from infections and cancer occurring in aged people. The decrease in IL-12 production may contribute to the dysregulation between the T-helper (TH)1 and TH2 subsets, characterized by a predominant production of TH2 cytokines, which has been described in the elderly [32, 34, 75].

Influenza virus-specific T-cell responses are decreased in the aged, and it is in part a result of defects in antigen presentation. The increased incidence of pneumococcal infections is a result of a defect in the production of antibodies to the capsular polysaccharide antigens, which are critical for killing of the bacteria by the phagocytic cells. This is in part a result of deficiencies in function [14].

Aged subjects are susceptible to infection with Streptococcus pneumoniaebacteria as a result of an inability to make antibodies to capsular polysaccharides. This is partly a result of decreased production of proinflammatory cytokines and increased production of IL-10 by mononuclear phagocytes. A major reason for the inability of macrophages from the aged to support B-cell responses to polysaccharide antigens is a result of a defect in secretion of IL-1 and IL-6. However, the cytokine secretion defect is not limited to IL-1 and IL-6, as other proinflammatory eytokines, such as IL-12 and TNF-α are also produced at lower levels by macrophages from the aged in comparison with young. To understand the molecular basis of cytokine dysregulation in aged mouse macrophages, Chelvarajan RL et al. [15] performed a microarray analysis on RNA from resting and LPS-stimulated macrophages from aged and control mice revealing that immune response (proinflammatory chemokines, cytokines, and their receptors) and signal transduction genes were specifically reduced in aged mouse macrophages following LPS stimulation. Accordingly, expression of IL-1 and IL-6 was reduced, and IL-l0 was increased. There was also decreased expression of IFN-γ. Genes in the Toll-like receptor-signaling pathway leading to nuclear factor-kB activation were also down-regulated by IL-1 receptor-associated kinase 3, a negative regulator of this pathway. An increase in expression of the gene for p38 MAPK was observed with a corresponding increase in protein expression and enzyme activity confirmed by Western blotting. Low doses of a p38 MAPK inhibitor enhanced proinflammatory cytokine production by macrophages and reduced IL-10 levels, indicating that increased p38 MAPK activity has a role in cytokine dysregulation in the aged mouse monocyte–macrophages [8, 19]. Macrophages from the aged were not defective in IL-10 production but produced more of this cytokine than macrophages from the young. Thus, the cytokine production is dysregulated in monocyte–macrophages from the aged following LPS stimulation.

A reduction in secretion of VEGF and expression of CAMs are thought to contribute to the delay in wound healing in the aged. In contrast, peritoneal macrophages from aged mice have been shown to produce more cyclooxygenase-2 (COX-2) and prostaglandin E_2 (PGE_2) in response to LPS stimulation. Moreover, the expression of a variety of TLRs, including TLR4, is decreased in the aged, which could be the reason for a decreased response of mononuclear phagocytes from aged mice to LPS [26].

LPS stimulation not only induces expression of many genes but also represses many genes that are constitutively expressed in mononuclear phagocytes [38]. Some of these repressed genes include PPAR-γ, CCL24, and CCR1. PPAR-γ has been shown to inhibit production of several inflammatory mediators such as TNF-α, IL-1, IL-6, and inducible nitric oxide synthase (NOS) and its suppression by LPS may be a prerequisite for the induction of the LPS-induced inflammatory phenotype [103, 104]. Macrophages from aged mice have a global defect in the TLR signaling pathway and in production of proinflammatory cytokines and chemokines, and the antiinflammatory cytokines are increased, such that the splenic macrophages in the aged have an antiinflammatory phenotype.

Kang et al. [105, 106] observed an age-related increase in COX-2 expression in monocytes. Cyclooxygenase catalyses the formation of prostanoids that are crucial in maintaining homeostasis and important in inflammation. The increased COX-2 in monocytes of older humans, which is mirrored in rats, may have downstream implications in atherosclerosis and cardiovascular risk as mononuclear prostanoids are implicated in atherosclerotic plaque stability. COX-2 is the major COX system in monocytes and monocytes-derived macrophages. Upon activation, these cells are responsible for production of COX-2-derived PGE_2, which is an important signaling molecule. Therefore, increased expression of COX-2 may lead to enhanced PGE_2 production, which is known to promote atherosclerotic plaque instability by stimulating MMP-2 and MMP-9 to degrade plaque architecture. It is interesting to note that in ageing rats, monocyte COX-2 expression increase in line with COX-2 levels in vascular smooth muscle and endothelial cells, indicating that these blood elements may be a predictor of systemic status [107].

The mechanism for an age-related change in COX formation is elusive. However, one mechanism could involve histones. When histones are acetylated by histone acetyltransferase, the DNA becomes more accessible to transcription factors. Also, age-linked increases in oxidative stress, proinflammatory agents (IL-1, IL-6), and total cholesterol levels could be involved [60].

There is some controversy concerning the basis for the decline in production of inflammatory cytokines and oxidative radicals in response to LPS stimulation. Renshaw et al.[28, 92] reported that the expression of TLR on macrophages was reduced with advancing age and that this was the basis for the reduced cytokine production upon stimulation with LPS. Boehmer et al. [9, 10] reported that TLR expression was not impacted by advanced age. The influence of aging appears to be selective. Macrophages from aged mice have increased levels of COX-2 and produce elevated levels of PGE2 upon stimulation with LPS [53, 113]. LPS induction of IL-10 production also appears to be elevated in macrophages from aged rodents and humans [96, 100]. It thus appears that aging selectively impacts LPS-induced signaling cascades such that some functions are depressed and others are elevated. Another example of a signaling deficiency that appears in advanced age is responsiveness to IFN-γ. Although expression of the receptor for IFN-γ appears to be normal, IFNγ-induced phosphorylation of MAPK and STAT-1 is reduced in aged rodents [27, 115]. Oxidative stress is hypothesized to alter transcription factors and nuclear receptors and thus alter the ability of macrophages to respond to inflammatory stimuli [68]. Antioxidants do seem to improve monocyte inflammatory function [87, 101, 114]. Neuroendocrine factors and stress hormones have also been hypothesized to contribute to the immunosenescence and decreased macrophage function. Haynes et al. [54], reported that administration of inflammatory cytokines of the innate immune system enhanced the adaptive immune response of aged mice, so that restoration of the functional balance of mononuclear phagocytes in the elderly will not only improve innate responses but, as a result, improve the function of the adaptive immune system, as well.

References

1. Agrawal A, Agrawal S, Cao JN et al (2007) Altered innate immune functioning of dendritic cells in elderly humans: a role of phosphoinositide 3-kinase-signaling pathway. J Immunol 178:6912–6922
2. Albright JW, Albright JF (1994) Ageing alters the competence of the immune system to control parasitic infection. Immunol Lett 40:279–285
3. Anderson CF, Mosser DM (2002) A novel phenotype for an activated macrophage: the type 2 activated macrophage. J Leukoc Biol 72:101–106
4. Antonini JM, Roberts JR, Clarke RW, Yang HM et al (2001) Effect of age on respiratory defense mechanisms: pulmonary bacterial clearance in Fischer 344 rats after intratracheal instillation of Listeria monocytogenes. Chest 120:240–249
5. Ahluwalia N, Mastro AM, Ball R et al (2001) Cytokine production by stimulated mononuclear cells did not change with aging in apparently healthy, well-nourished women. Mech Ageing Dev 122:1269–1279
6. Ashcroft GS, Horan MA, Ferguson MW et al (1998) Aging alters the inflammatory and endothelial cell adhesion molecule protiles during human cutaneous wound healing. Lab Invest 78:47–58
7. Bautmans L, Njemini R, Lambert M et al (2005) Circulating acute phase mediators and skeletal muscle performance in hospitalized geriatric patients. J Gerontol 60:361–367
8. Beutler B (2004) Inferences, questions and possibilities in Toll-like mceptor signaling. Nature 430:257–263
9. Boehmer ED, Goral J, Faunce DE, Kovacs EJ (2004) Age-dependent decrease in Toll-like receptor 4-mediated proinflammatory cytokine production and mitogen-activated protein kinase expression. J Leukoc Biol 75:342–349
10. Boehmer ED, Meehan MJ, Cutro BT, Kovacs EJ (2005) Aging negativrly skews macrophage TLR2- and TLR4-mediated pro-inflammatory responses without affecting the IL-2-stimulated pathway. Mech Ageing Dev 126:1305–1313
11. Bondada S, Wu H, Robertson DA, Chelvarajan RL (2000) Accessory cell defect in unresponsiveness of neonates and aged to polysaccharide vaccines. Vaccine 19:557–565
12. Bradley SF, Kauffman CA (1990) Aging and the response to Salmonella infection. Exp Gerontol 25:75–80

13. Castle SC (2000) Clinical relevance of age related immune dysfunction. Clin Infect Dise 31:578–585
14. Chelvarajan RL, Collins SM, Van Willigen JM, Bondada S (2005) The unresponsiveness of aged mice to polysaccharide antigens is a result of a defect in macrophage function. J Leukoc Biol 77:503–512
15. Chelvarajan RL, Liu Y, Popa D, Getchell ML et al (2006) Molecular basis of age-associated cytokine dysregulation in LPS-stimulated macrophages. J Leukoc Biol 79:1314–1327
16. Chinetti G, Fruchart JC, Staels B (2000) Peroxisome proliferator-activated receptors (PPARs): nuclear receptors at the crossroads between lipid metabolism and inflammation. Inflamm Res 49:497–505
17. Chiricolo M, Morini MC, Mancini R et al (1995) Cell adhesion molecules CD11a and CD18 in blood monocytes in old age and the consequences for immunological dysfunction. Preliminary results. Gerontology 41:227–234
18. Clark RB (2002) The role of PPARs in inflammation and immunily. J Leukoc Biol 21:388–400
19. Davis RJ (2000) Signal transduction by the JNK group of MAP kinases. Cell 103:239–252
20. de Fougerolles AR, Qin X, Springer TA (1994) Characterization of the function of intercellular adhesion molecule (ICAM)-3 and comparison with ICAM-1 and ICAM-2 in immune responses. J Exp Med 179:619–629
21. Della Bella S, Bierti L, Presicce P et al (2007) Peripheral blood dendritic cells and monocytes are differently regulated in the elderly. Clin Immunol 122:220–228
22. del Pozo MA, Pulido R, Munoz C, Alvarez V et al (1994) Regulation of ICAM-3 (CD50) membrane expression on human neutrophils through proteolytic shedding mechanism. Eur J Immunol 24:2586–2594
23. De Martinis M, Modesti M, Loreto MF et al (2000) Adhesion molecules on peripheral blood lymphocyte subpopulations in the elderly. Life Sci 68:139–151
24. De Martinis M, Modesti M, Ginaldi L (2004) Phenotypic and functional changes of circulating monocytes and polymorphonuclear leucocytes from elderly persons. Immunol Cell Biol 82:415–420
25. DeVeale B, Brummet TL, Seroude L et al (2004) Immunity and aging: the enemy within? Aging Cell 3:195–208
26. Dillon S, Agrawal A, Van Dyke T et al (2004) A Toll-like receptor 2 ligand stimulates Th2 responses in vivo, via induction of extracellular signal-regulated kinase mitogen-activated protein kinase and c-Fos in dendritic cells. J Immunol 172:4733–4743
27. Ding A, Hwang S, Schwab R (1994) Effect of aging on murine macrophages. Diminished response to IFNgamma for enhanced oxidative metabolism. J Immunol 153:2146–2152
28. Donnelly R P, Dickensheets H, Finbloom DS (1999) The interleukin-10 signal transduction pathway and regulation of gene expression in mononuclear phagocytes. J Interferon Cytokine Res 99:563–573
29. Donnini A, Argentati K, Mancini R et al (2002) Phenotype, antigen-presenting capacity, and migration of antigen-presenting cells in young and old age. Exp Gerontol 37:1097–1112
30. Elenkov IJ, Chrousos GP (2002) Stress hormones, proinflammatory and antiinflammatory cytokines, and autoimmunity. Ann N Y Acad Sci 966:290–303
31. Feart C, Pallet V, Boucheron C, Higueret D et al (2005) Aging affects the retinoic acid and the triiodothyronine nuclear receptor mRNA expression in human peripheral blood mononuclear cells. Eur J Endocrinol 152:449–458
32. Fernandez S, Jose P, Avdiushko MG et al (2004) Inhibition of IL-10 receptor function in alveolar macrophages by Toll-like receptor agonists. J Immunol 172:2613–2620
33. Fortunel NO, Hatzfeld A, Hatzfeld JA et al (2000) Transforming growth factor-β: pleiotropic role in the regulation of hematopoiesis. Blood 96:2022–2036
34. Franceschi C, Bonafe M, Valensin S et al (2000) Human immunosenescence: the prevailing of innate immunity, the failing of clonotypic immunity, and the filling of immunological space. Vaccine 18:1717–1720

35. Franceschi C, Bonafe M, Valensin S et al (2000) Inflammaging. An evolutionary perspective on immunosenescence. Ann N Y Acad Sci 908:244–254
36. Franceschi C, Bonafè M (2003) Centenarians as a model of healthy aging. Biochem Soc Transact 31:457–461
37. Friedman G, Ben-Yehuda A, Dabach Y et al (1997) Scavanger receptor activiry and expression of apolipoprotein E mRNA in monocyte derived macrophages of young and old healthy men. Atherosclerosis 128:67–73
38. Gao JJ, Diesl V, Wittmann T et al (2002) Regulation of gene expression in mouse macrophages stimulated with bacterial CpG-DNA and lipopolysaccharide. J Leukoc Biol 72:1234–1245
39. Garg M, Luo W, Kaplan AM, Bondada S (1996) Cellular basis of decreased immune responses to pneumococcal vaccines in aged mice. Infect Immun 64:4456–4462
40. Geiger H, Van Zant G (2002) Thc aging of lympho-hematopoietic stem cells. Nat Immunol 3:329–333
41. Geissmann F, Jung S, Littman DR (2003) Blood monocytes consist of two principal subsets with distinct migratory properties. Immunity 19:71–82
42. Ginaldi L, De Martinis M, D'Ostilio A et al (2001) Changes in the expression of surface receptors on lymphocyte subsets in the elderly: quantitative flow cytometry analysis. Am J Hematol 67:63–72
43. Ginaldi L, De Martinis M, D'Ostilio A et al (1999) The immune system in the elderly. III. Innate immunity. Immunol Res 20:117–126
44. Ginaldi L, De Martinis M, Modesti M et al (2000) Immunophenotypical changes of T lymphocytes in the elderly. Gerontology 46:242–248
45. Ginaldi L, Matutes E, Farahat N et al (1996) Differential expression of T cell antigens in normal peripheral blood lymphocytes: a quantitative analysis by flow cytometry. J Clin Pathol 49:539–544
46. Ginaldi L, Sternberg H (2003) The immune system. In: Timiras PS (ed) Physiological basis of aging and geriatrics, 3rd edn. CRC Press, NY, pp 265–283
47. Gordon S (2003) Alternative activation of macrophages. Nat Rev Immunol 3:23–35
48. Gratchev A, Schledzewski K, Guillot P, Goerdt S (2001) Alternatively activated antigen-presenting cells: molecular repertoire, immune regulation, and healing. Skin Pharmacol Appl Skin Physiol 14:272–279
49. Greiwe JS, Cheng B, Rubin DC et al (2001) Resistance exercise decreases skeletal muscle tumor necrosis factor alpha in frail elderly humans. FASEB J 15:475–482
50. Hakim FT, Flomerfelt FA, Boyiadiis M, Gress RE (2004) Aging, immunity and cancer. Curr Opin Immunol 16:151–156
51. Hamada K, Vannier E, Sacheck JM et al (2005) Senescence of human skeletal muscle impairs the local inflammatory cytokine response to acute eccentric exercise. FASEB J 19:264–266
52. Hausser G, Ludewig B, Gelderblom HR et al (1997) Monocyte-derived dendritic cells represent a transient stage of differentiation in the myeloid lineage. Immunobiology 197:534–542
53. Hayek MG, Mura C, Wu D et al (1997) Enhanced expression of inducible cyclooxygenase with age in murine macrophages. J Immunol 159:2445–2451
54. Haynes L, Eaton SM, Bums EM et al (2004) Inflammatory cytokines overcome age-related defects in CD4 T cell responses in vivo. J Immunol 172:5194–5199
55. Hsu HC, Scott DK, Mountz JD (2005) Impaired apoptosis and immune senescence-cause or effect? Immunol Rev 205:130–146
56. Iwama H, Ohyashiki JH, Hayashi S et al (1998) Telomeric length and telomerase activity vary with age in peripheral blood cells obtained from narmal individuals. Hum Genet 102:397–402
57. Iwasa H, Han J, Ishikawa F (2003) Mitogen-activated protein kinase p38 defines the common senescence-signaling pathway. Genes Cells 8:131–144
58. Janeway CA Jr (2002) Medzhitov R. Innate immune recognition. Annu Rev Immunol 20:197–216

59. Jozsi AC, Dupont-Versteegden EE, Taylor-Jones JM et al (2001) Molecular characteristics of aged muscle reflect an altered ability to respond to exercise. Int J Sport Nutr Exerc Metab 11:7–13

60. Kang Y-S, Kim JY, Bmening SA et al (2004) The C-type lectin SIGN-Rl mediates uptake of the capsular polysaccharide of Streptococcus pneumoniae in the marginal zone of mouse spleen. Proc Natl Acad Sci 101:215–220

61. Kang KB, Van Der Zypp A, Iannazzo L, Majewski H (2006) Age-related changes in monocyte and platelet cyclooxygenase expression in healthy male humans and rats. Transl Res 2006;148:289–294

62. Kessel JM, Hayflick J, Weyrich AS et al (1998) Coengagement of ICAM-3 and Fc receptors induces chemokine secretion and spreading by myeloid leucocytes. J Immunol 160:5579–5587

63. Kiertscher S, Luo J, Dubinett SM, Roth MD (2000) Tumors promote altered maturation and early apoptosis of monocyte-derived dendritic cells. J Immunol 164:1269–1276

64. Kohut ML, Senchina DS, Madden KS et al (2004) Age effects on macrophage function vary by tissue site, nature of stimulant, and exercise behavior. Exp Gerontol 39:1347–1360

65. Krabbe KS, Pedersen M, Bruunsgaard H (2004) Inflammatory mediators in the elderly. Exp Gerontol 39:687–699

66. Kurt I, Abasli D, Cihan M et al (2007) Chitotriosidase levels in healthy elderly subjects. Ann N Y Acad Sci 1100:185–188

67. Lang R, Patel D, Moms JJ, Rutschman RL, Murray PJ (2002) Shaping gene expression in activated and resting primary macrophages by IL-10. J Immunol 169:2253–2263

68. Lavrovsky Y, Chatterjee B, Clark RA, Roy AK (2000) Role of redox-regulated transcription factors in inflammation, aging and age-related diseases. Exp Gerontol 35:521–532

69. Le Morvan C, Cogne M, Drouet M (2001) HLA-A and HLA-B transcription decrease with ageing in peripheral blood leukocytes. Clin Exp Immunol 125:245–250

70. Lloberas J, Celada A (2002) Effect of aging on macrophage function. Exp Gerontol 37:1323–1329

71. Ma J, Chen T, Mandelin J et al (2003) Regulation of macrophage activation. Cell Mol Life Sci 40:2334–2346

72. Malm C, Sjodin TL, Sjoberg B et al (2004) Leukocytes, cytokines, growth factors and hormones in human skeletal muscle and blood after uphill or downhill running. J Physiol 556:983–1000

73. Mancuso P, McNish RW, Peters-Golden M, Brock TG (2001) Evaluation of phagocytosis and arachidonate metabolism by alveolar macrophages and recruited neutrophils from F344xBN rats of different ages. Mech Ageing Dev 122:1899–1913

74. Meydani SN, Han SN, Wu D (2005) Vitamin E and immune response in the aged: molecular mechanisms and clinical implications. Immunol Rev 205:269–284

75. Mills CD, Kincaid K, Alt JM et al (2000) M-1/M-2 macrophages and the Thl/Th2 paradigm. J Immunol 164:6166–6173

76. Moffatt OD, Devitt A, Bell ED (1999) Simmons DL, Gregory CD. Macrophage recognition of ICAM-3 on apoptotic leukocytes. J Immunol 162:6800–6810

77. Monti D, Salvioli S, Capri M et al (2000) Decreased susceptibility to ozidative stress-induced apoptosis of peripheral blood mononuclear cells from healthy elderly and centenarians. Mech Ageing Dev 121:239–250

78. Montoya MC, Sancho D, Bonello G et al (2002) Role of ICAM-3 in the initial interaction of T lymphocytes and APCs. Nat Immunol 3:159–168

79. Mosser DM (2003) The many faces of macrophage activation. J Leukoc Biol 73:209–212

80. Njemini R, Lambert M, Demanet C, Mets T (2006) The effect of aging and inflammation on heat shock protein 27 in human monocytes and lymphocytes. Exp Gerontol 41:312–319

81. Ogawa T, Kitagawa M, Hirokawa K et al (2000) Age-related changes of human bone marrow: a histometric estimation of proliferative cells, apoptotic cells, T cells, B cells and macrophages. Mech Ageing Dev 117:57–68

82. Ortega E, Garcia JJ, De la FM (2000) Modulation of adherence and chemotaxis of macrophages by norepinephrine. Influence of ageing. Mol Cell Biochem 203:113–117
83. Pascual V, Banchereau J, Palucka AK (2003) The central rote of dendritic cells and interferon-alpha in SLE. Curr Opin Rheumatol 15:548–556
84. Plackett TP, Boehmer ED, Faunce DE, Kovacs EJ (2004) Aging and innate immune cells. J Leukoc Biol 76:291–299
85. Pietschmann P, Hahn P, Kudlacek S et al (2000) Surface markers and transendothelial migration of dendritic cells from elderly subjects Exp Gerontol 35:213–224
86. Plowden J, Renshaw-Hcelscher M, Engleman C et al (2004) Innate immunity in aging: impact on macrophage funclion. Aging Cell 3:161–167
87. Poynter ME, Daynes RA (1998) Peroxisome proliferator-activated receptor alpha activation modulates cellular redox status, represses nuclear factor-kappaB signaling, and reduces inflammatory cytokine production in aging. J Biol Chem 273:32833–32841
88. Przybyla B, Gurley C, Harvey JF et al (2006) Aging alters macrophage properties in human skeletal muscle both at rest and in response to acute resistance exercise. Exp Gerontol 41:329–370
89. Pulsatelli L, Meliconi R, Mazzetti I et al (2000) Chemokine production by peripheral blood mononuclear cells in elderly subjects. Mech Ageing Dev 20:89–100
90. Rainer TH, Lam N, Cocks RA (1999) Adrenaline upregulates monocyte L-selectin in vitro. Resuscitation 43:47–55
91. Rao KMK (2001) MAP kinase activation in macrophages. J Leukoc Biol 69:3–10
92. Renshaw M, Rockwell J, Engleman C et al (2002) Cutting edge: impaired Toll-like receptor expression and function in aging. J Immunol 169:4697–4701
93. Reuben DB, Cheh AL, Harris TB et al (2002) Peripheral blood markers of inflammation predict mortality and functional decline in high-functioning community-dwelling older persons. J Am Geriatr Soc 50:638–644
94. Ricote M, Valledor AF, Glass CK (2004) Decoding transcriptional programs regulated by PPARs and LXRs in the macrophage: effects on lipid homeostasis, inflammation, and atherosclerosis. Arterioscler Thromb Vasc Biol 24:230–239
95. Rossi M, Young JW (2005) Human dendritic cells: potent antigen presenting cells at the crossroads of innate and adaptive immunity. J Immunol 175:1373–1381
96. Sadeghi HM, Schnelle JF, Thoma JK et al (1999) Phenotypic and functional characteristics of circulating monocytes of elderly persons. Exp Gerontol 34:959–970
97. Saurwein-Teissl M, Blasko I, Zisterer K et al (2000) An imbalance between pro- and anti-inflammatory cytokines, a characteristic feature of old age. Cytokine 12:1160–1161
98. Sebastian C, Espia M, Serra M et al (2005) MacrophAging: a cellular and molecular review. Immunobiology 210:121–126
99. Shortman K, Wu L (2004) Are dendritic cells end cells? Nat Immunol 5:1105–1106
100. Spencer NF, Norton SI, Harrison LL et al (1996) Dysregulation of IL-10 production with aging: possible linkage to the age-associated decline in DHEA and its sulfated derivative. Exp Gerontol 31:393–408
101. Spencer NF, Poynter ME, Im SY, Daynes RA (1997) Constitutive activation of NF-kappa B in an animal model of aging. Int Immuuol 9:1581–1588
102. Springer TA (1994) Traffic signals for lymphocyte recirculation and leukocyte emigration: the multistep paradigm. Cell 76:301–314
103. Starr R, Willson TA, Viney EM et al (1997) A family of cytokine-inducible inhibitors of signaling. Nature 387:917–921
104. Stout RD, Jiang C, Matta B et al (2005) Macrophages sequentially change their functional phenotype in response to changes in micrcenvironmental influences. J Immunol 175:342–349
105. Stout RD, Suttles J (2005) Immunosenescence and macrophage functional plasticity: dysregulation of macrophage function by age-associated microenvironmental changes. Immunol Rev 205:60–71
106. Swift ME, Bums AL, Gray KL, DiPietro LA (2001) Age-related alterations in the inflammatory response to dermal injury. J Invest Dermatol 117:1027–1035

107. Tracy RP (2003) Emerging relationships of inflammation, cardiovascular disease and chronic diseases of aging. Int J Obes Relat Metab Disord 27:29–34

108. Uyemura K, Castle SC, Makinodan T (2002) The frail elderly: role of dendritic cells in the susceptibility of infection. Mech Ageing Dev 123:955–962

109. Visser M, Pahor M, Taaffe DR et al (2002) Relationship of interleukin-6 and tumor necrosis factor-alpha with muscle mass and muscle strength in elderly men and women: the health ABC study. J Gerontol 57:326–332

110. Walrand S, Guillet C, Boirie Y, Vasson MP (2006) Insulin differentially regulates monocyte and polymorphonuclear neutrophil functions in healthy young and elderly humans. J Clin Endocrinol Metab 91:2738–2748

111. Weng N (2001) Intetplay between telomere length and telomerase in human leukocyte differentiation and aging. J Leukoc Biol 70:861–867

112. Williams JC, Fotherby MD, Foster LA et al (2000) Mononuclear cell adhesion to collagen ex vivo is related to pulse pressure in elderly subjects. Atherosclerosis 151:463–469

113. Wu D, Meydani SN (2004) Mechanism of age-associated upregulation in macrophage PGE2 synthesis. Brain Behav Immun 18:487–494

114. Wu D, Mura C, Beharka AA et al (1998) Age-associated increase in PGE2 synthesis and COX activity in murine macrophages is reversed by vitamin E. Am J Physiol 275:661–668

115. Yoon P, Keylock KT, Hartman ME et al (2004) Macrophage hypo-responsiveness to interferon-gamma in aged mice is associated with impaired signaling through Jak-STAT. Mech Ageing Dev 125:137–143

116. Zhang Y, Blattman JN, Kennedy NJ et al (2004) Regulation of innate and adaptive immune responses by MAP kinase phosphatase 5. Nature 430:793–797

117. Zhang M, Tang H, Guo Z et al (2004) Splenic stroma drives mature dendritic cells to differentiate into regulatory dendritic cells. Nat Immunol 5:1124–1133

118. Zissel G, Schlaak M, Muller-Quemheim J (1999) Age-related decrease in accessory cell function of human alveolar macrophages. J Investig Med 47:51.

Cellular Immunosenescence - NK and NKT Cells

NK Cells in Human Ageing

Raquel Tarazona, Inmaculada Gayoso, Corona Alonso, M. Luisa Pita, Esther Peralbo, Javier G. Casado, Beatriz Sánchez-Correa, Sara Morgado and Rafael Solana

Contents

Abstract: NK cells are cytotoxic lymphocytes that are involved in the early defense against virus infected and tumor cells. NK cells exhibit the capacity to distinguish normal and damaged cells as well as self- and foreign cells. Besides their cytotoxic capacity NK cells also regulate the immune response by producing cytokines and chemokines that directly participate in the elimination of pathogens or activate other cellular components of immunity. NK cells express a broad range of activating receptors and their function is controlled by inhibitory receptors specific for the MHC class I molecules that are ubiquitously expressed on target cells.

Several alterations have been described in human NK cell function with advancing ageing, therefore contributing to immunosenescence. Thus whereas healthy elderly, including centenarians, have preserved NK cell number and function, a decrease in NK cell activity is associated to increased incidence of infectious and inflammatory diseases and to increased risk of death due to infection. Here, we describe recent data about the effects of ageing on NK cells.

Keywords: Ageing • Immunosenescence • NK cells • Cytokines • NK cell ceptors

R. Solana (✉) · I. Gayoso · C. Alonso · M. L. Pita · E. Peralbo
Department of Immunology
Reina Sofia University Hospital
University of Córdoba, Spain
E-mail: rsolana@uco.es

R. Tarazona · J. G. Casado · B. Sánchez-Correa · S. Morgado
Immunology Unit
Department of Physiology
University of Extremadura, Cáceres, Spain

T. Fulop et al. (eds.), *Handbook on Immunosenescence*,
DOI 10.1007/978-1-4020-9062-2_27, © Springer Science+Business Media B.V. 2009

1 Introduction

Although it had been generally accepted that some aspects of innate immunity, are well preserved in ageing (Pawelec et al. 1998), cumulative evidences in the last decade support the existence of age-associated changes in the cellular components of the innate immune system, including NK cells, that are important in the increased susceptibility of elderly individuals to infectious diseases (Delarosa et al. 2006; Solana et al. 2006).

2 Natural Killer Cells

Natural killer (NK) cells are bone marrow-derived lymphocytes that participate in the early defense against intracellular pathogens and tumor cells. NK cells are part of the innate immunity arsenal and have been defined as cytotoxic non-T lymphocytes. The most important characteristic that distinguishes T-cells from NK cells is the T-cell antigen receptor (TcR) which is made from rearranging genes and is clonally expressed (Parham 2006). NK cells act within hours of infection in contrast to T-cells that require several days to arise. NK cells are characterized by the expression of CD56, an isoform of the neural cell adhesion molecule (N-CAM) and/or CD16, the low-affinity IgG Fc receptor (FcγRIIIa). The discovery on NK cells of receptors for polymorphic major histocompatibility complex (MHC) class I molecules has contributed to better understanding of NK cell biology. In spite of this, NK and T-cells have much in common: cell-surface molecules, effector functions as cytokine secretion and cytotoxicity. Many of the cell surface molecules we called NK cell associated receptors (NKR) are also expressed by subpopulations of T-cells and NKR expression on T-cells has been associated to memory/effector cells (Tarazona et al. 2002, 2004; Vallejo et al. 2004; Abedin et al. 2005; Casado et al. 2005; Delarosa et al. 2006; Michel et al. 2006; Gayoso et al. 2007; Solana et al. 2007; Lemster et al. 2008).

Although NK cells have been considered for many years as being a simple, homogenous and unspecific population in comparison with T- or B cells of adaptive immunity, different subsets have been defined according to the expression of NK markers and their capacity to kill or produce cytokines. Thus, human NK cells can be divided into two functional subsets based on their cell surface density of CD56, CD56^{bright} immunoregulatory cells and CD56^{dim} cytotoxic cells. Both subsets have been characterized extensively regarding their different functions, phenotype, and tissue localization. The CD56^{bright} NK cell subset has a distinctive role in the innate immune response as the primary source of NK cell-derived immunoregulatory cytokines (Cooper et al. 2001; Farag et al. 2003; Wendt et al. 2006). CD56^{dim} and CD56^{bright} subsets also differ in the expression of chemokine receptors that may contribute to cell trafficking (Cooper et al. 2001; Fehniger et al. 2003; Berahovich et al. 2006).

NK cells were long thought to respond directly to tumor or infected cells, but recent data show that NK cells acquire functionality through priming by dendritic cells (DC; Zitvogel et al. 2006; Long 2007; Lucas et al. 2007). This cross-talk between NK cells and myeloid DC also leads to DC maturation and may determine the quality and strength of the adaptive immunity responses (Vitale et al. 2005; Moretta et al. 2006).

NK cells exhibit the capacity to distinguish normal and damaged cells as well as self- and foreign cells. NK cell function is controlled by inhibitory receptors for the MHC class I molecules that are ubiquitously expressed on target cells (Table 1). In consequence, MHC class I positive targets are more resistant to NK mediated lysis. Human receptors for HLA class I molecules can be included into two structural types, those with immunoglobulin (Ig)-type domains (killer Ig-like receptors (KIR) and leukocyte immunoglobulin-like receptor) and those with lectin-like domains called CD94/NKG2 receptors. Inhibitory and activating forms of KIR and CD94/NKG2 receptors have been described. The ligands for KIRs are polymorphic determinants of HLA-A, HLA-B and HLA-C molecules whereas the ligands for the human CD94/NKG2 receptor are complexes of HLA-E bound to peptides derived from the leader sequences of other HLA class I molecules (Borrego et al. 2002; Lopez-Botet et al. 2004; Lanier 2005; Guma et al. 2006). HLA-G, a non-classical MHC class I molecule, is recognized by Leukocyte immunoglobulin-like receptor subfamily B member 1 (LILRB1/LIR1/ILT2/CD85j) and member 2 (LILRB2/LIR2/ILT4/CD85d) and KIR2DL4 (Shiroishi et al. 2006). Inhibitory receptors play a role in "missing-self" recognition, that confers to NK cells the capacity to attack cells that lose or downregulate the expression of MHC class I molecules. However, the expressions of inhibitory receptors on NK cells is not uniform and are germline-encoded by a set of polymorphic genes that segregate independently from MHC genes. Therefore, how NK cell self-tolerance arises in vivo is still poorly understood.

Licensing of NK cells by self-MHC class I has been proposed as a mechanisms for NK cell tolerance to self. This process takes place during NK cell maturation and involves inhibitory receptors that recognize target cell MHC class I molecules. This process results in two types of tolerant NK cells: functionally competent (licensed) NK cells, whose effector responses are inhibited by self-MHC class I molecules through the same receptors that conferred licensing, and functionally incompetent

Table 1 HLA class I specific inhibitory receptors expressed on human peripheral blood NK cells

Receptor	Ligand
KIR2DL1	HLA-C group 2
KIR2DL2/3	HLA-C group 1
KIR3DL1	HLA-B alleles
KIR3DL2	HLA-A alleles
CD94/NKG2A	HLA-E
KIR2DL4	HLA-G
ILT-2/CD85j	HLA-G and other HLA class I molecules
ILT-4/CD85d	HLA-G and other HLA class I molecules

(unlicensed) NK cells. Although this process has been defined for mouse NK cells several findings suggest that human NK cells also undergo this maturation process termed licensing (Kim et al. 2005; Parham 2006; Raulet 2006; Raulet and Vance 2006; Yokoyama and Kim 2006). Once NK cells acquire functional competence through "licensing" by self-MHC molecules, the result of effector-target interactions is governed by the integration of inhibitory and activating signals that determines whether the NK cell is finally activated, secretes cytokines and lyses target cells (Gasser and Raulet 2006).

NK cells recognize infected cells or tumor cells by using different types of activating receptors (Table 2) that may act in synergy to enhance cytotoxicity or cytokine release after activation (Bryceson et al. 2006). Activating receptors expressed by NK cells include besides the well characterized receptor CD16 that binds FcγRIIIa, NKG2D, CD244, NKp80 and the natural cytotoxicity receptors (NCR) NKp30, NKp46, NKp44. Ligands for activating receptors comprise both non-self ligands and self proteins up-regulated on damaged cells.

The C-type lectin-like receptor NKG2D is unique among activating receptors in that it recognizes a wide range of ligands some of which are primarily expressed in "stressed" tissues or on tumor cells. Human NKG2D ligands are the MHC class I chain related (MIC) proteins MICA and MICB and the UL-16 binding proteins ULBP-1, ULBP-2, ULBP-3 and ULBP-4 (Eagle and Trowsdale 2007; Mistry and O'Callaghan 2007).

NKp30 and NKp46 are constitutively expressed in NK cells and NKp44 is induced after activation (Arnon et al. 2006; Bryceson et al. 2006; Gasser and Raulet 2006). The NKp46 and NKp44 receptors recognize viral haemagglutinins (Draghi et al. 2007; Ho et al. 2008; Cagnano et al. 2008) and NKp30 has been shown to bind a still undefined ligand on DCs. This binding can be inhibited by

Table 2 Activating receptors expressed on human peripheral blood NK cells

Receptor	Ligand
CD16	IgG
NKp30	Unknown
NKp46	Viral haemaglutinin
NKp44*	Viral haemaglutinin
KIR2DS1	HLA-C group 2
KIR2DS2	HLA-C group 1
KIR2DS3	Unknown
KIR3DS1	HLA-Bw4?
CD94/NKG2C	HLA-E
NKG2D	MICA/B, ULBP1-4
CD244 (2B4)	CD48
DNAM-1	CD155, CD112
CRACC	CRACC
NTB-A	NTB-A

* Induced after activation

the main tegument protein of human cytomegalovirus, pp65 (Arnon et al. 2005, 2006).

Along with CD244, that binds CD48, other members of the signaling lymphocytic activating molecule (SLAM) family of NK cell receptors have been identified: NTB-A and CRACC, which bind NTB-A and CRACC, respectively.

Strong stimulatory signaling resulting from increased levels of stimulatory ligands can often overcome inhibitory signals provided by MHC class I molecules expressed on target cells (Bauer et al. 1999; Cerwenka et al. 2000; Diefenbach et al. 2000).

3   Effect of Ageing on NK Cell Number and Kinetics

Several alterations have been described in NK cells with advancing age, both in animals and humans. In old humans, contradictory data exist due mainly to the different selection criteria of the elderly populations studied, a common problem when comparing studies by different research groups. Thus, whereas there are studies showing that overall NK cell number and cytotoxicity is not significantly affected in very healthy elderly people including centenarians, in other studies that have not used the same strict selection criteria, the number or functions of these cells from elderly subjects are decreased (Table 3).

In a recent study it has been shown that ageing has an impact on NK cell kinetics (Zhang et al. 2007). The analysis of NK cell homeostasis using deuterium-enriched glucose has shown that these cells are in a state of dynamic homeostasis consistent with a model of postmitotic maturation preceding circulation and with a turnover time in blood of about 2 weeks. In young healthy individuals the proliferation rate is $4,3\pm2,4\%$/day, equivalent to a doubling time of 16 days, the total production rate is $15\pm7\times10^6$ cells/l/day and the half-life is approximately 10 days. However in NK cells from healthy elderly subjects the proliferation and production rates are significantly lower ($2,5\pm1,0\%$/day and $7,3\pm3,7\times10^6$ cells/l/day, respectively; Zhang et al. 2007). This study demonstrates that NK cell numbers are well preserved in healthy ageing, in spite of evidences for a reduction in total NK cell production rates of about 50%. These results suggest an increased proportion of long-lived NK cells in the elderly subjects. This may be related to the increased proportion of CD56[dim] cells, as previously reported in elderly subjects (Borrego et al. 1999).

The decreased proliferation and production rates of NK cells in the elderly can be associated to the telomere shortening observed in the elderly. Thus it has been shown that NK lymphocytes show an age-associated loss of telomeres together with an age-associated reduction of telomerase activity that was evident in individuals over 80 years of age in particular in the oldest individuals and in those with increased NK cell numbers (Mariani et al. 2003a, b).

Table 3 Effect of ageing on the NK cell compartment

	Decreased	Preserved	Increased
Percentage of NK cells			Facchini et al. 1987; Mariani et al. 1994; Borrego et al. 1999; Lutz et al. 2005
Number of NK cells			Borrego et al. 1999; Di Lorenzo G. et al. 1999
CD56 dim subset			Krishnaraj 1997; Borrego et al. 1999
CD56 bright subset	Krishnaraj 1997; Borrego et al. 1999		
Perforin content	Rukavina et al. 1998	Mariani et al. 1996	
Cytotoxicity	Facchini et al. 1987; Mariani et al. 1990; Solana and Mariani 2000; Ogata et al. 2001	Sansoni et al. 1993; Kutza and Murasko 1994, 1996	
Intracellular signaling	Mariani et al. 1998a		
ADCC		Sansoni et al. 1993; Mariani et al. 1998a; Solana and Mariani 2000; Plackett et al. 2004; Lutz et al. 2005	
Response to cytokines	Dussault and Miller 1994; Borrego et al. 1999; Murasko and Jiang 2005		
Cytokine and chemokine production	Mariani et al. 2001 2000a, 2000b; Mocchegiani and Malavolta 2004		
In vivo proliferation and production rates	Zhang et al. 2007		

4 NK Cells and Health Status in the Elderly

An extensive analysis of NK cell number and function in elderly individuals strengthens the significance of NK cell activity in healthy ageing and longevity. Thus a decreased NK cell function in old individuals is associated with an increased incidence of infectious diseases and death due to infection in elderly humans (Ogata et al. 1997, 2001) and elderly people (aged >85 years) with low numbers of NK cells were reported to have three times the mortality risk in the first two years of follow-up than those with high NK cell numbers (Remarque and Pawelec 1998). It has been also reported that decreased NK cell activity in the elderly is also associated with increased frequency of disorders as atherosclerosis

(Bruunsgaard et al. 2001). In a similar way it has been shown that a preserved NK function is related to better health status and lower incidence of respiratory tract infections in elderly individuals and to a better response to influenza vaccination (Mysliwska et al. 2004). Additional evidences supporting the significance of NK cells in healthy ageing come from studies in centenarians, that, in general, have a very well preserved NK cell cytotoxicity (Sansoni et al. 1992, 1993; Franceschi et al. 1995). Furthermore, when NK cells are studied in nonagenarians and centenarians the results show that higher NK cell numbers and NK cytolytic activity were associated with better retained ability to maintain an autonomous life style. These parameters were also associated with higher serum vitamin D levels, a well-nourished status and balanced basal metabolism, indicating the impact of hormonal and nutritional variables on NK cell function in elderly people and again emphasizing that results on NK cells may depend to a much greater extent than T-cells on the state of health of the individual (Mariani et al. 1998b; Pawelec et al. 1998). Moreover, the percentage of NK cells has been shown to correlate with serum zinc and selenium concentrations, and with plasma vitamin E and ubiquinone-10 concentrations, confirming that micronutrients may affect the number and function of NK cells in old age (Mariani et al. 1998b; Ravaglia et al. 2000). This suggests that any analysis of biomarkers of immunosenescence must of necessity take these variables into account.

Together, these results support the fact that preserved NK cytotoxicity can be considered a marker of healthy ageing, whereas low NK cytotoxicity is a predictor of increased morbidity and mortality due to infections.

5 Effect of Ageing on the Expression and Function of NK Cell Receptors

Although the overall NK cell cytotoxicity seems not to be significantly affected in the very healthy elderly donors, it has been demonstrated that, even in these donors, there is a decreased cytotoxicity per NK cell, associated with defective signal transduction (Table 3; Mariani et al. 1998a; Solana and Mariani 2000). Thus, the maintenance of NK cell activity is probably due to a compensatory increase in the number of NK cells to accommodate a possible decrement of NK cell cytotoxicity (Mariani et al. 1994). This increased cell number has been related to a higher number of $CD56^{dim}$ rather than $CD56^{bright}$ subset containing the most cytotoxic NK cells (Borrego et al. 1999; Solana et al. 1999). Neither the binding of effector cells to the target cells nor the perforin content of NK cells is significantly different in the old and young groups. On the contrary the defective NK cell cytotoxicity is associated with a decreased capacity of NK cells to release IP3 after interacting with the target cells and a delayed hydrolysis of PIP2, indicating that the PKC-dependent pathway is affected as a consequence of ageing (Mariani et al. 1998a). However NK activation and cytotoxic granule release induced by CD16 crosslinking is not affected by ageing (Pawelec et al. 1998; Solana et al. 1999; Solana and Mariani 2000; Bruunsgaard et al. 2001; Lutz et al. 2005).

Furthermore the PI-3-kinase pathway coupled to CD16 triggering is not significantly affected in NK cells from elderly people, indicating that the transduction pathways involved in natural or CD16-dependent NK cytotoxicity are differentially affected by ageing (Mariani et al. 1998a; Solana and Mariani 2000).

Despite the maintenance of CD16-mediated killing, the decreased per-cell NK cytotoxicity against the classic target cell line K562 suggests that the expression and/or the functionality of other NK activating receptors are likely to be defective in the elderly. Very little is known about the effects of senescence on the function of NK receptors, and discrepant results have been reported in this context. Whereas it was reported that the expression of HLA-specific killer immunoglobulin-like receptors is not significantly affected in NK cells from elderly compared to young donors (Mariani et al. 1994), other study has shown that NK cells present an age-related increase in KIR expression and a reciprocal decrease in CD94/NKG2A expression, although the CD94/NKG2A inhibitory signaling pathway is intact (Lutz et al. 2005).

In relation with the expression of other NK receptors involved in NK cell cytotoxicity, our results show that NK cells from elderly donors have a decreased expression of the activating receptor NKp30 (Fig. 1). NKp30 mediates the crosstalk between NK and DCs via the recognition of an unknown ligand expressed on DCs. As summarized on Figure 1 the engagement of the NKp30 receptor can lead either to a direct killing of DCs by NK cells, or to the secretion of IFN-gamma and TNF-alpha and the subsequent maturation of DCs. Therefore NK-activated DCs loaded with tumor or virally derived antigen have an increased capacity to prime T-cells. In return, activated DCs release Th1 cytokines that further enhances NK activation (Arnon et al. 2005, 2006). The decreased expression of this receptor on NK cells

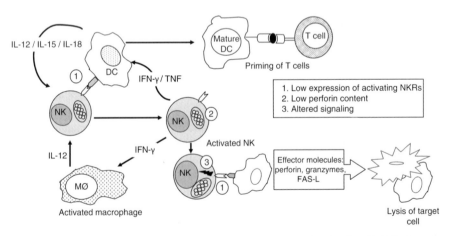

Fig. 1 Effect of human ageing on NK cell function. Cross-talk of NK cells with DCs through NKp30 receptor interaction with its unknown ligand results in inducing DCs maturation and NK cell activation. Whereas DCs collaborate with T-cells in the initiation of adaptive response, activated NK cells produce cytokines and kill target cells. Age-associated alterations in NK cell include: (1) Low expression of activating NKRs that could result in defective cross-talk with dendritic cells and defective recognition of target cells, (2) low perforin content, and (3) altered signal transduction

from elderly individuals should also affect the interaction between these cells leading to a decreased capacity to collaborate in the initiation of the adaptive immune response against virus infected or tumor cells (Fig. 1).

6 Effect of Ageing on NK Cell Response to Cytokines

Cytokine activation of NK cells results in enhanced cytotoxicity and in the synthesis and release of cytokines and chemokines. The enhancement of the cytotoxic activity of NK cells in response to IL-2, IL-12 or IFN-α and γ is well preserved in the healthy elderly. However, the capacity of these cytokine-activated killer cells to lyse the NK-resistant Daudi cell line is significantly decreased in the elderly (Kutza and Murasko 1994, 1996; Murasko and Jiang 2005). A major effect of ageing on cytokine and chemokine production by NK cells is a marked early decrease in IFN-γ secretion in response to IL-2, which can be overcome by increasing the incubation time (Murasko and Jiang 2005). In a similar way the production of MIP-1α, Rantes

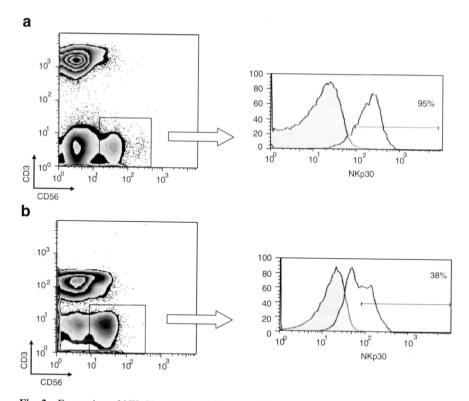

Fig. 2 Expression of NKp30 on NK cells from healthy young (a) and elderly (b) individuals. Peripheral blood lymphocytes were labeled with monoclonal antibodies against CD3, CD56 and NKp30. Results were analysed with a FACSCanto cytometer. Reduction of percentage and mean fluorescence channel of NKp30 was observed in elderly individuals

and IL-8 chemotactic cytokines by NK cells is decreased both in elderly subjects in response to IL-2 and in nonagenarians in response to IL-2 or IL-12 although these cells express the corresponding chemokine receptors. Because of the co-stimulatory role of chemokines on NK cell responses, the decreased production of chemokines can be involved in the defective functional activity of NK cells from old subjects (Mariani et al. 2001, 2002a, b).

Ageing also affects the response of NK cells to IFN-α/β both in mice and humans. This decreased response could be related to the delay in virus clearance observed in aged mice (Murasko and Jiang 2005). These results suggest that NK cells do show an age-associated defect in their response to cytokines, with a subsequent detriment both in their capacity to kill target cells and synthesize cytokines and chemokines.

7   Conclusions and Perspectives

NK cells are a key component of innate immunity in the elimination of virus infected or tumor cells. Recent evidences also support their significance in the initiation of adaptive responses by their crosstalk with DCs and subsequent activation of T-cells. NK cells can be affected by ageing, although several studies have shown a good correlation between the number and/or function of NK cells and the maintenance of an adequate health status in elderly and very elderly people (including nonagenarians and centenarians). On the contrary a decreased NK cell function is associated to increased risk of infectious diseases and risk of death due to infections, supporting the importance of the altered functions of NK cells in the age-associated deterioration of the immune system called immunosenescence.

Our recent finding that NK cells from healthy elderly individuals have a decreased expression of NKp30 receptor, important not only in NK cytotoxicity but also in regulating their cross-talk with DCs strongly support that the alterations in NK cells by ageing may have important consequences that may help to explain the association between a preserved NK cell function and the maintenance of a healthy status. Further studies on the effect of ageing on all NK cell subsets, on the expression and function of activating and inhibitory receptors and a more profound study of the molecular mechanisms involved in these processes are required to better understand the contribution of NK cell ageing to immunosenescence. Considering the increasing advances in the understanding of the mechanisms involved in NK cell interactions not only with tumor and virus infected target cells but also with other cells of the immune system the analysis of how ageing affect these different processes is mandatory.

References

Abedin S, Michel JJ, Lemster B, Vallejo AN (2005) Diversity of NKR expression in aging T cells and in T cells of the aged: the new frontier into the exploration of protective immunity in the elderly. Exp Gerontol 40:537–548

Arnon TI, Achdout H, Levi O, Markel G, Saleh N, Katz G, Gazit R, Gonen-Gross T, Hanna J, Nahari E, Porgador A, Honigman A, Plachter B, Mevorach D, Wolf DG, Mandelboim O (2005) Inhibition of the NKp30 activating receptor by pp65 of human cytomegalovirus. Nat Immunol 6:515–523

Arnon TI, Markel G, Mandelboim O (2006) Tumor and viral recognition by natural killer cells receptors. Semin Cancer Biol 16:348–358

Bauer S, Groh V, Wu J, Steinle A, Phillips JH, Lanier LL, Spies T (1999) Activation of NK cells and T cells by NKG2D, a receptor for stress-inducible MICA. Science 285:727–729

Berahovich RD, Lai NL, Wei Z, Lanier LL, Schall TJ (2006) Evidence for NK cell subsets based on chemokine receptor expression. J Immunol 177:7833–7840

Borrego F, Alonso MC, Galiani MD, Carracedo J, Ramirez R, Ostos B, Pena J, Solana R (1999) NK phenotypic markers and IL2 response in NK cells from elderly people. Exp Gerontol 34:253–265

Borrego F, Kabat J, Kim DK, Lieto L, Maasho K, Pena J, Solana R, Coligan JE (2002) Structure and function of major histocompatibility complex (MHC) class I specific receptors expressed on human natural killer (NK) cells. Mol Immunol 38:637–660

Bruunsgaard H, Pedersen AN, Schroll M, Skinhoj P, Pedersen BK (2001) Decreased natural killer cell activity is associated with atherosclerosis in elderly humans. Exp Gerontol 37:127–136

Bryceson YT, March ME, Ljunggren HG, Long EO (2006) Activation, coactivation, and costimulation of resting human natural killer cells. Immunol Rev 214:73–91

Cagnano E, Hershkovitz O, Zilka A, Bar-Ilan A, Golder A, Sion-Vardy N, Bogdanov-Berezovsky A, Mandelboim O, Benharroch D, Porgador A (2008) Expression of ligands to NKp46 in benign and malignant melanocytes. J Invest Dermatol 128:972–979

Casado JG, Soto R, Delarosa O, Peralbo E, del CM-V, Rioja L, Pena J, Solana R, Tarazona R (2005) CD8 T cells expressing NK associated receptors are increased in melanoma patients and display an effector phenotype. Cancer Immunol Immunother 54:1162–1171

Cerwenka A, Bakker AB, McClanahan T, Wagner J, Wu J, Phillips JH, Lanier LL (2000) Retinoic acid early inducible genes define a ligand family for the activating NKG2D receptor in mice. Immunity 12:721–727

Cooper MA, Fehniger TA, Caligiuri MA (2001) The biology of human natural killer-cell subsets. Trends Immunol 22:633–640

Delarosa O, Pawelec G, Peralbo E, Wikby A, Mariani E, Mocchegiani E, Tarazona R, Solana R (2006) Immunological biomarkers of ageing in man: changes in both innate and adaptive immunity are associated with health and longevity. Biogerontology 7:471–481

Di Lorenzo G., Balistreri CR, Candore G, Cigna D, Colombo A, Romano GC, Colucci AT, Gervasi F, Listi F, Potestio M, Caruso C (1999) Granulocyte and natural killer activity in the elderly. Mech Ageing Dev 108:25–38

Diefenbach A, Jamieson AM, Liu SD, Shastri N, Raulet DH (2000) Ligands for the murine NKG2D receptor: expression by tumor cells and activation of NK cells and macrophages. Nat Immunol 1:119–126

Draghi M, Pashine A, Sanjanwala B, Gendzekhadze K, Cantoni C, Cosman D, Moretta A, Valiante NM, Parham P (2007) NKp46 and NKG2D recognition of infected dendritic cells is necessary for NK cell activation in the human response to influenza infection. J Immunol 178:2688–2698

Dussault I, Miller SC (1994) Decline in natural killer cell-mediated immunosurveillance in aging mice—a consequence of reduced cell production and tumor binding capacity. Mech Ageing Dev 75:115–129

Eagle RA, Trowsdale J (2007) Promiscuity and the single receptor: NKG2D. Nat Rev Immunol 7:737–744

Facchini A, Mariani E, Mariani AR, Papa S, Vitale M, Manzoli FA (1987) Increased number of circulating Leu 11+ (CD 16) large granular lymphocytes and decreased NK activity during human ageing. Clin Exp Immunol 68:340–347

Farag SS, VanDeusen JB, Fehniger TA, Caligiuri MA (2003) Biology and clinical impact of human natural killer cells. Int J Hematol 78:7–17

Fehniger TA, Cooper MA, Nuovo GJ, Cella M, Facchetti F, Colonna M, Caligiuri MA (2003) CD56bright natural killer cells are present in human lymph nodes and are activated by T cell-derived IL-2: a potential new link between adaptive and innate immunity. Blood 101:3052–3057

Franceschi C, Monti D, Sansoni P, Cossarizza A (1995) The immunology of exceptional individuals: the lesson of centenarians. Immunol Today 16:12–16

Gasser S, Raulet DH (2006) Activation and self-tolerance of natural killer cells. Immunol Rev 214:130–142:130–142

Gayoso I, Pita ML, Peralbo E, Alonso C, Dela RO, Casado JG, Tarazona R, Solana R (2007) Remodelling of the CD8 T cell compartment in the elderly: expression of NK associated receptors on T cells is associated to the expansion of the effector memory subset. In Pawelec G (ed) T cells in ageing, Landes: Austin, TX

Guma M, Angulo A, Lopez-Botet M (2006) NK cell receptors involved in the response to human cytomegalovirus infection. Curr Top Microbiol Immunol 298:207–223

Ho JW, Hershkovitz O, Peiris M, Zilka A, Bar-Ilan A, Nal B, Chu K, Kudelko M, Kam YW, Achdout H, Mandelboim M, Altmeyer R, Mandelboim O, Bruzzone R, Porgador A (2008) H5-type influenza virus hemagglutinin is functionally recognized by the natural killer-activating receptor NKp44. J Virol 82:2028–2032

Kim S, Poursine-Laurent J, Truscott SM, Lybarger L, Song YJ, Yang L, French AR, Sunwoo JB, Lemieux S, Hansen TH, Yokoyama WM (2005) Licensing of natural killer cells by host major histocompatibility complex class I molecules. Nature 436:709–713

Krishnaraj R (1997) Senescence and cytokines modulate the NK cell expression. Mech Ageing Dev 96:89–101

Kutza J, Murasko DM (1994) Effects of aging on natural killer cell activity and activation by interleukin-2 and IFN-alpha. Cell Immunol 155:195–204

Kutza J, Murasko DM (1996) Age-associated decline in IL-2 and IL-12 induction of LAK cell activity of human PBMC samples. Mech Ageing Dev 90:209–222

Lanier LL (2005) NK cell recognition. Annu Rev Immunol 23:225–274

Lemster BH, Michel JJ, Montag DT, Paat JJ, Studenski SA, Newman AB, Vallejo AN (2008) Induction of CD56 and TCR-independent activation of T cells with aging. J Immunol 180:1979–1990

Long EO (2007) Ready for prime time: NK cell priming by dendritic cells. Immunity 26:385–387

Lopez-Botet M, Angulo A, Guma M (2004) Natural killer cell receptors for major histocompatibility complex class I and related molecules in cytomegalovirus infection. Tissue Antigens 63:195–203

Lucas M, Schachterle W, Oberle K, Aichele P, Diefenbach A (2007) Dendritic cells prime natural killer cells by trans-presenting interleukin 15. Immunity 26:503–517

Lutz CT, Moore MB, Bradley S, Shelton BJ, Lutgendorf SK (2005) Reciprocal age related change in natural killer cell receptors for MHC class I. Mech Ageing Dev 126:722–731

Mariani E, Mariani AR, Meneghetti A, Tarozzi A, Cocco L, Facchini A (1998a) Age-dependent decreases of NK cell phosphoinositide turnover during spontaneous but not Fc-mediated cytolytic activity. Int Immunol 10:981–989

Mariani E, Meneghetti A, Formentini I, Neri S, Cattini L, Ravaglia G, Forti P, Facchini A (2003a) Different rates of telomere shortening and telomerase activity reduction in CD8 T and CD16 NK lymphocytes with ageing. Exp Gerontol 38:653–659

Mariani E, Meneghetti A, Formentini I, Neri S, Cattini L, Ravaglia G, Forti P, Facchini A (2003b) Telomere length and telomerase activity: effect of ageing on human NK cells. Mech Ageing Dev 124:403–408

Mariani E, Meneghetti A, Neri S, Ravaglia G, Forti P, Cattini L, Facchini A (2002a) Chemokine production by natural killer cells from non-agenarians. Eur J Immunol 32:1524–1529

Mariani E, Monaco MC, Cattini L, Sinoppi M, Facchini A (1994) Distribution and lytic activity of NK cell subsets in the elderly. Mech Ageing Dev 76:177–187

Mariani E, Pulsatelli L, Meneghetti A, Dolzani P, Mazzetti I, Neri S, Ravaglia G, Forti P, Facchini A (2001) Different IL-8 production by T and NK lymphocytes in elderly subjects. Mech Ageing Dev 122:1383–1395

Mariani E, Pulsatelli L, Neri S, Dolzani P, Meneghetti A, Silvestri T, Ravaglia G, Forti P, Cattini L, Facchini A (2002b) RANTES and MIP-1alpha production by T lymphocytes, monocytes and NK cells from non-agenarian subjects. Exp Gerontol 37:219–226

Mariani E, Ravaglia G, Meneghetti A, Tarozzi A, Forti P, Maioli F, Boschi F, Facchini A (1998b) Natural immunity and bone and muscle remodelling hormones in the elderly. Mech Ageing Dev 102:279–292

Mariani E, Roda P, Mariani AR, Vitale M, Degrassi A, Papa S, Facchini A (1990) Age-associated changes in CD8+ and CD16+ cell reactivity: clonal analysis. Clin Exp Immunol 81:479–484

Mariani E, Sgobbi S, Meneghetti A, Tadolini M, Tarozzi A, Sinoppi M, Cattini L, Facchini A (1996) Perforins in human cytolytic cells: the effect of age. Mech Ageing Dev 92:195–209

Michel JJ, Turesson C, Lemster B, Atkins SR, Iclozan C, Bongartz T, Wasko MC, Matteson EL, Vallejo AN (2006) CD56-expressing T cells that have features of senescence are expanded in rheumatoid arthritis. Arthritis Rheum 56:43–57

Mistry AR, O'Callaghan CA (2007) Regulation of ligands for the activating receptor NKG2D. Immunology 121:439–447

Mocchegiani E, Malavolta M (2004) NK and NKT cell functions in immunosenescence. Aging Cell 3:177–184

Moretta L, Ferlazzo G, Bottino C, Vitale M, Pende D, Mingari MC, Moretta A (2006) Effector and regulatory events during natural killer-dendritic cell interactions. Immunol Rev 214:219–228:219–228

Murasko DM, Jiang J (2005) Response of aged mice to primary virus infections. Immunol Rev 205:285–296

Mysliwska J, Trzonkowski P, Szmit E, Brydak LB, Machala M, Mysliwski A (2004) Immunomodulating effect of influenza vaccination in the elderly differing in health status. Exp Gerontol 39:1447–1458

Ogata K, An E, Shioi Y, Nakamura K, Luo S, Yokose N, Minami S, Dan K (2001) Association between natural killer cell activity and infection in immunologically normal elderly people. Clin Exp Immunol 124:392–397

Ogata K, Yokose N, Tamura H, An E, Nakamura K, Dan K, Nomura T (1997) Natural killer cells in the late decades of human life. Clin Immunol Immunopathol 84:269–275

Parham P (2006) Taking license with natural killer cell maturation and repertoire development. Immunol Rev 214:155–160.:155–160

Pawelec G, Solana R, Remarque E, Mariani E (1998) Impact of aging on innate immunity. J Leukoc Biol 64:703–712

Plackett TP, Boehmer ED, Faunce DE, Kovacs EJ (2004) Aging and innate immune cells. J Leukoc Biol 76:291–299

Raulet DH (2006) Missing self recognition and self tolerance of natural killer (NK) cells. Semin Immunol 18:145–150

Raulet DH, Vance RE (2006) Self-tolerance of natural killer cells. Nat Rev Immunol 6:520–531

Ravaglia G, Forti P, Maioli F, Bastagli L, Facchini A, Mariani E, Savarino L, Sassi S, Cucinotta D, Lenaz G (2000) Effect of micronutrient status on natural killer cell immune function in healthy free-living subjects aged >/=90 y. Am J Clin Nutr 71:590–598

Remarque E, Pawelec G (1998) T cell immunosenescence and its clinical relevance in man. Rev Clin Gerontol 8:5–14

Rukavina D, Laskarin G, Rubesa G, Strbo N, Bedenicki I, Manestar D, Glavas M, Christmas SE, Podack ER (1998) Age-related decline of perforin expression in human cytotoxic T lymphocytes and natural killer cells. Blood 92:2410–2420

Sansoni P, Brianti V, Fagnoni F, Snelli G, Marcato A, Passeri G, Monti D, Cossarizza A, Franceschi C (1992) NK cell activity and T-lymphocyte proliferation in healthy centenarians. Ann N Y Acad Sci 663:505–507

Sansoni P, Cossarizza A, Brianti V, Fagnoni F, Snelli G, Monti D, Marcato A, Passeri G, Ortolani C, Forti E (1993) Lymphocyte subsets and natural killer cell activity in healthy old people and centenarians. Blood 82:2767–2773

Shiroishi M, Kuroki K, Rasubala L, Tsumoto K, Kumagai I, Kurimoto E, Kato K, Kohda D, Maenaka K (2006) Structural basis for recognition of the non-classical MHC molecule HLA-G by the leukocyte Ig-like receptor B2 (LILRB2/LIR2/ILT4/CD85d). Proc Natl Acad Sci U S A 103:16412–16417

Solana R, Alonso MC, Pena J (1999) Natural killer cells in healthy aging. Exp Gerontol 34:435–443

Solana R, Casado JG, Delgado E, Delarosa O, Marin J, Duran E, Pawelec G, Tarazona R (2007) Lymphocyte activation in response to melanoma: interaction of NK-associated receptors and their ligands. Cancer Immunol Immunother 56:101–109

Solana R, Mariani E (2000) NK and NK/T cells in human senescence. Vaccine 18:1613–1620

Solana R, Pawelec G, Tarazona R (2006) Aging and innate immunity. Immunity 24:491–494

Tarazona R, Casado JG, Soto R, Delarosa O, Peralbo E, Rioja L, Pena J, Solana R (2004) Expression of NK-associated receptors on cytotoxic T cells from melanoma patients: a two-edged sword? Cancer Immunol Immunother 53:911–924

Tarazona R, Delarosa O, Casado JG, Torre-Cisneros J, Villanueva JL, Galiani MD, Pena J, Solana R (2002) NK-associated receptors on CD8 T cells from treatment-naive HIV-infected individuals: defective expression of CD56. AIDS 16:197–200

Vallejo AN, Weyand CM, Goronzy JJ (2004) T-cell senescence: a culprit of immune abnormalities in chronic inflammation and persistent infection. Trends Mol Med 10:119–124

Vitale M, Della CM, Carlomagno S, Pende D, Arico M, Moretta L, Moretta A (2005) NK-dependent DC maturation is mediated by TNFalpha and IFNgamma released upon engagement of the NKp30 triggering receptor. Blood 106:566–571

Wendt K, Wilk E, Buyny S, Buer J, Schmidt RE, Jacobs R (2006) Gene and protein characteristics reflect functional diversity of CD56dim and CD56bright NK cells. J Leukoc Biol 80:1529–1541

Yokoyama WM, Kim S (2006) Licensing of natural killer cells by self-major histocompatibility complex class I. Immunol Rev 214:143–154.:143–154

Zhang Y, Wallace DL, de Lara CM, Ghattas H, Asquith B, Worth A, Griffin GE, Taylor GP, Tough DF, Beverley PC, Macallan DC (2007) In vivo kinetics of human natural killer cells: the effects of ageing and acute and chronic viral infection. Immunology 121:258–265

Zitvogel L, Terme M, Borg C, Trinchieri G (2006) Dendritic cell-NK cell cross-talk: regulation and physiopathology. Curr Top Microbiol Immunol 298:157–174

Natural Killer Cells and Human Longevity

Hideto Tamura and Kiyoyuki Ogata

Contents

Abbreviations

NK	Natural killer
DCs	Dendritic cells
PB	Peripheral blood
ADCC	Antibody-dependent cellular cytotoxicity
LNs	Lymph nodes
MHC	Major histocompatibility complex
IL	Interleukin
KIR	Killer Ig-like receptor
BM	Bone-marrow
Flt3	Fms tyrosine kinase 3
IFN	Interferon
NKRs	NK cell receptors
HLA	Human leukocyte antigen
MIC	MHC-I polypeptide-related sequence
TLR	Toll-like receptors
HIV	Human immunodeficiency virus
TNF	Tumor necrosis factor
GM-CSF	Granu locyte macrophage colony-stimulating factor
IHLs	Intrahepatic lymphocytes

K. Ogata (✉) · H. Tamura
Division of Hematology
Department of Medicine
Nippon Medical School
1-1-5 Sendagi, Bunkyo-ku, Tokyo 113-8603, Japan
Tel.: +81-3-3822-2131
Fax: +81-3-5685-1793
E-mail: ogata@nms.ac.jp

T. Fulop et al. (eds.), *Handbook on Immunosenescence,*
DOI 10.1007/ 978-1-4020-9062-2_28, © Springer Science+Business Media B.V. 2009

HCV	Hepatitis C virus
CMV	Cytomegalovirus
MDS	Myelodysplastic syndromes
LU	Lytic units
PCNK	NK activity on a per-cell basis
PS	Performance status

Abstract: Natural killer (NK) cells are a lymphocyte subset in the innate immune system. These cells not only mount an early immune response to infections and neoplasia but also affect the adaptive immune system by communicating with dendritic cells. In this chapter, we review basic findings on NK-cells and then information from 1) rare patients with isolated NK-cell deficiency, 2) patients with certain malignant neoplasia, and 3) healthy middle-aged and elderly individuals. Those findings indicate that NK-cells are crucial immune components for sustaining life. With increasing age, numbers of T- and B-lymphocytes decline while the number of NK-cells increases. This is especially marked in centenarians. In terms of reduced tolerance to stress such as infections in the elderly, the power of early responders in the immune system including NK-cells may be especially important.

Keywords: Natural killer cells • Longevity • Infection • Neoplasia

1   Introduction

Studies examining healthy people showed that among the various components in the human immune system, natural killer (NK) cells are well maintained throughout life, even in centenarians. This is sharp contrast to the decline in T- and B-cell numbers with increasing age. Therefore, it is hypothesized that well-preserved NK-cell function is essential for longevity. In this chapter, we summarize basic findings on NK-cells, including recent understanding of the interaction between NK-cells and dendritic cells (DCs), and then review information so far obtained on the role of NK-cells in human longevity.

2   Overview of NK–cells

2.1   NK-cell Subsets

NK-cells were originally identified as a population of large granular lymphocytes and once considered to be a homogenous subset of lymphocytes in the peripheral blood (PB). However, NK-cells consist of heterogeneous populations. They can be divided into two subsets by the expression levels of CD56 (neural cell adhesion molecule, NCAM) and the presence or absence of CD16 antigen (FcγRIIIA), which binds the Fc portion of IgG and mediates antibody-dependent cellular cytotoxicity (ADCC) by binding to opsonized cells [18, 43]. These two subsets, CD56[bright]CD16- cells and CD56[dim]CD16+ cells, differ in their homing capabilities, i.e., CD56[bright]CD16- NK-cells largely predominate in the lymph nodes (LNs) and comprise circa 10% of PB NK-cells, as well as in other functions including cytolytic activities, cytokine production and ability to proliferate. It was reported that the CD56[bright]CD16- subset potently induces cytokine secretion, is a cytokine-responsive NK-cell subset, but has low intrinsic cytotoxicity, whereas the CD56[dim]CD16+ subset has little intrinsic secretory capability, but potent cytolytic activity [18, 56]. These subsets also express different receptors for chemokines, cytokines, and major histocompatibility complex (MHC) Class I ligands [67]. CD56[bright]CD16- NK-cells constitutively express interleukin (IL)-2 receptors with high and intermediate affinity and increase in response to low doses of IL-2. On the contrary, CD56[dim]CD16+ NK-cells proliferate weakly in vitro in response to high doses of IL-2 [12]. Finally, resting CD56[bright]CD16- NK-cells are large granular cells and express high levels of the CD94/NKG2 family and very low levels of the killer Ig-like receptor (KIR) family, while resting CD56[dim]CD16+ NK-cells contain numerous cytolytic granules in the cytoplasm and express both KIR and CD94/NKG2 receptor at relatively high levels [39].

2.2 NK-cell Development and Related Cytokines

NK-cells share a common lymphoid progenitor with thymocytes and B-cells [17]. In both humans and mice, early NK progenitors appear to be bone-marrow (BM)-derived CD34+ cells, which express receptors for the *fms* tyrosine kinease 3 (Flt3) ligand, c-kit ligand, and IL-2 receptor β chain (CD122) shared with the trimeric receptor for IL-15, and the BM microenvironment is necessary for complete maturation of NK-cells. BM stroma-derived IL-15 in cooperation with c-kit ligand and Flt-3 ligand is a critical factor for the development of mature NK-cells from NK progenitors in the BM [22, 27]. IL-15, which is reported to protect NK-cells from IL-2 activation-induced cell death, is also important for the maintenance of NK-cells [55, 68, 79]. NK progenitors respond to early-acting, stromal cell-derived growth factors such as the c-kit and Flt3 ligands and develop into NK precursors with the CD34+IL-2/IL-15Rβ+CD56- phenotype. IL-15 matures these NK precursors into functional CD56[bright] NK-cells [28]. However, further studies are required to understand the regulation of CD56[dim] NK-cell differentiation.

IL-21, another cytokine that can bind the common γ-chain shared with IL-2, IL-4, IL-7, IL-9, and IL-15, plays a role in the proliferation and maturation of NK-cells [63]. IL-7 is an early-acting cytokine responsible for the generation of immature CD56[bright] NK-cells [86]. IL-2 is a growth factor for NK progenitors and mature NK-cells. In addition, IL-2 induces the production of NK effector molecules and enhances the lytic activity of NK-cells. IL-12 and IL-18 are NK-activating cytokines during late NK-cell differentiation and synergistically enhance the cytotoxicity of and interferon (IFN)-γ production by NK-cells [34, 44]. IL-1 and IL-18 potentiate the effects of IL-12 by upregulating IL-12 receptors on NK-cells.

2.3 NK-cell Receptors

NK-cell receptors (NKRs) can be classified as inhibitory and activating [10, 53]. The MHC Class I-specific inhibitory receptors were first identified in both mice and humans. It is well known that NK-cells are able to lyse MHC Class I-negative tumors and infected cells, which are not recognized by the inhibitory receptors on NK-cells. Several inhibitory types of receptors exist, including the two main groups consisting of the KIR family (KIR2DL, KIR3DL, etc.) and the heterodimeric, C-type lectin receptors CD94-NKG2A/B, which bind to MHC Class I molecules and human leukocyte antigen (HLA)-E, respectively [10, 11]. HLA-E is a nonclassical, Class Ib molecule for which surface expression requires binding of peptides derived from the leader sequences of different HLA Class I molecules. The lack of even a single MHC Class I allele, which is a frequent event in cancer, sensitizes HLA-E to NK-cell cytotoxicity [53].

NK-cell cytotoxicity is also triggered by activating receptors including MHC Class I-specific receptors, i.e., KIR (KIR2DS, KIR3DS, etc.), C-type lectin receptor CD94/NKG2C, and non-MHC Class I-specific receptors such as natural cytotoxicity receptors, NKG2D, leukocyte adhesion molecule, and DNAX accessory molecule-1 (DNAM-1, CD226). NKG2D and DNAM-1 can recognize stress-induced ligands expressed by several tumor cell lines, such as MHC-I polypeptide-related sequence A (MICA), MHC-I polypeptide-related sequence B (MICB), and UL-16-binding protein (NKG2D ligands), and poliovirus receptor (CD155) and Nectin-2 (CD112, DNAM-1 ligands) [15, 64, 66]. Natural cytotoxcity receptors such as NKp46, NKp44, and NKp30, for which the host ligands remain unknown, mediate the lysis of many types of cancer cells. Additional receptors of NK-cell activation also comprise a series of coreceptors including 2B4, NTB-A, and NKp80 coreceptors, CD18/CD11 (β2 integrins), CD2 adhesion molecules, and Toll-like receptors (TLR) [51, 72]. NK-cell activation depends on the expression of these ligands on the target cells. These receptors provide both inhibitory and activating signals, and the balance between them determines NK-cell activation, proliferation, and effector functions.

2.4 NK-cell Function

The main function of NK-cells is host defense against tumors and infections. NK-cells can directly kill infected cells or tumor cells that have lost the expression of MHC Class I molecules. NK cytotoxicity can be triggered by viral and bacterial products directly binding to surface TLR3 and TLR9 [52, 72]. NK-cells also act as the conductor for the activation of the immune defense along with T- and B-cells, macrophages, and immune effector cells in local sites.

NK-cells can respond to infections directly by recognizing infected cells, and indirectly by cytokine secretion and interaction with DCs expressing TLR. It has been reported that NK-cells play an important role in antiviral defense, especially in controlling the severity of Herpes virus, Hepatitis, and Human immunodeficiency virus (HIV) infections [7]. To perform this role, NK-cells require the activation of multiple effector pathways including direct cytotoxicity and the release of cytokines and chemokines. Viral infection immediately induces macrophages to produce cytokines such as tumor necrosis factor (TNF)-α, IL-12 and IFN-γ. Activated NK-cells can also secrete several cytokines, i.e., IFN-γ, granulocyte macrophage colony-stimulating factor (GM-CSF), M-CSF, TNF-α, IL-5, IL-10, and IL-13, to control the growth and spread of pathogens and tumors. Furthermore, many of the cytokines produced by NK-cells can affect the initiation and maintenance of adaptive immune responses. Although NK-cells are activated and kill virus-infected cells immediately, it takes 1-2 weeks after infection to activate adaptive immune responses, such as pathogen-specific killer T-cells and antibodies produced by B-cells.

Intrahepatic lymphocytes (IHLs) contain 37% NK-cells and that percentage in the IHL pool may increase to 90% in hepatic disease [23]. Infection with hepatotropic viruses such as Hepatitis C virus (HCV) activate liver NK-cells that play a crucial role in the recruitment of virus-specific T-cells to the liver and in inducing antiviral immunity in the site. Activated NK-cells can kill virus-infected cells by a cytolytic mechanism via the perforin/granzyme and FasL pathways and produce proinflammatory cytokines that can induce an antiviral state in host cells. Compromised NK-cell functions have been reported in chronic HCV-infected patients. To control mouse cytomegalovirus (CMV) infection, NK-cells use two main effector mechanisms: the secretion of IFN-γ and direct lysis of infected cells by exocytosis of granules that contain perforin and granzymes. TLR9 recognizes unmethylated CpG DNA, a component of bacterial and viral DNA, and delivers signals for cellular activation through the adaptor protein MyD88. TLR9-deficient or MyD88-deficient mice show an increased susceptibility to mouse CMV, indicating an important role of TLR9 and MyD88 in protection against mouse CMV [3, 20, 42, 74]. In human CMV infection, activated NK-cells produce IFN-γ and secrete lymphotoxin-α and TNF, which contributes to the NF-κB-dependent release of IFN-β from infected cells. IFN-γ and IFN-β work together to inhibit CMV replication [38].

NK-cell-produced IFN-γ might contribute to protecting humans from Influenza A and Sendai viruses. Contact between NK-cells and virus-infected macrophages induces IFN-γ production. Furthermore, the expression of MICB, a ligand for the NKG2D receptor, was up-regulated in virus-infected macrophages, suggesting the role of MICB in the activation of the IFN-γ gene in NK-cells [71]. In HIV infection, the number of CD3$^-$CD56$^+$ NK-cells in the PB was dramatically reduced in patients with ongoing viral replication compared with uninfected or aviremic patients. Therefore, NK-cells play an important role in controlling HIV infection. NK-cells obtained from viremic patients produce more IFN-γ and TNF-α than NK-cells from aviremic patients [2]. A recent study has shown that the decrease in MHC Class I molecules on T-cell blasts infected with certain HIV strains was selective. The expression of HLA-A and -B was decreased in infected cells, whereas HLA-C and -E remained on the surface. HLA-C and -E bind to the KIR and CD94-NKG2A receptors, respectively, on NK-cells, resulting in inhibition of NK-cell-mediated killing of HIV-infected cells [8].

NK-cells are also activated during parasitic and bacterial infections. NK-cells produce IFN-γ in response the infection of red blood cells with *Plasmodium falciparum*, the causative agent of malaria [4]. The importance of NK-cells in protecting against bacterial infection has been controversial and may depend upon the site of infection or type of inflammatory response elicited. The expression of the activating receptors NKp30, NKp46, and NKG2D was enhanced in NK-cells after exposure to monocytes infected with the intracellular pathogen *Mycobacterium tuberculosis*. The infected monocytes upregulated the expression of the NKG2D ligand ULBP1 through TLR2 activation, and NK-cells lysed infected monocytes through NKG2D- and NKp46-dependent mechanisms [75].

2.5 Localization and Trafficking of NK-cells

NK-cells comprise approximately 5–20% of lymphocytes in the spleen, liver, and PB, and are present at lower levels in the BM, thymus, and LNs [31, 45]. Although NK-cell trafficking is not understood in detail, it was reported that chemokine secretion and chemokine receptor expression by NK-cells are dynamically regulated, and that some chemoattractants and chemokines can induce the migration of NK-cells to inflammation sites [67]. It is possible that changes in key adhesion molecules may induce the physical movement of NK-cells into sites of infection. $CD56^{bright}CD16^-$ NK-cells express CCR5 and CCR7 as well as L-selectin, which can attract T-cells to LNs, and $CD56^{dim}CD16^+$ NK-cells express CX3CR1. In addition, both of these NK subsets express CXCR3 and CXCR4 [13, 32, 67].

2.6 NK-DC Interactions

The crosstalk between NK-cells and myeloid DCs leads to NK-cell activation and DC maturation. Activated NK-cells can kill DCs that fail to undergo proper maturation; this phenomenon is called "DC editing" [53]. In vitro studies showed that NK-cells activated by IL-2 can kill immature DCs by ligation between NK-activating receptors, mainly NKp30 on NK-cells, and still unidentified cellular ligands on DCs [30, 65]. Consistent with these data, NK-cells derived from patients with acute myeloid leukemia, who frequently exhibit downregulation of NKp30 surface expression, have impaired killing of immature DCs [19, 29]. Furthermore, the NK-cell-mediated DC killing was inhibited by transforming growth factor-β, which can downregulate the surface expression of NKp30 [14]. Recently, DNAM-1 has been shown to cooperate with NKp30 in the NK-cell-mediated lysis of DCs [64]. The expression of Nectin-2, one of the DNAM-1 ligands, is increased on immature DCs. Studies using immuno-histochemistry and confocal microscopy showed that DNAM-1 ligands are expressed by DCs present in normal LNs. In general, the function of activating NKRs is under the control of inhibitory NKRs specific for HLA Class I [54]. However, immature DCs do not follow this rule. Analysis of NK clones showed that an NK subset, which lacks KIR specific for HLA Class I alleles and expresses HLA-E-specific CD94/NKG2A receptors (the KIR⁻NKG2A^{dull} phenotype), can kill immature DCs [21]. The DC editing mediated by NK-cells might be important in the selection of appropriate DCs in conjunction with the removal of DCs that fail to perform optimal antigen presentation and T-cell priming. NK-cells are not able to kill mature DCs, mainly because mature DCs express higher levels of HLA-E than immature ones.

During NK-DC interaction, NK-cells can induce DC maturation mediated by TNF-α and IFN-γ, which are released upon engagement of the NKp30 triggering receptor [77]. Semino et al showed that NK-DC interaction results in IL-18 secretion by DCs and then IL-18-activated NK-cells secrete the proinflammatory cytokine high mobility group B1 (HMGB1) [70]. HMGB1 can induce DC maturation and protect DCs from lysis. These data suggest that NK-cells mediate DC maturation by several pathways. NK-cells kill tumor cells and virus-infected cells, and subsequently prime DCs with the killed cell-derived antigens to induce specific CD8⁺ T-cell responses [49, 50, 87]. After antigen uptake, DCs undergo maturation and release several cytokines, including IL-12, that enhance NK functions. NK-DC interactions also induce primary tumor rejection and long-term cytotoxic T-lymphocyte memory, bypassing the requirement for CD4⁺ helper T-cells [1].

3   Contribution of NK-cells to Human Longevity

To gain insight into role of NK-cells in human longevity, we review findings 1) from patients with isolated NK-cell deficiency, 2) on the relationship between NK-cells and the development and progression of malignancies in humans, and 3) on NK-cells in the healthy elderly.

3.1   Isolated NK-cell Deficiency in Humans

Various isolated defects in human immune system have been reported, which provide valuable information on the function and importance of each component of the immune system [57]. However, primary isolated NK-cell deficiency, in which other immunologic functions are normal and which occurs in the absence of other immunocompromising conditions, is very rare. Moreover, in some reported cases, the distinction between NK-cells and T-cells expressing NK-cell markers was unclear. The rarity of isolated NK-cell deficiency may imply the critical role of NK-cells in human life. Another explanation is that because NK-cells are an early responder in the immunogic defense system and communicate with late components in the immune system, another immune component(s) is often secondarily impaired in isolated NK-cell deficiency. In this chapter, we do not discuss patients in whom both NK-cells and other immunlogic components were compromised or unexamined [46, 82].

A girl reported in 1989 by researchers at the University of Massachusetts Medical School is probably the best-known patient with isolated NK-cell deficiency [6]. She had experienced recurrent otitis media since infancy and at the age of 13 years developed severe varicella infection and polymicrobial sepsis with *Haemophilus influenzae*, *Streptococcus pneumoniae*, and *Staphylococcus aureus* infection. Four years later, she again developed sepsis with *S. aureus* infection and interstitial pneumonia due to CMV. CD56+ and CD16+ cells were completely absent in her PB, along with an almost complete absence of NK-cell cytotoxicity and ADCC. She later developed aplastic anemia and died after undergoing stem cell transplantation [62]. The second patient was a 23-year-old woman who had recurrent condylomata due to human papilloma virus [5]. Her peripheral blood lacked NK (CD3-CD56+) cells but showed an increase in CD3+CD56+ cells. NK cytotoxicity was almost completely absent, which was only slightly augmented by the administration of IL-2. However, this patient appeared not to have experienced devastating infections. The third patient was a 5-year-old girl, who experienced repeated otitis media and Herpes virus infections, requiring acyclovir prophylaxis for the latter [40]. Examination of her PB showed a profoundly reduced number of NK (CD3-CD56+) cells and reduced NK cytotoxicity but normal ADCC. The fourth was a 2-year-old girl with recurrent, ultimately fatal, varicella infection [25]. Her PB also contained a markedly decreased number of NK (CD3-CD56+) cells and showed reduced NK cytotoxicity.

Another group of patients reported in the literature had a normal number of NK-cells but defective NK-cell functions. Two brothers (6 and 12 years of age), who experienced recurrent upper respiratory tract infections and otitis media, had nearly normal numbers of CD56+ and CD16+ cells in their PB, but NK cytotoxicity was almost completely absent, which was not improved by incubating cells with IL-2 or IFN-α [41]. A recent report has suggested that overexpression of inhibitory killer receptors is a possible underlying mechanism in such patients [33].

Information from the above patients indicates that NK-cells are important in the in vivo defense against viruses mainly in the family Herpesviridae. In patients who lack NK-cells, infections with Herpes viruses are usually life-threatening. Even in healthy individuals, an initial Herpes virus infection may be followed by latency with subsequent reactivation and, in some cases, cause malignancies including lymphoma, nasopharyngeal cancer, and Kaposi's sarcoma. Therefore, it is concluded that NK-cell deficiency in humans is associated with life-threatening diseases caused by Herpes viruses and therefore affects life span. The association between NK-cells and other viral and bacterial infections in vivo is less clear. All four reported patients who lacked NK-cells were women. Further accumulation of such patients and research on their pathophysiology including genetics will be important to understand this association.

3.2 Relationship between NK-cells and the Development and Progression of Malignancies

NK-cells may contribute to human longevity by controlling neoplastic cells in patients with malignancies. An example of data supporting this hypothesis comes from studies of myelodysplastic syndromes (MDS). MDS are malignant disorders of hematopoietic stem cells and predominantly occur in the elderly [58]. A well-designed study in the UK found that in the population aged 70 years and older, more than 50 new MDS patients are diagnosed annually per 100,000 persons [84]. MDS are composed of various subtypes and can be grouped into early-stage and advanced-stage MDS based on the percentage of neoplastic myeloblasts in the BM and PB. It is also believed that early-stage MDS is often overlooked due to the absence of specific signs and symptoms of the disorder [58]. A substantial proportion of patients with early-stage MDS progress to advanced-stage MDS and then to acute myeloid leukemia by mechanisms that have not been thoroughly clarified. MDS patients often have dysfunction in a variety of immunologic components including NK-cells [35]. NK-cell cytotoxicity, which may or may not be stimulated by IL-2 in vitro, is preserved in early-stage MDS but decreases with disease progression [24, 60]. The elevation in levels of circulating soluble IL-2 receptor [85], which can neutralize endogenous IL-2, and reduced expression of activating NK receptors such as NKG2D in NK-cells [24] may contribute to the reduced NK-cell cytotoxicity in advanced-stage MDS patients. These data suggest that NK-cells contribute to controlling disease progression in MDS and thus may affect longevity because of the high prevalence of MDS in the elderly. Similarly, NK-cells may prolong the life span of patients with other cancers by inhibiting disease progression [16, 37, 76].

Meanwhile, it is known that NK-cell activity varies significantly among healthy individuals. The question is whether differences in NK-cell activity in healthy people are involved in the development of malignancies and thus contribute to longevity. Imai et al examined NK-cell cytotoxicity in 3625 healthy Japanese, mainly in the 40-69-year-old age-group, living in Saitama prefecture [36]. They followed the cohort for 11 years to investigate cancer incidence and death from any cause. They recorded 154 cases of cancer (most frequent sites were the stomach, lung, and intestine) in the study period and found that reduced NK-cell cytotoxicity was a statistically significant risk factor for the development of cancer.

3.3 NK-cells in the Healthy Elderly

NK-cells in the healthy elderly have been examined in many studies. Sansoni et al carefully selected 138 healthy individuals, ranging in age from 4 to 106 years, and examined their immunologic parameters including lymphocyte subsets and NK-cell cytotoxicity [69]. They found that although the number of T- and B-cells declined with increasing age, the number of cells with NK markers did not undergo an age-related decline. Instead, the number of CD16+ cells and CD57+ cells increased with age. Moreover, centenarians had well-preserved NK-cell activity expressed in lytic units (LU), the magnitude of which was comparable to that in healthy young people and higher than that in the healthy middle-aged.

We also selected 82 healthy individuals, aged 30 to 99 years, and investigated their immunologic parameters [61]. We confirmed that the number of T-cells declined and the number of CD56+ cells increased with age and that NK-cell activity expressed as LU was maintained throughout this age range. In addition, because the number of total lymphocytes was found to decrease with age in most studies including ours, we calculated the index of absolute in vivo NK-cell activity (ALU = LU x mononuclear cell count per microliter of PB) and found that the ALU decreased as age increased. Moreover, the cytotoxic activity exerted by one NK-cell (NK activity on a per-cell basis, PCNK) decreased as age increased. When we retrospectively examined the medical records of the elderly in our cohort, it was found that low ALU and PCNK values correlated with a past history of severe infection. Therefore, we proposed that human NK-cells do not escape the aging process and that low NK-cell function is corrrelated with the development of severe infections, which may be fatal, in the elderly. Similarly, several other studies of the healthy elderly showed that the T-cell population declines while the NK-cell population increases in the PB and that the PCNK decreases [9, 26, 47, 48]. In particular, data from centenarians are striking. Miyaji et al reported that roughly 50% of lymphocytes were CD56+ cells in centenarians in contrast to about 11% in the middle-aged [48]. However, it has not been fully clarified whether the NK-cell increase in the very old indicates that NK-cells result in longevity or longevity resulting from other factors causes an increase in the number of NK-cells.

Based on the above findings, we conducted a prospective study to examine whether differences in NK-cell function among the healthy elderly is related to the development of infection and infectious death [59]. Our subjects were 108 immunologically normal elderly people aged 63–99 (mean 81) years residing in nursing homes due to impaired performance status (PS). We determined counts of lymphocytes, monocytes, and neutrophils, serum albumin value, percentage and absolute number of various lymphocyte subsets (CD3+, CD4+, CD8+, CD25+, CD56+, CD3+HLA·DR+, CD3+CD56+, and CD3·CD56+ cells), and NK-cell activity. The interassay variation in NK-cell activity was minimized by examining the same control cells in each assay. We then followed the cohort and analyzed the correlation between the development of infection during the first 12 months of follow-up and the predetermined parameters as well as age and PS. Using univariate logistic regression analysis, poor PS, low albumin value, old age, and low NK-cell activity correlated significantly with the development of infection. Multivariate logistic regression analysis showed that low NK-cell activity, poor PS score, and older age were independent variables associated with the development of infection. The odds ratio for the development of infection increased with the decrease in NK-cell activity. We next analyzed correlations between the predetermined parameters and the time until death due to infection in the 108 individuals. Eleven died of infection (all due to pneumonia) during the follow-up period. Univariate Cox proportional-hazards regression analysis showed that poor PS, high CD8[+] T-cell count, and low NK-cell activity correlated significantly with short survival time due to infection. Multivariate Cox proportional-hazards regression analysis showed that low NK-cell activity was an independent variable associated with short survival time due to infection. Other independent variables for short survival due to infection were poor PS and a high CD8[+] T-cell count. These findings support the hypothesis that well-preserved NK-cell activity is important for human longevity, at least in part because of its antiinfectious effect. The association between a high CD8[+] T-cell count and short survival time after infection deserves further discussion. A previous study also suggested an association between a high CD8[+] T-cell count and high mortality rate in the elderly [83]. One proposed explanation for this association is that clonal expansions of CD8[+] T-cells, which are often observed in the healthy elderly [78], are exaggerated in those with a high CD8[+] T-cell count. This clonal expansion probably reduces the naive repertoire of CD8[+] T-cells, which impairs T-cell responses and thus may be associated with vulnerability to infections.

Meanwhile, a functional relationship exists between NK-cells and T-cells. In a typical viral infection, NK-cell responses against the virus are observed during the first 1–3 days of infection [80]. These are gradually replaced with viral antigen-specific T-cell responses. When T-cell responses do not occur, as in severe combined immunodeficient mice and athymic nude mice, the increased NK-cell response is maintained for a prolonged period to defend the host [73, 81]. Considering the functional link between NK- and T-cells and the reduced T-cell count commonly observed in elderly people, the role of NK-cells in protecting against infections may be more important in the elderly than in younger individuals.

4 Concluding Remarks

NK-cells are a lymphocyte subset in the innate immune system which are early responders to infections and neoplasia. Data from isolated NK-cell deficiency, certain patients with malignant neoplasia, and healthy individuals all indicate that NK-cells are crucial immune components for sustaining life. In middle-aged people in developed countries who can overcome common infections, NK-cells may be important for defending against malignancies. In elderly people, common infections can cause significant morbidity and mortality. In terms of weakened T- and B-cell immunology as well as reduced tolerance of stress such as infections in the elderly, the strength of the early immune system response including that of NK-cells appears especially important. The role of NK-cells throughout the human life span should be studied further to confirm this hypothesis.

References

1. Adam C, King S et al (2005) "DC-NK cell cross talk as a novel CD4+ T-cell-independent pathway for antitumor CTL induction." Blood 106(1):338–344
2. Alter G, Malenfant JM et al (2004) "Increased natural killer cell activity in viremic HIV-1 infection." J Immunol 173(8):5305–5311
3. Andoniou CE, van Dommelen SL et al (2005) "Interaction between conventional dendritic cells and natural killer cells is integral to the activation of effective antiviral immunity." Nat Immunol 6(10):1011–1019
4. Artavanis-Tsakonas K, Riley EM (2002) "Innate immune response to malaria: rapid induction of IFN-gamma from human NK cells by live Plasmodium falciparum-infected erythrocytes." J Immunol 169(6):2956–63
5. Ballas ZK, Turner JM et al (1990) "A patient with simultaneous absence of "classical "natural killer cells (CD3-, CD16+, and NKH1+) and expansion of CD3+, CD4-, CD8-, NKH1+ subset." J Allergy Clin Immunol 85(2):453–459
6. Biron CA, Byron KS et al (1989) "Severe herpesvirus infections in an adolescent without natural killer cells." N Engl J Med 320(26):1731–1735
7. Biron CA, Nguyen KB et al (1999) "Natural killer cells in antiviral defense: function and regulation by innate cytokines." Annu Rev Immunol 17:189–220
8. Bonaparte MI, E Barker (2004) "Killing of human immunodeficiency virus-infected primary T-cell blasts by autologous natural killer cells is dependent on the ability of the virus to alter the expression of major histocompatibility complex class I molecules." Blood 104(7):2087–2094
9. Borrego F, Alonso MC et al (1999) "NK phenotypic markers and IL2 response in NK cells from elderly people." Exp Gerontol 34(2):253–265
10. Bottino C, Moretta L et al (2004) "Learning how to discriminate between friends and enemies, a lesson from Natural Killer cells." Mol Immunol 41(6–7):569–575
11. Braud VM, Allan DS et al (1998) "HLA-E binds to natural killer cell receptors CD94/NKG2A, B and C." Nature 391(6669):795–799
12. Caligiuri MA (1993) "Low-dose recombinant interleukin-2 therapy: rationale and potential clinical applications." Semin Oncol 20(6 Suppl 9):3–10
13. Campbell JJ, Qin S et al (2001) "Unique subpopulations of CD56+ NK and NK-T peripheral blood lymphocytes identified by chemokine receptor expression repertoire." J Immunol 166(11):6477–6482
14. Castriconi R, Cantoni C et al (2003) "Transforming growth factor beta 1 inhibits expression of NKp30 and NKG2D receptors: consequences for the NK-mediated killing of dendritic cells." Proc Natl Acad Sci U S A 100(7):4120–4125
15. Cerwenka A, LL Lanier (2003) "NKG2D ligands: unconventional MHC class I-like molecules exploited by viruses and cancer." Tissue Antigens 61(5):335–343
16. Coca S, Perez-Piqueras J et al (1997) "The prognostic significance of intratumoral natural killer cells in patients with colorectal carcinoma." Cancer 79(12):2320–2328
17. Colucci F, Caligiuri MA et al (2003) "What does it take to make a natural killer?" Nat Rev Immunol 3(5):413–425
18. Cooper MA, Fehniger TA et al (2001) "The biology of human natural killer-cell subsets." Trends Immunol 22(11):633–640
19. Costello RT, Sivori S et al (2002) "Defective expression and function of natural killer cell-triggering receptors in patients with acute myeloid leukemia." Blood 99(10):3661–3667
20. Delale T, Paquin A et al (2005) "yD88-dependent and -independent murine cytomegalovirus sensing for IFN-alpha release and initiation of immune responses in vivo." J Immunol 175(10):6723–6732
21. Della Chiesa M, Vitale M et al (2003) "The natural killer cell-mediated killing of autologous dendritic cells is confined to a cell subset expressing CD94/NKG2A, but lacking inhibitory killer Ig-like receptors." Eur J Immunol 33(6):1657–1666

22. Di Santo JP, Vosshenrich CA (2006) "Bone marrow versus thymic pathways of natural killer cell development." Immunol Rev 214:35–46

23. Doherty DG, C O'Farrelly (2000) "Innate and adaptive lymphoid cells in the human liver." Immunol Rev 174:5–20

24. Epling-Burnette PK, FBai et al (2007) "Reduced natural killer (NK) function associated with high-risk myelodysplastic syndrome (MDS) and reduced expression of activating NK receptors." Blood 109(11):4816–4824

25. Etzioni A, Eidenschenk C et al (2005) "Fatal varicella associated with selective natural killer cell deficiency." J Pediatr 146(3):423–425

26. Facchini A, Mariani E et al (1987) "Increased number of circulating Leu 11+ (CD 16) large granular lymphocytes and decreased NK activity during human ageing." Clin Exp Immunol 68(2):340–347

27. Farag SS, MA Caligiuri (2006) "Human natural killer cell development and biology." Blood Rev 20(3):123–37

28. Farag SS, Fehniger TA et al (2002) "Natural killer cell receptors: new biology and insights into the graft-versus-leukemia effect." Blood 100(6):1935–1947

29. Fauriat C, Moretta A et al (2005) "Defective killing of dendritic cells by autologous natural killer cells from acute myeloid leukemia patients." Blood 106(6):2186–2188

30. Ferlazzo G., Tsang ML et al (2002) "Human dendritic cells activate resting natural killer (NK) cells and are recognized via the NKp30 receptor by activated NK cells." J Exp Med 195(3):343–351

31. Ferlazzo G, C Munz (2004) "NK cell compartments and their activation by dendritic cells." J Immunol 172(3):1333–1339

32. Frey M, Packianathan NB et al (1998) "Differential expression and function of L-selectin on CD56bright and CD56dim natural killer cell subsets." J Immunol 161(1):400–408

33. Gazit R, Garty BZ et al (2004) "Expression of KIR2DL1 on the entire NK cell population: a possible novel immunodeficiency syndrome." Blood 103(5):1965–1966

34. Golab J (2000) "Interleukin 18–interferon gamma inducing factor–a novel player in tumour immunotherapy?" Cytokine 12(4):332–338

35. Hamblin TJ (1996) "Immunological abnormalities in myelodysplastic syndromes." Semin Hematol 33(2):150–162

36. Imai K, Matsuyama S et al (2000) "Natural cytotoxic activity of peripheral-blood lymphocytes and cancer incidence: an 11-year follow-up study of a general population." Lancet 356(9244):1795–1799

37. Ishigami S, Natsugoe S et al (2000) "Prognostic value of intratumoral natural killer cells in gastric carcinoma." Cancer 88(3):577–583

38. Iversen AC, Norris PS et al (2005) "Human NK cells inhibit cytomegalovirus replication through a noncytolytic mechanism involving lymphotoxin-dependent induction of IFN-beta." J Immunol 175(11):7568–7574

39. Jacobs R, Hintzen G et al (2001) "CD56bright cells differ in their KIR repertoire and cytotoxic features from CD56dim NK cells." Eur J Immunol 31(10):3121–3127

40. Jawahar S, Moody C et al (1996) "Natural Killer (NK) cell deficiency associated with an epitope-deficient Fc receptor type IIIA (CD16-II)." Clin Exp Immunol 103(3):408–413

41. Komiyama A, Kawai H et al (1990) "Natural killer cell immunodeficiency in siblings: defective killing in the absence of natural killer cytotoxic factor activity in natural killer and lymphokine-activated killer cytotoxicities." Pediatrics 85(3):323–330

42. Krug A, French AR et al (2004) "TLR9-dependent recognition of MCMV by IPC and DC generates coordinated cytokine responses that activate antiviral NK cell function." Immunity 21(1):107–119

43. Lanier LL, Le AM et al (1986) "The relationship of CD16 (Leu-11) and Leu-19 (NKH-1) antigen expression on human peripheral blood NK cells and cytotoxic T lymphocytes." J Immunol 136(12):4480–4486

44. Lauwerys BR, Garot N et al (2000) "Cytokine production and killer activity of NK/T-NK cells derived with IL-2, IL-15, or the combination of IL-12 and IL-18." J Immunol 165(4):1847–1853
45. Lian RH, V Kumar (2002) "Murine natural killer cell progenitors and their requirements for development." Semin Immunol 14(6):453–460
46. Lopez C, Kirkpatrick D et al (1983) "Correlation between low natural killing of fibroblasts infected with herpes simplex virus type 1 and susceptibility to herpesvirus infections." J Infect Dis 147(6):1030–1035
47. McNerlan SE, Rea IM et al (1998) "Changes in natural killer cells, the CD57CD8 subset, and related cytokines in healthy aging." J Clin Immunol 18(1):31–38
48. Miyaji C, Watanabe H et al (2000) "Functional alteration of granulocytes, NK cells, and natural killer T cells in centenarians." Hum Immunol 61(9):908–916
49. Mocikat R, Braumuller H et al (2003) "Natural killer cells activated by MHC class I(low) targets prime dendritic cells to induce protective CD8 T cell responses." Immunity 19(4):561–569
50. Moretta A (2002) "Natural killer cells and dendritic cells: rendezvous in abused tissues." Nat Rev Immunol 2(12):957–964
51. Moretta L, Bottino C et al (2006) "Surface NK receptors and their ligands on tumor cells." Semin Immunol 18(3):151–158
52. Moretta L, Ferlazzo G et al (2006) "Effector and regulatory events during natural killer-dendritic cell interactions." Immunol Rev 214:219–228
53. Moretta L, A Moretta (2004) "Killer immunoglobulin-like receptors." Curr Opin Immunol 16(5):626–633
54. Moretta L, A Moretta (2004) "Unravelling natural killer cell function: triggering and inhibitory human NK receptors." Embo J 23(2):255–259
55. Mrozek E, Anderson P et al (1996) "Role of interleukin-15 in the development of human CD56+ natural killer cells from CD34+ hematopoietic progenitor cells." Blood 87(7):2632–2640
56. Nagler A, Lanier LL et al (1989) "Comparative studies of human FcRIII-positive and negative natural killer cells." J Immunol 143(10):3183–3191
57. Notarangelo L, Casanova JL et al (2004) "Primary immunodeficiency diseases: an update." J Allergy Clin Immunol 114(3):677–687
58. Ogata K (2006) "Myelodysplastic syndromes: recent progress in diagnosis and understanding of their pathophysiology." J Nippon Med Sch 73(6):300–307
59. Ogata K, An E et al (2001) "Association between natural killer cell activity and infection in immunologically normal elderly people." Clin Exp Immunol 124(3):392–397
60. Ogata K, Yokose N et al (1994) "Assessment of therapeutic potential of interleukin 2 for myelodysplastic syndromes." Br J Haematol 86(3):562–567
61. Ogata K, Yokose N et al (1997) "Natural killer cells in the late decades of human life." Clin Immunol Immunopathol 84(3):269–275
62. Orange JS (2002) "Human natural killer cell deficiencies and susceptibility to infection." Microbes Infect 4(15):1545–1558
63. Parrish-Novak J, Dillon SR et al (2000) "Interleukin 21 and its receptor are involved in NK cell expansion and regulation of lymphocyte function." Nature 408(6808):57–63
64. Pende D, Castriconi R et al (2006) "Expression of the DNAM-1 ligands, Nectin-2 (CD112) and poliovirus receptor (CD155), on dendritic cells: relevance for natural killer-dendritic cell interaction." Blood 107(5):2030–2036
65. Pende D, Parolini S et al (1999) "Identification and molecular characterization of NKp30, a novel triggering receptor involved in natural cytotoxicity mediated by human natural killer cells." J Exp Med 190(10):1505–1516
66. Pende D, Rivera P et al (2002) "Major histocompatibility complex class I-related chain A and UL16-binding protein expression on tumor cell lines of different histotypes: analysis of tumor susceptibility to NKG2D-dependent natural killer cell cytotoxicity." Cancer Res 62(21):6178–6186
67. Robertson MJ (2002) "Role of chemokines in the biology of natural killer cells." J Leukoc Biol 71(2):173–183

68. Rodella L, Zamai L et al (2001) "Interleukin 2 and interleukin 15 differentially predispose natural killer cells to apoptosis mediated by endothelial and tumour cells." Br J Haematol 115(2):442–450

69. Sansoni P, Cossarizza A et al (1993) "Lymphocyte subsets and natural killer cell activity in healthy old people and centenarians." Blood 82(9):2767–2773

70. Semino C, Angelini G. et al (2005) "NK/iDC interaction results in IL-18 secretion by DCs at the synaptic cleft followed by NK cell activation and release of the DC maturation factor HMGB1." Blood 106(2):609–616

71. Siren J, Sareneva T et al (2004) "Cytokine and contact-dependent activation of natural killer cells by influenza A or Sendai virus-infected macrophages." J Gen Virol 85(Pt 8):2357–2364

72. Sivori S, Carlomagno S et al (2006) "Comparison of different CpG oligodeoxynucleotide classes for their capability to stimulate human NK cells." Eur J Immunol 36(4):961–967

73. Su H C, Ishikawa R et al (1993) "Transforming growth factor-beta expression and natural killer cell responses during virus infection of normal, nude, and SCID mice." J Immunol 151(9):4874–4890

74. Tabeta K, Georgel P et al (2004) "Toll-like receptors 9 and 3 as essential components of innate immune defense against mouse cytomegalovirus infection." Proc Natl Acad Sci U S A 101(10):3516–3521

75. Vankayalapati R, Garg A et al (2005). "Role of NK cell-activating receptors and their ligands in the lysis of mononuclear phagocytes infected with an intracellular bacterium." J Immunol 175(7):4611–4617

76. Villegas FR, Coca S et al (2002) "Prognostic significance of tumor infiltrating natural killer cells subset CD57 in patients with squamous cell lung cancer." Lung Cancer 35(1):23–28

77. Vitale M, Della Chiesa M et al (2005) "NK-dependent DC maturation is mediated by TNFalpha and IFNgamma released upon engagement of the NKp30 triggering receptor." Blood 106(2):566–571

78. Wack A, Cossarizza A et al (1998) "Age-related modifications of the human alphabeta T cell repertoire due to different clonal expansions in the CD4+ and CD8+ subsets." Int Immunol 10(9):1281–1288

79. Waldmann TA, Dubois S et al (2001) "Contrasting roles of IL-2 and IL-15 in the life and death of lymphocytes: implications for immunotherapy." Immunity 14(2):105–110

80. Welsh RM (1981) "Natural cell-mediated immunity during viral infections." Curr Top Microbiol Immunol 92:83–106

81. Welsh RM, Brubaker JO et al (1991) "Natural killer (NK) cell response to virus infections in mice with severe combined immunodeficiency. The stimulation of NK cells and the NK cell-dependent control of virus infections occur independently of T and B cell function." J Exp Med 173(5):1053–1063

82. Wendland T, Herren S et al (2000) "Strong alpha beta and gamma delta TCR response in a patient with disseminated Mycobacterium avium infection and lack of NK cells and monocytopenia." Immunol Lett 72(2):75–82

83. Wikby A, Maxson P et al (1998) "Changes in CD8 and CD4 lymphocyte subsets, T cell proliferation responses and non-survival in the very old: the Swedish longitudinal OCTO-immune study." Mech Ageing Dev 102(2–3):187–198

84. Williamson PJ, Kruger AR et al (1994) "Establishing the incidence of myelodysplastic syndrome." Br J Haematol 87(4):743–745

85. Yokose N, Ogata K et al (1994) "Elevated plasma soluble interleukin 2 receptor level correlates with defective natural killer and CD8 +T-cells in myelodysplastic syndromes." Leuk Res 18(10):777–782

86. Zamai L, Ponti C et al (2007) "NK cells and cancer." J Immunol 178(7):4011–4016

87. Zitvogel L (2002) "Dendritic and natural killer cells cooperate in the control/switch of innate immunity." J Exp Med 195(3):F9–F14

The Effects of Age on CD1d-restricted NKT-cells and Their Contribution to Peripheral T-cell Immunity

Douglas E. Faunce and Jessica L. Palmer

Contents

1 Introduction

Natural Killer T (NKT) cells are innate lymphocytes known for their roles in regulation of immune responses in cancer, autoimmunity, bacterial and viral infections, and the induction of immunologic tolerance [1–4]. Recently, our laboratory and others have also identified crucial roles for NKT-cells in the regulation of the host response to injury and sepsis [5–7]. As we will discuss further in this chapter, NKT-cells are now widely accepted as critical players in the initiation of maintenance of host defense, as they are uniquely poised to modulate multiple aspects of protective immunity. NKT-cells fill this position via their ability to rapidly produce significant quantities of immunomodulatory cytokines very early during the course of the immune response and can thereby influence the outcome of both innate and adaptive immune processes.

While a significant number of studies, described in this handbook and elsewhere, have identified both direct and indirect effects of advanced age on T-cells, B-cells, and cells of the innate immune system including macrophages, dendritic cells, granulocytes, etc., little is known of how NKT-cell populations might change with age and moreover, how the aging immune microenvironment affects NKT-cell function. Here, we will provide a brief overview of NKT-cells, their role in host defense, and review the limited information on the effects of age on NKT-cell biology.

D. E. Faunce (✉) · J. L. Palmer
Loyola University Medical Center
Bldg 110, Rm 4236
2160 South First Avenue
Maywood, IL 60153, USA
Tel: 708-327-2663,
Fax: 708-327-2813
E-mail: dfaunce@lumc.edu

T. Fulop et al. (eds.), *Handbook on Immunosenescence*,
DOI 10.1007/ 978-1-4020-9062-2_29, © Springer Science+Business Media B.V. 2009

2 NKT-cell Development and Restriction by CD1d, Antigen Specificity, and Tissue Distribution

Like virtually all T-lymphocytes, NKT-cells arise and differentiate from mainstream thymic precursors. Whereas conventional CD4+ and CD8+ T-cells differentiate and undergo negative and positive selection based upon thymic expression of self-peptide antigens and of MHC-II and MHC-I, NKT-cells on the other hand, acquire their differentiation signals and undergo thymic selection based upon thymic expression of self-lipid ligands presented on the MHC-I-like molecule, CD1d. NKT-cells arise from CD4+ CD8+ thymic precursors and express a canonical invariant $\alpha\beta$ TCR (Vα14-Jα18 in mouse and Vα24-Jα18 in human) that recognizes a self-lipid called isoglobotrihexosylceramide (iGb3), which is a breakdown product of the hexosaminadase-B pathway and is presented in the context of CD1d molecules expressed on thymic epithelia [8–10]. Upon engagement of the Vα14-Jα18 TCR with iGb3/CD1d complex, double positive NKT precursors down-regulate their expression of CD8. While some NKT precursors retain their expression of CD4 molecules, others eventually down regulate CD4 and become double-negative, invariant TCR-positive. As NKT-cells are so named, they acquire expression of NK lineage receptors including NK1.1, NKG2A/D, Ly49C/I in mouse and CD16, CD56, and CD161 in human.

NKT-cells are widely distributed throughout the body in both humans and mice and can be identified in the thymus, liver, spleen, lymph nodes, and circulation by either their co-expression of the invariant TCR and the above-mentioned NK associated markers or by their ability to bind lipid ligand-loaded CD1d tetramers or dimers [11, 12]. Overall, NKT-cells comprise approximately 0.5–1.0% of the entire T-lymphocyte pool. In the liver, they account for approximately 25–50% of lymphocytes (depending upon species, strain, etc.), in spleen they comprise approximately 2–3% of the lymphocyte population, while in the circulation and lymph nodes, NKT-cells make up only about 0.5–1.0% of circulating lymphocytes. Within the lymphoid compartment NKT-cells can be found in the splenic marginal zones, red pulp, PALS, and paracortical areas [13] (and Faunce et al, unpublished observations) and in the liver, they mainly accumulate in the liver sinusoids. Interestingly, the liver seems particularly adept for the recruitment and retention of NKT-cells, since they constitutively express CXCR6, the receptor for the chemokine CXCL16, which is expressed among other places on the surface of liver sinusoidal epithelium [14]. NKT-cells may also home to lymphoid organs or other sites of inflammation and immune responses via signals mediated through CCR1, CCR2, CCR4, CCR5, CCR6, and CXCR2 [13, 15].

3 CD1d Molecules and Lipid Antigens

Unlike conventional CD4+ and CD8+ T-cells that exhibit specificity for peptide antigens presented by MHC-II and MHC-I respectively, NKT-cells recognize glycolipid antigens presented in the context of the MHC-I-like molecule, CD1d

[1, 3, 16–18]. The CD1 family of cell surface glycoproteins is expressed by a variety of cell types, however, the CD1d isoform is expressed primarily on professional antigen presenting cells including macrophages, dendritic cells and B-cells and is expressed at the cell surface in conjunction with β2-microglobulin. In humans, five isoforms of CD1 exist, CD1a–e. In mice and rats however, only CD1d is expressed [1, 3, 16–18]. The invariant Vα14 (and Vα24) TCR only recognizes CD1d and not the other isoforms and it was the observation in the mid to late 1990's that minor T-cell subsets appeared restricted by CD1d for both function and development that led to the discovery that NKT-cells were indeed a unique subset with their own developmental restriction and antigen specificity [19–22]. Today, the CD1d-restriction of NKT-cells is exploited through the use of CD1d tetramers and dimers that are used for the specific recognition and identification of NKT-cells in both mice and humans [11, 12, 23–25].

As mentioned above, CD1d-restricted NKT-cells exhibit specificity for glycolipid antigens, rather than peptide antigens. The concept that CD1d presents lipid antigens to invariant TCRs was first considered when it was observed that the binding grooves of CD1d as well as the invariant TCR were extremely hydrophobic [20]. The first glycolipid identified as a specific activator of NKT-cells was alpha-galactosylceramide, a lipid isolate of the marine sponge *Agales mauritianus,* whose synthetic analogue KRN7000, exhibited potent anti-tumor immunity mediated by NKT-cells [24, 26–28] and is now known as a potent stimulator for NKT-cells both in vivo and in vitro [8,29–31]. More recently, it has been shown that specific microbial-derived lipids also are presented by CD1d to the invariant TCR for the activation of NKT-cells, including *Sphingomonas* GSL-1 [32], *Borrelia burgdorferi* alpha-glactosyldiacylglycerols [32], and mycobacterial phosphatidylinositolmannosides such as PIM-4 [33]. In addition to reactivity towards exogenous glycolipid antigens presented by CD1d, it is also well established NKT-cell development is restricted by thymic CD1d expression, thereby suggesting the requirement of a self-glycolipid during positive selection of NKT-cell precursors. Indeed, the glycosphingolipid isoglobotrihexosylceramide, or iGb3, appears to be a self-derived glycolipid ligand that is required for positive selection and expansion of NKT-cell precursors during development [10, 34], since β-hexosaminadase deficient mice, which as a result of this enzyme deficiency are unable to convert iGb4 to iGb3, almost completely lack invariant NKT-cells [34].

4   Effects of Age on NKT-cell Numbers and CD1d Expression

Clearly, age-related alterations in the number and/or function of NKT-cells could greatly influence the quality of the effector T-cell response. For the purposes of this chapter, we shall consider studies that have examined NKT-cell numbers and function in humans aged 59 and older and studies in mice of ages twelve months or older. Only a handful of reports have closely examined CD1d-restricted NKT-cell numbers in aged mice and humans and most agree that as age increases, so does the number of NKT-cells in the periphery [6, 35, 36]. It is not entirely clear whether the increase represents an accumulation of cells over time versus increased expansion of newly made cells. Increased frequency and numbers of NKT-cells could also result from increased recruitment or retention. In fact, it was recently reported by Berzins and colleagues that NKT-cells are comparatively long-lived (i.e., greater than one year in mice) and are retained for significantly greater periods of time in the thymus compared to conventional T-cells [37]. Some reports describe an increase in accumulated, longer-lived hepatic NKT-cells over time in both humans and mice [35, 36]. In mice, NKT-cell number increases 2-to-3-fold in the livers, spleens, and lymph nodes of aged animals [6, 38, 39]. It could be argued that older mice are slightly larger physically and therefore might have greater numbers of cells in general, however, the relative frequency of NKT-cells as compared to conventional T-cells is also 2-to-3-fold higher in aged mice as compared to young [6]. This increase could represent an unusual effect of aging, as most immune cell populations remain static or decrease in number. Some data suggests that this age-related increase in NKT-cells actually stems from newly made cells. Using 5'-bromo-2-deoxyuridine (BrdU) labeling, ligand-loaded CD1d dimer staining and flow cytometry, our laboratory observed that the spleens and lymph nodes of aged mice (18–22 months old) contained nearly 2.5-fold greater numbers of BrdU-positive NKT-cells (Palmer and Faunce, unpublished observations). BrdU is a thymidine analog that incorporates into the newly synthesized DNA, making it an effective marker to distinguish and track newly made cells. The precise mechanisms responsible for increased output of NKT-cells in aged mice remain to be elucidated. Likewise, the reasons for the potentially greater longevity of thymic NKT-cells also require further investigation.

While the majority of observations support the concept that NKT-cells increase with age, as with most topics, the opposite has been reported in that numbers of $V\alpha14$ and $V\alpha24$ NKT-cells were found to be decreased with advanced age, particularly in the liver [40, 41].

Since NKT-cells are stimulated by lipid ligands presented by the CD1d molecule on APCs, it follows that part of the aged-related breakdown could be attributed to transitions in CD1d expression or magnitude. However, CD1d magnitude and frequency of expression is similar on F4/80$^+$ monocyte/macrophages and CD11c$^+$ dendritic cells in aged and young mice [6]. This suggests that lipid antigen presentation to NKT-cells is intact in aged animals, so changes probably lie within altered responses from NKT-cells once they are activated by ligand-bearing APCs.

5   Aging, NKT-cell Function, and Peripheral T-cell Immunity

Few studies have directly addressed the effects of age on NKT-cell biology, however the topic has been briefly reviewed by others in the recent past [36, 42]. Similarly, very few studies have made direct comparisons of CD1d-restricted NKT-cell involvement in immune function between young and aged subjects, however based on what is known (again considering mice twelve months or older), it appears that NKT-cells modulate several aspects of T-cell function differently in aged mice compared to young. Recent studies by our laboratory demonstrated that in aged mice, NKT-cells contributed to the age-associated reduction of antigen-specific T-cell proliferation [6]. Removal of NKT-cells (Ly49C⁺ NK/NKT) from splenic T-cell preparations prior to stimulation restored the capacity of T-cells to proliferate in response to CD3ε ligation. The same observation was made for proliferation of peripheral lymph node T-cells. Importantly, comparable T-cell proliferation in aged and young mice could also be achieved among splenocyte preparations from young vs. aged mice given anti-CD1d monoclonal antibody systemically to block NKT-cell activation in vivo. Such observations implicated NKT-cells in the age-related suppression of the T-cell proliferative response to antigen. Perhaps the most compelling evidence for a direct connection between activated NKT-cells and suppression of T-cell effector function was demonstrated in a series of experiments conducted by our laboratory that utilized delayed type hypersensitivity (DTH) responses after immunization with ovalbumin in complete adjuvant as an index of antigen-specific effector T-cell response in vivo. From studies by our laboratory and others, it is known that aged mice exhibit blunted immune responses (including DTH) in vivo [6, 42–46]. However, we observed that while aged mice given control IgG mounted DTH responses that were 30–50% less in magnitude compared to young mice, aged mice treated systemically with anti-CD1d antibody to block the activation of NKT-cells in vivo, generated DTH responses that were remarkably similar to those seen in young mice [6]. Delayed-type hypersensitivity requires adequate generation of CD4⁺ effector T-cells during the priming phase in order for the effector arm of the response to proceed. Although aged mice and humans are known to possess fewer CD4⁺ T-cells and a contracted effector T-cell repertoire, our studies suggested that despite fewer CD4⁺ T-cell numbers overall, aged mice could generate adequate effector T-cell immunity in vivo when challenged with antigen and an adjuvant, provided NKT-cell activation was attenuated. The idea that blunted effector CD4⁺ T-cell immunity observed with aging can be overcome is also supported by studies from Haynes and colleagues that used a combination of adjuvant and inflammatory cytokines to achieve results similar to ours [44]. Taken together, the current observations suggest that the decline in the quality of protective T-cell immunity associated with aged animals may be due at least in part, to a CD1d-NKT dependent active suppression of effector T-cell function.

   In addition to changes in T-cell function and increased NKT-cell numbers, NKT-cell cytokine production also appears to change with increasing age. While this area of investigation needs to be explored much further, so far it has been shown that splenocytes activated by CD3ε mAb in vitro show increased IL-4 (both cytokine protein and mRNA) and diminished IL-2 output as compared to young, when measured by ELISA [6, 47]. It has also been demonstrated that CD1d-restricted NKT-cells from aged mice produce lower amounts of IFNγ both at basal levels and stimulation with IL-12 [36, 48]. This apparent NKT-cell dependent change in cytokine profile has been postulated to contribute to the overall decreased immunocompetence in aged animals although it has not been proven. Interestingly, systemic anti-CD1d treatment does not significantly decrease inducible IL-4 production [6] and it was found that in fact, memory T-cell subsets (CD44ʰⁱᵍʰCD445RBˡᵒʷNK1.1ⁿᵉᵍ) produce much of the age-associated IL-4 in response to CD3ε-stimulation, however, they do so in an NKT-cell-dependent fashion [38, 47]. Our laboratory also reported that IL-10 production among spleen cell populations is nearly 10 times higher than the amount produced by splenocyte cultures from young mice. Unlike IL-4, the age-related increase in inducible IL-10 was significantly diminished in splenocytes obtained from aged mice that were given systemic NKT-cell blockade. There is also evidence that NKT-cells from aged mice have impaired IFNγ production, since lower baseline levels and IL-12 induced production of this important cytokine have been noted with aging [36]. Although relatively meager, the current set of data collectively support the notion that as age advances, NKT-cells shift from a more protective, IFN-γ producing phenotype (Th1), to a suppressive (Th2) type phenotype in both mice and humans by increasing IL-4 and IL-10 output.

Lastly, in addition to age-related alterations in cytokine production, NKT-cells from aged mice have also been reported to exhibit decreased cytotoxic capabilities [40, 49]. However, whether this observation applies to all CD1d-restricted NKT-cells throughout the immune compartment vs. other CD1d-unrestricted NKT-cell populations, such as those that exist in the liver, remains to be determined.

6 Summary

In summary, the effects of age on conventional lymphocyte populations have been widely studied, but age-related alterations among innate lymphocytes including NKT-cells are not as well understood. From a thorough review of the current literature that examines elderly humans and truly gerontologic mice, it appears that as age advances, the number of NKT-cells increases and their functions, particularly cytokine production, deviate away from immune protection and more toward immune suppression. The mechanisms responsible for greater numbers of NKT-cells in aged mice is also unclear, but may result from dysregulated ontologic signals that control progenitor cell development and proliferation, cell death, and homeostatic proliferation. Additionally, the possibility exists that NKT-cells, like other cells of the innate immune system may exhibit comparatively greater longevity than conventional lymphocytes. What is clear is that given their potent regulatory capacity over immune and inflammatory processes, significantly more research is required with both human cells as well as mouse models to understand how age-related alterations in NKT-cell biology might contribute to either the age-related decline in immunity or development of cancers and autoimmunity.

References

1. Joyce S (2001) CD1d and natural T cells: how their properties jump-start the immune system. Cell Mol Life Sci 5:442
2. Bendelac A, MN Rivera, SH Park, JH Roark (1997) Mouse CD1-specific NK1 T cells: development, specificity, and function. Annu Rev Immunol 15:535

3. Bendelac A (1995) Mouse NK1⁺ T cells. Curr Opin Immunol 7:367
4. Stein-Streilein J, KH Sonoda, D Faunce, J Zhang-Hoover (2000) Regulation of adaptive immune responses by innate cells expressing NK markers and antigen-transporting macrophages. J Leukocyte Biol 67:488
5. Rhee RJ, S CArlton, JL Lomas, C Lane, L Brossay, WG Cioffi, A Ayala (2003) Inhibition of CD1d activation suppresses septic mortality: a role for NK-T cells in septic immune dysfunction. J Surg Res 115:74
6. Faunce DE, JL Palmer, KK Paskowicz, PL Witte, EJ Kovacs (2005) CD1d-restricted NKT cells contribute to the age-associated decline of T cell immunity. J Immunol 175:3102
7. Palmer JL, JM Tulley, EJ Kovacs, RL Gamelli, M Taniguchi, DE Faunce (2006) Injury-induced suppression of effector T cell immunity requires CD1d-positive APCs and CD1d-restricted NKT cells. J Immunol 177:92
8. Bendelac A, PB Savage, L Teyton (2007) The biology of NKT cells. Ann Rev Immunol 25:297
9. Savage PB, L Teyton, A Bendelac (2006) Glycolipids for natural killer T cells. Chem Soc Rev 35:771
10. Mattner J, KL Debord, N Ismail, RD Goff, C Cantu III, D Zhou, P Saint-Mezard, V Wang, Y Gao, N Yin, K Hoebe, O Schneewind, D Walker, B Beutler, L Teyton, PB Savage, A Bendelac (2005) Exogenous and endogenous glycolipid antigens activate NKT cells during microbial infections. Nature 434:525
11. Gumperz JE, S Miyake, T Yamamura, MB Brenner (2002) Functionally distinct subsets of CD1d-restricted natural killer T cells revealed by CD1d tetramer staining. J Exp Med 195:625
12. Matsuda JL, OV Naidenko, L Gapin, T Nakayama, C-R Wang, Y Koezuka, M Kronenberg (2000). Tracking the response of natural killer T cells to a glycolipid antigen using CD1d tetrameters. J Exp Med 192:741
13. Faunce DE, KH Sonoda, J Stein-Streilein (2001) MIP-2 recruits NKT cells to the spleen during tolerance induction. J Immunol 166:313
14. Geissmann F, TO Cameron, S Sidobre, N Manlongat, M Kronenberg, MJ Briskin, ML Dustin, DR. Littman 2005 Intravascular immune surveillance by CXCR6 +NKT cells patrolling liver sinusoids. Plos Biology 3:e113.
15. Kim CH (2002) Trafficking machinery of NKT cells: shared and differential chemokine receptor expression among Va24+VB11+ NKT cell subsets with distinct cytokine-producing capacity. Blood 100:11
16. Benlagha K, A Bendelac (2000) CD1d-restricted mouse V alpha 14 and human V alpha 24 T cells; lymphocytes of innate immunity. Semin Immunol 12:537
17. Brossay L, M Kronenberg (1999) Highly conserved antigen-presenting function of CD1d molecules. Immunogenetics 50:146
18. Prigozy TI, O Naidenko, P Qasba, D Elewaut, L Brossay, A Khurana, T Natori, Y Koezuka, A Kulkarni, M Kronenberg (2001) Glycolipid antigen processing for presentation by CD1d molecules. Science 291:664
19. Bendelac A, O Lantz, ME Quimby, JW Yewdell, JR Bennink, RR Brutkiewicz (1995) CD1 recognition by mouse NK1⁺ T lymphocytes. Science 268:863
20. Bendelac A (1995) CD1: presenting unusual antigens to unusual T lymphocytes. Science 269:185
21. Bendelac A, N Killeen, DR Littman, RH Scwartz (1994) A subset of CD4+ thymocytes selected by MHC class I molecule. Science 263:1774
22. Exley MA, J Garcia, SP Balk, S Porcelli (1997) Requirements for CD1d recognition by human invariant Valpha24 +CD4-CD8- T cells. J Exp Med 186:109
23. Kronenberg M, O Naidenko, F Koning (2001). Right on target: novel approaches for the direct visualization of CD1-specific T cell responses. Proc Nat Adac Sci U S A 98:2950
24. Naidenko OV, JK Maher, WA Ernst, T Sakai, RL Modlin, M Kronenberg (1999) Binding and antigen presentation of ceramide-containing glycolipids by soluble mouse and human CD1d molecules. J Exp Med 190:1069

25. Sidobre S, OV Naidenko, BC Sim, NR Gascoigne, KC Garcia, M Kronenberg (2002) The V alpha 14 NKT cell TCR exhibits high-affinity binding to a glycolipid/CD1d complex. J Immunol 169:1340

26. Morita M, K Motoki, T Akimoto, T Natori, T Sakai, E Sawa, K Yamaji, Y Koezuka, E Kobayashi, H Fukushima (1995) Structure-activity relationship of alpha-galactosylceramides against B16-bearing mice. J Med Chem 38:2176

27. Sakai T, OV Naidenko, H Iijima, M Kronenberg, Y Koezuka (1999) Syntheses of biotinylated alpha-galactosylceramides and their effects on the immune system and CD1 molecules. J Med Chem 42:1836

28. Kobayashi E, K Motoki, T Uchida, H Fukushima, Y Koezuka (1995) KRN7000, a novel immunomodulator, and its antitumor activities. Oncol Res 7:529

29. Kawakami K, Y Kinjo, S Yara, K Uezu, Y Koguchi, M Tohyama, M Azuma, K Takeda, S Akira, A Saito (2001) Enhanced gamma interferon production through activation of Valpha14(+) natural killer T cells by alpha-galactosylceramide in interleukin-18-deficient mice with systemic cryptococcosis. Infect Immun 69:6643.

30. Kawakami K, Y Kinjo, S Yara, Y Koguchi, UT Nakayama, M Taniguchi, A Saito (2001) Activation of Valpha14 +natural killer T cells by alpha-glactosylceramide results in development of Th1 response and local host resistance in mice infected with Cryptococcus neoformans. Infect Immun 69:213

31. Wu D, G Xing, MA Poles, A Horowitz, Y Kinjo, B Sullivan, V Bodmer-Narkevitch, O Plettenburg, M Kronenberg, M Tsuji, DD Ho, C Wong (2005) Bacterial glycolipids and analogs as antigens for CD1d-restricted NKT cells. Proc Natl Acad Sci U S A 102:1351

32. Kinjo Y, D Wu, G Kim, G-W Xing, MA Poles, DD Ho, M Tsuji, K Kawahara, C-H Wong, M Kronenberg (2005) Recognition of bacterial glycosphingolipids by natural killer T cells. pp 520

33. Fischer K, E Scotet, M Niemeyer, H Koebernick, J Zerrahn, S Maillet, R Hurwitz, M Kursar, M Bonneville, SH Kaufmann, UE Schaible (2004) Mycobacterial phosphatidylinositol mannoside is a natural antigen for CD1d-restricted T cells. Proc Natl Acad Sci U S A 101:10685

34. Zhou D, J Mattner, C Cantu, N Schrantz, N Yin, Y Gao, Y Sagiv, K Hudspeth, Y Wu, T Yamashita, S Teneberg, D Wang, RL Proia, SB Levery, PB Savage, L Teyton, A Bendelac (2004) Lysosomal glycoshingolipid recognition by NKT cells. Science 306:1786

35. Inui T, R Nakagawa, S Ohkura, Y Habu, Y Koike, K Motoki, N Kuranaga, M Fukasawa, N Shinomiya, S Seki (2002) Age-associated augmentation of the synthetic ligand- mediated function of mouse NK1.1 ag(+) T cells: their cytokine production and hepatotoxicity in vivo and in vitro. J Immunol 169:6127

36. Mocchegiani E, M Malavolta (2004) NK and NKT cell functions in immunosenescence. pp 177

37. Berzins SP, FW McNab, CM Jones, MJ Smyth, DI Godfrey (2006) Long-term retention of mature NK1.1+ NKT cells in the thymus. J Immunol 176:4059

38. Poynter ME, HH Mu, XP Chen, RA Daynes (1997) Activation of NK1.1+ T cells in vitro and their possible role in age-associated changes in inducible IL-4 production. Cell Immunol 179:22

39. Ishimoto Y, C Tomiyama-Miyaji, H Watanabe, H Yokoyama, K Ebe, S Tsubata, Y Aoyagi, T Abo (2004) Age-dependent variation in the proportion and number of intestinal lymphocyte subsets, especially natural killer T cells, double-positive CD4+ CD8+ cells and B220+ T cells, in mice. Immunology 113:371

40. Tsukahara A, S Seki, T Iiai, T Moroda, H Wantanabe, S Suzuki, T Tada, H Hiraide, K Hatakeyama, T Abo (1997) Mouse liver T cells: their change with aging and in comparison with peripheral T cells. Hepatology 26:301

41. DelaRosa O, R Tarazona, JG Casado, C Alonso, B Ostos, J Pena, R Solana (2002) Valpha24+ NKT cells are decreased in elderly humans. Exp Gerontol 37:213

42. Plackett TP, EM Schilling, DE Faunce, MA Choudhry, PL Witte, EJ Kovacs (2003) Aging enhances lymphocyte cytokine defects after injury. FASEB J 17:688

43. Kovacs EJ, TP Plackett, PL Witte (2004) Estrogen replacement, aging, and cell-mediated immunity after injury. J Leukocyte Biol 76:36

44. Haynes LES (2004) Inflammatory cytokines overcome age-related defects in CD4 T cell responses in vivo. J Immunol 172:5194

45. Eaton SM, EM Burns, K Kusser, TD Randall, L Haynes (2004) Age-related defects in CD4 T cellcognate helper function lead to reductions in humoral immune responses. J Exp Med 200:1616

46. Haynes L, SM Eaton, SL Swain (2000) The defects in effector generation associated with aging can be reversed by addition of IL-2 but not other related gamma(c)-receptor binding cytokines. Vaccine 18:1649

47. Dubey DP, Z Husain, E Levitan, D Zurakowski, N Mirza, S Younes, C Coronell, D Yunis, EJ Yunis (2000) The MHC influences NK and NKT cell functions associated with immune abnormalities and lifespan. Mech Ageing Dev 113:117

48. Mocchegiani E, L Santarelli, L Costarelli, C Cipriano, E Muti, R Giacconi, M Malavolta (2006) Plasticity of neuroendocrine-thymus interactions during ontogeny and ageing: role of zinc and arginine. Ageing Res Rev 5:281

49. Mocchegiani E, R Giacconi, C Cipriano, N Gasparini, G Bernardini, M Malavolta, M Menegazzi, E Cavalieri, M Muzzioli, AR Ciampa, H Suzuki (2004) The variations during the circadian cycle of liver CD1d-unrestricted NK1.1+TCR gamma/delta+ cells lead to successful ageing. Role of metallothionein/IL-6/gp130/PARP-1 interplay in very old mice. Exp Gerontol 39:775

Cellular Immunosenescence - Stem Cells

Lympho-Hematopoietic Stem Cells and Their Aging

Hartmut Geiger and Gary Van Zant

Contents

Abstract: The lympho-hematopoietic system is largely composed of cells with short lifespans (days) and thus requires continuous replenishment of the cells lost through hematopoietic stem and progenitor cells in a process called hematopoiesis. Experimental evidence from several laboratories clearly demonstrates that hematopoietic stem cells (HSCs) harvested from young and aged animals show functional differences that are intrinsic to HSCs, implying that also stem cells in the hematopoietic system can not defy aging. We will thus discuss in this chapter the cellular phenotypes and the possible molecular mechanisms associated with aged HSCs with respect to the specific properties stem cells are endowed with, and will

H. Geiger (✉)
Assistant Professor
Division of Experimental Hematology
TCHRF S7.601
Cincinnati Children's Hospital Medical Center
3333 Burnet Avenue
Cincinnati, OH 45229, USA
Tel.: 513 636 1338
Fax: 513 636 3768
E-mail: hartmut.geiger@cchmc.org

G. V. Zant
Department of Internal Medicine
University of Kentucky, Lexington
Kentucky, USA

T. Fulop et al. (eds.), *Handbook on Immunosenescence,*
DOI 10.1007/ 978-1-4020-9062-2_30, © Springer Science+Business Media B.V. 2009

investigate whether stem cell aging is inevitable or whether some of its aspects can be reverted or at least ameliorated.

Keywords: Stem cell • Aging • Hematopoiesis • Niche • DNA damage • Adhesion

1   Stem Cells

Organ or tissue attrition due to loss of cells by various means is inevitably associated with life. Thus to achieve tissue homeostasis for a long period of time, lost cells have to be replaced and/or renewed. Many, but perhaps not all tissues or organs, depend on undifferentiated stem cells to support the generation of novel differentiated cells for a given tissue. Many tissues of the major organ systems are thus composed of short-lived cells that require continuous replenishment like skin, intestine and the hematopoietic tissue as well as somatic stem cells (Potten and Morris, 1988; Morrison et al. 1995; Fuchs and Segre, 2000; Tani et al. 2000; Stappenbeck et al. 2003). Stem cells have been also identified in brain and heart, although their contribution to adult tissue homeostasis is still debated (McKay, 1997; Doetsch et al. 1999; Gage 2000; Beltrami et al. 2003; Oh et al. 2003).

Stem cells are commonly defined by two characteristics: their ability to either self-renew or to differentiate into most of the mature cells types that comprise a tissue (van der Kooy and Weiss 2000). Both processes are associated with the ability of stem cells to undergo symmetric versus asymmetric divisions (mode of the division). The regulation of the mode of division thus poses an important fundamental question in stem cell biology. The molecular determinants that influence symmetric versus asymmetric divisions of stem cells are not well understood, which still hinder rationale approaches to modulate the outcome of stem cell divisions for example for clinical purposes.

2   Hematopoiesis

The lympho-hematopoietic system is largely composed of cells with short lifespans (days) and thus requires continuous replenishment of the cells lost through stem and progenitor cells in a process called hematopoiesis. Hematopoiesis is in adults restricted mostly to the bone marrow (BM) cavities. Hematopoietic stem cells (HSCs) are the most primitive cells of the blood lineage and give, upon differentiation, rise to the entire panoply of mature blood cells. They are rare and comprise only about 0.01% of the BM cell population, but are a long-lived population that are normally not depleted during a lifetime.

The cellular differentiation pathway is organized in a functional hierarchy, in which HSCs differentiate upon an asymmetric division into progenitor cells (also called transient amplifying cells in other stem cell systems), which then differentiate upon multiple steps of additional asymmetric divisions into mature blood cells. Upon differentiation and further specification, hematopoietic progenitor cells (HPCs) lose their ability to self-renew forever, and thus only true HSCs are associated with unrestricted self-renewal capacity.

In addition to their self-renewal and differentiation capacity, HSCs are also endowed with a remarkable, but still not well understood mobilization and homing ability, meaning they are able to migrate out of the BM into the bloodstream and also are able to migrate with a relatively high efficiency and specificity from peripheral blood back into the BM and to their niche, where this self-renewal and differentiation takes place. The physiological role of HSCs found in the circulation has puzzled investigators for a long time. One explanation is that these circulating HSCs are a pool of cells that help distinct sites of hematopoiesis to communicate with each other (Wright et al. 2001). Another interesting recently published explanation is that HSCs apparently circulate into and out of the lymphatic system serving an immuno-surveillance role, and it is suggested that they can via this route survey peripheral organs and foster the local production of tissue-resident innate immune cells under both steady-state conditions and in response to inflammatory signals (Massberg et al. 2007).

Thus, due to these distinct abilities, the potential of hematopoietic stem cells can be tested in a transplantation assay, which is regarded as the gold standard for testing HSCs activity in vivo. In such an assay, syngeneic animals will be myeloablated or lethally irradiated, which opens up in both cases niches for HSCs in the BM. Subsequently, HSCs that are injected into the bloodstream of these recipient mice will home to these empty niches, undergo self-renewal and differentiation, and will consequently be able to contribute to the hematopoietic system of the animal for a lifetime. The relative or absolute ability of the transplanted

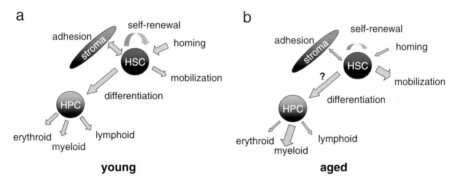

Fig. 1 Aging of hematopoietic stem cells. (a) Hematopoietic tem cells (HSCs) are defined by their ability to self-renew, to home to the bone marrow, to mobilize out of their niche into peripheral blood and their ability to adhere to stroma cells. In addition, HSCs will differentiate via hematopoietic progenitor cells (HPCs) in various distinct blood cell lineages. (b) Upon aging, HSCs present with reduced self-renewal activity, decreased homing but enhanced mobilization ability, which might be a result of the reduced ability of aged HSCs to adhere to stroma. Aged HSCs furthermore show a clear preference for myeloid over lymphoid and erythroid differentiation

stem cells to reconstitute the hematopoietic system of the recipient is regarded as a quantitative measurement of the stem cell potential.

3 How Do We Define and Isolate Hematopoietic Stem Cells?

Under a microscope, hematopoietic stem cell look actually identical to HPCs and similar to even some differentiated hematopoietic cells, including small- to medium-sized lymphocytes. So how do we identify and purify HSCs to study their biology? Over 50 years of intense research in the field of hematopoiesis and HSCs allow researchers now, at least in mice, to prospectively isolate the putative stem cells solely based on the inclusion or exclusion of distinct cell surface markers trough cell sorting via flow cytometry. HSC function and purity can then be subsequently verified in transplantation assays. Various distinct combinations of cell surface markers, which further evolved over time in complexity, but inversely resulted also in higher purity, have been used to identify HSCs. In aggregation of most of the literature, and most widely used by investigators at present, are three protocols to prospectively isolated stem cells, the LSK/CD34, the SLAM and the side population (SP) approach (Osawa et al. 1996; Kiel et al. 2005; Lin and Goodell 2006; Yilmaz et al. 2006). In the LSK/CD34 system, HSCs are defined as being negative for markers found on differentiated cells (lineage markers, and thus LIN- or L) as well as negative for CD34, but positive for the Sca-1 and the c-Kit epitopes. In the SLAM system, HSCs are defined as BM cells positive for CD150 while at the same time negative for CD48. Finally, in the SP approach a distinct cell population that does not retain the Hoechst dye 33342 (measured at two distinct emission wavelength) is highly enriched for HSCs. Although the purity of the presumed stem cell populations varies among these protocols, and each purification system might even enrich for slightly functionally distinct HSCs (Weksberg et al. 2008), all three are rigorously experimentally validated in terms of their ability to highly enrich for stem cells, and of course, there is major cell surface phenotype overlap among the purified populations (Kiel et al. 2005; Yilmaz et al. 2006; Weksberg et al. 2008).

3.1 The Aging of Hematopoietic Stem Cells

The aging process is probably best defined as a general loss in biological competence for both the individual cell and the organism as a whole. At the cellular level, it is expressed as decreasing replicative ability in proliferating cells and decreasing functional activity in postmitotic cells.

Stem cells were thought to be endowed with unlimited self-renewal capacity and thus assumed to be exempt from aging, which would result in functionally young stem cells in a chronologically aged animal. But evidence accumulating over the past decade has now proven that there is a measurable and successive functional decline in hematopoietic, intestinal and muscle stem cell replicative activity from adulthood to old age, resulting in a decline of stem cell function (Morrison et al. 1996b; Chen et al. 1999; Sudo et al. 2000; Geiger and Van Zant 2002; Kim et al. 2003; Van Zant and Liang 2003; Rossi et al. 2005; Chambers et al. 2007). As stem cell activity is necessary to replenish lost differentiated cells in a stem cell driven tissue, it has been hypothesized that aging of stem cells leads to reduced renewal and thus reduced tissue homeostasis in aged animals, probably most obvious under stress situations (Geiger et al. 2001b; Geiger and Van Zant 2002; Van Zant and Liang 2003; Sharpless and DePinho 2004; Torella et al. 2004).Ultimately, this may determine individual longevity, although so far no lifespan extension in response to stem cell therapy has been reported. This hypothesis though is supported for example by the fact that the function of the innate immune system, which depends on stem and progenitor cells activity, is compromised in aged individuals (Ginaldi et al. 1999; Butcher et al. 2001; Lord et al. 2001).

3.2   Defining Aging of Stem Cells

Stem cells are social entities that communicate and associate with supporting cells (called stroma) in a distinct 3 dimensional space (called niche). It is believed this niche is essential for stem cell regulation (Yin and Li 2006). So immediately the question arises whether stem cells age themselves (intrinsic aging) or the niche itself ages, which as a consequence impairs the function of an otherwise young and healthy stem cell occupying this niche (extrinsic aging). In case stem cell aging was mostly driven by extrinsic clues, we would anticipate that stem cells from aged animals, when transplanted into young niches (young animals), become functionally young again. Experimental evidence though from several laboratories clearly demonstrates that HSCs harvested from young and aged animals show functional differences that are intrinsic to HSCs (Geiger and Van Zant 2002; Geiger et al. 2005; Rossi et al. 2005) and less dependent on the microenvironment, although it does not exclude extrinsic influences on stem cell aging. These data thus allow us to refer to the cells as aged HSCs and young HSCs when the age refers to the animal from which the cells were harvested. Whether or not though stem cell aging in general is mostly driven by intrinsic mechanisms is still a matter of debate, as for example in muscle, aging of muscle progenitor cells is reverted by changes in the systemic environment and thus most likely dominated by extrinsic factors (Conboy et al. 2005).

   Various experimental approaches have been developed/employed to study causes and consequences of HSCs aging, and there seems to be a experimental duality in the field of aging research in general and also in the context of HSCs: Research on aging in a physiological environment and at a physiological pace in contrast to research on stem cell phenotypes in genetically modified animals which present with accelerated aging/stem cell aging. Let us have a short detour to the car repair shop to explain the differences in more detail.

We will start with describing the ailments of old cars (old stem cells) and just list all the problems a mechanic usually finds in them and which might be the reason for why the old car might not function very well anymore. We know that the mechanic's observations are correlative, but he will eventually replace/fix the worn out part(s) he was talking about and thus will subsequently test whether he was guessing right (causative approach).

Genetically modified animals on the other hand that present with phenotypes indicative of accelerated stem cell aging (either partial or in general) are more like cars in which we messed up on purpose with let's say the water pump and of course, over time the pump and subsequently the car will break. This tells us that the water pump is an essential part for the car, it does though not prove that in most cases in aged cars that is the part that will break, or whether preventing in general water pumps from braking in old cars will reduce the fragility of old cars. Only after the mechanic that usually sees all the old cars in the repair shop agrees that water pumps in old cars are an issue and tend to break, we are convinced about the relevance of our observations in the accelerated model [see also (Hasty and Vijg 2004; Miller 2004; Warner 2004)]. Although the authors do not imply that one approach might be superior over the other, it is still a good idea to differentiate between these experimental approaches. We will focus in the following paragraph primarily on physiological stem cell aging, and refer to premature aging systems whenever relevant.

There is still controversy on aspects of the phenotype and function of physiologically aged HSCs. The following phenotypes therefore represent commonly agreed phenotypes for aged HSCs and supported by research conducted by multiple independent investigators (canonical aging phenotypes). We suggest that the combination of these phenotypes comprise an physiologically aged HSCs, but that of course "partial" stem cell aging might be observed under given circumstances. Aged and young HSCs differ mostly in their function, and for HSCs, this function is best measured in transplantation assays. Consequently, most of the available data characterizing functional differences between aged and young stem cells has been generated by comparing young and aged HSCs in transplantation experiments.

3.3   Changes in Function Associated With Aged HSCs

In a competitive transplant setting, when stem cells from aged mice from the C57BL/6 inbred strain are transplanted along-side young cells into a lethally irradiated recipient animal, aged HSCs are less efficient in contributing to hematopoiesis (perturbed homeostasis) compared to young HSCs (Morrison et al. 1996b; Chen et al. 2000). Whether or not aged HSCs are also reduced in their ability to self-renew is still a matter of debate, although clearly aged HSCs are functionally impaired compared to young stem cells in serial transplantation assays.

Aging also affects the differentiation potential of HSCs (Rossi et al. 2005). Many studies have demonstrated that aged stem cells have a reduced ability to support the red blood cell system, and that aged HSCs do not efficiently generate both T- and B-lymphoid progeny, while they present with an increased ability to differentiate into the myeloid lineage [*see* (Linton and Dorshkind 2004) and references cited therein]. This difference in cell lineage self-renewal is emphasized by age-associated anemia and a decline in function of immune cells in aged individuals (Lipschitz and Udupa 1986; Lipschitz 1995; Ginaldi et al. 1999; Sudo et al. 2000; Butcher et al. 2001; Lord et al. 2001; Kim et al. 2003; Rossi et al. 2005). The generalized lymphoid defect has been at least in part attributed to an impaired ability of aged HSCs to differentiate into the common-lymphoid progenitor cell, the progenitor cells that will give rise to both the T- and the B-cell lineage. Thus aged HSCs are impaired in their ability to support the repopulation of the thymus and are less able to contribute to the B-cell as well as the T-cell lineage. Finally, aged HSCs are reduced in their ability to home from PB into the BM upon intravenous injection. A reduced ability to home to BM of aged HSCs was implied/speculated about in various publication and was recently experimentally confirmed by Liang et al. (Sudo et al. 2000; Kim et al. 2003; Liang et al. 2005; Rossi et al. 2005). The ability of HSCs to home to BM out of PB is clinically very important, as this is the first step to achieve successful engraftment in a HSC transplantation setting. Interestingly though, aged HSCs show enhanced mobilization proficiency upon G-CSF (Xing et al. 2006), which might in combination with the reduced homing indicate reduced cell–cell adhesion parameters for aged HSCs. Both impaired homing by old HSC and enhanced mobilization might imply "looser" niche association including dysregulated proteins involved in the HSC–niche interaction.

Comparing the engraftment properties of HSCs from various aged mouse inbred strains revealed that there are considerable differences in the rate of which stem cell self-renewal activity is reduced in aged animals, suggesting a strong genetic regulation of stem cell aging (Van Zant et al. 1990; Chen et al. 2000; Chen 2004; Geiger et al. 2005; Snoeck 2005;). Old C57BL/6 animals for example present with an increase in the number of phenotypically defined stem cells, although each of these stem cells has a clearly reduced potential upon transplantation, whereas old DBA/2 animals present with both, a reduced phenotypic number and a reduced function for aged HSCs. Thus, although overall the potential of the stem cell population decreases in the BM with aging independent of the strain, the pace with which this happens seem to be genetically restricted, adding another level of complexity to the determination of mechanisms that result in stem cell aging.

While the determination of stem cell function in the murine system via the transplantation assay can be relatively easily accomplished, our experimental tools to determine the function of human stem cells are understandably more limited. Thus investigations into the function of aged human HSCs are still in their infancy and more open to speculation, although both a reduced ability to support T-cell development as well as a reduced clonality and thus reduced stem cell number in aged humans has been so far identified [*see* for example (Wick et al. 1989; Abkowitz et al. 1998; Offner et al. 1999)]. In addition, elderly patients (similar to mice) frequently present with anemia. The mechanisms for this finding are mostly unexplained. (Balducci et al. 2006; Ferrucci et al. 2007).

3.4   Molecular Phenotypes Associated With Aged HSCs

What might be the molecular mechanisms responsible for the age-associated decrease in HSC function? As obvious from the previous paragraph, there are multiple phenotypes associated with aged stem cells. We thus do not assume that there is a single, unique molecular mechanism of stem cell aging, but rather that there are most likely multiple molecular pathways that result in these phenotypes, which we will address below.

3.5   Genome-Wide Gene Expression Profiling of Aged HSCs: Finding Pathways in Aging?

Several laboratories recently undertook a global approach to identify on the genome scale changes in the transcription level of genes associated with the young/aged transition of HSCs (Chambers et al. 2007; Rossi et al. 2005, Geiger and Van Zant, unpublished results). Unfortunately, each of these experiments were performed with HSCs purified according to a different scheme and analyzed with distinct microarrays, rendering a comparative approach almost impossible. In general though, genes associated with the stress response, cell adhesion, protein turnover and signal transduction dominated the up-regulated expression profile, while the down-regulated profile was marked by genes involved in the preservation of cell adhesion, genomic integrity and chromatin remodeling. So far though no specific pathway based on these RNA expression analyses could be identified based on the collections of these differentially expressed genes, emphasizing probably one more time the complexity of aging even at the single cell level. Interestingly though, in one set of these experiments, gene products associated with myeloid leukemia were markedly upregulated, which the authors interpreted in the way that aged stem cells might be, through their altered expression profile, already intrinsically prone to leukemia, although this hypothesis will require further experimental testing (Rossi et al. 2005).

3.6   The Role of Oxidative Damage in Stem Cell Aging

An important and probably universal mechanism that leads to a wide spectrum of intracellular damage during aging is extended exposure to reactive oxygen species (Hasty 2001). Long-term exposure to these metabolic byproducts leads to structural changes in a number of cellular macromolecules that impair their function. Such changes include the cross-linking of intracellular and intra-mitochondrial structural and functional proteins and carbohydrates, and the oxidation of fats and lipids in membranes as well as DNA damage. The multiple functional components a cell consists of form complex and interdependent physiological systems, making it difficult to determine which age-related change may be the primary cause of aging and which changes may be entrained by the primary event. Age-dependent changes in mitochondrial function and DNA integrity due to the accumulation of respiratory oxidative stress have also been reported for a variety of cell types, including liver, intestinal crypt and cardiac muscle cells (Bohr et al. 1998; Taylor et al. 2003). But the importance and frequency of mitochondrial mutations might have been overestimated compared with somatic mutations, as no increase in mitochondrial mutations in normally aged mice could be detected (Anson et al. 2000; Jacobs 2003; Khrapko and Vijg 2007; Vermulst et al. 2007). A role for reactive oxygen species and the p38 MAPK activity in limiting the self-renewal capacity and thus the lifespan of HSCs was recently experimentally demonstrated, as antioxidative treatment of HSCs resulted at least in partial reversion of the phenotypes associated with aged stem cells (Ito et al. 2006).

4   The Role of Telomere Length/Telomerase in Aging of HSCs

The hypothesis that cellular senescence is mediated via replicative exhaustion (Hayflick and Moorhead 1961; Barker et al. 1982) has received mechanistic support from the finding that telomeres may act as a mitotic clock (Vaziri et al. 1994; Greider 1998). Telomeres, the repetitive sequences at the chromosomal ends that provide chromosome stability, shorten with each round of cellular replication. When a critical short telomere length is reached, the cell enters a state of senescence or apoptoses. Some reports suggest a small, but significant decrease in telomere length in either human or murine HSCs upon aging or replicative stress post transplantation [(Vaziri et al. 1994; Brummendorf et al. 2001; Lansdorp 2008), and unpublished data Van Zant]. Since HSCs from laboratory mouse strains present with telomeres several times longer than human cells (Hemann and Greider 2000), and since stem cells synthesize telomerase to maintain telomeric length (Morrison et al. 1996a), whether natural telomere shortening by itself plays a role in HSC aging is still a matter of debate. These observations are further supported by the finding that although loss of telomerase activity clearly results in phenotypes associated with premature aging of stem cells, over-expression of telomerase in HSCs could so far not revert stem cell aging (Allsopp et al. 2003a, b).

5   The Role of DNA Damage in Aging of HSCs

A more likely cause for aging of stem cells in general, and HSCs in particular, might be age-dependent acquisition of defects in genomic DNA. HSC or intestinal stem cells show a high radiation sensitivity compared with most other cell types (Jacobson et al. 1949; Martin et al. 1998). This radio-sensitivity implies either a reduced ability of stem cells to repair even small amounts of DNA damage, stringent requirements on the DNA repair machinery for the maintenance of DNA fidelity, or increased rates of apoptosis. These various possibilities are not mutually exclusive. Moreover, brain, liver and muscle cells from old mice have a reduced ability to repair radiation-induced damage compared to young animals (Hamilton et al. 2001). Furthermore, Dolle et al. reported a general increase in the frequency of genomic mutations in old compared with young animals. Interestingly, small intestine, the only stem cell system with a high cell turnover analyzed in these experiments, showed the highest mutation frequency in 2.5-year-old animals among other tissues like heart, brain and liver (Vijg and Dolle 2002), although recent results indicated that the majority of this increase is attributed to a specific cell type in the organ/tissue, and thus does not affect all cells (Busuttil et al. 2007). Loss of DNA integrity with age as the major cause of stem cell aging is also compatible with the finding that aging of HSCs is mostly cell autonomous (van der Loo and Ploemacher 1995; Geiger et al. 2001a; Rossi et al. 2005; Rossi et al. 2007). Research to determine DNA-repair capacity in mammalian systems has mostly been concentrated on the quantification of DNA damage in whole tissues in response to induced damage by utilizing cell culture or animal models (Gaubatz and Tan 1994; Jeng et al. 1999; Goukassian et al. 2000; Doria and Frasca 2001; Zhao and Hemminki 2002; Beausejour et al. 2003; Chevanne et al. 2003; Parrinello et al. 2003; Scarpaci et al. 2003;). Although published results are contradictory, the majority of the data supports the notion that the DNA repair capacity declines with age and that aged HSC present with elevated levels of DNA damage (Mullaart et al. 1990; Rossi et al. 2007). HSC, similar to other types of stem cells, show an increased radiation sensitivity compared to mature cell types (Jacobson et al. 1949; Martin et al. 1998) and a distinct expression pattern of DNA-repair genes (Geiger lab, unpublished). Both facts imply that stem cells might use DNA repair pathways differently compared to well-studied pathways in differentiated cells or cell lines, a hypothesis supported by research on DNA repair pathways in ES cells (Cervantes et al. 2002; Hong and Stambrook 2004). In addition, the expression of the cyclin-dependent kinase inhibitor p16INK4a, a stress/DNA damage indicator, was found to be elevated in physiologically aged HSCs and this has been shown to be causative for reduced survival of aged HSCs under stress, as loss of p16 expression ameliorated stem cells aging (Janzen et al. 2006). Taken together, changes in the DNA repair system in HSCs, together with changes in cell cycle regulation due to DNA damage with age, might be an important cause for the decrease in the functional capacity of aged HSCs or in general aging of multiple tissue. Such a connection is further supported by comparative linkage analysis of hematopoietic stem cell traits and longevity (Geiger and Van Zant 2002). Loci mapped to chromosomes 2, 7 and 11 regulate DNA repair and aging of primitive hematopoietic cells and at the same time, longevity (Geiger et al. 2001a). As so far though only partial amelioration of HSCs aging could be achieved by altering expression of DNA repair genes or by antioxidative therapy, whether the DNA damage response plays the major role in stem cell aging will still be a matter of debate.

6   Altered Stem Cell–Niche Interactions in HSC Aging: A Novel Player in the Game

HSCs are entities that have social interactions. They reside in specialized three-dimensional microenvironments, or niches, in the BM. Cell-cell adhesion interactions between HSCs and stroma cells in the niche are believed to regulate HSC proliferation and differentiation. So far two niches, an endosteal and an endothelial niche, have been identified in the BM, and the distinct contribution of both of them to hematopoiesis is currently discussed [*see* for example (Adams and Scadden 2006; Kiel and Morrison 2006; Scadden 2006; Wilson and Trumpp 2006)]. Interactions of HSCs with stroma cells in the niche are consequently considered to be central to the biology of HSCs and have been therefore referred to as a stem cell synapses (similar to the immunological synapse; Adams and Scadden 2006; Scadden 2006; Yin and Li 2006). We recently reported that aged HSCs are impaired in their ability to strongly adhere to stroma cells [unpublished results and (Xing et al. 2006)]. This observation is supported by the fact that for example, the integrins $\alpha 4$ and $\alpha 5$ and the cell adhesion molecule VCAM-1 show lower expression on aged HSCs, whereas the expression of the adhesion molecule P-selectin and the $\alpha 6$ integrin are elevated in aged HSCs (Rossi et al. 2005; Xing et al. 2006). We could further demonstrate that physiologically aged primitive hematopoietic cells presented with elevated activity of the small Rho-GTPase CDC42, a protein tightly involved in regulating cellular adhesion (Van Hennik and Hordijk 2005; Wang et al. 2007; Yang et al. 2007). A distinct role for altered expression of adhesion molecules and thus altered adhesion in HSC differentiation was recently also suggested by Forsberg et al. (Forsberg et al. 2005), which supports a model in which unstable adhesion of aged HSCs to stroma might be causative for subsequent functional changes in aged HSCs. Whether the correlation between changes in expression of adhesion receptors and changes in the function of aged HSCs is also of mechanistic relevance though is not clear at the moment. We subsequently proposed that aged primitive hematopoietic cells are impaired in their ability to interact efficiently with stroma cells, which might result in the reduced self-renewal capacity as well as the altered differentiation ability associated with aged HSCs (Geiger et al. 2007). Elevated level of CDC42 activity detected in aged hematopoietic cells might be causative for these changes in cell–cell adhesion. These findings would further imply that also the stroma might play an important role in stem cell aging, as it too might be reduced in its ability to strongly interact with HSCs when aged. Molecular mechanisms that result in altered adhesion dynamics and altered function of aged HSCs might thus be tightly interconnected and result in an altered stem cell synapse for aged HSC. But as so many hypotheses linked to aging of stem cells, also this one is in critical need of additional experimental validation.

7 Amelioration/Prevention of Stem Cell Aging

Stem cell aging might be the underlying cause for dysregulated tissue homeostasis in aged individuals and consequently attenuation of stem cell aging will become a central to regenerative medicine. Identifying conditions under which in an aged organism aged stem cells are activated to be functionally equivalent to young stem cells could thus be a first step towards designing treatments to attenuate/revert the consequences of stem cell aging and consequently to improve age-associated imbalances in tissue homeostasis.

Studying muscle regeneration by muscle stem cells (satellite cells) in aged animals, Conboy et al. recently reported that aged muscle stem cells can be activated to repair/differentiate as efficiently as young muscle stem cells either by forced activation of Notch, or by systemic factors provided by serum from young animals (Conboy et al. 2003, 2005). They also identified that factors in serum from aged mice negatively affect muscle stem cell activation. As aging of HSCs is at least in part cell intrinsic, amelioration of HSCs aging might be more difficult to achieve. As mentioned above, loss of the p16 protein as well as antioxidative therapy both resulted in partial reversion of HSC aging. In addition, attenuation of HSC aging was also achieved by lifelong caloric restriction of mice from the BalbC inbred strain, without though further identification of a possible molecular mechanism underlying this stem cell response (Chen et al. 2003). These results are very promising and prove that it is possible to change the path of stem cell aging. More research though will be necessary to translate our knowledge on stem cell aging into therapies that promise a lifelong fountain of stem cell youth to all of us.

Acknowledgments   We apologize to the authors of all the references we forgot to cite or discuss due to space limitations in addition to aging of our neurons. Work in the laboratory of Dr. Geiger is supported by NIH grants DK077762 and HL076604. Work in the laboratory of Dr. Van Zant is supported by NIH Grants AG020917, AG022859, AG024950. Hartmut Geiger is a New Scholar in Aging of The Ellison Medical Foundation.

References

Abkowitz JL, Taboada M, Shelton GH, Catlin SN, Guttorp P, Kiklevich JV (1998) An X chromosome gene regulates hematopoietic stem cell kinetics. Proc Natl Acad Sci U S A 95:3862–3866

Adams GB, Scadden DT (2006) The hematopoietic stem cell in its place. Nat Immunol 7:333–337

Allsopp RC, Morin GB, DePinho R, Harley CB, Weissman IL (2003a) Telomerase is required to slow telomere shortening and extend replicative lifespan of HSCs during serial transplantation. Blood 102:517–520

Allsopp RC, Morin GB, Horner JW, DePinho R, Harley CB, Weissman IL (2003b) Effect of TERT over-expression on the long-term transplantation capacity of hematopoietic stem cells. Nat Med 9:369–371

Anson RM, Hudson E, Bohr VA (2000) Mitochondrial endogenous oxidative damage has been overestimated. FASEB J 14:355–360

Balducci L, Ershler WB, Krantz S (2006) Anemia in the elderly-clinical findings and impact on health. Crit Rev Oncol Hematol 58:156–165

Barker JE, McFarland EC, Bernstein SE (1982) The competitive ability of stem cells from mice with Hertwig's anemia. J Cell Physiol 113:257–260

Beausejour CM, Krtolica A, Galimi F, Narita M, Lowe SW, Yaswen P, Campisi J (2003) Reversal of human cellular senescence: roles of the p53 and p16 pathways. EMBO J 22:4212–4222.

Beltrami AP, Barlucchi L, Torella D, Baker M, Limana F, Chimenti S, Kasahara H, Rota M, Musso E, Urbanek K, Leri A, Kajstura J, Nadal-Ginard B, Anversa P (2003) Adult cardiac stem cells are multipotent and support myocardial regeneration. Cell 114:763–776

Bohr V, Anson RM, Mazur S, Dianov G (1998) Oxidative DNA damage processing and changes with aging. Toxicol Lett 102–103:47–52

Brummendorf TH, Rufer N, Baerlocher GM, Roosnek E, Lansdorp PM (2001) Limited telomere shortening in hematopoietic stem cells after transplantation. Ann N Y Acad Sci 938:1–7; discussion 7–8

Busuttil RA, Garcia AM, Reddick RL, Dolle ME, Calder RB, Nelson JF, Vijg J (2007) Intra-organ variation in age-related mutation accumulation in the mouse. PLoS ONE 2:e876

Butcher SK, Chahal H, Nayak L, Sinclair A, Henriquez NV, Sapey E, O'Mahony D, Lord JM (2001) Senescence in innate immune responses: reduced neutrophil phagocytic capacity and CD16 expression in elderly humans. J Leukoc Biol 70:881–886

Cervantes RB, Stringer JR, Shao C, Tischfield JA, Stambrook PJ (2002) Embryonic stem cells and somatic cells differ in mutation frequency and type. Proc Natl Acad Sci U S A 99:3586–3590.

Chambers SM, Shaw CA, Gatza C, Fisk CJ, Donehower LA, Goodell MA (2007) Aging hematopoietic stem cells decline in function and exhibit epigenetic dysregulation. PLoS Biol 5:e201

Chen J (2004) Senescence and functional failure in hematopoietic stem cells. Exp Hematol 32:1025–1032

Chen J, Astle CM, Harrison DE (1999) Development and aging of primitive hematopoietic stem cells in BALB/cBy mice. Exp Hematol 27:928–935

Chen J, Astle CM, Harrison DE (2000) Genetic regulation of primitive hematopoietic stem cell senescence. Exp Hematol 28:442–450

Chen J, Astle CM, Harrison DE (2003) Hematopoietic senescence is postponed and hematopoietic stem cell function is enhanced by dietary restriction. Exp Hematol 31:1097–1103

Chevanne M, Caldini R, Tombaccini D, Mocali A, Gori G, Paoletti F (2003) Comparative levels of DNA breaks and sensitivity to oxidative stress in aged and senescent human fibroblasts: a distinctive pattern for centenarians. Biogerontology 4:97–104

Conboy IM, Conboy MJ, Smythe GM, Rando TA (2003) Notch-mediated restoration of regenerative potential to aged muscle. Science 302:1575–1577

Conboy IM, Conboy MJ, Wagers AJ, Girma ER, Weissman IL, Rando TA (2005) Rejuvenation of aged progenitor cells by exposure to a young systemic environment. Nature 433:760–764

Doetsch F, Caille I, Lim DA, Garcia-Verdugo JM, Alvarez-Buylla A (1999) Subventricular zone astrocytes are neural stem cells in the adult mammalian brain. Cell 97:703–716

Doria G, Frasca D (2001) Age-related changes of DNA damage recognition and repair capacity in cells of the immune system. Mech Ageing Dev 122:985–998

Ferrucci L, Guralnik JM, Bandinelli S, Semba RD, Lauretani F, Corsi A, Ruggiero C, Ershler WB, Longo DL (2007) Unexplained anaemia in older persons is characterised by low erythropoietin and low levels of pro-inflammatory markers. Br J Haematol 136:849–855

Forsberg EC, Prohaska SS, Katzman S, Heffner GC, Stuart JM, Weissman IL (2005) Differential Expression of Novel Potential Regulators in Hematopoietic Stem Cells. PLoS Genet 1:e28.

Fuchs E, Segre JA (2000) Stem cells: a new lease on life. Cell 100:143–155

Gage FH (2000) Mammalian neural stem cells. Science 287:1433–1438

Gaubatz JW, Tan BH (1994) Aging affects the levels of DNA damage in postmitotic cells. Ann N Y Acad Sci 719:97–107

Geiger H, Koehler A, Gunzer M (2007) Stem Cells, Aging, Niche, Adhesion and Cdc42: A Model for Changes in Cell-Cell Interactions and Hematopoietic Stem Cell Aging. Cell Cycle 6

Geiger H, Rennebeck G, Van Zant G (2005) Regulation of hematopoietic stem cell aging in vivo by a distinct genetic element. Proc Natl Acad Sci U S A 102:5102–5107

Geiger H, True JM, de Haan G, Van Zant G (2001a) Age- and stage-specific regulation patterns in the hematopoietic stem cell hierarchy. Blood 98:2966–2972

Geiger H, True JM, De Haan G, Van Zant G (2001b) Longevity and stem cells: a genetic connection. Sci World J 1:77

Geiger H, Van Zant G (2002) The aging of lympho-hematopoietic stem cells. Nat Immunol 3:329-333

Ginaldi L, De Martinis M, D'Ostilio A, Marini L, Loreto MF, Quaglino D (1999) The immune system in the elderly: III. Innate immunity. Immunol Res 20:117–126

Goukassian D, Gad F, Yaar M, Eller MS, Nehal US, Gilchrest BA (2000) Mechanisms and implications of the age-associated decrease in DNA repair capacity. FASEB J 14:1325–1334

Greider CW (1998) Telomeres and senescence: the history, the experiment, the future. Curr Biol 8:R178–R181

Hamilton ML, Van Remmen H, Drake JA, Yang H, Guo ZM, Kewitt K, Walter CA, Richardson A (2001) Does oxidative damage to DNA increase with age? Proc Natl Acad Sci U S A 98:10469–10474

Hasty P (2001) The impact energy metabolism and genome maintenance have on longevity and senescence: lessons from yeast to mammals. Mech Ageing Dev 122:1651–1662

Hasty P, Vijg J (2004) Rebuttal to Miller: 'Accelerated aging': a primrose path to insight?' Aging Cell 3:67–69

Hayflick L, Moorhead P (1961) The serial cultivation of human diploid cell strains. Exp Cell Res 25:585

Hemann MT, Greider CW (2000) Wild-derived inbred mouse strains have short telomeres. Nucleic Acids Res 28:4474–4478

Hong Y, Stambrook PJ (2004) Restoration of an absent G1 arrest and protection from apoptosis in embryonic stem cells after ionizing radiation. Proc Natl Acad Sci U S A 101:14443–14448

Ito K, Hirao A, Arai F, Takubo K, Matsuoka S, Miyamoto K, Ohmura M, Naka K, Hosokawa K, Ikeda Y, Suda T (2006) Reactive oxygen species act through p38 MAPK to limit the lifespan of hematopoietic stem cells. Nat Med 12:446–451

Jacobs HT (2003) The mitochondrial theory of aging: dead or alive? Aging Cell 2:11–17

Jacobson LO, Marks EK, Robson MJ, Gaston EO, Zirkle RE (1949) Effect of spleen protection on mortality following x-irradiation. J Lab Clin Med 34:1538–1543

Janzen V, Forkert R, Fleming HE, Saito Y, Waring MT, Dombkowski DM, Cheng T, Depinho RA, Sharpless NE, Scadden DT (2006) Stem-cell ageing modified by the cyclin-dependent kinase inhibitor p16(INK4a). Nature 443:421–426

Jeng YW, Chao HC, Chiu CF, Chou WG (1999) Senescent human fibroblasts have elevated Ku86 proteolytic cleavage activity. Mutat Res 435:225–232

Khrapko K, Vijg J (2007) Mitochondrial DNA mutations and aging: a case closed? Nat Genet 39:445–446

Kiel MJ, Morrison SJ (2006) Maintaining Hematopoietic Stem Cells in the Vascular Niche. Immunity 25:862–864

Kiel MJ, Yilmaz OH, Iwashita T, Terhorst C, Morrison SJ (2005) SLAM family receptors distinguish hematopoietic stem and progenitor cells and reveal endothelial niches for stem cells. Cell 121:1109–1121

Kim M, Moon HB, Spangrude GJ (2003) Major age-related changes of mouse hematopoietic stem/progenitor cells. Ann N Y Acad Sci 996:195–208

Lansdorp PM (2008) Telomeres, stem cells, and hematology. Blood 111:1759–1766

Liang Y, Van Zant G, Szilvassy SJ (2005) Effects of aging on the homing and engraftment of murine hematopoietic stem and progenitor cells. Blood 106:1479–1487

Lin KK, Goodell MA (2006) Purification of hematopoietic stem cells using the side population. Methods Enzymol 420:255–264

Linton PJ, Dorshkind K (2004) Age-related changes in lymphocyte development and function. Nat Immunol 5:133–139

Lipschitz DA (1995) Age-related declines in hematopoietic reserve capacity. Semin Oncol 22:3–5

Lipschitz DA, Udupa KB (1986) Age and the hematopoietic system. J Am Geriatr Soc 34:448–454

Lord JM, Butcher S, Killampali V, Lascelles D, Salmon M (2001) Neutrophil ageing and immunesenescence. Mech Ageing Dev 122:1521–1535

Martin K, Potten CS, Roberts SA, Kirkwood TB (1998) Altered stem cell regeneration in irradiated intestinal crypts of senescent mice. J Cell Sci 111 (Pt 16):2297–2303

Massberg S, Schaerli P, Knezevic-Maramica I, Kollnberger M, Tubo N, Moseman EA, Huff IV, Junt T, Wagers AJ, Mazo IB, von Andrian UH (2007) Immunosurveillance by Hematopoietic Progenitor Cells Trafficking through Blood, Lymph, and Peripheral Tissues. Cell 131:994–1008

McKay R (1997) Stem cells in the central nervous system. Science 276:66–71

Miller RA (2004) Rebuttal to Hasty and Vijg: 'Accelerating aging by mouse reverse genetics: a rational approach to understanding longevity'. Aging Cell 3:53–54

Morrison SJ, Prowse KR, Ho P, Weissman IL (1996a) Telomerase activity in hematopoietic cells is associated with self-renewal potential. Immunity 5:207–216

Morrison SJ, Uchida N, Weissman IL (1995) The biology of hematopoietic stem cells. Ann Rev Cell Dev Biol 11:35–71

Morrison SJ, Wandycz AM, Akashi K, Globerson A, Weissman IL (1996b) The aging of hematopoietic stem cells [see comments]. Nat Med 2:1011–1016

Mullaart E, Lohman PH, Berends F, Vijg J (1990) DNA damage metabolism and aging. Mutat Res 237:189–210

Offner F, Kerre T, De Smedt M, Plum J (1999) Bone marrow CD34 cells generate fewer T cells in vitro with increasing age and following chemotherapy. Br J Haematol 104:801–808

Oh H, Bradfute SB, Gallardo TD, Nakamura T, Gaussin V, Mishina Y, Pocius J, Michael LH, Behringer RR, Garry DJ, Entman ML, Schneider MD (2003) Cardiac progenitor cells from adult myocardium: homing, differentiation, and fusion after infarction. Proc Natl Acad Sci U S A 100:12313–12318

Osawa M, Hanada K, Hamada H, Nakauchi H (1996) Long-term lymphohematopoietic reconstitution by a single CD34-low/negative hematopoietic stem cell. Science 273:242–245

Parrinello S, Samper E, Krtolica A, Goldstein J, Melov S, Campisi J (2003) Oxygen sensitivity severely limits the replicative lifespan of murine fibroblasts. Nat Cell Biol 5:741–747

Potten CS, Morris RJ (1988) Epithelial stem cells in vivo. J Cell Sci—Supplement 10:45–62

Rossi DJ, Bryder D, Seita J, Nussenzweig A, Hoeijmakers J, Weissman IL (2007) Deficiencies in DNA damage repair limit the function of haematopoietic stem cells with age. Nature 447:725–729

Rossi DJ, Bryder D, Zahn JM, Ahlenius H, Sonu R, Wagers AJ, Weissman IL (2005) Cell intrinsic alterations underlie hematopoietic stem cell aging. Proc Natl Acad Sci U S A 102:9194–9199

Scadden DT (2006) The stem-cell niche as an entity of action. Nature 441:1075–1079

Scarpaci S, Frasca D, Barattini P, Guidi L, Doria G (2003) DNA damage recognition and repair capacities in human naive and memory T cells from peripheral blood of young and elderly subjects. Mech Ageing Dev 124:517–524

Sharpless NE, DePinho RA (2004) Telomeres, stem cells, senescence, and cancer. J Clin Invest 113:160–168

Snoeck HW (2005) Quantitative trait analysis in the investigation of function and aging of hematopoietic stem cells. Methods Mol Med 105:47–62

Stappenbeck TS, Mills JC, Gordon JI (2003) Molecular features of adult mouse small intestinal epithelial progenitors. Proc Natl Acad Sci U S A 100:1004–1009

Sudo K, Ema H, Morita Y, Nakauchi H (2000) Age-associated Characteristics of Murine Hematopoietic Stem Cells. J Exp Med 192:1273–1280 [Record as supplied by publisher]

Tani H, Morris RJ, Kaur P (2000) Enrichment for murine keratinocyte stem cells based on cell surface phenotype. Proc Natl Acad Sci U S A 97:10960–10965

Taylor RW, Barron MJ, Borthwick GM, Gospel A, Chinnery PF, Samuels DC, Taylor GA, Plusa SM, Needham SJ, Greaves LC, Kirkwood TB, Turnbull DM (2003) Mitochondrial DNA mutations in human colonic crypt stem cells. J Clin Invest 112:1351–1360

Torella D, Rota M, Nurzynska D, Musso E, Monsen A, Shiraishi I, Zias E, Walsh K, Rosenzweig A, Sussman MA, Urbanek K, Nadal–Ginard B, Kajstura J, Anversa P, Leri A (2004) Cardiac Stem Cell and Myocyte Aging, Heart Failure, and Insulin-Like Growth Factor-1 Overexpression. Circ Res.

van der Kooy D, Weiss S (2000) Why stem cells? Science 287:1439–1441

van der Loo JC, Ploemacher RE (1995) Marrow- and spleen-seeding efficiencies of all murine hematopoietic stem cell subsets are decreased by preincubation with hematopoietic growth factors. Blood 85:2598–2606

Van Hennik PB, Hordijk PL (2005) Rho GTPases in hematopoietic cells. Antioxid Redox Signal 7:1440–1455

Van Zant G, Holland BP, Eldridge PW, Chen JJ (1990) Genotype-restricted growth and aging patterns in hematopoietic stem cell populations of allophenic mice. J Exp Med 171:1547–1565

Van Zant G, Liang Y (2003) The role of stem cells in aging. Exp Hematol 31:659–672

Vaziri H, Dragowska W, Allsopp RC, Thomas TE, Harley CB, Lansdorp PM (1994) Evidence for a mitotic clock in human hematopoietic stem cells: loss of telomeric DNA with age. Proc Natl Acad Sci U S A 91:9857–9860

Vermulst M, Bielas JH, Kujoth GC, Ladiges WC, Rabinovitch PS, Prolla TA, Loeb LA (2007) Mitochondrial point mutations do not limit the natural lifespan of mice. Nat Genet 39:540–543

Vijg J, Dolle ME (2002) Large genome rearrangements as a primary cause of aging. Mech Ageing Dev 123:907–915

Wang L, Yang L, Debidda M, Witte D, Zheng Y (2007) Cdc42 GTPase-activating protein deficiency promotes genomic instability and premature aging-like phenotypes. Proc Natl Acad Sci (accepted for publication)

Warner HR (2004) Head-to-head debate between Richard Miller and Paul Hasty/Jan Vijg. Aging Cell Vol. 3, Issue 2 (2004). Aging Cell 3:141–142

Weksberg DC, Chambers SM, Boles NC, Goodell MA (2008) CD150- side population cells represent a functionally distinct population of long-term hematopoietic stem cells. Blood 111:2444–2451

Wick M, Huber LA, Offner F, Winter U, Bock G, Schauenstein K, Jurgens G, Traill KN (1989) Immunodeficiency in old age. Curr Probl Dermatol 18:120–130

Wilson A, Trumpp A (2006) Bone-marrow haematopoietic-stem-cell niches. Nat Rev Immunol 6:93–106

Wright DE, Wagers AJ, Gulati AP, Johnson FL, Weissman IL (2001) Physiological migration of hematopoietic stem and progenitor cells. Science 294:1933–1936

Xing Z, Ryan MA, Daria D, Nattamai KJ, Van Zant G, Wang L, Zheng Y, Geiger H (2006) Increased hematopoietic stem cell mobilization in aged mice. Blood 108:2190–2197

Yang L, Wang L, Geiger H, Cancelas JA, Mo J, Zheng Y (2007) Rho GTPase Cdc42 coordinates hematopoietic stem cell quiescence and niche interaction in the bone marrow. Proc Natl Acad Sci U S A 104:5091–5096

Yilmaz OH, Kiel MJ, Morrison SJ (2006) SLAM family markers are conserved among hematopoietic stem cells from old and reconstituted mice and markedly increase their purity. Blood 107:924–930

Yin T, Li L (2006) The stem cell niches in bone. J Clin Invest 116:1195–1201

Zhao C, Hemminki K (2002) The in vivo levels of DNA alkylation products in human lymphocytes are not age dependent: an assay of 7-methyl- and 7-(2-hydroxyethyl)-guanine DNA adducts. Carcinogenesis 23:307–310

Implications of Developmental Switches for Hematopoietic Stem Cell Aging

Jens M. Nygren and David Bryder

Contents

Abstract: Each of the different hematopoietic cell types has their own properties and function, but only when they all act in tight synergy are they able to constitute a highly specific and efficient immune defense capable of efficient protection from invading pathogens and appropriate maintenance of blood clotting and oxygen transport functions.

All blood cell types are continuously produced in the bone-marrow by rare hematopoietic stem cells that persist throughout the life of the organism. These stem cells are influenced by their environment and developmental history and experience a range of cell intrinsic changes that over time alter their functional properties. These timed changes include alterations in fundamental processes such as self-renewal, proliferation, differentiation and gene expression, thereby being crucial for both normal maturation as well as hematopoietic aging.

Keywords: Aging • Developmental switch • Hematopoietic stem cell • Ontogeny • Quiescence

D. Bryder · J. M. Nygren (✉)
Stem Cell Aging, Department of Experimental Medical Science,
BMC D14, Lund University, 221 84 Lund, Sweden
Phone: +46 (0)46 22 20 313
Fax: +46 (0)46 22 24 218
E-mail: jens.nygren@med.lu.se

T. Fulop et al. (eds.), *Handbook on Immunosenescence*,
DOI 10.1007/ 978-1-4020-9062-2_31, © Springer Science+Business Media B.V. 2009

1   Introduction

The blood system produce hundred of millions of new blood cells everyday to maintain oxygen transport, blood clotting and immune function [Morrison et al. 1995b].
This process is highly conserved through evolution and therefore largely similar
between lower vertebrates and mammals [Laird et al. 2000; Zon 1995].

In the early 1960s, McCulloch and Till performed a series of ground breaking
experiments to search for multipotent and self-renewing hematopoietic stem cells
(HSC) that could sustain such extensive blood cell production throughout life. Bone-
marrow cells were injected intravenously into irradiated mice and the subsequent
engraftment of a rare fraction of these cells, as visible nodules in the spleens of the
recipients, were evaluated. From such experiments, it was established that nodules
appeared in proportion to the number of bone-marrow cells injected, and that individual nodules arose from single bone-marrow cells, named colony forming units spleen
(CFU-S) [McCulloch and Till 1960]. The ability of CFU-S to self-renew [Becker et al.
1963], a cardinal property of stem cell function, provided the first true evidence that
somatic HSC exists in the bone-marrow. Today, four decades later, we know that the
bone-marrow is the primary hematopoietic organ by the end of fetal maturation and
that seeding of HSC to the bone-marrow is a uniform process and results in homogeneous distribution to the different bone-marrow compartments, without spatial differences in hematopoiesis or HSC identity [Kiel et al. 2005]. The majority of cells in the
bone-marrow are maturing blood cells and their progenitors, and thus HSC constitute
a rare population of less than one in 15,000 bone-marrow cells [Lagasse et al. 2001].

2   Quiescent Hematopoietic Stem Cells

The identity of the bone-marrow HSC cannot be recognized by their morphology
and phenotype alone, but rather by their unique functional properties [Lagasse et al.
2001; Matsuzaki et al. 2004; Osawa et al. 1996]. Traditionally, function is evaluated
by the ability of cells to reconstitute the blood system following transplantation into
hosts in which endogenous HSC have been eradicated by a lethal dose of irradiation.
Similar to the CFU-S assay, reconstituting clones can be assayed by tissue sampling.
The progeny from reconstituting HSC are identified by monoclonal antibodies and
detected by flow cytometry to establish both level and quality of engraftment. With
this assay, HSC properties can be analyzed even at a clonal level by detection of the
descendants from single transplanted HSC [Osawa et al. 1996]. However, although
ultimately being capable of producing all blood cells, including phenocopies of
themselves, HSC remain low proliferative, presumably to limit divisional stress and
any intrinsic changes that comes with accumulated cell divisions and aging. The
mechanisms underlying such regulated quiescence is currently unknown but is one
of many features that take place throughout development which eventually lead to
the functional changes that are ascribed to the aging of HSC.

2.1 Quiescence and Cell Cycle Control

Adult HSC are largely quiescent in that their transit through the cell cycle is slow or even arrested at times. This is reflected by that as few as eight percent of the cells in the HSC pool enter cell cycle every day. Nonetheless, quiescence does not result in cell cycle arrest as most cells within a population of HSC have divided at least once within four to eight weeks [Bradford et al. 1997; Cheshier et al. 1999]. The series of events in an eukaryotic cell that are referred to as the cell cycle consists of distinct phases in which the cell undertakes sequential actions like growth and preparation of the chromosomes for replication (G_1 phase), DNA synthesis to duplicate the chromosomes (S phase), additional growth and preparation for cell division (G_2 phase) and finally, mitosis (M phase) during which the cell divides into 2 daughter cells [Steinman 2002]. This cyclic process is regulated at checkpoints [Mantel et al. 2001; Pardee 1989; Steinman 2002] during each phase-transition by cyclins that form complexes with cyclin-dependent kinases [Cheng 2004; Steinman 2002]. The cyclin-based surveillance system acts as a quality control that monitors the cell as it progresses through the cell cycle. Checkpoints can block progression through one phase if certain conditions are not met. For instance, mitosis is inhibited until DNA replication is completed or if not all chromosomes are attached to the mitotic spindle. A surveillance network of signaling molecules has been set up to instruct cells to stop dividing and to either repair the damage or initiate programmed cell death if necessary. For cells, like HSC, that persists and continues to proliferate throughout life, quiescence through tight negative control of cell cycle propagation and stringent surveillance of DNA integrity appears essential to minimize divisional stress and to ensure that damaged cells are not further propagated and do not progress into a cancerous state.

Some cells leave the cell cycle at the G_1 phase following a cell division and enter a nonproliferative G_0 stage [Pardee 1989]. Most often, G_0 cells are terminally differentiated and their exit from the cell cycle is thus permanent, whereas other cells, like HSC, are only temporally quiescent and can upon mitotic stimulation re-enter G_1 and prepare for additional cell cycles [Bradford et al. 1997]. HSC are relatively unresponsive to mitogenic stimuli [Bradford et al. 1997; Huang et al. 1999; Uchida et al. 2003] and this might reflect the fact that most cells in the HSC population are in a G_0 state. Thus, that HSC need a longer time and stronger stimulation than committed progenitor cells to respond to growth factors might reflect that they first need to get activated in order to reenter the cell cycle. Distinct regulation of the cell cycle activity of HSC by factors known to limit proliferation and differentiation [Cheng et al. 2000; Hock et al. 2004; Iwama et al. 2004; Lessard and Sauvageau 2003; Park et al. 2003; Walkley et al. 2005] is therefore presumably a key requirement to avoid exhaustion of the HSC compartment [Iscove and Nawa 1997] and should therefore represent a defining stem cell property. Active cell cycling have been suggested to exert negative effects on stem cell function [Fleming et al. 1993a; Glimm et al. 2000; Habibian et al. 1998; Jetmore et al. 2002; Orschell-Traycoff et al. 2000] although this can at least in part be an interpretation of experimental observations, as the design of such experiments have assumed both that dividing hematopoietic stem and progenitor cells have a similar cell cycle transit time and that HSC are identifiable by phenotype alone. Most likely, HSC in cycle are functionally normal but due to their quiescent state represents a rare fraction within populations of enriched HSC in $S/G_2/M$ stages. They are therefore outnumbered by nonquiescent and transiently reconstituting multipotent and lineage committed progenitor cells, which dominate most HSC enriched populations established to date [Nygren et al. 2006].

2.2   Quiescence but yet Hematopoiesis

As HSC divide, they can produce daughter cells of which at least one represent an identical replica of its ancestral HSC. Such self-renewing cell divisions are a hallmark of stem cells and necessary to maintain a constant HSC pool and lifelong production of all blood cell types [Becker et al. 1963]. Maintenance of the HSC pool can be the result of either asymmetrical cell divisions [Jan and Jan 1998] that results in one cell that is identical to the mother cell and one cell that is committed to differentiation, or of a balance of symmetrical cell divisions leading to either complete self-renewal or differentiation (i.e., result in either 2 HSC or 2 committed daughter cells). Nevertheless, asymmetric HSC divisions must occur at some point during cellular development and multilineage differentiation of committed cells [Takano et al. 2004] in order to appropriately generate progeny both for daily blood cell production as well as maintenance of a fairly constant number of slowly proliferating and inactive HSC. Daughter cells that do not inherit a stem cell identity loose the regulatory circuitry that limits proliferation by inhibiting mitogenic stimulation, and leave the quiescent state. Proliferation at the stages beneath the stem cells is likely to be an important regulator of differentiation as hematopoietic maturation requires signaling from the cyclin based surveillance system for proper influence on differentiation decisions [Ezoe et al. 2004].

The mechanisms that underlie and direct the multilineage commitment processes from HSC are still largely unknown, but several descriptive propositions of the differentiation processes has been established [Adolfsson et al. 2005; Katsura 2002; Kondo et al. 2001; Yang et al. 2004]. Common for these proposals is that self-renewing and multipotent long-term HSC exist throughout life as they throughout development maintain a quiescent state relative other hematopoietic cells [Nygren et al. 2006]. Their committed progeny irreversibly transit into short-term HSC that are also multipotent, but contribute to hematopoiesis for less than six to eight weeks, as such cells have lost the ability to extensively self-renew [Adolfsson et al. 2001; Yang et al. 2004]. Such transiently reconstituting HSC thereafter commit and enter progenitor states with restricted lineage potentials, to finally develop along certain cell lineage pathways with sequential restrictions in lineage potential and gene expression [Adolfsson et al. 2005; Akashi et al. 2003]. In light of the relatively short life span of a mouse (~2–3 years depending on strain), the low cell cycle activity among HSC, with a population turnover of several months [Cheshier et al. 1999], is remarkable. If the steady state is severely disrupted, for example following manipulative treatments such as myeloablation and bone-marrow transplantation, HSC react by rapid expansion in the recipient [Allsopp et al. 2001; Iscove and Nawa 1997; Plett et al. 2002] and under the influence of exogenous growth factors, commitment, migration or even self-renewal might occur [Bodine et al. 1993; Fleming et al. 1993b; Kronenwett et al. 2000]. This argues for that the activity of the HSC needs tight negative and intrinsic regulation to fulfill the requirements in different physiological conditions and for the entire life of the organism.

2.3   Quiescence Imposed by a Stem Cell Niche

It is currently unknown whether there is a default fate regarding aspects such as self-renewal or differentiation into individual lineages from HSC. Whereas coordinated and precise control of commitment and differentiation largely depends on soluble factors, originating from within and outside of the bone-marrow, maintenance of HSC identities is believed to be mainly achieved by delicate interactions of the stem cells and their microenvironment, often referred to as the HSC niche. Identification of the factors and their signaling pathways underlying such control has been a main focus of hematological research, as knowledge on such regulation would allow manipulation for therapeutic purposes.

Extrinsic factors produced either by the stem cells themselves or by surrounding stromal cells that bind to receptors on the cell membrane of the stem cell can exert their effects long range as soluble molecules, or locally through direct cell-to-cell contact between the stem cells and adjacent cells [Attar and Scadden 2004]. Stromal cells and their products are spatially distributed into niches that differ in their HSC maintenance capacity and therefore, homing of HSC and hematopoietic progenitor cells to different niches affects their fate and the regulation of hematopoiesis [Arai et al. 2004; Calvi et al. 2003; Zhang et al. 2003]. Under physiological conditions, but more pronounced during stress, HSC migrate in and out of the bone-marrow compartment [Dorie et al. 1979]. This occurs at a very low frequency [Abkowitz et al. 2003; Dorie et al. 1979; Wright et al. 2001] by a mechanism that can be stimulated by exogenous cytokine treatment [Kronenwett et al. 2000]. The purpose and regulation of this migratory activity is not completely understood but might play a role in the seeding of HSC to other niches within the bone-marrow [Abkowitz et al. 2003; Wright et al. 2001], secondary lymphoid organs, like the thymus [Schwarz and Bhandoola 2004] or other organs [McKinney-Freeman and Goodell 2004].

The best direct evidence for stem cell niches comes from work in the Drosophila testis, where germline stem cells surround apical hub cells at the tip of the testis, which provide self-renewing signals [Kiger et al. 2001; Tulina and Matunis 2001]. As the stem cells divide, the daughter cell that keeps contact with the hub cells, and thereby continues to receive self-renewing signals, retains a stem cell identity. The other daughter cell that is relocated away from the hub cells initiates differentiation.

In the bone-marrow, similar regional patterning of self-renewing signals has been found within the endosteal zone lining the bone surface in the marrow cavity [Arai et al. 2004; Calvi et al. 2003; Zhang et al. 2003], with a gradient decreasing toward the central zone of the marrow space. In support of this, the majority of hematopoietic stem and progenitor cells has long since been known to be distributed preferentially along the bone surface [Lambertsen and Weiss 1984; Lord and Hendry 1972; Lord et al. 1975]. These findings suggest that fate determination of HSC within the endosteal zone occurs in a similar fashion as for germline stem cells in Drosophila testes, where the fate of the 2 daughter cells from a dividing HSC at least in part is determined by their attachment to or displacement from the stem cell-supportive niche [Wilson and Trumpp 2006].

2.4 Regulating Quiescence or Commitment

Asymmetry of the daughter cells derived from HSC self-renewing divisions might be due to asymmetric distribution of intrinsic factors, such as transcription factors, cellular components or DNA during cell division [Enver et al. 1998; Takano et al. 2004]. However, HSC regulation is a complex process involving both intrinsic and extrinsic factors that can be both counteracting and synergistic and hence, asymmetric cell division through asymmetric distribution of intrinsic factors might be dependent on extrinsic signals that prime HSC for the subsequent intrinsic regulation. This might explain why extensive efforts to ex vivo expand HSC so far has, with some exceptions, been fruitless [Bryder and Jacobsen 2000; Glimm and Eaves 1999; Miller and Eaves 1997; Moore et al. 1997; Quesenberry et al. 2002; Sauvageau et al. 2004; Srour et al. 1999]. Regardless of the outcome from an asymmetric HSC division, the interaction of the 2 daughter cells with their environment results in fate decisions that determine the destiny of each particular cell and such interaction continues throughout the life of the cell. The newly formed cells can either return to a quiescent state as the parental HSC, carry on a second self-renewing asymmetric (or symmetric expanding) cell division, commit to differentiate along a certain lineage pathway or migrate to a distant site that offers suitable environment for either of the fates above [Wagers et al. 2002]. If the environment does not support any of these possibilities, the cell will due to the lack of instructive signals inevitably undergo apoptosis, a process that plays an important regulatory function for hematopoietic homeostasis [Domen and Weissman 2000; Wagers et al. 2002].

Regulation of these HSC fate decisions is most likely a combination of stochastic (random) events, mainly though intrinsic regulation at the time of cell division [Enver et al. 1998; Greaves et al. 2003; Ogawa 1999; Phillips et al. 1992; Till et al. 1964], and deterministic events, mainly due to extrinsic factors in the HSC niche, that can be either permissive or instructive in their action [Metcalf 1998; Morrison and Weissman 1994; Muller-Sieburg et al. 2002]. Eliminating single or multiple hematopoietic growth factors or signal transduction pathways by genetic engineering in mice, allows determination of the type of action a factor imposes on the

HSC. The action of some factors is redundant as their removal does not result in hematopoietic phenotypes and can be compensated for [Akashi et al. 1998; Metcalf 1993; Sitnicka et al. 2002] whereas others are indispensable for certain fates [Iwasaki et al. 2005]. The first case exemplifies permissive regulation, allowing cells to differentiate along a predestined differentiation pathway, and the latter instructive regulation, instructing cells toward a specific fate [Kondo et al. 2000].

A major group of extrinsic factors in hematopoiesis are cytokines that play an important role in regulation of hematopoiesis. Most such molecules are available both in soluble and cell membrane bound forms and interact by direct binding to cell membrane receptors on the hematopoietic cells or on intermediate cells with which the hematopoietic cells interact. The early acting cytokines Stem Cell Factor and Thrombopoietin are nonredundant regulators of the HCS-pool [Zhu and Emerson 2002]. Other cytokines act on more committed cells and drive differentiation along particular pathways, like Erythropoietin for erythroid cells, granulocyte-macrophage colony-stimulating factor (GM-CSF) and granulocyte colony-stimulating factor (G-CSF) for myeloid cells and interleukin 7 (IL-7) for B-cells [Ogawa 1993; Zhu and Emerson 2002]. Signaling from membrane bound receptors on HSC is propagated through elaborate intracellular signal transduction pathways to the nucleus, where they influence the activity of transcription factors. These bind to promoter elements on the DNA and regulate together with other regulatory molecules and DNA polymerases the transcription of target genes and ultimately, fate decisions. Several transcription factors have been implicated in the regulation of HSC self-renewal (ICN/CSL, Ikaros, HoxB4 and GATA-2), whereas others participate at more downstream cellular levels by inducing commitment toward individual hematopoietic lineages [Zhu and Emerson 2002].

3   Hematopoietic Stem Cell Developmental Switches

Development of a fully functional blood system occurs early in development and the hematopoietic system thereafter continuously changes to meet the demands on the organism at each stage of development. These changes mainly occur through alterations of identities and functions of the HSC through specific and seemingly irreversible switches that are mainly cell autonomous but depend on and are influenced by variation of the cellular environment of the HSC niches throughout ontogeny.

3.1   The Primitive to Definitive Switch

Onset of hematopoiesis is an early event in embryonic development and required to meet the demands of oxygen transportation as the embryo becomes larger and to provide an early defense against pathogens. In mouse development, gastrulation starts 7.5 days post conception (dpc) and leads to the formation of ectoderm, mesoderm and endoderm. During this process the extra- and intra-embryonic regions, the yolk sac and embryo proper, are established. In the yolk sac, cell aggregates called blood islands are formed and contain cells of both hematopoietic and endothelial lineages. These develop in close contact, and perhaps from a common progenitor cell known as the hemangioblast [Choi et al. 1998; Keller et al. 1999; Mikkola et al. 2003]. Commitment toward a hematopoietic fate occurs through the influence of various transcription factors, such as Tal-1/SCL, AML-1, Lmo2 and GATA-2, and results in the formation of committed primitive hematopoietic precursor cells [Zhu and Emerson 2002]. Such primitive precursors are primed towards myelo-erythroid lineages and mostly produce monocytes, for infectious defense in the placenta, and primitive erythrocytes, that are large, nucleated and produce embryonic globins [Weissman 2000]. This early burst of extra-embryonic erythrocyte production is necessary for oxygen transportation within the embryo at a time when oxygen diffusion from maternal circulation becomes insufficient [Cumano and Godin 2001]. The yolk sac remains a hematopoietic organ until the embryo itself can support blood cell production by around 11.5 dpc. Within the embryo, a region comprising the rudiments of the dorsal aorta and surrounding splanchnic mesoderm forms at around 8.5–10 dpc and at this site the development of definitive HSC initiates [Bertrand et al. 2005; de Bruijn et al. 2002; Godin et al. 1999]. The region, named the para-aortic splanchnopleura (P-Sp), later develops into the aorta gonad and mesonephros (AGM) at 10–12 dpc. Hematopoietic precursor cell activity can be identified by 10.5 dpc in a region of the mesenchyme surrounding and within the dorsal side of the aorta [Bertrand et al. 2005; de Bruijn et al. 2002; Godin et al. 1999]. These precursors develop into the HSC that support definitive hematopoiesis yielding small enucleated erythrocytes that express adult globins. The intra-embryonic definitive HSC are the sole precursors of the adult HSC that supply HSC activity throughout life [Cumano and Godin 2001], thus no further HSC are generated during late fetal and neonatal stages of development [Gothert et al. 2005]. The origin of the intra-embryonic definitive HSC has been under debate as to whether they really are descendants from the primitive yolk sac derived precursors or originate independently from definitive hematopoietic precursors. Studies by Moore and Metcalf in 1970 suggested that the yolk sac is required for both primitive and definitive hematopoiesis in mice [Moore and Metcalf 1970]. Culture of precirculation 7 dpc embryos from which the yolk sac had been removed developed without blood cell formation, whereas culture of 7 dpc yolk sac alone yielded abundant hematopoietic colonies. Although challenged over the years [Cumano et al. 2001; Medvinsky and Dzierzak 1996], this concept was recently confirmed by noninvasive labeling of progenitors of definitive hematopoiesis, expressing Runx1 in the yolk sac blood islands at 7.5 dpc, establishing that intra-embryonic definitive HSC can originate from extra-embryonic primitive precursors in the yolk sac of the developing embryo.

As definitive HSC in the AGM mature, they migrate and enter the blood circulation [Christensen et al. 2004; Delassus and Cumano 1996] to colonize the liver [Morrison et al. 1995a]. In the fetal liver environment, such cells gain properties changing their identity from being nonproliferating, nondifferentiating and nontransplantable, to cells that can rapidly proliferate and self-renew to expand their numbers to meet the growing requirements of the hematopoietic system [Ikuta and Weissman 1992; Lansdorp et al. 1993; Rebel et al. 1996b]. The capacity of the fetal liver HSC for multipotent blood cell production and long-term repopulation when transplanted into lethally irradiated hosts is extensive and unprecedented throughout ontogeny [Jordan et al. 1995; Rebel et al. 1996a; Rebel et al. 1996b]. With emergence of fetal liver hematopoiesis, the necessity of yolk sac erythropoiesis (12–14 dpc) decreases and leads to disappearance of yolk sac hematopoietic precursors. However, as yolk sac and fetal liver HSC display similar globin switching, these events are unlikely to be the result of alternating cell populations, but rather represent the outcome of developmental switches of primitive to definitive hematopoiesis and thereby changes in transcription. By the end of pregnancy, hematopoiesis in the liver transfers through the migration of HSC to the bone-marrow [Christensen et al. 2004; Delassus and Cumano 1996; Potocnik et al. 2000], which remains the main hematopoietic organ throughout life [Morrison et al. 1995b]. During these developmental processes, mesenchymal progenitor cells (with osteogenic, adipogenic and chondrogenic potential) in parallel home to and develop niches supporting self-renewal in the primary hematopoietic organs (fetal liver, bone-marrow and spleen) as these tissues develop in the fetus [Christensen et al. 2004; Mendes et al. 2005; Palis et al. 2001; Potocnik et al. 2000]. Whether the colonization of niches supporting hematopoiesis during midgestation is a multiwave process or the result of a constant flow of rare HSC in the fetal blood is currently unclear [Christensen et al. 2004; Delassus and Cumano 1996; Potocnik et al. 2000]. It appears likely that low numbers of HSC are constantly circulating both before and after their expansion and maturation in the fetal liver, until a suitable environment for hematopoiesis has developed in the bone-marrow.

The distinct developmental fates of extra- and intra-embryonic progenitors in extra- and intra-embryonic niches [Matsuoka et al. 2001; Orkin and Zon 2002; Walker et al. 2001; Yoder et al. 1997] thus require intrinsic developmental switches that alter lineage priming, gene expression, function, cell cycling and the phenotype of HSC. As transplantation of primitive extra-embryonic progenitors to intra-embryonic sites directs these cells to adopt a definitive fate, it appears as appropriate instruction is also contingent on environmental cues [Turpen et al. 1997].

3.2   Fetal to Adult Switch

Both embryonic and adult hematopoiesis is hierarchical, with differentiation occurring through distinct and sequential progenitor subsets [Kondo et al. 2003]. This suggests that the molecular mechanisms underlying cell fate decisions are conserved from embryo to adult. Despite of this similarity, the properties of fetal liver HSC that migrate to the bone-marrow by the end of gestation are in many aspects different from when they have adopted adult properties and fates in the bone-marrow [Jordan et al. 1995; Rebel et al. 1996a; Rebel et al. 1996b]. This fetal to adult developmental switch occurs in the bone-marrow during the first weeks after birth in a precise manner and involves coordinated alterations in the abilities to self-renew, proliferate, differentiate as well as in regulation of gene expression, suggesting cell intrinsic regulation rather than random environmental changes [Bowie et al. 2007b; Kikuchi and Kondo 2006].

Expansion of HSC numbers in the fetal liver occurs with cell cycle kinetics that are significantly different from those of adult HSC in the steady state bone-marrow [Nygren et al. 2006]. Following lodging to the bone-marrow environment, there is a need for reduction of the extended proliferative activity and hence switching of the regulatory circuitry into a more quiescent state [Bowie et al. 2006]. Such transformation seems to occur during neonatal week three to four after birth and completely alters the cycling behavior from a fetal high proliferative into an adult quiescent state that is maintained throughout adulthood [Bowie et al. 2006]. Fetal liver HSC have a dominating lymphoid potential [Morrison et al. 1996], differ in the factor dependence for their differentiation compared to adult HSC [Kikuchi and Kondo 2006] and support differentiation to B- and T-cell subtypes that are distinct in function and phenotype and normally not present in adults [Hayakawa and Hardy 2000; Ikuta et al. 1990]. These differences in lineage priming are changed upon adoption of adult HSC properties during the first week after birth. Whether the effects of these switches are reversible remains to be determined, but as HSC of fetal type undergo similar changes with analogous kinetics following transplantation into an adult environment they must involve intrinsic and, at least during steady state conditions, irreversible changes of the fetal HSC [Bowie et al. 2007b]. This change could involve components of c-kit signaling [Bowie et al. 2007b], in accordance with the role of the c-kit receptor in control of self-renewal in HSC [Bowie et al. 2007a]. Shorter cell cycle passage time of fetal HSC might be due to intrinsic proliferative control that favors symmetric self-renewing cell divisions. Similar intrinsic changes occurs in otherwise quiescent adult HSC that are exposed to an environment that demands a high degree of self-renewing cell divisions, for instance following serial transplantation [Allsopp et al. 2001]. That self-renewing cell divisions dominates fetal HSC cell divisions is not only reflected by an increased proliferative activity in vivo compared to adult bone-marrow HSC but also an enhanced capacity to long term repopulate the blood system of lethally irradiated recipient mice [Rebel et al. 1996a]. This can not be correlated with differences in the ability of transplanted cells to migrate to and engraft in the host bone-marrow, as fetal HSC transplanted together with a population of competitive adult counterparts maintain this property. Cells from both origins engraft similarly well in the adult recipients but the fetal donor cells out competes adult cells over time. Although fetal HSC transferred to an adult environment undergo developmental switching into an adult state, they maintain an enhanced capacity to proliferate with extended and preserved self-renewing abilities compared to adult cells having developed normally [Bowie et al. 2007b; Bowie et al. 2006; Rebel et al. 1996a]. As transition into an adult stage seems to occur with precise timing, it appears as cell autonomous molecular switches tightly regulate lineage priming during fetal and adult hematopoiesis, but depend on proper development with sequential changes of fate that cannot be sidestepped.

3.3   The Adult to Old Switch

Upon the fetal to adult developmental switch, HSC persists throughout adulthood in a relatively quiescent state compared to their progeny [Nygren et al. 2006], with more or less maintained properties and regulatory control. However, randomly occurring events impose direct wear and tear on HSC during their life span and as such changes can accumulate over time due to the self-renewal capability of HSC, it appears reasonable that they can result in phenotypic and functional changes and even a reduced capacity to maintain cellular homeostasis and survival. However, gene expression patterns of aged HSC have revealed that, compared to post-mitotic cells in other tissues, stress induced damage does not seem to play a major role on HSC aging in steady-state [Rossi et al. 2005]. This might be a result of a unique ability of HSC to maintain a quiescent state relative to their down stream progeny throughout ontogeny [Nygren et al. 2006] which would allow HSC to escape from much of the negative stress associated with life long and continuous proliferation. Furthermore, not all observed changes of HSC during aging appears to be attributed to macromolecular damage, suggesting contributions of cell autonomous changes through internal molecular switches [Rossi et al. 2007b]. In line with this, loss of immune function of aged HSC is likely due to cell autonomous changes that results in altered gene expression favoring myeloid specific genes, resulting in lineage skewing towards a myeloid fate [Rossi et al. 2005]. Thus, reduced competence of the adaptive immune system appears to be a result of an increased myeloid progenitor cell capacity, at the expense of lymphoid developmental potential. Phenotypical and functional evaluations have shown that the numbers of HSC in the aged bone-marrow are significantly increased [Rossi et al. 2005; Sudo et al. 2000]. Transplantation of HSC from young and old donors into young recipients showed that the elevated numbers of HSC in old mice were due to cell autonomous changes in the HSC leading to a higher incidence of self-renewing cell divisions with HSC aging.

Taken together, HSC that until recently were assumed to be exempt from aging show progressive alterations in many aspects upon reaching advanced age. Such changes however does not seem to occur in an as controlled and defined way as for the developmental switches that occur during early development. Although the cellular changes act in a cell autonomous manner, the actual switching of a cell from young to adult might indeed be triggered by environmental cues. Such factors would be linked to aging of the cellular environment of HSC, thereby altering the regulatory circuitry that controls on demand production of HSC progeny and in maintenance of their own quiescence. In support of this, aged HSC have been suggested to be affected by changes of the interaction with the supporting HSC niches in the bone-marrow, with a reduced ability for adhesion to stromal cells, impaired homing to the bone-marrow following transplantation and increased responsiveness to mobilizing factors [Liang et al. 2005; Xing et al. 2006]. Thus, intrinsic and environmental changes that occur within the pool of HSC collectively sets the prerequisite for cellular deterioration. With this interpretation, the developmental history of each individual cell establishes how and when the aging process will begin.

Such processes seem to be irreversible and unaffected by environmental factors once initiated, as the transfer of aged HSC to a young environment does not change their adult identity [Rossi et al. 2005; Sudo et al. 2000].

4 Aging of Hematopoietic Stem Cells

Aging are generally though of as the sum of the deteriorative effects on a cellular identity or function that accumulates over time and eventually reaches a state that leads to tissue failure. However, for the hematopoietic system it is doubtful whether the consequences of aging are attributed to changes of the actual HSC due to accumulation of wear and tear or environmental signals. Instead, many changes on function and identity of HSC might in fact constitute normal developmental steps that occur through controlled and evolutionary conserved switches. Such adaptation to changes in environment and requirement imposed in the system, begin in the developing embryo and continue throughout ontogeny.

4.1 Aging as the Result of Environment

As described earlier in this chapter, HSC are exposed to dramatically different environments during their maturation. Commitment towards hematopoiesis occur outside the embryo in the yolk sac blood islands, transit through the AGM region and fetal liver for developmental switching and expansion, and by the end of fetal development find their home in the bone-marrow where they, except from rare and transient migration into the blood system for relocation, stay throughout adult life. During this process, wear and tear of the most primitive HSC do occur but the extent of this and the importance it plays for their function remains largely unknown. Throughout adulthood, it has been proposed that the main site that supports maintenance of HSC is the endosteal bone-marrow niche, providing a sanctuary with limited damage to proteins, membranes and DNA imposed by the environment. The cell layers that comprise the endosteal zone are highly hypoxic, suggesting that it provides an environment with low pressure of cellular damage derived from reactive oxygen species [Parmar et al. 2007]. Furthermore, hypoxic conditions might be important for optimal stimulation of self-renewal and quiescence and thereby play an important role in avoiding accumulation of cellular damage by limiting proliferation [Tothova et al. 2007]. Hypoxic conditions could be entertained by a low flow of extra-cellular fluids in the HSC niche, thereby also limiting exposure to toxins, metabolic by products and toxic compounds from immune responses as seen elsewhere in the organism.

As HSC by definition persist for the lifetime of an organism, developmental marks should be accumulating and with time reach levels influencing cellular function thereby imposing changes on HSC stem cell identity. Recent studies have however underscored that environmental influences plays a minor role in the specification of these cells as transferring of aged cells to an young environment does not alter their identity or function [Rossi et al. 2005]. This argues for that environmental cues can not alter cell intrinsic changes of HSC once established or modify the genetic control that regulate the kinetics of this process [Phillips et al. 1992]. However, environmental factors such as toxins, inflammatory cytokines and DNA interfering compounds might well act over long time to impose some of the cellular changes accompanying age. Many of these are closely linked to metabolic and proliferative activities, emphasizing the importance of avoiding such influence on HSC by maintaining quiescence at all times, including during stress responses and extensive self-renewal [Nygren et al. 2006]. As all other cells, the bone-marrow stromal cells that constitute the HSC microenvironment age and undergo changes that might affect its HSC supporting capacity [Liang 2005 #646]. An increasing number of senescent stromal cells might be one important factor that through deteriorated HSC supportive function fails to prevent or possibly by themselves drive HSC aging.

4.2   Avoiding Aging by Quiescence

Downstream progenitor cell populations that have committed to individual hematopoietic lineages consist of a limited number of clones with an extensive capacity to produce mature effector cells of each lineage. The high degree of multiplying and differentiating cell divisions that take place within these populations impose a high degree of divisional stress on each cell. However, as progenitor cells lack extensive self-renewing properties, any damage on cells or their genetic material can only spread within the progeny of that clone and will disappear as it reaches its proliferative limit [Hayflick 1965; Lemischka et al. 1986]. In contrast, HSC, which through their asymmetric cell divisions can generate all different progenitor cell subsets, must find means to avoid such accumulation of damage as they will be carried on and amplified at progenitor cell stages for the rest of the life of that HSC clone. It therefore appears likely that HSC have adapted a regulatory circuitry that limits proliferation at the HSC stage.

In vivo labeling with the thymidine analogue BrdU into the DNA of proliferating cells have established that although all HSC constantly divide and participate in hematopoiesis, they are generally quiescent, with a population turnover that is distinguishable from that of the downstream progenitor cells even during stress or extensive expansion [Bradford et al. 1997; Cheshier et al. 1999; Nygren et al. 2006]. To expand the numbers of progeny generated from each clone, a finite but extensive proliferative capacity instead occurs at downstream progenitor cell levels. Thus, clonal stability of rare HSC seems to be the general incidence, whereas clonal succession occurs within all hematopoietic progenitor cell populations as each progenitor cell has a limited life span and is eventually succeeded by a new progenitor cell.

When studying hematopoiesis during aging, any cell type will however eventually reach its end point and succumb or perhaps enter senescence. As new HSC clones are not formed after midgestation embryogenesis [Gothert et al. 2005] loss of HSC clones can not be replenished but only substituted by expansion of similarly old clones that will eventually reach senescence or die. Senescent cells are metabolically active but have a changed pattern of gene expression and an irreversible loss of proliferative capacity. HSC senescence should normally represent a minor problem, if occurring at all, as HSC can be propagated for as long as four times the normal life span of a mouse through serial transplantation into sequential recipients [Harrison 1979]. The elements that are involved in avoiding senescence of HSC are not known but through studies of different mice strains, several genetic elements has been identified that are indispensable for controlling proliferation and thereby preservation of the HSC pool [Chen et al. 2000]. Although HSC appears to have found means to escape from proliferative stress such as through lodging to a hypoxic environment with low degree of oxidative stress [Parmar et al. 2007; Tothova et al. 2007], efficient exclusion of toxic components taken up from the environment by multidrug resistance membrane transporters [Zhou et al. 2002] and limiting genetic deterioration from repeated explicative stress [Nijnik et al. 2007; Rossi et al. 2007a], complete protection from these effects is unlikely. An example of this is the shortening of the critical telomere elements at the ends of the chromosomes following extensive proliferation.

Telomeres are the regions of highly repetitive DNA at the end of the chromosomes and functions as a disposable buffer of genetic material. Every time chromosomes are replicated, DNA polymerase complexes are incapable of continuing replication all the way to the end of the DNA strand of each chromosome, thereby leading to a gradual loss of nucleotides with each mitosis. This ultimately results in a genome with an increased chromosomal instability and, as a cellular defense mechanism, an increased predisposition to enter senescence or cell death. In some cells, including somatic stem cells, telomerase extend telomeres by adding extra repetitive DNA elements constituting telomeric sequences. However although genetic instability and functional impairment of HSC coincides with telomere shortening following extensive proliferative stress and following genetic alteration of telomerase function [Allsopp et al. 2001; Allsopp et al. 2003a; Samper et al. 2002], maintenance of telomeres is likely not sufficient by itself to avoid stem cell exhaustion [Allsopp et al. 2003b].

4.3 Avoiding Aging by Asymmetry

The quiescent stem cell specific asymmetric partitioning of cell fate during cell division of HSC into either preserved stem cell identity, or loss of such and commitment towards differentiation, limits the proliferative tension on the stem cell clone by allowing one of the daughter cells to maintain quiescence. Which elements that are unequally distributed to the daughter cells and how such partitioning takes place is not fully understood. However, displacement from a certain stem cell supporting environment within the niche might play a role [Kiger et al. 2001; Tulina and Matunis 2001; Wilson and Trumpp 2006] as well as regulated or stochastic distribution of transcription factions, organelles, receptors and other cellular constituents and biomolecules into gradients that establish differences in cell fate [Arai et al. 2004; Rusan and Peifer 2007; Yamashita et al. 2007; Zhang et al. 2003]. It would therefore seem reasonable that partitioning of cell fates by asymmetric cell divisions might play a role for avoiding aging of the HSC clone that strive for persistence throughout life. During stem cell divisions, centrosomes can be asymmetrically inherited with mother centrosomes that always ends in the daughter cell with remained stem cell identity, arguing that also genetic material could be passed on from stem cell to stem cell in a similar fashion. The concept of such partitioning of the DNA have been hypothesized and could explain how long lived cells that proliferate extensively avoid accumulation of genetic defects acquired during replication [Nijnik et al. 2007] by using the same DNA strand as template for DNA polymerase replication and passing it along into the daughter cell that inherit stemness, whereas the newly replicated strand ends up in the daughter cell with lost stem cell capacity [Cairns 1975]. Retaining the same set of template DNA strands throughout development could help preventing adult stem cells from accumulating mutations arising from errors in DNA replication. Instead, randomly occurring mutations during replication within a HSC clone are passed on to nonstem cell daughters that soon terminally differentiate. Such mechanism would reduce the rate of accumulation of mutations in HSC that would otherwise eventually lead to serious genetic disorders or aging [Rossi et al. 2007a]. The idea of an immortal strand in HSC has however to be strengthened by experimental data, and if present, it has to be established how such stem cell specific partitioning of immortal template and mortal copy strands take place. All definitive HSC clones are established during midgestation embryogenesis and thereafter no new clones are born. Thus expansion of the HSC pool thereafter can only occur through multiplication of such HSC clones. Depending on when immortal templates would be established, not all HSC necessarily need to have the capacity to partition DNA into mother and daughter cells following replication. Similarly, asymmetric distribution of proteins and cellular constituents, an event that plays important roles in specifying asymmetry of the daughter cells from asymmetric cell divisions [Enver et al. 1998; Takano et al. 2004], could be speculated to also be operational to specify fates at a HSC level, although to date representing an under explored mechanisms to these processes.

Chromatin remodeling is critical for regulating transcription, replication, recombination and segregation of the chromosomes. Histone complexes organize chromatin and play a major role in epigenetic imprinting of the DNA, and a critical role in HSC biology for the polycomb protein Bmi-1, a transcriptional repressor that maintain repression of genes after a cell division and thereby maintain epigenetic memory, was suggested [Lessard and Sauvageau 2003; Park et al. 2003]. It appears likely that such processes play key roles in determination of stemness of daughter cells from self-renewing HSC cell divisions, although the order of such events remain currently unknown. However, as epigenetic imprinting of DNA has to be replicated onto the daughter chromatin following each cell division, it appears reasonable that accumulated numbers of cell divisions might lead to functional changes, including reductions in self-renewing ability.

4.4   Genetic Control of Aging

Aging is a multi parameter sequence of events controlled by both environmental factors and the genetic composition of the individual. As outlined above, environmental factors can influence on normal wear and tear of HSC and their development, but seem to have a subordinate role for establishing the transcriptional networks that specifies developmental switches and aging. Although the molecular mechanisms have not been elucidated in detail, it is clear that various genetic traits are involved in the modulation of life span [de Haan et al. 2002; Geiger et al. 2005; Rossi et al. 2007a]. Such modulation in HSC involves reduction of damage to the cell and its genetic components over time, and is crucial to avoid premature ageing and senescence. Damage control is not mainly supplied by repair systems that maintain the integrity of proteins, DNA and cellular components, but also accomplished through preventing metabolic stress and genetic instabilities acquired from extended divisional activity. This provides a strategy to limit the number of deleterious actions occurring within the limited and irreplaceable HSC pool, and is mainly accomplished by an in nature unique ability to constantly participate in the process of hematopoiesis, while still maintaining proliferative quiescence over time [Nygren et al. 2006].

Several genes involved in maintaining HSC quiescence and the action of their protein products have been characterized. These components form a network that signals to the stem cell to maintain stem cell properties through self-renewing cell divisions [Reya et al. 2003; Willert et al. 2003] and is believed to transfer epigenetic memory that identifies stemness to at least one of the daughter cells [Lessard and Sauvageau 2003; Park et al. 2003]. The process of self-renewal however needs to be restricted and factors are needed that interfere with cell cycle control to restrict proliferation [Hock et al. 2004] and maintain and strengthen adhesive interaction of the HSC with the niche supporting quiescence [Wilson et al. 2004; Yang et al. 2007]. However, although many components of the circuitry that signals self-renewal and quiescence in the HSC and their niche have been postulated, little direct mechanistic insights have so far been provided.

Genes and genetic elements that have a general effect on the life span of an organism suggests that molecular machineries can be activated to ensure that homeostasis is maintained at various situation of stress, thereby putting some sort of break to the aging process. Genetic information located in the mitochondria has been identified as one major heritable component involved in aging. Instabilities of the mitochondrial DNA due to damages or replication can lead to mitochondrial dysfunction, increased oxidative stress and cellular senescence emphasizing the importance of long lived cells to limit metabolic activity and proliferation [Cadenas and Davies 2000]. Studies of cellular processes in mice have been standardized to involve only a limited number of inbred mouse stains. In these a varying degree of effects on HSC function have been observed during aging, however generally HSC does not seem to loose regenerative capacity as they age [Rossi et al. 2005]. This is further supported by studies demonstrating maintenance of hematopoiesis during conditions and time spans that by far extends the normal life expectancy of the organism [Ross et al. 1982].

5 Conclusion

The constant ongoing process of cell replacement in the hematopoietic system imposes a strong degenerative stress on the cellular elements that participate in these processes. Luckily, many of these adverse effects from prolonged regeneration disappear upon cellular differentiation and are therefore present only transiently. However, as stem cells are maintained throughout life, accumulation of any damage or other heritable cellular traits that occurs along these processes and its regulatory networks will have dramatic effects due to the hierarchical structure of hematopoietic development. Limiting metabolic and divisional stress in hematopoietic stem cells is therefore key for maintaining their appropriate lifelong function and to avoid proliferative exhaustion or leukemic transformation with age.

References

Abkowitz JL, Robinson AE, Kale S, Long MW, Chen J (2003). Mobilization of hematopoietic stem cells during homeostasis and after cytokine exposure. Blood 102:1249–1253

Adolfsson J, Borge OJ, Bryder D, Theilgaard-Monch K, Astrand-Grundstrom I, Sitnicka E, Sasaki Y, Jacobsen, SE (2001). Upregulation of Flt3 expression within the bone marrow Lin(-)Sca1(+)c- kit(+) stem cell compartment is accompanied by loss of self-renewal capacity. Immunity 15:659–669

Adolfsson J, Mansson R, Buza-Vidas N, Hultquist A, Liuba K, Jensen CT, Bryder D, Yang L, Borge OJ, Thoren LA, et al (2005) Identification of Flt3 +lympho-myeloid stem cells lacking erythro-megakaryocytic potential a revised road map for adult blood lineage commitment. Cell 121:295–306

Akashi K, He X, Chen J, Iwasaki H, Niu C, Steenhard B, Zhang J, Haug J, Li L (2003) Transcriptional accessibility for genes of multiple tissues and hematopoietic lineages is hierarchically controlled during early hematopoiesis. Blood 101:383–389

Akashi K, Kondo M, Weissman IL (1998) Role of interleukin-7 in T-cell development from hematopoietic stem cells. Immunol Rev 165:13–28

Allsopp RC, Cheshier S, Weissman IL (2001) Telomere shortening accompanies increased cell cycle activity during serial transplantation of hematopoietic stem cells. J Exp Med 193:917–924

Allsopp RC, Morin GB, DePinho R, Harley CB, Weissman IL (2003a) Telomerase is required to slow telomere shortening and extend replicative lifespan of HSC during serial transplantation. Blood 27:27

Allsopp RC, Morin GB, Horner JW, DePinho R, Harley CB, Weissman IL (2003b) Effect of TERT over-expression on the long-term transplantation capacity of hematopoietic stem cells. Nat Med 9:369–371

Arai F, Hirao A, Ohmura M, Sato H, Matsuoka S, Takubo K, Ito K, Koh GY, Suda T (2004) Tie2/angiopoietin-1 signaling regulates hematopoietic stem cell quiescence in the bone marrow niche. Cell 118:149–161

Attar EC, Scadden DT (2004) Regulation of hematopoietic stem cell growth. Leukemia 18:1760–1768

Becker AJ, Mc CE, Till JE (1963) Cytological demonstration of the clonal nature of spleen colonies derived from transplanted mouse marrow cells. Nature 197:452–454

Bertrand JY, Giroux S, Golub R, Klaine M, Jalil A, Boucontet L, Godin I, Cumano A (2005) Characterization of purified intraembryonic hematopoietic stem cells as a tool to define their site of origin. Proc Natl Acad Sci U S A 102:134–139

Bodine D, Seidel N, Zsebo K, Orlic D (1993) In vivo administration of stem cell factor to mice increases the absolute number of pluripotent hematopoietic stem cells. Blood 82:445–455

Bowie MB, Kent DG, Copley MR, Eaves CJ (2007a) Steel factor responsiveness regulates the high self-renewal phenotype of fetal hematopoietic stem cells. Blood

Bowie MB, Kent DG, Dykstra B, McKnight KD, McCaffrey L, Hoodless PA, Eaves CJ (2007b) Identification of a new intrinsically timed developmental checkpoint that reprograms key hematopoietic stem cell properties. Proc Natl Acad Sci U S A 104:5878–5882

Bowie MB, McKnight KD, Kent DG, McCaffrey L, Hoodless PA, Eaves CJ (2006) Hematopoietic stem cells proliferate until after birth and show a reversible phase-specific engraftment defect. J Clin Invest 116:2808–2816

Bradford GB, Williams B, Rossi R, Bertoncello I (1997) Quiescence, cycling, and turnover in the primitive hematopoietic stem cell compartment. Exp Hematol 25:445–453

Bryder D, Jacobsen SE (2000) Interleukin-3 supports expansion of long-term multilineage repopulating activity after multiple stem cell divisions in vitro. Blood 96:1748–1755

Cadenas E, Davies KJ (2000) Mitochondrial free radical generation, oxidative stress, and aging. Free Radic Biol Med 29:222–230

Cairns J (1975) Mutation selection and the natural history of cancer. Nature 255:197–200

Calvi LM, Adams GB, Weibrecht KW, Weber JM, Olson DP, Knight MC, Martin RP, Schipani E, Divieti P, Bringhurst FR, et al (2003) Osteoblastic cells regulate the haematopoietic stem cell niche. Nature 425:841–846

Chen J, Astle CM, Harrison DE (2000) Genetic regulation of primitive hematopoietic stem cell senescence. Exp Hematol 28:442–450

Cheng T (2004) Cell cycle inhibitors in normal and tumor stem cells. Oncogene 23:7256–7266

Cheng T, Rodrigues N, Shen H, Yang Y-G, Dombkowski D, Sykes M, Scadden DT (2000) Hematopoietic Stem Cell Quiescence Maintained by p21cip1/waf1. Science 287:1804–1808

Cheshier SH, Morrison SJ, Liao X, Weissman IL (1999) In vivo proliferation and cell cycle kinetics of long-term self- renewing hematopoietic stem cells. Proc Natl Acad Sci U S A 96:3120–3125

Choi K, Kennedy M, Kazarov A, Papadimitriou JC, Keller G (1998) A common precursor for hematopoietic and endothelial cells. Development 125:725–732

Christensen JL, Wright DE, Wagers AJ, Weissman IL (2004) Circulation and chemotaxis of fetal hematopoietic stem cells. PLoS Biol 2:E75

Cumano A, Ferraz JC, Klaine M, Di Santo JP, Godin I (2001) Intraembryonic, but not yolk sac hematopoietic precursors, isolated before circulation, provide long-term multilineage reconstitution. Immunity 15:477–485

Cumano A, Godin II (2001) Pluripotent hematopoietic stem cell development during embryogenesis. Curr Opin Immunol 13:166–171

de Bruijn MF, Ma X, Robin C, Ottersbach K, Sanchez MJ, Dzierzak E (2002) Hematopoietic stem cells localize to the endothelial cell layer in the midgestation mouse aorta. Immunity 16:673–683

de Haan G, Bystrykh LV, Weersing E, Dontje B, Geiger H, Ivanova N, Lemischka IR, Vellenga E, Van Zant G (2002) A genetic and genomic analysis identifies a cluster of genes associated with hematopoietic cell turnover. Blood 100:2056–2062

Delassus S, Cumano A (1996) Circulation of hematopoietic progenitors in the mouse embryo. Immunity 4:97–106

Domen J, Weissman IL (2000) Hematopoietic stem cells need two signals to prevent apoptosis; BCL-2 can provide one of these, Kitl/c-Kit signaling the other. J Exp Med 192:1707–1718

Dorie MJ, Maloney MA, Patt HM (1979) Turnover of circulating hematopoietic stem cells. Exp Hematol 7:483–489

Enver T, Heyworth CM, Dexter TM (1998) Do Stem Cells Play Dice? Blood 92:348–351

Ezoe S, Matsumura I, Satoh Y, Tanaka H, Kanakura Y (2004) Cell cycle regulation in hematopoietic stem/progenitor cells. Cell Cycle 3:314–318

Fleming WH, Alpern EJ, Uchida N, Ikuta K, Spangrude GJ, Weissman IL (1993a) Functional heterogeneity is associated with the cell cycle status of murine hematopoietic stem cells. J Cell Biol 122:897–902

Fleming WH, Alpern EJ, Uchida N, Ikuta K, Weissman IL (1993b) Steel factor influences the distribution and activity of murine hematopoietic stem cells in vivo. Proc Natl Acad Sci U S A 90:3760–3764

Geiger H, Rennebeck G, Van Zant G (2005) Regulation of hematopoietic stem cell aging in vivo by a distinct genetic element. Proc Natl Acad Sci U S A 102:5102–5107

Glimm H, Eaves CJ (1999). Direct evidence for multiple self-renewal divisions of human in vivo repopulating hematopoietic cells in short-term culture. Blood 94:2161–2168

Glimm H, Oh IH, Eaves CJ (2000). Human hematopoietic stem cells stimulated to proliferate in vitro lose engraftment potential during their S/G(2)/M transit and do not reenter G(0). Blood 96:4185–4193

Godin I, Garcia-Porrero JA, Dieterlen-Lievre F, Cumano A (1999) Stem cell emergence and hemopoietic activity are incompatible in mouse intraembryonic sites. J Exp Med 190:43–52

Gothert JR, Gustin SE, Hall MA, Green AR, Gottgens B, Izon DJ, Begley CG (2005). In vivo fate-tracing studies using the Scl stem cell enhancer: embryonic hematopoietic stem cells significantly contribute to adult hematopoiesis. Blood 105:2724–2732

Greaves MF, Maia AT, Wiemels JL, Ford AM (2003) Leukemia in twins: lessons in natural history. Blood 102:2321–2333

Habibian HK, Peters SO, Hsieh CC, Wuu J, Vergilis K, Grimaldi CI, Reilly J, Carlson JE, Frimberger AE, Stewart FM, Quesenberry PJ (1998) The fluctuating phenotype of the lymphohematopoietic stem cell with cell cycle transit. J Exp Med 188:393-398

Harrison DE (1979) Mouse erythropoietic stem cell lines function normally 100 months: loss related to number of transplantations. Mech Ageing Dev 9:427–433

Hayakawa K, Hardy RR (2000) Development and function of B-1 cells. Curr Opin Immunol 12:346–353

Hayflick L (1965) The Limited In Vitro Lifetime Of Human Diploid Cell Strains. Exp Cell Res 37:614–636

Hock H, Hamblen MJ, Rooke HM, Schindler JW, Saleque S, Fujiwara Y, Orkin SH (2004) Gfi-1 restricts proliferation and preserves functional integrity of haematopoietic stem cells. Nature

Huang S, Law P, Francis K, Palsson BO, Ho, AD (1999) Symmetry of initial cell divisions among primitive hematopoietic progenitors is independent of ontogenic age and regulatory molecules. Blood 94:2595–2604

Ikuta K, Kina T, MacNeil I, Uchida N, Peault B, Chien YH, Weissman IL (1990) A developmental switch in thymic lymphocyte maturation potential occurs at the level of hematopoietic stem cells. Cell 62:863–874

Ikuta K, Weissman IL (1992) Evidence that hematopoietic stem cells express mouse c-kit but do not depend on steel factor for their generation. Proc Natl Acad Sci U S A 89:1502–1506

Iscove NN, Nawa K (1997) Hematopoietic stem cells expand during serial transplantation in vivo without apparent exhaustion. Curr Biol 7:805–808

Iwama A, Oguro H, Negishi M, Kato Y, Morita Y, Tsukui H, Ema H, Kamijo T, Katoh-Fukui Y, Koseki H, et al (2004) Enhanced self-renewal of hematopoietic stem cells mediated by the polycomb gene product Bmi-1. Immunity 21:843–851

Iwasaki H, Somoza C, Shigematsu H, Duprez EA, Iwasaki-Arai J, Mizuno S, Arinobu Y, Geary K, Zhang P, Dayaram T, et al (2005) Distinctive and indispensable roles of PU.1 in maintenance of hematopoietic stem cells and their differentiation. Blood 106:1590–1600

Jan YN, Jan LY (1998) Asymmetric cell division. Nature 392:775–778

Jetmore A, Plett PA, Tong X, Wolber FM, Breese R, Abonour R, Orschell-Traycoff CM, Srour EF (2002) Homing efficiency, cell cycle kinetics, and survival of quiescent and cycling human CD34(+) cells transplanted into conditioned NOD/SCID recipients. Blood 99:1585–1593

Jordan CT, Astle CM, Zawadzki J, Mackarehtschian K, Lemischka IR, Harrison DE (1995) Long-term repopulating abilities of enriched fetal liver stem cells measured by competitive repopulation. Exp Hematol 23:1011–1015

Katsura Y (2002) Redefinition of lymphoid progenitors. Nat Rev Immunol 2:127–132

Keller G, Lacaud G, Robertson S (1999) Development of the hematopoietic system in the mouse. Exp Hematol 27:777–787

Kiel MJ, Iwashita T, Yilmaz OH, Morrison SJ (2005) Spatial differences in hematopoiesis but not in stem cells indicate a lack of regional patterning in definitive hematopoietic stem cells. Dev Biol 283:29–39

Kiger AA, Jones DL, Schulz C, Rogers MB, Fuller MT (2001) Stem cell self-renewal specified by JAK-STAT activation in response to a support cell cue. Science 294:2542–2545

Kikuchi K, Kondo M (2006) Developmental switch of mouse hematopoietic stem cells from fetal to adult type occurs in bone marrow after birth. Proc Natl Acad Sci U S A 103:17852–17857

Kondo M, Scherer DC, King AG, Manz MG, Weissman IL (2001) Lymphocyte development from hematopoietic stem cells. Curr Opin Genet Dev 11:520–526

Kondo M, Scherer DC, Miyamoto T, King AG, Akashi K, Sugamura K, Weissman IL (2000) Cell-fate conversion of lymphoid-committed progenitors by instructive actions of cytokines. Nature 407:383–386

Kondo M, Wagers AJ, Manz MG, Prohaska SS, Scherer DC, Beilhack GF, Shizuru JA, Weissman IL (2003) Biology of hematopoietic stem cells and progenitors: implications for clinical application. Annu Rev Immunol 21:759–806

Kronenwett R, Martin S, Haas R (2000) The role of cytokines and adhesion molecules for mobilization of peripheral blood stem cells. Stem Cells 18:320–330

Lagasse E, Shizuru JA, Uchida N, Tsukamoto A, Weissman IL (2001) Toward regenerative medicine. Immunity 14:425–436

Laird DJ, De Tomaso AW, Cooper MD, Weissman IL (2000) 50 million years of chordate evolution: seeking the origins of adaptive immunity. Proc Natl Acad Sci U S A 97:6924–6926

Lambertsen RH, Weiss L (1984) A model of intramedullary hematopoietic microenvironments based on stereologic study of the distribution of endocloned marrow colonies. Blood 63:287–297

Lansdorp P, Dragowska W, Mayani H (1993) Ontogeny-related changes in proliferative potential of human hematopoietic cells. J Exp Med 178:787–791

Lemischka IR, Raulet DH, Mulligan RC (1986) Developmental potential and dynamic behavior of hematopoietic stem cells. Cell 45:917–927

Lessard J, Sauvageau G (2003) Bmi-1 determines the proliferative capacity of normal and leukaemic stem cells. Nature 423:255–260

Liang Y, Van Zant G, Szilvassy SJ (2005) Effects of aging on the homing and engraftment of murine hematopoietic stem and progenitor cells. Blood

Lord BI, Hendry JH (1972) The distribution of haemopoietic colony-forming units in the mouse femur, and its modification by x rays. Br J Radiol 45:110–115

Lord BI, Testa NG, Hendry JH (1975) The relative spatial distributions of CFUs and CFUc in the normal mouse femur. Blood 46:65–72

Mantel CR, Braun SE, Lee Y, Kim YJ, Broxmeyer HE (2001) The interphase microtubule damage checkpoint defines an S-phase commitment point and does not require p21(waf-1). Blood 97:1505–1507

Matsuoka S, Tsuji K, Hisakawa H, Xu M, Ebihara Y, Ishii T, Sugiyama D, Manabe A, Tanaka R, Ikeda Y, et al (2001) Generation of definitive hematopoietic stem cells from murine early yolk sac and paraaortic splanchnopleures by aorta-gonad-mesonephros region-derived stromal cells. Blood 98:6–12

Matsuzaki Y, Kinjo K, Mulligan R, Okano H (2004) Unexpectedly efficient homing capacity of purified murine hematopoietic stem cells. Immunity 20:87–93

McCulloch EA, Till JE (1960) The radiation sensitivity of normal mouse bone marrow cells, determined by quantitative marrow transplantation into irradiated mice. Radiat Res 13:115–125

McKinney-Freeman S, Goodell MA (2004) Circulating hematopoietic stem cells do not efficiently home to bone marrow during homeostasis. Experimental Hematology 32:868–876

Medvinsky A, Dzierzak E (1996). Definitive hematopoiesis is autonomously initiated by the AGM region. Cell 86:897–906

Mendes SC, Robin C, Dzierzak E (2005) Mesenchymal progenitor cells localize within hematopoietic sites throughout ontogeny. Development 132:1127–1136

Metcalf D (1993) Hematopoietic regulators: redundancy or subtlety? Blood 82:3515–3523

Metcalf D (1998) Lineage Commitment and Maturation in Hematopoietic Cells: The Case for Extrinsic Regulation. Blood 92:345b–347

Mikkola HK, Fujiwara Y, Schlaeger TM, Traver D, Orkin SH (2003) Expression of CD41 marks the initiation of definitive hematopoiesis in the mouse embryo. Blood 101:508–516

Miller C L, Eaves CJ (1997) Expansion in vitro of adult murine hematopoietic stem cells with transplantable lympho-myeloid reconstituting ability. Proc Natl Acad Sci U S A 94:13648–13653

Moore KA, Ema H, Lemischka IR (1997) In vitro maintenance of highly purified, transplantable hematopoietic stem cells. Blood 89:4337–4347

Moore MA, Metcalf D (1970) Ontogeny of the haemopoietic system: yolk sac origin of in vivo and in vitro colony forming cells in the developing mouse embryo. Br J Haematol 18:279–296

Morrison SJ, Hemmati HD, Wandycz AM, Weissman IL (1995a) The purification and characterization of fetal liver hematopoietic stem cells. Proc Natl Acad Sci U S A 92:10302–10306

Morrison S J, Uchida N, Weissman I L (1995b) The biology of hematopoietic stem cells. Annu Rev Cell Dev Biol 11:35–71

Morrison SJ, Wandycz AM, Akashi K, Globerson A, Weissman IL (1996) The aging of hematopoietic stem cells. Nat Med 2:1011–1016

Morrison SJ, Weissman IL (1994) The long-term repopulating subset of hematopoietic stem cells is deterministic and isolatable by phenotype. Immunity 1:661–673

Muller-Sieburg CE, Cho RH, Thoman M, Adkins B, Sieburg HB (2002) Deterministic regulation of hematopoietic stem cell self-renewal and differentiation. Blood 100:1302–1309

Nijnik A, Woodbine L, Marchetti C, Dawson S, Lambe T, Liu C, Rodrigues NP, Crockford TL, Cabuy E, Vindigni A, et al (2007) DNA repair is limiting for haematopoietic stem cells during ageing. Nature 447:686–690

Nygren JM, Bryder D, Jacobsen SE (2006) Prolonged cell cycle transit is a defining and developmentally conserved hematopoietic stem cell property. J Immunol 177

Ogawa M (1993) Differentiation and proliferation of hematopoietic stem cells. Blood 81:2844–2853

Ogawa M (1999) Stochastic model revisited. Int J Hematol 69:2–5

Orkin SH, Zon LI (2002) Hematopoiesis and stem cells: plasticity versus developmental heterogeneity. Nat Immunol 3:323–328

Orschell-Traycoff CM, Hiatt K, Dagher RN, Rice S, Yoder MC, Srour EF (2000) Homing and engraftment potential of Sca-1(+)lin(-) cells fractionated on the basis of adhesion molecule expression and position in cell cycle. Blood 96:1380–1387

Osawa M, Hanada K, Hamada H, Nakauchi H (1996) Long-term lymphohematopoietic reconstitution by a single CD34- low/negative hematopoietic stem cell. Science 273:242–245

Palis J, Chan RJ, Koniski A, Patel R, Starr M, Yoder MC (2001) Spatial and temporal emergence of high proliferative potential hematopoietic precursors during murine embryogenesis. Proc Natl Acad Sci U S A 98:4528–4533

Pardee AB (1989) G_1 Events and Regulation of Cell Proliferation. Science 246:603–608

Park IK, Qian D, Kiel M, Becker MW, Pihalja M, Weissman IL, Morrison SJ, Clarke MF (2003) Bmi-1 is required for maintenance of adult self-renewing haematopoietic stem cells. Nature 423:302–305

Parmar K, Mauch P, Vergilio JA, Sackstein R, Down JD (2007) Distribution of hematopoietic stem cells in the bone marrow according to regional hypoxia. Proc Natl Acad Sci U S A 104:5431–5436

Phillips RL, Reinhart AJ, Van Zant G (1992) Genetic control of murine hematopoietic stem cell pool sizes and cycling kinetics. Proc Natl Acad Sci U S A 89:11607–11611

Plett PA, Frankovitz SM, Orschell-Traycoff CM (2002) In vivo trafficking, cell cycle activity, and engraftment potential of phenotypically defined primitive hematopoietic cells after transplantation into irradiated or nonirradiated recipients. Blood 100:3545–3552

Potocnik AJ, Brakebusch C, Fassler R (2000) Fetal and adult hematopoietic stem cells require beta1 integrin function for colonizing fetal liver, spleen, and bone marrow. Immunity 12:653–663

Quesenberry PJ, Colvin GA, Lambert JF (2002) The chiaroscuro stem cell: a unified stem cell theory. Blood 100:4266–4271

Rebel V, Miller C, Eaves C, Lansdorp P (1996a) The repopulation potential of fetal liver hematopoietic stem cells in mice exceeds that of their liver adult bone marrow counterparts. Blood 87:3500–3507

Rebel VI, Miller CL, Thornbury GR, Dragowska WH, Eaves CJ, Lansdorp PM (1996b) A comparison of long-term repopulating hematopoietic stem cells in fetal liver and adult bone marrow from the mouse. Exp Hematol 24:638–648

Reya T, Duncan AW, Ailles L, Domen J, Scherer DC, Willert K, Hintz L, Nusse R, Weissman IL (2003) A role for Wnt signalling in self-renewal of haematopoietic stem cells. Nature 423:409–414

Ross EA, Anderson N, Micklem HS (1982) Serial depletion and regeneration of the murine hematopoietic system. Implications for hematopoietic organization and the study of cellular aging. J Exp Med 155:432–444

Rossi DJ, Bryder D, Seita J, Nussenzweig A, Hoeijmakers J, Weissman IL (2007a) Deficiencies in DNA damage repair limit the function of haematopoietic stem cells with age. Nature 447:725–729

Rossi DJ, Bryder D, Weissman IL (2007b) Hematopoietic stem cell aging: mechanism and consequence. Exp Gerontol 42:385–390

Rossi DJ, Bryder D, Zahn JM, Ahlenius H, Sonu R, Wagers AJ, Weissman IL (2005) Cell intrinsic alterations underlie hematopoietic stem cell aging. Proc Natl Acad Sci U S A 102:9194–9199

Rusan NM, Peifer M (2007) A role for a novel centrosome cycle in asymmetric cell division. J Cell Biol 177:13–20

Samper E, Fernandez P, Eguia R, Martin-Rivera L, Bernad A, Blasco MA, Aracil M (2002) Long-term repopulating ability of telomerase-deficient murine hematopoietic stem cells. Blood 99:2767–2775

Sauvageau G, Iscove NN, Humphries, RK (2004) In vitro and in vivo expansion of hematopoietic stem cells. Oncogene 23:7223–7232

Schwarz BA, Bhandoola A (2004) Circulating hematopoietic progenitors with T lineage potential. Nat Immunol 5:953–960

Sitnicka E, Bryder D, Theilgaard-Monch K, Buza-Vidas N, Adolfsson J, Jacobsen SE (2002) Key Role of flt3 Ligand in Regulation of the Common Lymphoid Progenitor but Not in Maintenance of the Hematopoietic Stem Cell Pool. Immunity 17:463

Srour EF, Abonour R, Cornetta K, Traycoff CM (1999) Ex vivo expansion of hematopoietic stem and progenitor cells: are we there yet? J Hematother 8:93–102

Steinman RA (2002) Cell cycle regulators and hematopoiesis. Oncogene 21:3403–3413

Sudo K, Ema H, Morita Y, Nakauchi H (2000) Age-associated characteristics of murine hematopoietic stem cells. J Exp Med 192:1273–1280

Takano H, Ema H, Sudo K, Nakauchi H (2004) Asymmetric Division and Lineage Commitment at the Level of Hematopoietic Stem Cells: Inference from Differentiation in Daughter Cell and Granddaughter Cell Pairs. J Exp Med 199:295–302

Till JE, McCulloch EA, Siminovitch L (1964) A Stochastic Model of Stem Cell Proliferation, Based on the Growth of Spleen Colony-Forming Cells. Proc Natl Acad Sci U S A 51:29–36

Tothova Z, Kollipara R, Huntly BJ, Lee BH, Castrillon DH, Cullen DE, McDowell EP, Lazo-Kallanian S, Williams IR, Sears C, et al (2007). FoxOs are critical mediators of hematopoietic stem cell resistance to physiologic oxidative stress. Cell 128:325–339

Tulina N, Matunis E (2001) Control of stem cell self-renewal in Drosophila spermatogenesis by JAK-STAT signaling. Science 294:2546–2549

Turpen JB, Kelley CM, Mead PE, Zon LI (1997) Bipotential primitive-definitive hematopoietic progenitors in the vertebrate embryo. Immunity 7:325–334

Uchida N, Dykstra B, Lyons KJ, Leung FY, Eaves CJ (2003) Different in vivo repopulating activities of purified hematopoietic stem cells before and after being stimulated to divide in vitro with the same kinetics. Exp Hematol 31:1338–1347

Wagers AJ, Christensen JL, Weissman IL (2002) Cell fate determination from stem cells. Gene Ther 9:606–612

Walker L, Carlson A, Tan-Pertel HT, Weinmaster G, Gasson J (2001) The notch receptor and its ligands are selectively expressed during hematopoietic development in the mouse. Stem Cells 19:543–552

Walkley CR, Fero ML, Chien WM, Purton LE, McArthur, GA (2005) Negative cell-cycle regulators cooperatively control self-renewal and differentiation of haematopoietic stem cells. Nat Cell Biol 7:172–178

Weissman IL (2000) Stem cells: units of development, units of regeneration, and units in evolution. Cell 100:157–168

Willert K, Brown JD, Danenberg E, Duncan AW, Weissman IL, Reya T, Yates JR, Nusse R (2003) Wnt proteins are lipid-modified and can act as stem cell growth factors. Nature 423:448–452

Wilson A, Murphy MJ, Oskarsson T, Kaloulis K, Bettess MD, Oser GM, Pasche AC, Knabenhans C, Macdonald HR, Trumpp A (2004) c-Myc controls the balance between hematopoietic stem cell self-renewal and differentiation. Genes Dev18:2747–2763

Wilson A, Trumpp A (2006) Bone-marrow haematopoietic-stem-cell niches. Nat Rev Immunol 6:93–106

Wright DE, Wagers AJ, Gulati AP, Johnson FL, Weissman IL (2001) Physiological migration of hematopoietic stem and progenitor cells. Science 294:1933–1936

Xing Z, Ryan MA, Daria D, Nattamai KJ, Van Zant G, Wang L, Zheng Y, Geiger H (2006) Increased hematopoietic stem cell mobilization in aged mice. Blood 108:2190–2197

Yamashita YM, Mahowald AP, Perlin JR, Fuller MT (2007) Asymmetric inheritance of mother versus daughter centrosome in stem cell division. Science 315:518–521

Yang L, Bryder D, Adolfsson J, Nygren J, Mansson R, Sigvardsson M, Jacobsen SE (2004) Identification of Lin-Sca1+kit+CD34+Flt3- short-term hematopoietic stem cells capable of rapidly reconstituting and rescuing myeloablated recipients. Blood

Yang L, Wang L, Geiger H, Cancelas JA, Mo J, Zheng Y (2007) Rho GTPase Cdc42 coordinates hematopoietic stem cell quiescence and niche interaction in the bone marrow. Proc Natl Acad Sci U S A 104:5091–5096

Yoder MC, Hiatt K, Dutt P, Mukherjee P, Bodine, DM, Orlic D (1997) Characterization of definitive lymphohematopoietic stem cells in the day 9 murine yolk sac. Immunity 7:335–344

Zhang J, Niu C, Ye L, Huang H, He X, Tong WG, Ross J, Haug J, Johnson T, Feng JQ, et al (2003). Identification of the haematopoietic stem cell niche and control of the niche size. Nature 425:836–841

Zhou S, Morris JJ, Barnes Y, Lan L, Schuetz JD, Sorrentino BP (2002) Bcrp1 gene expression is required for normal numbers of side population stem cells in mice, and confers relative protection to mitoxantrone in hematopoietic cells in vivo. Proc Natl Acad Sci U S A 99:12339–12344

Zhu J, Emerson SG (2002) Hematopoietic cytokines, transcription factors and lineage commitment. Oncogene 21:3295–3313

Zon LI (1995) Developmental biology of hematopoiesis. Blood 86:2876–2891

Cellular Immunosenescence - Genetics

Associations of Cytokine Polymorphisms with Immunosenescence

Elissaveta Naumova and Milena Ivanova

Contents

Abstract: Deterioration of the immune system with aging is associated with an increased susceptibility to infectious diseases, cancer and autoimmune disorders. It has been demonstrated that immunosenescence is associated with chronic, low-grade inflammatory activity. The aging process is very complex and longevity is a multifactorial trait, which is determined by genetic and environmental factors, and the interaction of "disease" processes with "intrinsic" ageing processes. It is hypothesized that the level of immune response as well as possibly longevity could be associated with genes regulating immune functions. It is further hypothesized that the diversity of these genes might influence successful aging and longevity by modulating an individual´s response to life-threatening disorders. Several studies have focused on the role of genes encoding molecules with immune functions. In this chapter we will review the data on the role of cytokine gene polymorphisms in human longevity.

Keywords: Cytokines • Cytokine   gene   polymprphisms • Immunosenescence Longevity

E. Naumova (✉) · M. Ivanova
Central Laboratory of Clinical Immunology
University Hospital "Alexandrovska"
1.G. Sofiisky str., 1431 Sofia, Bulgaria
Tel: +3952 9230 690
Fax: +3592 9230 496
E-mail: immun@alexandrovska-hospital.bg

T. Fulop et al. (eds.), *Handbook on Immunosenescence*,
DOI 10.1007/978-1-4020-9062-2_32, © Springer Science+Business Media B.V. 2009

1   Introduction

Aging is a universal phenomenon affecting all animal species. This physiological process could be characterized as: inevitable consequence of being a multicellular organism; associated with a random passive decline in function; leading to a global loss of homeostasis over time and mortality increasing with aging (Helfand and Rogina, 2003). Aging is determined by a complex interaction of genetic, epigenetic and environmental factors, but a strong genetic component appears to have an impact on survival to advanced age. Among the several theories of aging proposed, the genetic theory suggests that several genes are involved in longevity (Kirkwood, 2002; Browner et al. 2004). Additionally, studies of Mitchell et al. indicated that up to 25% of the variation in human lifespan is heritable (Mitchell et al. 2001). The genetics of human longevity is quite peculiar in a context where antagonistic pleiotropy can play a major role and genes can have different biological role at different ages. Data of several studies imply that aging process may be associated with alterations in the immune system, suggesting that genetic determinants of senescence also resides in those polymorphisms for the immune system genes that regulate immune responses. Genes, encoding molecules involved in the development of protective immunity are highly polymorphic, present significant variation possibly resulting from an evolutionary adaptation of the organism facing an ever evolving environment. These genes include: HLA genes; genes encoding "unusual" HLA-like molecules (CD1); killer cell immunoglobulin-like receptor genes (KIR); leukocyte Fcγ receptor genes; cytokine and cytokine receptor genes; Toll-like receptor gene family; TNF- receptor associated factors. Several studies have focused on the role of cytokine gene polymorphisms for human longevity. The diversity of these genes might influence successful aging and longevity by modulating an individual´s response to life-threatening disorders.

In this chapter we summarize present knowledge on the role of cytokines in human longevity. Cytokines are an internal part of the immune response stimulated by antigen presentation in the context of HLA. Many studies have shown that the pathology of some infectious, autoimmune and malignant diseases is influenced by the profiles of cytokine production in pro-inflammatory (Th1) and anti-inflammatory (Th2) T cells. Additionally some authors have shown differences in cytokine levels in elderly and possible association with age-related diseases. Pro-inflammatory cytokines play a role in chronic inflammation, a phenomenon proposed to call "inflammaging" (Salvioli et al. 2006). People genetically predisposed to develop weak inflammatory activity seems to have fewer chances of developing cardiovascular diseases and subsequently live longer if they do not become affected by serious infectious diseases. Ferrucci et al. 1999, Harris et al. 1999 demonstrated that increased IL-6 serum levels could be a marker for functional disability and predictor of mortality in elderly. Increased expression levels of IL-6 were observed also in stress conditions, one of the characteristics of ageing (Heinrich et al. 2003). Elevated levels of this cytokine associated with development of frailty and susceptibility to diseases in elderly were also observed (Forsey et al. 2003). This inflammatory marker could be involved in low-grade inflammatory that develops with age (Cohen et al. 1997; Bruunsgaard et al. 1999; Ershler and Keller 2000). Dysredulation of IL-6 has been thought to be involved in the pathogenesis of a variety of age-related diseases, such as diabetes and atherosclerosis, which have a substantial inflammatory pathogenesis (Chamorro 2004; Dandona et al. 2004). IL-8 is also considered to be a potent inflammatory agent. However, IL-8 has also been reported to serve as an organ protective factor. It seems possible that an association of an increased serum level of IL-8 and a low level of IL-6 is related to longevity (Wieczorowska-Tobis et al. 2006). Additionally in elderly was observed a decreased capacity to produce IFN-γ, IL-2, IL-4 upon stimulation (Franceschi et al. 2000). The higher levels of TNF-α also correlate with functional status and decreased chance of long-life survival in elderly (Ferrucci 1999; Harris et al. 1999; Ershler et al. 2000; Forsey et al. 2003). Moreover, dysregulation and, in particular, overproduction of TNF has been implicated in a variety of human diseases including sepsis, cerebral malaria, and autoimmune diseases such as multiple sclerosis, rheumatoid arthritis (RA), systemic lupus erythematosus, and Crohn disease, as well as cancer. Interestingly, in a very large

Table 1 Gene polymorphisms of pro-inflammatory cytokines associated with aging

Cytokine gene polymorphism	Effect	Population	References
IL-2 (-330 T/C)	No association in elderly	Irish	Ross et al. 2003
	Increased (T-low) marginally in centenarians	Italian	Scola et al. 2005
IL-6 (-174 C/G)	Increased (C-low) in male centenarians	Italian	Bonafe et al. 2001
	No association	Sardinia, Southern Italy	Capurso, 2004; Pes et al. 2004
	Decreased (G/G-high) in octogenarians and nonagenerians	Irish	Rea et al. 2003; Ross O et al. 2003
	No association in nonagenarians	Finish	Wang X et al. 2001
	Increased G allele in elderly survivors	Finish	Harume et al. 2005
	Increased (GG) in elderly	Danish	Christiansen L et al. 2004
	No association	Bulgarian	Naumova et al. 2004
IFN-G (+874 T/A)	Increased (T/T-high) in female centenarians	Italian	Lio D et al. 2002
	No associations	Bulgarian	Naumova et al. 2004
TNF-A (-308 G/A)	Decreased (A-high) in centenarians	Danish	Buunsgaard H et al. 2004
	No association in nonagenarians	Finish	Wang X et al. 2001
	No association in centenarians	Italian	Lio D et al. 2003
	No association in elderly	Bulgarians	Naumova et al. 2004

study in Italian population IL-1Ra plasma levels were increased with age in both male and female subjects (Cavallone et al. 2003). Because of the pivotal role of anti-inflammatory cytokines TGF-β1 and IL-10 in regulation of immune responses, the variability of their levels may affect low grade inflammation that develops with age. It has been shown that the elevated level of anti-inflammatory cytokines IL-10 and TGF-β in serum of elderly is associated with increased resistance against septic shock (Forsey et al. 2003). Increased ex vivo capacity of macrophages from elderly to produce anti-inflammatory IL-10 was also found. Intriguingly, the existence of "risk immunological phenotype," probably associated with lack of tight control in systemic inflammation was also discussed.

Similarly to other genes, coding molecules with immune functions, cytokine genes are highly polymorphic. Most of the polymorphic sites identified so far are located in the noncoding regions, containing regulatory sequences, while exon sequences are highly conserved. Three main forms of polymorphisms were identified in cytokine genes: single nucleotide polymorphisms (SNPs) (Kruglyak et al. 1999), variable number of tandem repeats and micro-satellites (Weber and May 1989; Bidwell et al. 2001). Although still controversial, polymorphic variants observed for some cytokine genes have been correlated to the level of gene expression. Thus the cytokine gene polymorphism may be responsible for observed inter-individual differences in cytokine production and may be one possible mechanism for perturbation of the Th1/Th2 balance. Some polymorphisms may have a functional significance by altering directly or indirectly the level of genes expression and/or its function, others may only be useful for the determination of genetic linkage to a particular haplotype associated in turn with a given clinical condition (Bidwell et al. 1999, 2001).

Although the data are limited and controversial (Caruso et al. 2000) and many discrepancies are reported likely due to population-specific interactions between gene pool and environment, interleukins could be considered as putative "longevity genes. " It has been hypothesized that longevity could be associated with cytokine gene polymorphism correlated with different level of cytokine expression and modulating immune response to several diseases (Ershler et al. 2000; Bruunsgaard et al. 2001; Volpato et al. 2001). Taking into account the internal part of cytokine genes in immune response, the regulation of cytokine expression level and their polymorphic nature, investigation the genetic variations of these loci with functional significance could be appropriate immunogenetic candidate markers implicated in the mechanism of successful aging and longevity.

Genetic variations correlating with elevated levels of pro-inflammatory cytokines have been negatively associated with ageing (Bhojak et al. 2000). Several studies showed that cytokine polymorphisms related to different level of secretion were associated with longevity. Genetic polymorphisms, associated with high level of IL-10 expression were increased (Lio et al. 2003), while polymorphisms possibly related to increased expression of proinflammatory cytokines - IFN-γ, TNF-α and IL-6 were decreased in elderly individuals (Lio et al. 2002; Bruunsgaard et al. 2004). These data confirmed the hypothesis that longevity is related to antiinflammatory genotype profile. Additionally, the pro-inflammatory cytokine profile was correlated with decreased life span in elderly. However, in elderly with different eth-nical background, investigations reported contradicting results on associations with cytokine gene polymorphism (Bonafe et al. 2001; Lio et al. 2002). Additionally, the majority of data were associated with investigation of single polymorphisms in single cytokine genes. The analysis of extended haplotypes which include several polymorphisms in the cytokine gene, as well as haplotypes which consist of SNPs in different cytokine genes will help to determine the precise immunogenetic basis of longevity.

2 Gene Polymorphism of Proinflammatory Cytokines and Aging

2.1 IL-2

IL-2 is a proinflammatory cytokine, which plays a central role in activation of T-cell mediated immune response and defects in IL-2 mediated activation induce severe immune deficiency (Demoulin and Renauld, 1998). Several polymorphisms in the promoter (position -330) and coding (position +166 and exon 1) regions were described in IL-2 gene. A promoter polymorphism -330 T/C was shown to influence IL-2 production in anti-D3/CD28-stimulated peripheral blood lymphocytes. T-lym-phocytes from -330 CC homozygous subjects are able to produce higher amount of IL-2 than heterozygous or -330 TT homozygous individuals (Hoffmat et al. 2001).

Age-related decline in IL-2 production has been recognized since the early work of Gillis et al. Subsequent studies showed that IL-2 is reduced in aged subjects with associated effects on intracellular activation on nuclear transcription pathways (Rea et al. 1996; Pawelec et al. 2002). In humans, high IL-2 serum levels characterize subjects affected by Alzheimer's disease. Resent study in Italian (Scola et al. 2005) and Irish (Ross et al. 2003) elderly subjects did not showed a statistically significant effect of IL-2 -330 polymorphism in aging. However, a T allele associated with IL-2 low producer genotype was discussed to be marginally associated with aging (Scola et al. 2005). Data suggested that the genetic background favoring an increased IL-2 production might be detrimental for longevity.

2.2 IL-6

IL-6 is a pleotropic growth factor involved in different physiological and pathologi-cal processes. IL-6 is considered to be a potent inflammatory agent. It was found also to inhibit neutrophil apoptosis, suggesting that there is an autocrine or para-crine antiapoptotic role for IL-6 (Lindermans et al. 2006).

The human IL-6 gene is mapped to chromosome 7p21–24. Different studies identified three SNPs (−597G/A, −572G/C и −174G/C) and one AT polymorphism (−373(A)n(T)m) in 5′ regulatory region in the gene (Fishman et al. 1998; Terry et al. 2000; Georges et al. 2001). It was demonstrated that IL-6–174C allele was significantly associated with lower plasma concentrations of this cytokine (Terry et al. 2000).

Despite of the significant number of studies on possible role of IL-6 gene polymorphisms in different diseases, the associations still remain to be clarified (Rauramaa et al. 2000; Terry et al. 2000; Humphries et al. 2001; Nauck et al. 2002). Great amount of papers reported a positive association between some polymorphic markers of IL-6 gene and human longevity, and capacity of producing low levels of IL-6 thought life-span appears to be beneficial for longevity (Wright et al. 2003; Christiansen, 2004; Franceschi et al. 2005; Hurme et al. 2005) Most studies focused on IL-6 -174 C/G polymorphism and susceptibility to common causes of morbidity and mortality among elderly, such as type 2 diabetes, cardiovascular diseases, and dementia. IL-6-174 C/G polymorphism is predictive for longevity (Salvioli et al. 2006) Data on centenarians and elderly individuals from Italy showed increased frequency of C alleles in male centenarians and it seemed to be a gender specific effect on longevity (Bonafe et al. 2001). Correlations with the serum levels showed that men carrying the GG genotype had higher IL-6 serum levels in respect to subjects with CC or CG genotypes. The authors hypothesized that individuals predisposed to produce high level of IL-6 (men carrying GG) have a reduced capacity to reach the extreme limits of human life-span. Additionally, authors demonstrated that age-related increase of IL-6 serum levels in women is quite independent from -174 C/G genotype. It has also been shown that the proportion of IL-6 high producers (GG genotypes) was increased by individuals affected by age-related diseases with inflammatory pathogenesis—diabetes, atherosclerosis, osteoporosis, and neurodegenerative diseases. Similarly, Rea et al. (2003), Ross et al. (2003) reported decreased frequency of IL-6 -174 GG carriers in Irish octogenarian and nonagenarian subjects from the BELFAST elderly longitudinal ageing study. However, in Finish nonagenerians analysis on IL6-174, IL1a-889, IL1b-511, IL1Ra VNTR, IL10-1082, and TNFa-308 did not show any associations, alone or in combinations (Wang et al. 2001). It appears that IL-6 polymorphism does not affect life expectancy neither in the Sardinian population, nor in people from southern Italy, suggesting that the effect of IL-6 polymorphism on longevity might be population specific and dependent on gene – environment interactions (Capurso, 2004; Pes et al. 2004). Similar lack of association of IL-6 gene polymorphism with longevity was observed in the Bulgarian population (Naumova et al. 2004). These controversial data could be partly explained by population specific factors including genetic background, environmental factors and life stile. Most of studies analyzed the effect of isolated polymorphisms and this could partly contribute to the contradicting results. Recently, Terry et al. (Rauramaa et al. 2000) demonstrated that haplotype combination of promoter polymorphisms in IL-6 gene is more informative marker associated with the level of gene expression, compared with the influence of −174 G/C in isolation. Additionally, studies have demonstrated that CC or CG carriers have an increased risk of Alzheimer disease (AD) and cardiovascular diseases (Zhang et al. 2004).

2.3 IFN-γ

IFN-γ is one of the most representative type 1 cytokines, which plays a pivotal role in defense against viruses and intracellular pathogens and the induction of immune-mediated inflammatory responses. Taking into account the key role of this cytokine, its genetically controlled production is focused on investigation in several studies associated with longevity. Among numerous intronic polymorphisms in the IFN-γ gene, a variable length CA repeat sequence and polymorphism in the intron 1 at position +874 relative to the transcriptional start site has been implicated to influence the level of gene expression in vitro (Pravica et al. 1999). The single nucleotide polymorphism +874 T/A is one well-known single-nucleotide polymorphism at the 5' end of the CA repeat region in the first intron of the IFN-γ gene. Specific binding of the nuclear transcription factor-κB to the DNA sequence containing the +874 T allele has been reported and it could have functional consequences for the transcription of the IFN-γ gene and could then influence the rate of expression. Studies in Italian centenarians showed increased frequency of +874 T/T in female centenarians. On the other hand, investigations in elderly individuals from the Bulgarian population did not show significant differences in IFN-γ (+874) allele distribution compared to young controls (Naumova et al. 2004).

2.4 TNF-α

TNF-α is a pro-inflammatory cytokine involved in the immune response. This pleiotropic cytokine plays a wide variety of functions in many cell types.

The gene for TNF-α is located within the class III region of the major histocompatibility complex, which is a highly polymorphic region and its expression is tightly controlled at the transcriptional and posttranscriptional level. Several biallelic polymorphisms have been described within the TNF-α gene, including six in the promoter region at positions -1031T>C, -863C>A, -857C>T, -376G>A, -308G>A and -238G>A. Moreover, a number of studies have shown that the TNF-α promoter polymorphisms have a significant effect on transcriptional activity. Susceptibility to many diseases is thought to have a genetic basis, and the TNF gene is considered a candidate-predisposing gene. However, unraveling the importance of genetic variation in the TNF locus to disease susceptibility or severity is complicated by its location within the MHC and the strong linkage disequilibrium with other genes. Several investigations reported associations of MHC haplotypes with different TNF-α phenotypes: DR3 and DR4 haplotypes were correlated with high level of TNF-α (Jacob et al. 1990; Abraham et al. 1993), while DR2 haplotypes were associated with low expression (Bendtzen et al. 1988; Jacob et al. 1990). These finding proposed the existence of functional polymorphism involved in the regulation of TNF-α production. SNPs at position -308 have been commonly studied with respect to their influence on TNF-α expression. Transfection studies

Table 2   Gene polymorphisms of anti-inflammatory cytokines associated with aging

Cytokine gene polymorphism	Effect	Population	References
TGF-B1 (915 C/G)	Decreased C allele and C/G genotype in centenarians	Italian	Carrieri G et al. 2004
TGF-B1 (cdns 10, 25)	No associations in elderly	Bulgarians	Naumova et al. 2004
IL-10 (-1082 A/G)	Increased (G/G-high) in male centenarians	Italians	Lio D et al. 2002
	No association with longevity	Finish	Wang X et al. 2001
	No association with longevity	Irish	Ross O et al. 2003
	No association with longevity	Sardinian	Pes G et al. 2004
IL-10 (-819 C/T)	No association with longevity	Italian	Lio D et al. 2002
IL-10 (-592 C/A)	No association with longevity	Italian	Lio D et al. 2002
IL-10 (-1082G,-819C,-592C)	Increased in elderly	Italian	Lio D et al. 2002
IL-10 (-1082G,-819C,-592C)	Increased in elderly	Bulgarians	Naumova et al. 2004
IL-10 (-1082A,-819T,-592A)	Decreased in elderly	Bulgarians	Naumova et al. 2004

in human B-cell lines showed that the presence of rare TNF2 allele (A at position -308) results in higher constitutive and inducible levels of TNF expression compared with a common TNF1 allele (G at position -308), confirming the importance of this site in the transcriptional regulation of the TNF gene (Wilson et al. 1997; Makhatadze et al. 1998; Lio et al. 2001; Hajeer, 2001). The functional relevance of this SNP has been confirmed by its involvement in determining susceptibility to immune-inflammatory diseases (Makhatadze, 1998; Lio et al. 2001; Hajeer and Hutchinson 2001; Dalziel et al. 2002; Heijmans et al. 2002; O'Keefe et al. 2002; Sakao et al. 2002; Witte et al. 2002). Although the polymorphism -308 G/A associated with different gene expression is one of the most widely investigated in different diseases, no correlation of this SNP and longevity was found in centenarians from the Finnish and the Italian population (Wang et al. 2001; Lio et al. 2003). Similar results were observed for elderly individuals from the Bulgarian population (Naumova et al. 2004). In the Danish population, however decreased frequency of A allele was observed among centenarians. Positive association with the process of successful ageing was observed also in men centenarians from Italian population when the two SNPs -308 G/A from TNFA gene and -1082 G/A SNP from IL10 gene were analyzed simultaneously (Wang et al. 2001). The group of Lio D et al. reported that an anti-inflammatory genotype TNFA GG (low)/ IL10 GG (high) has a protective role in longevity. TNF-A and IL-10 have complex and opposing roles, and an autoregulatory loop appears to exist (Candore et al. 2002).

3 Gene Polymorphism of Antiinflammatory Cytokines and Aging

3.1 TGF-B1

TGF-B1 is a multifunctional cytokine that regulates cell proliferation, differentiation, and migration, and it was considered as an aniinflammatory molecule (Wright et al. 2003). In the study of Carrieri et al, the plasma levels of biologically active TGF-B1 were significantly increased in the elderly group, independently from TGF-B1 genotypes (Carrieri et al. 2004). The TGF-β1 gene consists of 7 exons and 6 introns. Until now, eight polymorphisms in the promoter (-509 C→T, -800 G→ A and -988 C→T), coding (+896 T→C, +915 G→C, +788 C→T, +652 C→T and +673 T→C) regions end one deletion (713 del C) in inton 4 of the TGF-β1 gene were discovered. Polymorphisms +896 (codon 10) and +915 (codon 25), associated with different level of expression are the most commonly studied. For polymorphism +915 G/C, the presence of C allele is generally associated with lower TGF-β synthesis in vitro and in vivo. Association between the presence of particular TGF-β1 allele and the level of the product indicates that the G-800 A and C-509 T polymorphisms may also be involved in the modulation of expression of the TGF-β1 gene. The -509 T allele - has been reported to be associated with marginally higher transcriptional activity of TGF-β compared to the -509C allele. TGF-β -800 G→A polymorphism is in a consensus CREB (cAMP response element-binding protein) shalf-site. The presence of A allele was suggested to have reduced affinity for the CREB family of transcription factors, resulting in a lower level of total TGF-β1 in the circulation. Analysis of these three SNPs +915 G→C, -509 C→T and -800 G→ A by the group of Carrieri G et al. observed that only +915 C allele and GC genotype with significantly lower frequency, compared to controls. Additionally they found also decreased frequency of extended haplotype G -800/C -509/C 869/C 915 and elevated level of TGF-β1 in elderly, but correlation with investigated genotypes in TGF-B1 gene was not found (Carrieri et al. 2004). Similarly no associations of TGF-B1 codons 10 and 25 genotypes with longevity were observed in Bulgarians (Naumova et al. 2004). It has been hypothesized that genetic determined cytokine profiles of TGF-β1 could be involved in mechanism of successful ageing but more data are need to confirm this results.

3.2 IL-10

IL-10 is a powerful cytokine that inhibits lymphocyte repeication and secretion of inflammatory cytokines (My-Chan Dang et al. 2006). Since one of the main functions of IL-10 is to limit inflammatory responses (Moore et al. 2001), polymorphisms in the regulatory region of this gene could be possibly related to longevity. Stimulation of human blood samples with bacterial lipopolysaccharide showed variation of IL-10 production, suggesting a genetic component of approximately 75% (Westendorp et al. 1997). Inter person differences in the regulation of IL-10 production may be critical with respect to the final outcome of an inflammatory response.

The IL-10 gene is located on chromosome 1 at q31–32. Several polymorphisms in the human IL-10 5' flanking region and two microsatelites associated with differential IL-10 production have been identified. The most extensively investigated SNPs are in the promoter region at position -1082, -819 and -592 (Turner et al. 1997, D'Alfonso et al. 2000; Kube et al. 2001) correlating with different transcriptional activity. The three dimorphisms appear in three potential haplotypes: GCC, ACC and ATA (G/A at position -1082, C/T at position -819 and C/A at -592 correspondingly) related to different level of gene expression. The ability of individuals to produce high levels of IL-10 is evidently controlled by a G at position -1082, as this variant is found in the highest producers (Turner et al. 1997; Eskdale et al. 1998; Crawley et al. 1999; D'Alfonso et al. 2000; Kube et al. 2001; Lio et al. 2002). Several studies reported the linkage between the sites -819 and -592. The A allele of the -592 SNP was found to be associated with lower stimulated IL-10 release. In the presence of allele -1082A, stimulation of lymphocytes with concanavalin A resulted in lower IL-10 production than in allele -1082A negative cells (Turner et al. 1997; Hutchinson et al. 1999). The functional relevance of this SNP has been shown by its involvement in determining susceptibility to immune-inflammatory diseases (Hajeer et al. 1998; Crawley et al. 1999; Tagore et al. 1999; Howell et al. 2001; Girndt et al. 2002; Shoskes et al. 2002; Wu et al. 2002) The two dimorphisms -819 and -592 exhibit strong linkage disequilibrium.

The IL-10 -1082 A/G polymorphism has been reported to be a male-specific marker for longevity (Lio et al. 2002), while no differenced were found regarding the -819 and -592 polymorphisms. The -1082GG genotype, associated with high IL-10 production, was argued to confer an anti-inflammatory status (Lio et al. 2002). Studies in Bulgarians demonstrated significant differences for two IL-10 haplotypes: one of them (-1,082A,-819T,-592A), possibly associated with the low level of gene expression was decreased in elderly, while the other (-1,082G,-819C,-592C) associated with high level of cytokine gene expression was significantly more frequent among healthy elderly compared to young controls. This effect was more pronounced in GCC homozygous individuals as indicated by the analysis of IL-10 genotypes. However, studies in two other populations— Irish nonagenarians (Ross et al. 2003) and Finish nonagenarians (Wang et al. 2001) did not show any association with longevity. A possible explanation for the negative results in the Irish and Finnish studies could be the younger age of the old subjects investigated in comparison with the Italian study. Interestingly to note that the IL-10 -1082 GG genotype is much less frequent in patients affected by Alzheimer's disease (Lio et al. 2003).

In summary, the capability to maintain a lower production of pro-inflammatory cytokines appears to be favorable for reaching the extreme limits of human life span in good health conditions and could be genetically controlled. Cytokine genes related to inflammation seems particularly relevant taking into account that the innate immunity is more involved during inflammation, and a chronic inflammatory status appears to be the major component of the most common age-related diseases, including cardiovascular diseases and infections. The emerging data on the pivotal role of additional interactions in affecting expression of some relevant cytokines (for example zinc–gene interactions) and studies in populations with different environmental background will allow to clarify further the role of cytokines in aging.

References

Abraham LJ, French MA, Dawkins RL (1993) Polymorphic MHC ancestral haplotypes affect the activity of tumour necrosis factor-alpha. Clin Exp Immunol 92:14–18

Bendtzen K, Morling N, Fomsgaard A et al (1988) Association between HLA-DR2 and production of tumour necrosis factor alpha and interleukin 1 by mononuclear cells activated by lipopolysaccharide. Scand J Immunol 28:599–606

Bhojak TJ, DeKosky ST, Ganguli M et al (2000) Genetic polymorphisms in the cathespin D and interleukin-6 genes and the risk of Alzheimer's disease. Neurosci Lett 288:21–24

Bidwell J, Keen L, Gallagher G et al (1999) Human cytokine gene nucleotide sequence alignments: supplement 1. Eur J Immunogenet 26:135–223

Bidwell J, Keen L, Gallagher G et al (2001) Cytokine gene polymorphism in human disease: on-line databases, supplement 1. Genes Immun 2:61–70

Bonafe M, Olivieri F, Cavallone L et al (2001) A gender-dependent genetic predisposition to produce high levels of IL-6 is detrimental for longevity. Eur J Immunol 31:2357–2361

Browner WS, Kahn AJ, Ziv E, Reiner AP, Oshima, J, Cawthon RM, Hsueh WC, Cummings SR (2004) The genetics of human longevity. Am J Med 117:851–860

Bruunsgaard H, Benfield TL, Andersen-Ranberg K et al (2004) The tumor necrosis factor alpha -308G>A polymorphism is associated with dementia in the oldest old. J Am Geriatr Soc 52:1361–1366

Bruunsgaard H, Pedersen M, Pedersen BK (2001) Aging and proinflammatory cytokines. Curr Opin Hematol 8:131–136

Bruunsgaard H, Skinhoj P, Qvist J et al. 1999. Elderly humans show prolonged in vivo inflammatory activity during pneumococcal infections. J Infect Dis. 180, 551–554

Candore G, Lio D, Colonna Romano G, Caruso C (2002) Pathogenesis of autoimmune diseases associated with 8.1ancestral haplotype: Effect of multiple gene interactions. Autoimmun Rev 1:29–35

Capurso C, Solfrizzi V, D'Introno A, Colacicco AM, Capurso SA, Semeraro C, Capurso A, Panza F (2004) Interleukin 6-174 G/C promoter gene polymorphism in centenarians: No evidence of association with human longevity or interaction with apolipoprotein E alleles. Exp Gerontol 39:1109–1114

Carrieri G, Marzi E, Olivieri F, Marchegiani F, Cavallone L, Cardelli M, Giovagnetti S, Stecconi R, Molendini C, Trapassi C, De Benedictis G, Kletsas D, Franceschi C (2004) The G/C915 polymorphism of transforming growth factor beta1 is associated with human longevity: A study in Italian centenarians. Aging Cell 3:443–448

Caruso C, Candore G, Colonna Romano G et al (2000) HLA, aging, and longevity: a critical reappraisal. Hum Immunol 61:942–949

Cavallone L, Bonafe M, Olivieri F et al (2003) The role of IL-1 gene cluster in longevity: a study in Italian population. Mech Ageing Dev 124:533–538

centenarians. Aging Clin Exp Res 16:244–248

Chamorro A (2004) Role of inflammation in stroke and atherothrombosis. Cerebrovasc Dis 7 (Suppl 3):1–5

Christiansen L, Bathum L, Andersen-Ranberg K, Jeune B, Christensen K (2004) Modest implication of interleukin-6 promoter polymorphisms in longevity. Mech Ageing Dev 125:391–395

Cohen HJ, Pieper CF, Harris T et al (1997) The association of plasma IL-6 levels with functional disability in community-dwelling elderly. J Gerontol A Biol Sci Med Sci 52:201–208

Crawley E, Kay R, Sillibourne J et al (1999) Polymorphic haplotypes of the interleukin-10 5' flanking region determine variable interleukin-10 transcription and are associated with particular phenotypes of juvenile rheumatoid arthritis. Arthritis Rheum 42:1101–1108

D'Alfonso S, Rampi M, Rolando V et al (2000) New polymorphisms in the IL-10 promoter region. Genes Immun 1:231–3

Dalziel B, Gosby AK, Richman R et al (2002) Association of the TNF-alpha -308 G/A promoter polymorphism with insulin resistance in obesity. Obes Res 10:401–7

Dandona P, Aljada A, Bandyopadhyay A (2004) Inflammation: the link between insulin resistance, obesity and diabetes. Trends Immunol 25:4–7

Demoulin JB and Renauld JC (1998). Signalling by cytokines interacting with the interleukin-2 receptor gamma chain. Cytokines Cell Mol Ther:243–256

down-regulates expression of chemokine stromal cell-derived factor-1: Functional consequences in cell migration and adhesion. Blood 102:1978–1984

Ershler WB, Keller ET (2000) Age-associated increased interleukin-6 gene expression, late-life diseases, and frailty. Annu Rev Med 51:245–270

Eskdale J, Gallagher G, Verweij C et al (1998) Interleukin 10 secretion in relation to human IL-10 locus haplotypes. Proc Natl Acad Sci U S A 95:9465–9470

Ferrucci L, Harris TB, Guralnik JM et al (1999) Serum IL-6 level and the development of disability in older persons. J Am Geriatr Soc 47:639–646

Fishman D, Faulds G Jeffery R et al (1998) The effect of novel polymorphisms in the interleukin-6 (IL-6) gene on IL-6 transcription and plasma IL-6 levels, and an association with systemic-onset juvenile chronic arthritis. J Clin Invest 102:1369–76

Forsey RJ, Thompson J, Ernerudh J et al (2003) Plasma cytokine profiles in elderly humans. Mech Ageing Dev 124:487–493

Franceschi C, Bonafe M, Valensin S et al (2000) Inflamm-aging. An evolutionary perspective on immunosenescence. Ann N Y Acad Sci 908:244–54

Franceschi C, Olivieri F, Marchegiani F, Cardelli M, Cavallone L, Capri M, Salvioli S, Valensin S, De Benedictis G, Di Iorio A, Caruso C, Paolisso G, Monti D (2005) Genes involved in immune response/inflammation, IGF1/insulin pathway and response to oxidative stress play a major role in the genetics of human longevity: The lesson of centenarians. Mech Ageing Dev 126:351–361

Georges JL, Loukaci V, Poirier O et al (2001) Interleukin-6 gene polymorphisms and susceptibility to myocardial infarction: the ECTIM study. Etude Cas-Temoin de l'Infarctus du Myocarde. J Mol Med 79:300–5

Girndt M, Kaul H, Sester U et al (2002) Anti- inflammatory interleukin-10 genotype protects dialysis patients from cardiovascular events. Kidney Int 62:949–55

Hajeer AH, Hutchinson IV (2001) Influence of TNF alpha gene polymorphisms on TNF alpha production and disease. Hum Immunol 62:1191–1199

Hajeer AH, Lazarus M, Turner D et al (1998) IL-10 gene promoter polymorphisms in rheumatoid arthritis. Scand J Rheumatol 27:142–145

Harris TB, Ferrucci L, Tracy RP et al (1999) Associations of elevated interleukin-6 and C-reactive protein levels with mortality in the elderly. Am J Med 106:506–512

Heijmans BT, Westendorp RG, Droog S et al (2002) Association of the tumour necrosis factor alpha -308G/A polymorphism with the risk of diabetes in an elderly population-based cohort. Genes Immun 3:225–228

Heinrich PC, Behrmann I, Haan S et al (2003) Principles of interleukin (IL)-6-type cytokine signalling and its regulation. Biochem J 374:1–20

Helfand SL, Rogina B (2003). Molecular genetics of aging in the fly: is this the end of the beginning? Bioessays 25:134–141

Hoffmann SC, Stanley EM, Darrin Cox E, Craighead N, DiMercurio BS, Koziol DE, Harlan DM, Kirk AD and Blair PJ (2001) Association of cytokine polymorphic inheritance and in vitro cytokine production in anti-CD3/CD28-stimulated peripheral blood lymphocytes. Transplantation 8:1444–1450

Howell WM, Turner SJ, Bateman A et al (2001) IL-10 promoter polymorphisms influence tumour development in cutaneous malignant melanoma. Genes Immun 2:25–31

Humphries SE, Luong LA, Ogg M et al (2001) The interleukin-6 -174 G/C promoter polymorphism is associated with risk of coronary heart disease and systolic blood pressure in healthy men.Eur Heart J 22:2243–52

Hurme M, Lehtimaki T, Jylha M, Karhunen PJ, Hervonen A (2005) Interleukin-6-174G/C polymorphism and longevity: A follow-up study. Mech Ageing Dev 126:417–418

Hutchinson IV, Pravica V, Perrey C et al (1999) Cytokine gene polymorphisms and relevance to forms of rejection. Transplant Proc 31:734–736

Jacob CO, Fronek Z, Lewis G et al 1990. Heritable major histocompatibility complex class II-associated differences in production of tumor necrosis factor alpha: relevance to genetic predisposition to systemic lupus erythematosus. Proc Natl Acad Sci U S A 87:1233–1237

Kirkwood TB (2002) Evolution of ageing. Mech. Ageing Dev 123:737–745

Kruglyak L (1999) Prospects for whole-genome linkage disequilibrium mapping of common disease genes. Nat Genet 22:139–144

Kube D, Rieth H, Eskdale J et al (2001) Structural characterisation of the distal 5' flanking region of the human interleukin-10 gene. Genes Immun 2:181–190

Lindemans CA, Coffer PJ, Schellens IM, de Graaff PM, Kimpen JL, Koenderman L (2006) Respiratory syncytial virus inhibits granulocyte apoptosis through a phosphatidylinositol 3-kinase and NF-kappaB-dependent mechanism. J Immunol 176:5529–5537

Lio D, Candore G, Colombo A et al (2001) A genetically determined high setting of TNF-alpha influences immunologic parameters of HLA-B8,DR3 positive subjects: implications for autoimmunity. Hum Immunol 62:705–713

Lio D, Scola L, Crivello A et al (2002) Gender-specific association between -1082 IL-10 promoter polymorphism and longevity. Genes Immun 3:30–33

Lio D, Scola L, Crivello A et al (2002) Allele frequencies of +874T–>A single nucleotide polymorphism at the first intron of interferon-gamma gene in a group of Italian centenarians. Exp Gerontol 37:315–319

Lio D, Scola L, Crivello A et al (2002) Gender-specific association between -1082 IL-10 promoter polymorphism and longevity. Genes Immun 3:30–3

Lio D, Scola L, Crivello A et al (2003) Inflammation, genetics, and longevity: further studies on the protective effects in men of IL-10 -1082 promoter SNP and its interaction with TNF-alpha -308 promoter SNP. J Med Genet 40:296–299

Makhatadze NJ (1998) Tumor necrosis factor locus: genetic organisation and biological implications. Hum Immunol 59:571–579

Mitchell BD, Hsueh WC, King TM, Pollin TI, Sorkin J, Agarwala R, Schaffer AA, Shuldiner AR (2001) Heritability of life span in the Old Order Amish. Am J Med Genet 102:346–352

Moore KW, de Waal Malefyt R, Coffman RL et al (2001) Interleukin-10 and the interleukin-10 receptor. Annu Rev Immunol 19:683–765

My-Chan Dang P, Elbim C, Marie JC, Chiandotto M, Gougerot-Pocidalo MA, El-Benna J (2006) Anti-inflammatory effect of interleukin-10 on human neutrophil respiratory burst involves inhibition of GM-CSF-induced p47PHOX phosphorylation through a decrease in ERK1/2 activity. FASEB 23

Nauck M, Winkelmann BR, Hoffmann M et al (2002) The interleukin-6 G(-174)C promoter polymorphism in the LURIC cohort: no association with plasma interleukin-6, coronary artery disease, and myocardial infarction. J Mol Med 80:507–513

Naumova E, Mihaylova A, Ivanova M et al (2004) Immunological markers contributing to sucsessful aging in Bulgarians. Exp Gerontol 39:637–644

O'Keefe GE, Hybki DL, Munford RS (2002) The G A single nucleotide polymorphism at the -308 position in the tumor necrosis factor-alpha promoter increases the risk for severe sepsis after trauma. J Trauma 52:817–825

Pawelec G, Barnett Y, Forsey R, Frasca D, Globerson A, McLeod J, Caruso C, Franceschi C, Fulop T, Gupta S, Mariani E, Mocchegiani E, Solana R (2002) T cells and aging Front. Bioscience 7:1056–1183

Pes G, Lio D, Carru C, Deiana L, Baggio G, Franceschi C, Ferrucci L, Oliveri F, Scola L, Crivello A, Candore G, Colonna-Romano G, Caruso C (2004) Association between longevity and cytokine gene polymorphisms. A study in Sardinian

Pravica V, Asderakis A, Perrey C et al (1999) In vitro production of IFN-gamma correlates with CA repeat polymorphism in the human IFN-gamma gene. Eur J Immunogenet 26:1–3

Rauramaa R, Vaisanen SB, Luong LA et al (2000) Stromelysin-1 and interleukin-6 gene promoter polymorphisms are determinants of asymptomatic carotid artery atherosclerosis. Arterioscler Thromb Vasc Biol 20:2657–2662

Rea IM, Ross OA, Armstrong M et al (2003) Interleukin-6-gene C/G 174 polymorphism in nonagenarian and octogenarian subjects in the BELFAST study. Reciprocal effects on IL-6, soluble IL-6 receptor and for IL-10 in serum and monocyte supernatants. Mech Ageing Dev 124:555–561

Rea IM, Stewart M, Campbell P, Alexander HD, Crockard AD, Morris TC (1996) Changes in lymphocyte subsets, interleukin 2, and soluble interleukin 2 receptor in old and very old age. Gerontology 42:69–78

Ross OA, Curran MD, Meenagh A et al (2003) Study of age-association with cytokine gene polymorphisms in an aged Irish population. Mech Ageing Dev 124:199–206

Sakao S, Tatsumi K, Igari H et al (2002) Association of tumor necrosis factor-alpha gene promoter polymorphism with low attenuation areas on high-resolution CT in patients with COPD. Chest 122:416–420

Salvioli S, Olivieri F, Marchegiani F, Cardelli M, Santoro A, Bellavista E, Mishto M, Invidia L, Capri M, Valensin S, Sevini F, Cevenini E, Celani L, Lescai F, Gonos E, Caruso C, Paolisso G, De Benedictis G, Monti D, Franceschi C (2006) Genes, ageing and longevity in humans: Problems, advantages and perspectives. Free Radic Res 40:1303–1323

Scola L, Candore G, Colonna-Romano G, Crivello A, Forte G, Paolisso G, Franceschi C, Lio D, Caruso C (2005). Biogerontology 6:425–429

Shoskes DA, Albakri Q, Thomas K et al (2002) Cytokine polymorphisms in men with chronic prostatitis/chronic pelvic pain syndrome: association with diagnosis and treatment response. J Urol 168:331–335

Tagore A, Gonsalkorale WM, Pravica V et al (1999) Interleukin-10 (IL-10) genotypes in inflammatory bowel disease. Tissue Antigens 54:386–390

Terry CF, Loukaci V, Green FR (2000) Cooperative influence of genetic polymorphisms on interleukin 6 transcriptional regulation. J Biol Chem 275:18138–18144

Turner DM, Williams DM, Sankaran D et al (1997) An investigation of polymorphism in the interleukin-10 gene promoter. Eur J Immunogenet 24:1–8

Volpato S., Gyralink J, Ferrucci L et al. 2001. Cardiovascular disease, interleukin-6, and risk of mortality in older women: the women's health and aging study. Circulation. 103:947–953

Wang XY, Hurme M, Jylha M et al (2001). Lack of association between human longevity and polymorphisms of IL-1 cluster, IL-6, IL-10 and TNF-alpha genes in Finnish nonagenarians. Mech Ageing Dev 123:29–38

Weber JL, May PE (1989) Abundant class of human DNA polymorphisms which can be typed using the polymerase chain reaction. Am J Hum Genet 44:388–396

Westendorp RG, Langermans JA, Huizinga T et al (1997) Genetic influence on cytokine production in meningococcal disease. Lancet 349:1912–1913

Wieczorowska-Tobis K, Niemir Z, Podkywka R, Korybalska K, Mossakowska M, Bręborowicz A (2006) Can an increased level of circulating IL-8 be a predictor of human longevity? Med Sci Monit 12(3) :CR118–CR121

Wilson AG, Symons JA, McDowell T et al (1997) Effects of a polymorphism in the human tumor necrosis factor alpha promoter on transcriptional activation. Proc Natl Acad Sci U S A 94:3195–9

Witte JS, Palmer LJ, O'Connor R et al (2002) Relation between tumour necrosis factor polymorphism TNFalpha-308 and risk of asthma. Eur J Hum Genet 10:82–5

Wright N, de Lera TL, Garcia-Moruja C, Lillo R, Garcia-Sanchez F, Caruz A, Teixido J (2003) Transforming growth factorbeta1 down-regulates expression of chemokine stromal cell-derived factor-1: Functional consequences in cell migration and adhesion. Blood 102:1978–1984

Wright N, de Lera TL, Garcia-Moruja C, Lillo R, Garcia-Sanchez F, Caruz A, Teixido J (2003) Transforming growth factorbeta1

Wu MS, Huang SP, Chang YT et al (2002) Tumor necrosis factor-alpha and interleukin-10 promoter polymorphisms in Epstein-Barr virus-associated gastric carcinoma. J Infect Dis 2002 185:106–9

Zhang Y, Hayes A, Pritchard A et al (2004) Interleukin-6 promoter polymorphism: risk and pathology of Alzheimer's disease. Neurosci Lett 362:99–102

Cytokine Polymorphisms and Immunosenescence

Owen A. Ross, Kelly M. Hinkle and I. Maeve Rea

Contents

Abstract: The influence of genetics on immunosenescence is still to be resolved. Common genetic variants (polymorphism) that reside within the genes encoding cytokines are candidates to positively or negatively affect immunosenescence. Cytokines regulate the type and magnitude of the immune function. Polymorphism can influence the expression level of the cytokine protein which can subsequently cause an imbalance in the cytokine cascade.

Herein we examine the current literature with respect to cytokine polymorphisms in ageing and the age-related neurodegenerative disorder, Parkinson's disease.

O. A. Ross (✉) · K. M. Hinkle
Molecular Genetics Laboratory and Core
Mayo Clinic, Department of Neuroscience
4500 San Pablo Road, Jacksonville, FL 32224, USA
Tel: (904)-953-0963
Fax: (904)-953-7370
E-mail: ross.owen@mayo.edu

I. M. Rea
Department of Geriatric Medicine, School of Medicine
Dentistry and Biomedical Science, Queens University
Belfast, Northern Ireland

T. Fulop et al. (eds.), *Handbook on Immunosenescence*,
DOI 10.1007/ 978-1-4020-9062-2_33, © Springer Science+Business Media B.V. 2009

Ageing studies have identified two cytokine promoter polymorphisms that have shown repeated associations IL-6 (-174) and IL-10 (-1082). Others have failed to confirm these associations. This is due in part to studies of limited sample sizes examining a restricted number of cytokine polymorphisms. The inflammatory processes that characterize the cell death that is the hallmark of neurodegenerative disorders such as Parkinson's disease, may also be influenced by cytokine polymorphisms. However as with ageing, the results to date have been inconsistent although a number of studies have suggested the IL-1β (-511) and TNF-α (-308) show significant association with Parkinson's disease susceptibility.

Given the complexity of the cytokine network, and the dynamic interplay between anti and proinflammatory aspects, cross-sectional studies examining many cytokine variants in large sample series are now warranted. Genome-wide association studies may hold promise in resolving the role of cytokine polymorphisms in the inflammatory processes in both disease and ageing.

1   Introduction

Ageing is a complex, multifactorial process which can be defined as a progressive, generalized impairment of function resulting in a loss of adaptive response to stress and an increasing risk of age-associated disease [44, 45, 51–53]. Although the specific biological basis of ageing remains obscure, molecular investigations over the last 50 years have led to a cluster of theories that attempt to resolve ageing across species. However the complexity of the ageing process has only been reflected in the numerous hypotheses that have been proposed [72].

There is increasing evidence from a growing number of studies that longevity has heritability in families. However, a familial history of longevity could also be caused by a shared environment. A study of Danish twins noted only modest heritability in the ability to reach the septuagenarian years and above; no evidence for an effect of shared family environment was found [47]. Other studies show that siblings of centenarians are shown to have a 4-fold higher survival rate to ages above 85 years compared to siblings of persons who died at the age of <75 years [89, 90]. Whereas the twin study examined correlations of age at death in those of old age, the latter study focused on those who survive to extreme old age, and was therefore more likely to detect a stronger effect if genetic factors play a role in longevity.

As the world of scientific research moves into a new era beginning with the publication of the human genome and the continual description of novel variations in genes, the prospect of greater resolution to the question of ageing is at hand. The draft publication of the human genome was released on February 16th 2001, on the day when one of the pioneers of modern science, Charles Darwin, would have reached the ripe old age of 192 years. The human genome is composed of 46 chromosomes that are estimated to encode for between twenty and thirty thousand genes (approximately 40% of which are functionally unresolved) [56, 117]. Extensive variation has also been observed at the nucleotide level. DNA sequence variants are estimated to occur in one in every three to five hundred base pairs and are linked with a large diversity of phenotypes, ranging from variation in traits e.g., eye colour, height, susceptibility to disease and even the variation in the rate of ageing.

Polymorphism, literally translated "multiple forms", is the term used to describe the DNA variants that exist within a species. Polymorphism in a gene may result in increased/reduced protein production or affect the level of the abnormal proteins generated, through directly influencing gene transcription [115]. There is increasing evidence to show that gene expression is regulated by complex interplay, from simple polymorphic variants in regulatory regions such as the promoter or 3' untranslated regions, to the presence of microRNA species that can work through a negative/positive feedback mechanism.

At the recent 55th American Society of Human Genetics (2005) meeting held in Salt Lake City, the International HapMap project released its Phase I data. This project's major aim was to help identify linkage disequilibrium patterns traversing the entire human genome and facilitate the identification of haplotype "tagging" single nucleotide polymorphisms (SNPs) [2, 22]. In 2006, public databases (such as dbSNP) housed data on more than nine million candidate human SNPs for which genotype data is available for nearly two and a half million of them [2]. These vast volumes of data, coupled with the incredible advances in genotyping and DNA sequencing technologies, create a situation whereby the geneticist can pinpoint a trait loci [68, 114]. Genome-wide association studies are being proclaimed as the latest, and perhaps most powerful, tool in the mapping of causative/modifying genetic loci in complex disorders such as ageing [101].

The human genome displays a considerable level of inter-individual variability from simple SNPs and short repeats to large-scale deletions, multiplications and rearrangements. Recent studies have demonstrated that large gene copy number variations (CNVs) occur frequently in the general population with for the most part no determinable disadvantage to carriers. However this phenomenon can be pathogenic and in rare cases result in severe disease phenotypes [99, 111, 121]. The severe disease state is usually caused through either a "gain or loss of function" that occurs from an altered balance in the level of the essential protein. However, the presence of variants that give rise to much milder phenotypes and produce a fractional increase/decrease in gene expression may result in the slow, progressive manner of symptoms that typify both the ageing process itself and also the numerous age-related diseases, including cardiovascular disease, cancer and neurodegenerative disorders.

Human longevity appears to be inextricably linked with optimal functioning of the immune system, suggesting that specific genetic determinants may reside in polymorphic loci in genes that regulate immune response. The deterioration of the immune system due to "immunosenescence" (age-associated immune deficiency), coupled with the associated increase in the susceptibility to infectious disease, cancer and autoimmune disorders has restricted the potential human lifespan [14, 32, 34]. However this deterioration of the immune function accompanied by an increased risk of morbidity and mortality observed in the noncentenarian elderly is in sharp contrast to the more intact immune function of centenarians [33]. Profound and complex changes within the humoral, cellular, and innate immune responses occur during the ageing process, therefore immunosenescence is reflected in the sum of dysregulations of the immune system and its interactions with the other major systems in the human body.

Cytokines are proteins that have a key function, as intercellular messengers, during immune responses and in tissue remodelling. The cytokine network plays a pivotal role in the regulation of the specific type and magnitude of immune and inflammatory response. Consistent with the "remodelling theory" of immunosenescence, differing levels of cytokine production are reported in the elderly and centenarians [8, 9, 96–98]. A potent inflammatory response is vital in the defense against pathogens throughout life and may positively influence reproductive success, but chronic inflammation appears to be a common component in the development of major age-related diseases. This "trade-off" effect is largely predictable since advanced age does not seem to have been foreseen by evolution [14]. Many age-related diseases display altered cytokine profiles, suggesting that an inflammatory pathogenesis may be at the basis of these common causes of morbidity and mortality among elderly. It may be expected that people reaching the extreme limits of human lifespan, having escaped from major-age-related diseases, i.e. healthy centenarians, will be characterized by having genotypic combinations that produce "optimal" pro/antiinflammatory activity [32].

2   Cytokine Polymorphism in Immunosenescence

In several cytokine genes, polymorphism (mostly SNPs or microsatellites) located within the critical promoter or other regulatory regions, is reported to affect gene transcription resulting in inter-individual variation in levels of cytokine production (Table 1). Any qualitative or quantitative effect on cytokine production will ineluctably impinge upon the synthesis and secretion of effector molecules downstream in the cytokine cascade and may therefore alter the immune response. The polymorphic nature of the cytokine genes may confer flexibility on the immune response with certain alleles promoting differential production of cytokines. These then may

Table 1   Position and polymorphisms in selected cytokine genes

Cytokine	Nucleotide position	Polymorphism
IL-1α	-889	C/T
IL-1β	-551	C/T
	+3953	C/T
IL-2	-330	T/G
IL-6	-174	C/G
IL-8	-251	A/T
IL-10	-1082	G/A
IFN-γ	Intron 1	(CA)n
	+874	A/T
TNF-α	-308	G/A
TNF-β	+252	A/G
TGF-β	-800	G/A
	-509	C/T
	+869	T/C
	+915	G/C

Table 2 Positive studies on cytokine gene polymorphisms in young, elderly and centenarians

Study	Gene polymorphism	Cente-narians	Elderly (age)	Young (age)	Population	Results
Bonafe et al. (2001)	IL-6 –174 C/G	68 M	150M(60-99)		Italian	↓ GG
Rea et al. (2003)	IL-6 –174 C/G		58 M(80-97)	75 M (19-45)	Irish	↓ GG
Christiansen et al. (2004)	IL-6 –174 C/G	178	1058 (60-95)	474 (18-59)	Danish	↑ GG
Lio et al. (2002)	IL-10 –1082A/G	31 M		161 M (18-60)	Italian	↑ GG
Lio et al. (2003)	IL-10 –1082A/G	72 M		115 M (22-60)	Italian	↑ GG
Lio et al. (2004)	IL-10 –1082A/G	54 M		110 M (18-60)	Italian	↑ GG
	IFN-γ +847T/A	142 F		90 F (19-45)	Italian	↑ A

↑ and ↓ represent a statistically significant ($p < 0.05$) increase or decrease of alleles or genotypes respect to control population.
M=male; F=female.

influence the outcome of viral and bacterial infections and/or increase susceptibility/resistance to autoimmune disorders. In summary, cytokines are essential in all areas of the immune response, so any age-related variation may be of crucial importance in determining whether intact immune function remains preserved. Herein we examine the current literature available investigating the frequency of cytokine polymorphism in ageing (Table 2 and 3).

2.1 Tumor Necrosis Factor Gene Cluster

The human leukocyte antigen (HLA) has been described as a gene system that regulates both the immune system and the ageing process. The HLA plays a central role in antigen presentation and immunosurveillence, and a number of studies have been carried out to investigate whether there is evidence of polymorphic association with immunosensecence [15, 16]. Studies have shown that the HLA-A1, B8, DR3 ancestral haplotype (8.1 AH) is associated with a variety of immune dysfunctions, autoimmune diseases and displays gender specific longevity association [15, 86]. Also of interest, the 8.1 AH is associated with variant immune responses and altered cytokine secretion patterns [15]. This HLA haplotype is also associated with a genetically-determined, high production setting for tumor necrosis factor-α (TNF-α) [60].

The *TNF* gene locus is found within the central HLA Class III region and determines the strength, effectiveness and duration of local and systemic inflammatory responses, as well as repair and recovery from infectious and toxic agents. *TNF* genes show strong linkage disequilibrium with HLA Class I and II genes, and with other genes in the HLA region that are factors in immunoregulation [58]. The multiple pro and antiinflammatory activities of TNF-α and related cytokines in the *TNF*

Table 3 Selected negative studies on cytokine gene polymorphisms in young, elderly and centenarians

Study	Gene polymorphism	Population	Centenarians	Elderly (age range)	Young (age range)
Wang et al. 2001	IL-1α -889 C/T	Finnish		52 M (90)	400 (18-60)
	IL-1α -889 C/T	Finnish		198 F (90)	
Cavallone	IL-1α -889C/T	Italian	40 M	160M(65-99)	478 M (19-65)
et al. 2003	IL-1α -889C/T	Italian	94 F	149F(65-99)	210 F (19-65)
	IL-1β -511C/T	Italian	40 M	160M(65-99)	478 M (19-65)
	IL-1β -511C/T	Italian	94 F	149F(65-99)	210 F (19-65)
Wang et al.	IL-1β -511 C/T	Finnish		52 M (90)	400 (18-60)
2001	IL-1β -511 C/T	Finnish		198 F (90)	400 (18-60)
	IL-1β +3953	Finnish		52 M (90)	400 (18-60)
	IL-1β +3953	Finnish		198 F (90)	
	IL-1raVNTR86bp	Finnish		52 M (90)	
	IL-1raVNTR86bp	Finnish		198 F (90)	
Cavallone	IL-1raVNTR86bp	Italian	40 M	160M(65-99)	478 M (19-65)
et al. 2003	IL-1raVNTR86bp	Italian	94 F	149F(65-99)	210 F (19-65)
Ross et al.	IL-2 – 330 T/G	Irish		28M (80-97)	41 M (19-45)
2003	IL-2 - 330 T/G	Irish		65 F(80-97)	59 F (19-45)
Scola et al.	IL-2 - 330 T/G	Italian	168		214
2005					
Wang et al.	IL-6 –174 C/G	Finnish		52 M (90)	400 (18-60)
2001	IL-6 –174 C/G	Finnish		198 F (90)	
Bonafe et al.	IL-6 –174 C/G	Italian	255 F	227F(60-99)	
2004					
Ross et al.	IL-6 –174 C/G	Irish		55 M(80-97)	69 M (19-45)
2003	IL-6 –174 C/G	Irish		127F(80-97)	120 F (19-45)
	IL-6 –174 C/G	Irish		135F(80-97)	107 F (19-45)
Capurso et al.	IL-6 –174 C/G	Italian	19 M		44 M (19-73)
2004	IL-6 –174 C/G	Italian	62 F		78 F (18-73)
Pes et al.	IL-6 –174 C/G	Italian	36 M		68 M (60)
2004	IL-6 –174 C/G	Italian	76 F		68 F (60)
Ross et al.	IL-8 -251 A/T	Irish		28 M(80-97)	41M (19-45)
2003	IL-8-251 A/T	Irish		65 F(80-97)	59 F (19-45)
	IL-10 –1082A/G	Irish		28 M(80-97)	41 M (19-45)
	IL-10 –1082A/G	Irish		65 F(80-97)	59 F (19-45)
Wang et al.	IL-10 –1082A/G	Finnish		52 M (90)	400 (18-60)
2001	IL-10 –1082A/G	Finnish		198 F (90)	
Lio et al.	IL-10 –1082A/G	Italian	159 F		99 F (18-60)
2002					
Lio et al.	IL-10 –1082A/G	Italian	102 F		112 F (22-60)
2003					
Pes et al.	IL-10 –1082A/G	Italian	32 M		31 M (60)
2004	IL-10 –1082A/G	Italian	55 F		54 F (60)
Ross et al.	IL-12 exon8 A/C	Irish		28 M(80-97)	41 M (19-45)
2003	IL-12 exon8 A/C	Irish		65 F(80-97)	59 F (19-45)
	IFN-γ intron 1	Irish		28 M(80-97)	41 M (19-45)
	IFN-γ intron 1	Irish		65 F(80-97)	59 F (19-45)
Lio et al.	IFN-γ +847T/A	Italian	32 M		158 M (19-45)
2002					
Pes et al.	IFN-γ +847T/A	Italian	32 M		36 M (19-45)
2004	IFN-γ +847T/A	Italian	64 F		58 F (19-45)
Wang et al.	TNF-α -308G/A	Finnish		52 M (90)	400 (18-60)
2001	TNF-α -308G/A	Finnish		198 F (90)	
Lio et al.	TNF-α -308G/A	Italian	72 M		115 M (18-60)
2003	TNF-α -308G/A	Italian	102 F		112 F (18-60)

Table 3 (continued)

Study	Gene polymorphism	Population	Centenarians	Elderly (age range)	Young (age range)
Ross et al. 2003	TNF-α -308G/A	Irish		28 M(80-97)	41 M (19-45)
	TNF-α -308G/A	Irish		65 F(80-97)	59 F (19-45)
	TNF-β +252A/G	Irish		28 M(80-97)	41 M (19-45)
	TNF-β +252A/G	Irish		65 F(80-97)	59 F (19-45)
Carrieri et al. 2004	TGF-β1 –800G/A	Italian	50 M		94 M (20-60)
	TGF-β1 -800G/A	Italian	122 F		153 F (20-60)
	TGF-β1 -509C/T	Italian	50 M		94 M (20-60)
	TGF-β1 -509C/T	Italian	122 F		153 F (20-60)
	TGF-β1 +869C/G	Italian	50 M		94 M (20-60)
	TGF-β1 +869C/G	Italian	122 F		153 F (20-60)
	TGF-β1 +915C/G	Italian	50 M		94 M (20-60)
	TGF-β1 +915C/G	Italian	122 F		153 F (20-60)

cluster make them attractive candidates along with other HLA genes for unravelling the molecular mechanism(s) underlying the development of ageing and related diseases.

The TNF cluster, containing both TNF-α and TNF-β genes, has numerous polymorphisms that may have an effect on transcription and ultimately protein levels. The TNF-α-308A/G polymorphism has been investigated in four studies that were aimed to assess its association, if any, with longevity. In studies of elderly and young subjects from Finland and Sweden there were no differences regarding the frequency of the TNF-α-308A/G polymorphism between the two age groups [19, 119]. In an Italian study, the frequency of this polymorphism did not vary between centenarians and younger subjects, and no significant gender difference emerged [63]. Likewise, the frequency of TNF-α -308A/G polymorphism in a study with Irish nonagenarians was not different compared to younger controls [105]. In the same study, no significant frequency difference for the TNF-β +252 A/G polymorphism between Irish nonagenarians and young control subjects was found either. Thus, these 4 studies appear to demonstrate that the TNF-α -308A/G polymorphism does not have a major independent effect on longevity.

2.2 Transforming Growth Factor-β

The cytokine transforming growth factor-β (TGF-β) has been shown to have an essential role in inflammation and in maintenance of immune response homeostasis. TGF-β belongs to the group of cytokines with antiinflammatory effects, due to its deactivating properties regarding macrophages [57, 120]. TGF-gene overexpression has been observed in human fibroblasts that displayed a senescent-like phenotype after exposure to oxidative stress [37]. Polymorphisms in the TGF-β gene influencing the cytokine production have been identified and subsequently linked to age-related pathologies, such as Alzheimer's disease [66].

A study by Carrieri et al. (2004) analyzed 419 subjects from Northern and Central Italy, including 172 centenarians and 247 younger controls, to examine the hypothesis that variability of the *TGF*-β gene affects successful aging and longevity [12]. The level of the active cytokine increased with age, and significant differences were found between the age groups for the genotype and allele frequencies at the +915 site but no differences were found for the other tested variants (the -800 G/A, -509 C/T and +869 C/G loci). As this +915 C/G polymorphism results in an arginine to proline substitution at codon 25 within the signal peptide that is cleaved from the TGF-β precursor, it is possible that the substitution could play a role in the efficient production of the mature growth factor or misdirection of the protein. Since TGF-β is immunosuppressive, the age-related increase of the active cytokine suggests that it could counteract/counterbalance the harmful effects of inflamm-ageing.

2.3   Interleukin-1 Gene Cluster

The interleukin-1 (*IL-1*) gene cluster is located on chromosome 2q13 and is an important mediator of systemic inflammatory responses. Genetic variation of three genes (*IL-1α*, *IL-1β*, and *IL-1Ra*) in the cluster has been investigated in ageing. Three studies to date have examined the frequency of *IL-1* variants in Finnish, Italian and Swedish populations [18, 19, 119]. These studies failed to show any association with either centenarians or elderly individuals in comparison to young controls. Promoter SNPs in this gene cluster are reported to alter gene expression and may therefore give rise to a different expression profile. Also, *IL-1* gene cluster polymorphisms are implicated in a number of age-related pathologies including neurodegenerative disorders such as Alzheimer's and Parkinson's disease [81, 95].

2.4   Interleukin-2

Interleukin-2 (IL-2) cytokine plays a pivotal role in cellular immunity by regulating the activation, differentiation and proliferation of T-lymphocytes during an immune response. In the elderly, decreased levels of proinflammatory IL-2 production and secretion have been reported, leading to a situation of limited T-lymphocyte proliferation and thus inhibited cellular response [13]. A promoter variant of the *IL-2* gene at position -330 T/G has been shown to negatively affect expression levels, demonstrating that the more common T-allele has a higher level of expression. Two studies have examined the frequency of the *IL-2* promoter polymorphism -330G in ageing populations. The first study by Ross et al. did not identify any frequency difference with this SNP and successful ageing in the Irish population [104]. The second study with Italian centenarians supported the lack of association. However, a trend was observed suggesting that the -330G allele is increased in frequency in the second study's centenarian cohort and thus decreased levels of the proinflammatory IL-2 cytokine promotes successful ageing [109]. Interestingly, although decreased IL-2 production was reported during the ageing process, increased levels of interleukin-6 (IL-6) were found [78].

2.5 Interleukin-6

The interleukin-6 (IL-6) protein is arguably the best cytokine candidate to act as a potential marker for the overall health status of an individual [27, 67]. This is partly due to the fact that IL-6 plays a major role in inflammation and in the humoral immune response. It has been reported that healthy elderly individuals and centenarians exhibit a proinflammatory status, with a distinctive increase in IL-6 production [32]. There is increasing evidence for directly proportional association of the *IL-6* -174 C/G promoter polymorphism (Fig. 1) with production levels of the cytokine and with age [7, 30, 85].

Bonafe and colleagues (2001) published that the homozygous -174GG genotype was a disadvantage for longevity in men, reporting associated higher IL-6 serum levels. The findings of Ross et al. that an overall decrease in the -174GG in a cohort of Irish octo/nonagenarians from the Belfast Elderly Longitudinal Free-living Ageing Study (BELFAST) study group and with particular respect to the total males in comparison to the controls during the study would appear to concur with the findings by Bonafe et al. However, Olivieri and colleagues (2002) reported that their subjects containing the -174C allele showed a significant age-related increase in the capability to produce IL-6, even though this genotype is supposed to predispose these individuals to be low producers [85]. Another study by Wang et al. in Finland detected no significant change in *IL-6* frequencies

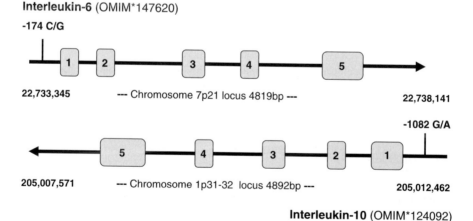

Interleukin-6 (OMIM*147620)

-174 C/G

1 2 3 4 5

22,733,345   --- Chromosome 7p21 locus 4819bp ---   22,738,141

-1082 G/A

5 4 3 2 1

205,007,571   --- Chromosome 1p31-32 locus 4892bp ---   205,012,462

Interleukin-10 (OMIM*124092)

Fig. 1 Genomic structures of IL-6 and IL-10

between nonagenarians and blood donors, though a reduction of 2% was noted in –174GG frequency in comparison with their age-selected younger control group [119]. This trend for a reduction in –174GG homozygosity in elderly males in 3 countries across Europe seems intriguing since it appears to confirm in different study populations and with alternate study designs like the earlier findings obtained in the Italian population.

In later studies, there was no difference in the *IL-6* -174 C/G promoter allelic and genotypic frequencies between centenarians and controls, but the number of subjects enrolled in these studies was low [10]. A modest but significant increase in the frequency of *IL-6* –174 GG homozygotes with age was noted in a group of Danish subjects, though no analysis was carried out for gender [20]. This discrepancy may be due to racial/genetic as well as lifestyle and ethnic/cultural differences between these populations.

A total of 9 studies have now looked at *IL-6* polymorphism with respect to ageing [11, 19]. IL-6 looks like the most interesting cytokine with respect to longevity studies, separate Caucasian European elderly populations and with different selection criteria, appear to demonstrate a decrease in the *IL-6*-174GG homozygote frequency with extreme old age. Italian researchers additionally demonstrated a reduction in *IL-6* high producer allele frequency for male centenarians which was not seen in females. In conclusion, large scale studies on many diverse racial and ethnic populations are needed to clarify this important topic.

2.6 Interleukin-8

Interleukin-8 (IL-8) is defined as a "chemokine" due to the observed chemotactic activity for specific types of leukocytes. It is produced by most cell types and is important for the activation of the inflammatory response and acts as a costimulatory factor for T-lymphocyte responses. IL-8 is also a potent neutrophil chemokine that facilitates the movement of neutrophils to inflammatory sites where they limit and contain the infection. As serious infections are more common in the elderly, it has been postulated that aspects of neutrophil function might be comprised with increasing age [23]. Recently, varied levels of IL-8 production by T- and natural killer (NK)-lymphocytes were reported in an elderly Italian population [69]. Only one study to date has examined the frequency of the functional *IL-8* -251 A/T promoter variant in ageing, though the researchers did not identify any association with either allele [104].

2.7 Interleukin-10

Antiinflammatory interleukin-10 (IL-10), which affects both the T- and B-lymphocyte responses, has been reported at an increased level in the elderly [88]. IL-10 is a potent proliferation and differentiation factor for B-lymphocytes and prevents production of proinflammatory cytokines such as IL-6 and IL-8. Along with significantly increased IL-6 and IL-10 levels, Rink and colleagues (1998) reported significantly increased production of IL-8 by leukocytes from the elderly. In the same paper, significantly decreased levels of IL-2 and interferon-γ (IFN-γ) were also reported [100]. A number of studies have investigated the association of ageing with the *IL-10* -1082 A/G promoter SNP (Fig. 1), and although the studies have not found any evidence for this, three reported an increase of *IL-10* -1082GG homozygous carriers in elderly males of Italian descent [59, 62, 63]. This may highlight a population-specific effect, although it is noteworthy that this association was not confirmed in other European Caucasian populations [91, 104, 119].

2.8   Interleukin-12

NK-lymphocytes play a central role in the innate immune response against bacterial or viral infections and tumors, and the NK-lymphocyte activities are highly regulated by numerous cytokines, particularly interleukin-12 (IL-12). IL-12 is secreted during the earliest stages of infection and inflammatory response, acting as the key immunoregulatory molecule in cellular immune responses. The critical action of IL-12 at the interface between innate and adaptive immune responses means that any age-associated alterations in expression levels are likely to have crucial functional consequences in vivo [96]. Increased levels of total IL-12, due to higher levels of the p40 subunit, are reported in the aged Irish population [96]. In the paper looking at *IL-12* polymorphisms and ageing by Ross et al., similar frequencies of the *IL-12* +16,974 A/C polymorphism in aged versus control subjects were observed. Although there was a trend for AA homozygotes to be underrepresented in elderly males with a 7% decrease in the A allele in elderly males, neither of these decreases achieved significance. Likewise, no apparent difference was present for old and young female subjects.

2.9   Interleukin-18 and Interleukin-19

Interleukin-18 (IL-18) is a proinflammatory cytokine that plays a vital role in both innate and acquired immune response [48]. IL-18 has been shown to induce IFN- γ and is implicated in a number of inflammatory diseases and neurodegenerative disorders [29, 83]. IL-18 serum concentrations are reported to be higher in centenarians compared to the younger population [38]. Frayling and colleagues (2007) reported an association of an *IL-18* SNP (rs5744292) on serum concentrations of the cytokine product and correlated these with physical functionality in the elderly [36]. These findings suggest a possible genetic association of *IL-18* with successful ageing and warrants further investigation.

Interleukin (IL)-19 belongs to the IL-10 family of cytokines, functioning to stimulate the expression of IL-10 (and the gene locus is adjacent to the *IL-10* gene). To date only one study has examined polymorphism of *IL-19* and its association, if any, to ageing. Okayam and colleagues (2007) investigated the frequency of four SNPs in the *IL-19* gene in the Japanese population. The results showed a significant association with age using logistic regression analysis. This preliminary finding requires independent replication to prove its validity.

2.10   Interferon-γ

Interferon-γ synthesis by T- and NK-lymphocytes and play a decisive role in defense against parasitic/viral infections and intracellular pathogens [82]. Proinflammatory IFN-γ was initially recognized for its antiviral activity but has since established itself as a multifunctional cytokine playing an important role in modulating almost all phases of the immune response, particularly the inflammatory response [4].

In centenarians, Lio and colleagues first reported that possession of the IFN-γ +874A allele (+847 SNP T/A is in linkage with a CA repeat microsatellite allele) was associated with longevity in Italian centenarian females likely by controlling inflammatory status [61]. Subsequently, Ross et al. could not be replicate this observation in nearly 200 Irish nonagenarians reporting similar frequencies for the CA 12 allele repeat in control and aged subjects [104]. The small decrease in the CA 12 repeat in aged, Irish, female nonagenarians was not significant but does demonstrate a similar trend to the findings in the Italian centenarian female cohort suggesting a gender-specific effect in *IFN-γ* genotypes. In Ross et al. the CA 13 repeat allele of *IFN-γ* microsatellite was similarly represented between Irish aged and young groups with no gender difference. The study also commented on a notable trend showing a decrease in the frequency of the heterozygote 12, 13 genotype within the aged subjects in comparison to the young controls (which was observed to be independent of gender).

In the aforementioned Italian study, trend of a decrease in the *IFN-γ* + 874T allele was observed among female Sardinian centenarians, however these results relate to only a relatively small number of Sardinian female centenarians, which may limit the statistical power of the study [91]. Thus, the *IFN-γ* high producer haplotype 12 CA/+874T showed a decrease in centenarian Italian females with a trend for the same change in Irish nonagenarians and Sardinian centenarians. These findings certainly warrant further replication studies and gender differences also need to be taken into account.

2.11   Gender Bias

It is postulated that cytokine allele frequencies are possibly gender- and geographically-specific, similarly to what has been proposed for other polymorphic systems such as the human leukocyte antigen [16]. Franceschi and colleagues (2000) have postulated that gender is a variable concerning the genetics of ageing, proposing that men and women follow different pathways to extreme longevity [35]. This postulate has been demonstrated in Italian centenarian studies for the *IL-6* -174 G/C, *IL-10* -1082 G/A and *IFN-γ* +874 T/A polymorphisms, where significant frequency differences have been identified when the data was analyzed on the basis of gender [7, 62, 85].

The *IL-6* -174GG genotype frequency is reported to be decreased in elderly males in two independent studies in Italian and Irish populations [7, 104]. The *IL-10* -1082 G/A and *IFN-γ* +874 T/A polymorphism have also been reported to be gender-specific markers for longevity [61, 62]. Lio and colleagues (2002) reported an increased frequency of the homozygote *IL-10* −1082GG genotype in Italian centenarian men, and this genotype is associated with high IL-10 cytokine production, conferring an anti-inflammatory status which is postulated to increase the possibility of extreme longevity [62]. The *IFN-γ* +874T allele is reported to be in absolute correlation with the 12 CA repeat allele, where the latter is associated with increased IFN-γ production [61, 93, 94]. The group reported that possession of the *IFN-γ* +874A allele, particularly in females, conferred an overall antiinflammatory status promoting longevity.

2.12   Cytokine Polymorphism Conclusions

Due to the intricate nature of the cytokine cascade and the perpetual interaction of cytokines within the immune function, a situation is created where the overexpression of one cytokine may be either compensated for or enhanced by another. This complexity, coupled with the difficulty of clearly defining cytokine activity as anti or proinflammatory, may well have confounded the groups whose studies are reviewed in this chapter [17]. The aforementioned studies also highlight the importance of validation of significant results in either a second subgroup or independent cohort of subjects. There is also need to identify such variables as race/ethnicity, gender and age when endeavouring to fully ascertain the role(s) of cytokine polymorphisms in immunosenescence.

Genetic variants in immune response genes are certainly attractive candidates to study in the attempt to elucidate the molecular mechanism(s) that occur during immunosenescence. However, the absence of age-association for many of the cytokine gene variants, even those associated with changing expression levels, would indicate the complexity of the cytokine cascade can not be truly reflected by a small number of polymorphic markers. Future studies concentrating on compiling a genetic cytokine profile that encompasses the overall network (and working in tandem with expression levels) will aid in the resolution of the role(s) of cytokines in the aged immune function/longevity.

3 Age-related Disorders

Identification of major genetic variants affecting population mortality and extreme longevity may spur the characterization of pathways high in the hierarchy of the physiological processes that influence the onset of common age-related diseases [46]. Conversely, the study of age-related disease may provide greater insight into the molecular mechanism(s) that contribute to the ageing process. For example, Parkinson's disease (PD) is one of the most prevalent age-related neurodegenerative disorders, with approximately 1% of the population older than 50 years being affected. The question that must be asked is whether age-related disorders such as PD are a direct cause or a result of the ageing process. Unlike the study of progeriod syndromes (which are characterized by accelerated ageing), age-related disorders require more focused attention to particular aspects of the disease that mimic, or contrast with, healthy ageing.

With increasing knowledge of the complexity of the biological pathways of the brain there is growing evidence to suggest that there is an active, endogenous immune system. Glia cells are one of the most numerous cell types in the brain, and a subgroup, microglia, form the tissue macrophage population. The microglia play an important role in the growth and survival of neurons and are also critical in the inflammatory response of the brain through the production and secretion of cytokines [21]. Inflammation of the brain is postulated to contribute to the pathogenesis of a number of neurodegenerative disorders including multiple sclerosis, Alzheimer's disease and PD. The pathological, neuroinflammatory damage that is observed in these diseases has led researchers to generate hypotheses regarding their progression and susceptible neuronal populations. This hallmark neuroinflammation also provides groups with a possible avenue for therapeutic intervention and implicates DNA variants that regulate the inflammatory response in disease pathogenesis. This next section of the chapter will focus on the role of cytokine polymorphisms in PD and how genetic findings in this complex disorder can help guide future studies regarding the mechanisms influencing ageing.

3.1 Parkinson's Disease Background

The renowned French neurologist Jean Martin Charcot (1825–1893) defined the clinical syndrome "maladie de Parkinson" that has since become known as Parkinson's disease. First described by the English physician James Parkinson (1755–1824) in his milestone 1817 publication "An Essay on the Shaking Palsy", parkinsonism is characterized by the triad of tremor, rigidity and bradykinesia. PD is the most common cause of parkinsonism and the second most frequent neurodegenerative disorder, after Alzheimer's disease. Neuropathological findings in PD are loss of pigmented neurons in the brain stem, *substantia nigra* and *locus coeruleus*, with intracellular Lewy body inclusions found within surviving neurons.

Historically PD was thought to have no genetic basis and epidemiological data appeared to support this view. Cross-sectional studies by Tanner et al. and Wirdefeldt et al. suggested that either there is no genetic basis or that it is only evident in early-onset PD (age of onset <50 years), although to date twin studies have been underpowered to refute incompletely penetrant genetic causes of PD [112]. Differing disease concordance rates between monozygotic and dizygotic twins in longitudinal studies (including those using 18F-dopa positron emission tomography; PET) do support heritability in PD [92]. In fact, many clinical reports note that familial aggregation of parkinsonism and a family history of disease is the second most significant risk factor after age [110].

The etiology and pathogenesis of PD remains unclear, however, it has been suggested that PD, like ageing, may be a multifactorial disorder caused by a combination of age, genetic and environmental factors. During the last decade, contention regarding the importance of genetics in PD was challenged by the identification of several large pedigrees in which parkinsonism appeared to have a monogenic, Mendelian pattern of inheritance (either autosomal dominant, autosomal recessive or X-linked) [28, 106]. However, research studies that have analyzed PD families with classical linkage methods have given rise to data which allowed the subsequent nomination of 13 regions of the human genome, where pathogenic mutations since been identified in five genes (*α-synuclein, parkin, DJ-1, PINK1 and LRRK2*), thus confirming the role of genetics in PD.

The identification of *LRRK2* pathogenic mutations as a cause of autosomal dominant parkinsonism which is clinically indistinguishable from sporadic PD has once again revolutionized this research field. The *LRRK2* c.6055G>A (Gly2019Ser) mutation has become renowned for its high frequency in specific racial groups (e.g., ~40% of PD patients of Berber Arab ethnicity) and appears to be present in most Caucasian populations. The *LRRK2* variant c.7153G>A (Gly2385Arg) may be the most frequent genetic risk factor the development of PD to date, but it appears to be restricted to those individuals of Chinese descent [107]. The reduced penetrance observed for *LRRK2* mutations accounts for the presence of these variants in healthy control subjects and is reflected in the diversity of the age at symptomatic onset of disease in patients. Likewise, even individuals within the same family carrying the same *LRRK2* mutation can present with symptoms decades apart with regards to age. These observations suggest that *LRRK2*-associated disease is regulated by important environmental and/or genetic modifiers [103].

3.2 PD and Cytokines

Evidence has also been accumulating over the last decade to indicate that chronic inflammation of the brain may be one of these possible disease modifiers and play a crucial role in the pathognomic dopaminergic neuronal death of PD [1, 71]. In support of this theory, proinflammatory cytokines, such as TNF-α, IL-2 and IL-6, are shown to be markedly up-regulated in the brain or the cerebrospinal fluid in PD patients [6, 24,

74, 75, 77]. Despite the potentially important role the inflammatory response, directed by cytokines, may play in the pathogenesis of PD, only a limited number of studies have been performed to assess if there is an underlying genetic influence (Table 4).

In 2000, Kruger and colleagues performed one of the first studies investigating the possible role of cytokine polymorphisms regarding susceptibility to and the pathogenesis of PD [55]. This study identified significant associations between two genes in the *TNF* pathway (*TNF-α* and *TNFR1*). These findings implicated the proinflammatory pathway in promoting the dopaminergic neuronal cell death that typifies PD. Between 2000 and 2003 further studies were performed in the Japanese and Finnish PD populations [70, 79–81]. Nishimura and colleagues investigated the frequency of variants in *TNF-α*, *IL-1ß*, chemokine monocyte chemoattractant protein

Table 4 Positive studies on cytokine gene polymorphisms in Parkinson's disease

Study	Population	Gene polymorphism	Patients	Controls	Results
Kruger et al. 2000	German	TNF-α -308 G/A	264 (114F 148M)	198	↑GA
Wahner et al. 2007	US	TNF-α -308 G/A	289 (133F 156M)	269 (130F 139M)	↑ 2°
Wu et al. 2007	Taiwanese	TNF-α -863 C/A	369 (173F 196M)	326 (143F 183M)	↑AA
Nishimura et al. 2001	Japanese	TNF-α -1031 C/T	172 (103F 69M)	157 (98F 59M)	↑ C
Wu et al. 2007	Taiwanese	TNF-α -1031 C/T	369 (173F 196M)	326 (143F 183M)	↑ CC
Kruger et al. 2000	German	TNFR1 -609 G/T	264 (114F 148M)	198	↓ B/2
Kruger et al. 2000	German	TNFR1 +36 A/G	264 (114F 148M)	198	↓ B/2
Nishimura et al. 2000	Japanese	IL-1β -511 C/T	122	112	↑1° 1° (AAO)
Schulte et al. 2002	German	IL-1β -511 C/T	295 (123F 172M)	270 (130F 140M)	↑ T
McGeer et al. 2002	Canadian	IL-1β -511 C/T	100	100	↑ T
Mattila et al. 2002	Finnish	IL-1β -511 C/T*	52 (27F 25M)	73 (34F 39M)	↓ 2° 2°
Wahner et al. 2007	US	IL-1β -511 C/T	289 (133F 156M)	269 (130F 139M)	↑ 2°
Hakansson et al. 2005	Swedish	IL-6 -174 G/C	265	308	↑ GG
Ross et al. 2003	Irish	IL-8 -251 A/T	90 (41F 49M)	93 (65F 28M)	↑ AT
Hakansson et al. 2005	Swedish	IL-10 -1082 G/A	265	308	↑ GG (AAO)
Nishimura et al. 2003	Japanese	MCP-1 -2518 A/G	329 (200F 129M)	340 (190F 150M)	↑ AA (AAO)

↑ and ↓ represent a statistically significant (p < 0.05) increase or decrease of alleles or genotypes respect to PD patients.

M =male; F =female. 1° =allele 1; 2°=allele 2. AAO= affects age-at-onset of symptoms.

This table highlights the inconsistency in results (*is inversely associted compared to other studies) and nomenclature that is used to describe each cytokine polymorphism.

(*MCP-1*), and chemokine receptor-2 (*CCR-2*) in the Japanese population. Mattila et al. investigated the *IL-1* gene cluster, including *IL-1α*, -ß and *IL-1RN* along with a SNP in the intercellular adhesion molecule 1 (*ICAM1*). The results of both studies supported the hypothesis that genetic variation of proinflammatory cytokine genes may influence PD with SNPs in the *TNF-α* and *IL-1β* genes associated (Fig. 2). However, a number of the SNPs examined showed no association with PD susceptibility.

A study in the German population also found no evidence of association with the *IL-1α* (-889 C/T) SNP with risk of PD [76]. Ross and colleagues (2004) investigated a cross-section of promoter variants in proinflammatory cytokine genes *IL-2* (-330 T/G), *IL-6* (-174 C/G), *IL-8* (-251 A/T) and *TNF-α* (-308 G/A) [108]. Although no association was observed for the variants of *IL-2*, *IL-6* and *TNF-α*, a significant decrease in the number of TT homozygous carriers for the *IL-8* gene was observed in the PD patients. Interestingly, IL-8 is also known as CXCL8 and belongs to the specific group of cytokines known as chemokines.

The cells of the brain, particularly neurons, are believed to possess a wide range of chemokine receptors [73]. Neurological injury and PD are often associated with the increase of nitric oxide and free radicals from glial cells in the brain [64, 113]. At sites of inflammation, brain cells are exposed to high concentrations of reactive oxygen species and reactive nitrogen intermediates (produced by activated neutrophils, macrophages and T-cells) as a normal part of the immune response. A potential variation in IL-8 expression in PD subjects may facilitate the influx of neutrophils, immune and activated glial cells to sites of damage and inflammation, resulting in increased oxidative damage and cell death. However when Huerta and colleagues (2004) examined the frequency of polymorphic variants in four chemokine genes, *RANTES*, *MCP-1*, *CCR2* and *CCR5*, no significant associations with PD were observed in the Spanish population studied [49]. These results support earlier results for *MCP-1* and *CCR2* observed by Nishimura et al. in the Japanese population.

In two Swedish studies by Hakansson and colleagues the frequency of several cytokine polymorphisms were studied [42]. No association with PD was observed for variants in the *IFN-γ*, *IFN-γR2*, platelet-activating factor acetylhydrolase and

Interleukin-1 Gene Cluster OMIM*147760 (α); *147720 (β)

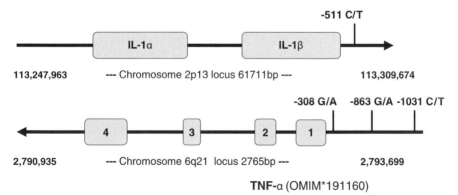

TNF-α (OMIM*191160)

Fig. 2 Genomic structures of IL-1cluster and TNF-α

ICAM1 genes. Likewise, a promoter SNP in the *IL-10* gene did not demonstrate any association with susceptibility to PD, however it did appear to affect the age-at-onset with a significantly higher frequency of the A-allele in early-onset PD patients. Interestingly, the *IL-6* (-174 G/C) promoter SNP did show association with PD with an increased number of -174 GG carriers in the PD patients. The authors further suggest this association is stronger when interactions with a SNP in the *estrogen receptor*-β gene were considered [41].

The latest two papers on this topic have looked at the primary genes that were implicated in PD pathogenesis, *TNF*-α and *IL-1*β [118, 122]. Wu et al. (2007) investigated 4 -promoter SNPs of the *TNF*-α gene (-308, -857, -863 and -1031) in their Taiwanese samples and identified a significant association for the -863 and -1031 SNPs, which were found to be in high linkage disequilibrium in the study. The strongest association was observed with an increased frequency of the -1031 CC genotype in PD patients, and these results concur with the earlier Japanese study by Nishimura et al. (2001) where an increase in this allele with early-onset PD was observed. Wahner et al. (2007) examined the *TNF*-α (-308 G/A) and the *IL-1*β (-511 C/T) SNPs in a US PD patient-control series and observed a significant association with both SNPs, suggesting each SNP individually increased the risk of PD by two-fold and when combined three-fold (Fig. 2).

3.3 Age-Related Disorders Conclusions

It is possible that cytokine polymorphism and genetic variants influence susceptibility to the development of parkinsonism symptoms. Given this hypothesis, it is then even more likely that these variants will influence pathogenesis of the disease affecting age-at-onset, progression and severity of symptoms. The complex nature of this devastating disease is indicative of a multifactorial disorder that is influenced by environmental agents (e.g., infection) acting on a genomic background of susceptibility. The hypothesis that neuroinflammation enhances the degenerative processes involved in PD implies that anti-inflammatory therapeutics may slow disease progression. The use of nonsteriodal antiinflammatory drugs (NSAIDs) has shown some promise in both PD and Alzheimer's disease [3, 54]. At present the only symptomatic relief comes from dopamine replacement (levodopa) and dopamine agonists, as research into the genetics of PD is still a relatively young field. In conclusion, further studies of cytokine polymorphism and genetic variants within genes of the proinflammatory network in PD are certainly warranted.

4 Perspectives

The first century of this new millennium will bear witness to a new era in both ageing research and clinical practice. We are moving into the postgenomic era and the beginning of individualized medicine and treatment. This holds great promise for the study of complex disorders such as ageing. The field of longevity genetics ("Longevics") will mature, and the identification of mutations that affect the immune system and prolong life will once again revolutionize our views of the ageing process [102]. A strong immune response is clearly important for survival, however this double-edged sword can also increase morbidity. The studies described in this chapter on cytokine gene polymorphisms and ageing certainly suggest that further work is warranted in order to achieve a greater understanding of the complex mechanism(s) underlying longevity.

The intricate nature of the cytokine cascade suggests that any imbalance may be detrimental to the individual. This possible imbalance may be due to an aberrant genomic background of the cytokine network and may be exaggerated by external forces such as infection, stress, smoking and/or diet. Many researchers support the pleiotrophic effect hypothesis as to why immunosenescence occurs by the immune system/response. To elaborate on this concept, it is thought that a proinflammatory genome-genotype ("genomotype") is beneficial in early-childhood and development when the individual is prone to infection. However as we survive past our optimal age and generalized degeneration begins, the proinflammatory genomotype becomes detrimental thus causing damage and promoting autoimmune disorders. Therefore what this phenomenon suggests is that each individual's inflammatory genomotype may behave either as a positive or negative influence on lifespan and this outcome is ultimately determined by the individual's specific environment.

By necessity, both the immune response and the ageing process are determined by genetic, environmental and stochastic factors. Each component is thought to produce a different size effect on a single biological pathway and therefore comparisons are extremely difficult to make. Therefore, the identification of genetic and environmental factors involved in regulating the cytokine response will help highlight other biological pathways that are important in maintaining a healthy immune system. A further confounding effect is gender, as a consistent increased number of females are becoming centenarians than males. The reason(s) for this difference remain unresolved, although studies suggest that gender may effect a differential immune responsiveness which then leads to an inflammatory phenotype. This observation of a gender-bias is supported by similar findings in age-related diseases such as PD, which is more prevalent in males.

Given the complexity previously described, how can one objectively measure the contribution of cytokine genetics to immunosenescence? This question is of course applicable to every pathway postulated to have an effect on the ageing process. Likewise, the underlying answer may also be the same being that one must measure the genetic influence(s) of the overall pathways. To date, as reviewed in this chapter, most studies have examined a small number of variants in one or two cytokine genes and observed inconsistent associations. This has in part been due to small sample sizes and financial restraints. However, the advances that are being made in molecular genetic techniques (including large-scale, rapid genotyping and direct DNA sequencing) will allow objective measurements of cytokine genetics with respect to immunosenescence to be ascertained. This means there is an unprecedented opportunity now available to help unravel the mechanism(s) of the immune system regarding ageing and age-related disorders.

Genome-wide association studies provide an objective measure of genetic variations and are an extension of the classical patient-control studies. These studies are now common-place in leading scientific journals (Nature, Science and the New England Journal of Medicine). Recent genome-wide association studies have identified polymorphisms of cytokine genes as being involved in numerous age-related disorders, like multiple sclerosis [5, 25, 26, 39, 40, 43, 65, 84, 116]. It remains to be seen if these types of association studies will lead to the identification of those genetic factors which influence ageing. These studies will likely require a large collaborative effort to obtain the necessary numbers of aged individuals that will provide the statistical power needed to observe moderate "effect sizes". The Genetics of Healthy Ageing (GEHA) is a current European study of nonagenarian sibling pairs which should have the statistical power to elucidate whether the earlier suggestive changes in cytokine polymorphisms in relation to age and perhaps gender have any coherence, across heterogeneous populations of nonagenarian siblings [31].

Ageing research is becoming of greater interest and importance. The average human lifespan continues to be increased, which has resulted in an expanding proportion of elderly people in society. The developments in molecular, gerontological research have created the potential for survival beyond that of centenarians. The development of stem cell research alone could allow for the generation of completely new cells and organs. In the case of PD, mouse embryonic stem (ES) cells have been used for cell replacement therapy in an animal model of PD [50, 87]. From cultured ES cells, Kim and colleagues (2002) were able to generate a supply of neurons that produce dopamine. The neurons functioned normally and gave clear behavioural responses when grafted into the brains of rats that model PD. The potential benefits of revolutionary experiments like this regarding the treatment and possible prevention of age-related pathologies and perhaps even the rate of ageing itself mean that the deteriorative processes of ageing may no longer be the scourge of mankind.

Acknowledgments OAR is funded by an APDA research grant and a Rapid Response Award from the Michael J. Fox Foundation. We are grateful to our Research Nurse Anne Murphy and to Department of Health and Social Services Northern Ireland and the Wellcome Trust for funding towards the Belfast Elderly Longitudinal Free-living Ageing Study (BELFAST). This chapter is dedicated to the memory of Donna J. Hinkle (1948–2007).

References

1. Allan SM, Rothwell NJ (2001) Cytokines and acute neurodegeneration. Nat Rev Neurosci 2:734–744
2. Altshuler D, Brooks LD, Chakravarti A, Collins FS, Daly MJ, Donnelly P (2005) A haplotype map of the human genome. Nature 437:1299–1320
3. Asanuma M, Miyazaki I (2007) Common anti-inflammatory drugs are potentially therapeutic for Parkinson's disease? Exp Neurol 206:172–178
4. Awad M, Pravica V, Perrey C, El Gamel A, Yonan N, Sinnott PJ, Hutchinson IV (1999) CA repeat allele polymorphism in the first intron of the human interferon-gamma gene is associated with lung allograft fibrosis. Hum Immunol 60:343–346

5. Baldassano RN, Bradfield JP, Monos DS, Kim CE, Glessner JT, Casalunovo T, Frackelton EC, Otieno FG, Kanterakis S, Shaner JL, Smith RM, Eckert AW, Robinson LJ, Onyiah CC, Abrams DJ, Chiavacci RM, Skraban R, Devoto M, Grant SF, Hakonarson H (2007) Association of Variants of the Interleukin-23 Receptor Gene With Susceptibility to Pediatric Crohn's Disease. Clin Gastroenterol Hepatol 5:972–976

6. Blum-Degen D, Muller T, Kuhn W, Gerlach M, Przuntek H, Riederer P (1995) Interleukin-1 beta and interleukin-6 are elevated in the cerebrospinal fluid of Alzheimer's and de novo Parkinson's disease patients. Neurosci Lett 202:17–20

7. Bonafe M, Olivieri F, Cavallone L, Giovagnetti S, Mayegiani F, Cardelli M, Pieri C, Marra M, Antonicelli R, Lisa R, Rizzo MR, Paolisso G, Monti D, Franceschi C (2001) A gender-dependent genetic predisposition to produce high levels of IL-6 is detrimental for longevity. Eur J Immunol 31:2357–2361

8. Bruunsgaard H, Pedersen BK (2003) Age-related inflammatory cytokines and disease. Immunol Allergy Clin North Am 23:15–39

9. Bruunsgaard H, Pedersen M, Pedersen BK (2001) Aging and proinflammatory cytokines. Curr Opin Hematol 8:131–136

10. Capurso C, Solfrizzi V, D'Introno A, Colacicco AM, Capurso SA, Semeraro C, Capurso A, Panza F (2004) Interleukin 6-174 G/C promoter gene polymorphism in centenarians: no evidence of association with human longevity or interaction with apolipoprotein E alleles. Exp Gerontol 39:1109–1114

11. Capurso C, Solfrizzi V, D'Introno A, Colacicco AM, Capurso SA, Semeraro C, Capurso A, Panza F (2007) Interleukin 6 Variable Number of Tandem Repeats (VNTR) Gene Polymorphism in Centenarians. Ann Hum Genet

12. Carrieri G, Marzi E, Olivieri F, Marchegiani F, Cavallone L, Cardelli M, Giovagnetti S, Stecconi R, Molendini C, Trapassi C, De Benedictis G, Kletsas D, Franceschi C (2004) The G/C915 polymorphism of transforming growth factor beta1 is associated with human longevity: a study in Italian centenarians. Aging Cell 3:443–448

13. Caruso C, Candore G, Cigna D, DiLorenzo G, Sireci G, Dieli F, Salerno A (1996) Cytokine production pathway in the elderly. Immunol Res 15:84–90

14. Caruso C, Candore G, Colonna-Romano G, Lio D, Franceschi C (2005) Inflammation and life-span. Science 307:208–209; author reply 208–209

15. Caruso C, Candore G, Colonna Romano G, Lio D, Bonafe M, Valensin S, Franceschi C (2000) HLA, aging, and longevity: a critical reappraisal. Hum Immunol 61:942–949

16. Caruso C, Candore G, Romano GC, Lio D, Bonafe M, Valensin S, Franceschi C (2001) Immunogenetics of longevity. Is major histocompatibility complex polymorphism relevant to the control of human longevity? A review of literature data. Mech Ageing Dev 122:445–462

17. Cavaillon JM (2001) Pro- versus anti-inflammatory cytokines: myth or reality. Cell Mol Biol (Noisy-le-grand) 47:695–702

18. Cavallone L, Bonafe M, Olivieri F, Cardelli M, Marchegiani F, Giovagnetti S, Di Stasio G, Giampieri C, Mugianesi E, Stecconi R, Sciacca F, Grimaldi LM, De Benedictis G, Lio D, Caruso C, Franceschi C (2003) The role of IL-1 gene cluster in longevity: a study in Italian population. Mech Ageing Dev 124:533–538

19. Cederholm T, Persson M, Andersson P, Stenvinkel P, Nordfors L, Madden J, Vedin I, Wretlind B, Grimble RF, Palmblad J (2007) Polymorphisms in cytokine genes influence long-term survival differently in elderly male and female patients. J Intern Med 262:215–223

20. Christiansen L, Bathum L, Andersen-Ranberg K, Jeune B, Christensen K (2004) Modest implication of interleukin-6 promoter polymorphisms in longevity. Mech Ageing Dev 125:391–395

21. Czlonkowska A, Kurkowska-Jastrzebska I, Czlonkowski A, Peter D, Stefano GB (2002) Immune processes in the pathogenesis of Parkinson's disease - a potential role for microglia and nitric oxide. Med Sci Monit 8:RA165–RA177

22. de Bakker PI, Yelensky R, Pe'er I, Gabriel SB, Daly MJ, Altshuler D (2005) Efficiency and power in genetic association studies. Nat Genet 37:1217–1223

23. Di Lorenzo G, Balistreri CR, Candore G, Cigna D, Colombo A, Romano GC, Colucci AT, Gervasi F, Listi F, Potestio M, Caruso C (1999) Granulocyte and natural killer activity in the elderly. Mech Ageing Dev 108:25–38

24. Dobbs RJ, Charlett A, Purkiss AG, Dobbs SM, Weller C, Peterson DW (1999) Association of circulating TNF-alpha and IL-6 with ageing and parkinsonism. Acta Neurol Scand 100:34–41

25. Duerr RH (2007) Genome-wide association studies herald a new era of rapid discoveries in inflammatory bowel disease research. Gastroenterology 132:2045–2049

26. Duerr RH, Taylor KD, Brant SR, Rioux JD, Silverberg MS, Daly MJ, Steinhart AH, Abraham C, Regueiro M, Griffiths A, Dassopoulos T, Bitton A, Yang H, Targan S, Datta LW, Kistner EO, Schumm LP, Lee AT, Gregersen PK, Barmada MM, Rotter JI, Nicolae DL, Cho JH (2006) A genome-wide association study identifies IL23R as an inflammatory bowel disease gene. Science 314:1461–1463

27. Ershler WB (1993) Interleukin-6: a cytokine for gerontologists. J Am Geriatr Soc 41:176–181

28. Farrer MJ (2006) Genetics of Parkinson disease: paradigm shifts and future prospects. Nat Rev Genet 7:306–318

29. Felderhoff-Mueser U, Sifringer M, Polley O, Dzietko M, Leineweber B, Mahler L, Baier M, Bittigau P, Obladen M, Ikonomidou C, Buhrer C (2005) Caspase-1-processed interleukins in hyperoxia-induced cell death in the developing brain. Ann Neurol 57:50–59

30. Fishman D, Faulds G, Jeffery R, Mohamed-Ali V, Yudkin JS, Humphries S, Woo P (1998) The effect of novel polymorphisms in the interleukin-6 (IL-6) gene on IL-6 transcription and plasma IL-6 levels, and an association with systemic-onset juvenile chronic arthritis. J Clin Invest 102:1369–1376

31. Franceschi C, Bezrukov V, Blanche H, Bolund L, Christensen K, de Benedictis G, Deiana L, Gonos E, Hervonen A, Yang H, Jeune B, Kirkwood TB, Kristensen P, Leon A, Pelicci PG, Peltonen L, Poulain M, Rea IM, Remacle J, Robine JM, Schreiber S, Sikora E, Slagboom PE, Spazzafumo L, Stazi MA, Toussaint O, Vaupel JW (2007) Genetics of healthy aging in Europe: the EU-integrated project GEHA (GEnetics of Healthy Aging). Ann N Y Acad Sci 1100:21–45

32. Franceschi C, Bonafe M, Valensin S, Olivieri F, De Luca M, Ottaviani E, De Benedictis G (2000) Inflamm-aging. An evolutionary perspective on immunosenescence. Ann N Y Acad Sci 908:244–254

33. Franceschi C, Monti D, Sansoni P, Cossarizza A (1995) The immunology of exceptional individuals: the lesson of centenarians. Immunol Today 16:12–16

34. Franceschi C, Motta L, Motta M, Malaguarnera M, Capri M, Vasto S, Candore G, Caruso C (2007) The extreme longevity: The state of the art in Italy. Exp Gerontol

35. Franceschi C, Motta L, Valensin S, Rapisarda R, Franzone A, Berardelli M, Motta M, Monti D, Bonafe M, Ferrucci L, Deiana L, Pes GM, Carru C, Desole MS, Barbi C, Sartoni G, Gemelli C, Lescai F, Olivieri F, Marchegiani F, Cardelli M, Cavallone L, Gueresi P, Cossarizza A, Troiano L, Pini G, Sansoni P, Passeri G, Lisa R, Spazzafumo L, Amadio L, Giunta S, Stecconi R, Morresi R, Viticchi C, Mattace R, De Benedictis G, Baggio G (2000) Do men and women follow different trajectories to reach extreme longevity? Italian Multicenter Study on Centenarians (IMUSCE). Aging (Milano) 12:77–84

36. Frayling TM, Rafiq S, Murray A, Hurst AJ, Weedon MN, Henley W, Bandinelli S, Corsi AM, Ferrucci L, Guralnik JM, Wallace RB, Melzer D (2007) An interleukin-18 polymorphism is associated with reduced serum concentrations and better physical functioning in older people. J Gerontol A Biol Sci Med Sci 62:73–78

37. Frippiat C, Dewelle J, Remacle J, Toussaint O (2002) Signal transduction in H2O2-induced senescence-like phenotype in human diploid fibroblasts. Free Radic Biol Med 33:1334–1346

38. Gangemi S, Basile G, Merendino RA, Minciullo PL, Novick D, Rubinstein M, Dinarello CA, Lo Balbo C, Franceschi C, Basili S, E DU, Davi G, Nicita-Mauro V, Romano M (2003) Increased circulating Interleukin-18 levels in centenarians with no signs of vascular disease: another paradox of longevity? Exp Gerontol 38:669–672

39. Graham RR, Kyogoku C, Sigurdsson S, Vlasova IA, Davies LR, Baechler EC, Plenge RM, Koeuth T, Ortmann WA, Hom G, Bauer JW, Gillett C, Burtt N, Cunninghame Graham DS, Onofrio R, Petri M, Gunnarsson I, Svenungsson E, Ronnblom L, Nordmark G, Gregersen

PK, Moser K, Gaffney PM, Criswell LA, Vyse TJ, Syvanen AC, Bohjanen PR, Daly MJ, Behrens TW, Altshuler D (2007) Three functional variants of IFN regulatory factor 5 (IRF5) define risk and protective haplotypes for human lupus. Proc Natl Acad Sci U S A 104:6758–6763

40. Hafler DA, Compston A, Sawcer S, Lander ES, Daly MJ, De Jager PL, de Bakker PI, Gabriel SB, Mirel DB, Ivinson AJ, Pericak-Vance MA, Gregory SG, Rioux JD, McCauley JL, Haines JL, Barcellos LF, Cree B, Oksenberg JR, Hauser SL (2007) Risk alleles for multiple sclerosis identified by a genomewide study. N Engl J Med 357:851–862

41. Hakansson A, Westberg L, Nilsson S, Buervenich S, Carmine A, Holmberg B, Sydow O, Olson L, Johnels B, Eriksson E, Nissbrandt H (2005) Interaction of polymorphisms in the genes encoding interleukin-6 and estrogen receptor beta on the susceptibility to Parkinson's disease. Am J Med Genet B Neuropsychiatr Genet 133:88–92

42. Hakansson A, Westberg L, Nilsson S, Buervenich S, Carmine A, Holmberg B, Sydow O, Olson L, Johnels B, Eriksson E, Nissbrandt H (2005) Investigation of genes coding for inflammatory components in Parkinson's disease. Mov Disord 20:569–573

43. Hampe J, Franke A, Rosenstiel P, Till A, Teuber M, Huse K, Albrecht M, Mayr G, De La Vega FM, Briggs J, Gunther S, Prescott NJ, Onnie CM, Hasler R, Sipos B, Folsch UR, Lengauer T, Platzer M, Mathew CG, Krawczak M, Schreiber S (2007) A genome-wide association scan of nonsynonymous SNPs identifies a susceptibility variant for Crohn disease in ATG16L1. Nat Genet 39:207–211

44. Harman D (1991) The aging process: major risk factor for disease and death. Proc Natl Acad Sci U S A 88:5360–5363

45. Harman D (2006) Free radical theory of aging: an update: increasing the functional life span. Ann N Y Acad Sci 1067:10–21

46. Heijmans BT, Westendorp RG, Slagboom PE (2000) Common gene variants, mortality and extreme longevity in humans. Exp Gerontol 35:865–877

47. Herskind AM, McGue M, Holm NV, Sorensen TI, Harvald B, Vaupel JW (1996) The heritability of human longevity: a population-based study of 2872 Danish twin pairs born 1870–1900. Hum Genet 97:319–323

48. Hoshino T, Kawase Y, Okamoto M, Yokota K, Yoshino K, Yamamura K, Miyazaki J, Young HA, Oizumi K (2001) Cutting edge: IL-18-transgenic mice: in vivo evidence of a broad role for IL-18 in modulating immune function. J Immunol 166:7014–7018

49. Huerta C, Alvarez V, Mata IF, Coto E, Ribacoba R, Martinez C, Blazquez M, Guisasola LM, Salvador C, Lahoz CH, Pena J (2004) Chemokines (RANTES and MCP-1) and chemokine-receptors (CCR2 and CCR5) gene polymorphisms in Alzheimer's and Parkinson's disease. Neurosci Lett 370:151–154

50. Kim JH, Auerbach JM, Rodriguez-Gomez JA, Velasco I, Gavin D, Lumelsky N, Lee SH, Nguyen J, Sanchez-Pernaute R, Bankiewicz K, McKay R (2002) Dopamine neurons derived from embryonic stem cells function in an animal model of Parkinson's disease. Nature 418:50–56

51. Kirkwood TB (1991) The biology of aging science 252:1864–1865

52. Kirkwood TB (2005) Understanding the odd science of aging. Cell 120:437–447

53. Kirkwood TB, Austad SN (2000) Why do we age? Nature 408:233–238

54. Klegeris A, McGeer EG, McGeer PL (2007) Therapeutic approaches to inflammation in neurodegenerative disease. Curr Opin Neurol 20:351–357

55. Kruger R, Hardt C, Tschentscher F, Jackel S, Kuhn W, Muller T, Werner J, Woitalla D, Berg D, Kuhnl N, Fuchs GA, Santos EJ, Przuntek H, Epplen JT, Schols L, Riess O (2000) Genetic analysis of immunomodulating factors in sporadic Parkinson's disease. J Neural Transm 107:553–562

56. Lander ES, Linton LM, Birren B, Nusbaum C, Zody MC, Baldwin J, Devon K, Dewar K, Doyle M, FitzHugh W, Funke R, Gage D, Harris K, Heaford A, Howland J, Kann L, Lehoczky J, LeVine R, McEwan P, McKernan K, Meldrim J, Mesirov JP, Miranda C, Morris W, Naylor J, Raymond C, Rosetti M, Santos R, Sheridan A, Sougnez C, Stange-Thomann N, Stojanovic N, Subramanian A, Wyman D, Rogers J, Sulston J, Ainscough R, Beck S, Bentley D, Burton J, Clee C, Carter N, Coulson A, Deadman R, Deloukas P, Dunham A, Dunham I, Durbin R, French L, Grafham D, Gregory S, Hubbard T, Humphray S, Hunt A, Jones M, Lloyd C,

McMurray A, Matthews L, Mercer S, Milne S, Mullikin JC, Mungall A, Plumb R, Ross M, Shownkeen R, Sims S, Waterston RH, Wilson RK, Hillier LW, McPherson JD, Marra MA, Mardis ER, Fulton LA, Chinwalla AT, Pepin KH, Gish WR, Chissoe SL, Wendl MC, Delehaunty KD, Miner TL, Delehaunty A, Kramer JB, Cook LL, Fulton RS, Johnson DL, Minx PJ, Clifton SW, Hawkins T, Branscomb E, Predki P, Richardson P, Wenning S, Slezak T, Doggett N, Cheng JF, Olsen A, Lucas S, Elkin C, Uberbacher E, Frazier M, Gibbs RA, Muzny DM, Scherer SE, Bouck JB, Sodergren EJ, Worley KC, Rives CM, Gorrell JH, Metzker ML, Naylor SL, Kucherlapati RS, Nelson DL, Weinstock GM, Sakaki Y, Fujiyama A, Hattori M, Yada T, Toyoda A, Itoh T, Kawagoe C, Watanabe H, Totoki Y, Taylor T, Weissenbach J, Heilig R, Saurin W, Artiguenave F, Brottier P, Bruls T, Pelletier E, Robert C, Wincker P, Smith DR, Doucette-Stamm L, Rubenfield M, Weinstock K, Lee HM, Dubois J, Rosenthal A, Platzer M, Nyakatura G, Taudien S, Rump A, Yang H, Yu J, Wang J, Huang G, Gu J, Hood L, Rowen L, Madan A, Qin S, Davis RW, Federspiel NA, Abola AP, Proctor MJ, Myers RM, Schmutz J, Dickson M, Grimwood J, Cox DR, Olson MV, Kaul R, Raymond C, Shimizu N, Kawasaki K, Minoshima S, Evans GA, Athanasiou M, Schultz R, Roe BA, Chen F, Pan H, Ramser J, Lehrach H, Reinhardt R, McCombie WR, de la Bastide M, Dedhia N, Blocker H, Hornischer K, Nordsiek G, Agarwala R, Aravind L, Bailey JA, Bateman A, Batzoglou S, Birney E, Bork P, Brown DG, Burge CB, Cerutti L, Chen HC, Church D, Clamp M, Copley RR, Doerks T, Eddy SR, Eichler EE, Furey TS, Galagan J, Gilbert JG, Harmon C, Hayashizaki Y, Haussler D, Hermjakob H, Hokamp K, Jang W, Johnson LS, Jones TA, Kasif S, Kaspryzk A, Kennedy S, Kent WJ, Kitts P, Koonin EV, Korf I, Kulp D, Lancet D, Lowe TM, McLysaght A, Mikkelsen T, Moran JV, Mulder N, Pollara VJ, Ponting CP, Schuler G, Schultz J, Slater G, Smit AF, Stupka E, Szustakowski J, Thierry-Mieg D, Thierry-Mieg J, Wagner L, Wallis J, Wheeler R, Williams A, Wolf YI, Wolfe KH, Yang SP, Yeh RF, Collins F, Guyer MS, Peterson J, Felsenfeld A, Wetterstrand KA, Patrinos A, Morgan MJ, de Jong P, Catanese JJ, Osoegawa K, Shizuya H, Choi S, Chen YJ (2001) Initial sequencing and analysis of the human genome. Nature 409:860–921

57. Letterio JJ, Roberts AB (1998) Regulation of immune responses by TGF-beta. Annu Rev Immunol 16:137–161

58. Lio D, Candore G, Colombo A, Colonna Romano G, Gervasi F, Marino V, Scola L, Caruso C (2001) A genetically determined high setting of TNF-alpha influences immunologic parameters of HLA-B8,DR3 positive subjects: implications for autoimmunity. Hum Immunol 62:705–713

59. Lio D, Candore G, Crivello A, Scola L, Colonna-Romano G, Cavallone L, Hoffmann E, Caruso M, Licastro F, Caldarera CM, Branzi A, Franceschi C, Caruso C (2004) Opposite effects of interleukin 10 common gene polymorphisms in cardiovascular diseases and in successful ageing: genetic background of male centenarians is protective against coronary heart disease. J Med Genet 41:790–794

60. Lio D, Candore G, Romano GC, D'Anna C, Gervasi F, Di Lorenzo G, Modica MA, Potestio M, Caruso C (1997) Modification of cytokine patterns in subjects bearing the HLA-B8,DR3 phenotype: implications for autoimmunity. Cytokines Cell Mol T 3:217–224

61. Lio D, Scola L, Crivello A, Bonafe M, Franceschi C, Olivieri F, Colonna-Romano G, Candore G, Caruso C (2002) Allele frequencies of +874T-1502; A single nucleotide polymorphism at the first intron of interferon-gamma gene in a group of Italian centenarians. Exp Gerontol 37:315–319

62. Lio D, Scola L, Crivello A, Colonna-Romano G, Candore G, Bonafe M, Cavallone L, Franceschi C, Caruso C (2002) Gender-specific association between -1082 IL-10 promoter polymorphism and longevity. Genes Immun 3:30–33

63. Lio D, Scola L, Crivello A, Colonna-Romano G, Candore G, Bonafe M, Cavallone L, Marchegiani F, Olivieri F, Franceschi C, Caruso C (2003) Inflammation, genetics, and longevity: further studies on the protective effects in men of IL-10 -1082 promoter SNP and its interaction with TNF-alpha -308 promoter SNP. J Med Genet 40:296–299

64. Liu B, Gao HM, Wang JY, Jeohn GH, Cooper CL, Hong JS (2002) Role of nitric oxide in inflammation-mediated neurodegeneration. Ann N Y Acad Sci 962:318–331

65. Lowe CE, Cooper JD, Brusko T, Walker NM, Smyth DJ, Bailey R, Bourget K, Plagnol V, Field S, Atkinson M, Clayton DG, Wicker LS, Todd JA (2007) Large-scale genetic fine mapping and genotype-phenotype associations implicate polymorphism in the IL2RA region in type 1 diabetes. Nat Genet 39:1074–1082

66. Luedecking EK, DeKosky ST, Mehdi H, Ganguli M, Kamboh MI (2000) Analysis of genetic polymorphisms in the transforming growth factor-beta1 gene and the risk of Alzheimer's disease. Hum Genet 106:565–569

67. Maggio M, Guralnik JM, Longo DL, Ferrucci L (2006) Interleukin-6 in aging and chronic disease: a magnificent pathway. J Gerontol A Biol Sci Med Sci 61:575–584

68. Margulies M, Egholm M, Altman WE, Attiya S, Bader JS, Bemben LA, Berka J, Braverman MS, Chen YJ, Chen Z, Dewell SB, Du L, Fierro JM, Gomes XV, Godwin BC, He W, Helgesen S, Ho CH, Irzyk GP, Jando SC, Alenquer ML, Jarvie TP, Jirage KB, Kim JB, Knight JR, Lanza JR, Leamon JH, Lefkowitz SM, Lei M, Li J, Lohman KL, Lu H, Makhijani VB, McDade KE, McKenna MP, Myers EW, Nickerson E, Nobile JR, Plant R, Puc BP, Ronan MT, Roth GT, Sarkis GJ, Simons JF, Simpson JW, Srinivasan M, Tartaro KR, Tomasz A, Vogt KA, Volkmer GA, Wang SH, Wang Y, Weiner MP, Yu P, Begley RF, Rothberg JM (2005) Genome sequencing in microfabricated high-density picolitre reactors. Nature 437:376–380

69. Mariani E, Pulsatelli L, Meneghetti A, Dolzani P, Mazzetti I, Neri S, Ravaglia G, Forti P, Facchini A (2001) Different IL-8 production by T and NK lymphocytes in elderly subjects. Mech Ageing Dev 122:1383–1395

70. Mattila KM, Rinne JO, Lehtimaki T, Roytta M, Ahonen JP, Hurme M (2002) Association of an interleukin 1B gene polymorphism (-511) with Parkinson's disease in Finnish patients. J Med Genet 39:400–402

71. McGeer EG, McGeer PL (2007) The role of anti-inflammatory agents in Parkinson's disease. CNS Drugs 21:789–797

72. Medvedev ZA (1990) An attempt at a rational classification of theories of ageing. Biol Rev Camb Philos Soc 65:375–398

73. Miller RJ, Meucci O (1999) AIDS and the brain: is there a chemokine connection? Trends Neurosci 22:471–479

74. Mogi M, Harada M, Kondo T, Riederer P, Nagatsu T (1996) Interleukin-2 but not basic fibroblast growth factor is elevated in parkinsonian brain. Short communication. J Neural Transm 103:1077–1081

75. Mogi M, Harada M, Riederer P, Narabayashi H, Fujita K, Nagatsu T (1994) Tumor necrosis factor-alpha (TNF-alpha) increases both in the brain and in the cerebrospinal fluid from parkinsonian patients. Neurosci Lett 165:208–210

76. Moller JC, Depboylu C, Kolsch H, Lohmuller F, Bandmann O, Gocke P, Du Y, Paus S, Wullner U, Gasser T, Oertel WH, Klockgether T, Dodel RC (2004) Lack of association between the interleukin-1 alpha (-889) polymorphism and early-onset Parkinson's disease. Neurosci Lett 359:195–197

77. Muller T, Blum-Degen D, Przuntek H, Kuhn W (1998) Interleukin-6 levels in cerebrospinal fluid inversely correlate to severity of Parkinson's disease. Acta Neurol Scand 98:142–144

78. Mysliwska J, Bryl E, Foerster J, Mysliwski A (1998) Increase of interleukin 6 and decrease of interleukin 2 production during the ageing process are influenced by the health status. Mech Ageing Dev 100:313–328

79. Nishimura M, Kuno S, Mizuta I, Ohta M, Maruyama H, Kaji R, Kawakami H (2003) Influence of monocyte chemoattractant protein 1 gene polymorphism on age at onset of sporadic Parkinson's disease. Mov Disord 18:953–955

80. Nishimura M, Mizuta I, Mizuta E, Yamasaki S, Ohta M, Kaji R, Kuno S (2001) Tumor necrosis factor gene polymorphisms in patients with sporadic Parkinson's disease. Neurosci Lett 311:1–4

81. Nishimura M, Mizuta I, Mizuta E, Yamasaki S, Ohta M, Kuno S (2000) Influence of interleukin-1beta gene polymorphisms on age-at-onset of sporadic Parkinson's disease. Neurosci Lett 284:73–76

82. Novelli F, Casanova JL (2004) The role of IL-12, IL-23 and IFN-gamma in immunity to viruses. Cytokine Growth Factor Rev 15:367–377
83. Ojala J, Alafuzoff I, Herukka SK, van Groen T, Tanila H, Pirttila T (2007) Expression of interleukin-18 is increased in the brains of Alzheimer's disease patients. Neurobiol Aging
84. Oliver J, Rueda B, Lopez-Nevot MA, Gomez-Garcia M, Martin J (2007) Replication of an Association Between IL23R Gene Polymorphism With Inflammatory Bowel Disease. Clin Gastroenterol Hepatol 5:977–981 e972
85. Olivieri F, Bonafe M, Cavallone L, Giovagnetti S, Marchegiani F, Cardelli M, Mugianesi E, Giampieri C, Moresi R, Stecconi R, Lisa R, Franceschi C (2002) The -174 C/G locus affects in vitro/in vivo IL-6 production during aging. Exp Gerontol 37:309–314
86. Papasteriades C, Boki K, Pappa H, Aedonopoulos S, Papasteriadis E, Economidou J (1997) HLA phenotypes in healthy aged subjects. Gerontology 43:176–181
87. Parish CL, Arenas E (2007) Stem-cell-based strategies for the treatment of Parkinson's disease. Neurodegener Dis 4:339–347
88. Pawelec G, Solana R (1997) Immunosenescence. Immunol Today 18:514–516
89. Perls T, Kunkel LM, Puca AA (2002) The genetics of exceptional human longevity. J Am Geriatr Soc 50:359–368
90. Perls TT, Bubrick E, Wager CG, Vijg J, Kruglyak L (1998) Siblings of centenarians live longer. Lancet 351:1560
91. Pes GM, Lio D, Carru C, Deiana L, Baggio G, Franceschi C, Ferrucci L, Oliveri F, Scola L, Crivello A, Candore G, Colonna-Romano G, Caruso C (2004) Association between longevity and cytokine gene polymorphisms. A study in Sardinian centenarians. Aging Clin Exp Res 16:244–248
92. Piccini P, Burn DJ, Ceravolo R, Maraganore D, Brooks DJ (1999) The role of inheritance in sporadic Parkinson's disease: evidence from a longitudinal study of dopaminergic function in twins. Ann Neurol 45:577–582
93. Pravica V, Asderakis A, Perrey C, Hajeer A, Sinnott PJ, Hutchinson IV (1999) In vitro production of IFN-gamma correlates with CA repeat polymorphism in the human IFN-gamma gene. Eur J Immunogenet 26:1–3
94. Pravica V, Perrey C, Stevens A, Lee JH, Hutchinson IV (2000) A single nucleotide polymorphism in the first intron of the human IFN-gamma gene: absolute correlation with a polymorphic CA microsatellite marker of high IFN-gamma production. Hum Immunol 61:863–866
95. Rainero I, Bo M, Ferrero M, Valfre W, Vaula G, Pinessi L (2004) Association between the interleukin-1alpha gene and Alzheimer's disease: a meta-analysis. Neurobiol Aging 25:1293–1298
96. Rea IM, McNerlan SE, Alexander HD (2000) Total serum IL-12 and IL-12p40, but not IL-12p70, are increased in the serum of older subjects; relationship to CD3(+)and NK subsets. Cytokine 12:156–159
97. Rea IM, Ross OA, Armstrong M, McNerlan S, Alexander DH, Curran MD, Middleton D (2003) Interleukin-6-gene C/G 174 polymorphism in nonagenarian and octogenarian subjects in the BELFAST study. Reciprocal effects on IL-6, soluble IL-6 receptor and for IL-10 in serum and monocyte supernatants. Mech Ageing Dev 124:555–561
98. Rea IM, Stewart M, Campbell P, Alexander HD, Crockard AD, Morris TC (1996) Changes in lymphocyte subsets, interleukin 2, and soluble interleukin 2 receptor in old and very old age. Gerontology 42:69–78
99. Redon R, Ishikawa S, Fitch KR, Feuk L, Perry GH, Andrews TD, Fiegler H, Shapero MH, Carson AR, Chen W, Cho EK, Dallaire S, Freeman JL, Gonzalez JR, Gratacos M, Huang J, Kalaitzopoulos D, Komura D, MacDonald JR, Marshall CR, Mei R, Montgomery L, Nishimura K, Okamura K, Shen F, Somerville MJ, Tchinda J, Valsesia A, Woodwark C, Yang F, Zhang J, Zerjal T, Zhang J, Armengol L, Conrad DF, Estivill X, Tyler-Smith C, Carter NP, Aburatani H, Lee C, Jones KW, Scherer SW, Hurles ME (2006) Global variation in copy number in the human genome. Nature 444:444–454

100. Rink L, Cakman I, Kirchner H (1998) Altered cytokine production in the elderly. Mech Ageing Dev 102:199–209

101. Risch NJ (2000) Searching for genetic determinants in the new millennium. Nature 405:847–856

102. Ross OA (2006) Longevics: genetic lessons for the ages. Ir J Med Sci 175:82

103. Ross OA (2007) Lrrking in the background: common pathways of neurodegeneration. J Am Geriatr Soc 55:804–805

104. Ross OA, Curran MD, Meenagh A, Williams F, Barnett YA, Middleton D, Rea IM (2003) Study of age-association with cytokine gene polymorphisms in an aged Irish population. Mech Ageing Dev 124:199–206

105. Ross OA, Curran MD, Rea IM, Hyland P, Duggan O, Barnett CR, Annett K, Patterson C, Barnett YA, Middleton D (2003) HLA haplotypes and TNF polymorphism do not associate with longevity in the Irish. Mech Ageing Dev 124:563–567

106. Ross OA, Farrer MJ (2005) Pathophysiology, pleiotrophy and paradigm shifts: genetic lessons from Parkinson's disease. Biochem Soc Trans 33:586–590

107. Ross OA, Farrer MJ, Wu RM (2007) Common variants in Parkinson's disease. Mov Disord 22:899–900

108. Ross OA, O'Neill C, Rea IM, Lynch T, Gosal D, Wallace A, Curran MD, Middleton D, Gibson JM (2004) Functional promoter region polymorphism of the proinflammatory chemokine IL-8 gene associates with Parkinson's disease in the Irish. Hum Immunol 65:340–346

109. Scola L, Candore G, Colonna-Romano G, Crivello A, Forte GI, Paolisso G, Franceschi C, Lio D, Caruso C (2005) Study of the association with -330T/G IL-2 in a population of centenarians from centre and south Italy. Biogerontology 6:425–429

110. Semchuk KM, Love EJ, Lee RG (1993) Parkinson's disease: a test of the multifactorial etiologic hypothesis. Neurology 43:1173–1180

111. Simon-Sanchez J, Scholz S, Fung HC, Matarin M, Hernandez D, Gibbs JR, Britton A, Wavrant de Vrieze F, Peckham E, Gwinn-Hardy K, Crawley A, Keen JC, Nash J, Borgaonkar D, Hardy J, Singleton A (2006) Genome-wide SNP assay reveals structural genomic variation, extended homozygosity and cell-line induced alterations in normal individuals. Hum Mol Genet

112. Simon DK, Lin MT, Pascual-Leone A (2002) "Nature versus nurture" and incompletely penetrant mutations. J Neurol Neurosurg Psychiatry 72:686–689

113. Soliman MK, Mazzio E, Soliman KF (2002) Levodopa modulating effects of inducible nitric oxide synthase and reactive oxygen species in glioma cells. Life Sci 72:185–198

114. Syvanen AC (2005) Toward genome-wide SNP genotyping. Nat Genet 37 Suppl:S5–10

115. van Deventer SJ (2000) Cytokine and cytokine receptor polymorphisms in infectious disease. Intensive Care Med 26 Suppl 1:S98–102

116. van Heel DA, Franke L, Hunt KA, Gwilliam R, Zhernakova A, Inouye M, Wapenaar MC, Barnardo MC, Bethel G, Holmes GK, Feighery C, Jewell D, Kelleher D, Kumar P, Travis S, Walters JR, Sanders DS, Howdle P, Swift J, Playford RJ, McLaren WM, Mearin ML, Mulder CJ, McManus R, McGinnis R, Cardon LR, Deloukas P, Wijmenga C (2007) A genome-wide association study for celiac disease identifies risk variants in the region harboring IL2 and IL21. Nat Genet 39:827–829

117. Venter JC, Adams MD, Myers EW, Li PW, Mural RJ, Sutton GG, Smith HO, Yandell M, Evans CA, Holt RA, Gocayne JD, Amanatides P, Ballew RM, Huson DH, Wortman JR, Zhang Q, Kodira CD, Zheng XH, Chen L, Skupski M, Subramanian G, Thomas PD, Zhang J, Gabor Miklos GL, Nelson C, Broder S, Clark AG, Nadeau J, McKusick VA, Zinder N, Levine AJ, Roberts RJ, Simon M, Slayman C, Hunkapiller M, Bolanos R, Delcher A, Dew I, Fasulo D, Flanigan M, Florea L, Halpern A, Hannenhalli S, Kravitz S, Levy S, Mobarry C, Reinert K, Remington K, Abu-Threideh J, Beasley E, Biddick K, Bonazzi V, Brandon R, Cargill M, Chandramouliswaran I, Charlab R, Chaturvedi K, Deng Z, Di Francesco V, Dunn P, Eilbeck K, Evangelista C, Gabrielian AE, Gan W, Ge W, Gong F, Gu Z, Guan P, Heiman TJ, Higgins

ME, Ji RR, Ke Z, Ketchum KA, Lai Z, Lei Y, Li Z, Li J, Liang Y, Lin X, Lu F, Merkulov GV, Milshina N, Moore HM, Naik AK, Narayan VA, Neelam B, Nusskern D, Rusch DB, Salzberg S, Shao W, Shue B, Sun J, Wang Z, Wang A, Wang X, Wang J, Wei M, Wides R, Xiao C, Yan C, Yao A, Ye J, Zhan M, Zhang W, Zhang H, Zhao Q, Zheng L, Zhong F, Zhong W, Zhu S, Zhao S, Gilbert D, Baumhueter S, Spier G, Carter C, Cravchik A, Woodage T, Ali F, An H, Awe A, Baldwin D, Baden H, Barnstead M, Barrow I, Beeson K, Busam D, Carver A, Center A, Cheng ML, Curry L, Danaher S, Davenport L, Desilets R, Dietz S, Dodson K, Doup L, Ferriera S, Garg N, Gluecksmann A, Hart B, Haynes J, Haynes C, Heiner C, Hladun S, Hostin D, Houck J, Howland T, Ibegwam C, Johnson J, Kalush F, Kline L, Koduru S, Love A, Mann F, May D, McCawley S, McIntosh T, McMullen I, Moy M, Moy L, Murphy B, Nelson K, Pfannkoch C, Pratts E, Puri V, Qureshi H, Reardon M, Rodriguez R, Rogers YH, Romblad D, Ruhfel B, Scott R, Sitter C, Smallwood M, Stewart E, Strong R, Suh E, Thomas R, Tint NN, Tse S, Vech C, Wang G, Wetter J, Williams S, Williams M, Windsor S, Winn-Deen E, Wolfe K, Zaveri J, Zaveri K, Abril JF, Guigo R, Campbell MJ, Sjolander KV, Karlak B, Kejariwal A, Mi H, Lazareva B, Hatton T, Narechania A, Diemer K, Muruganujan A, Guo N, Sato S, Bafna V, Istrail S, Lippert R, Schwartz R, Walenz B, Yooseph S, Allen D, Basu A, Baxendale J, Blick L, Caminha M, Carnes-Stine J, Caulk P, Chiang YH, Coyne M, Dahlke C, Mays A, Dombroski M, Donnelly M, Ely D, Esparham S, Fosler C, Gire H, Glanowski S, Glasser K, Glodek A, Gorokhov M, Graham K, Gropman B, Harris M, Heil J, Henderson S, Hoover J, Jennings D, Jordan C, Jordan J, Kasha J, Kagan L, Kraft C, Levitsky A, Lewis M, Liu X, Lopez J, Ma D, Majoros W, McDaniel J, Murphy S, Newman M, Nguyen T, Nguyen N, Nodell M, Pan S, Peck J, Peterson M, Rowe W, Sanders R, Scott J, Simpson M, Smith T, Sprague A, Stockwell T, Turner R, Venter E, Wang M, Wen M, Wu D, Wu M, Xia A, Zandieh A, Zhu X (2001) The sequence of the human genome. Science 291:1304–1351

118. Wahner AD, Sinsheimer JS, Bronstein JM, Ritz B (2007) Inflammatory cytokine gene poly-morphisms and increased risk of Parkinson disease. Arch Neurol 64:836–840

119. Wang XY, Hurme M, Jylha M, Hervonen A (2001) Lack of association between human longevity and polymorphisms of IL-1 cluster, IL-6, IL-10 and TNF-alpha genes in Finnish nonagenarians. Mech Ageing Dev 123:29–38

120. Weiss JM, Cuff CA, Berman JW (1999) TGF-beta downmodulates cytokine-induced mono-cyte chemoattractant protein (MCP)-1 expression in human endothelial cells. A putative role for TGF-beta in the modulation of TNF receptor expression. Endothelium 6:291–302

121. Wong KK, Deleeuw RJ, Dosanjh NS, Kimm LR, Cheng Z, Horsman DE, Macaulay C, Ng RT, Brown CJ, Eichler EE, Lam WL (2007) A comprehensive analysis of common copy-number variations in the human genome. Am J Hum Genet 80:91–104

122. Wu YR, Feng IH, Lyu RK, Chang KH, Lin YY, Chan H, Hu FJ, Lee-Chen GJ, Chen CM (2007) Tumor necrosis factor-alpha promoter polymorphism is associated with the risk of Parkinson's disease. Am J Med Genet B Neuropsychiatr Genet 144:300–304

Role of TLR Polymorphisms in Immunosenescence

Carmela Rita Balistreri, Giuseppina Candore, Giuseppina Colonna-Romano, Maria Paola Grimaldi, Domenico Lio, Florinda Listì, Sonya Vasto, Letizia Scola and Calogero Caruso

Contents

Abstract: Innate immunity provides a first line of host defense against infection through microbial recognition and killing while simultaneously activating a clonotypic immune response. Toll-like receptors (TLRs) are principal mediators of rapid microbial recognition and function mainly by detection of pathogen-associated molecular patterns (PAMPs) that do not exist in the host. The different members of TLRs recognize several PAMPs, such as peptidoglycan for TLR2, lipopolysaccharide (LPS) for TLR4, flagellin for TLR5, and CpGDNA-repeats for TLR9. Several endogenous ligands of various TLRs have been also identified in the host. In this chapter, we describe the involvement of TLR-4 polymorphisms in immunosenescence, and in particular in age-related diseases, suggesting the crucial role of molecules of innate immunity on these diseases pathophysiology. Hence, we observed that proinflammatory alleles may be related to unsuccessful aging as atherosclerosis and Alzheimer's disease; reciprocally, controlling inflammatory status by antiinflammatory alleles may allow to better attain successful aging.

Keywords: Alzheimer's disease • Atherosclerosis • Longevity • TLR4

C. R. Balistreri (✉) · G. Candore · G. Colonna-Romano · M. P. Grimaldi ·
D. Lio · F. Listì · S. Vasto · L. Scola · C. Caruso
Gruppo di Studio sull'Immunosenescenza
Dipartimento di Biopatologia e Metodologie Biomediche
Università di Palermo, Corso Tukory 211
90134 Palermo, Italy
Tel.: +390916555911
Fax: +390916555933
E-mail: marcoc@unipa.it or crbalistreri@unipa.it

T. Fulop et al. (eds.), *Handbook on Immunosenescence*,
DOI 10.1007/ 978-1-4020-9062-2_34, © Springer Science+Business Media B.V. 2009

1 Introduction

Ageing and longevity are due to a complex interaction of genetic, epigenetic and environmental factors [1]. The genetic component seems to have a relevant role in the attainment of longevity, because it is involved in cell maintenance systems, including immune system. An optimal performance of the both innate and clonotypic branches of immune system has been correlated with survival to extreme ages [2]. The ageing of immune system, known as immunosenescence, is the consequence of changes of clonotypic and innate immune cells caused by lymphoid tissue involution and chronic antigenic overload. The antigenic stress affects the immune system thorough out life with a progressive activation and generation of inflammatory responses involved in the pathophysiology of age-related diseases. Most of the parameters influencing immunosenescence appear to be under genetic control, and immunosenescence fits with the basic assumptions of evolutionary theories of aging, such as antagonistic pleiotropy. Accordingly, the innate immune system, by neutralizing infectious agents, plays a beneficial role until the time of reproduction and parental care, but, by determining a chronic inflammation, can play a detrimental one late in life, in a period largely not foreseen by evolution. In contrast, the clonotypic immune system, with advancing age, shows an exhaustion, due to accumulation of memory cells, which fill the immunological space [2]. As already mentioned, the genetic background seems to modulate the functionality of innate/inflammatory and clonotypic responses and consequently the inflammatory state occurring with advancing age [1, 2]. So, genes encoding molecules involved in innate/clonotypic immunity might influence the susceptibility to age-related diseases and the survival to extreme ages. In other words, the presence of pro/antiinflammatory genotypes might determine a negative or positive control of inflammation, influencing the susceptibility to age-related diseases and/or promoting longevity [2].

In this chapter, we describe the involvement of Toll-like receptor (TLR) 4 polymorphisms in immunosenescence, and in particular in age-related diseases, suggesting the crucial role of molecules of innate immunity on these diseases pathophysiology. Hence, we observed that proinflammatory alleles may be related to unsuccessful aging as atherosclerosis and Alzheimer's disease (AD); reciprocally, controlling inflammatory status by anti-inflammatory alleles may allow to better attain successful aging.

2 TLR4

The innate immune system is the first line of the defensive mechanisms that protect host from invading microbial pathogens. Host cells express various pattern recognition receptors (PRRs) that sense diverse pathogen-associated molecular patterns (PAMPs), ranging from lipids, lipoproteins, proteins and nucleic acids [3, 4].

Recognition of PAMPs by PRRs activates intracellular signaling pathways that culminate in the induction of inflammatory cytokines, chemokines, interferons (IFNs) and upregulation of co-stimulatory molecules. To date, it has been identified three families of PRRs, usually defined as "the trinity of pathogen sensors": Toll-like receptors (TLRs), NOD-like receptors and RIG-like receptors (RLR). NLRs with known functions detect bacteria, and RLRs are antiviral [3, 4].

TLRs family include, in human beings, 10 members that trigger innate immune responses through nuclear factor-κB (NF-κB)- dependent and IFN-regulatory factor (IRF)-dependent signaling pathways [4, 5]. TLRs are evolutionarily conserved molecules and were originally identified in vertebrates on the basis of their homology with Toll, a molecule that stimulates the production of antimicrobial proteins in *Drosophila melanogaster* [6, 7].

Some molecules of this family are expressed at the cell surface, whereas others are expressed on the membrane of endocytic vesicles or other intracellular organelles (Fig. 1). The structure of these receptors is quaternary and they are composed of an ectodomain of leucine-rich repeats n (LRRs), which are involved directly or through accessory molecules in ligand binding, and a cytoplasmic Toll/interleukin(IL)-1 receptor (TIR) domain that interacts with TIR-domain-containing adaptor molecules (Fig. 2) [8]. The different members of TLRs recognize several PAMPs, such as peptidoglycan for TLR2, lipopolysaccharide (LPS) for TLR4, flagellin for TLR5, and CpGDNA-repeats for TLR9 (Fig. 1) [9–12]. Several endogenous ligands of various TLRs have been also identified in the host [13].

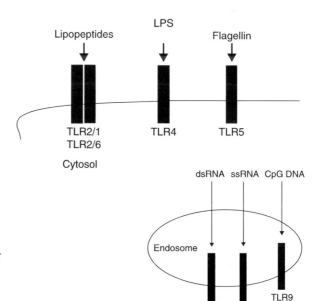

Fig. 1 The members of TLR family are expressed at the cell surface and on the membrane of endocytic vesicles or other intracellular organelles. They recognize several microbial molecules, as shown in the figure.

Fig. 2 The TLR structure is composed of an ectodomain of LRRs, which are involved directly or through accessory molecules in ligand binding, and a cytoplasmic Toll/inter-leukin-1 (IL-1) receptor (TIR) domain that interacts with TIR-domain-containing adaptor molecules.

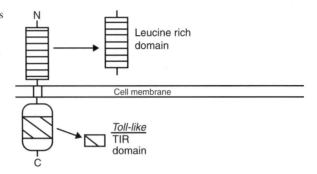

Taking into account their ability to link several molecules, it has been postulated that the genes encoding TLRs receptors would be subject to diversifying selection [14] This is because the proteins are in direct contact with molecules of microbial origin, which might change in structure to evade immune detection. In fact, weak purifying selection seems to apply in the case of the TLRs [14, 15]. Furthermore, the need for detection of various signature molecules seems to come and go in evolution. For example, while some invertebrates are highly sensitive to LPS, most invertebrates are not [16–19]. Drosophila exhibits no response to pure LPS or lipid A at all. Similarly, most vertebrates (fish, amphibians, reptiles, and birds) are at least relatively insensitive to LPS, if not entirely unresponsive [14]. In the case to Danio rerio and Gallus gallus, it is clear that TLR4 encoding genes are represented in the genome. However, in fish and in birds, these TLR4 homologs evidently to not trigger the same set of events as witnessed in mammals. Besides, among mammals, sensitivity to LPS is quite variable, depending upon which endpoint is examined. Humans, anthropoid apes, ungulates, and rabbits are highly sensitive to LPS; mice, rats, and baboons are comparatively resistant [14].

To date, it is possible to suggest that TLRs receptors are the key molecules of natural responses and they also provide a link between innate and clonotypic immunity [20–22]. These evidences have also opened inquiries into previously unknown disease mechanisms [23–25]. Their ability to detect different PAMPs gives a link between infection and various human diseases [23–25]. In fact, members of TLR family have been involved in the pathogenesis of several diseases by studies of people analyzing the incidence of diseases having different polymorphisms in genes encoding TLRs. So, it has been evidenced the crucial role of well-known component of TLR family, the TLR4, in some diseases, as atherosclerosis and AD [24–26].

TLR4 has been identified as the first human homologue of the Drosophila Toll [6, 7]. The extracellular domain of TLR4 that contain over 600 amino acids is highly polymorphic compared with the transmembrane and intracellular domain of the protein [5, 18]. This TLR4 polymorphism contributes to species-specific differences in recognition of LPS, the prototypic TLR4 ligand [5, 19]. The intracellular TIR domain, which is composed of three highly conserved regions, contains

150 amino acids [5, 20]. The TIR domain modulates protein–protein interactions between the TLRs and signal transduction elements [5, 20]. As already mentioned, TLR4 has been shown to be involved in the recognition of LPS, a major cell wall component of Gram negative bacteria [14]. In addition to LPS, TLR4 recognizes several endogenous ligands, such as oxidized-LDL (ox-LDL), lipoteichoic acid, heat-shock proteins (HSP), fibronectin and Aβ amyloid peptide of AD. Its activation by induction of NF-kB and mitogen dependent protein kinase pathways determines the production of cytokines, chemokines, other inflammatory mediators (Fig. 3) [13]. Therefore, it has been suggested that activated TLR4 triggers not only innate immunity but also clonotypic immunity. TLR4 activation on dendritic cells induces the expression of costimulatory molecules and production of inflammatory cytokines [22]. Then, activated dendritic cells present microorganism derived peptide antigens expressed on the cell surface with Major Histocompatibility Complex class II antigen to naive T-cells, thereby initiating an antigen-specific clonotypic immune response [20–22].

TLR4 activity and function may be modulated by genetic polymorphisms (for the most part, single nucleotide polymorphisms, SNPs), prevalently presented in extracellular domain. It has been identified a functional SNP in the human TLR4 gene, an A-G base transition at position +896 base pairs from the transcriptional start site, resulting in an aspartic acid to glycine exchange at position 299 in the amino-acid sequence (referred to as Asp299Gly or +896A/G) [27, 28]. This SNP

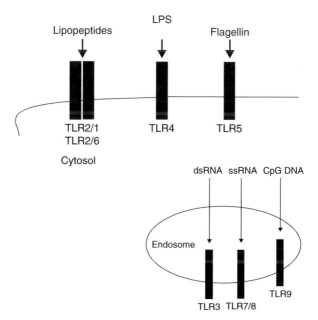

Fig. 3 Activation of TLR4 receptor by LPS (or other agents, as endogenous molecules-as shown in the figure) induces transmembrane signals that activate NF-kB and mitogen dependent protein kinase pathways, determining the expression of a wide number of genes encoding proteins, such as cytokines, with regulatory functions upon leukocyte activation and tissue inflammation.

causes hyporesponsiveness to LPS as well as an increased risk and susceptibility to Gram-negative infections both in human and experimental animals. Recently, it has been suggested that this SNP plays a role in a variety of human diseases, ranging from infectious and inflammatory diseases to cancer [23–26]. So, TLR4 plays a key role in both innate and clonotypic immunity to Gram-negative bacteria and to other agents and it seems to be the hub of inflammatory pathophysiology of age-related diseases, as atherosclerosis and AD [23–26].

3   Involvement of TLR4 in Age-Related Diseases: Its Role in Atherosclerosis, AD, and Cancer

By now, evidence is accumulating that TLR4 could affect atherosclerosis in multiple ways [24, 25, 28–35]. The association between TLR4 and atherosclerosis is consistent with findings showing that TLR4 mRNA and protein are more abundant in atherosclerosis lesions than in unaffected vessels [24, 25, 30]. Furthermore, cultured human vascular endothelial cells express little TLR4 under baseline conditions, and they express high levels of TLR4 on stimulation with proinflammatory cytokines [29]. Among cellular components presented in atherosclerotic plaques are several TLR4-expressing cells, including macrophages, endothelial cells, smooth muscle cells, T-cells and dendritic cells [24, 25, 28–35]. It is largely accepted that ox-LDL as well as other endogeneous ligands, that are expressed during arterial injury, as HSP are responsible for TLR4 ligation and activation. However, taking into account the role of life-long pathogen load on the development of elderly inflammatory status and atherosclerosis, PAMPs should also be involved in TLR4 activation (Fig. 4) [2, 28–37].

To date, there is a large body of genetic data pointing the involvement of Asp299Gly SNP in atherosclerosis development. Ultrasound analysis of carotid arteries in a large Italian population showed that the Asp299Gly was found less frequently in people with progressive lesions representing carotid atherosclerosis, compared with a control group. These results were confirmed by other studies that found a protective effect of the TLR4 variants on acute coronary events. However, other studies investigating a potential association of this SNP with cardiovascular diseases (CVD), as myocardial infarction (MI), did not yield significant results (Table 1) [28, 36–46]. On the other hand, association studies are influenced by a number of possible confounding factors, like the total number of patients and controls and the homogeneity of the population in term of geographical origin among others. Artefacts might occur if the controls are not ethnically matched with the patients.

Literature data have also recently demonstrated the involvement of TLR4 receptor in neurodegeneration. It is now known the role of innate immunity, and precisely of microglial cells, in the inflammatory pathogenesis of AD, as stated by the amyloid cascade/neuroinflammation hypothesis. The former is responsible for the production of the neurotoxic substances, such as reactive oxygen and nitrogen

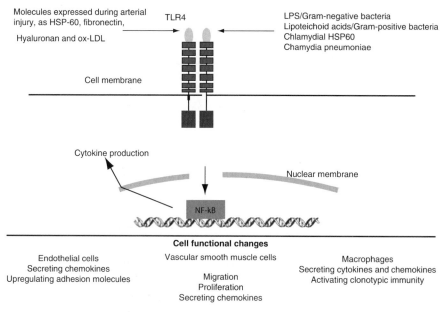

Fig. 4 TLR4 signaling pathway and its relation with atherosclerosis. Both endogenous and exogenous ligands can activate TLR4 on cells, such as endothelial cells, vascular smooth muscle cells, adventitial fibroblasts, dendritic cells and macrophages. Activated TLR4 lead to activation of the NF-KB. This activated transcription factor mediates the expression of several genes and the secretion of proinflammatory cytokines and chemokines, and it also induces expression of adhesion molecules. Ultimately, these processes might initiate or promote atherosclerotic lesions.

species, proinflammatory cytokines, complement proteins and other inflammatory mediators that bring important neurodegenerative changes. Some studies have suggested that activation of microglial cells may be induced throughout the binding of Aβ peptides. Several membrane proteins expressed on microglial cells seem to be implicated in Aβ peptides binding. It has been demonstrated that TLR4 receptor binds highly hydrophobic Aβ peptides aggregates suggesting the production of neurotoxic substances. A further, not mutually, alternative explanation on the key role of microglial activation may be related to the role of TLR4 as LPS receptor. In fact, also in AD life-long pathogen burden has been linked to the pathophysiology of the disease. So it should to be biologically plausible that functional variation in the TLR4 gene might influence the susceptibility to sporadic AD [47–56].

This might be the case for the allelic variants of TLR4 gene, as Asp299Gly SNP, associated, as above described, with an attenuated receptor signaling and a blunted inflammatory response. Association between this polymorphism and AD has been described by Minoretti et al. [57] in an Italian population sample. Our preliminary results of a recent study have confirmed that Asp299Gly polymorphism of TLR4 gene is associated with AD [56].

It has been also suggested the involvement of TLR4 receptor in cancer [23]. It is known the involvement of inflammation, as an etiological factor in several human cancer. Growing evidence suggests that the chronic inflammation induced

Table 1   Summary of studies investigating the potential association of Asp299Gly **TLR4SNP** with cardiovascular diseases

References	Association studies	Results	P-value
Kiechl et al[28]	Carotid stenosis	Participants with SNP have lower incidence of carotid stenosis	0.05
Ameziane et al[38]	Acute coronary events	Participants with SNP have lower incidence of coronary events	0.037
Balistreri et al[39]	MI	Patients (men) with SNP have lower incidence of MI	0.002
Edfeldt et al[40]	MI	Men with SNP have increased incidence of MI	0.004
Zee et al[41]	MI and stroke	Not significant	0.25
Yang et al[42]	Coronary artery stenosis	Participants with SNP have not lower risk of stenosis	0.9
Labrum et al[43]	Carotid events	There was no association between SNP and baseline intima-media thickness (IMT) or progression of IMT over the 3-year follow up	Not significant
O'Halloran et al[44]	Coronary artery disease	There was no evidence overall that the resistance alleles cumulatively influenced the risk of CVD compared to controls or stable angina patients	0.12, and 0.40, respectively
Vainas et al[45]	Peripherical arterial disease	Among patients affected by peripheral arterial disease, TLR4 +896 G allele carriership was univariantly associated with extensive (more than two vascular territories affected) atherosclerotic disease	0.02
Nebel et al[46]	MI	Patients (men) with SNP have not lower incidence of MI	0.36

by different pathogens may also play a role in pathophysiology of some cancer, as gastric cancer [23, 58–62]. Considering that genetic susceptibility is a major risk factor for this disease, it has been hypothesized that sequence variants in genes that regulate inflammatory response may modify individual susceptibility to cancer. So, some studies have analyzed the relationship between the associations of several functional polymorphisms in genes involved in LPS signaling variants and risk of cancer. Garza-Gonzales et al. [59] have investigated the association of Asp299Gly TLR4 SNP and distal gastric cancer in a Mexican population. The results obtained have not demonstrated any association between this SNP and distal gastric cancer, suggesting that it do not contribute to the development to disease. The same data have been obtained in a study performed in a Venezuelan population [60]. In another study, it has been investigated the role of different SNPs of some inflammatory genes, as Asp299Gly of TLR4 gene, in 377 patients affected by colorectal cancer and 326 controls from Spain [61]. There was no statistically significant association between this SNP and colorectal cancer risk. However, different results have been found in a study performed in 710 patients affected by lymphoma [62]. In fact, the TLR4 Asp299Gly variant was positively associated with the risk of mucosa-associated lymphoid tissue lymphoma (OR=2.76, 95% CI=1.12–6.81) and Hodgkin's lymphoma (OR=1.80, 95% CI=0.99–3.26). Hence, this study suggests an effect of this SNP in factors of the innate immune response in the etiology of some lymphoma subtypes.

4   Conclusions

Genetic factors play an important role in the ability to achieve exceptional old age, theoretically two class of genes can be considered to be at play [1]. On the one hand, individuals with a genetic make-up useful to achieve extreme old age most likely present with mutations that significantly increase the risk of premature death by lethal, age, and nonage-associated diseases. On the other hand, it has been suggested that genetic variants conferring protection against basic mechanisms of aging and/or age-related illnesses also might exist [1, 2].

To discover the gene factors that let an organism to survive beyond its reproductive age, it is necessary to use an extreme phenotype. From this perspective, the centenarians are the good choice as they represent the survived tail of a very special segment of population. They comprise a cohort of living people who celebrate today the 100th birthday and escaped neonatal mortality, preantibiotic era, fatal outcomes of age-related complex diseases. A small number of centenarians is in quite good heath (in "*good robustness*"), defined as "group A" by Franceschi et al., "escapers" by Evert et al., and "exceptionals" by Gondo et al. [63–65]. The centenarians also represent that segment of population who better adapted and readapted from both biological and non-biological point of view. Centenarians, as representative of longevity, consent to understand the role played by genetic structure of population on the onset of phenotype and the historical dynamism of the longevity trait from a demographic point of view. So, they are the best model for studying the genetics of longevity, and for identifying the genetic factors involved in age-related diseases, since the centenarians represent selected survivors who have clearly delayed or in some cases even escaped age-related diseases, that affect old people and are responsible their morbidity and mortality [66]. Hence, centenarians are a human model of disease-free [67]. In addition, centenarian offspring have increased likelihood of surviving to 100 years and show a reduced prevalence of age-associated diseases, as CVD and less prevalence of cardiovascular risk factors [68, 69]. So, genes involved in CVD may play an opposite role in human longevity, as Asp299Gly SNP. In particular, we have postulated that alleles associated to CVD susceptibility should not be included in the genetic background favoring longevity. So, the genetic background promoting pro-inflammatory responses may play an opposite roles in CVD and in longevity [37, 70–72].

Following a novel approach to study genes involved in CVD and reciprocally in longevity, we have recently demonstrated that antiinflammtory allele of Asp299Gly SNP of TLR4 gene, +896G, is overrepresented in male Sicilian centenarians and underrepresented in men affected by MI, with intermediate values in control population [37]. Thus, our results suggest a role of the innate immune defense system and particularly TLR4 in CVD, and our comparison with the oldest old may help elucidate the role of genetics in age-associated diseases characterized by a multifactorial etiology [39]. Accordingly, TLR4 polymorphisms, which attenuate receptor signaling, enhance the risk of infections, but decrease that of atherogenesis, presumably by limiting inflammatory responses [27, 28]. Hence, the mutation might result in an increased chance of longevity in a modern environment with reduced pathogen load and improved control of severe infections by antibiotics.

However, a recent study has excluded a noteworthy influence of Asp299Gly SNP upon human longevity or MI in German men [46]. The causes of the discrepancies seem be not clear, but the inclusion criteria, the studied populations, and the measured endpoint differed substantially among the studies. Further, it is claimed that results obtained on human populations should always be replicated. Indeed, association with particular genetic polymorphisms and longevity is reported for some population but not for others. However, this is not strange because, as underlined by Capri et al. [73] human populations are characterized by specific gene pools that arise from the particular group's history in terms of chance (genetic drift) and environment (natural selection). Hence, replication cannot reasonably be expected for longevity in light of the considerations discussed in that study.

The suggestion that enhanced male life expectancy is associated with anti-inflammatory TLR4 SNP is interesting in view of the role of TLR-4 proinflammatory allele in the control of infectious diseases [25]. In order to rationalize these two seemingly conflicting situations, it might be argued that males carriers of the antiinflammatory allele who are lucky enough not to contact serious bacterial infection earlier in life may have an increased chance of long life survival (trade-off). However the same appears not to be true for female life expectancy [74].

References

1. Capri M, Salvioli S, Sevini F, et al (2006) The genetics of human longevity. Ann N Y Acad Sci 1067:252–263
2. Candore G, Colonna-Romano G, Balistreri CR, et al (2006) Biology of longevity: role of the innate immune system. Rejuvenation Res 9:143–148
3. Janeway CA Jr, Medzhitov R (2002) Innate immune recognition. Annu Rev Immunol 20:197–216
4. Uematsu S, Akira S (2006) PRRs in pathogen recognition. Cent Eur J Biol 1: 299–331
5. Uematsu S, Akira S (2006) Toll-like receptors and innate immunity. J Mol Med 84:712–725
6. Hashimoto C, Hudson KL, Anderson KV (1988) The toll gene of Drosophila, required for dorsal-ventral embryonic polarity, appears to encode a transmembrane protein. Cell 52:269–79
7. Medzhitov R, Preston-Hurlburt P, Janeway CA Jr (1997) A human homologue of the Drosophilatoll protein signals activation of adaptive immunity. Nature 388:394–397

8. Means TK, Golenbock DT, Fenton MJ (2000) The biology of toll-like receptors. Cyt Growth Fact Rev 11:219–232

9. Yoshimura A, Lien E, Ingalls RR et al (1999) Cutting edge. Recognition of Gram-positive bacterial cell wall components by the innate immune system occurs via Toll-like receptor 2. J Immunol 163:1–5

10. Qureshi ST, Lariviere L, Leveque G et al (1999) Endotoxin-tolerant mice have mutations in the TLR4 gene. J Exp Med 189:615–625

11. Hayashi F, Smith KD, Ozinsky A, et al (2001) The innate immune response to bacterial flagellin is mediated by Toll-like receptor 5. Nature 410:1099–1103

12. Hemmi H, Takeuchi O, Kawai T et al (2000) A Toll-like receptor recognizes bacterial DNA. Nature 408:740–745

13. Tsan MF, Gao B (2004) Endogenous ligands of Toll-like receptors. J Leukoc Biol 76:514–519

14. Beutler B (2005) The Toll-like receptors: analysis by forward genetic methods. Immunogenetics 57:385–392

15. Smirnova I, Poltorak A, Chan EKL et al (2000) Phylogenetic variation and polymorphism at the Toll-like receptor 4 locus (TLR4). Genome Biol 1:1–10

16. Biswas C, Mandal C (1999) The role of amoebocytes in endotoxinmediated coagulation in the innate immunity of Achatina fulica snails. Scand J Immunol 49:131–138

17. Iwanaga S (2002) The molecular basis of innate immunity in the horseshoe crab. Curr Opin Immunol 14:87–95

18. Smirnova I, Poltorak A, Chan EK et al (2000) Phylogenetic variation and polymorphism at the toll-like receptor 4 locus (TLR4). Genome Biol 1:1–10

19. Hajjar AM, Ernst RK, Tsai JH et al (2002) Human Toll-like receptor 4 recognizes host-specific LPS modifications. Nat Immunol 3:354–359

20. O'Neill LA, Dinarello CA (2000) The IL-1 receptor/toll-like receptor superfamily: crucial receptors for inflammation and host defense. Immunol Today 21:206–209

21. Akira S, Takeda K, Kaisho T (2001) Toll like receptors: critical proteins linking innate and acquired immunity. Nat Immunol 2:675–680

22. Reis e Sousa C (2001) Dendritic cells as sensors of infection. Immunity 14:495–498

23. Karin M, Lawrence T, Nizet V (2006) Innate immunity gone away: linking microbial infections to chronic inflammation and cancer. Cell 124:823–835

24. Cook DN, Pisetsky DS, Schwartz DA (2004) Toll-like receptors in the pathogenesis of human disease. Nat Immunol 5:975–979

25. Schroder NW, Schumann RR (2005) Single nucleotide polymorphisms of Toll-like receptors and susceptibility to infectious disease. Lancet Infect Dis 5:156–164

26. Lehnardt S, Massillon L, Follett P, et al (2003) Activation of innate immunity in the CNS triggers neurodegeneration through a Toll-like receptor 4-dependent pathway. Proc Natl Acad Sci U S A 100:8514–8519

27. Arbour NC, Lorenz, E, Schutte BC, et al (2000) TLR4 mutations are associated with endotoxin hyporesponsiveness in humans. Nat Genet 25:187–191

28. Kiechl S, Lorenz E, Reindl M, et al (2002) Toll-like receptor 4 polymorphisms and atherogenesis. N Engl J Med 347:185–192

29. Faure E, Thomas L, Xu H et al (2001) Bacterial lipopolysaccharide and IFN-gamma induce toll-like receptor 2 and toll-like receptor 4 expression in human endothelial cells: role of NF kappa B activation. J Immunol 166:2018–2024

30. Vink A, de Kleijn DP, Pasterkamp G (2004) Functional role for toll-like receptors in atherosclerosis and arterial remodeling. Curr Opin Lipidol 15:515–521

31. Pasterkamp G, Van Keulen JK, De Kleijn DP (2004) Role of Toll-like receptor 4 in the initiation and progression of atherosclerotic disease. Eur J Clin Invest 34:328–334

32. Bjorkbacka H (2006) Multiple roles of Toll-like receptor signaling in atherosclerosis. Curr Opin Lipidol 17:527–533

33. Mullick AE, Tobias PS, Curtiss LK (2006) Toll-like receptors and atherosclerosis: key contributors in disease and health? Immunol Res 34:193–209

34. Michelsen KS, Doherty TM, Shah PK, et al (2004) TLR signaling: an emerging bridge from innate immunity to atherogenesis. J Immunol 173:5901–5907
35. Michelsen KS, Doherty TM, Shah PK, et al (2004) Role of Toll-like receptors in atherosclerosis. Circ Res 95:e96–e97
36. Stoll LL, Denning GM, Weintraub NL (2006) Endotoxin, TLR4 signaling and vascular inflammation: potential therapeutic targets in cardiovascular disease. Curr Pharm Des 12:4229–4245
37. Vasto S, Candore G, Balistreri CR, et al (2007) Inflammatory networks in ageing, age-related diseases and longevity. Mech Ageing Dev 128:83–91
38. Ameziane N, Beillat T, Verpillat P, et al (2003) Association of the Toll-like receptor 4 gene Asp299Gly polymorphism with acute coronary events. Arterioscler Thromb Vasc Biol 23:e61–e64
39. Balistreri CR, Candore G, Colonna-Romano G, et al (2004) Role of Toll-like receptor 4 in acute myocardial infarction and longevity. JAMA 292:2339–2340
40. Edfeldt K, Bennet AM, Eriksson P, et al (2004) Association of hypo-responsive toll-like receptor 4 variants with risk of myocardial infarction. Eur Heart 25:1447–1453
41. Zee RY, Hegener HH, Gould J, et al (2005) Toll-like receptor 4 Asp299Gly gene polymorphism and risk of atherothrombosis. Stroke 36:154–157
42. Yang IA, Holloway JW, Ye S (2003) TLR4 Asp299Gly polymorphism is not associated with coronary artery stenosis. Atherosclerosis 170:187–190
43. Labrum R, Bevan S, Sitzer M, et al (2007) Toll receptor polymorphisms and carotid artery intima-media thickness. Stroke 38:1179–1184
44. O'Halloran AM, Stanton A, O'Brien E, et al (2006) The impact on coronary artery disease of common polymorphisms known to modulate responses to pathogens. Ann Hum Genet 70:934–945
45. Vainas T, Stassen FR, Bruggeman CA, et al (2006) Synergistic effect of Toll-like receptor 4 and CD14 polymorphisms on the total atherosclerosis burden in patients with peripheral arterial disease. J Vasc Surg 44:326–332
46. Nebel A, Flachsbart F, Schafer A, et al (2007) Role of the toll-like receptor 4 polymorphism Asp299Gly in longevity and myocardial infarction in German men. Mech Ageing Dev 128:409–411
47. Lehnardt S, Massillon L, Follett P, et al (2003) Activation of innate immunity in the CNS triggers neurodegeneration through a Toll-like receptor 4-dependent pathway. Proc Natl Acad Sci U S A 100:8514–8519
48. Lotz M, Ebert S, Esselmann H, et al (2005) Amyloid beta peptide 1-40 enhances the action of Toll-like receptor-2 and -4 agonists but antagonizes Toll-like receptor-9-induced inflammation in primary mouse microglial cell cultures. J Neurochem 94:289–298
49. Akiyama S, Barger S, Barnum B, et al (2000) Inflammation and Alzheimer's disease. Neurobiol Aging 21:383–421
50. Streit WJ (2004) Microglia and Alzheimer's disease pathogenesis. J Neurosci Res 77:1–8
51. Fassbender K, Walter S, Kuhl S, et al (2004) The LPS receptor (CD14) links innate immunity with Alzheimer's disease. FASEB J 18:203–215
52. Eikelenboom P, Bate C, Van Gool WA, et al (2002) Neuroinflammation in Alzheimer's disease and prion disease. Glia 40:232–239
53. Bsibsi M, Ravid R, Gveric D, et al (2002) Broad expression of Toll-like receptors in the human central nervous system. J Neuropathol Exp Neurol 61:1013–1021
54. Lucas SM, Rothwell NJ, Gibson RM (2006) The role of inflammation in CNS injury and disease. Br J Pharmacol 147 (Suppl 1):S232–S240
55. Finch CE, Morgan TE (2007) Systemic inflammation, infection, ApoE alleles, and Alzheimer disease: a position paper. Curr Alzheimer Res 4:185–189
56. Candore G, Balistreri CR, Grimaldi MP, et al (2007) Polymorphisms of pro-inflammatory genes and Alzheimer's disease risk: a pharmacogenomic approach. Mech Ageing Dev 128:67–75

57. Minoretti P, Gazzaruso C, Vito CD, et al (2006) Effect of the functional toll-like receptor 4 Asp299Gly polymorphism on susceptibility to late-onset Alzheimer's disease. Neurosci Lett 391:147–149

58. Caruso C, Lio D, Cavallone L, Franceschi C. (2004) Aging, longevity, inflammation, and cancer. Ann N Y Acad Sci 1028:1–13

59. Garza-Gonzalez E, Bosques-Padilla FJ, Mendoza-Ibarra SI et al (2007) Assessment of the toll-like receptor 4 Asp299Gly, Thr399Ile and interleukin-8 -251 polymorphisms in the risk for the development of distal gastric cancer. BMC Cancer 7:70

60. Kato I, Canzian F, Plummer M et al (2007) Polymorphisms in genes related to bacterial lipopolysaccharide/peptidoglycan signaling and gastric precancerous lesions in a population at high risk for gastric cancer. Dig Dis Sci 52:254–261

61. Landi S, Gemignani F, Bottari F (2006) Polymorphisms within inflammatory genes and color-ectal cancer. J Negat Results Biomed 5:15

62. Nieters A, Beckmann L, Deeg E et al (2006) Gene polymorphisms in Toll-like receptors, inter-leukin-10, and interleukin-10 receptor alpha and lymphoma risk. Genes Immun 7:615–624

63. Franceschi C, Motta L, Valensin S et al (2000) Do men and women follow different trajecto-ries to reach extreme longevity? Italian Multicenter Study on Centenarians (IMUSCE). Aging (Milano) 12:77–84

64. Evert J, Lawler E, Bogan H et al (2003) Morbidity profiles of centenarians: survivors,delayers, and escapers. J Gerontol A Biol Sci Med Sci 58:232–237

65. Gondo Y, Hirose N, Arai Y et al (2006) Functional status of centenarians in Tokyo, Japan: developing better phenotypes of exceptional longevity. J Gerontol A Biol Sci Med Sci 61:305–310.

66. De Benedictis G, Franceschi C (2006) The unusual genetics of human longevity. Sci Aging Knowledge Environ 10:pe20

67. Franceschi C, Bonafe M (2003) Centenarians as a model for healthy aging. Biochem Soc Trans 31:457–461

68. Perls T, Terry D (2003) Genetics of exceptional longevity. Exp Gerontol 38:725–730

69. Terry DF, Wilcox M, McCormick MA et al (2003) Cardiovascular advantages among the off-spring of centenarians. J Gerontol A Biol Sci Med Sci 58:425–431

70. Lio D, Candore G, Crivello A, et al. (2004) Opposite effects of interleukin 10 common gene polymorphisms in cardiovascular diseases and in successful ageing: genetic background of male centenarians is protective against coronary heart disease. J Med Genet 41:790–794

71. Nuzzo D, Vasto S, Balistreri CR, et al (2006) Role of proinflammatory alleles in longevity and atherosclerosis: results of studies performed on -1562C/T MMP-9 in centenarians and myocardial infarction patients from Sicily. Ann N Y Acad Sci.1089:496–501

72. Candore G, Balistreri CR, Grimaldi MP et al (2006) Opposite role of pro-inflammatory alleles in acute myocardial infarction and longevity: results of studies performed in a Sicilian popula-tion. Ann N Y Acad Sci 1067:270–5

73. Capri M, Salvioli S, Monti D et al (2007) Human longevity within an evolutionary perspec-tive: The peculiar paradigm of a post-reproductive genetics. Exp Gerontol 43:53–60

74. Balistreri CR, Candore G, Lio D, Colonna-Romano G et al (2005) Role of TLR4 receptor polymorphisms in Boutonneuse fever. Int J Immunopathol Pharmacol 18:655–660

Part III
Mechanisms - Receptors and Signal Transduction

Signal Transduction Changes in T-cells with Aging

Tamas Fulop, Gilles Dupuis, Carl Fortin and Anis Larbi

Contents

Abstract: There are several functions of T-lymphocytes which are altered with aging. The cause is not exactly known. However the changes in T-lymphocyte activation could be caused by the altered T-cell receptor (TCR) signaling after ligation. The recently described membrane lipid rafts (MR) are critical to the assembly of the TCR, the CD28 coreceptor and the IL-2 receptor signaling machinery. The defect in IL-2 production by CD4⁺ T-cells with aging is not due to lower levels of expres-

T. Fulop (✉)
Research Center on Aging, Department of Medicine
Immunology Graduate Programme, Faculty of Medicine
University of Sherbrooke, Sherbrooke, Quebec, Canada
E-mail: tamas .fulop@usherbrooke.ca

G. Dupuis
Clinical Research Center, Department of Biochemistry
Immunology Graduate Programme, Faculty of Medicine
University of Sherbrooke, Sherbrooke, Quebec, Canada

C. Fortin
Clinical Research Center, Immunology Graduate Programme, Faculty of Medicine
University of Sherbrooke, Sherbrooke, Quebec, Canada

A. Larbi
Center for Medical Research
Section for Transplant-Immunology and Immuno-Hematology
Tuebingen Aging and Tumor Immunology group
University of Tuebingen, Germany

T. Fulop et al. (eds.), *Handbook on Immunosenescence,*
DOI 10.1007/ 978-1-4020-9062-2_35, © Springer Science+Business Media B.V. 2009

sion of the TCR, CD28 or intracellular signaling molecules. However, there is a direct correlation between the activation of p56^{Lck} and LAT at the cellular level and their association/recruitment with the lipid raft fractions of CD4$^+$ and CD8$^+$ T-cells. p56^{Lck}, LAT and Akt/PKB are weakly phosphorylated in MR of stimulated CD4$^+$ T-cells of elderly as compared to young donors. Moreover, MR undergo changes in their lipid composition (ganglioside M1, cholesterol) with aging. There exists a differential role for lipid rafts in CD4$^+$ and CD8$^+$ T-cell activation with aging and consequently a differential localization of CD28 which may explain disparities in response to stimulation in human aging, mainly affecting the CD4$^+$ T-lymphocyte population.

Keywords: T-cells • CD4+ T-cells • CD8+ T-cells • Lipid rafts • Signal transduction • Aging Cholesterol • CD28 Coreceptor

1 Introduction

Most of the cell functions occur through specific receptors triggered by various ligands. T-cells possess several receptors which lead to their activation and to the maintenance of their activation status. Antigenic recognition by the T-cell receptor (TCR) triggers a series of biochemical events that result in the expression of a range of genes that are essential to T-cell responses, expansion and effector functions [1]. In addition, ligation of costimulatory CD28, that is required for interleukin-2 production and commitment to proliferation [2], enhances lipid raft polarization [3, 4]. Thus, CD28 triggering is essential for sustained T-cell activation [2]. Once IL-2 is secreted it will act in a paracrine manner on T-cells to trigger their clonal expansion via the IL-2 receptors. Membrane lipid rafts (MR) are dynamic structures and the time-dependent recruitment or exclusion of signaling proteins in these MR control T-cell activation and immune responses [5]. Moreover, lipid rafts are dynamic structures whose composition and function may vary according to cell types and cell subsets, especially in the case of T-lymphocytes [6]. Heterogeneity in MR composition and function may explain disparities in lymphocyte subset functions [7].

2 Signaling via TCR, CD28 and IL-2 Receptors and Their Changes with Aging

2.1 Receptors Involved in T-Lymphocyte Activation

The encounter of pathogens with lymphocytes will initiate their activation resulting in clonal expansion. The cascade of signaling molecules initiated by the stimulation of specific surface receptors results in the activation of several transcription factors. The most important receptors implicated in the clonal expansion of T-cells are the

TCR, the coreceptors including CD28 and the IL-2 cytokine receptor (IL-2R). These receptors function via an intracellular signaling cascade assuring the specificity and the fidelity of the expected response. T-cells need a first signal (signal 1) priming them to the possibility to respond by a clonal expansion to a specific antigen presented in the frame of a major histocompatibility complex (MHC) by an antigen-presenting cell (APC). This will assure that the whole membrane and the early signaling machinery is readily assembled to proceed toward the next stage, that is, the progression toward the full, sustained response. This is ensured by various coreceptors among which the most important is CD28, which represents signal 2. Signals transmitted by this receptor assure that the clonal expansion occurs via a sustained activation by the creation of the immune synapse (IS). Finally, as the concerted CD28 activation leads to the production of IL-2, it should also efficiently stimulate T-cells, representing signal 3. Altogether these receptors act for a complete response of T-cells assuring an adequate response to a specific antigen. With aging several studies have shown that the number of TCR is not changed. The CD28 number, claimed as a biomarker of aging, seems to decrease mainly in the case of a specific T-cell subpopulation, the memory CD8+ T-cells. These cells seem to represent a very late differentiated population characterizing immunosenescence [8]. These cells are the result of continuous chronic stimulations by antigens probably of viral origin including cytomegalovirus (CMV) and other herpes viruses, as similar changes were observed during CMV infection [9]. They are also the result of the low-grade chronic inflammation, however, the inflam-aging theory could not be validated in SENIEUR donors. One naturally arising question is whether this is a normal process related to aging, whether related to age-related disease processes or to the progressing frailty syndrome occurring in certain groups of elderly subjects. Our works suggest that in case of CD4+ T-cells the number of CD28 co-receptor is not decreasing, while it is decreasing in the CD8+ T-cell subpopulation [10]. Whether, the expression of IL-2R change during aging is still controversial, however, our work suggests a maintained expression in healthy elderly individuals. The TCR and CD28 are signaling via two specific cascades, however, there are more and more data suggesting that a cross-talk could exist between these two major pathways. We will describe these signaling pathways individually and in their cross-talk with a special emphasis on changes occurring with aging. However, first we will discuss MR and their role in signaling with special emphasis on the age-related changes.

2.2   Membrane Lipid Raft Function and Composition

One of the most important advances in membrane biology and consequently in the signaling field was the discovery of the existence of lipid rafts in the cell membrane that are now called membrane rafts (MR) [11]. These microdomains are composed mainly of satured lipids, cholesterol, glycosphyngolipids, GPI-anchored proteins, and posttranslationally modified proteins. These high-melting sphingolipids packed with cholesterol generate a liquid-ordered phase (lo) arrangement. This composition forms an efficient signaling platform necessary for an adequate signaling and cell response.

TCR ligation induces a redistribution of phosphorylated proteins into MR, which are highly compact relatively small domains (20–200 nM). The saturation of the lipids as well as the enrichment in cholesterol both allow the rafts to move through the membrane as discrete units. Their movement will be differentially segregated to the various poles of the cell depending on their main specific component, such as ganglioside M1 (GM1), GM3, or flotillin. The consequence of cell polarity is the asymmetric localization of membrane receptors and signaling molecules between the leading edge (at the cell front) and the uropod at the rear edge [12] This cell polarity will also influence the protein composition and the protein–protein interactions into the rafts. Data support the role of MR in the asymmetric distribution of membrane proteins during cell polarization. There is still a debate on which interactions direct and determine the MR movements and functions, and whether they involve cholesterol, membrane proteins, or both [13]. Experimental data seem to indicate that there could be several types of rafts playing different roles [14]. Furthermore, the role of MR is not limited to signal transduction, but also to lipid transport, virus entry, cell movement, as well as cell–cell communication. The accumulation or clusters of signaling molecules via MR initiate the formation of a signaling platform, which increases the efficiency of signaling. T-cell activation is the consequence of the interaction between the TCR and specific antigen presented by the APC. Signal 1 is occurring over a time frame of a few seconds but the interaction between T-cells and APC can be sustained for many hours. This prolonged interaction leads to the formation of the supramolecular activation cluster (SMAC) at the immunological synapse (IS). Thus, the sustained T-cell activation via organized MR signaling ultimately leads to the formation of a mature IS needed to achieve full T-cell activation through the contribution of CD28. The organization and composition of the membrane will directly modulate the formation of such a signaling platform, which ultimately influences cellular activation and functions. Thus, MR play a very important role in signaling by the formation of the signalosome, which are multicomponent transduction complexes. The correlation between the capacity of a molecule to be recruited into the IS and its preference for being linked to membrane rafts is still debated. However, very recent experimental evidence suggest that dynamic rafts reorganization at the IS favor T-cell activation by generating an environment where signal transduction is protected and essentially amplified [12]. Thus, the recruitment and clustering of MR within the IS segregate negative and positive actors of T-cell activation and protect TCR signaling.

Furthermore, the localization of molecules throughout the membrane is dependent on posttranslational modifications including acylation, farnesylation, and palmitoylation. Recently, it was demonstrated that LAT phosphorylation was not optimal in antigen-primed anergic CD4+ T-cells after TCR ligation [15]. It is of interest that LAT association with membrane rafts was defective in these CD4+ T-cells and this was partly explained by the impaired palmitoylation of LAT. It can be supposed that the posttranslational lipidation of the signaling molecules targeting them to MR under stimulation is altered with aging. In T-cells some of the signaling machinery is constitutively included in MR, such as the TCR, Lck, while other molecules are recruited during activation, such as CD28, IL-2R, LAT, PI3K. It is of note that we presented evidence that CD4+ and CD8+ T-cells require differential activation [10].

The signaling machinery in CD4+ T-cells relies on MR for its assembly, while in CD8+ T-cells a certain preassembly of the signalosome decreases the necessity of MR for adequate signaling. This could be perhaps explained by the differential fate of these two T-cell subpopulations. There are still numerous questions to answer on the role of MR in T-cell activation and IS formation, nevertheless, a consensus exists, which states that in a way or another MR participate in T-cell activation.

2.3 The Contribution of Membrane Lipid Rafts to the Altered-T-Lymphocyte Functions with Aging

We have reported an alteration in the function of MR with aging. MR poorly coalesce in CD4$^+$ T-cells of elderly subjects [10] although the alterations are less pronounced in the case of CD8$^+$ T-cells. We have also reported alterations in the recruitment and activation of Lck and LAT into MR of T-cells from aged humans [16]. One important finding was that CD28 and IL-2R were weakly recruited to MR in CD4$^+$T-cells of elderly subjects. In contrast, these proteins were already located to MR in CD8$^+$ T-cells from elderly subjects prior to stimulation. These observations suggested that the assembly of the signaling machinery in CD4$^+$ T-cells relies largely on MR, whereas in CD8$^+$ T-cells a preassembly of the signalosome has been suggested by us [10] and by others [6, 7].

Moreover, MR of CD4$^+$ and CD8$^+$ T-cells behave differently in polarization experiments induced by anti-TCR/CD28-coated beads. While the beads induced MR polarization to the region of contact in CD4$^+$ T-cells of young and elderly individuals, the beads failed to induce coalescence in CD8$^+$ T-cells of both groups of donors. Recently, it was supposed that the expression of CD8 gives to the cell a "dominant-negative" phenotype towards MR polarization [6] as it occurred in immature CD4$^+$CD8$^+$ T-cells [18]. Thus, MR functions may be settled on during T-cell selection by an unknown mechanism. Altogether these data suggest that CD4$^+$ T-cells heavily rely on MR to reach a full state of activation, while CD8$^+$ T-cells due to their pre-existing signalosome could circumvent "lipid rafting." This raised the possibility that similar age-related changes in MR cholesterol composition may affect differentially CD4$^+$ and CD8$^+$ T-cells, the former being much more affected.

To further support the hypothesis that the properties of the signalosome in CD8$^+$ T-cells differ from that of CD4$^+$ T-cells we assessed the effect of MR disruption on T-cell proliferation. Data revealed that CD8$^+$ T-cells were less sensitive to a low concentration (0.5 mM) of β-methyl cyclodextrin, a MR disrupting agent, as compared to CD4$^+$ T-cells. Whereas the proliferative response of CD4$^+$ T-cells of young and elderly donors was completely abolished, there still remained a partial response of CD8$^+$ T-cells to TCR/CD28 stimulation. These observations suggested differential intrinsic properties of MR in CD4$^+$ T-cells as compared to CD8$^+$ T-cells which may result in a differential mode of signaling. These data may also explain the differential kinetic of IL-2 production by CD4$^+$ and CD8$^+$ T-cells.

One key component of MR is cholesterol which serves to stabilize their structure and to modulate their fluidity [19]. The concentration of cholesterol was 1.6-fold higher in MR fractions from CD4+ and CD8+ T-cells of elderly subjects as compared to young individuals. The anisotropy of CD4+ and CD8+ T-cells and MR fractions prepared from these cells was increased by approximately 10% in the case of elderly donors, suggesting an inverse correlation between MR cholesterol content and plasma membrane fluidity. The cause of the increase in the concentration of cholesterol in resting T-cells with aging is not known but may be the result of an imbalance in cellular cholesterol metabolism. Preliminary data from our laboratories indicate that significant changes occur with aging in the HDL-mediated reverse cholesterol transport. This mechanism is membrane raft-dependent [20] and suggests that its deregulation may contribute to the elevated plasma membrane cholesterol content in T-lymphocytes from normolipemic elderly humans. Altogether the increased cholesterol content and decreased fluidity of the membrane found here in both T-cells subsets reinforce our previous data in T-cells [21], contributing to functional decrease, however can not give an explanation for the differential functional behavior between these T-cells subsets. In this context another question arises concerning the properties of the lipids ordering the lipid rafts. We showed a quantitative increase in rafts cholesterol with aging but changes in oxidative status should alter MR properties and functioning as well. Since CD8+ T-cells possess a cytotoxic activity via their granules, they may be gifted with a higher potency towards oxidation and other aggressions than CD4+ T-cells also explaining why they were less affected by immune senescence. Moreover, unsatured fatty acids were shown to inhibit T-cells activation and functions by selectively displacing signaling molecules from MR. Thus, changes in fatty acids composition may also explain discrepancies between young and elderly donors as well as between CD4+ and CD8+ T-cells from the same donor. We are currently addressing these questions.

In view of the alterations in plasma membrane cholesterol concentration in MR, we also analyzed the distribution of the GM1. The GM1 fluorescence intensity in CD4+ and CD8+ T-cells of elderly individuals was more than two-fold than that measured in the corresponding T-cells of young donors. The increase in GM1 may have critical effects on T-cell functions that depend on MR, namely the recruitment of proteins involved in the early events of signaling. In this connection, it has been reported that over-expression of membrane microdomains constituent such as GM1 in PC12 cells can suppress nerve growth factor signals by modulating signal-transducing molecules localization and plasma membrane fluidity [22]. As a corollary, high levels of GM1 in MR of resting CD4+ T-cells of elderly individuals may interfere with GM1 turnover [23] resulting in defects in early T-cell signaling as well as in IL-2 production.

The end-point of MR function is to induce the formation of the IS via SMAC [24, 25]. The data of O'Keefe et al. [26] showed that the formation of SMAC is not required for activation of naïve CD8+ T-cells, giving support to the differential sensitivity of activation between CD4+ and CD8+ T-lymphocytes. This reinforces our hypothesis that CD4+ T-cells did not behave in the same manner as CD8+ T-cells in aging due do their differential mode of signalling. The triggering of CD28 is a critical step for MR polarization which results in SMAC formation leading ultimately to IL-2 production [27]. Differential alterations in the CD28 signaling between CD4+ and CD8+ T-cells subsets may clearly explain the functional alterations of MR with aging leading to altered signaling and function mainly in CD4+ T-cells, as will be described below.

2.4   T-cell Receptor Signalling and its Changes with Aging

T-lymphocyte activation culminates in cell proliferation and differentiation into effector and memory cells. The engagement of the receptors by duly presented antigens leads to a specific response driven by the signaling cascade. At the very early step of T-cell activation there are several key events that determine the specificity and the intensity of T-cell response. The first step in TCR-mediated signaling is the activation of different tyrosine kinases, leading to the tyrosine phosphorylation of several downstream molecules. The first signal through the TCR induces the phosphorylation of Lck, via recruitment of ZAP-70 leading to LAT phosphorylation (see Figure 1) which becomes a scaffold for the recruitment of multiple partners including other adaptor proteins and enzymes involved in phospholipid metabolism such as phosphatidyli-nositol-3-kinase (PI3K) and phospholipase-Cγ1 (PLC-γ1). A host of experimental data support the view that many proteins involved in T-cell signaling such as p56^{Lck}, LAT, SLP-76, protein kinase-Cθ and Gads are recruited in MR, whereas others such as CD45 are excluded [28] or transiently associated as in the case of CD4 [29].

The activation of Lck is a very tightly controlled process, which involves phosphatases, such as CD45 and the tyrosine kinases Csk, as well as regulatory molecules, such as Cbp/PAG and FynT. The control of Lck activation involves the tyrosine phosphatase CD45 and the PTK Csk which is regulated by the MR-resident Cbp/PAG and FynT, as well as the CaMKII substrate, cytosolic resident C3BP [30–32]. Csk is a ubiquitously expressed cytosolic PTK; it plays a negative regulatory role in cells by inhibiting intracellular processes induced by Src tyrosine kinases. The Csk SH2 domain interacts specifically with several tyrosine phosphorylated molecules and among them with the recently identified adaptor-Csk-binding protein/phosphoprotein associated with glycosphyngolipid-enriched microdomains (Cbp/PAG). Cbp/PAG has been shown to be palmitoylated and targeted to rafts. In resting human T-cells Cbp/PAG is constitutively phosphorylated and this results in recruitment of Csk to the rafts. This interaction increases the catalytic activity of Csk on its substrate, thereby inhibiting Src tyrosine kinases activity. However, this interaction is reversible. The dephosphorylation of Cbp/PAG releases Csk and promotes the activation of Src kinases upon TCR stimulation. This represents a sort of threshold regulator in T-cell activation. So far, no data exist concerning the activity of these factors with aging. However, it can be hypothesized that the interaction between Cbp/PAG and Csk is altered, therefore affecting the release of Csk.

With aging there is a well-known deregulation of the immune response. This deregulation is mainly the reflection of alterations in the cellular immune response mediated by T-lymphocytes. The main alterations are the decreased proliferation due to reduced IL-2 production leading to altered clonal expansion. The causes of this decline are not well understood, however, many explanations have been proposed.

One hypothesis to explain this observation suggests alterations in TCR-dependent signaling. During the past few years our laboratory has greatly contributed to the elucidation of the multiple changes in TCR signal transduction [16]. We and others have shown that several steps of the signaling cascade following TCR ligation are altered with aging [33]. However, much effort has focused on downstream events of T-cell signaling and less attention has been given to possible alterations in upstream events [34, 35], including the assembly of signaling molecules in MR. Recently, we have presented evidence that the age-related alterations in T-cell activation are linked to changes in MR composition and function [16]. It is now well documented that other early events related to protein tyrosine phosphorylation following TCR activation are altered in T-cells with aging, such as the generation of myoinositol 1, 4, 5-trisphosphate, intracellular free calcium mobilization, and PKC translocation to the membrane. It was also shown that defects in translocation of PKC following TCR stimulation are present in T-cells of old humans [15] and mice. Recently, our work showed that the activation, that is, tyrosine phosphorylation of the upstream molecules, such as Lck and LAT was also altered with aging. Thus, with aging we observe an alteration in all activation phases of T-cell signaling. This activation via the intermediate signaling events finally should lead to the activation of NFAT and NF-kB for the production of IL-2, which is consequently also altered with aging (Fig.1).

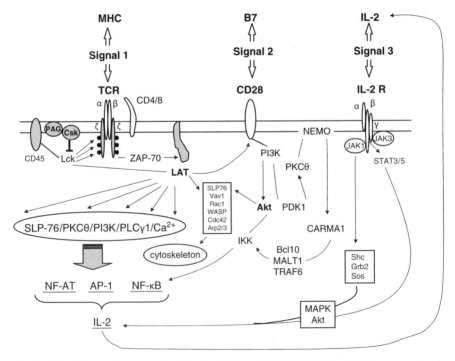

Fig. 1 Signalling pathways involved in signal 1, 2, and 3. TCR, CD28 and IL-2 receptor signalling is shown. The signalling events shown here are described and quoted throughout this review

Recently, data clearly showed that changes in MR machinery also occur in autoimmune diseases such as in systemic lupus erythematosus (SLE). Jury et al. [36, 37] demonstrated in their paper that p56^{Lck} was over-associated in MR of CD3$^+$ T-cells explaining the hyperactivity of these cells in SLE patients. Based on the data presented, we suggest that the changes in MR composition and functions lead to impaired p56^{Lck} activation and may be the main cause of the alterations in CD4$^+$ T-cell functions and consequently in immune senescence.

2.5   CD28 Dependent Signaling and Their Changes with Aging

For an efficient T-lymphocyte activation, the T-cell co-receptors (e.g., CD28, ICOS) should also be activated by their ligands (e.g., CD80/CD86) expressed on antigen presenting cells (APC) [38–41]. Certain pathways seem to be privileged and among them the phophatidylinositol 3-kinase (PI-3K; *See* Fig. 1). The main components of the PI-3K pathway include the following molecules PI-3K→Akt→IKK→NF-κB and PI-3K→PDK-1→PKCθ→IKK→NF-κB from which certain are recruited to MR. Interestingly, the CD28 pathway also activates the Lck, LAT, SLP-76, Grb2/GADS, Vav and the protein phosphatase PP2A [42–45]. Ultimately this co-stimulatory pathway regulate the translocation of NF-AT and NF-κB [46, 47]. The cytoplasmic tail of CD28 is phosphorylated by Lck which in turn initiate the recruitment and activation of PI-3K [48]. PI-3K initiates the translocation of Akt (PKB) in MR following its phosphorylation by PDK1. PDK1 is inserted in MR and phosphorylates PKCθ which leads to the activation of the latter molecule. The activated PKCθ recruit NEMO to MR and activates, via CARMA1 (CARD11), the complex Bcl10/MALT1/ TRAF6 [43–45]. This complex induces the ubiquitination of IKK, its degradation by the proteasome and, finally the activation of NF-kB and the translocation of the Rel proteins to the nucleus. Thus, PI-3K and Akt are the essential early components for the induction of T-lymphocytes functions by the concurrent and/or individual activation of TCR et CD28 [45, 49]. All these events assure that IL-2 will be produced and secreted. As the level of CD28 expression is decreasing with aging this could contribute to the diminished production of IL-2 via an altered T-lymphocyte signaling, leading ultimately to a decreased T-lymphocyte clonal expansion.

Our recent work indicates that CD28 signaling leading to the phosphorylation of Akt is decreased mainly in CD4$^+$ T-cells from aged individuals. Akt was weakly activated in CD4$^+$ T-cells of elderly subjects but not in the case of CD8$^+$ T-cells. These data indicate a critical alteration in CD28 signaling in CD4$^+$ T-cells of elderly subjects, which can not be explained by the slight change in CD28 expression. Paradoxically, the marked increase in CD28^{low} CD8$^+$ T-cells did not affect Akt activation. This further contributes to the decrease of NF-κB activation in mice and in humans already shown to be due to a decreased inactivation of IκB by the proteasome. Moreover, in view of the pleiotropic effects of Akt, its decreased activation also suggested that in CD4$^+$ T-cells, downstream signaling events including the up-regulation of the transcription factors, NF-kB and NF-AT, would be impaired and that would result in defects in cytoskeletal rearrangements, cell cycling and ultimately in a decreased production of IL-2 in T-cells. We have also demonstrated that the CD28 number only partly explains the inability to activate adequately T-cells as Akt activation was more efficient in CD8[+] T-cells, having reduced CD28 co-receptors, compared to CD4[+] T-cells, having relatively conserved CD28 co-receptor number with aging. Our most recent results seemed to suggest that this is not the decreased number of CD28 co-receptors which plays the crucial role but the altered CD28 localization as a determinant factor of the immunosenescence [10]. Thus, changes in the CD28 co-receptor signaling might have far reaching consequences on T-cell functions in aging.

These findings explain one very important finding in immunosenescence which is the differential sensitivity of CD4[+] and CD8[+] T-cells towards activation induced cell death (AICD). CD4[+] T-cells are more susceptible to AICD than CD8[+] T-cells [50]. This can be explained by the differential signaling of CD28 towards Akt activation as this pathway mediates the survival/apoptosis of T-cells. Moreover, we already published data showing that the level of expression of a special receptor is not the best marker for cellular function but its differential membrane localization, such as for Toll-like receptors [51] and/or signaling molecules will ultimately influence cell fate and this immune function.

2.6   Convergence of TCR/CD28 Signaling Pathways in T-cells Activation and Their Changes with Aging

The signaling pathways elicited by TCR and CD28 converge for inducing the translocation of NF-κB and initiate the transcription of the IL-2 gene. It was suggested that the amplification of the signaling cascade initiated by the TCR is mainly dependent on CD28 for the polarization of MR [47]. Indeed, the engagement of CD28 induces the redistribution of MR enriched in GM1 at the site of TCR contact with APC. CD28 generates a favorable environment where the signals are protected, segregated and amplified. This prolonged physical stability between the T-lymphocyte and APC is fundamental to the production of IL-2 and to the clonal expansion of T-lymphocytes [40]. The IS formation is occurring after the MR polarization. The IS is a special spatial region highly organized containing signaling proteins, adhesion and cytoskeleton molecules [3, 24, 52, 53]. In this context, it is of note that the activation of CD4[+] and CD8[+] lymphocytes differ in their dynamics. The CD4[+] necessitate a prolonged activation to be able to proliferate, while a hour contact is enough in case of CD8[+] lymphocytes [54]. Three different studies including our suggest a differential role for MR in the activation of CD4[+] and CD8[+] cells [6, 10, 17] as described above.

In summary, with aging, there is an alteration of T-cell signaling either in signal 1 or signal 2 or both. As already described there are many alterations in the signaling cascade of T-cells, including calcium metabolism, tyrosine kinases phosphorylation, and PKC translocation to the membrane. Moreover, it is now well accepted that there are alterations in the very early stages of the signaling cascade, that is, in the composition and function of MR. There is an increase in cholesterol and sphingolipid content, while a decrease in Lck and LAT tyrosine phosphorylation was observed. Not only was the composition of membrane raft found altered but also their functions. With aging MR polarize much less than do those of young subjects. These changes, taking into account what was described above concerning the role of MR in IS formation, underline the functional changes observed in T-cells with aging. It is of note that various subpopulations of T-cells are differently affected. CD4+ cells are most affected by these signal transduction changes with aging, whereas although CD8+ T-cells are also affected, their reactivity is better maintained than that of CD4+ T-cells. Nevertheless, one should also consider the changes within CD8 and CD4 susbets, i.e., naïve versus memory cells. This will need further investigations to identify whether the loss of cellular functions and signaling are only due to loss of CD28 expression (in the memory cells) or has another origin.

2.7   IL-2 Signalling and its Changes with Aging

IL-2 is one of the most important cytokine for T-cells representing the "signal 3" for the efficient clonal expansion of T-cells under antigenic stimulation [55]. IL-2 receptor is composed of several subunits having specific role, however only the β subunit is involved in the signaling initiation [56, 57]. Whether this subunit is associated with MR for effective signaling is still controversial. Nevertheless, the signaling cascade is well known. The ligand attachment to the IL-2 receptor is initiating the activation by tyrosine phosphorylation of Janus kinases 3 (JAK3), which in turn activates the signal transducer and activator of transcription 3 and 5 (STAT3 and STAT5) [58, 59]. This results in the translocation to the nucleus of these transcription factors which initiates the cellular response of proliferation [60]. The Jak/STAT pathway is a rapid intracellular communication system used by many cytokines and growth factors to mediate signals from the plasma membrane to the nucleus in order to regulate proliferation and differentiation of most tissue types (See Fig. 1). These pathways play a crucial role in the induction of the T-cell response to these cytokines namely clonal expansion [60, 61]. Many factors are controlling the Jak/STAT pathways which are also zinc dependent [62]. Furthermore, the Jak/STAT is one of the signaling pathway which is sensitive to redox conditions [63, 64].

In T-cells from elderly individuals we reported recently an alteration in IL-2 receptor signal transduction resulting in decreased JAK3 and STAT3/5 activation [65]. Thus, aging is accompanied with a signaling defect of the cytokine receptors IL-2 independently of the receptor number, as was already demonstrated [21] except for the very elderly aged over 90 years. This latter phenomenon seems to be in accordance with studies demonstrating less immune dysfunction in old old compared to young old individuals suggesting a contribution of an intact immune system to longevity. It is of note that zinc supplemented at physiological doses could not modulate the altered IL-2 signaling of individuals aged up to 90 years old. This suggests that either the normal zinc levels in T-cells are not sensitive to a supplementation or that the zinc mediated processes including anti-oxidant, anti-inflammatory, membrane physiology maintenance are not major players in the altered signaling. Indeed, as we have shown, one of the basic age-related alterations affects the membrane composition [10]. In contrast, over 90 years old, the zinc could reverse the negative signaling effect of IL-2 indicating that the physiological behavior of T-cells of old–old individuals is fundamentally different. This needs further studies to determine the mechanism by which zinc is acting but it can be hypothesized that the inhibitory molecules like Protein inhibitor of activated STATs (PIAS) can be more efficiently modulated at this age [66]. This indicates that in T-lymphocyte activation one should always take into account the negative regulatory factors too.

3 Membrane Lipid Rafts and Cytoskeleton

T-cell activation involves F-actin rearrangements. Several molecules which are associated with DRM participate in tethering DRM to the actin cytoskeleton. Actin polymerization is regulated by the RhoGTPase Rac1 which activates WASP and Cdc42 which upreglulates the activity of Scar/WAVE. Activation of WASP and WAVE stimulates F-actin branching by upregulating the activity of the Arp2/3 complex [67]. The interaction between DRM and the actin cytoskeleton works in two directions: DRM-associated proteins regulate F-actin rearrangements whereas the actin cytoskeleton serves to induce and sustain DRM polarization in activated cells. During the formation of IS, CD28 is responsible for actin rearrangement and the coalescence of DRM. In addition, the adaptors Vav1 and Slp76 are key regulators of actin rearrangements required for the accumulation of signaling molecules/DRM at the T-cell/APC interface. The upregulation of Vav1 activity by CD28 is achieved through Lck. Thus, Lck is involved in CD28-related actin remodeling, MR coalescence and T-cell activation. A decade ago, it was found that F-actin polymerization was altered in T-cells of elderly under stimulation. No data in relation to MR exist, however, considering the alterations found in their composition and function in T-cells with aging we can suggest that the F-actin rearrangements could also be deficient in aging. Taken together, it can be concluded that with aging there is an alteration in T-cell activation due to a deregulation of the intracellular signaling pathways via an alteration of the T-cell membrane composition leading to altered functions, such as proliferation and IL-2 production. Although F-actin polymerization has been reported to be altered in lymphocytes of aged mice [68], there are no data in T-cells with respect to actin reorganization in young or elderly subjects and the relationship to MR.

4 Negative Regulation of T-Lymphocyte Activation and its Changes with Aging

Lymphocytes are not only positively activated by kinases but also negatively. This can be at the level of various molecules of the signaling cascade or the termination of the activation process. One way to negatively regulate T-lymphocyte activation is through protein phosphatases (PPases). In addition to the kinase component of T-cell activation, it exists other enzymes which intervene in the negative regulation of the signaling cascade such as the PPases and the phosphatidylinositol (PtdIns) phosphatases [69, 70]. The most important targets of PPases are the activation pathways of Lck and PI-3K. SHP-1 dephosphorylates and inhibits PI-3K [47, 71]. The PPase SHIP and the PtdIns phosphatase PTEN converge for the negative regulation of PI-3K. While SHIP hydrolyses the phosphate groups on phosphotyrosine residues of PI-3K, the PTEN cut the phosphate groups in position 3 of PtdIns-3, 4, 5 trisphosphates, destroying recognition site by the PH domain of PI-3K [71–73]. The activity of PPases, which is as finely regulated as that of protein kinases, ultimately also depends on their interaction with MR. This is clearly demonstrated for the modulation of CD45 activity [74–76] and as we have demonstrated for the PPase SHP-1 [77]. CD45, when located in MR has a positive effect on Lck activation, while when CD45 is displaced, such as in the quiescent state, Lck is inactivated. We have recently shown a similar phenomenon for SHP-1 in neutrophils [77]. There is more and more experimental evidence that the balance between tyrosine kinases and phosphatases is essential for the maintenance of the resting status and for activation, which can predict alterations with aging. Only a few data exist concerning phosphatase activity in T-cells with aging. CD45 is a receptor-like phosphatase expressed on all nucleated hematopoietic cells. One key function of CD45 is to serve as a positive regulator of Src tyrosine kinases, by opposing Csk function, and dephosphorylating the negative regulatory C terminal tyrosine of Src tyrosine kinases. CD45-protein tyrosine phosphatase activity in old T-cells was found to be decreased compared to young cells [78]. However, it may be necessary to reassess the behavior of CD45 under activation in terms of its involvement in the IS, from which it is usually excluded upon T-cell activation. Our own studies using cholesterol repletion of T-cells from young subjects, being a partial aging model of T-cells, suggest alterations in phosphatase activities (our unpublished data). Furthermore, because in neutrophils which are very short-lived cells important alterations were found for SHP-1 activity, it can be suggested that phosphatase activities might also be altered with aging in long-lived cells such as T-cells. Our very recent data indicate that there is much more SHP-1 content in the membrane of T-cells from elderly compared to young subjects [79]. The activity of SHP-1 is also increased in T-cells of elderly as determined by tyrosine phosphorylation following anti-CD3 and anti-CD28 stimulations compared to identical conditions in T-cells of young subjects. The exact significance of this increased activity is not well understood, but could have a negative effect on Lck activation [80]. Altogether, there are interestingly very few data concerning the phosphatase activity in relation to TCR activation. Certainly, no data exist concerning their association/recruitment to MR. This should be further explored in the future.

The other way to negatively regulate T-lymphocyte activation is by scaffold Homer proteins. The Homer proteins are composed of three members. These proteins expressed in several tissues were found in MR of glial cells. These Homer proteins were, until very recently, associated to Ca^{2+} mobilization, following their interaction with TRP canonics (TRPC) [81]. However a recent publication of Huang and al [82] clearly demonstrate that Homer2 and Homer3 are negative regulators of lymphocyte activation. These proteins compete with calcineurin for NF-AT. This competition stops the calcineurin-dependent dephosphorylation of NF-AT and its subsequent translocation to the nucleus. These results raise the possibility that Homer (1, 2 ou 3) could be differentially recruited in MR of lymphocytes in elderly subjects. A preferential and sustained recruitment of Homer in MR could contribute to the diminution of the immune response of elderly subjects.

Thus, most of the early signaling events were shown to be altered with aging in human T-cells especially in CD4[+] T-cells. Thus, it would be very difficult to assign the alteration in T-cell activation to any of the participating signaling molecules. Then, what can be the cause of these signaling alterations in T-cells occurring during immunosenescence? Could a common change explain this signaling alteration in T-cells upon activation? Investigations in the late 1980s already suggested that biochemical and biophysical alterations of the cell membrane could be responsible for the altered immune response with aging. Alterations in the lipid composition and fluidity of the cell membrane were found [83]. One explanation that is naturally emerging is the changes at the membrane level either qualitatively or quantitatively.

5   Membrane Composition Changes with Aging: Role of Cholesterol

It was suggested several decades ago that the T-cell membrane from elderly subjects is more rigid than that of young subjects [83]. We recently presented evidence that an increase in free cholesterol could explain these physicochemical changes observed about 20 years ago [19]. There is a twofold increase in the T-cell membrane cholesterol content with aging. Cholesterol is an essential component of the membrane as it maintains a certain order in the plasma membrane structure, as it is now well recognized, through the MR (*See* Fig. 2). This increase in cholesterol content leads to the contention that if we can extract the overcharge we would be able to restore T-cell functions. Unfortunately, until now only partial restoration of the functions was obtained. Methyl-β-cyclodextrin (MBCD) used in small quantities has so many other membrane disturbing effects that no functional improvement was observed in T-cells of elderly [21, 84]. Statin (which inhibits cholesterol synthesis via the inhibition of the HMG-CoA reductase) used at high concentrations necessary to see a reduction in cellular cholesterol levels in Jurkat cells resulted in apoptotic death [51]. The only known physiological cholesterol extracting agent is high-density lipoprotein (HDL). HDL via the reverse transport of cholesterol is able to decrease the membrane cholesterol content very rapidly, but it was much less efficient in case of T-cells of elderly (our unpublished data). Nevertheless, the proliferation and IL-2 production of T-cells of elderly were slightly improved.

The other way to assess the role of cholesterol is to replenish the membrane of T-cells of young subjects with cholesterol to the level observed in T-cells of elderly subjects. Our results with the replenishment with free cholesterol have shown a decrease in proliferation and IL-2 secretion, such as observed in immunosenescence. Thus, increased cholesterol in the membrane of T-cells from young subjects

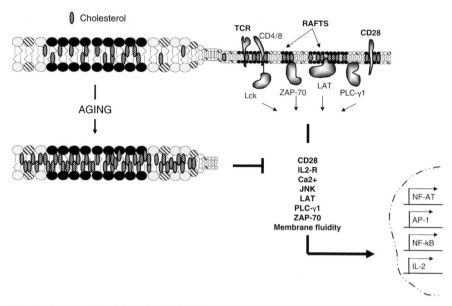

Fig. 2 Age-associated alterations in TCR signaling. TCR signaling events which are altered with aging are depicted here. Non-cited molecules or pathways are not changing with age. The relevant reference can be find throughout this review

rendered them functionally aged. In the mean time the GM-1 content in the membrane is increased. There is no explanation why the cholesterol is increasing as the serum cholesterol content is remaining unchanged in elderly subjects. It could be that the cholesterol uptake is dysregulated, the intracellular cholesterol production via the HMG-CoA reductase can be increased, or that the reverse cholesterol transport assured by HDL is deficient. Our recent experimental data seem to indicate that the reverse transport of cholesterol by HDL is indeed altered in T-cells with aging.

6   Do Membrane Rafts Properties Contribute to Human Immunosenescence?

Considering all the changes described above the question naturally arises what is the role of MR and could changes in their composition and in their function contribute to the altered T-cell activation observed during immunosenescence? The experimental data presented so far seem to support a positive answer to this question. With aging, as described above, we demonstrated an alteration in the function of the MR as they are almost unable to coalesce in CD4+ T-cells with aging. The alterations are less dramatic for CD8+ T-cells. We have demonstrated an alteration in the recruitment and activation of Lck and LAT into MR. In this context one of the most important findings is that the CD28 as well as the IL-2R cannot be recruited to the membrane rafts in CD4+ T-cells of elderly subjects explaining the alteration of the signaling of these receptors with aging. In contrast, in CD8$^+$ T-cells these receptors are already recruited to the MR. Thus, the age-associated alterations in their properties include the increase in cholesterol content, impaired coalescence, and selective differences in the recruitment of key proteins involved in TCR signaling. It can be thus hypothesized taking into account these experimental data that the increased rigidity of the membrane following the increase in cholesterol content limits MR functionality. This loss of function leads to the inability to recruit to the IS the necessary machinery or alternatively to exclude the nonparticipating molecules to reach an adequate activation, which is a hallmark of immunosenescence.

7   Conclusion

With aging we observe an alteration of the immune response collectively designated as immunosenescence. One of its most striking aspects is the altered T-cell activation for clonal expansion by specific antigens. The causes of this decreased activation are not completely known. Recent studies shed light on the role of signaling alterations following TCR and CD28 ligation. The final outcome of protein rafting is the formation of the IS, which is needed to sustain the activation, which will result in a proper immune response. We can document changes in molecular events with aging, but we are not yet able to explain these changes. The ultimate defect in signaling can be explained by the newly discovered membrane rafts alterations in composition, function, and size with aging. These functional and physicochemical properties are influenced by intrinsic as well as extrinsic factors. Understanding the events that lead to changes in the TCR signaling cascade would be of great benefit considering the large number of diseases in which MR dysfunction is thought to play a role. Altogether these data suggest that MR alterations in T-cells do contribute to immunosenescence.

Acknowledgments   This work was partly supported by a grant-in aid from the Canadian Institute of Health Research (No 63149), Research Center on Aging, the Faculty of Medicine of the University of Sherbrooke, ZINCAGE project (EU contract n. FOOD-CT-2003-506850), T-cells and Aging "T-CIA" (QLK6-CT-2002 02283), the Deutsche Forschungsgemeinschaft (DFG PA 361/11-1 and SFB 685-B4), the Fortune Program (of Tübingen University Medical School). We thank the Clinical Research Center for assistance and access to microscopes.

References

1. Margulies DH (1997) Interactions of TCRs with MHC-peptide complexes: a quantitative basis for mechanistic models. Curr Opin Immunol 9:390–395
2. Wells AD, Gudmundsdottir H, Turka LA, J (1997) Following the fate of individual T-cells throughout activation and clonal expansion. Signals from T-cell receptor and CD28 dif-

ferentially regulate the induction and duration of a proliferative response. Clin Invest 100:3173–3183

3. Viola A, Schroeder S, Sakakibara Y, Lanzavecchia A (1999) T-lymphocyte costimulation mediated by reorganization of membrane microdomains. Science 283:680–682

4. Marmor MD, Julius M (2001) Role for lipid rafts in regulating interleukin-2 receptor signaling Blood 98:1489–1497

5. Alonso MA, Millan J (2001) The role of lipid rafts in signalling and membrane trafficking in T lymphocytes. J Cell Sci 114:3957–3965

6. Kovacs B, Maus MV, Riley JL, Derimanov GS, Koretzky GA, June CH, Finkel TH (2002) Human CD8+ T-cells do not require the polarization of lipid rafts for activation and proliferation. Proc Natl Acad Sci 99:15006–15011

7. Pike LJ (2004) Lipid rafts: heterogeneity on the high seas. Biochem J 378:281–292

8. Effros RB (2004) Replicative senescence of CD8 T-cells: effect of human aging. Exp Gerontol 39:517–524

9. Koch S, Larbi A, Ozcelik D, Solana R, Gouttefangeas C, Attig S, Wikby A, Strindhall J, Franceschi C, Pawelec G (2007) Cytomegalovirus infection: a driving force in human T-cell immunosenescence. Ann N Y Acad Sci 1114:23–35

10. Larbi A, Dupuis G, Khalil A, Douziech N, Fortin C, Fülöp T Jr (2006) Differential role of lipid rafts in the functions of CD4+ and CD8+ human T lymphocytes with aging. Cell Signal 18:1017–1030

11. Hanzal-Bayer MF, Hancock JF (2007) Lipid rafts and membrane traffic. FEBS Lett 581:2098–104

12. Manes S, Viola A (2006) Lipid rafts in lymphocytes activation and migration. Molec Membr Biol 23:59–69

13. Douglass AD, Vale RD (2005) Single-molecule microscopy reveals plasma membrane microdomains created by protein-protein networks that exclude or trap signaling molecules in T-cells. Cell 121:937–950

14. Mishra S, Joshi PG (2007) Lipid raft heterogeneity: an enigma. J Neurochem 103 (Suppl 1):135–42

15. Hundt M, Tabata H, Jeon MS, Hayashi K, Tanaka Y, Krishna R, De Giorgio L, Liu YC, Fukata M, Altman A (2006) Impaired activation and localization of LAT in anergic T-cells as a consequence of a selective palmitoylation defect. Immunity 24:513–522

16. Larbi A, Douziech N, Dupuis G, Khalil A, Pelletier H, Guerard KP Jr, Fülöp T (2004) Age-associated alterations in the recruitment of signal-transduction proteins to lipid rafts in human T lymphocytes. J Leukoc Biol 75:373–381

17. de Mello Coelho V, Nguyen D, Giri B, Bunbury A, Schaffer E, Taub DD (2005) Quantitative differences in lipid raft components between murine CD4+ and CD8+ T-cells. BMC Immunol 5:2–10

18. Ebert PJ, Baker JF, Punt JA (2000) Immature CD4+CD8+ thymocytes do not polarize lipid rafts in response to TCR-mediated signals. J Immunol 165:5435–5442

19. Silvius JR (2003) Role of cholesterol in lipid raft formation: lessons from lipid model systems. Biochim Biophys Acta 1610:174–183

20. Gaus K, Kritharides L, Schmitz G, Boettcher A, Drobnik W, Langmann T, Quinn CM, Death A, Dean W, Jessup RT (2004) Apolipoprotein A-1 interaction with plasma membrane lipid rafts controls cholesterol export from macrophages. FASEB J 18:574–576

21. Larbi A, Douziech N, Khalil A, Dupuis G, Gherairi S, Guerard KP, Fülöp T Jr (2004) Effects of methyl-beta-cyclodextrin on T lymphocytes lipid rafts with aging. Exp Gerontol 39:551–558

22. Nishio M, Fukumoto S, Furukawa K, Ichimura A, Miyazaki H, Kusunoki S, Urano T, Furukawa K (2004) Overexpressed GM1 suppresses nerve growth factor (NGF) signals by modulating the intracellular localization of NGF receptors and membrane fluidity in PC12 cells. J. Biol Chem 279:33368–33378

23. Tuosto L, Parolini I, Schröder S, Sargiacomo M, Lanzavecchia A, Viola A (2001) Organization of plasma membrane functional rafts upon T-cell activation. Eur J Immunol 31:345–349

24. Burack WR, Lee KH, Holdorf AD, Dustin ML, Shaw AS (2002) Cutting edge: quantitative imaging of raft accumulation in the immunological synapse. J Immunol 169:2837–2841
25. Dustin ML, (2002) J. Membrane domains and the immunological synapse: keeping T-cells resting and ready. Clin Invest 109:155–160
26. O'Keefe JP, Blaine K, Alegre ML, Gajewski TF (2004) Formation of a central supramolecular activation cluster is not required for activation of naive CD8+ T-cells. Proc Natl Acad Sci 101:9351–9356
27. Sadra A, Cinek T, Imboden JB (2004) Translocation of CD28 to lipid rafts and costimulation of IL-2. Proc Natl Acad Sci 101:11422–11427
28. Drevot P, Langlet C, Guo XJ, Bernard AM, Colard O, Chauvin JP, Laserre R, He HT (2002) TCR signal initiation machinery is pre-assembled and activated in a subset of membrane rafts. EMBO J 21:1899–1908
29. Krummel MF, Sjaastad MD, Wulfing C, Davis MM (2000) Differential clustering of CD4 and CD3zeta during T-cell recognition. Science 289:1349–1352
30. Davidson D, Bakinowski M, Thomas ML, Horejsi V, Veillette A (2003) Phosphorylation-dependent regulation of T-cell activation by PAG/Cbp, a lipid raft-associated transmembrane adaptor. Mol Cell Biol 23:2017–2028
31. Tasken K, Ruppelt A (2006) Negative regulation of T-cell receptor activation by the cAMP-PKA-Csk signalling pathway in T-cell lipid rafts. Front Biosci 11:2929–2939
32. Davidson T, Schraven B, Veiette A (2007) PAG-associated FynT regulates calcium signalling and promotes anergy in T lymphocytes. Mel Cell Biol 27:1960–1973
33. Pawelec G, Hirokawa K, Fülöp T Jr (2001) Mechanical altered T-cell signalling in ageing. Ageing Dev. 122:1613–1637
34. Grossmann A, Ledbetter JA, Rabinovitch PS (1989) Reduced proliferation in T lymphocytes in aged humans is predominantly in the CD8+ subset, and is unrelated to defects in transmembrane signaling which are predominantly in the CD4+ subset. Exp. Cell Res. 180:367–382
35. Laux I, Khoshnan A, Tindell C, Bae D, Zhu X, June CH, Effros RB, Nel A (2000) Response differences between human CD4(+) and CD8(+) T-cells during CD28 costimulation: implications for immune cell-based therapies and studies related to the expansion of double-positive T-cells during aging. Clin Immunol 96:187–197
36. Jury EC, Kabouridis PS, Flores-Borja F, Mageed RA, Isenberg DA (2004) Altered lipid raft-associated signaling and ganglioside expression in T lymphocytes from patients with systemic lupus erythematosus. J Clin Invest 113:1176–1187
37. Jury EC, Flores-Borja F, Kabouridis PS (2007) Lipid rafts in T-cell signalling and disease. Semin Cell Dev Biol 18:608–15
38. Li SP, Cai Z, Shi W, Brunmark A, Jackson M, Linton PJ (2002) Early antigen-specific response by naive CD8 T-cells is not altered with aging. J Immunol 168:6120–6127
39. Ward SG (1996) CD28: a signalling perspective. Biochem J 318:361–377
40. Ghosh P, Buchholz MA, Yano S, Taub DD, Longo, DL (2002) Effect of rapamycin on the cyclosporin A-resistant CD28-mediated costimulatory pathway. Blood 99:4517–4524
41. Pizzo P, Giurisato E, Bigsten A, Tassi M, Tavano R, Shaw A, Viola A (2004) Physiological T-cell activation starts and propagates in lipid rafts. Immunol Lett 91:3–9
42. Martin M, Schneider H, Azouz A. Rudd EC (2001) Cytotoxic T lymphocyte antigen 4 and CD28 modulate cell surface raft expression in their regulation of T-cell function. J Exp Med 194:1675–1681
43. Lee KY, D'Aquisto F, Hayden MS, Shim JH, Ghosh S (2005) PDK1 nucleates T-cell receptor-induced signaling complex for NF-kappaB activation. Science 308:114–118
44. Matsumoto R, Wang D, Blonska M, Li H, Kobayashi M, Pappu B, Chen Y, Wang D, Lin X (2005) Phosphorylation of CARMA1 plays a critical role in T-cell receptor-mediated NF-kappaB activation. Immunity 23:575–585
45. Sommer K, Guo B, Pomerantz JL, Bandaranayake AD, Moreno-Garcia ME, Ovechkina YL, Rawlings DJ (2005) Phosphorylation of the CARMA1 linker controls NF-κB activation. Immunity 23:561–574

46. Schmitz ML, Krappmann D (2006) Controlling NF-1547;B activation in T-cells by costimulatory receptors. Cell Death Differ 13:834–842
47. Wang S, Chen L (2004) Co-signaling molecules of the B7-CD28 family in positive and negative regulation of T lymphocyte responses. Microbes Infections 6:759–766
48. Rudd CE, Schneider H (2003) Unifying concepts in CD28, ICOS and CTLA4 co-receptor signalling. Nature Immunol 3:544–556
49. Cantrell D (2002) Protein kinase B (Akt) regulation and function in T lymphocytes. Sem Immunol 14:19–26
50. Gupta S (2005) Molecular mechanisms of apoptosis in the cells of the immune system in human aging. Immunol Rev 205:114–129
51. Larbi A, Muti E, Giacconi R, Mocchegiani E, Fülöp T (2006) Role of lipid rafts in activation-induced cell death: the fas pathway in aging. Adv Exp Med Biol 584:137–55
52. Monks CR, Freiberg BA, Kupfer H, Sciaky N, Kupfer A (1998) Three-dimensional segregation of supramolecular activation clusters in T-cells. Nature 395:82–86
53. Dustin ML, Shaw AS (1999) Costimulation: building an immunological synapse. Science 283:649–650
54. Pawelec G, Mariaini M, Barnett R, Forsey Y, Larbi A, Solana R, Fülöp T Jr, Simoneri T (2006) Human T-cell clones in long-term culture as models for the impact of chronic antigenic stress In: Conn M (ed) Textbook of models for the study of human aging. Academic Press, New York, pp 781–793
55. Santoro TJ, Malek TR, Rosenberg YJ, Morse HC 3rd, Steinberg AD (1984) Signals required for activation and growth of autoimmune T lymphocytes. J Mol Cell Immunol 1:347–56
56. Schmandt R, Fung M, Arima N, Zhang N, Leung B, May C, Gibson S, Hill M, Green W, Mills GB (1992) T-lymphocyte proliferation: tyrosine kinases in interleukin 2 signal transduction. Baillieres Clin Haematol 5:551–73
57. Minami Y, Kono T, Miyazaki T, Taniguchi T (1993) The IL-2 receptor complex: its structure, function, and target genes. Annu Rev Immunol 11:245–268
58. Farrar WL, Ferris DK (1989) Two-dimensional analysis of interleukin 2-regulated tyrosine kinase activation mediated by the p70-75 beta subunit of the interleukin 2 receptor. J Biol Chem 264:12562–12567
59. Miyazaki T, Kawahara A, Fujii H, Nakagawa Y, Minami Y, Liu ZJ, Oishi I, Silvennoinen O, Witthuhn BA, Ihle JN (1994) Functional activation of Jak1 and Jak3 by selective association with IL-2 receptor subunits. Science 266:1045–1047
60. Nakajima H, Liu XW, Wynshaw-Boris A, Rosenthal LA, Imada K, Finbloom DS, Hennighausen L, Leonard WJ (1997) An indirect effect of Stat5a in IL-2-induced proliferation: a critical role for Stat5a in IL-2-mediated IL-2 receptor alpha chain induction. Immunity 7:691–701
61. Lin JX, Leonard WJ (2000) The role of Stat5a and Stat5b in signaling by IL-2 family cytokines. Oncogene.19:566–2576
62. Du JX, Yun CC, Bialkowska A, Yang VW (2007) Protein inhibitor of activated STAT1 interacts with and up-regulates activities of the pro-proliferative transcription factor Krüppel-like factor 5. J Biol Chem 282:4782–4793
63. Duhé RJ, Evans GA, Erwin RA, Kirken RA, Cox GW, Farrar WL (1998) Nitric oxide and thiol redox regulation of Janus kinase activity. Proc Natl Acad Sci U S A 95:126–131
64. Kaur N, Lu B, Monroe RK, Ward SM, Halvorsen SW (2005) Inducers of oxidative stress block ciliary neurotrophic factor activation of Jak/STAT signaling in neurons. J Neurochem 92:1521–1530
65. Fulop T, Larbi A, Douziech N, Levesque I, Varin A, Herbein G (2006) Cytokine receptor signalling and aging. Mech Ageing Dev 127:526–537
66. Tan JA, Hall SH, Hamil KG, Grossman G, Petrusz P, French FS (2002) Protein inhibitors of activated STAT resemble scaffold attachment factors and function as interacting nuclear receptor coregulators. J Biol Chem 277:16993–17001
67. Zeng R, Cannon JL, Abraham RT, Way M, Billadeau DD, Bubeck-Wardenberg J, Burkhardt JK (2003) SLP-76 coordinates Nck-dependent Wiskott-Aldrich syndrome protein recruitment

with Vav-1/Cdc42-dependent Wiskott-Aldrich syndrome protein activation at the T-cell-APC contact site. J Immunol 171:1360–1368

68. Brock MA, Chrest F (1993) Differential regulation of actin polymerization following activation of resting T lymphocytes from young and aged mice. J Cell Physiol 157:367–378

69. Hermiston ML, Xu Z, Majeti R, Weiss A (2002) Reciprocal regulation of lymphocyte activation by tyrosine kinases and phosphatases. J Clin Invest 109:9–14

70. Mustelin T, Tasken K (2003) Positive and negative regulation of T-cell activation through kinases and phosphatases. Biochem J 371:15–27

71. Kilgore NE, Carter JD, Lorenz U, Evavold BD (2003) Cutting edge: dependence of TCR antagonism on Src homology 2 domain-containing protein tyrosine phosphatase activity. J Immunol 170:4891–4895

72. Seminario MC, Wange RL (2003) Lipid phosphatases in the regulation of T-cell activation: living up to their PTEN-tial. Immunol Rev 192:80–97

73. Horn S, Endl E, Fehse B, Weck MM, Mayr GW, Jucker M (2004) Restoration of SHIP activity in a human leukemia cell line downregulates constitutively activated phosphatidylinositol 3-kinase/Akt/GSK-3beta signaling and leads to an increased transit time through the G1 phase of the cell cycle. Leukemia 18:1839–1849

74. Alexander DR (2000) The CD45 tyrosine phosphatase: a positive and negative regulator of immune cell function. Semin Immunol 12:349–359

75. Johnson KG, Bromley SK, Dustin ML, Thomas, ML (2000) A supramolecular basis for CD45 tyrosine phosphatase regulation in sustained T-cell activation. Proc Natl Acad Sci U S A 97:10138–10143

76. Irles C, Symons A, Michel F, Bakker TR, Van Der Merwe PA, Acuto O (2003) CD45 ectodomain controls interaction with GEMs and Lck activity for optimal TCR signaling. Nat Immunol 4:189–197

77. Fortin CF, Larbi A, Lesur O, Douziech N, Fulop T (2006) Impairment of SHP-1 down-regulation in the lipid rafts of human neutrophils under GM-CSF stimulation contributes to their age-related, altered functions. J Leukoc Biol 79:1061–1072

78. Rider DA, Sinclair AJ, Young SP (2003) Oxidative inactivation of CD45 protein tyrosine phosphatase may contribute to T lymphocyte dysfunction in the elderly. Mech Ageing Dev 124:191–198

79. Tomoiu A, Larbi A, Fortin C, Dupuis G, Fulop T Jr (2007) Do membrane rafts contribute to human immunosenescence? Ann N Y Acad Sci 1100:98–110

80. Methi T, Ngai J, Mahic M, Amarzguioui M, Vang T, Tasken K (2005) Short-interfering RNA-mediated Lck knockdown results in augmented downstream T-cell responses. J Immunol 175:7398–7406

81. Worley PF, Zeng W, Huang G, Kim JY, Shin DM, Kim MS, Yuan JP, Kiselyov K, Muallem S. Homer proteins in Ca2 +signaling by excitable and non-excitable cells. Cell Calcium 42:363–371

82. Huang GN, Huso DL, Bouyain S, Tu J, McCorkell KA, May MJ, Zhu Y, Lutz M, Collins S, Dehoff M, Kang S, Whartenby K, Powell J, Leahy D, Worley PF (2008) NFAT binding and regulation of T-cell activation by the cytoplasmic scaffolding Homer proteins. Science 319:476–481

83. Rivnay B, Bergman S, Shinitzky M, Globerson A (1980) Correlations between membrane viscosity, serumcholesterol, lymphocyte activation and aging in man. Mech Ageing Dev 12:119–126

84. Fulop T, Douziech N, Goulet AC, Desgeorges S, Linteau A, Lacombe G, Dupuis G (2001) Cyclodextrin modulation of T lymphocyte signal transduction with aging. Mech Ageing Dev 122:1413–1430

Molecular Signaling of CD95- and TNFR-Mediated Apoptosis in Naïve and Various Memory Subsets of T-Cells

Sudhir Gupta and Ankmalika Gupta

Contents

Abstract: There are multiple ways for cells to die, including necrosis, apoptosis, and autophagy. Apoptosis or programmed cell death or suicidal cell death is a physiological form of cell death, which is critical in cellular homeostasis. Apoptosis occurs in almost all cell types in the body and begins as early as eight cell embryo stage and continues throughout the lifespan of the organism, albeit at different rate. There are multiple roads to apoptotic cell death, including extrinsic or death receptor-mediated and intrinsic, which may be mediated via mitochondrial pathway and the endoplasmic reticulum pathways. Most of apoptotic cell death are mediated by serine proteases, the caspases, which cleave a number of target substrates, including enzymes, transcription factors, and structural proteins. However, apoptosis may also be mediated by caspase-independent pathways. In this review we will discuss molecular signaling and regulation of death receptor pathways, particularly CD95- and TNFR- mediated apoptosis, in naïve and various memory subsets of T-cells, and changes during human aging.

Keywords: CD95 • Caspases • NF-κB • FLIP • TNF • TNF receptors

S. Gupta (✉) · A. Gupta
Medical Sciences I, C-240
University of California, Irvine
Irvine, CA 92697
Tel.: (949) 824-5818
Fax: (949) 824-4362
E-mail: sgupta@uci.edu

T. Fulop et al. (eds.), *Handbook on Immunosenescence*,
DOI 10.1007/ 978-1-4020-9062-2_36, © Springer Science+Business Media B.V. 2009

1   Introduction

Life requires death; without cell death many of us may have been borne with chromosomal defects. There is an evidence to suggest at even at 8 cell stage of embryo, 2 cells that display chromosomal abnormalities are deleted by apoptosis. In postnatal life, apoptosis plays a critical role in cellular homeostasis and removal of mutated or undesired cells. In the immune system, apoptosis plays an important role in selection of T-cell repertoire, killing of target cells by cytotoxic T-cells (CTL) and natural killer cells, removal of effector cells at the termination of an immune response, immune privilege, and lymphocyte homeostasis. One of the major players in the execution of apoptosis is a group of cysteine proteases, the caspases; though under certain conditions, and in certain cell types, apoptosis may be mediated by a caspase-independent pathway (Loeffler et al. 2001). Apoptosis signals may be mediated via extrinsic or death receptor pathway (Ashkanazi and Dixit 1998; Gupta 2001, 2002; Larvik and Krammer 2005; Gupta and Gupta 2007), and intrinsic pathway, which is mediated via mitochondria and the endoplasmic reticulum (ER) (Ferri and Kroemer 2001; Gupta 2000; Gupta and Gupta 2007; Green and Evan 2002; Kroemer and Reed 2000; Martnou and Green 2001; Zamzami and Kroemer 2001). In all 3 pathways, a set of distinct initiator or proximal caspases are activated, which then activate common effector or executioner caspases to induce morphological and biochemical features of apoptosis (Gupta 2002). All caspases are produced as catalytically inactive zymogens and undergo proteolytic activation. Initiator caspases (caspase-8 and caspase-10) are activated in a large membrane death-inducing signaling complex (DISC). Initiator caspases are characterized by the presence of 80–100 amino acid death domain (DD). DD superfamily is comprised of subfamily of DD, death effector domain (DED), and the caspase-recruiting domain (CARD), which facilitates the recruitment of initiator caspases into the DISC. Initiator caspases undergo autoproteolytic activation following homodimerization. Activated initiator caspases cleave and activate executioner caspases, primarily caspase-3, caspase-6, and caspase-7. Activated executioner caspases cleave a number of cell-death substrates, including actin, lamin, inhibitor of caspase-activated DNAse (ICAD), plectin, RAS homologue-associated coiled-coil containing protein kinase 1 (ROCK1) and gelsolin, DNA-repair enzymes, and survival transcription factors to induce apoptosis (Gupta 2002; Igney and Krammer 2002). The apoptotic cells express several "eat-me" signals including phosphatidyl serine and different surface sugars which allow them to be engulfed by neighboring phagocytic cells. More recently, certain caspases have shown to be involved the activation and proliferation of T-cells. However, these mechanisms will not be discussed in this review.

2   Death Receptor Signaling Pathways of Apoptosis

In the death receptor pathway, apoptosis cascade is triggered by signals via cell surface death receptors, which belong to a large superfamily of tumor necrosis factor receptors (TNFR), and are characterized by the presence of DD in their cytoplasmic tail. They include TNFR1, CD95, TNF-related apoptosis-inducing ligand receptor-1 (TRAILR1), TRAILR2, death receptor 3 (DR3) and DR6 (Krammer et al. 2007). In this review we will discuss two prototype death receptors, the CD95 and TNFR.

2.1   CD95-mediated Apoptosis Signaling (Fig. 1)

Ligation of CD95 with CD95 ligand (CD95L) or anti-CD95 antibodies triggers the recruitment of a set of adaptor molecules and procaspases (due to homotypic interactions between their DD and DED) resulting in the formation of DISC. DISC

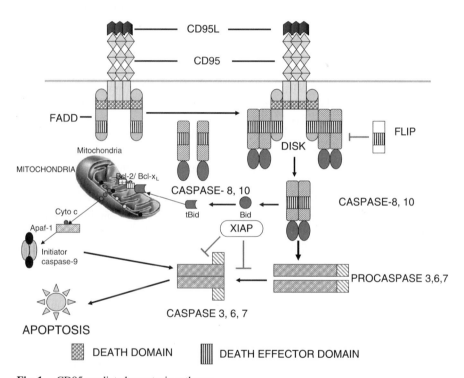

Fig. 1   CD95-mediated apoptosis pathway
Upon ligation with CD95 ligand (CD95L), CD95 undergoe oligomerization of its death doman (DD), which recruits am adaptor Fas-associated death domain (FADD) and then by homotypic protein-protein interaction between their death effector domain (DED), it recruits initiator procaspases (-8, -10) forming a death-inducing signal complex (DISC) as a platform for initiation of apoptosis, Procaspase-8, -10 are activated by homodimerization and axtive caspase-8, -10 are released from the DISC into the cytoplasm where they cleave executioner caspases to form homodimetic active executioner caspases to induce apoptosis. When caspase-8 at the DISC is low, it cleaves Bid to generate truncated Bid (tBid), which is translocated to the mitochondria where it promotes apoptosis by releasing cytocrome c. Cytochrome c binds to Apaf-1 and recruits procaspase-9 to form an Apoptosome. Active caspases-9 activates effector caspases resulting in apoptosis. XIAP inhibits the activation and activity of caspase-3.

contains oligomerized/trimerized CD95, Fas-associated death domain (FADD), 2 isoforms of procaspase-8, procasapse-8a (FLICE or MACHα1) and procaspase-8 (MACHα2), procaspase-10, and cellular FLICE inhibitory protein (FLIP). The formation of DISC results in autoproteolytic activation of initiator caspases, procaspase-8 and procaspase-10. The activation of procaspase-8 is dependent upon its local concentrations (high concentrations favor) for autoproteolytic activation. The homodimers of procaspase-8 have proteolytic activity and proteolytic process appears to occur at the DISC by 2 cleavage events, resulting the generation of an active caspase-8 tetramer (Chang et al. 2003), which is subsequently released from the DISC into the cytosol to activate effector procaspases to induce apoptosis. Procaspase-10 forms active heterodimer at the DISC; however, whether caspase-10 can trigger CD95-induced apoptosis in the absence of caspase-8 is controversial; levels of procaspase-10 at the DISC are not sufficient to trigger apoptosis alone (Kischkel et al. 2001; Sprick et al. 2002). Based upon the concentration of caspase-8 at the DISC CD95-mediated apoptosis signaling pathway is divided into 2 types (Scaffidi et al. 1998). Active caspase-8 concentration at the DISC is high in Type-I cells. In these cells, active caspase-8 activates effector caspase-3, caspase-6, and caspase-7. In contrast, Type-II cells are characterized by low levels of active caspase-8 at the DISC and requires additional amplifying mechanism to induce apoptosis. It involves cleavage of BH3-interacting-domain death agonist (BID) by active caspase-8 to generate truncated BID (tBID), which induces aggregation of Bcl-2-associated X protein (Bax) at the mitochondria and release of cytochrome c. In the cytosol cytochrome c binds to adapter Apaf-1 (Apoptosis-activating factor) to form large protein complex, apoptosome, along with procaspase-9. This is followed by activation of procaspase-9 to active caspase-9, which in turn activate effector caspase-3, caspase-6, and caspase-7 to induce apoptosis. Type-II signaling is blocked by Bcl-2 and Bcl-x$_L$, whereas Type-I signaling cannot be blocked by Bcl-2 or Bcl-x$_L$ (Scaffidi et al. 1998). CD95-mediated apoptosis in T-cells is predominantly mediated via Type-I signaling.

2.2 TNFR-mediated Apoptosis Signaling

TNF-α exerts a variety of biological effects, including production of inflammatory cytokines, proliferation, differentiation, and cell death (Ashkanazi and Dixit 1998; Gupta 2000, 2001, 2002; Hsu et al. 1996). While pleiotropic effects of TNF-α are mediated by binding to type I and type II receptors (TNFR-I and TNFR-II), the death-inducing signal is predominantly mediated via TNFR-I; however, TNFR-II have been shown to participate indirectly in TNF-α-induced cell death via regulating apoptosis mediated by TNFR-I (Declercz et al. 1998; Haridas et al. 1998; Locksley et al. 2001; Pimentel-Muinos and Seed 1999; Screaton G and Xu 2000; Tartaglia et al. 1993; Thomas et al. 1990; Vandenabeele et al. 1995; Weiss et al. 1998). Both cell survival and cell death signals mediated by TNFR require distinct sets of adapters and other downstream signaling molecules. Steps of TNF-α -induced signaling are reviewed [33,34] and shown in Fig. 2.

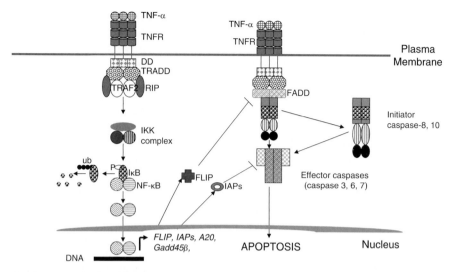

Fig. 2 TNF-TNFR signaling pathway
Upon ligation with TNF-α, TNFR-I mediates both survival signal and death signal by recruitment of different set of adapter proteins (TRAF-2/RIP and FADD).

Upon interaction with TNF-α, TNFR-I undergoes trimerization of its receptor death domains, which in turn recruit an adaptor protein, TNFR-associated death domain (TRADD). In order to induce death signal, TRADD recruits FADD. Therefore, for death inducing signaling via CD95 or TNFR, FADD serves as a common conduit. The remaining downstream signaling steps are similar to those described above for CD95-mediated apoptosis. Alternatively, for the survival and other biological function of TNF-α, TRADD recruits distinct sets of adapter proteins, the TRAF-2 (TNFR-associated factor-2) and receptor interactive protein (RIP). TRAF-2 and RIP stimulate pathways leading to activation of MAP kinase and NFκB. Both NF-κB (Ghosh and Karin 2002; Karin and Lin 2002) and transient activation of (mitogen-activated protein kinases) MAPK induce survival signals (Natoli et al. 1997), whereas prolonged activation of MAPK promote apoptosis (Hacki et al. 2000). MAPK is a family of proteins, including p38, MAPK, and extracellular signal regulatory kinase 1 and 2 (ERK). The antiapoptotic genes that are up-regulated by NF-κB activation include *cIAP1, cIAP2, XIAP, Gadd45β, Bcl-X$_L$, A20, TRAF-1, TRF-2 and FLIP* (Chen et al. 2000; DeSmaele et al. 2001; Ghosh and Karin 2002; Tang et al. 2001).

3   Regulation of Death Receptor-mediated Apoptosis

3.1   cFLIP Proteins

A role of cFLIP proteins in the inhibition of extrinsic pathway of apoptosis is well established (Golks et al. 2005; Thome and Tschopp 2001). Three alternatively spliced forms of cFLIPs (cFLIP$_L$, cFLIPs, cFLIP$_R$) have been described. All 3 isoforms contain 2 DED with homology to n-terminal domain of procaspase-8 and are recruited to the CD95 DISC by protein-protein interactions via their DED. Both cFLIPs and cFLIP$_R$ are structurally related and block activation of procaspase-8 at the DISC; however, the role of cFLIP$_L$ is more complex. At high level cFLIP$_L$ blocks the activation of procaspase-8 at the DISC by blocking its processing, whereas at low concentration of cFLIP$_L$ at the DISC promotes the cleavage of procaspase-8 resulting in the formation of cFLIP$_L$—procaspase-8 heterodimer resulting in facilitating apoptosis. Therefore, cFLIP$_L$ based upon its concentration at the CD95 DISC may serve as antiapoptotic or proapoptotic molecule. Both cFLIPs and cFLIP$_R$ rescue T-cells from activation-induced cell death (AICD). A role of cFLIP in T-cell activation has been supported in FLIP transgenic and knock out mice, as well as by an overexpression of cFLIP$_L$ (Dohrman et al. 2005; Thome and Tschopp 2001).

In addition to 3 spliced isoforms, 2 N-terminal cleavage products of cFLIP, p43-FLIP and p22-FLIP have been reported, which promote survival via activation of NF-κB (Golks et al. 2005; Kataoka and Tschopp 2004). P43-FLIP (a cleaved form of FLIP$_L$) activates NF-κB via its interaction with TRAF1, TRAF2 and RIP-1, which together activate NF-κB. Since FLIPs does not associate with this complex, it appears that caspase-like domain of cFLIPl is essential in the activation of NF-κB via TRF2/RIP pathway. P22-FLIP, which is generated by N-terminal cleavage by caspase-8, activates NF-κB by directly interacting with IKK complex via IKKγ. The ratio between procaspase-8 to cFLIP is critical in determining the amount of p22-FLIP generation and therefore, activation of NF-κB. Though described originally as an inhibitor of CD95-mediated apoptosis, it is apparent that cFLIP proteins also regulate TNFR-mediated apoptosis.

3.2   NF-κB

The predominant form of NF-κB in lymphocytes is a heterodimer comprising of p50 and p65. In unstimulated cells, NF-κB is kept in the cytoplasm through interaction with the inhibitory proteins termed as IκB (inhibitor κB) (Ghosh and Karin 2002; Karin and Lin 2002). When cells are exposed to TNF-α, IκB is phosphorylated followed by ubiquitination and degradation of IκB by the 26S proteosome. Free NF-κB dimers are released and translocated to the nucleus, where they activate transcription of a number of target genes, including anti-apoptotic genes *cIAP1, cIAP2, XIAP, Gadd45β, Bcl-X$_L$, A20, TRAF-1, TRF-2 and FLIP*.

3.3   A20 and Gadd45β

TNFR-mediated apoptosis is also regulated by A20 and gadd45β (De Smaele et al. 2001; Opipari et al. 1992). A20 is a ring finger protein, which has dual activity in that it inhibits apoptosis as well as inhibits NF-κB activation (Heyninck and Beyaert 2005; Opipari et al. 1992).These activities of A20 are cell type specific. A20 inhibits NF-κB activation and therefore promotes apoptosis by first deubiquitination of K^{63} RIP (which activates NF-κB) and subsequent K^{48} ubiquitination of RIP rendering RIP susceptible to S26 proteasomal degradation. In contrast, A20 inhibits apoptosis, at least partially, by binding to TXBP151, which inhibits TNF-α-induced apoptosis. Furthermore, A20 and cIAP interact with a common region in TRAF2. Therefore, A20 releases cIAP from the TRAF2-signaling complex, thereby allowing cIAPs to exert their antiapoptotic effects. Gadd45β inhibits TNF-α-induced apoptosis by inhibiting prolonged activation of MAPK (De Smaele et al. 2001).

3.4 IAP Proteins

IAP family proteins, which were originally identified in the genome of baculovirus, have a key role in the negative regulation of caspase-dependent apoptosis mediated by death receptor, the ER pathway, and mitochondrial pathway (reviewed in Salvesen and Duckett 2004). The cIAP-1 and cIAP-2, two structurally homologous proteins were initially isolated by their interaction with TRAF-1 and TRAF-2 in the TNF-RII complex. cIAP1 is also recruited to DISK of TNF-RI by TRAF-2. In addition to cIAP1 and cIAP2, XIAP have a conserved COOH-terminal RING finger, zinc-binding domain (Liston et al. 1996). Among these IAPs XIAP suppresses apoptosis by preventing the activation of procaspases9-and caspase-3 and by inhibiting directly the enzyme activity of mature caspases. TRAF-2-IAP complex inhibits caspases-8 activation by an unknown mechanism.

4 Apoptosis in Naïve and Memory Subsets of CD4+ and CD8+ T-cells in Aging

4.1 T-cell Differentiation into Memory Subsets

Recent work has suggested that following virus infection or antigen stimulation, naïve T-cells (T_N) undergo a series of proliferative and differentiation steps ultimately culminating in an acquisition and maintenance of memory for a particular antigen/pathogen (Gupta et al. 2004; Kataoka et al. 2001; Sallusto et al. 2004; Tomiyama et al. 2002; Weninger et al. 2001). The memory T-cells display differential expression of adhesion molecules (CD62L) and chemokine receptors (CCR-7). CCR7+ and CD62^{high} T-cells are found in lymph nodes, whereas CCR7- and CD62L^{low} are found in extranodal sites such as liver and lung. Based upon these adhesion molecules and chemokine receptors, memory CD8+ T-cells have been divided into "central" memory (T_{CM}) T-cells for those that are found in lymphoid organs and

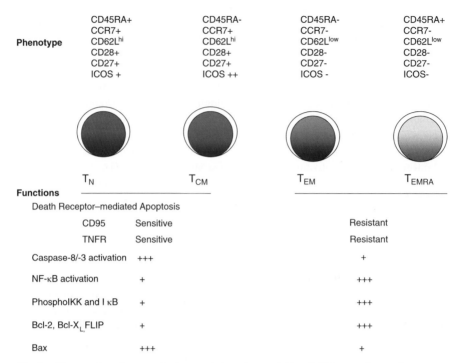

Phenotype	CD45RA+ CCR7+ CD62L^{hi} CD28+ CD27+ ICOS +	CD45RA- CCR7+ CD62L^{hi} CD28+ CD27+ ICOS ++	CD45RA- CCR7- CD62L^{low} CD28- CD27- ICOS -	CD45RA+ CCR7- CD62L^{low} CD28- CD27- ICOS-
	T_N	T_{CM}	T_{EM}	T_{EMRA}

Functions			
Death Receptor–mediated Apoptosis			
CD95	Sensitive		Resistant
TNFR	Sensitive		Resistant
Caspase-8/-3 activation	+++		+
NF-κB activation	+		+++
PhosphoIKK and I κB	+		+++
Bcl-2, Bcl-X$_L$ FLIP	+		+++
Bax	+++		+

Fig. 3 Phenotypic and apoptosis characteristics of naïve (T_N) and different subsets of memory T-cells (T_{CM}= central memory; T_{EM} and T_{EMRA}= two types of effector memory)

"effector" memory (T_{EM}) cells that are found in peripheral nonlymphoid tissues and mucosal sites. Furthermore, effector memory CD8+ T-cells in humans (not in mice) have been further subdivided, based upon the expression or lack of CD45RA, into CD8+CD28-CCR7-CD62^{low} CD45RA- (T_{EM}) and CD8+CD28-CCR7-CD62^{low} CD45RA+ (T_{EMRA}). These subsets have been extensively characterized (Gupta et al. 2004, 2006) and shown in Fig. 3.

4.2 Apoptosis of Naïve and Memory Subsets and Effect of Age

We have reported that T_N and T_{CM} T cell subsets (T_{CM}>T_N) are sensitive to TNF-α-induced (Gupta and Gollapudi 2006, 2006a; Gupta and Gupta 2007), where as T_{EM} and T_{EMRA} cells are resistant to apoptosis. Similar observations have been made with CD95-mediated poptosis (Gupta et al. 2008), and oxidative stress-induced apoptosis (Gupta et al. 2007). We have also defined various molecular mechanisms responsible for such differential sensitivity to TNF-α-induced apoptosis (Gupta et al. 2006). Several investigators have reported increased apoptosis in T-cells and CD4+ and CD8+ T-cells in aged humans (Aggarwal and Gupta 1998;

Aggarwal et al. 1999; Gupta 2000; Gupta 2002; Gupta 2002a; Gupta et al. 2003; Lechner et al. 1996; Phelouzat et al. 1996, 1997). We and others have reported increased susceptibility of aged T-cells and CD4+ and CD8+ T-cells to activation-induced apoptosis and Fas (CD95)-induced apoptosis (Aggarwal and Gupta 1998; Aggarwal and Gupta 1999; Iwai et al. 1994; Lechner et al. 1996; Miyawaki et al. 1992; Phelouzat et al. 1997; Shinohara et al. 1995), which is associated with increased caspase activation (Aggarwal and Gupta 1999). Furthermore, we have demonstrated that FADD plays an important role in increased sensitivity of aged T-cells to apoptosis (Gupta et al. 2004). We have also demonstrated that TNF-α-mediated apoptosis is increased in both CD4+ and CD8+ T-cells in aged humans [Aggarwal et al. 1999; Gupta 2002; Gupta et al. 2003]. Increased apoptosis is associated with decreased expression of Bcl-2 and TRAF-2. We have demonstrated that both up-regulation of FADD and decreased NF-κB activity play an important role in increased sensitivity of aged T-cells to TNF-α-induced apoptosis. Recently, we have observed that T_N and T_{CM} CD8+ T-cells and CD4+ in aging are more sensitive to TNF-α induced [Aggarwal and Gupta 1998; Gupta 2002a; Gupta and Gollapudi 2006a; Kataoka and Tschopp 2004; Phelouzat et al. 1997], and anti-CD95-induced apoptosis (Gupta et al. 2008) as compared to young subjects. Therefore, increased sensitivity of T_N and T_{CM} CD8+ T-cells is not unique to TNF-α. We have also shown that T_{EM} and T_{EMRA} CD8+ and CD4+ T-cells in aged humans are equally resistant to apoptosis as that of young subjects, suggesting that the accumulation of T_{EM} and T_{EMRA} during aging is not due to alterations in apoptosis (Gupta and Gollapudi 2006, 2006a).

We and others have investigated various mechanisms, which may be associated with increased apoptosis of T-cell subsets in aged humans, especially TNF-α-induced apoptosis. NF-κB is an important regulator of TNF-α-induced apoptosis. Pahlvani and Harris (1996) reported decreased NF-κB DNA binding activity in nuclear extracts of concanavalin A-stimulated splenic lymphocytes from old Fischer rats as compared to young rats. Whisler et al. (1996) reported decreased levels of NF-κB in unstimulated and PHA, PMA and anti-CD3-stimulated T-cells from a small number of aged humans as compared to young subjects. Trebilcock and Ponnappan (1996) demonstrated decreased induction of NF-κB in response to PMA and TNF-α. These authors suggested that decreased induction of NF-κB could be due to decreased proteosome-mediated degradation of IκB (Ponnappan et al. 1999). We have investigated TNF-α signaling pathway of apoptosis in aged subsets in detail and observed that TNF-α-induced activation of NF-κB in T_N and T_{CM} is significantly decreased as compared to young subjects (manuscript in preparation). Furthermore, aged T_N and T_{CM} CD8+ T-cells display decreased activation of IKKα/β, and decreased phosphorylation of IκB as compared to T_N and T_{CM}. We have also demonstrated that an overexpression of IKKβ that resulted in the upregulation of NF-κB corrected increased sensitivity of aged T-cells to TNF-α-induced apoptosis (Gupta et al. 2005). Therefore, establishes a role of decreased NF-κB in increased sensitivity of aged T-cells to TNF-α-induced apoptosis.

5 Naïve, Central Memory and Effector Memory CD8+ T-cells in Aging

In aging, there is a significant reduction in naïve CD8+ T-cells (Fagnoni et al. 2002) and CD8+ CD28+ T-cells, which contain both naïve and central memory CD8+ T-cells (Brzeznska et al. 2004). In addition, there is an accumulation of CD8+CD28- T-cells, which are oligoclonal and show characteristics of cellular senescence (i.e., short telomere length indicative of long replicative history), and increased IFN-γ production [Bandres et al. 2000; Effros. 1994; Monteiro et al. 1996; Nociari et al. 1999; Posnett et al. 1994; Saurwein-Teissl et al. 2002]. These CD28- CD8+ T-cells are comprised of 2 subpopulations of effector memory CD8+ T-cells, namely T_{EM} and T_{EMRA} CD8+ T-cells. Our study shows a marked decrease in the proportions of naïve CD8+ T-cells and an increase in T_{EM} and T_{EMRA} CD8+ T-cells. However, when data were analyzed for absolute numbers, a significant decrease in T_N and T_{CM} a significant increase in T_{EMRA} CD8+ T-cells was observed (Gupta 2005). Fagnoni et al (2002) also observed an increase in primed CD8+CD28-CD45RA+ (equivalent to T_{EMRA}) in aged humans.

6 Apoptosis of Naïve, Central Memory and Effector Memory T-Cell Subsets in Aging

Herndon et al. (Herndon et al. 1997) have provided evidence of increased AICD of naïve T (CD45RO-) cells in aged humans and suggested its role in age-associated T-cell deficiency. However, they did not investigate apoptosis in memory T-cells. Brezinska et al. (2004) concluded that AICD (as measured by DNA content and caspasese-3 activation) in CD8+CD28+ (containing T_N and T_{CM}) and CD8+CD28- (containing T_{EM} and T_{EMRA}) was comparable. However, these investigators presented data from a single middle aged individual.

We have reported that in aged humans, both CD45RA+ (naïve) and CD45RO+ (memory) CD4+ and CD8+ T-cells were more sensitive to anti-CD95-induced apoptosis as compared to young subjects (Brzezinska et al. 2004). Furthermore, CD45RO+ displayed greater sensitivity to anti-CD95-induced apoptosis as compared to CD45RA+ CD4+ and CD8+ T-cells in both young and aged subjects. Miyawaki et al. (1992) also reported that healthy adult memory T-cells are more susceptible to anti-CD95-induced apoptosis as compared to naïve T-cells. We reported decreased expression of Bcl-2 in both CD4+ and CD8+ T-cells from aged humans as compared to young subjects; however, we did not examine Bcl-2 expression in naïve and memory subsets (Aggarwal and Gupta 1998). Shinohara et al. (1995) demonstrated decreased Bcl-2 expression in memory subsets of CD4+ and CD8+ T-cells in healthy adults. This would be consistent with our observation of increased sensitivity of memory T-cell subsets to death-receptor-mediated apoptosis as compared to naïve T-cell subsets. Although a role of Bcl-2 family protein in death receptor pathway has been argued, Iwai et al. (1994) and Yoshina et al. (1994) have demonstrated that Bcl-2 blocks anti-CD95-induced apoptosis in mitogen-activated T-cells. Therefore, it is likely that decreased Bcl-2 expression in aging may play a role in increased sensitivity of T-cell subsets in aged humans. However, experiments of Bcl-2 overexpression need to performed to define a definitive role of decreased Bcl-2 in increased susceptibility of aged naïve and memory subsets to death-receptor-mediated apoptosis.

We have also examined TNF-α-induced apoptosis in both naïve and memory subsets of CD4+ and CD8+ T-cells, using TUNEL assay and flow cytometry and observed that both CD45RA+ naïve and CD45RA- memory CD4+ and CD8+ T-cells from aged individuals were more sensitive to TNF-α-induced apoptosis (Aggarwal and Gupta 1998).

As discussed above, naïve T-cells, as defined by the presence of CD45RA contain T_{EMRA} CD8+ T-cells (and a very small population of T_{EMRA} CD4+ T-cells), and CD45RA- (CD45RO+) contain both T_{CM} and T_{EM} CD8+ T-cells. Therefore, we have examined the relative sensitivity of T_N and T_{CM}, T_{EM} and T_{EMRA} CD8+ and CD4+ T-cell subsets to TNF-α-induced apoptosis. Naïve CD8+ T-cells and central memory CD8+ T-cells are more sensitive to death-receptor and oxidative stress-induced apoptosis, whereas effector memory CD8+ T-cells are resistant to apoptosis (manuscript in preparation). In aged humans we observed that naïve and central memory CD8+ T-cells displayed increased TNF-α-induced apoptosis as compared to young subjects, which is associated with increased caspase-8 and caspase-3 activation. In contrast, effector memory subsets are resistant to TNF-α-induced apoptosis and display minimal caspase activation in both young and aged subjects. Therefore, it appears that during aging decrease in naïve CD8+ T-cells is due to both decreased thymic output as well as increased apoptosis. We have also observed increased apoptosis in T_N and T_{CM} (T_{CM} > T_N) CD4+ T-cells in aged humans as compared to young subjects; however, no significant difference was observed in the apoptosis of T_{EM} and T_{EMRA} CD4+ T-cells between aged and young humans; both were resistant to apoptosis (Gupta and Gollapudi 2006).

There are several possible mechanisms to explain differential sensitivity of various memory subsets to apoptosis. Since T_{CM} cells have high a replicative property (more than T_N cells), increased apoptosis may be critical to make niche for new T_{CM} CD4+ and CD8+ T-cells and to maintain homeostasis of T_{CM} cells. It is known that IL-7 and IL-15 provide survival signals in maintaining memory T-cells (Schluns and Defracois 2003; Alpdogan and van den Brink 2005). Furthermore, we have observed that IL-7 serves as an important preferential survival factor for T_{CM} cells, whereas, IL-15 provides preferential survival signal for T_{EM} and T_{EMRA} T-cells (Personal unpublished observations). A decreased IL-7 in aging may contribute to increased apoptosis of T_{CM} cells in aging. The low replicative property of T_{EM} and T_{EMRA} cells, which does not allow for the creation of an "immunological nitch" may be responsible for relative resistance of T_{EM} and T_{EMRA} cells to apoptosis. A large number of studies have been reported on CD8+CD28- T-cells generated after repeated stimuli (as a model of aging) and reported features of replicative senescence (low proliferative potentials and resistance to apoptosis). However,

Brzezinska et al. (2004) have reported that aged CD8+CD28- proliferate more than adult counterparts. We have observed that both T_{EM} and T_{EMRA} CD8+ T-cells from young and aged subjects can proliferate well in the presence of exogenous IL-2 and IL-15 (unpublished observation). We have also observed increased expression of IL-15 gene in CD8+ T-cells from aged humans (by gene array). These observations suggest that CD8+CD28- T-cells generated by repeated activation in vitro are not a true model for CD8+CD28- T-cells in aged humans. Furthermore, increased accumulation of CD8+CD28- T-cell population in aged humans may be due to an increased growth provided by increased IL-15 in aging.

Acknowledgment   Part of work cited was supported by USPHS grant AG-18313.

References

Aggarwal S, Gupta S (1998) Increased apoptosis of T cell subsets in aging humans: Altered expression of Fas (CD95), Fas ligand, Bcl-2, and Bax. J Immunol 160:1627–1637

Aggarwal S, Gupta S (1999) Increased activity of caspase-3 and caspase-8 during Fas-mediated apoptosis in lymphocytes from aging humans. Clin Exp Immunol 117:285–290

Aggarwal S, Gollapudi S, Gupta S (1999) Increased TNF-α-induced apoptosis in lymphocytes from aged humans: changes in TNF-α receptor expression and activation of caspases. J Immunol 162:2154–2161

Alpdogan O, Van Den Brink MRM (2005) IL-7 and IL-15: therapeutic cytokines for immunodeficiency. Trends Immunol 26:56–64

Ashkanazi A, Dixit VM (1998) Death receptors: signaling and modulation. Science 281:1305–1308

Bandres E, Merino J, Vazquez S et al (2000) The increase of IFN-γ production through aging correlates with the expanded CD8+CD28-CD57+ subpopulation. Clin Immunol 96:230–235

Brzezinska A, Magalska A, Szybinska A et al (2004) Proliferation and apoptosis of human CD8+CD28+ and CD8+CD28- lymphocytes during aging. Exp Gerontol 39:539–544

Chang DW, Xing Z, Capacio VL et al (2003) Interdimer processing mechanism of procaspase-8 activation. EMBO 22:4132–4142

Chen C, Edelstein LC, Gelinas C (2000) The Rel/ NF-κB family directly activates expression of the apoptotic inhibitor Bcl-x (L). Mol Cell Biol 20: 2687–2695

Declercq W, Denecker G, Fiers W et al (1998) Cooperation of both TNF receptors in inducing apoptosis: involvement of the TNF receptor-associated factor binding domain of the TNF receptor 75. J Immunol 161:390–399

De Smaele E, Zazzeroni F, Papa S et al (2001) Induction of gadd45β by NF-κβ downregulates proapoptotic JNK signaling. Nature 414:308–313

Dohrman A,Kataoka T, Cuenin S et al (2005) Cellular FLIP (long form) regulates CD8+ T cell activation through caspase-8-dependent NF-κB activation. J Immunol 174:5270–5278

Effros RB, Boucher N, Porter V et al (1994) Decline in CD28 +T cells in centenarians and in long-term T cell cultures: A possible cause of both in vivo and in vitro immunosenescence. Exp Gerontol 29:601–609

Fagnoni FF, Vescovini R, Paserri G et al (2002) Shortage of circulating naïve CD8+ T cells provides new insights on immunodeficiency in aging. Blood 95:2860–2868

Ferri KF, Kroemer G (2001) Organelle-specific initiation of cell death pathways. Nat Cell Biol 3: E255–E266

Ghosh S, Karin M (2002) Missing pieces in the NF-kB puzzle. Cell 109:S81–S96

Golks A, Brenner D, Krammer PH et al (2005) The c-FLIP NH2 terminus (p22-FLIP) induces NF-κB activation. J Exp Med 203:1295–1305

Golks A, Brenner D, Fritsch C et al (2005) cFLIP$_R$ a new regulator of death receptor-induced apoptosis. J Biol Chem 280:14507–14513

Green DR, Evan GI (2002) A matter of life and death. Cancer Cell 1:19–30

Gupta S (2000) Molecular steps of death receptor and mitochondrial pathways of apoptosis. Life Sci 69:2957–2964

Gupta S (2000) Molecular and biochemical pathways of apoptosis in lymphocytes from aged humans. Vaccine 18:1596–1601

Gupta S (2001) Molecular steps of TNF receptor-mediated apoptosis. Curr Mol Med 1:299–306

Gupta S (2002) Decision between life and death during TNF-induced signaling. J Clin Immunol 22:270–278

Gupta S (2002a) Tumor necrosis factor-a-induced apoptosis in T cells from aged humans: a role of TNFR-I and downstream signaling molecules. Exp Gerontol 37:293–299

Gupta S (2005) Death of lymphocytes: A clue to immune deficiency in human aging. Discov Med 5:298–302

Gupta S, Bi R, Su K et al (2004) Characterization of naïve, memory, and effector CD8+ T cells: Effect of age. Exp Gerontol 39:545–550

Gupta S, Bi R, Kim C et al (2005) A role of NF-κB signaling pathway in increased tumor necrosis factor-α-induced apoptosis of lymphocytes in aged humans. Cell Death Differ 12:177–183

Gupta S, Bi R, Gollapudi S (2006) Differential sensitivity of naïve and memory subsets of human CD8+ T cells to TNF-α-induced apoptosis. J Clin Immunol 26:193–203

Gupta S, Chiplunkar S, Kim C et al (2003). Effect of age on molecular signaling of TNF-α-induced apoptosis in human lymphocytes. Mech. Ageing Dev 124:503–509

Gupta S, Gollapudi S (2006) Molecular Mechanisms of TNF-α-induced apoptosis in naïve and memory T cell subsets. Autoimmun Rev 5:264–268

Gupta S, Gollapudi S (2006a) TNF-α-induced apoptosis in human naïve and memory CD8+ T cells in aged humans. Exp Gerontol 41:69–77

Gupta S, Gupta A (2007) Death of memory T cell subsets in humans: changes during aging. Expert Rev Clin Immunol 3:637–45

Gupta S, Young T, Yel L et al (2007) Differential sensitivity of naïve and subsets of memory CD4+ and CD8+ T cells to hydrogen peroxide-induced-apoptosis. Genes Immun 1–10

Gupta S, Bi R, Su H et al (2008) CD95-mediated apoptosis in naïve, and central and effector memory subsets of CD4+ and CD8+ T cells in aged humans. Ex Gerontol 43:266–274

Hacki J, Egger L, Monney L et al (2000) Apoptotic cross talk between the endoplasmic reticulum and mitochondria controlled by Bcl-2. Oncogene 19:2286–2295

Haridas V, Darnay BG, Natrajan K et al (1998) Overexpression of the p80 TNFR leads to TNF-dependent apoptosis, nuclear factor-kappa B activation. J Immunol 160:3152–3162

Herndon FJ, Hsu HC, Mountz JD (1997) Increased apoptosis of CD45RO- T cells with aging. Mech Ageing Dev 194:123–134

Heyninck K, Beyaert R (2005) A20 inhibits NF-kB activation by dual ubiquitin-editing functions. Trends Biochem Sci 30:1–4

Hsu H, Shu HB, Pan MG et al (1996) TRADD-TRAF2 and TRADD-FADD interactions define two distinct TNF receptor 1 signal transduction pathways. Cell 84:299–308

Igney FH, Krammer PH (2002) Immune escape of tumors: apoptosis resistance and counterattack. J Leukocyte Biol 71:907–920

Iwai K, Miyawaki T, Takizawa T et al (1994) Differential expression of *bcl-2* and susceptibility to anti-Fas-mediated death in peripheral blood lymphocytes, monocytes and neutrophils. Blood 84:1201–1208

Karin M, Lin A (2002) NF-κB at the crossroads of life and death. Nature Immunol 3:221–227

Kataoka T, Tschopp J (2004) N-terminal fragment of c-FLIP, process by caspase-8 specifically interacts with TRAF2 and induces activation of the NF-κB. Mol Cell Biol 24:2627–2636

Kataoka T, Budd RC, Holler N et al Preferential localization of effector memory cells in nonlymphoid tissue. Science 291:2413–2417

Kischkel FC, Lawrence DA, Tinel A et al (2001). Death receptor recruitment of endogeneous caspase-10 and apoptosis initiation in the absence of caspase-8. J Biol Chem 276:46639–46646

Krammer PH, Arnold R, Lavrik I (2007) Life and Death in peripheral T cells. Nat Rev Immunol 7:532–542

Kroemer G, Reed JC (2000) Mitochondrial control of cell death. Nat Med 6:513–519

Larvik I, Golks A, Krammer PH (2005) Death receptor signaling. J Cell Sci 118:265–267

Lechner H, Amort M, Steger MM et al (1996) Regulation of CD95 (Apo-1) expression and the induction of apoptosis of human T cells: changes in old age. Int Arch Allergy Immunol 110:238–243

Liston P, Roy N, Tamai K et al (1996) Suppression of apoptosis in mammalian cells by NIAP and a related family of IAP genes. 379:349–353

Locksley RM, Kileen N, Lenardo MJ (2001) The TNF and TNF receptor superfamilies: interating mammalian biology. Cell 104:487–501

Loeffler M, Daugas E, Susin SA et al (2001) Dominant cell death induced by extramitochondrially targeted apoptosis-inducing factor. FASEB J.15:758–767

Martinou J-C, Green DR (2001) Breaking the mitochondrial barrier. Nat Rev Mol Cell Biol 2:63–67

Miyawaki T, Uehara T, Nabu R et al (1992) Differential expression of apoptosis-related Fas antigen on lymphocyte subpopulations in human peripheral blood. J Immunol 49:3753–3758

Monteiro J, Baltiwala F, Ostrer H et al (1996) Shortened telomeres in clonally expanded CD28-CD8+ T cells imply a replicative history that is distinct from their CD28+CD8+ counterparts. J Immunol 156:3587

Natoli G, Costanzo A, Ianni A et al (1997) Activation of SAPK/JNK by TNF receptor 1 through a noncytotoxic TRAF-2-dependent pathway. Science 275:200–203

Nociari MM, Telford W, Russo C (1999) Postthymic development of CD28-CD8+ T cell subset: age-associated expansion and shift from memory to naïve phenotype. J Immunol 162:3327–3335

Opipari AW Jr, Hu HM, Yabkowitz R et al (1992) The A20 zinc finger protein protects cells from tumor necrosis factor cytotoxicity. J Biol Chem 267:12424–12427

Orrenius S, Zhivotovsky B, Nicotera P (2003) Regulation of cell death: the calcium-apoptosis link. Nat Rev Mol Cell Biol 4:552–564

Pahlavani M, Harris MD (1996) The age-related changes in DNA binding activity of AP-1, NF-κB, and Oct-1 transcription factors in lymphocytes from rats. Age 19:45–54

Phelouzat MA, Arbogast A, Laforge T et al (1996) Excessive apoptosis of mature T lymphocytes is a characteristic feature of human immune senescence. Mech Ageing Dev 88:25–38

Phelouzat MA, Laforge T, Abrogast A et al (1997) Susceptibility to apoptosis of T lymphocytes from elderly humans is associated with increased in vivo expression of functional fas receptors. Mech Ageing Dev 96:35–46

Pimentel-Muinos FX, Seed B (1999) Regulated commitment of TNF receptor signaling: a molecular switch for death or activation. Immunity 11:783–793

Posnett DN, Sinha R, Kabak S et al (1994) Clonal populations of T cells in normal elderly humans: The cell equivalent to "benign monoclonal gammopathy" J Exp Med 179:609–618

Ponnappan U, Zhong M, Trebilcock GU (1999) Decreased proteosome-mediated degradation in T cells from the elderly: A role in immune senescence. Cell Immunol 192:167–174

Salvesen GS, Duckett CS (2004) IAP proteins: blocking the road to death's door. Nat Rev Mol Cell Biol 3:401–410

Sallusto F, Geginat J, Lanzavecchia A (2004) Central memory and effector memory T cell subsets: Function, generation, and maintenance. Annu Rev Immunol 22:745–763

Saurwein-Teissl M, Lung TL, Marx F et al (2002) Lack of antibody production following immunization in old age:Association with CD8+CD28- T cell clonal expansions and an imbalance in the production of Th1 and Th2 cytokines. J Immunol 168:5893–5899

Scaffidi C, Fulda S, Srinivasan A et al (1998) Two CD95 (APO-1/Fas) signaling pathways. EMBO J 17:1675–1687

Schluns KS, Lefrancois L (2003) Cytokine control of memory T cell development and survival. Nat Rev Immunol 3:269–279

Screaton G, Xu X-N (2000) T cell life and death signaling via TNF-receptor family members. Curr Opin Immunol 12:316–3222

Shinohara S, Sawada T, Nishioka Y et al (1995) Differential expression of Fas and Bcl-2 protein on CD4+ T cells, CD8+ T cells and monocytes. Cell Immunol 163:303–308

Sprick MR, Rieser E, Stahl H et al (2002) Caspase-10 is recruited to and activated at the native TRAL and CD95 death-inducing signaling complexes in FADD-dependent manner but cannot functionally substitute caspase-8. EMBO J 21:4520–4530

Tang G, Minemoto Y, Dibling B et al (2001) Inhibition of JNK activation through NF-κB target genes. Nature 414:313–317

Tartaglia L, Pennica D, Goddel DV (1993) Ligand passing: the 75-kDa tumor necrosis factor (TNF) receptor recruits TNF for signaling by the p55-kDa TNF receptor. J Biol Chem 268:18542–18548

Thomas B, Grell M, Pfizenmaier K et al (1990) Identification of a 60-kDa tumor necrosis factor (TNF) receptor as the major signal transducing component in TNF responses. J Exp Med 172:019–1023.

Thome M, Tschopp J (2001) Regulation of lymphocyte proliferation and death by flip. Nat Rev Immunol 1:50–58

Tomiyama H, Matsuda T, Takiguchi M (20020 Differentiation of CD8+ T cells from a memory to memory/effector phenotype. J Immunol 168:5538–5550

Trebilcock GU, Ponnappan U (1996) Evidence for lowered induction of nuclear factor kappa B in activated human T lymphocytes during aging. Gerontology 42:137–146

Vandenabeele P, Declercq W, Vanhaesebroeck B et al (1995) Both TNF receptors are required for TNF-mediated induction of apoptosis in PC60 cells. J Immunol 154:2904–2913

Weil R, Israel A (2006) Deciphering the pathway from the TCR to NF-κB. Cell Death Differ 13:826–833

Weiss T, Grell M, Siekienski K et al (1998) TNFR80-dependent enhancement of TNFR60-induced cell death is mediated by TNFR-associated factor 2 and is specific for TNFR60. J Immunol 161:3136–3142

Weninger W, Crowley MA, Manjunath N (2001) Migratory properties of naïve, effector, and memory CD8 (+) T cells. J Exp Med 194:953–966

Whisler RL, Beiqing L, Chen M (1996) Age-related decreases in IL-2 production by human T cells are associated with impaired activation of nuclear transcriptional factors AP-1 and NF-AT. Cell Immunol 169:185–195

Yoshino K, Kondo E, Cao L et al (1994) Inverse expression of Bcl-2 protein and Fas antigen in lymphoblasts in peripheral nodes and activated peripheral blood T and B lymphocytes. 83:1856–1861

Zamzami N, Kroemer G (2001) The mitochondrion in apoptosis: how pandora's box opens. Nat Rev Mol Cell Biol 2:67–71

Mechanisms - Mitochondria

Mitochondria and Immunosenescence

Pazit Beckerman and Arie Ben Yehuda

Contents

1 Introduction

The immune system undergoes age-associated changes, that affect its response to infections and cancer, and contributes to the organism's aging and its associated pathologies. An eminent hypothesis to explain the aging process, most supported by experimental data, is the mitochondrial free radical theory. Evidence is accumulating, linking mitochondrial oxidative damage and apoptosis to immunosenescence.

2 Mitochondria- Structure and Biology

Mitochondria are ubiquitous organelles that are intimately involved in many cellular processes. Its principal task is to provide the energy necessary for normal cell functioning and maintenance. Mitochondria are composed of several compartments, each with specific metabolic functions, including the inner and the outer membranes, the intermembrane space and the matrix. The inner membrane joins the mitochondrial cristae at specific junctions. The cristae contain the electron transport chain (ETC), phosphorylation apparatus, and membrane transporters [1].

The electron donors, NADH and $FADH_2$, provide reducing equivalents to the ETC. The ETC is composed of 4 multisubunit enzyme complexes. NADH is oxidized by complex I, reducing the lipid soluble mobile electron carrier coenzyme Q. Complex III oxidizes reduced coenzyme Q and in turn reduces the mobile carrier protein cytochrome c that donates its electron to cytochrome oxidase, complex IV, for the reduction of oxygen to water. The complexes of the ETC are likely to

P. Beckerman (✉) · A. B. Yehuda
University Hospital Kerem
The Department of Medicine
Hadassah Ein

T. Fulop et al. (eds.), *Handbook on Immunosenescence,*
DOI 10.1007/ 978-1-4020-9062-2_37, © Springer Science+Business Media B.V. 2009

be organized in larger supercomplexes, forming a respirasome, in order to optimize channeling of reducing equivalents. Electron transfer down the redox potential gradient is coupled to the active transport of hydrogen ions from the matrix to the cytosol. This process requires a tightly controlled permeability of the inner membrane to ions and small molecules.

The phosphorylation apparatus uses the inner membrane proton gradient to phosphorylate ADP by complex V. Complex V couples proton flow down the electrochemical gradient from outer aspect of the inner membrane to the matrix side and the energy is utilized to drive complex V resulting in ATP production.

Uncoupling of respiration from ADP phosphorylation is a mechanism of physiologic regulation of the rate of oxidative phosphorylation. Uncoupling of respiration in pathologic states occurs due to damage to either the integrity of the inner membrane or of complex V. Uncoupling of respiration in pathologic states is more likely to collapse the electrochemical gradient, impairing energy production and increasing the probability of mitochondrial permeability transition [1, 2].

3 Mitochondrial Diseases

The classic mitochondrial diseases result from mutations in mitochondrial DNA (mtDNA) or nuclear genes that disrupt mitochondrial respiratory functions. These disorders have brain and skeletal muscle manifestations, and are often referred to as mitochondrial encephalomyopathies. Hundreds of point mutations, deletions and rearrangements have been associated with these diseases. Since all of the mitochondrial diseases have a disrupted respiratory function, one might expect a similar phenotype. The clinical variability is large, however, with many disease exhibiting tissue specific manifestations.

The role of mitochondrial dysfunction in a number of common conditions including the process of aging is being slowly elucidated. Evidence is emerging to suggest that mitochondria play a key role in the etiology of neurological disorders.

Parkinson's disease is a chronic neurodegenerative condition. Mitochondrial dysfunction, and in particular oxidative stress, has been implicated in its pathogenesis. Deficiencies of complex I have been observed in some patients with Parkinson's disease [3, 4], in the substantia nigra and subsequently in the peripheral tissues. Complex I is the target of toxins known to produce parkinsonian features in humans, such as MPTP. Inhibition of complex I results in increased free radical generation and could contribute to the oxidative mediated damage seen in Parkinson's disease. Families with mtDNA mutations and Parkinsonism have been identified [5]. Several studies that have sequenced mtDNA in Parkinson's disease patients have not identified any consistent mutations, although none has focused on Parkinson's patients with complex I deficiency. Mitochondrial complex I deficiencies have been described not only in the brain but also in skeletal muscle, platelets and lymphocytes in Parkinson's disease [6]. The relation between mitochondrial dysfunction and Parkinson's disease has evoked an attempt to develop treatment that might improve disease progression, using coenzyme Q_{10}, that may enhance respiratory chain function [7].

Mutations in the genes for amyloid precursor protein are associated with Alzheimer's disease. Amyloid Aβ can inhibit oxidative phosphorylation in mitochondria [8]; impaired COX activity, reduced immunoreactive protein or decreased mRNA for mtDNA encoded proteins have been observed in the Alzheimer's disease brain; Aβ directly interacts with a mitochondrial enzyme, ABAD. ABAD is important in cell function, its inactivation results in a lethal phenotype, it is up regulated in Alzheimer's disease neurons and its coexpression with amyloid precursor protein exacerbates Aβ induced free radical mediated cell damage and death [9]. ABAD and Aβ colocalize in the mitochondria of Alzheimer's disease cortex and this interaction causes increased mitochondrial activity and apoptosis.

4 Mitochondria and Aging

The mitochondrial theory of aging states, that the original insult to mtDNA is induced by the continuous generation of reactive oxygen species (ROS) and other toxic species. mtDNA may be particularly susceptible to oxidative damage due to its lack of protective histones and its proximity to the inner mitochondrial membrane, where reactive oxygen species are produced. Some of the mutations in mtDNA impair respiratory chain function, leading to increased ROS production and further mtDNA damage, creating a vicious cycle. The positive feedback between mtDNA mutation and generation of ROS is thought to result in an increase in oxidative damage during aging, with eventual loss of cellular and tissue functions through a combination of energy insufficiency, signaling defects, apoptosis and replicative senescence.

Two mechanisms combine to increase ROS production from mitochondria in aged tissues. First, decreased flux through the electron transport chain increases the reduction of upstream complexes, especially complexes I and III, enhancing electron leak that generates ROS. Second, aging-induced modification of individual electron transport chain complexes can directly result in a greater fraction of electron leak.

Decreases in enzyme activity of an ETC complex can lower the rate of oxidative phosphorylation [1]. A decrease of 30-50% in activity is probably needed to result in a significant maximal rate lowering. The sites of greatest control of respiration are complex I in the ETC and the adenine nucleotide translocase and complex V in the phosphorylation apparatus. These sites require the least decrease in enzyme activity for decreases in the rate of oxidative phosphorylation to occur. Aging may alter the inner membrane, thereby impairing the activity of ETC complexes, or alter complex V, thereby slowing the rate or efficiency of phosphorylation.

Mitochondrial transmembrane potential is the driving force of cellular ATP formation, and its reduction can lead to ATP depletion and cell deenergization. Evidence show that oxidants may induce mitochondrial transmembrane potential reduction and mitochondrial depolarization by promoting mitochondrial permeability transition due to oxidation of mitochondrial pyridine nucleotides and glutathione [10].

In support of this hypothesis many studies have linked ROS production and oxidative stress to aging and longevity [11].

Many tissues from aged individuals have lower respiratory function compared to tissues from younger individuals. Many reports also demonstrate that the rate of production of ROS from mitochondria increases with age in mammalian tissues: an increase of ROS was found in hepatocytes from aged rats [12], higher levels of peroxide and increased peroxide production after an adriamycin-induced oxidative stress. ROS production was also shown to increase in senescent fibroblasts and aging skeletal muscle cells.

A strong negative correlation has been demonstrated between expected lifespan and metabolic rate and ROS production rate of different species [13], and between lifespan and membrane lipid saturation.

Interventions and mutations that prolong survival tend to decrease the production of ROS from mitochondria, providing further evidence to the connection between aging and mitochondrial function: Calorie restriction has been shown to extend longevity; it increases the life span of rodents and delayed autoimmunity and onset of malignancy in mice. Calorie restriction also reduces the over-production of various T-cells subsets while maintaining the capacity of cells to respond to mitogens. It also maintains appropriate levels of apoptosis, including responses to dexamethasone induced death. The potency of NK and cytolytic T-cells was also maintained for longer periods in calorie restricted mice [14]. Sohal et al. proposed that calorie restriction significantly reduces aging of the mitochondria and production of ROS [15]. It attenuates age related changes in lipid peroxidation. It also decreases mitochondrial ROS production at complex I and lowers mtDNA oxidative damage. The major impact of calorie restriction on mitochondrial respiration appears to be a modulation of state 4 respiration, which increases via an increase in uncoupling protein content. The decreased coupling of respiration results in a decreased production of ROS that is reversed by an increase in fat intake (reviewed in 1). Calorie restriction also seems to trigger an adaptive response protecting the most basic requirements of membrane integrity.

Antioxidants experimental effect on aging may also demonstrate the mitochondrial relation, since it has been suggested that improvement in the age-related decreases in mitochondrial oxidative phosphorylation caused by antioxidants, attenuates aging. Still, the role of antioxidants in longevity is disputed. Studies comparing constitutive antioxidant levels between mammalian species, and experiments increasing or decreasing their tissue antioxidant concentrations in different ways, indicate that antioxidants do not seem to control aging rate, although they can protect against different pathologies and early death (reviewed in 16).

ROS have been shown to target al.1 biomolecules in the cell, which undergo chemical modifications that accumulate with age- protein carbonylation and methionine oxidation, advanced glycation end-products, lipid peroxidation and nucleotide modifications [11].

Finally, mtDNA point mutations and deletions are more prevalent in aged tissues and cells. Numerous studies have documented the presence of large mtDNA deletions from muscle and brain from old individuals. A minimal threshold level of 90-95% of mutated mtDNA is usually necessary to impair respiratory chain function, depending on the type of mutation and the tissue affected. This may result from extensive fragmentation of mtDNA in minicircles in elderly subjects, increasing the amount of mtDNA mutations [17].

Two mouse models have further implicated mtDNA mutations in the aging process. Knockin mice have been developed by two research groups [18, 19]. These mice express a proofreading-deficient PolgA, the nuclear encoded catalytic subunit of the mtDNA polymerase, and acquire mtDNA mutations at a much higher rate than normal. The PolgA mutator mice accumulate mtDNA mutations in numerous tissues, reproducing the effect of aging. The mice have a phenotype consistent with premature aging, including osteoporosis, reduced activity, alopecia, reduced fertility, cardiac hypertrophy, and severe weight loss with decreased muscle mass and lipoatrophy. Interestingly, in spite of the widespread mutations, these mice do not appear to have any change in the levels of hydrogen peroxide or increased oxidative damage to DNA, proteins or lipids [19]. Still, evidence shows that mitochondrial but not cytosolic targeting of catalase, an antioxidant enzyme, over-expression enhances lifespan and reduces age-related cardiac pathology and cataracts. This further emphasizes the contribution of the mitochondrion to free radical mediated cellular damage and dysfunction in relation to aging [20].

Many tissues in error-prone PolgA mice described above contain increased levels of caspase-3. This increase in caspase-3 activation was also observed in tissues from normal aged mice. The mutant mice also showed increased TUNEL staining, an indication of the DNA fragmentation, a hallmark for apoptosis. Therefore, the diverse signs of aging in these mice may be due to apoptosis induction [19]. The induction of apoptosis may be related to the observation that patients carrying high loads of certain mtDNA mutations show a high degree of TUNEL-positive muscle fibers. Widespread apoptosis is also found in mouse embryos lacking mitochondrial transcription factor A, which is necessary for mtDNA expression and maintenance. These studies support the hypothesis that mtDNA mutations accumulation can induce the premature emergence of aging associated features (reviewed in 21). The role of mtDNA mutations in normal aging still remains to be elucidated.

5   Mitochondria and Immunosenescence

The mechanisms involved in immunosenescence have not been fully deciphered yet. The mitochondria could contribute to alteration of the age-related immunodeficiency by two mechanisms. First, like any eukaryote cell, lymphocytes require oxidoreductase processes by mitochondria, via the respiratory chain. Second, mitochondria are involved in apoptosis, a major process in T-cell death.

Mitochondrial modifications in the immune system cells are still largely obscure. Peripheral lymphocytes of 366 healthy individuals were examined by electron microscope. Ultrastructural mitochondrial damages increased from 50 years of age until 80 years, but after 80 years decreased [22]. The morphologic changed consisted of disappearance of the mitochondrial cristae, which were replaced by a lamellar structure, electron dense and electron opaque material, that was similar to lipofuscin.

With increasing age, human lymphocytes express reduced proliferation in response to mitogens [23], suggesting that the mitogenic stimulus induces stress which is better tolerated by cells from young, rather than from old individuals. It has been shown that antioxidants were able to recover the age dependent impairment of lymphocyte response to mitogens [24], which suggests an oxidative stress.

A few studies have evaluated the age dependent alterations of mitochondrial parameters in immune cells.

A clear cut delay of the increase in ATP following phytohemagglutinin stimulation has been shown in older human cells [25]. Also, a decrease of mitochondrial respiration with aging of mouse splenic lymphocytes was found [26].

Several studies have identified, using fluorescent probes specific for mitochondrial transmembrane potential, a decrease in respiratory activity of murine lymphocytes during aging [27]. The existence and maintenance of the lymphocyte transmembrane potential involves two main mechanisms: the active transport of monovalent cations, sodium and potassium, and their diffusion through membrane pores. The reduction in ATP-ase activity during aging may lead to the reduction in membrane potential.

Another study used two mitochondrial specific probes with a potential dependent or independent uptake, and found that the decline in the respiratory activity in the mouse occurred approximately six months prior to the decrease in mitochondrial membrane mass [28]. Respiratory activity of splenocytes decreased with age in animals older than six months to 50% of its initial level by 24 months. Mitochondrial membrane mass decreased after 12 months, by 25% up to 24 months. These results, with minor differences, were repeated in rat cells [29], showing that respiratory activity per unit of mitochondrial mass declined in an age dependent manner.

Rottenberg et al. showed that spleen lymphocytes from old mice had lower respiration rates than lymphocytes from young mice. Cyclosporine, an inhibitor of the mitochondrial permeability transition (PT), restored normal respiration rates to lymphocytes from old mice, suggesting enhanced susceptibility to mitochondrial permeability transition activation. By using DiOC6 as a probe for mitochondrial transmembrane potential, they showed that lymphocytes from old mice also had a lower mitochondrial membrane potential than lymphocytes from young mice, which was also restored by cyclosporine. Lymphocytes from old mice also exhibited a more oxidized state, as represented by the ratio FAD/FADH, a useful measure for the redox potential in mitochondria. It was suggested that enhanced generation of ROS leads to increased oxidative stress in lymphocytes from old mice, which renders their mitochondria more susceptible to PT activation [30].

These results were later demonstrated on leukocytes from healthy human volunteers of different age groups. Leukocytes were subjected to oxidative injuries by exposure to t-butylhydroperoxide, and were labeled with fluorochromes for measuring mitochondrial transmembrane potential, membrane peroxidation and mitochondrial oxidant formation. Mitochondrial transmembrane potential declined after t-butylhydroperoxide exposure, and the change was more prominent in leukocytes from older individuals. Cyclosporine A partially restored mitochondrial transmembrane potential, implying again the contribution role of PT. The mitochondrial depolarization was accompanied by increased oxidant formation and oxidation of pyridine nucleotides, which were more prominent in older individuals [31].

Studies of age-induced immune dysfunction suggest that the decline of the immune system response is largely due to T-cells dysfunction, which is associated with shifts in the composition of the T-cells population, specifically, a shift from a low memory to naïve ratio to a higher ratio [32]. One of the dysfunctions identified in T-cells from old rodents and humans is an attenuation of calcium signaling, which accompanies the expansion of memory T-cells [33]. Mather et al. review the changes in calcium signaling in aging T-cells [34]. Activation of TCR receptor induces a sustained elevation of calcium ions, which activated the nuclear factor of activated T-cells, transcription factors, and initiates the transcription of genes of the immune response. Ionomycin, a calcium ionophore that induces a sustained increase in calcium ions, induces T-cells proliferation, but is much less effective in raising calcium levels in T-cells from old mice, suggesting that calcium signaling mechanisms might be modulated in aging. The small fraction of ionomycin resistant cells in T-cells preparations from young mice, similar to the majority of cells from old mice, consists of memory cells.

Thapsigargin, an inhibitor of the endoplasmic reticulum Ca^{2+} ATPase releases calcium from internal stores and activates calcium release activated calcium channels in T lymphocytes. The thapsigargin-induced sustained calcium elevation was shown to depend critically on mitochondrial calcium uptake, which is driven by the mitochondrial transmembrane potential. The mitochondria remove Ca^{2+} from the vicinity of the calcium channels, thus preventing their activation. Inhibition of mitochondrial calcium uptake also inhibits the T-cell receptor-induced sustained elevation of calcium. Permeability transition (PT) is a large non specific channel that is activated by calcium and ROS. Its activation collapses the mitochondrial transmembrane potential, inhibits oxidative phosphorylation and calcium sequestration by mitochondria, and may induce apoptosis. Mather et al. showed that in T lymphocytes from young mice, the ionomycin-induced elevation of cell free calcium was inhibited by collapsing the mitochondrial membrane potential by uncouplers and ionophores, and activation of the PT. In T lymphocytes from old mice, ionomycin is ineffective in sustaining the calcium elevation, but treatment with cyclosporine A, which inhibits PT, restores the ionomycin-sustained calcium elevation. The enhanced activation of PT in T-cells from old mice was associated with enhanced oxidation of mitochondrial FAD, therefore aging may result in a reduction in mitochondrial transmembrane potential and enhanced oxidation of T-cell mitochondria, thereby activating PT and inhibiting calcium elevation, which affects T-cells proliferation [34].

Ayub et al. suggested that this change in calcium influx, whether mitochondria-mediated or not, is actually the result of activation of apoptotic pathways. Fas-stimulation of T-cells was shown to block calcium influx [35], a blockade that was specific for the fas-induced apoptosis route. A similar uncoupling of calcium influx from the calcium store release was observed in neutrophils [36]. The mechanism by which fas ligand uncouples calcium channel opening is not yet resolve, although the mechanism described above, including loss of mitochondrial membrane potential, is a possible explanation [37].

A number of studies measured the enzyme activity of individual electron transport chain complexes or oxygen consumption by leukocytes as an index of aging-related decrease in oxidative function of these cells.

Drouet et al. examined oxidative phosphorylation parameters with aging in lymphocytes [38]. Lymphocytes were retrieved from human volunteers, aged from 23 to 98 years, who were divided into two age groups, with average ages of 35 and 80.8 years. T-cells subpopulation analysis revealed a decline in absolute count of naïve cells in the elderly, whereas no significant change was observed in the percentage and absolute number of memory cells. Activity of complexes II, III, and IV of the respiratory chain was analyzed. Complex III activity did not change with aging, however, a significant decrease in complex II+III activity occurred in the elderly group. No difference was observed in complex IV activity between the groups.

The authors suggested that decline in complex II activity with aging could be secondary to a decline in the levels of active enzyme molecules per mitochondrion, or due to accumulation of altered molecules in the organelle. The decreased production of energy in the mitochondria, together with an increase of oxidative stress with aging, can activate the mitochondrial permeability transition pore and initiate apoptosis.

The sensitivity of lymphocytes in this study to specific inhibitors of respiratory chain complexes, such as rotenone and malonate, was high and unaffected by age, as opposed to an effect previously shown on human platelets.

Drouet et al. also examined the possibility that the decreases in respiratory chain activity could be secondary to mtDNA mutations, but found no mtDNA deletion, concluding that the dysfunction could be related to nuclear DNA damage, a suggestion that requires more investigation.

Sandhu et al. measured the activities of complexes I-V and CS [citrate synthase] in crude mitochondria fraction from four brain areas as well as from lymphocytes, from 1, 3-4, 12 and 24-month-old age group rats [39]. Age related alterations in mitochondrial electron transport chain complexes I-V and CS were observed. With the increasing age of the rats, a significant decline was seen in the specific activity of complexes I-V and CS. Since mtDNA encodes seven subunits of complex I and three subunits of complex IV, the authors suggest that the pattern of complex I and IV activities may be consistent with mtDNA deletions.

This study also correlated mitochondrial dysfunction with simultaneous aging in brain and immune cells. Interestingly, T-cells mediated immunity dysfunction has been implicated in the etiology of many of the chronic neurodegenerative diseases in the elderly. Several studies also give partial indication that lymphocyte analysis may provide an easy noninvasive method for investigating respiratory chain enzymes and assessing mitochondrial function in patients with neurodegenerative diseases.

6 Mitochondria and Apoptosis

Mitochondria play a central role in the regulation of programmed cell death.

Cells undergoing apoptosis exhibit a decrease in mitochondrial transmembrane potential that precedes nuclear signs of apoptosis. This applies to different cells types, including lymphocytes exposed to glucocorticoids or other lethal activation signals (40, 41). Apoptosis induced by pathologic stimuli is preceded by mitochondrial transmembrane potential dissipation. Both transcription of mitochondrial genome and synthesis of mitochondrial proteins are perturbed early during the apoptotic process. Loss of mitochondrial function is also observed in anucleate cells induced to undergo apoptosis, indicating that apoptotic alterations of mitochondrial function can occur in complete independence of the nucleus. Mitochondria are required in some cell free systems to induce nuclear apoptosis. Cyclosporine A, a PT inhibitor, efficiently prevents the apoptosis associated fall in mitochondrial transmembrane potential, which may indicate that apoptotic mitochondrial transmembrane potential reduction results from PT.

Direct induction of PT by protoporphyrin IX, which is well known for its PT-triggering capacity, induced mitochondrial transmembrane potential disruption, enhanced generation of superoxide anions, and increased signs of apoptosis in thymocytes and T-cells from mice, as evidenced by DNA hypoploidy and fragmentation and chromatin loss [42].

Regulation of T-cells apoptosis is essential for lymphocyte homeostasis and immune functions [43]. During an adaptive immune response naïve and memory T-cells proliferate and fulfill their effector function. This expansion phase is followed by the contraction phase, in which T-cells numbers decline and reach normal levels. This process is highly regulated and requires a switch from an apoptosis resistant towards an apoptosis sensitive state in T lymphocytes. T-cells homeostasis is basically controlled by two separate apoptosis pathways: activation induced cell death (AICD) and activated T-cells autonomous death (ACAD). In ACAD, cell death is determined by the ratio between anti- and pro-apoptotic Bcl-2 family members at the mitochondria. The intrinsic cell death pathway critically depends on permeabilization of the outer mitochondrial membrane for cell death execution. A number of apoptotic signals converge on mitochondria, such as oligomerization of the apoptotic Bax and Bak proteins, leading to permeabilization of the outer membrane and release of cytochrome c, apoptosis inducing factors and Smac/DIABLO into the cytoplasm. Cytochrome c binds to adaptor molecules, including apoptosis protease activating factor 1 (Apaf-1) and initiator pro-caspase proteins, forming an 'apopto-some', which leads to cleavage of pro-caspase-9 to active caspase 9, which can then activate downstream effector caspases 3 and 7, resulting in apoptosis. During ACAD, the pro-apoptotic Bcl-2 and Bcl-X_L are found in a constitutive association with Bim on the mitochondrial membrane, blocking the apoptotic function of Bim assuring cell survival. The ratio between Bcl-2 versus Bim regulates T-cells death. Mitochondria in apoptotic cells are also believed by some to release considerably more ROS.

7   Apoptosis and Immunosenescence

Apoptosis plays a key role in a variety of immune processes, including elimina-tion of potential anti-self clones, removal of faulty pre-B and pre-T-cells arising in the marrow and thymus, and also destruction of virally infected and tumorigenic cells by natural killer cells and cytolytic T-cells. Given the importance of apoptosis in the normal functioning of the immune system, immunosenescence itself could be altered by age related changes in apoptosis, including the mitochondrial path-way. Controversial data exist in the literature. Some investigators have reported a decrease of Fas/FasL-induced apoptosis in aged animals, and in human CD8+ T-cells reaching replicative senescence after multiple rounds of antigen-specific proliferation [44].

Increased resistance to apoptosis was found in cells from people chronically exposed to oxidative stress, as in patients affected by Fanconi's Anemia or uremia.

Monti et al. [45] examined peripheral blood mononuclear cells from three age groups of human donors. They induced apoptosis by 2-deoxy-D-ribose (dRib), an agent that induces apoptosis in mononuclear cells by interfering with cell redox status and mitochondrial membrane potential. They found an inverse correlation between the age of the donors and the propensity of their mononuclear cells to undergo apoptosis. Cells from old people showed an increased resistance to dRib-induced glutathione depletion and a decreased tendency to lose the mitochondrial membrane potential. No difference in Bcl-2 was found. This indicates a decreased tendency to undergo apoptosis in the old. Moreover, the increased resistance of dRib-induced apoptosis of mononuclear cells appeared to be related to glutathione depletion, but independent of Bcl-2 content, suggesting mitochondrial involvement that is age related.

On the other hand, others identified increased apoptosis in lymphocytes from elderly people following activation with anti-CD3, Phytohemagglutinin, Concana-valin, or activation with polyclonal mitogen plus anti-Fas treatment.

Gupta et al. [46] examined T-cells subsets of the aged (65-95 years) and the young (20-29 years) using peripheral blood T-cells. They found increased expres-sion of Fas and FasL on both CD4+ and CD8+ lymphocytes of the aged subjects.

They also compared naïve and memory cells. A decreased expression of Bcl-2 (anti apoptotic protein) and increased expression of Bax (pro apoptotic protein) was noted in naïve and memory T-cells of the aged [47-48].

Monti et al. [45] suggested that this apparent contradiction in results can be explained taking into account the experimental setting, and hypothesized that aging is characterized on one hand by an increased tendency to undergo apoptosis in activated lymphocytes, and on the other hand, by a decreased tendency to undergo apoptosis as a more general process of senescence.

These changes in aging T-cells could explain the reduced number of naïve T-cells produced in the elderly, and contribute to the early termination of immune responses in the elderly.

Another explanation to the different response of memory versus naïve cells was offered by Kim et al. They have demonstrated that splenic T lymphocytes from old mice exhibit a significant decline in mitochondrial membrane potential; yet despite this change, there is a lower rate of withdrawal apoptosis in the memory CD4$^+$ and CD8$^+$ T-cells. To explain the survival of the cells in spite of increased oxidative stress, the authors demonstrated increased glutathione production and phase II enzyme (antioxidants) expression, which protect the memory T-cells. Phase II enzymes play a role during aging, and age-related changes in their expression were shown in various tissues, including brain and liver. Kim et al. showed similar increases in memory T-cells, compared to naive cells. Moreover, compared with wild type mice, mice lacking the expression of NF-E2-related factor-2, the transcription factor that regulated phase II enzyme expression, had a significantly increased rate of apoptosis in response to an oxidative stress stimuli. These cells exhibit a greater decline in mitochondrial membrane potential and increased ROS production. The authors claim that this mechanism could contribute in part to the accumulation of memory T-cells during aging [49].

In summary, the aging process affects the function of multiple cells and organs in the human organism. One theory that explains the aging process, and supported by experimental data, is the mitochondrial free radical theory. According to this theory, ROS accumulate in the mitochondria, causing an oxidative damage to mitochondrial DNA and to the mitochondrial respiratory chain function, thereby causing the decrease in cellular function. A large body of evidence exists that supports this theory in different tissues, including heart, skeletal muscle and brain. Data is accumulating that similar processes also take place in the immune system. Studies on immune cells from humans and animals have shown age-related decreases in mitochondrial respiration, mitochondrial transmembrane potential, and respiratory chain complexes activity. Moreover, mitochondria are also involved in the apoptotic process, which in itself plays an important role in T-cells regulation and homeostasis, and is essential for immune system function. Changes in apoptotic processes have been shown to occur in cells of the aging immune system, thereby further emphasizing mitochondrial role in immunosenescence. Further studies are needed in order to understand to what extent mitochondrial changes with age influence the dysregulation of both innate and cognate immunity and what are the clinical consequences of such changes.

References

1. Lesnefsky EJ, Hoppel CL (2006) Oxidative phosphorylation and aging. Ageing Res Rev. 5(4):402–433
2. Weiss JN, Korge P, Honda HM, Ping P (2003) Role of the mitochondrial permeability transition in myocardial disease. Circ Res 93(4):292–301
3. Swerdlow RH, Parks JK, Miller SW, Tuttle JB, Trimmer PA, Sheehan JP, Bennett JP, Davis RE, Parker WD (1996) Origin and functional consequences of the complex I defect in Parkinson's disease. Ann Neurol 40(4):663–671
4. Schapira AH, Cooper JM, Dexter D, Jenner P, Clark JB, Marsden CD (1990) Mitochondrial complex I deficiency in Parkinson's disease. J Neurochem 54(3):823–827
5. Gu M, Cooper JM, Taanman JW, Schapira AH (1998) Mitochondrial DNA transmission of the mitochondrial defect in Parkinson's disease. Ann Neurol 44(2):177–186
6. Yoshino H, Nakagawa-Hattori Y, Kondo T, Mizuno Y (1992) Mitochondrial complex I and II activities of lymphocytes and platelets in Parkinson's disease. J Neural Transm Park Dis Dement Sect 4(1):27–34
7. Shults CW, Oakes D, Kieburtz K, Shults CW, Oakes D, Kieburtz K, Beal MF, Haas R, Plumb S, Juncos JL, Nutt J, Shoulson I, Carter J, Kompoliti K, Perlmutter JS, Reich S, Stern M, Watts RL, Kurlan R, Molho E, Harrison M, Lew M (2002) Parkinson Study Group. Effects of coenzyme Q10 in early Parkinson disease: evidence of slowing of the functional decline. Arch Neurol 59(10):1541–1550
8. Casley CS, Canevari L, Land JM, Clark JB, Sharpe MA (2002) Beta-amyloid inhibits integrated mitochondrial respiration and key enzyme activities. J Neurochem. 80(1):91–100
9. Schapira AH (2006) Mitochondrial disease. Lancet. 368(9529):70–82
10. Crompton M (1999) The mitochondrial permeability transition pore and its role in cell death. Biochem J. 341(2):233–249
11. Lenaz G, Baracca A, Fato R, Genova ML, Solaini G (2006) New insights into structure and function of mitochondria and their role in aging and disease. Antioxid Redox Signal 8(3-4):417–437
12. Cavazzoni M, Barogi S, Baracca A, Parenti Castelli G, Lenaz G (1999) The effect of aging and an oxidative stress on peroxide levels and the mitochondrial membrane potential in isolated rat hepatocytes. FEBS Lett 449(1):53–6
13. Barja G, Herrero A (2000) Oxidative damage to mitochondrial DNA is inversely related to maximum life span in the heart and brain of mammals. FASEB J 14(2):312–8
14. Fraker PJ, Lill-Elghanian DA (2004) The many roles of apoptosis in immunity as modified by aging and nutritional status. J Nutr Health Aging 8(1):56–63
15. Sohal R, Weindruch R (1996) Oxidative stress, caloric restriction, and aging. Science 273(5271):59–63
16. Sanz A, Pamplona R, Barja G (2006) Is the mitochondrial free radical theory of aging intact? Antioxid Redox Signal 8(3–4):582–599
17. Hayakawa M, Katsumata K, Yoneda M, Tanaka M, Sugiyama S, Ozawa T (1996) Age-related extensive fragmentation of mitochondrial DNA into minicircles. Biochem Biophys Res Commun 226(2):369–377
18. Trifunovic A, Wredenberg A, Falkenberg M, Spelbrink JN, Rovio AT, Bruder CE, Bohlooly YM, Gidlof S, Oldfors A, Wibom R, Tornell J, Jacobs HT, Larson NG (2004) Premature ageing in mice expressing defective mitochondrial DNA polymerase. Nature 429(6990):417–423
19. Kujoth GC, Hiona A, Pugh TD, Someya S, Panzer K, Wohlgemuth SE, Hofer T, Seo AY, Sullivan R, Jobling WA et al. (2005) Mitochondrial DNA mutations, oxidative stress, and apoptosis in mammalian aging. Science 309(5733):481–484
20. Schriner SE, Linford NJ, Martin GM, Treuting P, Ogburn CE, Emond M, Coskun PE, Ladiges W, Wolf N, Van Remmen H, Wallace DC, Rabinovitch PS (2005) Extension of murine life span by overexpression of catalase targeted to mitochondria. Science 308(5730):1909–1911

21. Chan DC (2006) Mitochondria: dynamic organelles in disease, aging, and development. Cell. 125(7):1241–1252
22. Beregi E, Regius O (1983) Relationship of mitochondrial damage in human lymphocytes and age. Aktuelle Gerontol 13(6):226–228
23. Murasko DM, Weiner P, Kaye D (1987) Decline in mitogen induced proliferation of lymphocytes with increasing age. Clin Exp Immunol 70(2):440–448
24. Chaudhri G, Clark IA, Hunt NH, Cowden WB, Ceredig R (1986) Effect of antioxidants on primary alloantigen-induced T cell activation and proliferation. J Immunol 137(8):2646–2652
25. Verity MA, Tam CF, Cheung MK, Mock DC, Walford RL (1983) Delayed phytohemagglutinin-stimulated production of adenosine triphosphate by aged human lymphocytes: possible relation to mitochondrial dysfunction. Mech Ageing Dev 23(1):53–65
26. Weindruch RH, Cheung MK, Verity MA, Walford RL (1980)Modification of mitochondrial respiration by aging and dietary restriction. Mech Ageing Dev 12(4):375–92
27. Witkowski J, Micklem HS (1985) Decreased membrane potential of T lymphocytes in ageing mice: flow cytometric studies with a carbocyanine dye. Immunology 56(2):307–313
28. Leprat P, Ratinaud MH, Julien R (1990) A new method for testing cell ageing using two mitochondria specific fluorescent probes. Mech Ageing Dev 52(2–3):149–167
29. Pieri C, Recchioni R, Moroni F (1993) Age-dependent modifications of mitochondrial transmembrane potential and mass in rat splenic lymphocytes during proliferation. Mech Ageing Dev 70(3):201–212
30. Rottenberg H, Wu S (1997) Mitochondrial dysfunction in lymphocytes from old mice: enhanced activation of the permeability transition. Biochem Biophys Res Commun 240(1):68–74
31. Tsai K, Hsu TG, Lu FJ, Hsu CF, Liu TY, Kong CW (2001) Age-related changes in the mitochondrial depolarization induced by oxidative injury in human peripheral blood leukocytes. Free Radic Res 35(4):395–403
32. Pawelec G, Adibzadeh M, Solana R, Beckman I (1997) The T cell in the ageing individual. Mech Ageing Dev 93(1–3):35–45
33. Sulger J, Dumais-Huber C, Zerfass R, Henn FA, Aldenhoff JB (1999 Mar) The calcium response of human T lymphocytes is decreased in aging but increased in Alzheimer's dementia. Biol Psychiatry 45(6):737–742
34. Mather MW, Rottenberg H (2002) The inhibition of calcium signaling in T lymphocytes from old mice results from enhanced activation of the mitochondrial permeability transition pore. Mech Ageing Dev 123(6):707–724
35. Lepple-Wienhues A, Belka C, Laun T, Jekle A, Walter B, Wieland U, Welz M, Heil L, Kun J, Busch G, Weller M, Bamberg M, Gulbins E, Lang F (1999) Stimulation of CD95 (Fas) blocks T lymphocyte calcium channels through sphingomyelinase and sphingolipids. Proc Natl Acad Sci U S A 96(24):13795–13800
36. Ayub K, Laffafian I, Dewitt S, Hallett MB (2004) Ca influx shutdown in neutrophils induced by Fas (CD95) cross-linking. Immunology 112(3):454–60
37. Ayub K, Hallett MB (2004) Signalling shutdown strategies in aging immune cells. Aging Cell 3(4):145-149
38. Drouet M, Lauthier F, Charmes JP, Sauvage P, Ratinaud MH (1999) Age-associated changes in mitochondrial parameters on peripheral human lymphocytes. Exp Gerontol. 34(7):843–852
39. Sandhu SK, Kaur G (2003) Mitochondrial electron transport chain complexes in aging rat brain and lymphocytes. Biogerontology 4(1):19–29
40. Zamzami NP, Marchetti P, Castedo M, Zanin C, Vayssiere JL, Petit PX, Kroemer G (1995) Reduction in mitochondrial potential constitutes an early irreversible step of programmed lymphocyte death in vivo. J Exp Med 181(5):1661–1672
41. Petit PX, LeCoeur H, Zorn E, Dauguet C, Mignotte B, Gougeon ML (1995) Alterations in mitochondrial structure, function are early events of dexamethasone-induced thymocyte apoptosis. J Cell Biol 130(1):157–567
42. Marchetti P, Hirsch T, Zamzami N, Castedo M, Decaudin D, Susin SA, Masse B, Kroemer G (1996) Mitochondrial permeability transition triggers lymphocyte apoptosis. J Immunol 157(11):4830–4836

43. Arnold R, Brenner D, Becker M, Frey CR, Krammer PH, (2006) How T lymphocytes switch between life and death. Eur J Immunol 36(7):1654–1658
44. Spaulding C, Guo W, Effros RB, et al. (1999) Resistance to apoptosis in human CD8+ T-cells that reach replicative senescence after multiple rounds of antigen-specific proliferation. Exp Gerontol 34(5):633–644
45. Monti D, Salvioli S, Capri M, Malorni W, Straface E, Cossarizza A, Botti B, Piacentini M, Baggio G, Barbi C, Valensin S, Bonafe M, Franceschi C (2000) Decreased susceptibility to oxidative stress-induced apoptosis of peripheral blood mononuclear cells from healthy elderly, centenarians. Mech Ageing Dev 121(1–3):239–250
46. Gupta S (2000) Molecular and biochemical pathways of apoptosis in lymphocytes from aged humans. Vaccine 18(16):1596–1601
47. Aggarwal S, Gupta S (1998) Increased apoptosis of T-cell subsets in aging humans: altered expression of Fas (CD95), Fas ligand, Bcl-2, Bax J Immunol 160(4):1627–1637
48. Gupta S, Gollapudi S (2006) Molecular mechanisms of TNF-alpha-induced apoptosis in naive, memory T cell subsets. Autoimmun Rev 5(4):264–268
49. Kim HJ, Nel AE (2005) The role of phase II antioxidant enzymes in protecting memory T-cells from spontaneous apoptosis in young and old mice. J Immunol 175(5):2948–59

Mechanism - Proteasome

Proteasome Activity and Immunosenescence

Bertrand Friguet

Contents

Abbreviations

G6PDH	glucose-6-phosphate dehydrogenase
HNE	4-hydroxy-2-nonenal
ROS	reactive oxygen species
RNS	reactive nitrogen species

Abstract: The proteasome is the main proteolytic system implicated in the removal of oxidatively damaged proteins, general turnover of intracellular proteins and targeted degradation of proteins that have been marked by poly-ubiquitination. Impairment of proteasome function has been associated with cellular aging in a variety of tissues and cell types including lymphocytes, and is believed to contribute to the age-related accumulation of oxidized proteins due to their decreased elimination by the proteasomal pathway. This chapter first summarizes the most relevant features of the proteasomal system and then expands on the current knowledge on the impact of aging on proteasome structure and function, taking in account the fate of proteasome upon oxidative stress situations. Finally, the possible implication of age-related alterations of the proteasomal system in the process of immunosenescence is presented.

Keywords: Proteasome • Aging • Protein oxidation • Damaged protein degradation • Immunosenescence

B. Friguet (✉)
Université Pierre et Marie Curie, Paris 6, UMR 7079
Case Courrier 256, 4 Place Jussieu, 75252 Paris cedex 05, France
Tel./Fax: 33 (0) 1 44 27 82 34
E-mail: bertrand.friguet@snv.jussieu.fr

T. Fulop et al. (eds.), *Handbook on Immunosenescence,*
DOI 10.1007/ 978-1-4020-9062-2_38, © Springer Science+Business Media B.V. 2009

1 Introduction

Aging is a complex process controlled by genetic and environmental factors, which is accompanied by the decline of different physiological functions of an organism during the last part of its life. Damage to macromolecules has been implicated in the cellular degeneration that occurs during aging and accumulation of oxidized proteins represents a hallmark of cellular aging (Beckman and Ames 1998; Berlett and Stadtman 1997). Indeed, proteins are targets for numerous posttranslational modifications such as oxidation, conjugation with lipid peroxidation products and glycoxidation, that have been shown to affect their biological function (Davies 1987, 1993; Stadtman 1990, 2006). In addition, calorie restriction, the only intervention known to slowdown aging, delays the age-related accumulation of oxidatively damaged proteins (Goto et al. 2002; Shibatani and Ward 1996) while long-lived transgenic animals were found to exhibit a decreased load of protein oxidative damage (Orr and Sohal 1994). Elimination of damaged protein and protein turnover is critical to preserve cell function and the main proteolytic system in charge of cytosolic protein degradation is the proteasome, a multicatalytic proteolytic complex that recognizes and selectively degrades oxidatively damaged and poly-ubiquitinated proteins (Coux et al. 1996; Davies 2001; Grune et al. 1997; Voges et al. 1999). Since accumulation of oxidized protein with age can be due to increased protein alteration, decreased elimination (i.e., repair and degradation) of oxidatively damaged protein or the combination of both phenomenons, one of the hypothesis put forward to explain oxidized protein build-up is a decrease of proteasome activity with age (Friguet 2006; Friguet et al. 2000; Gaczynska et al. 2001; Keller et al. 2000a). In fact, age-related impairment of proteasome has been documented in a variety of organs, tissues and cell types, which appears to be the result of numerous factors including decreased proteasome components expression, alteration and/or replacement of proteasome subunits and formation of inhibitory elements such as oxidatively modified cross-linked proteins. Since both age-related accumulation of damaged proteins and impairment of proteasome have been documented in lymphocytes (Beregi et al. 1991; Poggioli et al. 2002; Ponnappan et al. 1999; Sell et al. 1998), alterations of proteasome structure and function may therefore directly contribute to the complex process of immunosenescence.

2 Proteasomes

2.1 20S Proteasome Structure and Proteolytic Activity

The 20S proteasome is a high molecular weight multicatalytic proteolytic complex found in Archaebacteria and Eukaryotes that is implicated in the degradation of most of the intracellular proteins including oxidized and poly-ubiquitinated proteins (Coux et al. 1996; Davies 2001; Grune et al. 1997; Voges et al. 1999). This complex that has been first observed in erythrocytes by Harris in 1968 (Harris 1968), is ubiquitous in eukaryotic cells, in which it can represent up 1% of total soluble proteins (Tanaka et al. 1986). In mammalian cells, the proteasome constitutes the main nonlysosomal proteolytic system involved in protein degradation in the cytosol and in the nucleus. Besides acting as a housekeeping enzyme by eliminating abnormal and oxidized proteins, the proteasome is also implicated in a broad range of cellular functions through the selective degradation of ubiquitin-targeted regulatory proteins such as transcription factors, cyclins and rate-limiting enzymes in important metabolic pathways (Cie-chanover and Iwai 2004; Goldberg et al. 1997; King et al. 1996; Pajonk and McBride 2001). The 20S proteasome exhibits a cylinder shape of about 15 nm length and 11 nm diameter and is made up of four stacked rings of seven subunits classified as α or β subunits (Groll et al. 1997; Hegerl et al. 1991; Lowe et al. 1995). The seven α subunits form the apical rings of the complex while the seven β subunits form the inner rings and carry the catalytic activities. The two outer chambers are formed by the junction of one α ring and one β ring and the central catalytic chamber is made by the junction of the two β rings. The eukaryotic proteasome has only three catalytically active β subunits: β1 for the peptidyl glutamylpeptide hydrolase (or postacidic) activity, β2 for the trypsin-like activity and β5 for the chymotrypsin-like activity that cleave peptide bonds after an acidic, basic and hydrophobic aminoacid, respectively (Coux et al. 1996; Groll et al. 1997; Kisselev et al. 1999). The specificity pockets S1 have been described as positive, negative or neutral electrostatic potential surfaces (Borissenko and Groll 2007). Two copies of each subunit are present in the catalytic chamber that contains six active sites. These activities can be conveniently assayed using specific fluorogenic peptides. Proteasomes have the unique property to use a N-terminal threonine as a catalytic residue. A maturation step is needed to generate the N-terminal amino group which implicates intramolecular autolysis to remove the prosegments of the β-subunit precursors. The proteolytic mechanism was elucidated using crystal structures of yeast and bovine liver proteasomes (Groll et al. 1997; Unno et al. 2002) and site-directed mutagenesis (Ditzel et al. 1998; Groll et al. 1999). Interestingly, when cells are exposed to such stimuli as IFNγ, TNFα or LPS the subunit composition of the 20S proteasome is modified, as inducible homologous subunits are incorporated in the structure upon de novo synthesis: the iβ1, iβ2 and iβ5 subunits, respectively replace their β1, β2 and β5 constitutive counterparts to form the immunoproteasome (Fruh et al. 1994; Gaczynska et al. 1993; Tanaka 1994). Such replacement of proteasome subunits modify proteasome peptidase activities and lead to higher chymotrypsin-like and trypsin-like activities and lower peptidyl glutamylpeptide hydrolase activity, thus increasing production of peptides with higher affinity for MHC class I complex (Fruh et al. 1994; Gaczynska et al. 1993; Kloetzel 2004; Rivett and Hearn 2004; Rock and Goldberg 1999; Tanaka 1994).

2.2 20S Proteasome Inhibitors

The development of selective inhibitors of the proteasome has been very useful for deciphering the cellular functions of the proteasome. The majority of proteasome inhibitors are short peptides bearing a reactive group which creates a covalent bond with the catalytic N-terminal threonine such as peptide aldehydes (MG 132, Braun et al. 2005; Groll et al. 1997), peptide boronates (MG 262, bortezomib or Velcade™, Adams et al. 1998; Adams and Kauffman 2004) and peptide vinyl sulfones (Bogyo et al. 1997; Borissenko and Groll 2007). Epoxomicin is a peptide epoxyketone that is a natural molecule isolated from the actinomycete strain Q996-17. Epoxomicin preferentially inhibits the chymotrypsin-like activity and is characterized by its unique specificity for the proteasome (Elofsson et al. 1999). The natural β lactone lactacystin (Streptomyces sp.) is a nonpeptidic molecule that form covalent acyl ester bond with the N-terminal threonine (Borissenko and Groll 2007; Fenteany et al. 1995). Lactacystin in itself is not active against the proteasome but its spontaneous hydrolysis generates clasto-lactacystin β lactone (omularide) which binds specifically to the β5 subunit and inhibits the chymotrypsin-like activity. Noncovalent inhibitors of the proteasome have been investigated less extensively. The anti HIV protease Ritonavir and benzylstatine derivatives have been shown to inhibit the proteasome non-covalently (Furet et al. 2004; Schmidtke et al. 1999). The cyclic tripeptide TMC-95A, which is a metabolite of Apiospora montagnei, is a very potent inhibitor of all three peptidase activities of the proteasome (Koguchi et al. 2000). Non covalent binding of TMC-95A with the proteasome active sites has been demontrated by X-ray analysis (Groll et al. 2001). Other molecules have also been described as proteasome inhibitors such as gliotoxin (Kroll et al. 1999), lipopeptides (Basse et al. 2006), bi- or multivalent molecules (Loidl et al. 1999), ajoene (Xu et al. 2004), arecoline derivatives (Marastoni et al. 2004) and epigallocatechin-3-gallate analogs (Wan et al. 2005).

2.3   20S Proteasome Regulators and the 26S Proteasome

The eukaryotic 20S proteasome cylinder is closed in its latent form and can be switched to an active form under certain experimental conditions such as heat treatment, addition of fatty acids or detergent at low concentration (Ando et al. 2004; Dahlmann et al. 1985). In addition, the opening of the α rings can be promoted upon binding to the 20S proteasome of regulatory complexes such as PA700 (19S) or PA28 (11S), Dahlmann 2005). The 26S proteasome results from the ATP-dependent association with PA700 or 19S regulator and is an essential component of the ubiquitin–proteasome degradation pathway of poly-ubiquitinated proteins. The axial channel of the 20S proteasome is gated by the Rpt2 subunit of PA700 while PA28 stimulates 20S proteasome peptidase activities and may facilitate product release in vivo (Kohler et al. 2001). 20S proteasome can bind one or two 19S regulators resulting the formation of either "single-capped" or "double-capped" 26S proteasome. In addition, hybrid proteasome containing one PA28 and one PA700 complex associated at both end of the 20S proteasome can be formed (Tanahashi et al. 2000). The association of PA28 to the 20S proteasome is ATP-independent and results in an increase of proteasome peptidase activities while it does not improve protein degradation (Dubiel et al. 1992; Ma et al. 1992; Whitby et al. 2000). As for the immunoproteasome subunits, the expression of PA28 subunits is induced after treatment of cell by IFNγ. In the cytosol PA28 is composed of two types of subunits α and β of about 28 kDa forming hexa or heptameric rings α3β3 or α3β4 while in the nucleus PA28 is made of single type subunit γ (Ahn et al. 1995; Knowlton et al. 1997; Mott et al. 1994). The 19S regulator is composed of at least eigthteen subunits belonging to either the «lid» or the «base» of the complex. Six of the nine subunits of the base are ATPases exhibiting a chaperone-like activity and are believed to participate to the unfolding of the substrate protein prior to its entrance in the 20S proteasome catalytic chamber and its degradation (Braun et al. 1999; Hershko and Ciechanover 1998; Kloetzel 2001). The lid subunits are involved in the recognition of polyubiquitinated protein substrates and recycling the ubiquitin moiety through isopeptidase activity (Deveraux et al. 1994; Hershko and Ciechanover 1998). Polyubiquitination of a protein is a complex process that requires ATP and involves ubiquitin, a 76 amino acids protein, and three enzymes, E1 (ubiquitin-activating enzyme), E2 (ubiquitin-conjugating enzymes) and E3 (ubiquitin ligases), to ensure specific recognition of the protein substrate (Ciechanover and Iwai 2004; Finley et al. 2004; Weissman 2001).

3 Age-Associated Impairment of Proteasome Function

3.1 Accumulation of Oxidized Proteins

Protein are oxidized as a result of oxidative insult derived from the production of reactive oxygen species (ROS) and reactive nitrogen species (RNS), that includes superoxide anion, hydrogen peroxide, the hydroxyl radical, nitric oxide and peroxynitrite (Berlett and Stadtman 1997; Dean et al. 1997). These reactive species are produced in the cell during the aerobic metabolism at the level of organelles such as mitochondria and peroxisome and by other enzymatic or nonenzymatic pathways (Beckman and Ames 1998). Increased ROS production is also achieved during situations of oxidative stress such as UV irradiation or inflammation. Basal production of ROS is part of normal cellular redox homeostasis, and antioxidants (enzymatic and nonenzymatic) regulate their level. However, when the balance between ROS production and elimination is disrupted, increased damage to macromolecules (including lipids, nucleic acids and proteins) occurs, leading to both reversible and irreversible oxidative modifications (Hensley and Floyd 2002). Within a protein, all amino acids can be oxidized but sulfur-containing (cysteine and methionine) and aromatic (tryptophane and tyrosine) amino acids are the most susceptible to oxidation (Stadtman and Levine 2003). In addition, tyrosine is a target for the reactive nitrogen species peroxynitrite, giving rise to nitrotyrosine. Oxidation of cysteine leads to disulfide bridges, mixed disulfides and cysteic acids, i.e. cysteine sulfenic, sulfinic and sulfonic acids (Requena et al. 2003). Formation of disulfide bridges, mixed disulfides or cysteine sulfenic acids is reduced by the thioredoxin/thioredoxine reductase or the glutaredoxin/

glutathione/glutathione reductase systems (Holmgren 2000; Levine and Stadtman 2001; Poole et al. 2004). Oxidation of methionine into methionine sulfoxide can be reversed catalytically by the peptide methionine sulfoxide reductases system (Grimaud et al. 2001; Sharov et al. 1999).

Oxidation of other amino acids most often leads to the formation of hydroxyl and carbonyl derivatives. Thus, detection of protein-associated carbonyl groups has been widely used for assessing the extent of protein oxidation. Several methods aimed at quantitative measurement of carbonyl groups within proteins are based on their specific derivatization by 2, 4–dinitrophenylhydrazine and immunochemical detection of such derivatized carbonylated proteins can be achieved using an antidinitrophenyl antibody (Levine et al. 1994). Upon oxidation, proteins usually become less active, less thermostable and more hydrophobic (Davies 1987; Fisher and Stadtman 1992; Friguet et al. 1994b). Protein damage can also originate from oxidation-derived reactions of amino acids such as lysine, arginine, histine and cysteine with lipid peroxidation products (e.g., 4-hydroxy-2-nonenal, malondialdehyde) or with sugars or derived metabolites to form glycoxidation adducts (e.g., carboxymethyl lysine, pentosidine). The resulting adducts that are formed on the protein often bring in carbonyl groups and/or cross-links (Friguet and Szweda 1997; Szweda et al. 2002). The function of these modified proteins is generally impaired or even completely inactivated.

Age-related increases in protein carbonyl content, taken as a signature of oxidative modifications, have been widely documented in different tissues and organisms: human dermal fibroblasts, human epidermal cells, human lenses, human erythrocytes, human brain, rat hepatocytes and whole *Drosophila* (Levine and Stadtman 2001; Petropoulos et al. 2000). In human keratinocytes and lenses, we have shown that increased protein oxidation is associated with increased protein glycoxidation and conjugation by lipid peroxidation adducts (Petropoulos et al. 2000; Viteri et al. 2004). Such an increase in oxidatively damaged protein is believed to affect cellular integrity, since it is associated with the impairment of key enzymes. Recent data argue for an age-related increase in protein carbonyl content such that elderly individuals would have one-third of their proteins in average carrying this oxidative modification (Stadtman and Levine 2000). However, not all proteins are equally sensitive to oxidation and there are growing evidence that only a restricted set of proteins would be preferentially affected. Indeed, Sohal and colleagues have already reported that in aging flies, two mitochondrial enzymes, aconitase and adenine nucleotide translocase, are specific targets for oxidative modification (Yan et al. 1997; Yan and Sohal 1998) and we have recently shown that glutamate dehydrogenase and ornithine carbamoyl transferase are preferentially glycoxidized in the liver mitochondrial matrix of old rats (Hamelin et al. 2007). Moreover, based on a proteomic approach, we have previously reported that age-related increases in protein glycoxidation and modification by the lipid peroxidation product 4-hydroxy-2-nonenal (HNE) are also restricted to preferential target proteins in human peripheral blood lymphocytes (Poggioli et al. 2002, 2004).

3.2 Oxidized Protein Elimination

Since repair of oxidized proteins is limited to reduction in specific oxidation products of sulfur-containing amino acids, oxidation of all other amino acids within a protein will target it for degradation (Carrard et al. 2002; Friguet 2006). Upon mild oxidation, proteins become more prone to proteolysis, while highly oxidized proteins usually become resistant to proteolysis because of the formation of intra- and intermolecular cross-links (Friguet and Szweda 1997; Grune et al. 1997). Oxidized proteins represent good substrates for degradation by the proteasome in vitro, and oxidized proteins have been shown to be preferentially degraded by the 20S proteasome in an ATP- and ubiquitin-independent manner in a variety of cell types (Davies 2001; Shringarpure et al. 2003). However, certain studies have reported that the ubiquitin-26S proteasome pathway is involved in degradation of oxidized protein from lens cells (Shang et al. 2001). Moreover, ubiquitination of proteins carrying glycoxidation and lipid peroxidation adducts has also been documented (Bulteau et al. 2001b; Marques et al. 2004). The increased susceptibility of an oxidized protein to proteolysis has been correlated with exposure of hydrophobic amino acids at the surface of the protein that may represent a recognition signal for degradation by the 20S proteasome (Davies 2001; Grune et al. 1997). Alternatively, such exposure of residues that are normally hidden in the hydrophobic core of the protein may result from decreased thermodynamic stability of the oxidized protein that renders it more flexible, especially at the C-terminus and/or N-terminus end of the protein, hence making it more prone to progressive degradation by either the 20S or 26S proteasomes (Goldberg et al. 1997). Interestingly, recent evidence has been provided that chaperone-mediated autophagy of proteins carrying a KFERQ motif is activated upon oxidative stress, implying participation of this proteolytic pathway in elimination of some oxidized proteins (Kiffin et al. 2004). Moreover, it has been also recently reported that when proteasome capacity is exceeded, autophagin expression is induced suggesting a physiological link between the lysosomal and proteasomal degradation systems (Klionsky 2005).

The proteasome appears to be a key actor in damaged protein elimination and other regulatory processes, and oxidative damage to protein has been implicated in age- and disease-related impairment of cellular functions. Therefore, the fate of the proteasome during oxidative stress has received particular attention. Indeed, peptidyl glutamyl peptide hydrolase and trypsin-like activities are readily inactivated upon exposure of the 20S proteasome to metal-catalyzed oxidation in vitro (Conconi et al. 1996, 1998). However, these alterations depend on whether the proteasome is in its active or latent state, a finding that may be related to the differential susceptibility to oxidative stress of the 26S and 20S proteasomes (Reinheckel et al. 1998). Moreover, in vitro treatment of the 20S and 26S proteasomes with nitric oxide or HNE was found to inactivate certain peptidase activities (Conconi and Friguet 1997; Farout et al. 2006; Ferrington and Kapphahn 2004; Glockzin et al. 1999). In addition, the proteasome is a target for modifications by oxidative processes in vivo that can lead to either its transient or irreversible inactivation. We first reported that FAO hepatoma cells, treated with iron and ascorbate in order to promote metal-catalyzed oxidation, exhibited decreased peptidyl glutamyl peptide hydrolase and trypsin-like activities, indicating that the proteasome was a target for inactivation upon oxidative stress (Conconi et al. 1998). Interestingly, both α-crystallin and Hsp 90 were found to protect proteasomes against oxidative insults in vitro, while depletion or overexpression of Hsp 90 in FAO cells resulted in decreased or increased protection of proteasome trypsin-like activity, respectively. This chaperone-mediated protection of proteasome activity during oxidative stress may be related to other antioxidant properties described, especially for small heat shock proteins (Arrigo 2001). In addition, neural SH-SY5Y cells stably transfected with human HDJ-1, a member of the HSP40 family, were shown to retain a greater preservation of proteasome activity following oxidative injury (Ding and Keller 2001). Taken together the data suggest that heat shock proteins may confer resistance to oxidative stress, at least in part, by preserving proteasome function. Oxidative stress induced in vivo by treatment with ferric nitriloacetate in kidney and ischemia-reperfusion in brain induced impairment of proteasome function correlated with the appearance of HNE-modified proteasomes (Keller et al. 2000c; Okada et al. 1999). Upon coronary occlusion-reperfusion, inactivation of trypsin-like activity has been associated with specific modification by HNE of three proteasome subunits (Bulteau et al. 2001a). In contrast, upon UV irradiation of cultured keratinocytes leading to a decline in proteasome activity, no modification of the proteasome was observed when the proteasome was purified from irradiated cells (Bulteau et al. 2002a). Proteasome inhibition resulted from the UV-induced increased load of damaged proteins, such as HNE modified proteins. In neural cells, inhibition of mitochondrial complex I by rotenone and 1-methyl-4-phenylpyridinium was found to increase the production of ROS and to inactivate the proteasome, most likely through oxidative damage and ATP depletion (Hoglinger et al. 2003; Shamoto-Nagai et al. 2003). Upon treatment of neuroblastoma cells with rotenone, a drastic reduction in proteasome activity was observed and suggested to originate from direct modification of 20S proteasome subunits by acrolein while aggregated acrolein-modified proteins coimmunoprecipated with the proteasome (Shamoto-Nagai et al. 2003). Conversely, proteasome inhibition has been shown to decrease complex I and complex II activities and to increase oxygen free radical production, indicating that mitochondrial homeostasis is altered, oxidative stress is triggered, and cell vulnerability to oxygen free radicals is increased as a result of proteasome inhibition (Hoglinger et al. 2003; Sullivan et al. 2004). These findings underscore the critical importance of the interplay of the different protein maintenance systems implicated in cellular redox homeostasis, protection against oxidative stress and oxidized protein removal. Finally, it has been recently shown that both 26S and 20S proteasomes peptidase activities could be inhibited upon treatment with the prooxidant buthionine sulfoximine of T cells from young donors resulting in an increase in oxidized proteins and a decline in both activation-induced proliferation and degradation of the NκB inhibitor, IκB (Das et al. 2007).

3.3 Decreased Proteasome Activity with Age

The age-related accumulation of oxidatively modified and ubiquitinated proteins, and the general decline in protein turnover, have raised the possibility that proteasome function is impaired with age (Carrard et al. 2002; Friguet et al. 2000). Pioneering studies from our group and that of Ward indicated that proteasome proteolytic activity is affected with aging (Conconi et al. 1996; Shibatani and Ward 1996; Shibatani et al. 1996). Indeed, we showed that the 20S proteasome from rat liver exhibited a 50% decrease for the peptidyl glutamylpeptide hydrolase activity when purified from old animals compared with young ones, while Ward and collaborators reported a 40% decrease in the same peptidase activity when activated by SDS and assayed in crude homogenates (Conconi et al. 1996; Shibatani et al. 1996; Shibatani and Ward 1996). Interestingly, we also reported that decreased protein uptake upon dietary self-selection of nutriments, can compensate for the age-related decrease of 20S proteasome activity observed with standard diet in rat liver (Anselmi et al. 1998). This finding may be related to the beneficial effects associated with dietary restrictions in calories and proteins, including decreased macromolecular damage, increased expression of antioxidant enzymes and increased longevity. Subsequently, we and other groups have reported that proteasome activity declines with age in a variety of tissues (Bardag-Gorce et al. 1999; Bulteau et al. 2002b; Hayashi and Goto 1998; Keller et al. 2000a; Merker et al. 2000; Petropoulos et al. 2000; Ponnappan et al. 1999; Viteri et al. 2004), although some studies have shown that this decline may not be universal. Such a decline in proteasome activity is believed to contribute to the age-associated build up of oxidized protein.

We have shown that the age-related decline in proteasome activity might be explained by decreased expression of proteasome subunits in human keratinocytes (Petropoulos et al. 2000), human fibroblasts (Chondrogianni et al. 2000), and rat cardiomyocytes (Bulteau et al. 2002b). Interestingly, fibroblasts from healthy centenarians exhibited proteasome activity and proteasome subunit expression levels closer to those of younger individuals than older ones, suggesting that sustained proteasome activity could have contributed to the successful aging of these individuals (Chondrogianni et al. 2000). In a more recent study, the exhaustive analysis of proteasome subunit expression in senescent WI 38 human fibroblasts has indicated that only the expression of catalytic β-subunits is decreased, and that less 20S proteasome is assembled while certain α-subunits are found in a free state (Chondrogianni et al. 2003). Moreover, exposure of WI 38 young fibroblasts to sublethal doses of the proteasome inhibitor epoxomycin resulted in a senescent-like phenotype. Transcriptome analysis using microarrays performed on both mouse skeletal muscle and human fibroblasts has shown decreased expression of several 20S and 26S proteasome subunits (Lee et al. 1999; Ly et al. 2000). In both analyses, performed with either post-mitotic or mitotic cell types, fewer than 2% of the genes monitored showed age-related altered expression, with very little overlap except for proteasome components. The gene expression profile observed with dietary-restricted old animals led the authors to propose that the anti-aging effect associated with dietary restrictions may have originated from stimulation of protein turnover and decreased accumulation of macromolecular damage (Lee et al. 1999). Evidence for changes in the proteasome composition has been provided in certain age related neurode-generative diseases (Vigouroux et al. 2004). Of particular interest is the Huntington disease where a concomitant increased of chymotrypsin-like and trypsin-like activi-ties of the proteasome and an overexpression of the iβ1 and iβ5 inducible subunits were observed in the affected brain regions, indicating that changes in the 20S core particle subunit composition may play a role in neurodegeneration (Diaz-Hernan-dez et al. 2003, 2004). More recently Ferrington et al. reported in aged muscle a two to threefold increased of immunoproteasome whereas 20S proteasome expres-sion was decreased. Moreover the low proteasome activity was attributed to a 75% reduced amount of PA700 and PA28 complexes, suggesting that in aged muscle, the endogenous content of proteasome activators is inadequate for complete activation of the 20S proteasome (Ferrington et al. 2005).

In addition to decreased and/or modified proteasome subunits expression, as an explanation for the age-related decline in proteasome activity, our initial finding of decreased peptidyl glutamylpeptide hydrolase specific activity of proteasome purified from aged rat liver was indicative of direct inactivation of the proteasome (Anselmi et al. 1998; Conconi et al. 1996). Further studies on proteasome purified from rat liver or cardiomyocytes and human epidermis showed decreased protea-some proteolytic activity coupled with subunit replacement and/or posttranslational modifications, as evidenced by comparison of two-dimensional gel electrophoretic patterns of proteasome subunits (Anselmi et al. 1998; Bulteau et al. 2000; Bulteau et al. 2002b). In the spinal cord of Fisher 344 rats, the age related decrease of pro-teasome activity was associated with both a decreased level of proteasome expres-sion and an increased level of HNE modified β subunits (Keller et al. 2000b). In more recent studies, 26S proteasome was purified from human peripheral blood lymphocytes obtained from donors of different ages, and the patterns of proteasome subunits modified by either glycoxidation or conjugation with a lipid peroxidation product were analyzed by 2D gel electrophoresis followed by specific immunode-tection of the carboxymethyl lysine or HNE adducts (Carrard et al. 2003). These modifications were analyzed, since treatment of purified proteasome with either glyoxal or HNE can inactivate the proteasome (Bulteau et al. 2001b; Conconi and Friguet 1997). Interestingly, only a restricted number of 20S proteasome subunits were modified with age, while PA700 subunits were hardly modified (Carrard et al. 2003). The question as to why some proteasome subunits are more prone to modi-fications than others remains to be elucidated, but the age-related increased load of modifications in certain proteasome subunits might be related to the observed inactivation of proteasome peptidase activities. Finally, the fate of the proteasome was analyzed in the human eye lens and an age-related decline in all three peptidase activities was observed (Viteri et al. 2004). This finding was consistent with a pre-vious report from Wagner and Margolis indicating an age-related decline in pro-teasome peptidase activities in the bovine lens (Wagner and Margolis 1995). This decline could be explained, at least in part, by decreased proteasome content with age. However, among the three peptidase activities, the peptidylglutamyl peptide hydrolase activity was much more decreased than the other two, indicating that this peptidase activity has been targeted for inactivation. Although this finding was only correlative and may not be related to the observed inactivation, increased glycoxidative modifications of the proteasome were evidenced with age (Viteri et al. 2004).

Proteasome activity has been reported to be inhibited by highly modified proteins such as cross-linked proteins generated upon incubation with the lipid peroxidation product HNE (Friguet et al. 1994a). Indeed, in contrast to oxidized G6PDH that becomes more sensitive to degradation, when treated with HNE, the model protein glucose-6-phosphate dehydrogenase (G6PDH) becomes less susceptible to proteolysis by the 20S proteasome. Moreover, these cross-linked proteins were found to inhibit the degradation of an oxidized protein by the proteasome in a non-competitive manner (Friguet and Szweda 1997). Thus, if present in cellular extracts of elderly individuals, such cross-linked proteins could act as inhibitors of the proteasome. Evidence for such an inhibitory mechanism has been provided since introduction of artificial lipofuscin (a ceroid pigment that accumulates in aged cells) has been shown to inhibit proteasome function (Sitte et al. 2000). More recently, accumulation of lipofuscin has been shown to result in proteasome inhibition which can induce apoptosis through the increase of proteasome regulated proapoptotic proteins (Powell et al. 2005). Conversely, proteasome inhibition can promote lipofuscin formation, suggesting that insufficient proteasomal function may contribute to lipofuscinogenesis by a compensatory increase in the amount of proteins that are directed for lysosomal degradation (Terman and Sandberg 2002). Since proteasome inhibition also induces alteration of mitochondrial homeostasis in neural cell (Hoglinger et al. 2003; Sullivan et al. 2004), the appearance of increased level of lipofuscin suggest that impairments in mitochondrial turnover may occur following proteasome inhibition. Of additional interest is the observation that proteasome peptidase activities that were strongly inhibited in rat heart homogenates from old animals, were partially restored when assayed on the purified proteasome, suggesting that endogenous inhibitors were eliminated during the purification process (Bulteau et al. 2002b). Finally, depending on the cellular system investigated, the age-related decline in proteasome activity appears to be due, at least in part, to the combined effects of: (a) decreased proteasome subunits expression; (b) direct inactivation upon modification of proteasome subunits; and (c) the presence of endogenous inhibitors such as cross-linked proteins.

4 Proteasome and Immunosenescence

Proteasomal function is generally impaired with age. Indeed, an age-related decline of proteasomal function has been documented in a variety of tissues and cell types such as rat cardiomyocytes (Bulteau et al. 2002b), human keratinocytes (Petropoulos et al. 2000), human fibroblasts (Chondrogianni et al. 2000, 2003; Merker et al. 2000) and human lens (Viteri et al. 2004). In the immune system, aging is associated with significant deficits in immune function and a decline of proteasome proteolytic activity has been reported in lymphocytes with increasing age of human donors (Carrard et al. 2003; Ponnappan et al. 1999). It is commonly accepted that older individual fail to generate a vigorous immune response, particularly to antigens not previously encountered (Ginaldi et al. 2001; Webster 2000). This decline in immune responsiveness with age is due, at least in part, to loss of Th cell function which affect both cellular and humoral immunity (Gravekamp 2001; Weksler and Szabo 2000). Thus, the decreased B cell response to antigenic stimulation is related to Th cell deficiency and to alterations in B cell development (Kline et al. 1999). In addition to lower antigenic response, an increase in autoantigenic response is observed with advancing age (Stacy et al. 2002; Weksler and Szabo 2000). The overall decline of the immune system is linked to several pathologies such as higher susceptibility to infections, autoimmunity and cancer (Ben-Yehuda et al. 1998; Dunn and North 1991; Miller 2000). In the immune system, decreased proteasomal activity would be expected to contribute not only to accumulation of oxidized proteins but also to the lower activation of transcription factors such as NFκB, and most importantly to the lower production of antigenic peptides by the immunoproteasome for binding to MHC class I molecules.

Several studies have demonstrated the crucial role of the transcription factor NFκB in the activation of T cell through the activation of IL-2 and IL-2R genes (Pimentel-Muinos et al. 1994). The expression of the two latter have been shown to decline with age suggesting a default in their transcriptional activation. In the cytosol, NFκB is under an inactive form bound to its inhibitor IκB. The activation of NFκB occurs after stimulation by numerous agents such as cytokines (IL-1 and TNF-α), bacterial and viral infection (Ponnappan 1998). The stimulated-degradation of IκB by the proteasome declines with advancing age and results in the decreased induction of NFκB, hence contributing to the immune decline observed in the elderly (Ponnappan et al. 1999). Examination of stimulated phosphorylation and ubiquitination of IκB did not demonstrate any significant age-related alterations (Ponnappan et al. 1999). The lowered degradation of IκB was then associated to a decreased proteasome function in the elderly. Indeed, proteasome chymotrypsin-like activity was shown to decrease for T cell proteasome enriched fractions (Ponnappan 2002) and for purified 26S proteasome from human lymphocytes (Carrard et al. 2003). However, no evidence for 20S proteasome (Ponnappan et al. 1999) nor 26S proteasome (Carrard et al. 2003) decreased content was found in the elderly samples. Since the observed lower activity was not related to a decreased proteasome expression, we investigated the integrity of the proteasome structure during aging (Carrard et al. 2003). The 19S complex subunits were marginally altered upon aging since only two of its subunits, the ATPase subunits S4 and S7, were glycoxidized and/or conjugated with the lipid peroxidation product HNE. Nevertheless, it should be pointed out that S4 subunit has been implicated in 26S proteasome assembly in human cells (Mason et al. 1998). However, glycation of this subunit did not appear to affect the stability of the 26S proteasome complex, since no enhanced dissociation into 20S and 19S was observed with age. In contrast, the 20S core was much more prone to posttranslational modification during aging. Indeed, α and β subunits were overall more affected by glycation, conjugation with lipid peroxidation product and ubiquitination in the elderly. Those modifications could have a direct impact on proteasome stability or activity. Indeed, modifications of α subunits could interfere with the accessibility of the substrate to the catalytic chamber and/or impact catalytic activities by destabilizing the interaction between regulatory α and catalytic β subunits. For example, the $\alpha7$ subunit is thought to coordinate the assembly of the rest of the α subunits in human proteasome (Gerards et al. 1998) and was severely modified by glycation, conjugation with HNE and was ubiquitinated. Another interesting finding regarding lowered protease activity with age was the modification by both glycation and HNE conjugation of the $i\beta5$ catalytic subunit which carries the chymotrypsin-like peptidase activity. Despite glycation of $i\beta5$ in early ages, the chymotrypsin-like specific activity was not affected. However, this does not rule out the possibility that glycation occurring in samples from elderly donors may target more crucial lysine residues involved in the catalytic activity. In contrast, conjugation of $i\beta5$ with HNE resulted in a concomitant decreased chymotrypsin-like activity of the proteasome complex. The observed increased ubiquitination of $i\beta5$ with age may also contribute to proteasome inactivation. The specific modification of 26S proteasome subunits could be central in the defect of activation of transcriptional factors implicated in the immune response and in antigen processing. Indeed, age-related decline of proteasome in human T-lymphocytes has been recently attributed to both a lower expression of certain catalytic and structural proteasome subunits, including immunoproteasome subunits, and increased oxidative modification of proteasome subunits (Ponnappan et al. 2007). Consequently, a lower degradation of infectious protein agents by the 26S proteasome and immunoproteasome could then result directly in a higher infection level and indirectly in a lowered immune response of the elderly. An age-related up-regulation of immunoproteasome subunits has been documented in muscle and brain that could be associated with constant inflammation or oxidative stress (Diaz-Hernandez et al. 2004; Ferrington et al. 2005), while down-regulation of immunoproteasome subunits in certain tumor cells has been interpreted as an immunosurveillance escape mechanism (Kageshita et al. 1999; Meidenbauer et al. 2004; Murakami et al. 2001). Up-regulation of immunoproteasome subunits has also been documented upon treatment with oxidants arguing for the ability of the proteasome system to cope with stress and the immunoproteasome to be part of the anti-stress response (Ding et al. 2003). Interestingly, treatment of senescent fibroblasts with IFNγ, as opposed to young fibroblasts, failed to induce immunoproteasome subunits (Stratford et al. 2006). In addition, such polymorphisms of immunoproteasome subunits as the LMP2 ($i\beta1$) codon 60 (R60H) have been associated with certain autoimmune diseases like spondylo and rheumatoid arthritis, and insulin-dependent diabetes mellitus (Deng et al. 1995; Pryhuber et al. 1996; Vargas-Alarcon et al. 2004) while an influence on susceptibility to TNFα-induced apoptosis of this particular polymorphism was observed in peripheral blood lymphocytes (Mishto et al. 2002). Therefore, investigating the age-related status of the immunoproteasome may be of critical importance due to its pivotal role in the antigen presentation pathway and both quantitative and qualitative alterations of the immunoproteasome activity would be expected to have a strong influence on the quantity and quality of immunodominant epitopes presented to T-cell receptor of CD8+ lymphocytes, hence leading to subsequent modifications of the immune response against antigens.

Akcnowledgments The work in our laboratory is supported by funds from the MENRT and European Framework Program 6 and 7 (IP 518230, Proteomage -IP 200880,Mark-Age).

References

Adams J, Behnke M, Chen S, Cruickshank AA, Dick LR, Grenier L, Klunder JM, Ma YT, Plamondon L, Stein RL (1998) Potent and selective inhibitors of the proteasome: dipeptidyl boronic acids. Bioorg Med Chem Lett 8:333–338

Adams J, Kauffman M (2004) Development of the proteasome inhibitor Velcade (Bortezomib). Cancer Invest 22:304–311

Ahn JY, Tanahashi N, Akiyama K, Hisamatsu H, Noda C, Tanaka K, Chung CH, Shibmara N, Willy PJ, Mott JD, et al (1995) Primary structures of two homologous subunits of PA28, a gamma-interferon-inducible protein activator of the 20S proteasome. FEBS Lett 366:37–42

Ando H, Watabe H, Valencia JC, Yasumoto K, Furumura M, Funasaka Y, Oka M, Ichihashi M, Hearing VJ (2004) Fatty acids regulate pigmentation via proteasomal degradation of tyrosinase: a new aspect of ubiquitin-proteasome function. J Biol Chem 279:15427–15433

Anselmi B, Conconi M, Veyrat-Durebex C, Turlin E, Biville F, Alliot J, Friguet B (1998) Dietary self-selection can compensate an age-related decrease of rat liver 20 S proteasome ac tivity observed with standard diet. J Gerontol A Biol Sci Med Sci 53:B173–B179

Arrigo AP (2001) Hsp27: novel regulator of intracellular redox state. IUBMB Life 52:303–307

Bardag-Gorce F, Farout L, Veyrat-Durebex C, Briand Y, Briand M (1999) Changes in 20S proteasome activity during ageing of the LOU rat. Mol Biol Rep 26:89–93

Basse N, Papapostolou D, Pagano M, Reboud-Ravaux M, Bernard E, Felten AS, Vanderesse R (2006) Development of lipopeptides for inhibiting 20S proteasomes. Bioorg Med Chem Lett 16:3277–3281

Beckman KB, Ames BN (1998) The free radical theory of aging matures. Physiol Rev 78:547–581

Ben-Yehuda A, Danenberg HD, Zakay-Rones Z, Gross DJ, Friedman G (1998) The influence of sequential annual vaccination and of DHEA administration on the efficacy of the immune response to influenza vaccine in the elderly. Mech Ageing Dev 102:299–306

Beregi E, Regius O, Rajczy K (1991) Comparative study of the morphological changes in lymphocytes of elderly individuals and centenarians. Age Ageing 20:55–59

Berlett BS, Stadtman ER (1997) Protein oxidation in aging, disease, and oxidative stress. J Biol Chem 272:20313–20316

Bogyo M, McMaster JS, Gaczynska M, Tortorella D, Goldberg AL, Ploegh H (1997). Covalent modification of the active site threonine of proteasomal beta subunits and the Escherichia coli homolog HslV by a new class of inhibitors. Proc Natl Acad Sci U S A 94:6629–6634

Borissenko L, Groll M (2007). 20S proteasome and its inhibitors: crystallographic knowledge for drug development. Chem Rev 107:687–717

Braun BC, Glickman M, Kraft R, Dahlmann B, Kloetzel PM, Finley D, Schmidt M (1999) The base of the proteasome regulatory particle exhibits chaperone-like activity. Nat Cell Biol 1:221–226

Braun HA, Umbreen S, Groll M, Kuckelkorn U, Mlynarczuk I, Wigand ME, Drung I, Kloetzel PM, Schmidt B (2005) Tripeptide mimetics inhibit the 20 S proteasome by covalent bonding to the active threonines. J Biol Chem 280:28394–28401

Bulteau AL, Lundberg KC, Humphries KM, Sadek HA, Szweda PA, Friguet B, Szweda LI (2001a). Oxidative modification and inactivation of the proteasome during coronary occlusion/reperfusion. J Biol Chem 276:30057–30063

Bulteau AL, Moreau M, Nizard C, Friguet B (2002a) Impairment of proteasome function upon UVA- and UVB-irradiation of human keratinocytes. Free Radic Biol Med 32:1157–1170

Bulteau AL, Petropoulos I, Friguet B (2000) Age-related alterations of proteasome structure and function in aging epidermis. Exp Gerontol 35:767–777

Bulteau AL, Szweda LI, Friguet B (2002b) Age-dependent declines in proteasome activity in the heart. Arch Biochem Biophys 397:298–304

Bulteau AL, Verbeke P, Petropoulos I, Chaffotte AF, Friguet B (2001b). Proteasome inhibition in glyoxal-treated fibroblasts and resistance of glycated glucose-6-phosphate dehydrogenase to 20 S proteasome degradation in vitro. J Biol Chem 276:45662–45668

Carrard G, Bulteau AL, Petropoulos I, Friguet B (2002) Impairment of proteasome structure and function in aging. Int J Biochem Cell Biol 34:1461–1474

Carrard G, Dieu M, Raes M, Toussaint O, Friguet B (2003) Impact of ageing on proteasome structure and function in human lymphocytes. Int J Biochem Cell Biol 35:728–739

Chondrogianni N, Petropoulos I, Franceschi C, Friguet B, Gonos ES (2000). Fibroblast cultures from healthy centenarians have an active proteasome. Exp Gerontol 35:721–728

Chondrogianni N, Stratford FL, Trougakos IP, Friguet B, Rivett AJ, Gonos ES (2003) Central role of the proteasome in senescence and survival of human fibroblasts: induction of a senescence-like phenotype upon its inhibition and resistance to stress upon its activation. J Biol Chem 278:28026–28037

Ciechanover A, Iwai K (2004) The ubiquitin system: from basic mechanisms to the patient bed. IUBMB Life 56:193–201

Conconi M, Friguet B (1997). Proteasome inactivation upon aging and on oxidation-effect of HSP 90. Mol Biol Rep 24:45–50

Conconi M, Petropoulos I, Emod I, Turlin E, Biville F, Friguet B (1998) Protection from oxidative inactivation of the 20S proteasome by heat-shock protein 90. Biochem J 333 (Pt 2):407–415.

Conconi M, Szweda LI, Levine RL, Stadtman ER, Friguet B (1996) Age-related decline of rat liver multicatalytic proteinase activity and protection from oxidative inactivation by heat-shock protein 90. Arch Biochem Biophys 331:232–240

Coux O, Tanaka K, Goldberg AL (1996) Structure and functions of the 20S and 26S proteasomes. Annu Rev Biochem 65:801–847

Dahlmann B (2005) Proteasomes. Essays Biochem 41:31–48

Dahlmann B, Rutschmann M, Kuehn L, Reinauer H (1985) Activation of the multicatalytic proteinase from rat skeletal muscle by fatty acids or sodium dodecyl sulphate. Biochem J 228:171–177

Das R, Ponnappan S, Ponnappan U (2007) Redox regulation of the proteasome in T lymphocytes during aging. Free Radic Biol Med 42:541–551

Davies KJ (2001). Degradation of oxidized proteins by the 20S proteasome. Biochimie 83:301–310

Davies KJ (1987) Protein damage and degradation by oxygen radicals. I. general aspects. J Biol Chem 262:9895–9901

Davies KJ (1993) Protein modification by oxidants and the role of proteolytic enzymes. Biochem Soc Trans 21:346–353

Dean RT, Fu S, Stocker R, Davies MJ (1997) Biochemistry and pathology of radical-mediated protein oxidation. Biochem J 324 (Pt 1):1–18

Deng GY, Muir A, Maclaren NK, She JX (1995) Association of LMP2 and LMP7 genes within the major histocompatibility complex with insulin-dependent diabetes mellitus: population and family studies. Am J Hum Genet 56:528–534

Deveraux Q, Ustrell V, Pickart C, Rechsteiner M (1994) A 26 S protease subunit that binds ubiquitin conjugates. J Biol Chem 269:7059–7061

Diaz-Hernandez M, Hernandez F, Martin-Aparicio E, Gomez-Ramos P, Moran MA, Castano JG, Ferrer I, Avila J, Lucas JJ (2003). Neuronal induction of the immunoproteasome in Huntington's disease. J Neurosci 23:11653–11661

Diaz-Hernandez M, Martin-Aparicio E, Avila J, Hernandez F, Lucas JJ (2004) Enhanced induction of the immunoproteasome by interferon gamma in neurons expressing mutant Huntingtin. Neurotox Res 6:463–468

Ding Q, Keller JN (2001) Proteasome inhibition in oxidative stress neurotoxicity: implications for heat shock proteins. J Neurochem 77:1010–1017

Ding Q, Reinacker K, Dimayuga E, Nukala V, Drake J, Butterfield DA, Dunn JC, Martin S, Bruce-Keller AJ, Keller JN (2003) Role of the proteasome in protein oxidation and neural viability following low-level oxidative stress. FEBS Lett 546:228–232

Ditzel L, Huber R, Mann K, Heinemeyer W, Wolf DH, Groll M (1998) Conformational constraints for protein self-cleavage in the proteasome. J Mol Biol 279:1187–1191

Dubiel W, Pratt G, Ferrell K, Rechsteiner M (1992) Purification of an 11 S regulator of the multicatalytic protease. J Biol Chem 267:22369–22377

Dunn PL, North RJ (1991) Effect of advanced ageing on the ability of mice to cause tumour regression in response to immunotherapy. Immunology 74:355–359

Elofsson M, Splittgerber U, Myung J, Mohan R, Crews CM (1999) Towards subunit-specific proteasome inhibitors: synthesis and evaluation of peptide alpha',beta'-epoxyketones. Chem Biol 6:811–822

Farout L, Mary J, Vihn J, Szweda LI, Friguet B (2006). Inactivation of the Proteasome by 4-Hydroxy-2-nonenal is site specific and dependant on 20S proteasome subtypes. Arch Biochem Biophys (in press)

Fenteany, G., Standaert, R.F., Lane, W.S., Choi, S., Corey EJ, Schreiber SL (1995) Inhibition of proteasome activities and subunit-specific amino-terminal threonine modification by lactacystin. Science 268:726–731

Ferrington DA, Husom AD, Thompson LV (2005) Altered proteasome structure, function, and oxidation in aged muscle. FASEB J 19:644–646

Ferrington DA, Kapphahn RJ (2004) Catalytic site-specific inhibition of the 20S proteasome by 4-hydroxynonenal. FEBS Lett 578:217–223

Finley D, Ciechanover A, Varshavsky A (2004) Ubiquitin as a central cellular regulator. Cell 116: S29–S32, 2 p following S32

Fisher MT, Stadtman ER (1992) Oxidative modification of Escherichia coli glutamine synthetase. Decreases in the thermodynamic stability of protein structure and specific changes in the active site conformation. J Biol Chem 267:1872–1880

Friguet B (2006) Oxidized protein degradation and repair in ageing and oxidative stress. FEBS Lett 580:2910–2916

Friguet B, Bulteau AL, Chondrogianni N, Conconi M, Petropoulos I (2000) Protein degradation by the proteasome and its implications in aging. Ann N Y Acad Sci 908:143–154

Friguet B, Stadtman ER, Szweda LI (1994a) Modification of glucose-6-phosphate dehydrogenase by 4-hydroxy-2-nonenal. Formation of cross-linked protein that inhibits the multicatalytic protease. J Biol Chem 269:21639–21643

Friguet B, Szweda LI (1997) Inhibition of the multicatalytic proteinase (proteasome) by 4-hydroxy-2-nonenal cross-linked protein. FEBS Lett 405:21–25

Friguet B, Szweda LI, Stadtman ER (1994b) Susceptibility of glucose-6-phosphate dehydrogenase modified by 4-hydroxy-2-nonenal and metal-catalyzed oxidation to proteolysis by the multicatalytic protease. Arch Biochem Biophys 311:168–173

Fruh K, Gossen M, Wang K, Bujard H, Peterson PA, Yang Y (1994). Displacement of housekeeping proteasome subunits by MHC-encoded LMPs: a newly discovered mechanism for modulating the multicatalytic proteinase complex. EMBO J 13:3236–3244

Furet P, Imbach P, Noorani M, Koeppler J, Laumen K, Lang M, Guagnano V, Fuerst P, Roesel J, Zimmermann J, Garcia-Echeverria C (2004). Entry into a new class of potent proteasome inhibitors having high antiproliferative activity by structure-based design. J Med Chem 47:4810–4813

Gaczynska M, Osmulski PA, Ward WF (2001) Caretaker or undertaker? The role of the proteasome in aging. Mech Ageing Dev 122:235–254

Gaczynska M, Rock KL, Goldberg AL (1993) Gamma-interferon and expression of MHC genes regulate peptide hydrolysis by proteasomes. Nature 365:264–267

Gerards WL, de Jong WW, Bloemendal H, Boelens W (1998) The human proteasomal subunit HsC8 induces ring formation of other alpha-type subunits. J Mol Biol 275:113–121

Ginaldi L, Loreto MF, Corsi MP, Modesti M, De Martinis M (2001). Immunosenescence and infectious diseases. Microbes Infect 3:851–857

Glockzin S, von Knethen A, Scheffner M, Brune B (1999) Activation of the cell death program by nitric oxide involves inhibition of the proteasome. J Biol Chem 274:19581–19586

Goldberg AL, Akopian TN, Kisselev AF, Lee DH, Rohrwild M (1997) New insights into the mechanisms and importance of the proteasome in intracellular protein degradation. Biol Chem 378:131–140

Goto S, Takahashi R, Araki S, Nakamoto H (2002) Dietary restriction initiated in late adulthood can reverse age-related alterations of protein and protein metabolism. Ann N Y Acad Sci 959:50–56

Gravekamp C (2001) Tailoring cancer vaccines to the elderly: the importance of suitable mouse models. Mech Ageing Dev 122:1087–1105

Grimaud R, Ezraty B, Mitchell JK, Lafitte D, Briand C, Derrick PJ, Barras F (2001). Repair of oxidized proteins. Identification of a new methionine sulfoxide reductase. J Biol Chem 276:48915–48920

Groll M, Ditzel L, Lowe J, Stock D, Bochtler M, Bartunik HD, Huber R (1997) Structure of 20S proteasome from yeast at 2.4 A resolution. Nature 386:463–471

Groll M, Heinemeyer W, Jager S, Ullrich T, Bochtler M, Wolf DH, Huber R (1999) The catalytic sites of 20S proteasomes and their role in subunit maturation: a mutational and crystallographic study. Proc Natl Acad Sci U S A 96:10976–10983

Groll M, Koguchi Y, Huber R, Kohno J (2001) Crystal structure of the 20 S proteasome:TMC-95A complex: a non-covalent proteasome inhibitor. J Mol Biol 311:543–548

Grune T, Reinheckel T, Davies KJ (1997) Degradation of oxidized proteins in mammalian cells. FASEB J 11:526–534

Hamelin M, Mary J, Vostry M, Friguet B, Bakala H (2007) Glycation damage targets glutamate dehydrogenase in the rat liver mitochondrial matrix during aging. FEBS J 274:5949–5961

Harris JR (1968) Release of a macromolecular protein component from human erythrocyte ghosts. Biochim Biophys Acta 150:534–537

Hayashi T, Goto S (1998) Age-related changes in the 20S and 26S proteasome activities in the liver of male F344 rats. Mech Ageing Dev 102:55–66

Hegerl R, Pfeifer G, Puhler G, Dahlmann B, Baumeister W (1991) The three-dimensional structure of proteasomes from Thermoplasma acidophilum as determined by electron microscopy using random conical tilting. FEBS Lett 283:117–121

Hensley K, Floyd RA (2002) Reactive oxygen species and protein oxidation in aging: a look back, a look ahead. Arch Biochem Biophys 397:377–383

Hershko A, Ciechanover A (1998) The ubiquitin system. Annu Rev Biochem 67:425–479

Hoglinger GU, Carrard G, Michel PP, Medja F, Lombes A, Ruberg M, Friguet B, Hirsch EC (2003) Dysfunction of mitochondrial complex I and the proteasome: interactions between two biochemical deficits in a cellular model of Parkinson's disease. J Neurochem 86:1297–1307

Holmgren A (2000) Antioxidant function of thioredoxin and glutaredoxin systems. Antioxid Redox Signal 2:811–820

Kageshita T, Hirai S, Ono T, Hicklin DJ, Ferrone S (1999) Down-regulation of HLA class I antigen-processing molecules in malignant melanoma: association with disease progression. Am J Pathol 154:745–754

Keller JN, Hanni KB, Markesbery WR (2000a) Possible involvement of proteasome inhibition in aging: implications for oxidative stress. Mech Ageing Dev 113:61–70

Keller JN, Huang FF, Markesbery WR (2000b) Decreased levels of proteasome activity and proteasome expression in aging spinal cord. Neuroscience 98:149–156

Keller JN, Huang FF, Zhu H, Yu J, Ho YS, Kindy TS (2000c) Oxidative stress-associated impairment of proteasome activity during ischemia-reperfusion injury. J Cereb Blood Flow Metab 20:1467–1473

Kiffin R, Christian C, Knecht E, Cuervo AM (2004) Activation of chaperone-mediated autophagy during oxidative stress. Mol Biol Cell 15:4829–4840

King RW, Deshaies RJ, Peters JM, Kirschner MW (1996) How proteolysis drives the cell cycle. Science 274:1652–1659

Kisselev AF, Akopian TN, Castillo V, Goldberg AL (1999) Proteasome active sites allosterically regulate each other, suggesting a cyclical bite-chew mechanism for protein breakdown. Mol Cell 4:395–402

Kline GH, Hayden TA, Klinman NR (1999) B cell maintenance in aged mice reflects both increased B cell longevity and decreased B cell generation. J Immunol 162:3342–3349

Klionsky DJ (2005) The molecular machinery of autophagy: unanswered questions. J Cell Sci 118:7–18

Kloetzel PM (2001) Antigen processing by the proteasome. Nat Rev Mol Cell Biol 2:179–187

Kloetzel PM (2004) The proteasome and MHC class I antigen processing. Biochim Biophys Acta 1695:225–233

Knowlton JR, Johnston SC, Whitby FG, Realini C, Zhang Z, Rechsteiner M, Hill CP (1997) Structure of the proteasome activator REGalpha (PA28alpha). Nature 390:639–643

Koguchi Y, Kohno J, Nishio M, Takahashi K, Okuda T, Ohnuki T, Komatsubara S (2000) TMC-95A, B, C, and D, novel proteasome inhibitors produced by Apiospora montagnei Sacc. TC 1093. Taxonomy, production, isolation, and biological activities. J Antibiot (Tokyo) 53:105–109

Kohler A, Cascio P, Leggett DS, Woo KM, Goldberg AL, Finley D (2001) The axial channel of the proteasome core particle is gated by the Rpt2 ATPase and controls both substrate entry and product release. Mol Cell 7:1143–1152

Kroll M, Arenzana-Seisdedos F, Bachelerie F, Thomas D, Friguet B, Conconi M (1999) The secondary fungal metabolite gliotoxin targets proteolytic activities of the proteasome. Chem Biol 6:689–698

Lee CK, Klopp RG, Weindruch R, Prolla TA (1999) Gene expression profile of aging and its retardation by caloric restriction. Science 285:1390–1393

Levine RL, Stadtman ER (2001) Oxidative modification of proteins during aging. Exp Gerontol 36:1495–1502

Levine RL, Williams JA, Stadtman ER, Shacter E (1994) Carbonyl assays for determination of oxidatively modified proteins. Methods Enzymol 233:346–357

Loidl G, Groll M, Musiol HJ, Huber R, Moroder L (1999) Bivalency as a principle for proteasome inhibition. Proc Natl Acad Sci U S A 96:5418–5422

Lowe J, Stock D, Jap B, Zwickl P, Baumeister W, Huber R (1995) Crystal structure of the 20S proteasome from the archaeon T. acidophilum at 3.4 A resolution. Science 268:533–539

Ly DH, Lockhart DJ, Lerner RA, Schultz PG (2000) Mitotic misregulation and human aging. Science 287:2486–2492

Ma CP, Slaughter CA, DeMartino GN (1992) Identification, purification, and characterization of a protein activator (PA28) of the 20 S proteasome (macropain). J Biol Chem 267:10515–10523

Marastoni M, Baldisserotto A, Canella A, Gavioli R, Risi CD, Pollini GP, Tomatis R (2004) Arecoline tripeptide inhibitors of proteasome. J Med Chem 47:1587–1590

Marques C, Pereira P, Taylor A, Liang JN, Reddy VN, Szweda LI, Shang F (2004) Ubiquitin-dependent lysosomal degradation of the HNE-modified proteins in lens epithelial cells. FASEB J 18:1424–1426

Mason GG, Murray RZ, Pappin D, Rivett AJ (1998) Phosphorylation of ATPase subunits of the 26S proteasome. FEBS Lett 430:269–274

Meidenbauer N, Zippelius A, Pittet MJ, Laumer M, Vogl S, Heymann J, Rehli M, Seliger B, Schwarz S, Le Gal FA, Dietrich PY, Andreesen R, Romero P, Mackensen A (2004) High frequency of functionally active Melan-a-specific T cells in a patient with progressive immunoproteasome-deficient melanoma. Cancer Res 64:6319–6326

Merker K, Sitte N, Grune T (2000) Hydrogen peroxide-mediated protein oxidation in young and old human MRC-5 fibroblasts. Arch Biochem Biophys 375:50–54

Miller RA (2000) Effect of aging on T lymphocyte activation. Vaccine 18:1654–1660

Mishto M, Bonafe M, Salvioli S, Olivieri F, Franceschi C (2002) Age dependent impact of LMP polymorphisms on TNFalpha-induced apoptosis in human peripheral blood mononuclear cells. Exp Gerontol 37:301–308

Mott JD, Pramanik BC, Moomaw CR, Afendis SJ, DeMartino GN, Slaughter CA (1994) PA28, an activator of the 20 S proteasome, is composed of two nonidentical but homologous subunits. J Biol Chem 269:31466–31471

Murakami Y, Kanda K, Yokota K, Kanayama H, Kagawa S (2001) Prognostic significance of immuno-proteosome subunit expression in patients with renal-cell carcinoma: a preliminary study. Mol Urol 5:113–119

Okada K, Wangpoengtrakul C, Osawa T, Toyokuni S, Tanaka K, Uchida K (1999) 4-Hydroxy-2-nonenal-mediated impairment of intracellular proteolysis during oxidative stress. Identification of proteasomes as target molecules. J Biol Chem 274:23787–23793

Orr WC, Sohal RS (1994) Extension of life-span by overexpression of superoxide dismutase and catalase in Drosophila melanogaster. Science 263:1128–1130

Pajonk F, McBride WH (2001) The proteasome in cancer biology and treatment. Radiat Res 156:447–459

Petropoulos I, Conconi M, Wang X, Hoenel B, Bregegere F, Milner Y, Friguet B (2000) Increase of oxidatively modified protein is associated with a decrease of proteasome activity and content in aging epidermal cells. J Gerontol A Biol Sci Med Sci 55:B220–B227

Pimentel-Muinos FX, Mazana J, Fresno M (1994) Regulation of interleukin-2 receptor alpha chain expression and nuclear factor.kappa B activation by protein kinase C in T lymphocytes. Autocrine role of tumor necrosis factor alpha. J Biol Chem 269:24424–24429

Poggioli S, Bakala H, Friguet B (2002) Age-related increase of protein glycation in peripheral blood lymphocytes is restricted to preferential target proteins. Exp Gerontol 37:1207–1215

Poggioli S, Mary J, Bakala H, Friguet B (2004) Evidence of preferential protein targets for age-related modifications in peripheral blood lymphocytes. Ann N Y Acad Sci 1019:211–214

Ponnappan S, Ovaa H, Ponnappan U (2007) Lower expression of catalytic and structural subunits of the proteasome contributes to decreased proteolysis in peripheral blood T lymphocytes during aging. Int J Biochem Cell Biol 39:799–809

Ponnappan U (1998) Regulation of transcription factor NF kappa B in immune senescence. Front Biosci 3:d152–d168

Ponnappan U (2002) Ubiquitin-proteasome pathway is compromised in CD45RO+ and CD45RA+ T lymphocyte subsets during aging. Exp Gerontol 37:359–367

Ponnappan U, Zhong M, Trebilcock GU (1999) Decreased proteasome-mediated degradation in T cells from the elderly: A role in immune senescence. Cell Immunol 192:167–174

Poole LB, Karplus PA, Claiborne A (2004) Protein sulfenic acids in redox signaling. Annu Rev Pharmacol Toxicol 44:325–347

Powell SR, Wang P, Divald A, Teichberg S, Haridas V, McCloskey TW, Davies KJ, Katzeff H (2005) Aggregates of oxidized proteins (lipofuscin) induce apoptosis through proteasome inhibition and dysregulation of proapoptotic proteins. Free Radic Biol Med 38:1093–1101

Pryhuber KG, Murray KJ, Donnelly P, Passo MH, Maksymowych WP, Glass DN, Giannini EH, Colbert RA (1996) Polymorphism in the LMP2 gene influences disease susceptibility and severity in HLA-B27 associated juvenile rheumatoid arthritis. J Rheumatol 23:747–752

Reinheckel T, Sitte N, Ullrich O, Kuckelkorn U, Davies KJ, Grune T (1998) Comparative resistance of the 20S and 26S proteasome to oxidative stress. Biochem J 335 (Pt 3):637–642

Requena JR, Levine RL, Stadtman ER (2003) Recent advances in the analysis of oxidized proteins. Amino Acids 25:221–226

Rivett AJ, Hearn AR (2004) Proteasome function in antigen presentation: immunoproteasome complexes, Peptide production, and interactions with viral proteins. Curr Protein Pept Sci 5:153–161

Rock KL, Goldberg, AL (1999) Degradation of cell proteins and the generation of MHC class I-presented peptides. Annu Rev Immunol 17, 739–779

Schmidtke G, Holzhutter HG, Bogyo M, Kairies N, Groll M, de Giuli R, Emch S, Groettrup M (1999) How an inhibitor of the HIV-I protease modulates proteasome activity. J Biol Chem 274:35734–35740

Sell DR, Primc M, Schafer IA, Kovach M, Weiss MA, Monnier VM (1998) Cell-associated pentosidine as a marker of aging in human diploid cells in vitro and in vivo. Mech Ageing Dev 105:221–240

Shamoto-Nagai M, Maruyama W, Kato Y, Isobe K, Tanaka M, Naoi M, Osawa T (2003) An inhibitor of mitochondrial complex I, rotenone, inactivates proteasome by oxidative modification and induces aggregation of oxidized proteins in SH-SY5Y cells. J Neurosci Res 74:589–597

Shang F, Nowell TR Jr, Taylor A (2001) Removal of oxidatively damaged proteins from lens cells by the ubiquitin-proteasome pathway. Exp Eye Res 73:229–238

Sharov VS, Ferrington DA, Squier TC, Schoneich C (1999) Diastereoselective reduction of protein-bound methionine sulfoxide by methionine sulfoxide reductase. FEBS Lett 455:247–250

Shibatani T, Nazir M, Ward WF (1996) Alteration of rat liver 20S proteasome activities by age and food restriction. J Gerontol A Biol Sci Med Sci 51:B316–B322

Shibatani T, Ward WF (1996) Effect of age and food restriction on alkaline protease activity in rat liver. J Gerontol A Biol Sci Med Sci 51:B175–B178

Shringarpure R, Grune T, Mehlhase J, Davies KJ (2003) Ubiquitin conjugation is not required for the degradation of oxidized proteins by proteasome. J Biol Chem 278:311–318

Sitte N, Huber M, Grune T, Ladhoff A, Doecke WD, Von Zglinicki T, Davies KJ (2000). Proteasome inhibition by lipofuscin/ceroid during postmitotic aging of fibroblasts. FASEB J 14:1490–1498

Stacy S, Krolick KA, Infante AJ, Kraig E (2002) Immunological memory and late onset autoimmunity. Mech Ageing Dev 123:975–985

Stadtman ER (1990) Metal ion-catalyzed oxidation of proteins: biochemical mechanism and biological consequences. Free Radic Biol Med 9:315–325

Stadtman ER (2006) Protein oxidation and aging. Free Radic Res 40:1250–1258

Stadtman ER, Levine RL (2003) Free radical-mediated oxidation of free amino acids and amino acid residues in proteins. Amino Acids 25:207–218

Stadtman ER, Levine RL (2000) Protein oxidation. Ann N Y Acad Sci 899:191–208

Stratford FL, Chondrogianni N, Trougakos IP, Gonos ES, Rivett AJ (2006) Proteasome response to interferon-gamma is altered in senescent human fibroblasts. FEBS Lett 580:3989–3994

Sullivan PG, Dragicevic NB, Deng JH, Bai Y, Dimayuga E, Ding Q, Chen Q, Bruce-Keller AJ, Keller JN (2004). Proteasome inhibition alters neural mitochondrial homeostasis and mitochondria turnover. J Biol Chem 279:20699–20707

Szweda PA, Friguet B, Szweda LI (2002) Proteolysis, free radicals, and aging. Free Radic Biol Med 33:29–36

Tanahashi N, Murakami Y, Minami Y, Shimbara N, Hendil KB, Tanaka K (2000) Hybrid proteasomes. Induction by interferon-gamma and contribution to ATP-dependent proteolysis. J Biol Chem 275:14336–14345

Tanaka K (1994) Role of proteasomes modified by interferon-gamma in antigen processing. J Leukoc Biol 56:571–575

Tanaka K, Yoshimura T, Ichihara A, Kameyama K, Takagi T (1986) A high molecular weight protease in the cytosol of rat liver. II. Properties of the purified enzyme. J Biol Chem 261:15204–15207

Terman A, Sandberg S (2002) Proteasome inhibition enhances lipofuscin formation. Ann N Y Acad Sci 973:309–312

Unno M, Mizushima T, Morimoto Y, Tomisugi Y, Tanaka K, Yasuoka N, Tsukihara T (2002) The structure of the mammalian 20S proteasome at 2.75 A resolution. Structure 10:609–618

Vargas-Alarcon G, Gamboa R, Zuniga J, Fragoso JM, Hernandez-Pacheco G, Londono J, Pacheco-Tena C, Cardiel MH, Granados J, Burgos-Vargas R (2004) Association study of LMP gene polymorphisms in Mexican patients with spondyloarthritis. Hum Immunol 65:1437–1442

Vigouroux S, Briand M, Briand Y (2004). Linkage between the proteasome pathway and neurode-generative diseases and aging. Mol Neurobiol 30:201–221

Viteri G, Carrard G, Birlouez-Aragon I, Silva E, Friguet B (2004) Age-dependent protein modifications and declining proteasome activity in the human lens. Arch Biochem Biophys 427:197–203

Voges D, Zwickl P, Baumeister W (1999) The 26S proteasome: a molecular machine designed for controlled proteolysis. Annu Rev Biochem 68:1015–1068

Wagner BJ, Margolis JW (1995) Age-dependent association of isolated bovine lens multicatalytic proteinase complex (proteasome) with heat-shock protein 90, an endogenous inhibitor. Arch Biochem Biophys 323:455–462

Wan SB, Landis-Piwowar KR, Kuhn DJ, Chen D, Dou QP, Chan TH (2005) Structure-activity study of epi-gallocatechin gallate (EGCG) analogs as proteasome inhibitors. Bioorg Med Chem 13:2177–2185

Webster RG (2000) Immunity to influenza in the elderly. Vaccine 18:1686–1689

Weissman AM (2001) Themes and variations on ubiquitylation. Nat Rev Mol Cell Biol 2, 169–178

Weksler ME, Szabo P (2000) The effect of age on the B-cell repertoire. J Clin Immunol 20:240–249

Whitby FG, Masters EI, Kramer L, Knowlton JR, Yao Y, Wang CC, Hill CP (2000) Structural basis for the activation of 20S proteasomes by 11S regulators. Nature 408:115–120

Xu B, Monsarrat B, Gairin JE, Girbal-Neuhauser E (2004) Effect of ajoene, a natural antitumor small molecule, on human 20S proteasome activity in vitro and in human leukemic HL60 cells. Fundam Clin Pharmacol 18:171–180

Yan LJ, Levine RL, Sohal RS (1997) Oxidative damage during aging targets mitochondrial aconi-tase. Proc Natl Acad Sci U S A 94:11168–11172

Yan LJ, Sohal RS (1998) Mitochondrial adenine nucleotide translocase is modified oxidatively during aging. Proc Natl Acad Sci U S A 95:12896–12901

Mechanisms - Cytokines

Age-Related Changes in Type 1 and Type 2 Cytokine Production in Humans

Elizabeth M. Gardner and Donna M. Murasko

Contents

Abstract: Aging is accompanied by several changes in immunity; however, altered T-cell function is one of the most consistent and dramatic changes observed. Because of the key roles that cyokines play in modulating the immune response, investigators have hypothesized that these age-related changes in T-cell function are related to, at least in part, by alterations in cytokine production. While data from murine studies generally support an age-related shift form a Th1-like cytokine response to a Th2-like response, data in humans do not support this age-related shift in cytokine production. This review of several studies indicates that age-associated changes in cytokine productions in humans are inconsistent. Further, these age-associated changes in cytokine production do not necessarily induce a shift to a Type 2 cytokine response. This review highlights the variables that may contribute to the inconsistent results among studies. Additional studies in humans are both

E. M. Gardner (✉) · D. Murasko
Department of Bioscience and Biotechnology
Drexel University, Philadelphia
PA 19104, USA

E. M. Gardner
Department of Food Science and Human Nutrition
Michigan State University, East Lansing, MI 48824, USA
Fax: +1517-353-8963.
E-mail: egardner@msu.edu

T. Fulop et al. (eds.), *Handbook on Immunosenescence*,
DOI 10.1007/978-1-4020-9062-2_39, © Springer Science+Business Media B.V. 2009

critical and warranted to clearly identify the effect of altered cytokine production on age-associated changes in immune function.

Keywords: Aging • Cell-mediated response • Humans Humoral response • Immunity Type 1 cytokines • Type 2 cytokines

1 Introduction

It is well known that the incidence of cancer, infectious diseases, and autoimmune disorders increases with advancing age (Miller 1996). In addition, aging is accompanied by multiple changes in immune function, including decreased lymphoproliferative responses to both mitogens and antigens, reduced delayed type hypersensitivity reactions, and impaired antibody responses to both vaccination and infection (Miller 1996; Murasko and Gardner 2003). Thus, it has been postulated that these age-related diseases can be explained, at least in part, by an overall dysregulation in immune function (Shearer 1997).

The most consistent and dramatic age-related changes of the immune system have been demonstrated in the T-cell compartment (Miller, 1996; Murasko and Gardner 2003). Therefore, many studies have examined T-cell responses during aging to identify potential mechanism(s) responsible for these age-associated alterations in immune function. Investigators have postulated that altered cytokine production may contribute significantly to age-associated changes in immune function in both animal models and in humans. The best evidence for an age-associated dysregulation in cytokine production has been demonstrated in the mouse model. Most studies indicate that interleukin-2 (IL-2) production is consistently decreased, (Shearer 1997), while interleukin-4 (IL4) production is generally increased (Albright et al. 1995; Hobbs et al. 1993).

The above observations have led investigators to postulate that aging per se may induce a shift from a Type 1-like cytokine (IL-2, IFN-γ, IL-12) cell-mediated response to a predominantly Type 2-like cytokine (IL4, IL-5, IL-6, IL-10) response. While this hypothesis is generally supported in murine models, there is no conclusive evidence that such a shift to a dominant Th-2 response occurs in elderly humans. In fact, in 2002, we published a comprehensive review of the literature in humans to evaluate whether or not there were definitive and consistent changes in cytokine production in elderly subjects (Gardner et al. 2006). This survey of the literature did not support an age-related shift in cytokine production that favored a predominantly Th-2 response in the elderly. Since that review, little new information has emerged to support the hypothesis that there is a consistent age-related shift in cytokine production in elderly humans.

The purpose of the current review is not to reiterate our previous survey of the literature (Gardner and Murasko 2002), but rather to provide a concise summary of what is known about age-related changes in cytokine production in elderly humans, to suggest possible explanations for differences in outcomes of studies, and most important, to call for future studies to determine the impact of age-related changes on cytokine production on the immune response of the elderly.

2 Parameters that Confound Comparison of Results Among Human Studies

In our previous review (Gardner and Murasko 2002), we extensively described the various confounding variables that can influence the outcome of studies on age-related changes in human populations. These confounding variables are described briefly below and in Table 1 so that the reader is aware of possible factors that may influence the outcome of a study of immune function in elderly subjects.

2.1 Subject Populations

One of the major variables that may contribute to the outcomes of different studies is the age distribution of subjects in any given study. In order to evaluate whether or not cytokine production is altered in elderly humans, it is necessary to review the criteria utilized to select elderly subjects. First and foremost, the elderly must be at least 60 (preferably 65) years of age. It is equally important to design studies

Table 1 Parameters to consider when evaluating multiple studies on age-related changes in immune function of elderly subjects

Subject population	Advantages	Disadvantages
Age range Elderly: 60+ years of age Young: 18–40 years of age	Able to determine age-related changes in immune function in well-defined populations	Difficult to enroll both young and elderly subjects in the same study. Difficult to enroll elderly subjects
Health status Frail (nursing home) Elderly Healthy elderly Senieur (exceptional elderly)	Able to obtain information about the response of elderly populations with varying health status	Frail and Senieur elderly may not reflect age-related changes in immune function of general elderly population
Demographics Racial background Socioeconomic status	Similar demographics afford assessment of immune function in elderly reduces variability in subject population	Similar demographics may not reflect total elderly population, with different racial backgrounds or economic status
Sample sizes Large	Reduce possible skewed responses due to heterogeneity in immune response	Difficulty in enrolling a large sample number in a single study
Small	Enrollment and retention more likely	Response may be skewed and not reflect response of entire population

in which both young and elderly subjects are evaluated concurrently. Inclusion of both age groups in the same study enables investigators to clearly delineate the changes in immune function that can be attributed to old age, minimizing any variation due to assay conditions. Despite this, studies have utilized subjects who cannot be categorized as elderly (e.g., <60 years of age) and have not included a concurrent examination of young and elderly in the same study (Gardner and Murasko 2002). Therefore, the best design for assessing age-related changes in immune function, including cytokine production, is to choose subjects who meet the age requirement for elderly and to include both young and elderly individuals in the same study.

2.2   Health Status of the Subjects

A second critical component of any aging study is to clearly define the health status of the population to be evaluated in that given study. In general, human studies evaluate age-related changes in immune function in three classes of elderly: frail or nursing home elderly, exceptionally healthy (Senieur) elderly, or healthy elderly. Frail or nursing home elderly typically represents a population who is generally not in good health, having chronically debilitating disorders. Therefore, it is difficult to delineate changes in immune function that are due to age rather than to disease. However, it is still important to assess immune function in this population to identify strategies that may enhance the immune response or reduce the incidence and/or severity of infectious disease in this population. It is important to note that the changes that occur in immune function in the frail elderly may not reflect the changes seen in the healthy, free-living elderly population. The Senieur protocol was developed to limit the influence of chronic disease on age-related changes in the immune response of the elderly. The criteria employed for selection of elderly individuals in the Senieur protocol are described in detail (Ligthart et al. 1990). These Senieur elderly represents a group of individuals with exceptional health status, who are largely free from debilitating or chronic illnesses, which is not typical of the health status of the overall elderly population. Therefore, while this protocol is useful to elucidate changes in immune function that are primarily due to age and not to underlying disease, the data obtained may not be extended to the general elderly population. Finally, many studies enroll elderly who do not meet the criteria of the Senieur protocol, but whose health is generally good. In general, these individuals are independent, community-living individuals who do not have debilitating diseases, immune-related disorders or are taking chemotherapeutic agents. This population has the advantage of being more readily accessible for aging studies and results from this population are more representative of the response of the elderly population.

In summary, regardless of which population of elderly is employed in a study, it is critical to carefully define that population and to recognize the limitations of examining the chosen population for assessment of age-related changes in cytokine function.

2.3 Demographics of the Subject Population

Another consideration when evaluating age-related changes in the immune response of the elderly is the demographics of the population, which includes, but is not limited to, racial background and socioeconomic status. In order to limit variability of results, investigators typically assess age-related changes in a nearly homogeneous population of elderly. Thus, most if not all, of the subjects have the same racial (but not necessarily ethnic) background with similar socioeconomic status. While it may be argued that controlling for race and economic status can ultimately limit the variability of the results of the study, it is important to recognize that the results obtained from one subset of the elderly population may not reflect the diversity of responses within the elderly population at large. For example, most of the studies performed in the United States on age-related changes in the immune response have been generated in the Caucasian population; similiar studies in non-Caucasian elderly are seriously lacking (Marin et al. 2002; Sambamoorhi and Findley 2005).

It is recognized that subject recruitment is difficult under the best of circumstances. In fact, we recently reported strategies that we utilized to successfully enhance both recruitment and retention of elderly in human studies (Gonzales et al. 2007). The lack of data in non-Caucasian groups may not be intentional, but rather, may reflect the inability of investigators to gain access to these populations for their studies. Secondly, the under-representation of non-Caucasians may also reflect a lack of trust of elderly subjects at the time of recruitment (Gonzales et al. 2007). Our laboratory recently conducted a study to evaluate age-related changes in the immune response of a racially-diverse elderly population. The results of this study (Gardner et al. 2006), which will be discussed below, clearly indicate that immune response data generated from Caucasian elderly do not necessarily reflect the responses of subsets of non-Caucasian elderly. Therefore, additional studies in racially diverse populations are warranted to provide conclusive data regarding age-related changes in the elderly population at large.

2.4 Sample Size of the Population

We (Murasko et al. 1991) and others (Barcellini et al. 1988) have documented that the immune response of elderly subjects shows marked heterogeneity. It has been postulated that several factors may contribute to this heterogeneity and include factors such as health status, genetic variability, and behaviors, such as diet, smoking, level of physical activity, or cognitive status (Ritz and Gardner 2006). Although many studies have consistently shown that the mean proliferative responses to either nonspecific stimulation or antigenic stimulation are reduced in the elderly compared to young individuals (Bernstein et al. 1998; Gardner et al 2006); we have clearly shown that there are some elderly who produce responses that are nearly equivalent to those of young, while others produce responses that are only about

20% of the response of the young (Murasko et al. 1997). Therefore, it is necessary to employ large samples to control for this heterogeneity in the immune response of the elderly. However, many studies in the literature have assessed immune function on a small number of elderly. Therefore, it is plausible that small sample sizes may unintentionally select for responses that are either very high or very low. Thus, the data generated on a small cohort of elderly subjects may not be indicative of a larger elderly population and can contribute to differences in the outcomes of studies on age-related changes in the immune response even when other variables, such as health status, are controlled. Investigators should perform a statistical power analysis to determine the number of subjects needed to offset the expected heterogeneity of the immune response in an elderly population.

3   Age-Related Changes in Cytokine Production

Evaluation of age-related changes in cytokine production has been the focus of many studies in which both young and elderly individuals have been assessed concurrently. It would seem, therefore, that a comprehensive review of these reports should definitively answer the question of whether or not there is an age-associated dysregulation in cytokine production in elderly humans. Unfortunately, this has not been the case; differences in experimental conditions, such as the stimulating agent, the tissue employed, and the time points of evaluation, make it difficult to compare the results of all studies and to draw general conclusions from them.

Typically, cytokine production has been assessed in peripheral blood mononuclear cells (PBMC), but some investigations have utilized cultures of whole blood or have isolated specific subsets of lymphocytes for analysis. Likewise, some studies have evaluated cytokine production in response to a nonspecific stimulus, such as PHA, while others after specific stimulation, such as influenza. Clearly, differences in outcomes may reflect the tissue analyzed as well as the stimulating agent utilized to induce cytokine production. Both the time points and the methods of assessments vary considerably among studies. In most cases, cytokine production is measured at only one time point (e.g., 48 or 72 hrs after stimulation); therefore, it is possible that differences in outcomes of reports may simply reflect kinetic differences in the peak of the response to a particular cytokine. Finally, comparison of reports on age-related alterations in cytokine production is made more difficult by the various techniques used to quantitate cytokines. Some studies have measured cytokines in supernatants from stimulated cells by bioassays, while others have employed enzyme-linked immunosorbent assays (ELISA) or radioimmunoassays (RIA). Bioassays assess the functional activity of a sample using either growth or inhibition of growth of cell lines specifically responsive to that particular cytokine (e.g., IL-2, IL-4, IL-6) or inhibition of viral cytopathic effect (i.e., IFN). In contrast, both ELISA and RIA measure the total amount of a cytokine by using antibodies specific for antigenic determinants of the cytokine.

While ELISA and RIA are highly sensitive and specific in quantitating cytokine concentrations, they do not provide any information about the functional activity of the cytokines measured. Importantly, it is difficult to compare the results of studies on the same cytokine when one employed a bioassay and the other used ELISA since these results do not necessarily correlate (Murasko, unpublished data).

Some studies have evaluated cytokine mRNA produced by cells of young and elderly to avoid the problems of measuring proteins in the supernatants of stimulated cells. While the levels of mRNA provide useful information regarding age-associated alterations in transcription of cytokine genes, it is important to recognize that mRNA results do not always reflect the amount of protein produced and secreted. For example, we have reported previously (Gardner and Murasko 2002), elderly individuals who had increased levels of IFN-γ mRNA had comparable levels of biologically active IFN-γ relative to young controls.

It is, therefore, difficult to resolve disparities among studies when different methods of cytokine analyses have been employed. Clearly, the combination of these variations in experimental design could significantly contribute to the varying outcomes, even when all other parameters of the study population are controlled. It is quite possible that differences among studies of humans may reflect even subtle differences in experimental design.

In summary, appropriate evaluation of the current literature of changes in cytokine production with age requires careful consideration of the health of the subjects, the demographics of the population, the cell types and stimuli used, and the techniques employed to measure cytokines. Additional comprehensive evaluations in studies that utilize appropriate and well-controlled experimental designs are absolutely critical to identify the impact of altered cytokine production on immune function in the elderly.

4   Age-Related Changes in Type 1 and Type 2 Cytokines

In human studies, IL-2 and IFN-γ are the most frequently measured cytokines for characterization of Type 1 cytokine responses, while ILs-4, 6, and 10 are often employed to characterize Type 2 cytokine responses. In order to make general conclusions regarding the effect of cytokine dysregulation on age-associated changes in immune function, the data from several reports in which Type 1 or Type 2 cytokines were assessed from either healthy or Senieur elderly, along with young subjects in the same study, are summarized below. For simplicity and ease of comparison among studies, this review will mainly focus on studies in which cytokine production was assessed in PBMC after mitogenic or antigenic stimulation. However, when appropriate, a discussion of those studies in which cytokine production was assessed in isolated immune cells, whole blood, plasma, or sera will be included. These criteria regarding the studies reviewed in this chapter were selected in order to draw broad conclusions regarding cytokine dysregulation in the elderly.

5 Type 1 Cytokines

5.1 Interleukin-2

One of the most consistent age-related changes in immune function is decreased T-cell lymphoproliferative responses (Miller 1996; Murasko et al. 1987). Since interleukin-2 (IL-2) is necessary for the activation and proliferation of T lymphocytes (Janeway et al. 2005), it stands to reason that age-related changes in IL-2 production have been assessed in several studies in the elderly. Age-related changes in IL-2 production have been measured in elderly subjects under various culture conditions and in response to nonspecific stimulation or after stimulation with specific antigens, such as influenza.

The overall results of several studies in which IL-2 production was evaluated are summarized in Table 2. In a survey of fourteen studies, in which PBMC or whole blood from young and elderly subjects were stimulated with PHA, an age-related decrease was observed in eleven reports (Barcellini et al. 1988; Born et al. 1995; Gardner et al. 2000, 2006; Gillis et al. 1981, Murasko et al. 1991; Nagel et al. 1986; Orson et al. 1989; Song et al. 1993; Wu et al. 1994; Xu et al. 1993), while there was no age-related difference in three studies (Bruunsgaard et al. 2000; Sindermann et al. 1995; Weifang et al. 1996). However, the two studies (Bruunsgaard et al. 2000; Sindermann et al. 1995) reporting no change in IL-2 levels stimulated whole blood with PHA, rather than PBMC. Interestingly, in one of the more recent studies (Gardner et al. 2006), PHA-induced IL-2 production was assessed in PBMCs from a racially-diverse group of elderly, consisting of 33 Caucasians, 39 African Americans and 41 Latinos. This study demonstrated that IL-2 production was reduced in all elderly, regardless of racial background, relative to young controls assessed con-

Table 2 Summary of age-related changes in type 1 cytokines[a]

Cytokine	Assessment	Stimulus	Age-related Changes[b]
IL-2	PBMC	PHA	Decreased (11 reports) No change (1 reports)
	Whole Blood	PHA	No change (2 reports)
	PBMC	Trivalent influenza vaccine	Decrease (5 reports) No change (1 report Latino)
	PBMC	Live influenza virus	Decrease (2 reports) No change (2 reports)
IFN-γ	PBMC	PHA or ConA	Decreased (4 reports) No change (2 reports) Increased (1 report)
	Whole blood	PHA	No Change (2 reports)
	PBMC	Influenza vaccine	Decreased (4 reports) No change (1 reports)

[a] Adapted from (Gardner and Murasko 2006)
[b] Results are compared to young controls

Table 3 Summary of age-related changes in Type 2 Cytokines[a]

Cytokine	Assessment	Stimulus	Age-related changes[b]
IL-4	PBMC	PHA, ConA	No change (2 reports)
		Anti-CD2/Anti-CD28	Increased (1 report)
		Anti-CD3/PMA	Decreased (1 report)
	PBMC	Influenza vaccine	Undetectable (2 reports)
IL-6	PBMC	PHA or ConA	No change(3 reports)
			Increased (2 reports)
			Decreased (report)
	Serum	None	No change (3 reports)
	Plasma		Increased (2 reports)
IL-10	Blood	PHA	Decreased (1 report)
	PBMC	Influenza vaccine	Increase (1 report)
			Decreased (2 reports)
	PBMC	None	No change (2 reports)
	Serum	None	No change (1 report)

[a] Adapted from (Gardner and Murasko 2006)
[b] Results are compared to young controls

currently. This observation of decreased IL-2 production in non-Caucasian elderly has been confirmed in a subsequent study in our laboratory (Gardner and Murasko, unpublished data). Therefore, the majority, but not all, of studies demonstrate an age-related decrease in PHA-induced IL-2 production, relative to young controls.

Several studies (Gardner et al. 2006; McElhaney et al. 1990, 1992, 1995; Quyang et al. 2000) have also evaluated IL-2 production in the elderly after stimulation with influenza to determine the response to a specific antigen. In two reports (McElhaney et al. 1990, Quyang et al. 2000), when PBMC were stimulated with trivalent influenza vaccine, the elderly produced significantly less IL-2 after vaccination than did young controls. Interestingly, a more recent influenza study (Gardner et al. 2006) in a racially-diverse elderly population demonstrated that PBMC from elderly Caucasians and African Americans, but not from Latinos, produced significantly less IL-2 after influenza vaccination, relative to that produced by young controls. When various strains of live influenza virus were employed, mixed results were obtained. Studies have indicated that IL-2 production after stimulation of PBMCs with influenza virus was either reduced or unchanged (McElhaney et al. 1992, 1995), depending on the strain of influenza utilized, relative to the response of young controls.

Therefore, a careful review of current literature clearly suggests that while many elderly produce less IL-2 than young, not all elderly demonstrate an age-related decrease in IL-2 production. Importantly, recent data also suggests that racial background must be considered when evaluating age-related changes in IL-2 production. The reasons for these disparate results among studies are not clear. However, possible reasons include differences in sample numbers assessed within various studies, the overall heterogeneity in the immune response of the elderly, and the type of stimulus. Based upon this review, decreased in IL-2 production cannot be presented as a definitive age-associated alteration in humans.

6 Interferon-γ (IFN-γ)

IFN-γ is secreted mainly by T lymphocytes and NK cells and is known for inducing antiviral activity, upregulating MHC class I and II antigens, and activating macrophages (Janeway et al. 2005). Since IFN-γ is a strong inducer of cell-mediated immune (CMI) responses, investigators have hypothesized that age-related changes in IFN-γ may play a role in the decline of CMI with age (Shearer 1997).

There have been several reports that have assessed the effect of age on IFN-γ production in the elderly. The results of these studies are summarized in Table 2. When changes in IFN-γ production by PBMC after stimulation with either PHA or ConA were evaluated in young and elderly subjects, four studies reported an age-associated decrease (Born et al. 1995; Candore et al. 1993; Lio et al. 1998, 2000), two studies demonstrated no change (Hessen et al. 1991; Weifeng et al. 1986), and one showed an increase in IFN-γ (Murasko et al. 2001), relative to the response of young subjects. Two other studies in which cultures of blood were stimulated with PHA reported no differences in IFN-γ production between young and elderly individuals (Bruunsgaard et al. 2000; Sindermann et al. 1993). Although the exact reasons for the differences in outcomes among these reports are not clear, a review of these studies clearly indicates that the experimental designs among studies varied considerably. There were differences in length of stimulation in vitro (1–5 days) and in the techniques used to measure IFN-γ (bioassay versus ELISA). Therefore, the discrepancy among studies may simply reflect altered kinetics of IFN-γ production or variations in assays used for quantitation of IFN-γ.

Studies in which PBMC were incubated with specific stimuli using influenza antigen generally support an age-related decrease in IFN-γ. Five studies demonstrated decreased IFN-γ production to influenza virus in the elderly, relative to young controls (Bernstein et al. 1998, Gardner et al. 2006, McElhaney et al. 2006; Murasko et al. 2001; Quyang et al. 2000;). In one study (Bodnar et al. 1997), IFN-γ production by PBMC from elderly after stimulation with influenza showed a non-significant decrease relative to that produced by young subjects. This lack of statistical age-related decrease in the elderly was likely due to the small number of subjects included in the study. Our recent study (Gardner et al. 2006) in a racially-diverse elderly population also supports an age-related decrease in IFN-γ production, with both the total elderly, as well as all elderly subgroups, producing less IFN-γ after influenza vaccination compared young controls. However, an interesting observation that emerged from this study was that IFN-γ levels decreased from pre- to post-vaccination in elderly African Americans, but not in any of the other groups of elderly individuals or in the total elderly population. This observation was confirmed in a subsequent study (unpublished observations). These data suggest that racial background can influence age-related changes in the cell-mediated response. Importantly, these altered responses of elderly African Americans, relative to the total elderly population, may not have emerged had the elderly not been categorized by racial background. Future studies are necessary to validate these findings.

In a recent report, McElhaney et al. (2006) questioned whether or not indices of CMI could be utilized to distinguish between elderly individuals who did or did not develop laboratory diagnosed influenza (LDI). In this study, 90 elderly (60 years and older) and 10 healthy young adult controls were immunized with the 2003–2004 trivalent inactivated influenza vaccine. The study reported that 9 out of 90 elderly developed LDI during the course of the study. Before vaccination, subjects who developed LDI had 10-fold lower levels of IFN-γ after stimulation with live influenza virus compared to those elderly who did not develop LDI. Although the subjects without LDI showed no significant change in IFN-γ levels over the course of the study, the older adults who developed LDI showed significant increases in IFN-γ levels in influenza-stimulated PBMCs. The mean IFN-γ:IL-10 ratio in influenza-stimulated PBMC was 10-fold lower in LDI versus nonLDI subjects. These results are important because they correlate cytokine production with LDI in the elderly and also argue for altered Type 1 and Type 2 cytokine responses in the elderly. Clearly, future studies should confirm this observation in a larger population of elderly with or without LDI.

In summary, a careful review of the current reports suggest that there are no consistent age-related changes in IFN-γ production after non-specific stimulation, at least when PHA or ConA are utilized. Until additional studies that carefully compared dose and kinetics are performed, no definitive conclusions can be made. In contrast, the data to date are fairly consistent in demonstrating an age-associated decrease in IFN-γ production upon antigen-specific stimulation, at least when influenza is the antigen used.

7   Type 2 cytokines

7.1   Interleukin 4

IL-4 is a Type 2 cytokine secreted by T-cells, B cells, macrophages, mast cells, and basophils and induces B cell differentiation and antibody class switching (Janeway et al. 2005). It has been demonstrated that IL-4 plays a critical regulatory role in inhibiting the production of Type 1 cytokines, while stimulating the production of Type 2 cytokines (Shearer 1997).

Assessment of age-related changes in IL-4 production in humans in response to mitogenic stimulation is quite limited and the results of these studies are not consistent (Gardner and Murasko 2002). While two reports showed that stimulation with either PHA (Candore et al. 1993) or ConA (Bernstein et al. 1998) resulted in comparable IL-4 production by both young and elderly, there are reports to indicate either an age-related increase (Nijhuis et al. 1994); or decrease (Karanfilov et al. 1999) in IL-4 production. However, those studies indicating an age-related increase, measured IL-4 production by PBMCs after stimulation with a combination of anti-CD2/anti-CD28, whereas the report demonstrating an age-related increase utilized a combination of CD3 and PMA. Therefore, differences in IL-4 production after non-specific stimulation may be dependent on the agent used to induce the response.

Attempts have been made to evaluate the age-related changes in IL-4 production by PBMC after stimulation with specific antigens. When PBMCs from young or elderly subjects were stimulated with either trivalent whole inactivated influenza vaccine (Bodnar et al. 1997) or after stimulation of PBMC with trivalent influenza subvirion vaccine (Bernstein et al. 1998), IL-4 levels could not be detected. It is possible that increasing age has either no effect on IL-4 production or that the effect is not very robust, since variations in experimental design result in very different outcomes. Additional studies that address these experimental issues are necessary before the effect of age on IL-4 production can be ascertained.

7.2   Interleukin 6

IL-6 is a Type 2 cytokine that impacts both T and B cell responses, and is a major component of the acute phase inflammatory response. The major cells types that produce IL-6 include T-cells, monocytes, macrophages and mast cells (Janeway 2006). T-cell activation and differentiation, B cell differentiation and mucosal IgA responses are all induced by the production of IL-6.

IL-6 has been deemed a "gerontologist cytokine" because it has been postulated that advancing age is associated with increased IL-6 levels (Ershler et al. 1993). However, a careful review of the literature to date does not support this claim, at least in human studies. Several studies have assessed the impact of age-related changes on IL-6 production after stimulation of PBMC or whole blood with mitogens. Stimulation with PHA (Candore et al. 1993; Beharka et al. 2001) or a combination of PHA and PMA (Fagiolo et al. 1993) induced comparable IL-6 production from PBMC of elderly and young after 24 hrs of incubation. However, a longer stimulation with PHA and PMA induced higher levels of IL-6 in elderly at 48 and 72 hrs of stimulation, while IL-6 levels remained constant in the young from 24–72 hrs (Fagiolo et al. 1993). It is not certain if this age-related increase is due to the type of stimulus (e.g., the addition of PMA to the culture) or reflects actual kinetic differences between young and elderly. Clearly, measurement at later time points may indicate an age-related increase in IL-6. However, an additional study argues against age-related kinetic differences since whole blood incubated with PHA for 96 hrs induced comparable levels of IL-6 in young and elderly subjects. The possibility that the inducing agent influences IL-6 production can not be excluded. A well-defined study by Beharka and colleagues measured IL-6 production by PBMCs from the same individuals after stimulation with PHA or ConA in fetal bovine serum (FBS) or autologous plasma (AP). While PHA in AP, PHA in FBS, and ConA in FBS induced comparable levels of IL-6 in young and elderly, IL-6 was decreased when ConA in AP was utilized, relative to young controls. Collectively, it appears that kinetic differences as well as the stimulating agents influence IL-6 production after nonspecific stimulation. Future studies in which a detailed kinetic analysis is performed using the same stimulating agent are required to definitively determine the effects of age on IL-6 production.

The effect of age on IL-6 production by PBMC stimulated with specific antigen has only been evaluated in response to influenza vaccine (Bernstein et al. 1998). In this study, IL-6 production was comparable between young and elderly subjects when PBMCs were stimulated in vitro with trivalent influenza vaccine before and after influenza immunization. However, it is important to note that there was considerable heterogeneity in IL-6 responses in both young and elderly before and after influenza vaccination. Therefore, if small numbers of subjects are evaluated, it is possible that a higher IL6 response in the elderly may reflect a sampling error rather than true biologic differences.

It has been suggested that concentrations of IL-6 in plasma or serum increase with advancing age (Ershler et al. 1993; Kania et al. 1995). Although the investigators who support this hypothesis recognize that IL-6 is usually undetectable in the absence of inflammation, (Ershler 1993), they still believe that this increase is solely due to age and not symptomatic inflammation. However, this conclusion is difficult to support since the elderly subjects in these reports, although defined as healthy elderly, were not screened for inflammatory diseases, such as arthritis. We have found in a previous influenza study that IL-6 levels were significantly elevated in a subset of elderly individuals prior to vaccination with influenza (Bernstein et al. 1998). These individuals did not produce a significant increase in IL-6 after vaccination with influenza. When the health status of these individuals was analyzed retrospectively, those individuals with increased IL-6 levels had reported that they did have arthritic flare-ups (Bernstein et al. 1996). Three additional studies evaluating IL6 levels in plasma and sera have observed no age-associated difference (Beharka et al. 2001; James et al. 1997; Peterson et al. 1994). In one study (Beharka et al. 2001) it was reported that there was no age-associated increase in IL-6 among the elderly; interestingly, subjects that were in the 65–69 and 75–80 age groups had higher IL-6 levels than those in the 70–74 and > 80 age groups. Collectively, these studies suggest that both health status and genetic heterogeneity may be a major factor in the variation in IL6 production observed among studies.

Overall in the human system, the data for an age-related increase in IL-6 is not convincing. Studies using similar techniques and subject populations have reported contrasting results. While there is strong evidence for elevated levels of IL-6 in disease states (Ershler, 1993) that are associated with aging, in the absence of disease, the current data does not support an age-associated change in IL-6 production.

7.3 Interleukin-10

IL-10 is produced by T and B cells, monocytes, and macrophages and inhibits macrophage activity by inhibiting cytokine production and downregulating MHC class II antigen expression (Janeway 2006). Like IL-4, IL-10 plays a key regulatory role in inhibiting production of Type 1 cytokines (Shearer 1997), thus down-regulating CMI responses. Investigators have hypothesized that an age-related increase in IL-10 production may influence the age-related decrease in CMI. Recent data from McElhaney et al. (2006) support this hypothesis since IL-10 levels increased after ex vivo stimulation of PBMC with influenza following immunization of elderly subjects, regardless of whether or not they had LDI. However, LDI subjects had threefold higher levels of IL-10 production by PBMC after ex vivo stimulation with influenza, compared with non-LDI subjects. This suggests that those elderly who develop LDI may favor a more Th-2 like response due to altered IFN-γ:IL-10 ratios.

Earlier studies, however, have utilized a number of culture conditions to evaluate production of IL-10 by PBMC or whole blood. Basal IL-10 production by PBMC cultured for 24 hrs without stimulation showed comparable levels in young and elderly (Llorente et al. 1997). The only study examining IL-10 in serum found comparable levels in young and elderly subjects (Peterson et al. 1994). Stimulation of PBMCs with trivalent influenza vaccine prior to immunization (Bernstein et al. 1998) also demonstrated no age-related differences. However, production of IL-10 after stimulation of PBMC with trivalent influenza vaccine or influenza B after immunization resulted in significantly decreased IL-10 production in the elderly compared to young (Bernstein et al. 1998; Llorente et al. 1999). A similar age-associated decrease was observed after stimulation of whole blood with PHA for 24 hrs (Bruunsgaard et al. 2000).

Therefore, similar to the data with other cytokines, conflicting results have been observed with IL-10. The data on IL-10 production range from being decreased, unchanged or increased, and are influenced by the stimulus or tissue examined. The age-related changes in influenza vaccine-induced IL-10 production that is observed only after influenza vaccination indicate that altered IL-10 production in response to specific stimuli is subtle and may be unmasked only by in vivo immune challenges, such as illness or vaccination. However, due to the differences in stimuli and the limited number of studies, a definitive conclusion is not possible at this time.

8   Conclusions and Future Directions

It is well established that immune function declines with advancing age in both humans and in animal models. Since cytokines are key components in the regulatory communication that occurs among immune cell, it is likely that altered cytokine production may contribute to these age-associated changes in immune function. Murine models of aging have shown an age-regulated dysfunction in cytokine production, as evidenced by consistently decreased IL-2 and increased IL-4. These data, coupled with the increased incidence of cancer and virus infections in the elderly have led investigators to hypothesize that aging may favor a predominant Type 2 cytokine response. Therefore, the purpose of this chapter was to evaluate the current literature regarding age-related changes in cytokine production in the elderly to determine whether the preponderance of evidence supports this contention.

Our current review of the literature cannot support the contention that there is, in fact, an age-associated shift to a predominant Type 2 cytokine response in the elderly. Despite the large number of studies that have been conducted over the last several years, differences in experimental design make it extremely difficult to compare the data among studies. This review clearly shows that factors such as age, health status, genetic heterogeneity and the demographics of the elderly population, all influence the outcome of a study. Likewise, differences in stimulating agent, its dose, time points of assessments and method of assessment for cytokine production all greatly influence the results of human studies. Therefore, without some way to control for the confounding variations in experimental design, a definitive conclusion among studies cannot be made. In epidemiologic studies, a meta analysis of raw data from several studies is often employed to draw conclusions regarding a biologic outcome from studies that do not have the same design. Perhaps a meta analysis of the studies evaluating cytokine production in the elderly may reveal associations that have not been apparent by simply reviewing the published data.

In order to validate the contention of an age-related shift in cytokine production, it is necessary to assess both Type 1 and Type 2 cytokines concurrently in the same study. While this concurrent analysis has been done in some of the studies reviewed, it has not been reported in all of them. Likewise, it is not acceptable to measure only one cytokine falling into either category and suggest that a predominant Type 1 or 2 response has been achieved. Rather, it is necessary to measure a panel of cytokines that may be induced during the response being assessed. Such an analysis can easily be performed with the development of multiplex cytokine bead arrays, in which several cytokines can be assessed from the same sample.

In summary, based on the current data, the reader is left with more questions than answers regarding the effect of cytokine dysregulation on age-related changes in immune function. It is clear that there are age-related changes between young and elderly in cytokine production; however, more comprehensive studies are required to assess the influence of age-associated cytokine dysregulation on the immune response of the elderly. Further, while assessment in response to mitogens may reflect the potential of cells, it is the response to natural, environmental stimuli, such as infectious agents that are most important. Therefore, is important for these studies to focus on the immune response to infectious agents, rather than to nonspecific stimulation, so that effective cytokine treatments may be developed to enhance vaccination strategies and immunotherapeutic targets.

Acknowledgments We thank Dr. Barry W. Ritz for critical reading of the manuscript.

References

Beharka AA, Meydani M, Wu D, Leka LS, Meydani A, Meydani SN (2001) Interleukin-6 production does not increase with age. J Gerontol Biol Sci 56A:B81–B88
Bernstein ED, Murasko DM (1998) Effect of age on cytokine production in humans. Age 21:137–151

Bernstein ED, Gardner EM, Abrutyn E, Gross P, Murasko DM (1998) Cytokine production after influenza vaccination in a healthy elderly population. Vaccine 16:1722–1731

Bodnar Z, Steger MM, Saurwein-Teissl M, Maczek C, Grubeck Loebenstein B (1997) Cytokine production in response to stimulation with tetanus toxoid, mycobacterium tuberculosis and influenza antigens in peripheral blood mononuclear cells and T cell lines from healthy elderlies. Intern Arch Allergy Immunol 112:323–330

Born J, Uthgenannt D, Dodt C, Nunninghoff D, Ringvolt E, Wagner T, Fehm HL (1995) Cytokine production and lymphocyte subpopulations in aged humans. An assessment during nocturnal sleep. Mech Ageing Dev 84:113–126

Bruunsgaard H, Pedersen AN, Schroll M, Skinhoj P, Pedersen BK (2000) Proliferative responses of blood mononuclear cells (BMNC) in a cohort of elderly humans: role of lymphocyte phenotype and cytokine production. Clin Exp Immunol 119:433–440

Candore G, DiLorenzo G, Melluso M, Cigna D, Colucci AT, Modica MA, Caruso C (1993) > -interferon, interleukin-4 and interleukin-6 vitro production in old subjects. Autoimmunity 16:275–280

Castle S, Uyemura K, Wong W, Modlin R, Effros R (1997) Evidence of enhanced type 2 immune response and impaired upregulation of a type 1 response in frail elderly nursing home residents. Mech Ageing Dev 94:7–16

Castle SC, Uyemura K, Crawford W, Wong W, Klaustermeyer WB, Makinodan T (1999) Age-related impaired proliferation of peripheral blood mononuclear cells is associated with an increase in both IL-10 and IL-12. Exp Gerontol 34:243–252

Ershler WB (1993) Interleukin 6: a cytokine for gerontologists. J Am Ger Soc 41:176–181

Ershler WB, Sun WH, Binkley N, Gravenstein S, Volk MJ, Kamoske G, Klopp RG, Roecker EB, Daynes RA, Weindruch R (1993) Interleukin 6 and aging: blood levels and mononuclear cell production increase with advancing age and in vitro production is modifiable by dietary restriction. Lymph Cytokine Res 12:225–230

Fagiolo U, Cossarizza Am Scala E, Fanales-Belasio E, Ortolani C, Cozzi E, Monti D, Franceschi C, Paganelli R (1993) Increased cytokine production in mononuclear cells of healthy elderly people. Eur J Immunol 23:2375–2378

Gardner, EM, Bernstein, ED, Popoff, KA, Abrutyn E, Murasko, DM (2000) Immune response to influenza vaccine in healthy elderly: Lack of association with plasma β-carotene, retinol, α-tocopherol or zinc. Mech Ageing Dev 117;29–45

Gardner EM, Mursasko DM (2002) Age-related changes in Type 1 and Type 2 cytokine production in humans. Biogerontol 3:271–289

Gardner, EM, Gonzalez EW, Nogusa S, Murasko DM (2006) Age-related changes in the immune response to influenza vaccination in a racially-diverse, healthy elderly population. Vaccine 24:1609–1614

Gillis S, Koziak R, Durante M, Weksler ME (1981) Immunological studies of aging: Decreased production of and response to T cell growth factor by lymphocytes from aged humans. J Clin Invest 67:937–942

Gonzalez EW, Gardner EM, Murasko D. (2007) Recruitment and retention of older adults in influenza immunization study. J Cultural Diver (In Press)

Hobbs MV, Weigle WO, Noonan DJ, Torbett BE, McEvilly RJ, Koch RJ, Cardenas GJ, Ernst DN (1993) Patterns of cytokine gene expression by CD4 +from young and old mice. J Immunol 150:3602–3614

Janeway C, Travers, Walport, Shlomchik (2005) Immunobiology—The immune system in health and disease" 6th Ed.

Karanfilov CI, Liu B, Fox CC, Lakshmann RR, Whisler RL (1999) Age-related defects in Th1 and Th2 production by human T cells can be dissociated from altered frequencies of CD45RA+ and CD45R)+ T cell subsets. Mech Ageing Dev 109:97–112

Ligthart GJ, Coberand JX, Geertzen HGN, Meinders AE, Knook DL, Hijmins W (1990) Necessity of the assessment of healthy status in human immunogerontological studies: evaluation of the SENIEUR protocol. Mech Ageing Dev 55:89–105

Lio D, D'Anna C, Gervasi F, Schola L, Potestio M, DiLorenzo G, Listi F, Colombo A, Candore G, Caruso C (1998) Interleukin-12 release by mitogen-stimulated mononuclear cells in the elderly. Mech Ageing Dev 102:211–219

Lio D, Balistreri CR, Candore G, D'Anna C, DiLorenzo G, Gervasi F, Listi F, Schola L, Caruso C (2000) In vitro treatment with interleukin-2 normalizes type-1 cytokine production by lymphocytes from eldery. Immunopharmacol Immunotoxicol 22:195–203

Lombard PR, Steiner G (1992). Preliminary report on cytokine determination in human synovial fluids: a consensus study of the European Workshop for Rheumatology Research. Clin Exp Rheumat 10:515–520

Llorente L, Richaud-Patin Y, Alvarado C, Vidaller A, Jakez-Ocampo J (1997) Autoantibody production in healthy elderly people is not promoted by interleukin-10 although this cytokine is expressed in them by a peculiar CD8+CD3+ large granular cell subpopulation. Scand. J Immunol 45:401–407

Marine MG, Johnson WG, Salas-Lopez D (2002) Influenza vaccination among minority populations in the United States. Prev Med 34:235–241

McElhaney JE, Beattie BL, Devine R, Grynoch R, Toth EL, Bleackley RC (1990) Age-related decline in interleukin 2 production in response to influenza vaccine. J Am Ger Soc 38:652–658

McElhaney JE, Meneilly GS, Beattie BL, Helgason CD, Lee SF, Devine RD, Bleackley RC (1992) The effect of influenza vaccination on IL2 production in healthy elderly: implications for current vaccination practices. J Gerontol 47:M3–M8

McElhaney JE, Meneilly GS, Pinkoski MJ, Lechelt KE, Bleackley RC (1995) Vaccine-related determinants of the interleukin-2 response to influenza vaccination in healthy young and elderly adults. Vaccine 13:6–10

McElhaney JE, Xie D, Hager WD, Barry MB, Wang Y, Kleppinger A, Ewen C, Kane KP, Bleackley RC (2006) T cell responses are better correlates of vaccine protection in the elderly. J Immunol 176:6333–6339

Miller RA (1996) The aging immune system: primer and prospectus. Science 273:70–7

Molteni M, Della Bella S, Mascagni B, Coppola C, De Micheli V, Zulian C, Birindelli S, Vanoli M, Scorza R (1994) Secretion of cytokines upon allogeneic stimulation: effect of aging. J Biol Regul Homeostatic Agents 8:41–47

Murasko DM, Weiner P, Kaye D (1987) Decline in mitogen induced proliferation with increasing age. Clin Exp Immunol 70:440–448

Murasko DM, Goonewardene IM (1990) T-cell function in aging: mechanisms of decline. Ann Rev Gerontol Geriat 10:71–96

Murasko DM, Nelson BJ, Matour D, Goonewardene IM, Kaye D (1991) Heterogeneity of changes in lymphoproliferative ability with increasing age. Exper Gerontol 26:269–279

Murasko DM, Bernstein ED, Gardner EM, Gross P, Munk G, Dran S, Abrutyn E (2001) Role of humoral and cell-mediated immunity in protection from influenza disease after immunization of healthy elderly. Exp Gerontol 37:427–439

Murasko DM, Gardner EM (2003) Immunology of aging. In: Hazzard WR, Blass JP, Halter JB, Ouslander JG, Tinetti ME (eds) Principles of geriatric medicine and gerontology 5th edn New York, McGraw Hill, pp 35–52

Mysliwska J, Bryl E, Foerster J, Mysliwski A (1998) Increase of interleukin 6 and decrease of interleukin 2 production during the ageing process are influenced by the health status. Mech Ageing Dev 100:313–328

Nagel JE, Chopra RK, Chrest FJ, McCoy MT, Schneider EL, Holbrook NJ, Adler WH (1988) Decreased proliferation, interleukin 2 synthesis, and interleukin 2 receptor expression are accompanied by decreased mRNA expression in phytohemagglutinin-stimulated cells from elderly donors. J Clin Invest 81:1096–1102

Nijhuis EW, Remarque EJ, Hinloopen B, Van DerPouw-Kraan T, Van Lier RA, Ligthart GJ, Nagelkerken L (1994) Age-related increase in the fraction of CD27-CD4+ cells and IL-4 production as a feature of CD4+ T cell differentiation in vitro. Clin Exp Immunol 96:528–534

Orson FM, Saadeh CK, Lewis DE, Nelson DL (1989) Interleukin 2 receptor expression by T cells in human aging. Cell Immunol 124:278–291

Peterson PK, Chao CC, Carson P, Hu S, Nichol K, Janoff EN (1994) Levels of tumor necrosis factor, interleukin 6, interleukin 10, and transforming growth factor are normal in the serum of the healthy elderly. Clin Infect Dis 19:1158–1159

Quyang Q, Cicek G, Westendorp RGJ, Cools HJM, Van Der Klis RJ, Remarque EJ (2000) Reduced IFNγ production in elderly people following vitro stimulation with influenza vaccine and endotoxin. Mech Ageing Dev 121:131–137

Rabinowich H, Goses Y, Reshef T, Klajman A (1985) Interleukin-2 production and activity in aged humans. Mech Ageing Dev 32:213–226

Ritz BW, Gardner EM (2006) Protein-energy malnutrition and energy restriction differentially affect viral immunity. J Nutr 136:1141–1144

Salkind AR (1994) Influence of age on the production of Fos and Jun by influenza virus-exposed T cells. J Leuk Biol 56:817–820

Sambamoorhi U, Findley PA (2005) Who are the elderly who never receive influenza immunizations? Prev Med 40:468–478

Saurwein-Teissi M, Blasko I, Zisterer K, Neuman B, Lang B, Grubeck-Loebenstein B (2000) An imbalance between pro- and anti-inflammatory cytokines, a characteristic feature of old age. Cytokine 12:1160–1161

Scheffer C, Zawotzky R, Rink L (2000) Interferon-γ levels finally become stable with increasing age as revealed by using an ELISA corresponding to the bioactivity. Mech Ageing Dev 121:47–58

Shearer GM (1997) Th1/Th2 changes in aging. Mech Ageing Dev 94:1–5

Sindermann J, Kruse A, Frercks HJ, Schultz RM, Kirchner H (1993) Investigations of the lymphokine system in elderly individuals. Mech Ageing Dev 70:149–159

Weifeng C, Schulin L, Xinomei G, Xuewen F (1986) The capacity of lymphocyte production by peripheral blood lymphocytes from aged humans. Immunolog Invest 15:575–583

Weyand CM, Brandes JC, Schmidt D, Fulbright JW, Goronzy JJ (1998) Functional properties of CD4+ CD28- T cells in the aging immune system. Mech Ageing Dev 102:131–147

Wu D, Meydani SN, Sastre J, Hayek M, Meydani M (1994) In vitro glutathione supplementation enhances interleukin-2 production and mitogenic response of peripheral blood mononuclear cells from young and old subjects. J Nutr 124:655–663

Xu X, Beckman I, Bradley J (1993) Age-related changes in the expression of IL-2 and high- affinity IL-2-binding sites. Intern Arch Allergy Immunol 102:224–231

Yen CJ, Lin SL, Huang KT, Lin RH (2000) Age-associated changes in interferon-γ and interleukin-4 secretion by purified human CD4+ and CD8 +T cells. J Biomed Sci 7:317–321

Cytokine Expression and Production Changes in Very Old Age

Susan E. McNerlan, Marilyn Armstrong, Owen A. Ross and I. Maeve Rea

Contents

1   Introduction

Ageing is associated with various changes in immune parameters, alterations in lymphocyte subsets and cytokine dysregulation (Cossarizza et al. 1997). Cytokines are central to the regulation of the immune-inflammatory response in old age and so perhaps play a pivitol role in ageing and survival. But whether these alterations in cytokine expression and production are the secret of long life or are an indication of underlying disease, even in the apparently healthy, is uncertain. While studies of cytokine gene polymorphisms suggest that certain cytokine genotypes are associated with long life (Rea et al. 2006), cytokine levels have also been associated with various age-related diseases (Forsey et al. 2003). Studies of these parameters in very

I. M. Rea (✉) · S. E. McNerlan
Department of Geriatric Medicine
School of Medicine
Dentistry and Biomedical Sciences
Queen's University, Belfast
Whitla Medical Building
97 Lisburn Road
Belfast BT7 9AB, UK
E-mail: i.rea@qub.ac.uk; s.mcnerlan@qub.ac.uk

M. Armstrong
School of Medicine
Dentistry and Biomedical Sciences
Queen's University, Belfast

O. A. Ross
Mayo Clinic
Jacksonville, USA

T. Fulop et al. (eds.), *Handbook on Immunosenescence*,
DOI 10.1007/978-1-4020-9062-2_40, © Springer Science+Business Media B.V. 2009

elderly subjects, i.e., those who have aged successfully, are perhaps the most useful in determining the key to longevity.

Cytokines have been investigated extensively in elderly people, at times with conflicting results. This is possibly in part due to the number of different methodologies employed. Immunoassays have been used for the measurement of circulating cytokines in plasma. However, due to the detection limits of kits, and the presence of natural inhibitors, soluble receptors or antagonists, their presence in serum may be masked. Bioassays, involving in vitro stimulation of whole blood or separated mononuclear cells, have also been widely employed in the study of age-associated changes in cytokine production. However, the response of cells to stimulants in an unnatural environment may not reflect what occurs in vivo. Also neither bioassays or immunoassays give an indication of the exact cellular source of these growth factors. Intracellular cytokine detection is a relatively new methodology which enables detection of cytokines at a single cell level thereby identifying the specific cell subsets producing these mediators (Jason et al. 1997; Jung et al. 1993; Prussin et al. 1995). The technique is performed in whole blood so cells can be kept in their natural environment. Still, while each of these methodologies have their limitations, a great deal of information on the cytokine profile of very elderly subjects has still been and is continuing to be elucidated.

2   IL-6

Interleukin 6 (IL-6) has been described as a "cytokine for gerontologists" (Ershler, 1993). It plays a key role in the acute phase response and displays both proinflammatory and anti-inflammatory activities. It is normally present in low levels in the blood, with increased levels detected during infection or trauma. Interleukin 6 levels have been widely reported to be elevated in the serum of very elderly subjects (Cohen et al. 1997; Forsey et al. 2003; Giuliani et al. 2001; Wei et al. 1992). Giuliani et al, in a study of 220 women aged 25–104 years, including 22 centenarians, showed that serum IL-6 levels increased exponentially with age. In the same group, soluble IL-6 receptor, which enhances IL-6 activity, and soluble gp130, an IL-6 inhibitor, increased until the 7th decade of life before decreasing in the older age groups.

The mechanisms behind this increase in IL-6 levels with age, as well as the cellular sources are still not fully understood. IL-6 production by both stimulated and unstimulated leucocytes is increased in elderly subjects by both PBMN cells and monocytes (Rea et al. 1995; Rink et al. 1998; Roubenoff et al. 1998). Using the technique of intracellular cytokine detection by flow cytometry, O'Mahoney et al. (1998) showed a statistically significant increase in intracellular IL-6 production in CD3+ T-cells and an insignificant increase in monocytes.

A number of studies have linked IL-6 polymorphisms to longevity, however, results have been conflicting. In a study of Italian centenarians, the 174G/C promoter polymorphism in the IL-6 gene, the GG genotype was decreased in male centenarians and was associated with increased plasma IL-6 levels. This would suggest that those genotypes producing high levels of IL-6 appear to be detrimental to long life, at least in men; there was no difference detected in women (Bonafe et al. 2001). Studies of Irish octo- and nonagenarians have also shown the GG genotype to be decreased in the elderly (Rea et al. 2003; Ross et al. 2003a). Other studies, however, have shown no difference in genotype frequencies between centenarians and young controls (Carpurso et al. 2004; Pes et al. 2004). The reasons for these discrepancies are unclear, however, cultural and lifestyle differences between the populations studied may play a role.

This increase in IL-6 levels, rather than being the key to longevity, may instead be a reflection of an increased inflammatory state caused by underlying disease even in the apparently well elderly person. Elevated IL-6 levels have been reported to be associated with several age-related diseases including coronary heart disease, arthritis and osteoporosis (Forsey et al. 2003). High levels are also associated with a decline in function and cognitive ability and also in stroke (Barbieri et al. 2003; Cesari et al. 2004; Cohen et al. 1997; Ershler and Keller 2000). It has also been indicated as a strong predictor of mortality in elderly people (Bruunsgaard et al. 2003a; Harris et al. 1999; Volpato et al. 2001) but not in persons aged 100 years (Bruunsgaard et al. 2003b).

3   TNF-α

TNF-α is another pro-inflammatory cytokine and an important mediator of the immune response. It is widely reported as being elevated in the plasma of elderly people and levels have been found to correlate with IL-6, sTNFR and CRP in centenarians (Rea et al. 1999; Bruunsgaard et al. 1999, 2000, Sandmand et al. 2003). Increased production from unstimulated monocyte monlayers has also been reported (McNerlan et al. 1997), However, LPS stimulated leucocytes have yielded conflicting results (Bruunsgaard et al. 2003a).

Using intracellular cytokine detection by flow cytometry, the percentage and absolute counts of CD3+ T-cells producing TNF-α were significantly higher in a study of very healthy octo- and nona-genarians compared to young controls (McNerlan et al. 2002). In another study of slightly younger individuals, >62 years (mean age 73), there were significant increases in intracellular T-cell TNFα and an insignificant increase in monocyte TNF-α (O'Mahoney et al. 1998). However, a Danish study which showed increased circulating TNF-α with increasing age in a cohort including centenarians only found an increase in the percentage and number of T-cells expressing TNF-α in the group of 81 year olds but not in the centenarians, suggesting that T-cells contribute to the increased TNF-α levels in elderly subjects but other mechanisms must come into play in the much older individual (Sandmand et al. 2003).

Polymorphisms of the TNF-α gene do not appear to be associated with longevity (Rea et al. 2006). Three studies of Finnish nonagenarians, Italian centenarians and

Irish nonagenarians showed no difference in the frequency of the TNFα-308A/G polymorphism compared to young controls (Lio et al. 2003; Ross et al. 2003b; Wang et al. 2001). No significant sex differences emerged either. There is, however, a reported association with Alzheimers disease. A haplotype for TNFα associates in siblings with late onset AD and carriers of -308A show an earlier mean age at onset (Alvarez et al. 2002; Collins et al. 2000; McCusker et al. 2001). High plasma levels of TNF-α were found to be associated with moderate to severe dementia in a cohort of Danish centenarians (Bruunsgaard et al. 1999), however, it is unclear whether its role is causative or if it is the result of an increased immune activation caused by the underlying pathologic processes.

TNFα is evident in other disease processes associated with ageing. High levels of TNF-α were seen in a study of 130 octogenarians with atherosclerotic CVD (Bruunsgaard et al. 2000), and in a group of centenarians with generalized athero-sclerosis (Bruunsgaard et al. 1999). Higher levels of TNF-α were found in a study of 70-year-old men with type II diabetes mellitus compared to age-matched controls and levels were found to correlate with the severity of insulin resistance (Nilsson et al. 1998). High levels of both TNF-α and IL-6 were associated with lower muscle mass and muscle strength in older men and women (Visser et al. 2002).

In a study of 333 relatively healthy 80 year olds, TNF-α was found to be associated with mortality in men but not women (Bruunsgaard et al. 2003a), whereas in a group of centenarians, recruited around their 100th birthday, elevated TNF-α was associated with mortality in both men and women (Bruunsgaard et al. 2003b).

4   Other Pro-Inflammatory Cytokines

Ageing is characterized by a low grade increase in inflammatory markers. In addition to IL-6 and TNFα, another primary mediator of the inflammatory response is IL-1. Reports on the production of IL-1β from cells from elderly people have been conflicting with reports of increased, decreased and no difference (Krabbe et al. 2004). Differing results may be due to different cell populations (WB, PBMC, monocytes,etc.) and the stimulants used (LPS, PMA, etc.). The InCHIANTI Study of subjects >65 years of age found no relationship between serum levels of IL-1β and age but found levels were associated with heart failure and angina (Di Iorio et al. 2003).

IL-18 is another proinflammatory cytokine associated with various major disabling conditions, including ischemic disease. However, whether it is the cause or a byproduct of these events is uncertain. Serum IL-18 levels are higher in centenarians compared to a young control group and also compared to a group of patients with chronic ischemic syndromes (Gangemi et al. 2003). These authors also report a significant increase in circulating levels of IL-18 binding protein, a natural inhibitor, compared to the other 2 groups which would explain the apparent paradox of elevated IL-18 with no vascular disease in these centenarians. Another study of 1671 elderly subjects aged 65-80 years showed elevated IL-18 levels to be associated with a decline in physical function, and that a polymorphism in the IL-18 gene which reduces IL-18 serum concentration, was associated with improved walking speed (Frayling et al. 2007).

IL-8 is a neutrophil chemotactic factor and inflammatory cytokine which brings neutrophils to the site of inflammation to contain infection (Baggiolini, et al. 1992). Increased levels have been detected after LPS stimulation of leucocytes from elderly individuals (Rink et al. 1998). IL-8 has been proposed as a possible key to longevity in a small study of centenarians. A study of 30 young people (21–37 years), 30 healthy elderly (65–87 years) and 10 centenarians found levels of IL-8 to be elevated in the serum of the centenarians compared to the other two groups (Wieczorowska-Tobis et al. 2006), while IL-6 levels were unchanged. This might suggest that increased serum IL-8 alongside low IL-6 might be related to longevity, although larger studies are needed to confirm this finding. However, Ross et al. (2003a) found that while AA homozygotes of the IL-8 -251 A/T polymorphism are associated with higher production levels of IL-8, there was no significant difference in IL-8 -251 A/T polymorphisms in a group of nonagenarians compared to young controls, but the study was relatively small.

IL-12 is a central cytokine acting on T- and NK cells directing proliferation of activated T-cells towards a Th1 phenotype (Trinchieri 1993). It is an important cytokine in the early inflammatory response where it stimulates IFNγ production from T- and NK cells. It is a disulphide linked heterodimer composed of a p40 heavy chain and a p35 light chain. The heterodimer IL-12p70 equates with biological activity whereas the homodimer IL-12p40 acts as an IL-12 antagonist in vitro (Mattner et al. 1993). Several studies have investigated age-related IL-12 production by mitogen-stimulated PBMCs in elderly people but results have been conflicting (Tortorella et al. 2002). In a study of very elderly subjects there was no difference in the IL-12A/C polymorphisms with ageing (Ross et al. 2003a).

However, in a study of very elderly subjects (Irish octo/nonagenarians), serum levels of total IL-12, IL-12p40 and the IL12p40/IL-12 p70 ratio, but not IL-12p70, were increased significantly with age (Rea et al. 2000). This increase in total IL-12 and the p40 subunit may be part of the cytokine dysregulation evident in the elderly or there may be an age-related imbalance in the transcription of the p40 and p70 subunits which are encoded on different genes.

5   Anti-Inflammatory Cytokines

Antiinflammatory activity is also reportedly increased in the elderly. IL-10 has both anti-inflammatory and B-cell stimulatory activities. It is produced by activated T-cells, B-cells, monocytes/macrophages and dendritic cells and is thought to block the ability of monocytes etc to act as antigen presenting cells by down-regulating the MHC. IL-10 is an important anti-inflammatory cytokine, capable of inhibiting the synthesis of proinflammatory cytokines such as IFNγ, TNFα, IL-2 and IL-3 and is produced in higher amounts by stimulated leucocytes from elderly subjects compare to the young (Rink et al. 1998). IL-10 production by unstimulated monocyte monolayers was also found to be increased in a group of very elderly subjects and correlated with IL-6 production from the same monocytes (Rea et al. 1996a).

The GG 1082 allele of the IL-10 promoter polymorphism, a polymorphism associated with increased IL-10 production, was found to be increased in male centenarians compared to young controls, suggesting that an increased antiinflammatory state is the key to longevity in men (Lio et al. 2002). However, this was not found in Finnish or Irish nonagenarian studies (Rea et al. 2006). It also stands contrary to other findings where increased IL-10 production has not given survival advantage. Patients with meningococcal septicaemia who are high IL-10 producers have a 20-fold higher chance of a fatal outcome compared to low producers (Westendorp et al. 1997). Also children with sudden infant death tend to have high IL-10 levels or high IL-10 producer allele status (Summers et al. 2000). Therefore perhaps only homozygous GG 1082 men who have avoided serious bacterial infections earlier in life may have an increased chance of longevity. An antiinflammatory genotype might be advantageous later in life, when a chronic proinflammatory state appears to develop. This phenomenon is called Inflamm-ageing (Franceschi et al. 2000) and is more evident in males compared to females, which may explain the higher frequency of antiinflammatory genotype in very elderly males.

IL-19 is a relatively new member of the IL-10 family, whose full function remains to be elucidated. IL-19 induces the production of IL-10 and IL-19 from PBMCs (Jordan et al. 2005). It also stimulates production of IL-6 and TNFα from monocytes in vitro (Liao et al. 2002), suggesting it may exhibit pro-inflammatory activities. As increased production of both IL-6 and TNFα are reported in ageing, IL-19 may also play a role in the ageing process. To date there have been no reports of any age associated changes in IL-19 levels, however, a recent Japanese study of 500 subjects aged between 19 and 100 years has shown an association between IL-19 gene polymorphisms and age (Okayama et al. 2007).

TGFβ is another cytokine with anti-inflammatory activities which seems to have an important role in ageing. In a study of Italian centenarians the active cytokine was found to increase with age and there was a significant difference found for the genotype and allele frequencies at the +915 site on the TGFβ gene (Carrieri et al. 2004). This increase in the active anti-inflammatory cytokine may contribute to longevity by counteracting the harmful effects of the increased inflammatory activities seen in advanced age.

Cytokine antagonists also play a role in the anti-inflammatory response. IL-1 receptor antagonist (IL-1RA), produced by monocytes and macrophages, blocks the binding of IL-1 to its cell surface receptors. Also 2 distinct soluble forms of the TNF-receptor occur in the plasma of healthy individuals, where they bind TNF and act as physiological inhibitors of TNF activity (Seckinger et al. 1989). A study of elderly Italian subjects (mean age 79.6±5.8) found that plasma concentrations of both IL-1RA and sTNFr were greater in healthy aged subjects compared to young controls. Levels of plasma neopterin, a product of activated monocytes/macrophages, were also elevated and positively correlated with both IL-1RA and sTNFr, suggesting that the increase in these antagonists is due to monocyte activation in elderly people (Catania et al. 1997). Another Italian study of aged subjects (range 66–80 years old) and 20 centenarians also showed sTNFRI and sTNFRII to be significantly elevated in healthy old subjects compared to young controls, and even higher in centenarians (Gerli et al. 2000). Soluble CD30, another member of the TNF superfamily, was also increased in the plasma of centenarians compared to the young.

As cytokines do not work alone but are instead a part of a complex network, more studies are needed of the balance of the pro- and antiinflammatory cytokines in successful ageing. Lio et al. (2003) report that a combination of high IL-10 and low TNFα producer polymorphisms is a combination that favors longevity in males but not females. However, the number of males in the study was small. Further larger studies are therefore required into the balance of these systems in elderly subjects.

6   TH1/TH2 Cytokines

Helper T-cells (TH) in humans have been classified into either TH1 or TH2 cells depending on the cytokines they produce. IL-12, IL-2 and IFNγ are associated with TH1 responses while IL-10, IL-4, IL-6 and IL-13 are prominent TH2 cytokines (Mosmann et al. 1996). Altered cytokine production in elderly people has suggested that there is a shift towards a Type 2 cytokine profile. However, not all findings have been clear cut.

Most studies have shown that lymphocytes from elderly subjects produce significantly less IL-2, the most important T-cell growth factor, compared to the young (Caruso et al. 1996; Gillis et al. 1981; Rea et al. 1996b). Methodology of intracellular cytokine detection has shown no change in the proportion of IL-2+ve T-cells (McNerlan et al. 2002) or an increase (Pietschmann et al. 2003). IL-15, another stimulator, particularly of memory T-cells, has been found to be increased in the serum of centenarians compared to both young and old controls (Gangemi et al. 2005). Interestingly there was no significant difference between the young and the old. As IL-15 is an important stimulator of memory T-cell proliferation, this may explain the accumulation of memory T-cells in the very elderly individuals.

IFNγ is the major TH1 cytokine. Caruso et al. (1996) showed a significant decrease in both IFNγ and IL-2 production by mitogen-stimulated mononuclear cell cultures from elderly subjects but no significant difference in TNFα, IL-4 and IL-6. Rink et al. (1998) also reported that IFNγ is produced less by lymphocytes of elderly people.

However, several reports have shown, using intracellular cytokine detection methods, an increase in the percentage of IFNγ positive T-cells in aged subjects (McNerlan et al. 2002; Pietschmann et al. 2003; Sandmand et al. 2002). Sandmand and Rink also showed that IL-4 and IL-10 positive T-cells were increased in aged subjects. Pietschmann showed that some changes were gender-specific. In elderly women they showed an increase in the proportion of T-cells positive for IFNγ, IL-2,

IL-4, IL-10 and IL-13. In men they only saw an increase in IL-2, IL-4 and IL-13. Therefore changes in IFNγ and IL-10 seemed likely to be gender-specific.

Zanni et al. (2003) showed an increase in both type 1 (IFNγ, IL-2 and TNFα) and type 2 (IL-4, IL-6, IL-10) cytokines with age. Type 1 cytokine-positive cells in all three CD8+ subsets investigated (CD95-CD28+(naïve), CD95+CD28- (effector/cytotoxic) and CD95+CD28+ (memory)). An increase in type 2 producing cells was only seen in the memory CD8 cells.

7   Conclusions

Cytokine expression and production drives and modulates the inflammatory response through the complex network of activating and down-regulating interactions, always striving to achieve a homeostatic milieu after the "stress/danger" response, whether bacterial, viral or other, has been quenched.

As with other body systems, the homeostatic control, titration and modulation of immune responsiveness seems to become more fragile and less tightly focused with increasing age and this may explain some of the dissonance between the proinflammatory and anti-inflammatory control mechanisms and some of the elements of immune-ageing.

However, there is suggestive evidence that other factors both genetic and environmental, together with sex, are likely to have or have had an important influence on shaping the immune profile of our most aged people. In geographically separate populations, cytokine allele shift seems to have been shaped by different bacterial, viral or antigen exposure. Similarly in nonagenarians and centenarians, there is some suggestion of an allele frequency shift towards a more anti-inflammatory profile which may have a gender-weighted effect. It is not clear whether this is acquired or innate, or a "nature" or "nurture" effect. An interesting suggestion might be that survivors of the 1915 influenza pandemic, such as present-day nonagenarians, may carry a cytokine genotype profile which both facilitated their survival from the influenza epidemic but allowed survival to very old age, in an environment where antibiotic use could soften the need for an action-packed immune responsiveness.

Much research needs to be carried out to answer these very challenging but fascinating questions, which have an important role in helping us understand our immune systems better, the role which they have in protecting us from acute and chronic disease and improving the quality of our ageing. A large pan European study, such as is currently being carried out with the "platinum seniors" of Europe in European Union-funded Genetics of Healthy Ageing (GEHA) project, has the organizational breadth of ability and the statistical weight, to help answer some of these questions.

References

Alvarez V et al (2002) Association between the TNFalpha-308 A/G polymorphism and the onset-age of Alzheimer disease. Am J Med Genet 114:574

Baggiolini M et al (1992) Interleukin-8, a chemotactic and inflammatory cytokine. FEBS Lett 307:97.

Barbieri M et al (2003) Chronic inflammation and the effect of IGF-I on muscle strength and power in older persons. Am J Physiol Endocrinol Metab 284:E481

Bonafe M et al (2001) A gender-dependent genetic predisposition to produce high levels of IL-6 is detrimental for longevity. Eur J Immunol 31:2357

Bruunsgaard H et al (1999) A high plasma concentration of TNF-α is associated with dementia in centenarians. J Gerontol A Biol Sci Med Sci 54:M357–M364

Bruunsgaard H et al (2000) Ageing, TNF-α and atherosclerosis. Clin Exp Immunol 121:255

Bruunsgaard H et al (2003a) Predicting death from tumour necrosis factor-alpha and interleukin-6 in 80 year old people. Clin Exp Immunol 132:24

Bruunsgaard H et al (2003b) Elevated levels of tumour necrosis factor alpha and mortality in centenarians. Am J Med 115:278

Carpurso C et al (2004) Interleukin 6-174G/C promoter gene polymorphism in centenarians: no evidence of association with human longevity or interaction with apolipoprotein E alleles. Exp Gerontol 39:1109

Carrieri G et al (2004) The G/C915 polymorphism of transforming growth factor-beta 1 is associated with human longevity: a study in Italian centenarians. Aging Cell 3:443

Caruso C et al (1996) Cytokine production pathway in the elderly. Immune Res 15:84

Catania A et al (1997) Cytokine antagonists in aged subjects and their relation with cellular immunity. J Gerontol A Biol Sci Med Sci 52A:B93–B97

Cesari M et al (2004) Inflammatory markers and physical performance in older persons. The InCHIANTI Study. J Ger A Biol Sci Med Sci 59:242

Cohen HJ et al (1997) The association of plasma IL-6 levels with functional disability in community dwelling elderly. J Ger A Biol Sci Med Sci 52:201

Collins JS et al (2000) Association of a haplotype for tumour necrosis factor in siblings with late-onset Alzheimer disease. The NIMH Alzheimer Disease Genetics Initiative. Am J Med Genet 96:823

Cossarizza A et al (1997) Cytometric analysis of Immunosenescence. Cytometry 27:297

Di Iorio A et al (2003) Serum IL-1beta levels in health and disease: a population based study. 'The InCHIANTI Study'. Cytokine 22:198

Ershler WB (1993) Interleukin-6: a cytokine for gerontologists. J Am Geriatr Soc 41:176

Ershler WB, Keller ET (2000) Age-associated increased interleukin-6 gene expression, late-life diseases and frailty. Annu Rev Med 51:245

Forsey RJ et al (2003) Plasma cytokine profiles in elderly humans. Mech Ageing Dev 124:487

Franceschi C et al (2000) Inflamm-aging. An evolutionary perspective on immunosenescence. Ann N Y Acad Sci 908:244

Frayling TM et al (2007) An interleukin-18 polymorphism is associated with reduced serum concentrations and better functioning in older people. J Gerontol A Biol Sci Med Sci 62:73

Gangemi S et al (2003) Increased circulating interleukin-18 levels in centenarians with no sign of vascular disease: another paradox of longevity. Exp Gerontol 38:669

Gangemi S et al (2005) Age-related modifications in circulating IL-15 levels in humans. Mediators Inflamm 2005:245

Gerli R et al (2000) Chemokines, sTNF-Rs and sCD30 serum levels in healthy aged people and centenarians. Mech Ageing Dev 121:37

Gillis S et al (1981) Immunological studies of aging. Decreased production of and response to T cell growth factor by lymphocytes from aged humans. J Clin Invest 67:937

Giuliani N et al (2001) Serum interleukin-6, soluble interleukin-6 receptor and soluble gp130 exhibit different patterns of age- and menopause-related changes. Exp Gerontol 36:547

Harris TB et al (1999) Associations of elevated interleukin-6 and C-reative protein levels with mortality in the elderly. Am J Med 106:506

Jason J, Larned J (1997) Single cell cytokine profiles in normal humans: comparison of flow cytometric reagents and stimulation protocols. J Immunol Methods 207:13

Jordan WJ et al (2005) Human IL-19 regulates immunity through auto-induction of IL-19 production of IL-10. Eur J Immunol 35:1576

Jung T et al (1993) Detection of intracellular cytokines by flow cytometry. J Immunol Methods 159:197

Krabbe KS et al (2004) Inflammatory mediators in the elderly. Exp Gerontol 39:687

Liao YC et al (2002) IL-19 induces production of IL-6 and TNF-α and results in cell apoptosis through TNF-α. J Immunol 169:4288

Lio D et al (2002) Gender specific association between -1082 IL-10 promoter polymorphism and longevity. Genes Immun 3:30

Lio D et al (2003) Inflammation, genetics and longevity: further studies on the prospective effects in men of IL-10—1082 promoter SNP and its interaction with TNF-alpha -308 promoter SNP. J Med Genet 40:296

Mattner F et al (1993) The interleukin-12 subunit p40 specifically inhibits effects of the interleukin-12 heterodimer. Eur J Immunol 23:2202

McCusker SM et al (2001) Association between polymorphisms in regulatory region of gene encoding tumour necrosis factor α and risk of Alzheimer Disease and vascular dementia: a case-control study. Lancet 357:436

McNerlan SE et al (1997) TNF-α production from monocyte monolayers is increased in old age. Immunology 92(Suppl 1):107 (Abstract)

McNerlan SE et al (2002) A whole blood method for measurement of intracellular TNFα, IFNγ and IL-2 expression in stimulated CD3+ lymphocytes: differences between young and elderly subjects. Exp Gerontol 37:227

Mosmann TR, Sad S (1996) The expanding universe of T cell subsets, Th1, Th2 and more. Immunol Today 17:138

Nilsson J et al (1998) Relation between plasma tumour necrosis factor-α and insulin sensitivity in elderly men with non-insulin-dependent diabetes mellitus. Arterioscler Thromb Vasc Biol 18:1199

Okayama N et al (2007) Association of interleukin-19 gene polymorphisms with age. J Gerontol A Biol Sci Med Sci 62A:507

O'Mahoney L et al (1998) Quantitative intracellular cytokine measurement: age-related changes in proinflammatory cytokine production. Clin Exp Immunol 113:213

Pes GM et al (2004) Association between longevity and cytokine gene polymorphisms. A study in Sardinian centenarians. Ageing Clin Exp Res 16:244

Pietschmann P et al (2003) The effect of age and gender on cytokine production by human peripheral blood mononuclear cells and markers of bone metabolism. Exp Gerontol 38:1119

Prussin C, Metcalfe DD (1995) Detection of intracytoplasmic cytokines using flow cytometry and directly conjugated anti-cytokine antibodies. J Immunol Methods 188:117

Rea IM et al (1995) Increased IL-6 production from monocyte monolayers in octogenarian and nonagenarian subjects. Immunol 86(Suppl 1):58 (abstract)

Rea IM et al (1996a) IL-10 production from monocyte monolayers in very old age. Immunology 89(Suppl 1):68 Abstract

Rea IM et al (1996b) Changes in lymphocyte subsets, interleukin 2 and soluble interleukin 2 receptor in old and very old age. Gerontology 42:69

Rea IM et al (1999) CD69, CD25 and HLA-DR activation antigen expression on CD3+ lymphocytes and relationship to serum TNF-α, IFN-γ and sIL-2R levels in ageing. Exp Gerontol 34:79

Rea IM et al (2000) Serum IL-12 and IL12p40 but not IL-12p70 are increased in the serum of older subjects: relationship to CD3+ and NK subsets. Cytokine 12:156

Rea IM et al (2003) Interleukin-6-gene C/G 174 polymorphism in nonagenarian and octogenearian subjects in the BELFAST study. Reciprocal effects on IL-6, soluble IL-6 receptor and for IL-10 in serum and monocyte supernatants. Mech Ageing Dev 124:555

Rea IM et al (2006) Longevity. In: Vandenbroeck K (ed) Cytokine gene polymorphisms in multi-factorial conditions. CRC Press, p 379

Rink L et al (1998) Altered cytokine production in the elderly. Mech Ageing Dev 102:199

Ross OA et al (2003a) Study of age-association with cytokine gene polymorphisms in an aged Irish population. Mech Ageing Dev 124:199

Ross OA et al (2003b) HLA haplotypes and TNF polymorphism do not associate with longevity in the Irish. Mech Ageing Dev 124:563

Roubenoff R et al (1998) Monocyte cytokine production in an elderly population: effect of age and inflammation. J Ger A Biol Sci Med Sci 53:M20–M26

Sandmand M et al (2002) Is ageing associated with a shift in the balance between Type 1 and Type 2 cytokines in humans. Clin Exp Immunol 127:107

Sandmand M et al (2003) High circulating levels of TNF-α in centenarians is not associated with increased production in T-lymphocytes. Gerontol 49:155

Seckinger P et al (1989) Pruification and biological characterisation of a specific TNFα inhibitor. J Biol Chem 264:11966

Summers AM et al (2000) Association of IL-10 genotype with sudden infant death syndrome. Hum Immunol 61:1270

Tortorella C et al (2002) APC-dependent impairment of T cell proliferation in aging: role of CD28- and IL-12/IL-15-mediated signalling. Mech Ageing Dev 123:1389

Trinchieri G (1993) Interleukin-12 and its role in the generation of Th1 cells. Immunol Today 14:335

Visser M et al (2002) Relationship of interleukin-6 and tumour necrosis factor-α with muscle mass and muscle strength in elderly men and women: the Health ABC Study. J Gerontol A Biol Sci Med Sci 57:M326–M332

Volpato S et al (2001) Cardiovascular disease, interleukin-6 and risk of mortality in older women: the women's health and aging study. Circulation 103:947

Wang XY et al (2001) Lack of association between human longevity and polymorphisms of IL-1 cluster, IL-6, IL-10 and TNF-alpha genes in Finnish nonagenarians. Mech Ageing Dev 123:29

Westendorp RG et al (1997) Genetic influence on cytokine production in meningococcal disease. Lancet 348:1912

Wei J et al (1992) Increase of plasma IL-6 concentration with age in healthy subjects. Life Sci 51:1953

Wieczorowska-Tobis K et al (2006) Can an increased level of circulating IL-8 be a predictor of human longevity? Med Sci Monit 12:CR118–CR121

Zanni F et al (2003) Marked increase with age of type 1 cytokines within memory and effec-tor/cytotoxic CD8+ T cells in humans: a contribution to understand the relationship between inflammation and immunosenescence. Exp Gerontol 38:981

Mechanisms - Neuro-Endocrine-Immune Network

Neuro-Endocrine-Immune Network and its Age-Related Changes

K. Hirokawa and M. Utsuyama

Contents

1 Introduction

In living beings, external stimuli elicit a behavioral, verbal, or physiological response. The stimuli can be classified into 2 types: ordinary stimuli such as sound, smell, sight, and touch that are received by the sensory organs and pathological stimuli such as bacterial, viral, and fungal infections that are received by the immune system (Fig. 1).

Ordinary stimuli that are received by the sensory organs, perceived by the cerebral cortex, and recognized by the association cortex, stimulate the limbic system and finally reach the hypothalamus. In contrast, infections stimulate the cells of the immune system and induce the production of various cytokines that are transported via the blood stream to the brain and influence the function of the hypothalamus [1].

The hypothalamus has many centers that are responsible for various functions such as the regulation of pituitary secretion, sexual behavior, reproduction, water balance regulation, satiety, autonomic nerve regulation, feeding, circadian rhythms, aggressiveness, fighting behavior, drinking, exploration behavior, and heat conservation [2]. It is believed that the hypothalamus influences the functioning of the immune system via 1) pituitary-adrenal-gonad axis and 2) the innervation of lymphoid organs.

K. Hirokawa (✉)
Institute for Health and Life Sciences
Ascent Myogadani 4F, 4-4-22, Kohinata
Bunkyo-ku, Tokyo 112-0006, Japan
E-mail: hirokawa@h-ls.jp

T. Fulop et al. (eds.), *Handbook on Immunosenescence*,
DOI 10.1007/978-1-4020-9062-2_41, © Springer Science+Business Media B.V. 2009

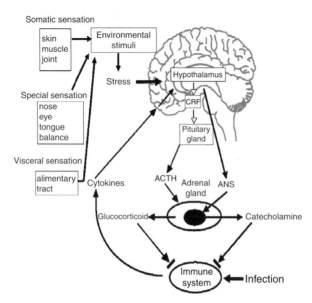

Fig. 1   Activation of the neuroendocrine-immune network by stress and infection. The various types of environmental stimuli that are received by sensory organs act as stress factors when they exceed normal physiological limits. This stress eventually stimulates the hypothalamus to secrete corticotropin releasing factor (CRF). CRF then stimulates the pituitary gland to secrete adrenocorticotropic hormone (ACTH), which in turn stimulates the adrenal cortex to secrete glucocorticoids. At the same time, the hypothalamus also stimulates,the autonomic nervous system (ANS), leading to the secretion of catecholamines by the adrenal medulla. Infections independently stimulate the immune system to produce various types of cytokines, most of which can enter the brain though areas where the blood-brain-barrier is weak, and stimulate the hypothalamus. This eventually results in the secretion of both glucocorticoids and catecholamines

Thus, all stimuli that are received by the body can reach the hypothalamus and influence its functions including the functions of the endocrine and immune systems. This consequently leads to the activation of the neuroendocrine-immune network.

Ordinary stimuli are essential for the normal development and growth of a living body. Physical stimuli help the development of normal body constitution. Visual and auditory stimuli including words and language promote the normal psychological and spiritual development of humans. Exposure to various infectious agents is also necessary for the normal development of the immune system.

It is not unusual for stimuli to exceed the normal physiological range. In such situations, these stimuli act as a source of stress for the body. In such cases, the hypothalamus plays a major role in the activation of the neuroendocrine-immune network for the maintenance of homeostasis. Homeostatic control involves the activation of the autonomic nervous system [3] and the hypothalamus-pituitary-adrenal axis. The former induces the production of catecholamines and the latter, glucocorticoids. These products are essential for the maintenance of homeostasis when the body is exposed to stress. However, both catecholamines and glucocorticoids have a suppressive effect on the immune system. This is a kind of physiological trade-off. In any event, stress downregulates the activity of the immune system.

It is important to note that the nervous, endocrine, and immune systems change with age, and thus, the action of the neuroendocrine-immune system against stress also changes with age. To put it plainly, the ability of the neuroendocrine-immune system to cope with stress declines with age [1]. This chapter will briefly summarize various neuroendocrine-immune interactions and the age-related changes in these interactions.

2   Neuroendocrine-immune Interactions at the Cellular Level

Lymphocytes can produce various hormones and neurotransmitters [4,5] and express receptors for these molecules. Table 1 shows the common mediators released by the cells of the immune and neuroendocrine systems. The cells of the immune system produce many interleukins (ILs). It has become apparent that the cells of the nervous and endocrine systems can also produce most of these ILs and express receptors for them. The right hand side of Table 1 lists the mediators originally produced by the cells of the neuroendocrine system. It is now commonly accepted that the cells of the immune system produce pituitary hormones and express their receptors. Fig. 2 shows the expression of hormones and neurotransmitter receptors in the splenic T-cells of mice, as determined by reverse transcription-polymerase chain reaction (RT-PCR). It is interesting to note that the expression levels of these receptors change in a variable pattern with age. Expression levels of mRNA of the glucocorticoid and thyroid stimulation hormone (TSH) receptors do not change greatly with age. The levels of the thyrotropin-releasing hormone receptor (TRH-R), adrenocorticotropin

Table 1   Common Mediators

Immune system	Neuroendocrine system
	Endorphin, Encephalin
	Somatostatins, Substance P
Interleukins	Catecholamine, Acetylcholine
Interferons	VIP
	GH, TSH, PRL, ACTH
	LH, TRH, CRH, LHRH
	Thyroxin
	Insulin
	Adrenal steroids
	Gonadal steroids
Serotonin*	
Histamine*	
Prostaglandin*	

Asterisk (*) indicates substances that were considered to be produced by both the immune and neuroendocrine systems.

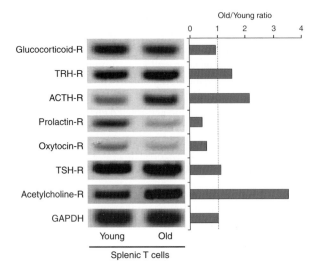

Fig. 2   The mRNA expression of various hormone and neurotransmitter receptors (R) in splenic T-cells from young and old mice. The columns indicate the ratio of old to young mice. The mRNA expression levels of thyrotropin-releasing hormone receptor (TRH-R), adrenocorticotropin receptor (ACTH-R), and acetylcholine receptor (acetylcholine-R) are increased in the T-cells from the old mice

receptor (ACTH-R), and the acetylcholine receptor (acetylcholine-R) increase with age while those of the prolactin receptor (prolactin-R) and the oxytocin receptor (oxytocin-R) decrease with age [1]. These facts suggest that interactions between the cells of the immune and neuroendocrine systems change with age.

3   Neuroendocrine-immune Interaction at the Organ Level

3.1   Hypothalamus-pituitary Axis and Immune System

The hypothalamus plays an important role in the control of both endocrine functions and the autonomic nervous system. Accordingly, it also operates as a control center for immune functions.

Thymic hypoplasia with T-cell-dependent immunodeficiencies was observed in Snell dwarf mice with congenital hypopituitarism [6]. This is consistent with the fact that the suppression of pituitary functions either by hypophysectomy [1] (Table 2) or the administration of antipituitary antibodies [7] results in a decrease in immune functions. Conversely, implanting growth hormone (GH)-producing cell lines in rats resulted in the reversal of the thymus atrophy and induced the thymus to regrow to a larger size [8]. The effects of GH in the thymus are mediated by insulin-like growth factor-1 (IGF-1), and thymic functions are actually under the control of

Table 2 Weight of organs after AHTL and hypophysectomy

Treatments	Thymus	Adrenal	Ovary	Hypophysis
Control +Sham-AHTL	314 ± 23	57 ± 3	99 ± 4	12 ± 1
Control +AHTL	423 ± 19	35 ± 3	61 ± 2	15 ± 1
Hypox +Sham-AHTL	128 ± 8	11 ± 1	12 ± 1	(–)
Hypox +AHTL	146 ± 15	12 ± 1	13 ± 1	(–)

Each group, 5 rats. Control group, sham operation of hypophysectomy.AHTL, lesioning of anterior hypothalamus. Sham-AHTL, sham operation of AHTL.Hypox, hypophysectomy. Data, mean ± 1 SEM.

GH/IGF-1-mediated circuits [9]. These findings taken together indicate that thymic size and function are dependent on the serum GH level.

Several reports have indicated that electronic lesions in the anterior hypothalamus resulted in a decrease in thymic weight [10,11], presumably by compromising pituitary function. Lesions in the ventromedial nucleus result in a significant decrease in pituitary and plasma GH levels [12]. We extended these earlier studies in rats by widening the area of destruction in the anterior portion of the hypothalamus, including the anterior hypothalamic nucleus, suprachiasmatic nucleus, and periventricular nucleus, (hereafter referred to as anterior hypothalamic lesioning, (AHTL)) and performed AHTL not only in young rats but also in aged rats with an atrophic thymus [1,13,14].

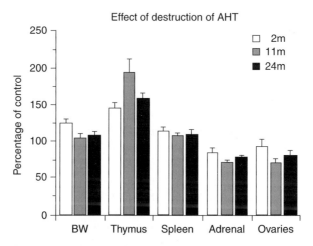

Fig. 3 Effect of destruction of the anterior portion of the hypothalamus (AHTL) in Wistar rats. AHTL was performed in rats at 2 months (open columns), 11 months (grey columns), and at 24 months of age (solid columns). Body weight and the weight of various organs were assessed 4 weeks after AHTL. The results are expressed as a percentage of the control age-matched rats that underwent a shamoperation. Vertical bars, 1 standard error of the mean

Contrary to the results of previous reports, AHTL resulted in thymic hypertrophy not only in young rats but also in middle-aged and old rats (Fig. 3). Interestingly, the magnitude of thymic hyperplasia after AHTL differed with age, indicating that the relationship between the hypothalamus and thymus changes during the course of aging. Furthermore, it was found that thymic hyperplasia did not occur in hypophysectomized rats (Table 2); thus, indicating that pituitary hormones regulate thymic hyperplasia.

Significant atrophy of the adrenal glands and gonads (testes or ovaries) was observed in rats subjected to AHTL, suggesting that ACTH and luteinizing hormone (LH) were not associated with thymic hyperplasia. High serum GH levels were noted in rats treated with AHTL, and these high levels were observed not only in young rats but also in middle-aged and old rats (Table 3). Since the secretion of GH is episodic, the single point sample data shown in Table 3 must be interpreted with caution. However, the rise in serum GH levels was consistent with the slightly hypertrophic pituitary gland in rats subjected to AHTL, i.e., the weight of the pituitary gland in the control and AHTL groups was 12 ± 1 mg and 15 ± 1 mg, respectively. Furthermore, high serum GH levels were not observed in adrenalectomized (adx) or ovariectomized (ovx) rats (Table 3).

We presume that a high serum GH level is necessary for thymic hyperplasia. When the serum GH levels of rats and mice at various ages were assessed, high serum GH levels were observed only at the newborn stage (Table 4). This is consistent with the results of a previous study [15] that reported profuse GH secretion in neonates. The fact that atrophy of thymus can be reversed and the thymus can be induced to regrow to a larger size by the administration of GH (8) suggests that the serum GH level shows a gradual decline with age. Actually, the fall in GH over

Table 3 Serum GH and LH levels in various experiments

Age	Treatments	GH(ng/ml)	LH(ng/ml)
6 weeks	Sham-AHTL	9.4 ± 2.2	6.8 ± 1.5
	AHTL	182.3 ± 7.0	4.0 ± 1.5
	Hypox + Sham	4.0 ± 0.9	2.4 ± 0.3
	Hypox + AHTL	3.1 ± 0.1	2.5 ± 0.6
2 months	Ovx	12.7 ± 1.7	14.1 ± 0.5
	Sham-Ovx	13.8 ± 1.4	3.7 ± 0.3
	Adx	15.6 ± 2.6	3.0 ± 0.1
	Sham-Adx	15.1 ± 4.6	3.3 ± 0.5
11 months	Sham-AHTL	26.9 ± 7.0	2.5 ± 0.2
	AHTL	176.0 ± 7.5	3.4 ± 0.3
24 months	Sham-AHTL	41.0 ± 18.4	2.8 ± 0.3
	AHTL	168.0 ± 0.7	3.0 ± 0.2

AHTL: lesioning of anterior hypothalamus. Sham-AHTL, shamoperation of AHTL. Ovx, ovariectomy. Sham-Ovx, sham operation of Ovx. Adx, adrenalectomy. Sham-Adx, sham operation of Adx.
Data, mean ± 1 SEM, obtained from 5 rats.

Table 4   Serum level of GH in mice and rats at various ages

Age	Rat	Mouse
18 fd	1.5	ND
NB	129.3 ± 5.4	141.7
1 month	3.9 ± 0.4	2.2 ± 0.6
3 months	14.0 ± 4.9	1.8 ± 0.4
6 months	12.3 ± 0.7	2.3 ± 0.3
12 months	10.4 ± 1.2	2.6 ± 0.1
18 months	8.8 ± 0.8	2.4 ± 0.2
24 months	12.0 ± 1.2	6.8 ± 2.5

Fd, fetal day. NB; Newborn Data: mean concentration of GH (ng/ml) ± SEM, obtained from 4 to 6 animals. Asterisk (*) indicates that the GH levels in samples pooled from several animals were assessed. ND, not done.

the life span is from 1200 μgm^{-2} in adolescents to 60 μm^{-2} in older individuals [15]. However, the most important point to be noted is that GH secretion appears to be extraordinarily high at the newborn stage in mice, rats, and humans and that this high level is necessary for thymic growth.

These findings collectively indicated that the serum GH level is dependent on the balance between positive and negative signals (growth-hormone-releasing hormone (GHRH) and growth-hormone-release-inhibiting hormone (GHRIH), respectively) or somatostatin (SST) in the hypothalamus. We examined the mRNA levels of these positive and negative signals in the mouse hypothalamus and found that the level of GHRH mRNA decreased with age while that of pre-pro-SST mRNA increased with age. In addition, we also analyzed the receptors for these signals in the pituitary glands and found that with age, the level of GHRH-receptor mRNA also decreased while that of the SST receptor increased (Utsuyama, personal communication). These observations are consistent with those of some previous reports. Florio et al. [17] reported that the pre-pro-SST mRNA levels in the hypothalamus of 25-month-old rats were slightly greater than those in younger rats. Furthermore, an age-related increase was observed in the levels of the SST receptor (sst2) in the pituitary gland of aging rats [18]. Based on the fact that high levels of serum GH are observed only at the newborn stage in rats and mice (Table 4), it can be assumed that hypothalamic positive signal is superior to hypothalamic negative signal, resulting in a high level of GH. However, at later stages of development, the negative signal becomes superior to the positive signal, leading to a decline in the secretion of GH (Fig. 4). This concept has been validated in aging humans; i.e., available clinical data have suggested that excessive SST release occurred with diminished GHRH secretion [19]. Thus, the destruction of the anterior portion of the hypothalamus, which contains the cells that produce SST (negative signal), shifts the balance between the positive and negative hypothalamic signals toward the predominance of the positive signal. This results in high serum GH levels even in the middle-aged and old rats, and eventually leads to thymic hyperplasia.

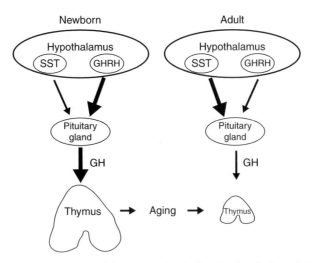

Fig. 4 Schematic representation of the control thymic function by the hypothalamus-pituitary axis. In newborn animals, the strength of the positive signal of growth hormone releasing hormone (GHRH) is greater than that of the negative signal of somatostatin (SST) in the hypothalamus, leading to an increased secretion of growth hormone (GH). In young adult animals, the strength of the negative signal is greater than that of the positive one, leading to a decrease in the secretion of GH. A decrease in the serum level of GH in the young adult results in to thymic involution

In addition to having various centers for the control of endocrine functions, the hypothalamus is closely related with the sympathetic nervous system (SNS). As the thymus is rich in nerve fibers [20], it is possible that the hypothalamus also influences thymic function through the sympathetic nerve fibers. To test this possibility, we examined the effect of AHTL on both the host thymus and the thymus implanted under the kidney capsule. Briefly, 2 lobes of a newborn thymus were implanted under the kidney capsule in young rats, and AHTL was performed on these rats after 1 month. One month after AHTL, the rats were sacrificed and the weight of the host and implanted thymuses was assessed. Contrary to our expectation, AHTL had no effect on the implanted thymus; although the host thymus, however, became hyperplastic. However, hypophysectomy greatly influenced both the host and implanted thymuses (Table 5). These results suggested that thymic hyperplasia after AHTL depends not on only the high serum GH levels but also on some unknown local requirement. The variation in the response could be attributed to the difference in autonomic innervation between the host and the implanted thymuses. The stimulation of the SNS is known to suppress immune function. Miles et al. [21] reported that ablation of the peripheral nervous system caused a significant increase in splenic T-cells. Earlier studies by Besedovsky et al. [22] reported that surgical denervation of the rat spleen resulted in an increase in the antibody-forming activity. Therefore, it is likely that AHTL affects the functions of the SNS, and alterations in the SNS around the host thymus might be essential for the development of thymic hyperplasia after AHTL in addition to the high serum GH levels. Furthermore, a decrease in serum GH levels by hypophysectomy leads to a significant atrophy of both the implanted and host

rtrt /5rt reason

Table 5 Effect of AHTL on the host and implanted thymuses in normal and hypophysectomized rats

Treatment	Host thymus	Implanted thymus	Adrenal gland
Sham-AHTL	304 ± 23	137 ± 11	57 ± 5
AHTL	441 ± 13	102 ± 21	36 ± 3
AHTL + Hypox	105 ± 11	47 ± 12	19 ± 5

A new-born thymus was grafted under the kidney capsule in 2-month-old normal rats or in hypophysectomized rats. One month after the implantation of the thymus, the rats underwent AHTL, and 1 month later, they were sacrificed for the assessment of organ weight. AHTL, lesioning of anterior hypothalamus. Sham-ATHT, sham operation of AHTL. Data, mean ± 1 SEM, obtained from 5 rats.

thymuses (Table 5). Further experiments are clearly necessary to clarify the relationship between nerve fibers, the thymus, and the hypothalamus.

3.2 Adrenal Glands and the Immune System

With the exception of erythrocytes, most cells have glucocorticoid receptors. Therefore, physiological and pharmacological effects of this hormone are very variable. Glucocorticoids are known to have distinct antiinflammatory, immunosuppressive, and oncostatic effects. Glucocorticoid immunosuppression is mediated by a direct cytolytic effect, through the inhibition of lymphocyte function, or indirectly through soluble suppressor mediators [23]. In vivo glucocorticoid administration results in pronounced thymic involution, and immunohistological analysis of the changes following glucocorticoid performed using the terminal deoxynucleotidyl transferase dUTP nick end labeling (TUNEL) method reveal the development of extensive apoptosis in the cortex [24].

Adrenal glands removal in mice leads to a significant increase in the weight of the thymus and spleen as well as in the number of splenic T-cells (Table 6). The effect is partly due to a decrease in the serum levels of glucocorticoids and partly due to an increase in the serum levels of the adrenocorticotropic hormone (ACTH) in the serum. These changes are mediated by a negative feed back reaction through the hypothalamic-pituitary axis. Interestingly, the thymus can also influence the function of the adrenal glands, i.e., it was observed that the implantation of a newborn thymus increased the weight of the adrenal glands in nude mice [25]. This increase in weight

Table 6 Effect of adrenalectomy on thymus and splenic T-cells in rats

Groups	Body weight	Thymus	Spleen	Splenic T cells
Sham	194 ± 4	233 ± 4	195±7	1.49 ± 0.12
Exp	192 ± 3	417 ± 19	549 ± 24	2.33 ± 0.44

Exp indicates adlenalectomy.

might be mediated by the secretion of ACTH by the T-cells following appropriate stimulation [26].

3.3 Gonads and the Immune System

Sex steroids are known to suppress immune functions [27]. We also reported that various steroids suppressed the in vitro proliferation of mouse spleen cells by mitogenic stimulation [28]. Physiological thymic involution that starts around puberty can be ascribed to the increased level of sex steroids. Interestingly, this thymic involution is not an irreversible phenomenon. In mice and rats, thymus atrophy at any age can be

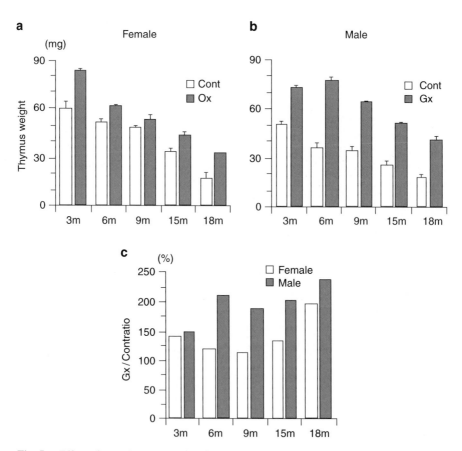

Fig. 5 Effect of gonadectomy on thymic weight in female (a) and male (b) C57BL/6 mice. Thymic weight was assessed 2 months after gonadectomy. Open columns, sham operation (Cont). Grey columns, gonadectomy (Gx). (c) Ratio of gonadectomized to control mice (Gx/Cont ratio). The magnitude of increase in thymic weight after Gx is more prominent in males than that in females, and thymic weight tends to increase with age

reversed, and the thymus can be induced to regrow to a larger size by the removal of testes or ovaries (Fig. 5a, Fig. 5b) [29–32]. It is important to note that the extent of thymic restoration after gonadectomy in our study was gender- and age-dependent. The size of the restored thymus was considerably larger in males than in females and in older mice than in younger mice (Fig. 5c). The restoration of thymic size after gonadectomy is temporary and is observed for several weeks. It differs from the long-term thymic hyperplasia observed after AHTL. Thymic restoration after gonadectomy may be simply due to the decreased suppressive effect of sex steroids on lymphocytes [30]. The decrease in the serum levels of sex steroids stimulates the hypothalamus-pituitary axis through negative feedback to secrete hormones capable of restoring thymic size and cellularity. This concept has been supported by the fact that thymic hyperplasia after gonadectomy does not occur in hypophysectomized rats [31].

4   Neuroimmune Interaction at the Time of Infection [33]

Overwhelming evidence suggests that various cytokines and their receptors are present in the brain and influence its functions. It was previously thought that large molecules such as cytokines are prevented from entering the brain by the blood-brain-barrier (BBB). However, it has been clearly shown that recombinant IL-2 injected into patients can enter the brain through areas where the BBB is weak, and exert a neuromodulatory effect [34].

Lipopolysaccharide (LPS) is known to trigger an acute-phase response and the synthesis of proinflammatory cytokines. LPS injection in experimental animals induces various neurological manifestations and physiological changes such as fever, hypotension, and the secretion of variable hormones and is therefore used to develop infection models.

During an infection, cytokines are mainly produced in the immune system and partly, to some extent, in the brain. Therefore, it is quite likely that cytokines produced in the immune system might influence the neurological and physiological functions of the brain.

It is interesting to note that the mRNA level of various cytokine receptors was found to be increased in the spleen of young mice but not old mice. A similar enhancement in the levels of cytokine receptor mRNA was also observed in the brain of mice after LPS stimulation, but the magnitude of this increase varied according to the type of cytokine receptor, the brain region, and the age of the mice [33].

Fig. 6 indicates the mRNA expression level of various cytokine receptors in the cerebral cortex after LPS injection in mice. In young mice, the mRNA levels of IL-1R1, IL-2Ra, IL-3R, and IL-6R peaked at 3 or 6 h after LPS injection. In old mice, the expression of IL-1R1 and IL-3R was delayed, definitely lower in IL-2Ra, and almost similar in IL-6R. However, the mRNA expression level of tumor necrosis factor (TNF)αR and interferon (IFN)γR was higher in the old mice than in the young mice.

In any event, cytokines produced by immune cells might directly or indirectly influence brain function through the various cytokine receptors expressed in the brain. Moreover, the interaction between the immune system and the brain during

Fig. 6 Changes in the mRNA level of various cytokine receptors in the frontal cortex of mice after lipopolysaccharide (LPS) injection (30 mg/mouse) The type of cytokine receptor is indicated in the upper right-hand corner of each graph. Open circles with solid line, young mice. Open circles with dotted line, old mice. Each point, average of 3 samples. Vertical bars, standard error of the mean. Ordinate, the ratio of the mRNA level after LPS injection to that before the injection

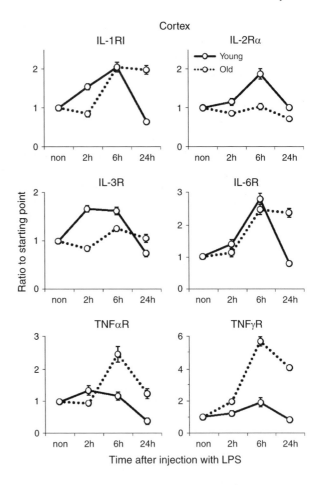

an infection is expected to be different in young and old mice because cytokine production changes with age as does the expression of cytokine receptors in the brain [35]. It is interesting to note that the mRNA levels of some cytokine receptors in old mice were higher than that in young mice after LPS stimulation. In other words, the neuroimmune interactions are subject to change with advancing age, and these changes could be responsible for the fact that the elderly are vulnerable to various physiological disorders during an infection.

5   Conclusion

All environmental stimuli including infection eventually reach the hypothalamus and influence its function. The hypothalamus has many centers, which are essential for the maintenance of the life. An important hypothalamic function is the control of the neuroendocrine-immune network. Therefore, all environmental stimuli are processed by the neuroendocrine-immune network. When the stimuli exceed the normal physiological range, the neuroendocrine-immune network plays a major role in the maintenance of the internal environment, which is known as homeostasis. With aging, however, the activity of the 3 systems, i.e., the nervous, endocrine, and immune systems, decline and so does the homeostatic capacity of the neuroendocrine-immune network. This chapter has shown several examples of age-related changes observed in the neuroendocrine-immune network at both the cellular as well as the organellar level. 1) The mRNA expression levels of hormone and neurotransmitter receptors in T-cells changes with age. 2) The destruction of the anterior portion of the hypothalamus causes thymic hyperplasia, and the extent of this hyperplasia varies with the age of the animal,. 3) Thymic involution is controlled by the hypothalamus. 4) Gonadectomy has a serious influence on thymic weight, and its effect varies with gender and age. 5) An intravenous injection of LPS induces an elevation in the mRNA levels of the receptors of various cytokines in the brain. The extent of this elevation varies with age and the brain region investigated. These findings indicate that the homeostatic control of the neuroendocrine-immune network is more efficient in young than in old individuals.

References

1. Hirokawa K, Utsuyama M, Makinodan T (2006). Immunity and aging. In: Pathy MSJ, Sinclair AJ, Morley JE (eds).Principles and practice of geriatric medicine. pp 19–36. John Wiley & Son
2. Kandel ER, Schwarz JH, Jessell TM (1991) Principles of neural science, Prentice-Hall International Inc
3. Downing JE, Miyan JA (2000) Neural immunoregulation: emerging roles for nerves in immune homeostasis and disease. Immunol Today 21:281–289
4. Blalock JE (2005) The immune system as the 6th sense. J Intern Med 257:126–138
5. Cotman CW, Brinton RE, Galaburda A, MeEwen B, Schneider DM (1985) The neuroimmune endocrine connection. Raven Press. pp1–150
6. Fabris N, Pierpaolii W, Sorkin E (1972) Lymphocytes, hormones, and ageing. Nature 240:557–559
7. Pierpaoli W, Sorkin E (1969) A study on antipituitary serum. Immunology 16:311–318
8. Kelly KW, Brief, S, Westly HJ, Novakofski J, Bechtel PJ, Simon J, Walker EB (1986) GH3 pituitary adenoma cells can reverse thymic aging in rats. Proc Natl Acad Sci U S A 83: 5663–5667
9. Savino W, de Mello-Coelho V, Dardenne M (1995) Control of thymic microenvironment by growth hormone/insulin-like growth factor I-mediated circuits. Neuroimmunumodulataion 2:313–318
10. Isakovic K, Jankovic BD (1973) Neuro-endocrine correlates of immune response. II. Changes in the lymphatic organs of brain-lesioned rats. Int Arch Allergy Immunol 45:373–384
11. Cross RJ, Markesbery WR, Brooks WH, Roszman TL (1984) Hypothalamic-immune interactions: neuromodulation of natural killer activity by lesioning of the anterior hypothalamus. Immunology 51:399–405
12. Frohman LA, Bernardis LL (1968) Growth hormone and insulin levels in weaning rats with ventromedial hypothalamic lesions. J Endocrinol 82:1125–1132

13. Paxinos G, Watson C (1986) In: The brain in stereotaxic coordinates. 2nd ed, Acad Press, Sydney
14. Utsuyama M, Kobayashi S, Hirokawa K (1997) Induction of thymic hyperplasia and suppression of splenic T cells by lesioning of anterior hypothalamus in Wistar rats. J Neuroimmunol 77:174–180
15. de Zegher F, Devlieger H, Eggermont E, Veldhuis JD (1993) Of growth hormone and prolactin hypersecretion by the human infant on the day of birth. J Clin Endocrinol Metab 76:1177–1181
16. Veldhuis JD, Bowers CY (2003) Human GH pulsatility : an ensemble property regulated by age and gender. J Endocrinol Invest 26:799–813
17. Florio T, Ventra C, Postiglione A, Schettini G (1991) Age-related alterations of somatostatin gene expression in different rat brain areas. Brain Res 557:64–68
18. Reed DK, Korytko AL, Hipkin R, Wehrenberg WB, Schonbrunn A, Cuttler L (1999) Pituitary somatostatin receptor (sst) 1-5 expression during rat development: Age-dependent expression of sst2. Endocrinology 140:4739–4744
19. Giustina A, Veldhuis JD (1998) Pathophysiology of the neuroregulation of growth hormone secretion in experimental animals and the human. Endocr Rev 19:717–797
20. Felten DL, Felten SY, Carlson SL, Olschowka JA, Livnat S (1985) Noradrenergic and peptidergic innervation of lymphoid tissue. J Immunol 135:S755–S765
21. Miles K, Chelmicka-Schorr E, Atweh S, Otten G, Amson BG (1985) Sympathetic ablation alters lymphocyte membrane properties. J Immunol 135:S797–S801
22. Besedovsky HO, del Rey A., Sorkin E, Da Prada M, Keller HH (1979) Immunoregulation mediated by the sympathetic nervous system. Cell Immunol 48:346–355
23. Munck A, Naray-Fejes-Toth A, Guyre PM (1987) Mechanism of glucocorticoid actions on the immune system. In: Berczi I and Kovacs K (eds) Hormones and Immunity pp.20–37
24. Ishiyama N, Kitagawa M, Kina I, Hirokawa K (1998) Expression of truncated VCAM-1 in thymocytes and its role during the process of apoptosis. Pathobiology 66:274–283
25. Hirokawa K, Sato K,, Makinodan T (1982) Influence of age of thymic graft on the differentiation of T cells in nude mice. Clin Immunol Immunop 24:251–262
26. Kruger TE, Smith LR, Harbour DV,, Blalock JE (1989) Thyrotropin: an endogenous regulator of the in vitro immune response. J Immunol 142:744–747
27. Grossman CJ (1985) Interaction between the gonadal steroids and the immune system. Science 227:255–261
28. Hirokawa K, Okayasu I, Hatakeyama S (1979) Effect of pregnancy and its related hormones on the in vitro proliferation of spleen cells. Acta Pathol Japon 29:837–844
29. Brunelli, R, Frasca D, Fattorossi A, Spano M, Baschieri S, D'Amelio R, Zichella L, Doria G (1991) Thymus regeneration induced by gonadectomy in old mice. Characterization of T cell phenotype and mitotic responsiveness. J Immunol Res 3:62–68
30. Greenstein BD, Fitzpatrick FTA, Adcock IM, Kendall MD, Wheeler MJJ (1986) Reappearance of the thymus in old rats after orchidectomy: Inhibition of regeneration by testosterone. J Endocrinol 110:417–422
31. Utsuyama M, Hirokawa K (1989) Hypertrophy of the thymus and restoration of immune functions in mice rats by gonadectomy. Mech Ageing Dev 47:175–185
32. Utsuyama M, Hirokawa K, Mancini C, Brunelli R, Leter G, Doria G (1995) Differential effects of gonadectomy on thymic stromal cells in promoting T cell differentiation in mice. Mech Ageing Dev 81:107–117
33. Utsuyama M, Hirokawa K (2002) Differential expression of various cytokine receptors in the brain after stimulation with LPS in young and old mice. Exp Gerontol 37: 411–420
34. Nistico G, De Sarro G (1991) Is interleukin 2 a neuromodulator in the brain. Trends Neurosci 14:146–150
35. Godbout JP, Johnson RW (2004) Interleukin-6 in the aging brain. J Neuroimmunol 147:141–144

Sex Hormones and Immunosenescence

Christian R. Gomez, Vanessa Nomellini and Elizabeth J. Kovacs

Contents

E. J. Kovacs (✉) · C. R. Gomez · V. Nomellini
Loyola University Medical Center
Bldg. 110, Room 4232
2160 South First Avenue
Maywood, IL 60153, USA
Phone: 708.327.2477
Fax: 708.327.2813
E-mail: ekovacs@lumc.edu

C. R. Gomez
Facultad de Ciencias de la Salud
Universidad Diego Portales
Ejército 141, Santiago, Chile

T. Fulop et al. (eds.), *Handbook on Immunosenescence,*
DOI 10.1007/ 978-1-4020-9062-2_42, © Springer Science+Business Media B.V. 2009

Abstract: Sex hormones impact a number of aspects of immunity. As a result of the aging process, dramatic changes occur in the endocrine system, including the levels of sex hormones. Thus, it is possible that the hormonal environment may play a role in the effects of aging on normal aspects of the aging immune system, as well as in immune responses to injury and infection. Although much has been discovered regarding age-related changes in the immune and the endocrine systems, the exact mechanism of the interplay between these factors has yet to be resolved. In this chapter, we explore each of these areas and investigate how sex hormones may be an important component to immunosenescence. Finally, both beneficial and adverse effects of hormone replacement therapy on the aging process are discussed. As age and gender are potential modifiers of the disease process, therapies targeted to the specific hormonal and immune status of an individual may prove to be most beneficial for optimal clinical outcomes.

1   Introduction

In studying human longevity, two observations clearly stand out: first, the highest increase in life expectancy recorded in history has occurred in the past century and [186], second, the average lifespan of women is almost 10% higher than men [227]. The fact that this sex difference occurs not only in humans but also in many mammalian species suggests that the hormonal environment plays a role in the aging process.

Among the prominent effects of sex on aging is the response of the immune system. While not as dramatic as the role that sex steroids (estrogens and androgens) play in sexual differentiation and reproduction [188, 248], their effects in immune function have been well documented [48, 188, 248]. Overall, females exhibit stronger humoral and cell-mediated immune responses than males [248]. For example, females in their reproductive years have higher plasma levels of immmonoglobulins (Ig), such as IgM and IgG, and mount more vigorous antibody responses than males after immunization or infection [reviewed in [10]]. Females also exhibit a more rapid allograft rejection compared to males [93]. As a result of this heightened immunity, females also have an increased susceptibility to various autoimmune diseases. Additionally, female to male incidence of developing of rheumatoid arthritis is 2–4:1, 5–13:1 for systemic lupus erythematosus and 25–50:1 for Hashimoto thyroiditis [10]. There are also sex differences in the response to injury [9, 96]. Among those sustaining most types of traumatic injury, male patients show increased mortality compared with female patients [82]. In addition, females have significantly higher infection and sepsis survival rates [33, 188, 215], and a lower risk for postinjury pneumonia [80]. Interestingly, unlike other forms of traumatic injury, females have greater mortality following burn injury than males [127]. This may be sex hormone mediated during reproductive years, but since it occurs over most of the life span, from ages 10–70 [127], factors other than sex hormones alone are likely to be involved.

While chromosomal effects may explain some of the sex differences in immunity, the hormonal environment seems to have the greatest influence [10]. As part of the normal aging process, changes occur in both the immune and endocrine systems. Since the endocrine system is an important component in the regulation of the immune system, it is possible that a more complex interplay between these two systems exists. Understanding the consequences of aging on immunity is further complicated by genetic background, mutations, oxidative damage, etc. [232]. In this chapter, we will first describe how sex hormones modulate the immune response. Next, we will examine how the endocrine system changes with age, focusing on the sex hormones. We will then describe specific manifestations of immunosenescence from a perspective involving age-associated changes in sex hormones. Finally, the therapeutic and adverse effects of sex hormone replacement on the aging process and on specific aspects of immunosenescence will be discussed. Although progress has been made with regard to the effects of age on the immune system and the endocrine system, the exact mechanism of the interaction between these systems in the elderly has yet to be resolved. In this review, we will explore each of these areas and investigate how sex hormones may be an important component of immunosenescence.

2   The Effects of Sex Hormones on the Immune Response

During reproductive years, females have a more robust humoral and cellular immune response compared to males [98]. Depending on the concentration of estrogen, it can either be immunostimulatory or immonosuppresive. *See* Figure 1 for the biosynthetic pathway of the sex hormones. At levels seen over the menstrual cycle (in particular proestrous levels of estrogen) boost immunity. However, in pregnancy higher levels of estrogen are immunosupresive [41, 233]. In contrast to estrogen, all concentrations of testosterone are though to be immunosupresive [35, 177]. Sex hormones modulate immune cell responses through direct and indirect actions on a series of targets, including lymphoid organs, T cells, B cells, natural killer (NK) cells, and macrophages. For instance, the number of $CD4^+$ lymphocytes is higher in females [178] and thymocytes and lymphocytes from female mice respond more vigorously to antigens than those from males [255]. In addition, the production of cytokines, such as interleukin (IL)-1β was higher in macrophages from females after in vitro stimulation [106]. In addition, the production of IL-4 [60] and interferon-gamma (IFN-γ) [214] was higher in splenocytes from females compared to males. Sex hormones also influence the immune system through their actions on the central nervous system, bones, endocrine organs, and nonlymphoid tissues (liver, kidney, complement producing cells, and mucosal epithelial cells) [48].

The immunomodulatory role of estrogen, particularly on lymphopoiesis and immune responses have been studied extensively (reviewed in [147, 233]). Periovulatory levels of estradiol have been shown to stimulate antibody production by

B cells [50, 76, 172, 190]. However, this increases the potential for autoimmune diseases [2, 182, 247]. In contrast, peri-ovulatory estradiol levels led to a suppression of B cell lineage precursors [111, 165]. Pregnancy levels of estrogen, on the other hand, suppressed the T cell-mediated delayed-type hypersensitivity (DTH) reaction [43, 64, 95] and inhibited the release of tumor necrosis factor-α (TNF-α). These high levels of estrogen also stimulated T cell-induced IL-4, IL-10, and IFN-γ secretion [123, 211]. In macrophages, late pregnancy levels of estrogen inhibited LPS-stimulated IL-6 secretion [56, 112] and TNF-α release [239, 268]. In addition, secreted IL-1β levels were increased at peri-ovulatory levels, but inhibited at high pregnancy levels [201, 221]. This biphasic effect of estrogen is especially relevant when considering proinflammatory diseases in pre and postmenopausal women, as will be discussed later.

Progesterone is a major gonadal hormone synthesized primarily by the corpus luteum, the testes, and the adrenal cortex [217]. Besides its well-known endocrine and neuroprotective effects [217], progesterone has been suggested to have an immunosuppressive role. This is thought to play a protective role in pregnancy [229]. The regulatory effects of progesterone on the immune system include blocking cytotoxic T cell activity [159], reducing NK cell activity [102], and modifying the cytokine response [46, 197, 198].

Testosterone also has many immunomodulatory roles [35, 177]. T cell apoptosis is decreased in males compared to females, as reflected in the decreased numbers in the periphery of men [164]. In B cells, testosterone inhibited IgG and IgM secretion [121]. In contrast, endotoxin-stimulated monocytes from males produced more TNF-α than females [14, 34, 218]. Whether this response to endotoxin is due to increased testosterone concentrations remains uncertain, though, since in vitro studies have not shown an effect of testosterone on TNF-α production [202]. In vivo and in vitro analysis of immune-endocrine interactions, including manipulation of testosterone levels through castration, have elucidated the differences between males and females in terms of immunocompetence [177]. These differential roles of sex hormones on the immune system have been proposed to be main determinants of male versus female responses to injury and infection. As a result of the aging process, dramatic changes occur in the endocrine system, including the sex hormones. Thus, it is possible that the hormonal environment may play a role in the effects of aging on the immune system.

3   Endocrine Changes with Aging

3.1   Overall Changes

As a normal part of aging, hormonal changes occur resulting from a decline in secretion of hormones and/or availability of target cells. Perhaps the most characterized hormone changes with age are the decline in secretion of estrogen in the ovaries (menopause) and testosterone in the testes (andropause) (all of the following hormonal changes with age are reviewed in [13, 44, 146]). As a result, the levels of luteinizing hormone (LH) and follicle-stimulating hormone (FSH) released by the pituitary gland are elevated, due to the lack of negative feedback by the gonadal hormones. Changes in the sex hormone environment occurring as a result of advanced age are summarized in Table 1. Other changes in the endocrine system seen with age include a decreased release of growth hormone causing a diminished production of insulin-like growth factor-1 (IGF-1) by the liver and other organs (somatopause) and a diminished production of the sex hormone precursor, dehydroepiandrosterone (DHEA) by the adrenal cortex (adrenopause). Altogether, both central (hypothalamic and pituitary) and peripheral (ovarian, testicular, and adrenal) components of the endocrine system are affected over time and have thus been linked with the aging process [146].

Table 1 Sex hormone environment in advanced age

Factor	Females	References	Males	References
Tropic hormones				
FSH	↑	[116, 223]	↑	[171]
LH	↑	[116, 223]	↑	[171]
Sex hormones				
Pregnenolone	↓	[103]	↓	[103, 174]
Estradiol	↓↓	[92, 107, 156,180]	↓	[73, 100, 242]
Progesterone	↓	[79, 107, 223, 228]	no change or ↓	[29, 187]
Testosterone	↓	[54, 145]	↓	[36, 61, 120, 166, 252]
DHT	↓	[145, 224]	no change or ↓↑	[52, 70, 94, 246]
Androsterodione	↓	[94]	↓	[94]
DHEA (S)	↓	[94, 124, 149, 189]	↓	[94, 124, 149, 189]
Sex hormone receptors				
Estrogen receptors	tissue specific	[37, 114, 222, 258]	↓	[222]
Progesterone receptors	tissue specific	[37, 45, 78, 226]	tissue specific	[37, 45, 78, 225]
Androgen receptor	↓	[238]	↓	[210, 261, 270]
Others				
SHBG	no change or ↓↑	[40, 54, 161]	↑	[241, 242]
Aromatase	↑	[109, 110, 204]	↑	[109, 241]
5 α-reductase			↓	[241]

Arrows indicate increase or decrease in aged subject relative to young. FSH follicle stimulating hormone, LH luteinizing hormone, DHT dihydrotestosterone, DHEA (S) dehydroepiandrosterone (sulfate), SHBG sex hormone binding globulin.

4 Menopause and Andropause

In women, the average onset of menopause is 51 years of age, and results in a postreproductive period that encompasses nearly a third of their lives [116]. For most women, menopause is accompanied by vasomotor symptoms, depressed mood, changes in body composition (such as increased body fat), and an elevated risk of coronary heart disease, myocardial infarction, and stroke [116]. The use of animal models has helped to uncover some of the mechanisms involved in reproductive aging like humans, female primates exhibit hormone cyclicity in that extensive menstrual bleeding and shedding of the endometrial lining occur similar to humans [260]. However, utilization of humans and nonhuman primates for experimentation purposes involves a series of complications, including their extended lifespan and excessive research cost [260]. As an alternative, rodent models have been used. The estrous cycle in female rodents can be divided into four stages: proestrus, estrus, metestrus, and diestrus, with ovulation normally occurring during estrus [148]. In female mice, advanced age correlates with progressively longer estrous cycles, characterized by lower levels of estrogen [181]. Eventually, this decline in estrogen leads to the absence of ovarian follicle development and low plasma estrogen and progesterone concentrations [181]. The effect of aging on the estrous cycle in female rats is different from mice, in that they have well defined estrous cycles [157]. However, irregular cycles emerge at middle age, in which ovulatory activity occurs at longer intervals. This period is chronologically followed either by constant estrus, irregular pseudopregnancies, and anestrus [72, 157]. Overall, the decline in ovarian function differs between rats and mice, as well as between strains, and may occur between 6 and 18 months of age, or even up to 24 months for some strains [72].

Andropause, on the other hand, is defined as the progressive decline (0.8–2% each year) in testosterone levels, beginning at middle-age [175]. Unlike women, men do not have a universally recognized "syndrome of andropause," as the decline occurs more gradually [195]. The clinical features associated with andropause include increased body fat, loss of muscle and bone mass, fatigue, depression, anemia, poor libido, erectile dysfunction, insulin resistance, and a higher risk of cardiovascular disease [124]. Andropause is also present in male rodents; however this is strain dependent in both mice [36, 61] and rats [120, 166, 252].

5 Specific Changes in Sex Hormones with Age

5.1 Pregnenolone

Pregnenolone is the precursor of all known steroid hormones [194]. In humans maximum serum pregnenolone levels are achieved between 25 and 30 years of age in both men and women [103]. After this time, women exhibit a gradual decline

[103], while men maintain constant levels up to approximately 52 years of age, followed by a continuous decrease [103, 174]. Since circulating pregnenolone is mostly, if not entirely, of adrenal origin [103], these results have raised the question of the contribution of the adrenal glands to the defective production of sex steroids during aging [103].

5.2 *Estradiol*

The most dramatic change with the onset of menopause in women is an abrupt decrease in circulating estradiol. By perimenopause, serum estrogen concentrations decline, FSH concentrations become augmented to levels higher than in younger women, but LH does not change [223]. Eventually, follicular activity ceases, estrogen concentrations fall, and LH and FSH rise above premenopausal levels [116]. After menopause, however, small quantities of estrone—an estradiol precursor synthesized from androsterodione in the cortex of the adrenal gland and in interstitial ovarian cells—are converted to estradiol (Fig. 1). Thus, estradiol is still present, but the normal cycling levels seen prior to menopause are replaced

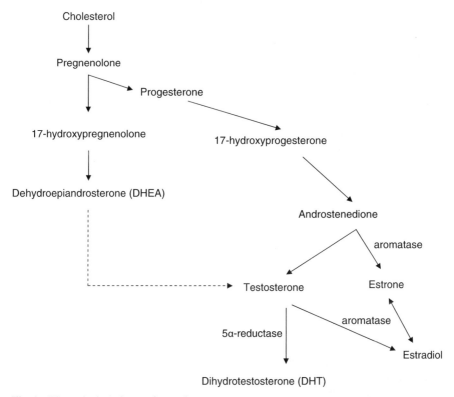

Fig. 1 Biosynthetic pathways for sex hormones

by levels that are much lower and do not fluctuate [156]. Similarly, during the period of lengthening cycles in female mice, a fall in circulating levels of estradiol can be measured [180]. In the phase of persistent diestrus, low plasma levels of estradiol were observed in conjunction with follicle-depleted ovaries [92], suggesting that ovarian aging in mice also contributes to the reproductive defect in estradiol production. Aged female rats, however, produced levels of estradiol at constant estrous levels, which are comparable to that of animals with regular cycles [107]. Since the ovaries of aged rats are capable of normal function under appropriate gonadotrophic stimulation, it has been hypothesized that altered hypothalamo–pituitary function is a major cause for cessation of regular estrous cycle in the female rat [107].

Estrogens in males, predominantly produced by peripheral aromatization of testicular and adrenal androgens, have diverse roles including spermatogenesis [185], sexual behavior [185], and development and maintenance of the skeleton [244]. As in women, serum concentrations of estradiol decrease in men [73]. This decrease in males has been attributed to a decline in free estradiol, or that which is unbound to sex hormone-binding globulin (SHBG)—the carrier protein used by estradiol and testosterone in the serum. Levels of the SHBG-bound fraction of estradiol, in contrast, increase with age [242]. With this estradiol reduction in men, a more pronounced decline in estrone is also observed [242]. Studies in rodents, on the other hand, have shown interesting results. Aged male Fisher 344 rats, which frequently have Leydig cell hyperplasia or develop testicular Leydig cell tumors, had augmented levels of estradiol, mainly at the testicular level [99]. On the contrary, male Brown Norway rats exhibited decreased circulating levels of estradiol with age, and orchidectomy produced a progressive decline in FSH and LH [100]. These findings suggest that aged male Brown Norway rats experience both primary and secondary testicular failure. Therefore, this strain is likely a better rat model for studying male reproductive aging, compared to Fisher 344 rats.

5.3   Estrogen Receptors

Estrogen receptor (ER)α and ERβ belong to the steroid/thyroid hormone superfamily of nuclear receptors [183]. These receptors are expressed in a variety of immune cells, including T cells and macrophages [233]. The decline in circulating estrogen associated with advanced age may also differentially modulate ER levels in males and females. ERα mRNA and protein levels were decreased and ERβ was virtually absent in uteri from aged mice [222]. Similarly, sex, age, and region-dependent expression of ERα and ERβ were found in rat brains [37,258]. However, ERα decreased in kidneys from aged males, but was augmented in those from aged females; ERβ, was not expressed in kidney [222]. The gender effects in the expression of ERs may contribute to sex specific pathology in the elderly [233].

5.4   Progesterone

In 30–49 year old women with normal cycles, progesterone levels are lower than those of younger females at the last stage of the estrus cycle [79]. This decrease seems to be more accentuated during the menopausal transition [79, 223, 228]. Similar to humans, middle-aged female rats experienced a reduction in the levels of progesterone compared to young rats [259]. In contrast, serum progesterone was much higher in aged Long-Evans female rats during the pseudopregnancy phase than in rats experiencing constant estrous or anestrous [107]. Thus, as discussed earlier in the context of estradiol, strain differences must be taken into account when trying to compare the altered rat hypothalamic–pituitary–gonadal axis of aging with that of humans.

Outside of the luteal phase in females, healthy adult men and women do not show significant differences in serum levels of progesterone [187] In two independent studies, no variation in serum progesterone was found with age in males [29, 187]. However, in one study, a progesterone derivative,17-hydroxyprogesterone (which is derived from progesterone via 17-hydroxylase, or from 17-hydroxypregnenolone) was significantly reduced with age [29]. Since most of the 17-hydroxyprogesterone in the male is synthesized in the testis, it has been hypothesized that this decrease probably may reflect a decrease in Leydig cell function [29].

5.5   Progesterone Receptors

The biological effects of progesterone are mediated through the progesterone receptor (PR), which has two isoforms (PR-A and PR-B) [217]. The changes in progesterone levels are associated with age and affect the number, activity, and distribution of PRs. In mammary glands, greater expression of PR was found with advanced age in 30–40-week-old ovariectomized mice in response to estradiol, compared to younger females. Similarly, aged (40-week-old) mice, relative to their younger (10 and 20 weeks old) counterparts, had higher expression of PR [226]. PR expression, on the other hand, was decreased in the rat penis and was linked to erectile dysfunction [225]. There appeared to be no global or marked decline in brain PR with age [37, 45, 78]. Overall, these results indicate that the effects of advanced age on PR expression are determined in a tissue specific manner.

5.6   Testosterone

As a result of abnormalities in the hypothalamic–pituitary–testicular axis during andropause, serum LH and FSH levels increase with age [171]. However, serum LH concentrations often do not parallel the decline in testosterone [171], as a result of impaired gonadotrophin-releasing hormone secretion and alterations in gonadal steroid feedback mechanisms [245]. In fact, since testosterone is synthesized from estradiol, decreases in total serum levels of testosterone observed in aged men have been explained by a reduction in the circulating levels of free (unbound) estradiol [242]. As noted earlier, some strains of male rodents also experience a decline in serum testosterone. For example, aged CBF1 male mice had decreased levels of testosterone, which was associated with reduced LH, but not FSH, relative to young animals [36]. In contrast, DBA/2J mice showed comparable levels of testosterone at all ages, while C57BL/6J male mice had a very slow rate of decline [61]. Similarly, many aged male rats exhibit a significant decrease in testosterone when compared to younger animals [120, 166, 252].

The mechanisms involved in the age-related decline in serum testosterone of males include primary structural gonadal impairment, degenerative modifications of the pituitary gland, and deficits of the neuro-hypothalamic system. In addition, alteration of peripheral components of the testosterone axis has been found, such as an increase in SHBG and aromatase [109, 241] (which causes the bioconversion of testosterone to estrogens), and a decrease in 5-α-reductase (which converts dihydrotestosterone (DHT) to the active form of testosterone) [241]. Unlike testosterone, DHT cannot be aromatized into estradiol. While these age-related observations are important, it is also crucial to consider the effect of other factors, such as genetics, chronic diseases, medications, obesity, alcohol consumption, smoking, diet, and stress [241].

Irrespective of age, androgens play an important role in women. In fact, female androgen insufficiency can lead to symptoms including fatigue, diminished sense of well-being, decreased libido, and reduction in bone mass, muscle strength, and memory [23]. A decline in total and free testosterone with age has been reported in women [54, 145]. However, reports are inconsistent regarding the levels of SHBG and the effect on testosterone levels in aged women [40, 161]. Using a larger number of subjects, no variation in SHBG with age was reported [54]. However, a more consistent increase in aromatase has been described [109, 110, 204]. The decline in testosterone in women is more pronounced in the early reproductive years, plateaus in midlife, and tends to increase slightly in the later years [54] In contrast, with the sharp decline in estradiol that occurs with menopause an effect on circulating testosterone may not be observed at this time [54].

5.7   Other Androgens

Aside from testosterone, additional androgens, including DHT, androstenedione, DHEA and its sulfated form (DHEAS), may be affected with increasing age. Nevertheless, information regarding age-associated changes of serum DHT in aging men is conflicting. Some have reported increases [70], while others have found no

changes [94, 246] or even decreases in serum levels of DHT [52]. Plasma androstenedione levels decline with age, both in males and in females [94]. Plasma levels
of DHEA and DHEAS, secreted mostly by the adrenal glands, are also reduced
in both males and females [94, 124, 189]. DHEAS peaked at 20–24 years in men
and at 15–19 years in women, then declined steadily in both sexes, though the levels were significantly higher in men than women at ages from 20 to 69 years old
[189]. In general, women show a more pronounced androgen decline in their early
reproductive years, and a plateau in midlife [54]. Menopause does not produce an
abrupt decline in androgens, as it does with estradiol.

5.8   Androgen receptors

The androgen receptor (AR) is a member of the steroid nuclear receptor superfamily
that is activated by testosterone and its derivatives [24]. To date, only one AR gene
has been identified in humans [158]. AR is mainly expressed in androgen target tissues, such as the prostate, skeletal muscle, the liver, and the central nervous system
(CNS). The highest expression levels are observed in the prostate, adrenal gland,
and epididymis [124]. It has been reported that aging is accompanied by a decrease
in AR concentration in different tissues from men [210] and rodents [31, 205]. In
support of the notion that decreased AR is biologically relevant, a CAG-repeat polymorphism of the AR that causes decreased androgen sensitivity has been associated
with reduced bone mineral density in men aged 20–50 years [270] and impaired
cognitive function in men as they age [261]. The amount of AR declined in the brain
cortex of mice of both sexes with advanced age [238]. However, the relative level
of AR phosphorylation was significantly higher in aged compared to adult, as well
as female relative to male, mice [238]. The significance of differences in the levels
of phosphorylation is not clearly understood, but it has been proposed that it might
lead to a transformation of AR into a tight nuclear binding form, which is required
for downstream hormone activity [238].

6   Changes in Sex Hormones Contribute to Immunosenescence
During Normal Aging

6.1   Sex Hormones and the Age-Associated Increase
in Circulating IL-6

The well described chronic proinflammatory state in aged individuals without
underlying disease [25, 38, 68, 75, 213], is characterized in part by circulating
levels of interleukin-6 (IL-6) [65-67]. This age-related increase of IL-6 in serum

begins as early as 30–40 years of age and is more prominent among men [265]. Population studies have identified serum IL-6 levels as a reliable predictor of disability among the elderly [74]. Genetic studies indicated that those who are predisposed to produce low levels of IL-6 during aging—for example, men positive for the polymorphic variant at the 174 C/G locus—appeared to have extended longevity [32]. Moreover, these same investigations indicated that later in life, women experience higher serum IL-6 levels compared to men, in a 174 C/G locus–independent manner [32]. These results suggest that genetics influence longevity in men more than in women. It is possible that environmental factors play a greater role in determining longevity in women or that genetic factors may become prominent later in their life [32].

The increase in circulating IL-6 associated with age can be explained, in part, by the decline in sex hormones, as has been suggested for estrogen, testosterone, and DHEA [231]. In vitro studies using cells obtained from humans and rodents showed that spontaneous increases in the expression and secretion of IL-6 and other proinflammatory cytokines (IL-1 and TNF-α) occurred in macrophages as a result of estrogen deficiency produced by natural [30, 191] or surgical menopause [115, 130, 133, 192, 193], or after discontinuation of estrogen replacement [30, 192]. In vivo cytokine increases, as a consequence of estrogen deficiency, have been more difficult to demonstrate because of technical limitations [196], but similar results to the in vitro observations have been found [42, 87]. In support of these observations, macrophages obtained from ovariectomized mice showed increased expression of components of the IL-6 receptor complex [154]. Since the IL-6 gene lacks the classical estrogen response elements (ERE) in its promoter [203], a mechanism other than direct transcriptional regulation must be present to explain the effects of estrogen on IL-6 production. Perhaps the best described mechanism involves the binding of estrogen-ER/NF-κB dimers to NF-κB binding sites, thereby preventing subsequent transcription [119]. Additionally, exposure to low proestrus levels of estrogen in vivo attenuated the activation of NF-κB in macrophages from young adult mice cultured ex vivo in a model of acute ethanol exposure followed by burn injury [167].

Similar to estrogen deficiency, the age-associated decline in androgens may also upregulate proinflammatory cytokines [196]. Testoterone deficiency induced IL-6 mRNA and protein synthesis in bone marrow cells obtained from young mice after orchidectomy [267]. In vitro, testosterone reduced IL-6 production in macrophages [121], osteoblasts [105], synoviocytes [150] and cell lines [125].

An inverse correlation has also been described for plasma DHEA and circulating IL-6 with age [113, 230]. After in vivo hormone supplementation with DHEA and DHEAS, circulating concentrations of IL-6 [55] and TNF-α were inhibited [131]. The effects of low levels of DHEA on IL-6 production have been observed in splenocytes [113, 128], monocytes [230] and macrophages [132]. However, it has yet to be established whether androgen effects on IL-6, such as testosterone and DHEAS, occur through downstream cell signaling or through indirect mechanisms.

6.2 Sex Hormones and the Age-Related Shift to a Th2 Immune Response

Lymphocytes from aged individuals have decreased proliferation and a decline in production of the Th1 cytokines, IL-2, IFN-γ and IL-12. In contrast, the production of the Th2 cytokines, IL-4, IL-5, IL-6 and IL-10, is increased [81]. These alterations in cytokine secretion produce a shift from a Th1/Th2 balance to a predominantly Th2-phenotype. This, in turn, results in altered immune responses and a higher susceptibility to bacterial and viral infections, as well as to neoplasias [208].

An important contributor to the development of the Th2 phenotype observed in aging is a result of augmented numbers of memory T cells over naive Tcells [169]. When pregnancy and aging were used as variables for different levels of sex hormones, having given birth, parous mice delayed their increase in splenic memory T cells. Also, they augmented the memory/naïve ratio in old mice [27]. In addition, the memory to naïve T cell ratio was lower in aged males [27]. Female mice which have produced offspring exhibited only a slight decrease in circulating IL-2 and an increase in IL-4, IFN-γ, and IL-6 compared with virgin females in association with advanced age [26]. Males, on the other hand, had a smaller decrease in IL-2 during adulthood and lower IFN-γ production with age [26]. From these data, it can be concluded that the onset, magnitude and kinetics of the age-related changes in Th1 and Th2 cytokine production are dependent on the sex hormone status.

6.3 Hormones, Other Major Information Exchange Systems, and Advanced Age

The endocrine, immune, and nervous systems communicate through the release of hormones, cytokines, and neurotransmitters. As aging modifies the functionality of each one of these information exchange systems, it is expected that the interaction between them will also be affected. Straub and collaborators have provided evidence that changes in sex hormones in conjunction with neurotransmitters can contribute to the Th2 shift associated with advanced age [232].

While not a sex hormone, the glucocorticoid cortisol increases the secretion of Th2 cytokines [243, 251] and reduces the production of Th1 cytokines [184, 249, 251]. Similarly, the neurotransmitter, norepinephrine, inhibits the production of Th1 cytokines [62, 71] and augments the levels of Th2 cytokines [62]. However, in contrast with sex hormones, advanced age is associated with a relative increase in cortisol [104, 149] and increased circulating levels of norepinephrine (10–15% per decade over the adult level) [219]. Thus, in addition to sex hormones, imbalances in neurotransmitters can further shift aged individuals towards a Th2 phenotype, perpetuating the defects associated with aging, such as autoimmune

Table 2 Involvement of sex hormones in the manifestation of some aberrant immune responses in advanced age

Condition	References
Normal aging	
Onset of IL-6 increase	[30, 42, 87, 105, 113, 115, 121, 125, 130, 133, 150, 154, 191–193, 196, 203, 230, 231, 267]
Th2 phenotype	[26, 27, 232]
Immune response after injury	
Trauma-hemorrhage	[9, 82, 83, 117, 118, 168]
Burn injury	[1, 90, 127, 138, 140, 155, 200, 240, 139]
Sepsis	[49, 51, 199]
Dermal wound healing	[15, 19–22, 85, 86, 144, 170, 173, 206, 263]

disease, tumor growth, and acceleration of atherosclerosis. The involvement of sex hormones in the manifestation of the aberrant immune responses in advanced age, during normal aging, is summarized in Table 2.

7 Specific Outcomes of Sex Hormone-Related Changes with Age

Independent of age, epidemiologic evidence indicates that sex is a risk factor for trauma and sepsis [reviewed in [7]]. For example, most injury victims are young males [136]. In addition, a higher incidence of bacteremic infections, as well as increased mortality, has been reported in male trauma patients compared with females [33, 162]. The major insults that result in systemic immune dysregulation and are affected by age and sex hormones are hemorrhagic shock, burn injury, and sepsis. After a review on each of these models, the long term effects of aging and sex hormones on wound healing will be discussed.

7.1 Trauma-Hemorrhage

Clinical and experimental studies demonstrated that age and sex are major determinants in the host response following traumatic injury, shock, and/or infection [9, 83, 168]. Following hemorrhagic trauma, female rodents had increased survival and improved cell-mediated immune responses compared to their male counterparts [3, 7, 135, 266]. Additional studies identified testosterone as mainly responsible for the depressed cell-mediated immune responses in males [4-6, 8, 256, 257] and estrogen in enhancement of cell-mediated immune responses in females [6, 8, 77, 134, 135, 262]. Interestingly, some studies showed a reversal of the pattern observed in the young. As opposed to younger injured animals, aged males exhibited enhanced immune responses following injury, when compared to aged females [82, 117]. In addition, macrophages obtained from young males secreted low levels of IL-1β and IL-6 and higher IL-10 than aged subjects Meanwhile, macrophages from aged males released higher levels of IL-1β and IL-6 and reduced IL-10 [117]. In contrast, macrophages isolated from young females following trauma-hemorrhage had enhanced IL-1β and suppressed IL-10 production. Unlike their aged male counterparts, aged females did not have differences in the production of IL-1β and IL-6, but released higher levels of IL-10 secretion [117]. In other studies, splenocyte responses, such as proliferation and the release of IL-2 and IFN-γ, declined in young males but were enhanced in young females after trauma-hemorrhage [118] These effects were reversed in aged animals [118]. Thus, in the trauma-hemorrhage model, the sexually dimorphic cellular response of macrophages and splenocytes in young males and females is reversed, as sex hormone levels decline with age.

7.2 Burn Injury

After burn injury, there is an enhanced systemic inflammatory response, characterized by higher levels of proinflammatory mediators, and defective immune responses, such as DTH and lymphocyte proliferation [59, 141, 269]. Epidemiological studies in burn patients have demonstrated higher mortality in females relative to males sustaining a similar sized burn injury [84, 127, 163, 209]. Similarly, after a 15% total body surface area (TBSA) burn, decreased survival was observed in female mice relative to males [97]. Interestingly, estrogen levels were significantly higher (10–15 fold over baseline) in females following burn injury [58], whereas concentrations of circulating testosterone were decreased [58, 152, 167] These observations suggest that significantly higher levels of estrogen may lead to an improper cell-mediated immune response. Further support for this idea is seen in experiments which show that proestrus levels of estradiol inhibited IL-6, whereas pregnancy levels of the hormone increased the expression of IL-6 [56, 97, 115, 167] Thus, the disparity in the sex-associated outcome between burn injury and hemorrhagic trauma may most likely be due to changes in circulating hormones present after injury.

Aged humans [127] and rodents show higher mortality following burn injury [137] After a 15% TBSA burn, aged mice had a higher mortality rate than young adult mice [137]. In addition, aged female burn–injured mice showed elevated circulating levels of IL-6 and Th2 cytokine production by lymphocytes, but significant decreased DTH response and Con A-stimulated splenocyte proliferation responses compared to young mice [200]. As low, proestrus levels of estrogen suppressed the production of proinflammatory cytokines [47, 95, 234], our laboratory tested the therapeutic efficacy of estrogen supplementation on the immune response following injury in aged female mice. In our studies, low, proestrus levels of estrogen resulted in a marked improvement in survival over a 10-day period after burn injury [90]. In addition, attenuated serum levels of IL-6 were observed, in conjunction with a partial restoration of the DTH response [140]. A recovery in IFN-γ, but not in IL-4 production, suggested a restoration of the Th1-Th2 shift, as a result of the estrogen treatment [139]. Overall, our results demonstrate that using the immunomodulatory properties of estradiol has beneficial effects in aged, injured subjects.

7.3 Sepsis

Retrospective studies indicate that men have increased morbidity and mortality from sepsis as compared to women [9, 33, 160, 215, 266]. After sepsis-induced cecal ligation and puncture in rodents, splenocytes from septic males exhibited reduced proliferative capacity and decreased production of IL-2 and IL-3, but not in those from female septic mice [266]. In similar studies, higher plasma levels of IL-1β were found in female mice versus male mice after LPS administration, as a model of the inflammatory response provoked during infection [153]. These data suggest that better cellular responses and higher levels of proinflammatory cytokines may contribute to the improved response in females relative to males during sepsis.

Infectious diseases comprise one of the ten major causes of death in the elderly [264]. Moreover, pneumonia, influenza, and complications of bacteremia in this age group are associated with a poor prognosis. Elderly patients hospitalized with *Streptoccocus pneumoniae* infection, had prolonged elevation of circulating proinflammatory cytokines [39], as do aged volunteers given endotoxin [142]. In animal models, aged mice given LPS were approximately six times more sensitive to the lethal toxicity than young mice [237]. In addition, LPS exposure induced higher serum and tissue levels of IL-6, IL-1β and TNF-α in aged mice as compared to young [88, 89, 169, 237].

The effect of age and sex on cytokine production has also been studied in peripheral blood mononuclear cells isolated from young and elderly subjects [199]. After in vitro stimulation with LPS, decreased intracellular levels of TNF-α and IL-6 were detected in monocytes from elderly women, relative to young women [199]. In contrast, monocytes from elderly males showed an elevated number of cells positive for both IL-1β and TNF-α after LPS stimulation [199]. In different analyses, spontaneous production of the chemokine IL-8, was decreased in macrophages obtained from elderly males, as compared to that of aged females [49]. Upon in vitro stimulation with LPS, production of IL-8 by macrophages from elderly males was increased over levels in young males. However, cells from aged females showed no change compared to cells from young donors [49]. The involvement of sex hormones in the response to LPS with aging was further supported by the observation that castrated young male rats exhibited similar macrophage function to aged male rats [51].

7.4 Wound healing

The process of wound healing can be separated into the following overlapping phases: hemostasis, inflammation, proliferation, and resolution [57]. These four phases have been studied in detail and exhibit impairment in association with aging [reviewed in [91]]. The detrimental effects of aging on the healing of acute wounds include a prolonged inflammatory response [18, 235], upregulation of protease activity [17], and reduced extracellular matrix deposition [16].

Elderly men heal more slowly than do elderly women. Interestingly, this is true even when both sexes receive estrogen treatments [19]. Estrogen treatment has been shown to accelerate the rate of acute healing in men, and particularly in elderly women, by reducing the inflammatory response [15]. On the contrary, testosterone significantly delayed acute healing in aged humans, as a result of an increased inflammatory response [21]. This suggests that, besides the alterations in immune status [168, 220], the age-associated decrease in sex hormones [86] may also contribute to sex differences in wound healing in the elderly.

The salutary effect of estrogen in wound healing includes lessened inflammatory cell infiltration [19, 170] and inhibition of the proinflammatory cytokines macrophage migration inhibitory factor (MIF) and TNF-α [22]. In addition, estrogen improved the rate of re-epithelialization [20], promoted angiogenesis [173], and stimulated wound contraction [206].

In elderly men, elevated serum testosterone levels correlated with delayed healing of excisional punch wounds [21]. The use of animal models has allowed us to gain a great deal of information regarding the mechanisms involved in this phenomenon. In mice, systemic administration with the AR antagonist, flutamide, improved wound repair, decreased DNA-binding activity of NF-κB, and lowered the production of TNF-α. In other studies, macrophages isolated from the wound site directly upregulated the proinflammatory cytokines, TNF-α [21] and IL-6 [85] in response to testosterone. This evidence suggests a possible role for the AR in impaired healing and increased wound inflammation [21]. However, careful interpretation of these results is required, as there is conflicting evidence showing both inhibitory and stimulatory effects of testosterone in the production of proinflammatory cytokines in vitro [86]. The participation of sex hormones in the manifestation of the aberrant immune responses in advanced age after injury is summarized in Table 2.

8 Therapeutic Benefits Versus Detrimental Effects of Hormone Replacement Therapies

As discussed in the previous pages, experimental research and observational clinical data have provided evidence for the beneficial effects of hormone replacement therapy (HRT) on the aging process. However, large trials have recently called into question whether the effects of some forms of HRT are truly advantageous, potential hazards and concerns have even been raised. In this section, we will briefly discuss the results of recent HRT trials.

8.1   Estrogen and Progesterone

As noted above there is a vast array of immunomodulatory properties of estrogen and progesterone [217]. Thus, the accumulation of basic and clinical data prompted the development of interventional studies to analyze the therapeutic effects of HRT. Postmenopausal estrogen therapy, alone and in combination with progestin, involves approximately 100 years of research and 75 years of clinical practice [254]. However, for the last few years, evidence has surfaced against the beneficial effects of estrogen replacement [129].

The Heart and Estrogen/Progestin Replacement Study (HERS) compared the effects of conjugated equine estrogens plus medroxyprogesterone acetate on cardiovascular function in 2,763 women with prior coronary disease. The results showed an increase in coronary heart disease in women taking HRT [108]. The Women's Estrogen for Stroke Trial (WEST), a randomized, double-blind, placebo-controlled trial, assessed the effects of estradiol therapy in 664 postmenopausal women (mean age, 71 years) who already had an ischemic stroke or transient ischemic attack. In this study, no benefit of estrogen treatment on cerebral stroke incidence was found and, in fact, an increased risk of fatal stroke was reported [250]. The Women's Health Initiative (WHI), a large, placebo-controlled trial involving more than 16,000 women aimed to study the effects of estrogen therapy alone or combined estrogen plus progestin. Benefits included decreased risks for colorectal cancer, beginning at 3 years, and for hip fracture over time [212]. This study was terminated in 2004 resulting from findings of an increased risk of breast cancer, cardiovascular complications, ischemic stroke, levels of inflammatory biomarkers, and dementia, including Alzheimer's disease (reviewed in [217]). Other studies have indicated that the greatest benefits of estrogen replacement are increased bone density and decreased risks of fractures [129]. Subsequent to these trials, many medical organizations recommend that estrogens should not be used in women over the age of 60 years [217]. Accordingly, the use of estrogen currently is recommended only temporarily for women who undergo surgical or natural premature menopause [129] and for short-term control of hot flashes at the beginning of menopause [69].

As an aftermath of the HERS, WEWT and WHI trials, the recommended dosages of estrogen and estrogen–progestin therapies have markedly decreased since they first were introduced. Data demonstrating that benefits in vasomotor and vulvovaginal symptoms, prevention of bone loss, and protection of the endometrium in association with aging can still be achieved with lower doses than the commonly prescribed ones [254].

8.2   Testosterone

Most of the information regarding the benefits of testosterone replacement therapy has been postulated from studies involving younger hypogonadal patients and animal models [236]. In younger men, the benefit to risk ratio is high. However in aged males, potential risks have not been assessed, so the benefit to risk ratio of testosterone replacement therapy in the aging male is still not known [124].

In older, hypogonadal males, continued testosterone therapy increases muscle mass [124, 129]. In one study, transdermal testosterone was administered to 123 subjects continuously for up to 42 months [253]. Continuous treatment normalized testosterone levels, increased the mean serum estradiol to testosterone ratio, and suppressed mean serum FSH and LH levels [253]. In addition, lean body mass augmented as early as 3 months, while fat mass decreased. These changes were maintained with treatment, but were not accompanied by significant increments in muscle strength [253]. As a caveat, however, this study was neither placebo-controlled nor powered to determine the effects of the treatment on prostate cancer risk.

Testosterone treatment has been shown to improve libido in both males and females [129]. However, information from controlled trials, specifically on sexual function in the elderly, remains scarce [28, 124]. In some small studies, parameters of sexual function in elderly men have been shown to be improved compared with placebo treatment [143, 179]. Nevertheless, a lack of an effect has been reported in trials using the anabolic androgen, oxandrolone [216], an aromatase inhibitor [151], or DHT [143]. Additional studies are needed to accurately make conclusions on the effects of androgen administration on sexual function in elderly men. In many short term studies, testosterone therapy has shown an improved, but rather modest, sexual function in elderly women compared with those on estrogen or placebo [reviewed in [28]]. However, secondary effects, such as supraphysiological and unpredictable levels of testosterone to an adverse lipid profile, have been observed. Thus, androgen replacement to improve sexual function in aged females may not be the best choice of therapy [28].

The effects of testosterone on cardiovascular disease include improvement of cardiovascular efficiency [63], reduced incidence of angina [63], and improved cardiac muscle remodeling and coronary artery vasodilation [122, 126]. However, when the effects of androgen therapy on cardiovascular risks have been analyzed, the findings have generally been unremarkable. This dampens the potential of using androgen therapy to prevent the occurrence or to improve the outcome of cardiovascular diseases in elderly men [124]. In addition, side effects can be seen with long term testosterone treatment using near physiologic doses. Polycythemia is the major side effect [129], but long term administration of testosterone or DHT may also increase the risk of prostatic carcinoma and benign prostatic hyperplasia [176]. Other side effects include sleep apnea, breast development in men, breast carcinoma, fluid retention, hypertension, alterations in the lipid profile, and atherosclerosis [101, 207].

8.3   DHEA

A great deal of information has been accumulated in recent years regarding the beneficial effects of pharmacological doses of DHEA. Potential benefits include cardioprotection, antiobesity, immunostimulation, and neuroprotection [129]. The effect of DHEA on the improvement of immune function in the elderly was evidenced by observations in aged mice showing that immunization shortly after an oral dose of DHEAS provided adjuvant effects that improve immunity against influenza [11, 12]. However, in a prospective randomized, double-blind study, in which participants received either DHEA for 4 consecutive days starting 2 days before immunization or placebo, there was no improvement in the age-related decrease response to immunization against influenza [53]. In conclusion, more studies are necessary to justify the use of DHEAS as an adjuvant for the elderly.

9   Conclusions

Analysis of the contribution of sex hormones to different aspects of imnunosenescence has been presented in this chapter. After a review of the enormous amount of literature on the field, one may conclude that changes in the sex hormone environment can contribute to immunosenescence. Thus, sex hormone status can help shape normal aspects of the aging immune system, as well as immune responses to injury and infection. Additionally, we can conclude that immunosenescence is a manifestation of the continuous interplay between the immune, the endocrine, and the nervous systems over time. Overall, when trying to determine the best treatment option for any number of pathological conditions, it is important to consider both age and sex as potential modifiers of the disease process. Thus, therapies targeted to the specific hormonal and immune status of an individual may prove to be of most benefit for optimal clinical outcomes.

Acknowledgments   The authors are indebted to Dr. Melanie Bird and Jessica L. Palmer for thoughtful discussions and critical review of this manuscript. This work was supported by the National Institutes of Health R01 AG018859 (EJK), R01 AA012034 (EJK), F30 AG029724 (VN), Illinois Excellence in Academic Medicine Grant (EJK), and Ralph and Marion C. Falk Research Trust (EJK).

References

1. ABA: National Burn Repository: 2002 Report. 2002
2. Ahmed SA, Aufdemorte TB, Chen JR, Montoya AI, Olive D, Talal N (1989) Estrogen induces the development of autoantibodies and promotes salivary gland lymphoid infiltrates in normal mice. J Autoimmun 2:543–552

3. Altura BM (1976) Sex and estrogens in protection against circulatory stress reactions. Am J Physiol 231:842–847

4. Angele MK, Ayala A, Cioffi WG, Bland KI, Chaudry IH (1998) Testosterone: the culprit for producing splenocyte immune depression after trauma hemorrhage. Am J Physiol 274: C1530–C1536

5. Angele MK, Ayala A, Monfils BA, Cioffi WG, Bland KI, Chaudry IH (1998) Testosterone and/or low estradiol: normally required but harmful immunologically for males after trauma-hemorrhage. J Trauma 44:78–85

6. Angele MK, Knoferl MW, Schwacha MG, Ayala A, Cioffi WG, Bland KI, Chaudry IH (1999) Sex steroids regulate pro- and anti-inflammatory cytokine release by macrophages after trauma-hemorrhage. Am J Physiol 277:C35–C42

7. Angele MK, Schwacha MG, Ayala A, Chaudry IH (2000) Effect of gender and sex hormones on immune responses following shock. Shock 14:81–90

8. Angele MK, Knoferl MW, Ayala A, Bland KI, Chaudry IH (2001) Testosterone and estrogen differently effect Th1 and Th2 cytokine release following trauma-haemorrhage. Cytokine 16:22–30

9. Angele MK, Frantz MC, Chaudry IH (2006) Gender and sex hormones influence the response to trauma and sepsis: potential therapeutic approaches. Clinics 61:479–488

10. Ansar Ahmed S, Penhale WJ, Talal N (1985) Sex hormones, immune responses, and autoimmune diseases. Mechanisms of sex hormone action. Am J Pathol 121:531–551

11. Araneo B, Dowell T, Woods ML, Daynes R, Judd M, Evans T (1995) DHEAS as an effective vaccine adjuvant in elderly humans. Proof-of-principle studies. Ann N Y Acad Sci 774:232–248

12. Araneo BA, Woods ML, 2nd, Daynes RA (1993) Reversal of the immunosenescent phenotype by dehydroepiandrosterone: hormone treatment provides an adjuvant effect on the immunization of aged mice with recombinant hepatitis B surface antigen. J Infect Dis 167:830–840

13. Arlt W, Hewison M (2004) Hormones and immune function: implications of aging. Aging Cell 3:209–216

14. Asai K, Hiki N, Mimura Y, Ogawa T, Unou K, Kaminishi M (2001) Gender differences in cytokine secretion by human peripheral blood mononuclear cells: role of estrogen in modulating LPS-induced cytokine secretion in an ex vivo septic model. Shock 16:340–343

15. Ashcroft GS, Dodsworth J, van Boxtel E, Tarnuzzer RW, Horan MA, Schultz GS, Ferguson MW (1997) Estrogen accelerates cutaneous wound healing associated with an increase in TGF-beta1 levels. Nat Med 3:1209–1215

16. Ashcroft GS, Horan MA, Ferguson MW (1997) Aging is associated with reduced deposition of specific extracellular matrix components, an upregulation of angiogenesis, and an altered inflammatory response in a murine incisional wound healing model. J Invest Dermatol 108:430–437

17. Ashcroft GS, Horan MA, Herrick SE, Tarnuzzer RW, Schultz GS, Ferguson MW (1997) Age-related differences in the temporal and spatial regulation of matrix metalloproteinases (MMPs) in normal skin and acute cutaneous wounds of healthy humans. Cell Tissue Res 290:581–591

18. Ashcroft GS, Horan MA, Ferguson MW (1998) Aging alters the inflammatory and endothelial cell adhesion molecule profiles during human cutaneous wound healing. Lab Invest 78:47–58

19. Ashcroft GS, Greenwell-Wild T, Horan MA, Wahl SM, Ferguson MW (1999) Topical estrogen accelerates cutaneous wound healing in aged humans associated with an altered inflammatory response. Am J Pathol 155:1137–1146

20. Ashcroft GS, Yang X, Glick AB, Weinstein M, Letterio JL, Mizel DE, Anzano M, Greenwell-Wild T, Wahl SM, Deng C et al (1999) Mice lacking Smad3 show accelerated wound healing and an impaired local inflammatory response. Nat Cell Biol 1:260–266

21. Ashcroft GS, Mills SJ (2002) Androgen receptor-mediated inhibition of cutaneous wound healing. J Clin Invest 110:615–624

22. Ashcroft GS, Mills SJ, Lei K, Gibbons L, Jeong MJ, Taniguchi M, Burow M, Horan MA, Wahl SM, Nakayama T (2003) Estrogen modulates cutaneous wound healing by downregulating macrophage migration inhibitory factor. J Clin Invest 111:1309–1318

23. Bachmann G, Bancroft J, Braunstein G, Burger H, Davis S, Dennerstein L, Goldstein I, Guay A, Leiblum S, Lobo R et al (2002) Female androgen insufficiency: the Princeton consensus statement on definition, classification, and assessment. Fertil Steril 77:660–665

24. Bain DL, Heneghan AF, Connaghan-Jones KD, Miura MT (2007) Nuclear receptor structure: implications for function. Annu Rev Physiol 69:201–220

25. Ballou SP, Lozanski FB, Hodder S, Rzewnicki DL, Mion LC, Sipe JD, Ford AB, Kushner I (1996) Quantitative and qualitative alterations of acute-phase proteins in healthy elderly persons. Age Ageing 25:224–230

26. Barrat F, Lesourd B, Boulouis HJ, Thibault D, Vincent-Naulleau S, Gjata B, Louise A, Neway T, Pilet C (1997) Sex and parity modulate cytokine production during murine ageing. Clin Exp Immunol 109:562–568

27. Barrat F, Lesourd BM, Louise A, Boulouis HJ, Vincent-Naulleau S, Thibault D, Sanaa M, Neway T, Pilet CH (1997) Surface antigen expression in spleen cells of C57B1/6 mice during ageing: influence of sex and parity. Clin Exp Immunol 107:593–600

28. Basaria S, Dobs AS (2006) Clinical review: Controversies regarding transdermal androgen therapy in postmenopausal women. J Clin Endocrinol Metab 91:4743–4752

29. Belanger A, Candas B, Dupont A, Cusan L, Diamond P, Gomez JL, Labrie F (1994) Changes in serum concentrations of conjugated and unconjugated steroids in 40- to 80-year-old men. J Clin Endocrinol Metab 79:1086–1090

30. Bismar H, Diel I, Ziegler R, Pfeilschifter J (1995) Increased cytokine secretion by human bone marrow cells after menopause or discontinuation of estrogen replacement. J Clin Endocrinol Metab 80:3351–3355

31. Blondeau JP, Baulieu EE, Robel P (1982) Androgen-dependent regulation of androgen nuclear receptor in the rat ventral prostate. Endocrinology 110:1926–1932

32. Bonafe M, Olivieri F, Cavallone L, Giovagnetti S, Mayegiani F, Cardelli M, Pieri C, Marra M, Antonicelli R, Lisa R et al (2001) A gender-dependent genetic predisposition to produce high levels of IL-6 is detrimental for longevity. Eur J Immunol 31:2357–2361

33. Bone RC (1992) Toward an epidemiology and natural history of SIRS (systemic inflammatory response syndrome). JAMA 268:3452–3455

34. Bouman A, Schipper M, Heineman MJ, Faas MM (2004) Gender difference in the non-specific and specific immune response in humans. Am J Reprod Immunol 52:19–26

35. Bouman A, Heineman MJ, Faas MM (2005) Sex hormones and the immune response in humans. Hum Reprod Update 11:411–423

36. Bronson FH, Desjardins C (1997) Reproductive failure in aged CBF1 male mice: interrelationships between pituitary gonadotropic hormones, testicular function, and mating success. Endocrinology 101:939–945

37. Brown TJ, MacLusky NJ, Shanabrough M, Naftolin F (1990) Comparison of age- and sex-related changes in cell nuclear estrogen-binding capacity and progestin receptor induction in the rat brain. Endocrinology 126:2965–2972

38. Bruunsgaard H, Andersen-Ranberg K, Jeune B, Pedersen AN, Skinhoj P, Pedersen BK (1999) A high plasma concentration of TNF-alpha is associated with dementia in centenarians. J Gerontol A Biol Sci Med Sci 54:M357–M364

39. Bruunsgaard H, Skinhoj P, Qvist J, Pedersen BK (1999) Elderly humans show prolonged in vivo inflammatory activity during pneumococcal infections. J Infect Dis 180:551–554

40. Burger HG, Dudley EC, Cui J, Dennerstein L, Hopper JL (2000) A prospective longitudinal study of serum testosterone, dehydroepiandrosterone sulfate, and sex hormone-binding globulin levels through the menopause transition. J Clin Endocrinol Metab 85:2832–2838

41. Calabrese EJ (2001) Estrogen and related compounds: biphasic dose responses. Crit Rev Toxicol 31:503–515

42. Cantatore FP, Loverro G, Ingrosso AM, Lacanna R, Sassanelli E, Selvaggi L, Carrozzo M (1995) Effect of oestrogen replacement on bone metabolism and cytokines in surgical menopause. Clin Rheumatol 14:157–160

43. Carlsten H, Verdrengh M, Taube M (1996) Additive effects of suboptimal doses of estrogen and cortisone on the suppression of T lymphocyte dependent inflammatory responses in mice. Inflamm Res 45:26–30

44. Chahal HS, Drake WM (2007) The endocrine system and ageing. J Pathol 211:173–180

45. Chakraborty TR, Gore AC (2004) Aging-related changes in ovarian hormones, their receptors, and neuroendocrine function. Exp Biol Med (Maywood) 229:977–987

46. Choi BC, Polgar K, Xiao L, Hill JA (2000) Progesterone inhibits in-vitro embryotoxic Th1 cytokine production to trophoblast in women with recurrent pregnancy loss. Hum Reprod 15 (Suppl 1):46–59

47. Christman JW, Holden EP, Blackwell TS (1995) Strategies for blocking the systemic effects of cytokines in the sepsis syndrome. Crit Care Med 23:955–963

48. Chrousos GP, Elenkov IJ (2006) Interactions of the endocrine and immune system. In De Groot LJJ Endocrinology, 5th edn, vol 1. Elsevier Saunders, pp 799–818

49. Clark JA, Peterson TC (1994) Cytokine production and aging: overproduction of IL-8 in elderly males in response to lipopolysaccharide. Mech Ageing Dev 77:127–139

50. Clerici E, Bergamasco E, Ferrario E, Villa ML (1991) Influence of sex steroids on the antigen-specific primary antibody response in vitro. J Clin Lab Immunol 34:71–78

51. Corsini E, Lucchi L, Meroni M, Racchi M, Solerte B, Fioravanti M, Viviani B, Marinovich M, Govoni S, Galli CL (2002) In vivo dehydroepiandrosterone restores age-associated defects in the protein kinase C signal transduction pathway and related functional responses. J Immunol 168:1753–1758

52. Couillard C, Gagnon J, Bergeron J, Leon AS, Rao DC, Skinner JS, Wilmore JH, Despres JP, Bouchard C (2000) Contribution of body fatness and adipose tissue distribution to the age variation in plasma steroid hormone concentrations in men: the HERITAGE Family Study. J Clin Endocrinol Metab 85:1026–1031

53. Danenberg HD, Ben-Yehuda A, Zakay-Rones Z, Gross DJ, Friedman G (1997) Dehydroepiandrosterone treatment is not beneficial to the immune response to influenza in elderly subjects. J Clin Endocrinol Metab 82:2911–2914

54. Davison SL, Bell R, Donath S, Montalto JG, Davis SR (2005) Androgen levels in adult females: changes with age, menopause, and oophorectomy. J Clin Endocrinol Metab 90:3847–3853

55. Daynes RA, Araneo BA, Ershler WB, Maloney C, Li GZ, Ryu SY (1993) Altered regulation of IL-6 production with normal aging. Possible linkage to the age-associated decline in dehydroepiandrosterone and its sulfated derivative. J Immunol 150:5219–5230

56. Deshpande R, Khalili H, Pergolizzi RG, Michael SD, Chang MD (1997) Estradiol downregulates LPS-induced cytokine production and NFkB activation in murine macrophages. Am J Reprod Immunol 38:46–54

57. Diegelmann RF, Evans MC (2004) Wound healing: an overview of acute, fibrotic and delayed healing. Front Biosci 9:283–289

58. Dolecek R (1989) Endocrine changes after burn trauma—a review. Keio J Med 38:262–276

59. Drost AC, Larsen B, Aulick LH (1993) The effects of thermal injury on serum interleukin 1 activity in rats. Lymphokine Cytokine Res 12:181–185

60. Dudley DJ, Chen CL, Mitchell MD, Daynes RA, Araneo BA (1993) Adaptive immune responses during murine pregnancy: pregnancy-induced regulation of lymphokine production by activated T lymphocytes. Am J Obstet Gynecol 168:1155–1163

61. Eleftheriou BE, Lucas LA (1974) Age-related changes in testes, seminal vesicles and plasma testosterone levels in male mice. Gerontologia 20:231–238

62. Elenkov IJ, Wilder RL, Chrousos GP, Vizi ES (2000) The sympathetic nerve—an integrative interface between two supersystems: the brain and the immune system. Pharmacol Rev 52:595–638

63. English KM, Steeds RP, Jones TH, Diver MJ, Channer KS (2000) Low-dose transdermal testosterone therapy improves angina threshold in men with chronic stable angina: A randomized, double-blind, placebo-controlled study. Circulation 102:1906–1911

64. Erlandsson MC, Gomori E, Taube M, Carlsten H (2000) Effects of raloxifene, a selective estrogen receptor modulator, on thymus, T cell reactivity, and inflammation in mice. Cell Immunol 205:103–109

65. Ershler WB (1993) Interleukin-6: a cytokine for gerontologists. J Am Geriatr Soc 41:176–181

66. Ershler WB, Sun WH, Binkley N, Gravenstein S, Volk MJ, Kamoske G, Klopp RG, Roecker EB, Daynes RA, Weindruch R (1993) Interleukin-6 and aging: blood levels and mononuclear cell production increase with advancing age and in vitro production is modifiable by dietary restriction. Lymphokine Cytokine Res 12:225–230

67. Ershler WB, Sun WH, Binkley N (1994) The role of interleukin-6 in certain age-related diseases. Drugs Aging 5:358–365

68. Ershler WB, Keller ET (2000) Age-associated increased interleukin-6 gene expression, late-life diseases, and frailty. Annu Rev Med 51:245–270

69. Estrogen and progestogen use in peri- and postmenopausal women: March 2007 position statement of The North American Menopause Society. Menopause 14:168–182

70. Feldman HA, Longcope C, Derby CA, Johannes CB, Araujo AB, Coviello AD, Bremner WJ, McKinlay JB (2002) Age trends in the level of serum testosterone and other hormones in middle-aged men: longitudinal results from the Massachusetts male aging study. J Clin Endocrinol Metab 87:589–598

71. Feldman RD, Hunninghake GW, McArdle WL (1987) Beta-adrenergic-receptor-mediated suppression of interleukin 2 receptors in human lymphocytes. J Immunol 139:3355–3359

72. Felicio LS, Nelson JF, Finch CE (1984) Longitudinal studies of estrous cyclicity in aging C57BL/6J mice: II. Cessation of cyclicity and the duration of persistent vaginal cornification. Biol Reprod 31:446–453

73. Ferrini RL, Barrett-Connor E (1998) Sex hormones and age: a cross-sectional study of testosterone and estradiol and their bioavailable fractions in community-dwelling men. Am J Epidemiol 147:750–754

74. Ferrucci L, Harris TB, Guralnik JM, Tracy RP, Corti MC, Cohen HJ, Penninx B, Pahor M, Wallace R, Havlik RJ (1999) Serum IL-6 level and the development of disability in older persons. J Am Geriatr Soc 47:639–646

75. Franceschi C, Bonafe M, Valensin S, Olivieri F, De Luca M, Ottaviani E, De Benedictis G: Inflamm-aging (2000) An evolutionary perspective on immunosenescence. Ann N Y Acad Sci 908:244–254

76. Franklin RD, Kutteh WH (1999) Characterization of immunoglobulins and cytokines in human cervical mucus: influence of exogenous and endogenous hormones. J Reprod Immunol 42:93–106

77. Friedman D, Netti F, Schreiber AD (1985) Effect of estradiol and steroid analogues on the clearance of immunoglobulin G-coated erythrocytes. J Clin Invest 75:162–167

78. Funabashi T, Kleopoulos SP, Brooks PJ, Kimura F, Pfaff DW, Shinohara K, Mobbs CV (2000) Changes in estrogenic regulation of estrogen receptor alpha mRNA and progesterone receptor mRNA in the female rat hypothalamus during aging: an in situ hybridization study. Neurosci Res 38:85–92

79. Furuhashi N, Suzuki M, Abe T, Yamaya Y, Takahashi K (1977) Changes of hypophysio-ovarian endocrinological function by aging in woman. Tohoku J Exp Med 121:231–238

80. Gannon CJ, Pasquale M, Tracy JK, McCarter RJ, Napolitano LM (2004) Male gender is associated with increased risk for postinjury pneumonia. Shock 21:410–414

81. Gardner EM, Murasko DM (2002) Age-related changes in Type 1 and Type 2 cytokine production in humans. Biogerontology 3:271–290

82. George RL, McGwin G, Jr., Metzger J, Chaudry IH, Rue LW 3rd (2003) The association between gender and mortality among trauma patients as modified by age. J Trauma 54:464–471

83. George RL, McGwin G Jr (2003) Windham ST, Melton SM, Metzger J, Chaudry IH, Rue LW, 3rd: Age-related gender differential in outcome after blunt or penetrating trauma. Shock 19:28–32

84. Germann G, Barthold U, Lefering R, Raff T, Hartmann B (1997) The impact of risk factors and pre-existing conditions on the mortality of burn patients and the precision of predictive admission-scoring systems. Burns 23:195–203

85. Gilliver SC, Ashworth JJ, Mills SJ, Hardman MJ, Ashcroft GS (2006) Androgens modulate the inflammatory response during acute wound healing. J Cell Sci 119:722–732

86. Gilliver SC, Ashworth JJ, Ashcroft GS (2007) The hormonal regulation of cutaneous wound healing. Clin Dermatol 25:56–62

87. Girasole G, Giuliani N, Modena AB, Passeri G, Pedrazzoni M (1999) Oestrogens prevent the increase of human serum soluble interleukin-6 receptor induced by ovariectomy in vivo and decrease its release in human osteoblastic cells in vitro. Clin Endocrinol (Oxf) 51:801–807

88. Gomez CR, Goral J, Ramirez L, Kopf M, Kovacs EJ (2006) Aberrant acute-phase response in aged interleukin-6 knockout mice. Shock 25:581–585

89. Gomez CR, Hirano S, Cutro BT, Birjandi S, Baila H, Nomellini V, Kovacs EJ (2007) Advanced age exacerbates the pulmonary inflammatory response after lipopolysaccharide exposure. Crit Care Med 35:246–251

90. Gomez CR, Plackett TP, Kovacs EJ: Aging and estrogen (2007) modulation of inflammatory responses after injury. Exp Gerontol 42:451–456

91. Gosain A, DiPietro LA (2004) Aging and wound healing. World J Surg 28:321–326

92. Gosden RG, Laing SC, Felicio LS, Nelson JF, Finch CE (1983) Imminent oocyte exhaustion and reduced follicular recruitment mark the transition to acyclicity in aging C57BL/6J mice. Biol Reprod 28:255–260

93. Graff RJ, Lappe MA, Snell GD (1969) The influence of the gonads and adrenal glands on the immune response to skin grafts. Transplantation 7:105–111

94. Gray A, Feldman HA, McKinlay JB, Longcope C (1991) Age, disease, and changing sex hormone levels in middle-aged men: results of the Massachusetts Male Aging Study. J Clin Endocrinol Metab 73:1016–1025

95. Gregory MS, Duffner LA, Faunce DE, Kovacs EJ (2000) Estrogen mediates the sex difference in post-burn immunosuppression. J Endocrinol 164:129–138

96. Gregory MS, Duffner LA, Hahn EL, Tai HH, Faunce DE, Kovacs EJ (2000) Differential production of prostaglandin E(2) in male and female mice subjected to thermal injury contributes to the gender difference in immune function: possible role for 15-hydroxyprostaglandin dehydrogenase. Cell Immunol 205:94–102

97. Gregory MS, Faunce DE, Duffner LA, Kovacs EJ (2000) Gender difference in cell-mediated immunity after thermal injury is mediated, in part, by elevated levels of interleukin-6. J Leukoc Biol 67:319–326

98. Grossman C (1989) Possible underlying mechanisms of sexual dimorphism in the immune response, fact and hypothesis. J Steroid Biochem 34:241–251

99. Gruenewald DA, Hess DL, Wilkinson CW, Matsumoto AM (1992) Excessive testicular progesterone secretion in aged male Fischer 344 rats: a potential cause of age-related gonadotropin suppression and confounding variable in aging studies. J Gerontol 47:B164–B170

100. Gruenewald DA, Naai MA, Hess DL, Matsumoto AM (1994) The Brown Norway rat as a model of male reproductive aging: evidence for both primary and secondary testicular failure. J Gerontol 49:B42–B50

101. Gruenewald DA, Matsumoto AM (2003) Testosterone supplementation therapy for older men: potential benefits and risks. J Am Geriatr Soc 51:101–115; discussion 115

102. Hansen KA, Opsahl MS, Nieman LK, Baker JR, Jr., Klein TA (1992) Natural killer cell activity from pregnant subjects is modulated by RU 486. Am J Obstet Gynecol 166:87–90

103. Havlikova H, Hill M, Hampl R, Starka L (2002) Sex- and age-related changes in epitestosterone in relation to pregnenolone sulfate and testosterone in normal subjects. J Clin Endocrinol Metab 87:2225–2231

104. Herbert J (1995) The age of dehydroepiandrosterone. Lancet 345:1193–1194

105. Hofbauer LC, Khosla S (1999) Androgen effects on bone metabolism: recent progress and controversies. Eur J Endocrinol 140:271–286

106. Hu SK, Mitcho YL, Rath NC (1988) Effect of estradiol on interleukin 1 synthesis by macrophages. Int J Immunopharmacol 10:247–252
107. Huang HH, Steger RW, Bruni JF, Meites J (1978) Patterns of sex steroid and gonadotropin secretion in aging female rats. Endocrinology 103:1855–1859
108. Hulley S, Grady D, Bush T, Furberg C, Herrington D, Riggs B, Vittinghoff E (1998) Randomized trial of estrogen plus progestin for secondary prevention of coronary heart disease in postmenopausal women. Heart and Estrogen/progestin Replacement Study (HERS) Research Group. JAMA 280:605–613
109. Ishunina TA, van Beurden D, Van Der Meulen G, Unmehopa UA, Hol EM, Huitinga I, Swaab DF (2005) Diminished aromatase immunoreactivity in the hypothalamus, but not in the basal forebrain nuclei in Alzheimer's disease. Neurobiol Aging 26:173–194
110. Ishunina TA, Swaab DF (2007) Alterations in the human brain in menopause. Maturitas 57:20–22
111. Islander U, Erlandsson MC, Hasseus B, Jonsson CA, Ohlsson C, Gustafsson JA, Dahlgren U, Carlsten H (2003) Influence of oestrogen receptor alpha and beta on the immune system in aged female mice. Immunology 110:149–157
112. Jain SK, Rogier K, Prouty L, Jain SK (2004) Protective effects of 17beta-estradiol and trivalent chromium on interleukin-6 secretion, oxidative stress, and adhesion of monocytes: relevance to heart disease in postmenopausal women. Free Radic Biol Med 37:1730–1735
113. James K, Premchand N, Skibinska A, Skibinski G, Nicol M, Mason JI (1997) IL-6, DHEA and the ageing process. Mech Ageing Dev 93:15–24
114. Jankowski M, Rachelska G, Donghao W, McCann SM, Gutkowska J (2001) Estrogen receptors activate atrial natriuretic peptide in the rat heart. Proc Natl Acad Sci U S A 98:11765–11770
115. Jilka RL, Hangoc G, Girasole G, Passeri G, Williams DC, Abrams JS, Boyce B, Broxmeyer H, Manolagas SC (1992) Increased osteoclast development after estrogen loss: mediation by interleukin-6. Science 257:88–91
116. Johnson SR (1998) Menopause and hormone replacement therapy. Med Clin North Am 82:297–320
117. Kahlke V, Angele MK, Ayala A, Schwacha MG, Cioffi WG, Bland KI, Chaudry IH (2000) Immune dysfunction following trauma-haemorrhage: influence of gender and age. Cytokine 12:69–77
118. Kahlke V, Angele MK, Schwacha MG, Ayala A, Cioffi WG, Bland KI, Chaudry IH (2000) Reversal of sexual dimorphism in splenic T lymphocyte responses after trauma-hemorrhage with aging. Am J Physiol Cell Physiol 278:C509–C516
119. Kalaitzidis D, Gilmore TD (2005) Transcription factor cross-talk: the estrogen receptor and NF-kappaB. Trends Endocrinol Metab 16:46–52
120. Kaler LW, Neaves WB (1981) The androgen status of aging male rats. Endocrinology 108:712–719
121. Kanda N, Tsuchida T, Tamaki K (1996) Testosterone inhibits immunoglobulin production by human peripheral blood mononuclear cells. Clin Exp Immunol 106:410–415
122. Kang SM, Jang Y, Kim JY, Chung N, Cho SY, Chae JS, Lee JH (2002) Effect of oral administration of testosterone on brachial arterial vasoreactivity in men with coronary artery disease. Am J Cardiol 89:862–864
123. Karpuzoglu-Sahin E, Zhi-Jun Y, Lengi A, Sriranganathan N, Ansar Ahmed S (2001) Effects of long-term estrogen treatment on IFN-gamma, IL-2 and IL-4 gene expression and protein synthesis in spleen and thymus of normal C57BL/6 mice. Cytokine 14:208–217
124. Kaufman JM, Vermeulen A (2005) The decline of androgen levels in elderly men and its clinical and therapeutic implications. Endocr Rev 26:833–876
125. Keller ET, Chang C, Ershler WB (1996) Inhibition of NFkappaB activity through maintenance of IkappaBalpha levels contributes to dihydrotestosterone-mediated repression of the interleukin-6 promoter. J Biol Chem 271:26267–26275
126. Kenny AM, Prestwood KM, Gruman CA, Fabregas G, Biskup B, Mansoor G (2002) Effects of transdermal testosterone on lipids and vascular reactivity in older men with low bioavailable testosterone levels. J Gerontol A Biol Sci Med Sci 57:M460–M465

127. Kerby JD, McGwin G Jr, George RL, Cross JA, Chaudry IH, Rue LW 3rd (2006) Sex differences in mortality after burn injury: results of analysis of the National Burn Repository of the American Burn Association. J Burn Care Res 27:452–456

128. Kim HR, Ryu SY, Kim HS, Choi BM, Lee EJ, Kim HM, Chung HT (1995) Administration of dehydroepiandrosterone reverses the immune suppression induced by high dose antigen in mice. Immunol Invest 24:583–593

129. Kim MJ, Morley JE (2005) The hormonal fountains of youth: myth or reality? J Endocrinol Invest 28:5–14

130. Kimble RB, Vannice JL, Bloedow DC, Thompson RC, Hopfer W, Kung VT, Brownfield C, Pacifici R (1994) Interleukin-1 receptor antagonist decreases bone loss and bone resorption in ovariectomized rats. J Clin Invest 93:1959–1967

131. Kimura M, Tanaka S, Yamada Y, Kiuchi Y, Yamakawa T, Sekihara H (1998) Dehydroepiandrosterone decreases serum tumor necrosis factor-alpha and restores insulin sensitivity: independent effect from secondary weight reduction in genetically obese Zucker fatty rats. Endocrinology 139:3249–3253

132. Kipper-Galperin M, Galilly R, Danenberg HD, Brenner T (1999) Dehydroepiandrosterone selectively inhibits production of tumor necrosis factor alpha and interleukin-6 [correction of interlukin-6] in astrocytes. Int J Dev Neurosci 1999, 17:765–775

133. Kitazawa R, Kimble RB, Vannice JL, Kung VT, Pacifici R (1994) Interleukin-1 receptor antagonist and tumor necrosis factor binding protein decrease osteoclast formation and bone resorption in ovariectomized mice. J Clin Invest 94:2397–2406

134. Knoferl MW, Jarrar D, Angele MK, Ayala A, Schwacha MG, Bland KI, Chaudry IH (2001) 17 beta-Estradiol normalizes immune responses in ovariectomized females after trauma-hemorrhage. Am J Physiol Cell Physiol 281:C1131–C1138

135. Knoferl MW, Angele MK, Schwacha MG, Bland KI, Chaudry IH (2002) Preservation of splenic immune functions by female sex hormones after trauma-hemorrhage. Crit Care Med 30:888–893

136. Kong LB, Lekawa M, Navarro RA, McGrath J, Cohen M, Margulies DR, Hiatt JR (1996) Pedestrian-motor vehicle trauma: an analysis of injury profiles by age. J Am Coll Surg 182:17–23

137. Kovacs EJ, Grabowski KA, Duffner LA, Plackett TP, Gregory MS (2002) Survival and cell mediated immunity after burn injury in aged mice. J Amer Aging Assoc 25:3–10

138. Kovacs EJ, Messingham KA, Gregory MS: Estrogen regulation of immune responses after injury. Mol Cell Endocrinol 2002, 193:129–135

139. Kovacs EJ, Duffner LA, Plackett TP (2004) Immunosuppression after injury in aged mice is associated with a TH1-TH2 shift, which can be restored by estrogen treatment. Mech Ageing Dev 125:121–123

140. Kovacs EJ, Plackett TP, Witte PL (2004) Estrogen replacement, aging, and cell-mediated immunity after injury. J Leukoc Biol 76:36–41

141. Kowal-Vern A, Walenga JM, Sharp-Pucci M, Hoppensteadt D, Gamelli RL (1997) Postburn edema and related changes in interleukin-2, leukocytes, platelet activation, endothelin-1, and C1 esterase inhibitor. J Burn Care Rehabil 18:99–103

142. Krabbe KS, Bruunsgaard H, Hansen CM, Moller K, Fonsmark L, Qvist J, Madsen PL, Kronborg G, Andersen HO, Skinhoj P et al (2001) Ageing is associated with a prolonged fever response in human endotoxemia. Clin Diagn Lab Immunol 8:333–338

143. Kunelius P, Lukkarinen O, Hannuksela ML, Itkonen O, Tapanainen JS (2002) The effects of transdermal dihydrotestosterone in the aging male: a prospective, randomized, double blind study. J Clin Endocrinol Metab 87:1467–1472

144. Kurokouchi K, Kambe F, Yasukawa K, Izumi R, Ishiguro N, Iwata H, Seo H (1998) TNF-alpha increases expression of IL-6 and ICAM-1 genes through activation of NF-kappaB in osteoblast-like ROS17/2.8 cells. J Bone Miner Res 13:1290–1299

145. Labrie F, Belanger A, Cusan L, Gomez JL, Candas B (1997) Marked decline in serum concentrations of adrenal C19 sex steroid precursors and conjugated androgen metabolites during aging. J Clin Endocrinol Metab 82:2396–2402

146. Lamberts SW, Van Den Beld AW, Van Der Lely AJ (1997) The endocrinology of aging. Science 278:419–424
147. Lang TJ (2004) Estrogen as an immunomodulator. Clin Immunol 113:224–230
148. Larsen PR, Kronenberg, H.M., Melmed, S., Polonsky, KS (2003) Williams Textbook of endocrinology, 10th edn. Saunders
149. Laughlin GA, Barrett-Connor E (2000) Sexual dimorphism in the influence of advanced aging on adrenal hormone levels: the Rancho Bernardo Study. J Clin Endocrinol Metab 85:3561–3568
150. Le Bail J, Liagre B, Vergne P, Bertin P, Beneytout J, Habrioux G (2001) Aromatase in synovial cells from postmenopausal women. Steroids 66:749–757
151. Leder BZ, Rohrer JL, Rubin SD, Gallo J, Longcope C (2004) Effects of aromatase inhibition in elderly men with low or borderline-low serum testosterone levels. J Clin Endocrinol Metab 89:1174–1180
152. Lephart ED, Baxter CR, Parker CR Jr (1987) Effect of burn trauma on adrenal and testicular steroid hormone production. J Clin Endocrinol Metab 64:842–848
153. Li P, Allen H, Banerjee S, Franklin S, Herzog L, Johnston C, McDowell J, Paskind M, Rodman L, Salfeld J et al (1995) Mice deficient in IL-1 beta-converting enzyme are defective in production of mature IL-1 beta and resistant to endotoxic shock. Cell 80:401–411
154. Lin SC, Yamate T, Taguchi Y, Borba VZ, Girasole G, O'Brien CA, Bellido T, Abe E, Manolagas SC (1997) Regulation of the gp80 and gp130 subunits of the IL-6 receptor by sex steroids in the murine bone marrow. J Clin Invest 100:1980–1990
155. Linn BS (1980) Age differences in the severity and outcome of burns. J Am Geriatr Soc 28:118–123
156. Longcope C, Hunter R, Franz C (1980) Steroid secretion by the postmenopausal ovary. Am J Obstet Gynecol 138:564–568
157. Lu KH, Hopper BR, Vargo TM, Yen SS (1979) Chronological changes in sex steroid, gonadotropin and prolactin secretions in aging female rats displaying different reproductive states. Biol Reprod 21:193–203
158. Lubahn DB, Joseph DR, Sullivan PM, Willard HF, French FS, Wilson EM (1988) Cloning of human androgen receptor complementary DNA and localization to the X chromosome. Science 240:327–330
159. Mannel DN, Falk W, Yron I (1990) Inhibition of murine cytotoxic T cell responses by progesterone. Immunol Lett 26:89–94
160. Martin GS, Mannino DM, Eaton S, Moss M (2003) The epidemiology of sepsis in the United States from 1979 through 2000. N Engl J Med 348:1546–1554
161. Maruyama Y, Aoki N, Suzuki Y, Sinohara H, Yamamoto T (1984) Variation with age in the levels of sex-steroid-binding plasma protein as determined by radioimmunoassay. Acta Endocrinol (Copenh) 106:428–432
162. McGowan JE Jr, Barnes MW, Finland M (1975) Bacteremia at Boston City Hospital: Occurrence and mortality during 12 selected years (1935–1972), with special reference to hospital-acquired cases. J Infect Dis 132:316–335
163. McGwin G Jr, George RL, Cross JM, Reiff DA, Chaudry IH, Rue LW 3rd (2002) Gender differences in mortality following burn injury. Shock 18:311–315
164. McMurray RW, Suwannaroj S, Ndebele K, Jenkins JK (2001) Differential effects of sex steroids on T and B cells: modulation of cell cycle phase distribution, apoptosis and bcl-2 protein levels. Pathobiology 69:44–58
165. Medina KL, Kincade PW (1994) Pregnancy-related steroids are potential negative regulators of B lymphopoiesis. Proc Natl Acad Sci U S A 91:5382–5386
166. Meites J (1982) Changes in neuroendocrine control of anterior pituitary function during aging. Neuroendocrinology 34:151–156
167. Messingham KA, Heinrich SA, Kovacs EJ (2001) Estrogen restores cellular immunity in injured male mice via suppression of interleukin-6 production. J Leukoc Biol 70:887–895
168. Miller RA (1996) The aging immune system: primer and prospectus. Science 273:70–74

169. Miller RA (1997) Age-related changes in T cell surface markers: a longitudinal analysis in genetically heterogeneous mice. Mech Ageing Dev 96:181–196

170. Mills SJ, Ashworth JJ, Gilliver SC, Hardman MJ, Ashcroft GS (2005) The sex steroid precursor DHEA accelerates cutaneous wound healing via the estrogen receptors. J Invest Dermatol 125:1053–1062

171. Mitchell R, Hollis S, Rothwell C, Robertson WR (1995) Age related changes in the pituitary-testicular axis in normal men; lower serum testosterone results from decreased bioactive LH drive. Clin Endocrinol (Oxf) 42:501–507

172. Mizoguchi Y, Ikemoto Y, Yamamoto S, Morisawa S (1985) Studies on the effects of estrogen on antibody responses in asymptomatic HB virus carriers and non-responders to HB vaccine inoculation. Gastroenterol Jpn 20:324–329

173. Morales DE, McGowan KA, Grant DS, Maheshwari S, Bhartiya D, Cid MC, Kleinman HK, Schnaper HW (1995) Estrogen promotes angiogenic activity in human umbilical vein endothelial cells in vitro and in a murine model. Circulation 91:755–763

174. Morley JE, Kaiser F, Raum WJ, Perry HM, 3rd, Flood JF, Jensen J, Silver AJ, Roberts E (1997) Potentially predictive and manipulable blood serum correlates of aging in the healthy human male: progressive decreases in bioavailable testosterone, dehydroepiandrosterone sulfate, and the ratio of insulin-like growth factor 1 to growth hormone. Proc Natl Acad Sci U S A 94:7537–7542

175. Morley JE, Kaiser FE, Perry HM 3rd, Patrick P, Morley PM, Stauber PM, Vellas B, Baumgartner RN, Garry PJ (1997) Longitudinal changes in testosterone, luteinizing hormone, and follicle-stimulating hormone in healthy older men. Metabolism 46:410–413

176. Morley JE (2000) Testosterone treatment in older men: effects on the prostate. Endocr Pract 6:218–221

177. Muehlenbein MP, Bribiescas RG (2005) Testosterone-mediated immune functions and male life histories. Am J Hum Biol 17:527–558

178. Muller D, Chen M, Vikingsson A, Hildeman D, Pederson K (1995) Oestrogen influences CD4 +T-lymphocyte activity in vivo and in vitro in beta 2-microglobulin-deficient mice. Immunology 86:162–167

179. Nankin HR, Lin T, Osterman J (1986) Chronic testosterone cypionate therapy in men with secondary impotence. Fertil Steril 46:300–307

180. Nelson JF, Felicio LS, Osterburg HH, Finch CE (1981) Altered profiles of estradiol and progesterone associated with prolonged estrous cycles and persistent vaginal cornification in aging C57BL/6J mice. Biol Reprod 24:784–794

181. Nelson JF, Felicio LS, Randall PK, Sims C, Finch CE (1982) A longitudinal study of estrous cyclicity in aging C57BL/6J mice: I. Cycle frequency, length and vaginal cytology. Biol Reprod 27:327–339

182. Nilsson N, Carlsten H (1994) Estrogen induces suppression of natural killer cell cytotoxicity and augmentation of polyclonal B cell activation. Cell Immunol 158:131–139

183. Nilsson S, Makela S, Treuter E, Tujague M, Thomsen J, Andersson G, Enmark E, Pettersson K, Warner M, Gustafsson JA (2001) Mechanisms of estrogen action. Physiol Rev 81:1535–1565

184. Norbiato G, Bevilacqua M, Vago T, Taddei A, Clerici (1997) Glucocorticoids and the immune function in the human immunodeficiency virus infection: a study in hypercortisolemic and cortisol-resistant patients. J Clin Endocrinol Metab 82:3260–3263

185. O'Donnell L, Robertson KM, Jones ME, Simpson ER (2001) Estrogen and spermatogenesis. Endocr Rev 22:289–318

186. Oeppen J, Vaupel JW (2002) Demography. Broken limits to life expectancy. Science 296:1029–1031

187. Oettel M, Mukhopadhyay AK (2004) Progesterone: the forgotten hormone in men? Aging Male 7:236–257

188. Olsen NJ, Kovacs WJ (1996) Gonadal steroids and immunity. Endocr Rev 17:369–384

189. Orentreich N, Brind JL, Rizer RL, Vogelman JH (1984) Age changes and sex differences in serum dehydroepiandrosterone sulfate concentrations throughout adulthood. J Clin Endocrinol Metab 59:551–555

190. Paavonen T, Andersson LC, Adlercreutz H (1981) Sex hormone regulation of in vitro immune response. Estradiol enhances human B cell maturation via inhibition of suppressor T cells in pokeweed mitogen-stimulated cultures. J Exp Med 154:1935–1945

191. Pacifici R, Rifas L, McCracken R, Vered I, McMurtry C, Avioli LV, Peck WA (1989) Ovarian steroid treatment blocks a postmenopausal increase in blood monocyte interleukin 1 release. Proc Natl Acad Sci U S A 86:2398–2402

192. Pacifici R, Brown C, Puscheck E, Friedrich E, Slatopolsky E, Maggio D, McCracken R, Avioli LV (1991) Effect of surgical menopause and estrogen replacement on cytokine release from human blood mononuclear cells. Proc Natl Acad Sci U S A 88:5134–5138

193. Passeri G, Girasole G, Jilka RL, Manolagas SC (1993) Increased interleukin-6 production by murine bone marrow and bone cells after estrogen withdrawal. Endocrinology 133:822–828

194. Payne AH, Hales DB (2004) Overview of steroidogenic enzymes in the pathway from cholesterol to active steroid hormones. Endocr Rev 25:947–970

195. Perry HM, 3rd: The endocrinology of aging. Clin Chem 1999, 45:1369–1376

196. Pfeilschifter J, Koditz R, Pfohl M, Schatz H (2002) Changes in proinflammatory cytokine activity after menopause. Endocr Rev 23:90–119

197. Piccinni MP, Giudizi MG, Biagiotti R, Beloni L, Giannarini L, Sampognaro S, Parronchi P, Manetti R, Annunziato F, Livi C, et al (1995) Progesterone favors the development of human T helper cells producing Th2-type cytokines and promotes both IL-4 production and membrane CD30 expression in established Th1 cell clones. J Immunol 155:128–133

198. Piccinni MP, Scaletti C, Vultaggio A, Maggi E, Romagnani S (2001) Defective production of LIF, M-CSF and Th2-type cytokines by T cells at fetomaternal interface is associated with pregnancy loss. J Reprod Immunol 52:35–43

199. Pietschmann P, Gollob E, Brosch S, Hahn P, Kudlacek S, Willheim M, Woloszczuk W, Peterlik M, Tragl KH (2003) The effect of age and gender on cytokine production by human peripheral blood mononuclear cells and markers of bone metabolism. Exp Gerontol 38:1119–1127

200. Plackett TP, Schilling EM, Faunce DE, Choudhry MA, Witte PL, Kovacs EJ (2003) Aging enhances lymphocyte cytokine defects after injury. FASEB J 17:688–689

201. Polan ML, Daniele A, Kuo A (1988) Gonadal steroids modulate human monocyte interleukin-1 (IL-1) activity. Fertil Steril 49:964–968

202. Posma E, Moes H, Heineman MJ, Faas MM (2004) The effect of testosterone on cytokine production in the specific and non-specific immune response. Am J Reprod Immunol 52:237–243

203. Pottratz ST, Bellido T, Mocharla H, Crabb D, Manolagas SC (1994) 17 beta-Estradiol inhibits expression of human interleukin-6 promoter-reporter constructs by a receptor-dependent mechanism. J Clin Invest 93:944–950

204. Purohit A, Reed MJ (2002) Regulation of estrogen synthesis in postmenopausal women. Steroids 67:979–983

205. Rajfer J, Namkung PC, Petra PH (1980) Identification, partial characterization and age-related changes of a cytoplasmic androgen receptor in the rat penis. J Steroid Biochem 13:1489–1492

206. Rappolee DA, Mark D, Banda MJ, Werb Z (1988) Wound macrophages express TGF-alpha and other growth factors in vivo: analysis by mRNA phenotyping. Science 241:708–712

207. Rhoden EL, Morgentaler A (2004) Risks of testosterone-replacement therapy and recommendations for monitoring. N Engl J Med 350:482–492

208. Rink L, Cakman I, Kirchner H (1998) Altered cytokine production in the elderly. Mech Ageing Dev 102:199–209

209. Rodriguez JL, Miller CG, Garner WL, Till GO, Guerrero P, Moore NP, Corridore M, Normolle DP, Smith DJ, Remick DG (1993) Correlation of the local and systemic cytokine response with clinical outcome following thermal injury. J Trauma 34:684–694; discussion 694–685

210. Roehrborn CG, Lange JL, George FW, Wilson JD (1987) Changes in amount and intracellular distribution of androgen receptor in human foreskin as a function of age. J Clin Invest 79:44–47

211. Roggia C, Tamone C, Cenci S, Pacifici R, Isaia GC (2004) Role of TNF-alpha producing T cells in bone loss induced by estrogen deficiency. Minerva Med 95:125–132

212. Rossouw JE, Anderson GL, Prentice RL, LaCroix AZ, Kooperberg C, Stefanick ML, Jackson RD, Beresford SA, Howard BV, Johnson KC et al (2002) Risks and benefits of estrogen plus progestin in healthy postmenopausal women: principal results From the Women's Health Initiative randomized controlled trial. JAMA 288:321–333

213. Salvioli S, Capri M, Valensin S, Tieri P, Monti D, Ottaviani E, Franceschi C (2006) Inflamm-aging, cytokines and aging: state of the art, new hypotheses on the role of mitochondria and new perspectives from systems biology. Curr Pharm Des 12:3161–3171

214. Sarvetnick N, Fox HS (1990) Interferon-gamma and the sexual dimorphism of autoimmunity. Mol Biol Med 7:323–331

215. Schroder J, Kahlke V, Staubach KH, Zabel P, Stuber F (1998) Gender differences in human sepsis. Arch Surg 133:1200–1205

216. Schroeder ET, Zheng L, Ong MD, Martinez C, Flores C, Stewart Y, Azen C, Sattler FR (2004) Effects of androgen therapy on adipose tissue and metabolism in older men. J Clin Endocrinol Metab 89:4863–4872

217. Schumacher M, Guennoun R, Ghoumari A, Massaad C, Robert F, El-Etr M, Akwa Y, Rajkowski K, Baulieu EE (2007) Novel perspectives for progesterone in hormone replacement therapy, with special reference to the nervous system. Endocr Rev 28:387–439

218. Schwarz E, Schafer C, Bode JC, Bode C (2000) Influence of the menstrual cycle on the LPS-induced cytokine response of monocytes. Cytokine 12:413–416

219. Seals DR, Esler MD (2000) Human ageing and the sympathoadrenal system. J Physiol 528:407–417

220. Shallo H, Plackett TP, Heinrich SA, Kovacs EJ (2003) Monocyte chemoattractant protein-1 (MCP-1) and macrophage infiltration into the skin after burn injury in aged mice. Burns 29:641–647

221. Shanker G, Sorci-Thomas M, Register TC, Adams MR (1994) The inducible expression of THP-1 cell interleukin-1 mRNA: effects of estrogen on differential response to phorbol ester and lipopolysaccharide. Lymphokine Cytokine Res 13:1–7

222. Sharma PK, Thakur MK (2004) Estrogen receptor alpha expression in mice kidney shows sex differences during aging. Biogerontology 5:375–381

223. Sherman BM, West JH, Korenman SG (1976) The menopausal transition: analysis of LH, FSH, estradiol, and progesterone concentrations during menstrual cycles of older women. J Clin Endocrinol Metab 42:629–636

224. Shifren JL, Schiff I (2000) The aging ovary. J Womens Health Gend Based Med 9 (Suppl 1): S3–S7

225. Shirai M, Yamanaka M, Shiina H, Igawa M, Fujime M, Lue TF, Dahiya R (2003) Down-regulation of androgen, estrogen and progesterone receptor genes and protein is involved in aging-related erectile dysfunction. Int J Impot Res 15:391–396

226. Shyamala G, Chou YC, Louie SG, Guzman RC, Smith GH, Nandi S (2002) Cellular expression of estrogen and progesterone receptors in mammary glands: regulation by hormones, development and aging. J Steroid Biochem Mol Biol 80:137–148

227. Statistics and indicators on women and men (2007), URL http://unstats.un.org/unsd/demographic/products/indwm/tab3a.htm. United Nations Statistics Division 2006 Accession date Sept 13, 2007

228. Stein DG (2005) The case for progesterone. Ann N Y Acad Sci 1052:152–169

229. Stites DP, Siiteri PK (1983) Steroids as immunosuppressants in pregnancy. Immunol Rev 75:117–138

230. Straub RH, Konecna L, Hrach S, Rothe G, Kreutz M, Scholmerich J, Falk W, Lang B (1998) Serum dehydroepiandrosterone (DHEA) and DHEA sulfate are negatively correlated with serum interleukin-6 (IL-6), and DHEA inhibits IL-6 secretion from mononuclear cells in

man in vitro: possible link between endocrinosenescence and immunosenescence. J Clin Endocrinol Metab 83:2012–2017

231. Straub RH, Hense HW, Andus T, Scholmerich J, Riegger GA, Schunkert H (2000) Hormone replacement therapy and interrelation between serum interleukin-6 and body mass index in postmenopausal women: a population-based study. J Clin Endocrinol Metab 85:1340–1344

232. Straub RH, Cutolo M, Zietz B, Scholmerich J (2001) The process of aging changes the interplay of the immune, endocrine and nervous systems. Mech Ageing Dev 122:1591–1611

233. Straub RH (2007) The complex role of estrogens in inflammation. Endocr Rev 28:521–574

234. Strong VE, Mackrell PJ, Concannon EM, Naama HA, Schaefer PA, Shaftan GW, Stapleton PP, Daly JM (2000) Blocking prostaglandin E2 after trauma attenuates pro-inflammatory cytokines and improves survival. Shock 14:374–379

235. Swift ME, Burns AL, Gray KL, DiPietro LA (2001) Age-related alterations in the inflammatory response to dermal injury. J Invest Dermatol 117:1027–1035

236. Tan RS, Culberson JW (2003) An integrative review on current evidence of testosterone replacement therapy for the andropause. Maturitas 45:15–27

237. Tateda K, Matsumoto T, Miyazaki S, Yamaguchi K (1996) Lipopolysaccharide-induced lethality and cytokine production in aged mice. Infect Immun 64:769–774

238. Thakur MK, Asaithambi A, Mukherjee S (2000) Synthesis and phosphorylation of androgen receptor of the mouse brain cortex and their regulation by sex steroids during aging. Mol Cell Biochem 203:95–101

239. Tomaszewska A, Guevara I, Wilczok T, Dembinska-Kiec A (2003) 17beta-estradiol- and lipopolysaccharide-induced changes in nitric oxide, tumor necrosis factor-alpha and vascular endothelial growth factor release from RAW 264.7 macrophages. Gynecol Obstet Invest 56:152–159

240. Tran DD, Groeneveld AB, Van Der Meulen J, Nauta JJ, Strack van Schijndel RJ, Thijs LG (1990) Age, chronic disease, sepsis, organ system failure, and mortality in a medical intensive care unit. Crit Care Med 18:474–479

241. Valenti G (2005) The pathway of partial androgen deficiency of aging male. J Endocrinol Invest 28:28–33

242. Van Den Beld AW, de Jong FH, Grobbee DE, Pols HA, Lamberts SW (2000) Measures of bioavailable serum testosterone and estradiol and their relationships with muscle strength, bone density, and body composition in elderly men. J Clin Endocrinol Metab 85:3276–3282

243. Van Der Poll T, Barber AE, Coyle SM, Lowry SF (1996) Hypercortisolemia increases plasma interleukin-10 concentrations during human endotoxemia—a clinical research center study. J Clin Endocrinol Metab 81:3604–3606

244. Vanderschueren D, Vandenput L, Boonen S, Lindberg MK, Bouillon R, Ohlsson C (2004) Androgens and bone. Endocr Rev 25:389–425

245. Veldhuis JD, Zwart A, Mulligan T, Iranmanesh A (2001) Muting of androgen negative feedback unveils impoverished gonadotropin-releasing hormone/luteinizing hormone secretory reactivity in healthy older men. J Clin Endocrinol Metab 86:529–535

246. Vermeulen A, Kaufman JM, Giagulli VA (1996) Influence of some biological indexes on sex hormone-binding globulin and androgen levels in aging or obese males. J Clin Endocrinol Metab 81:1821–1826

247. Verthelyi D, Ahmed SA (1994) 17 beta-estradiol, but not 5 alpha-dihydrotestosterone, augments antibodies to double-stranded deoxyribonucleic acid in nonautoimmune C57BL/6J mice. Endocrinology 135:2615–2622

248. Verthelyi D (2001) Sex hormones as immunomodulators in health and disease. Int Immunopharmacol 1:983–993

249. Vieira PL, Kalinski P, Wierenga EA, Kapsenberg ML, de Jong EC (1998) Glucocorticoids inhibit bioactive IL-12p70 production by in vitro-generated human dendritic cells without affecting their T cell stimulatory potential. J Immunol 161:5245–5251

250. Viscoli CM, Brass LM, Kernan WN, Sarrel PM, Suissa S, Horwitz RI (2001) A clinical trial of estrogen-replacement therapy after ischemic stroke. N Engl J Med 345:1243–1249

251. Visser J, van Boxel-Dezaire A, Methorst D, Brunt T, de Kloet ER, Nagelkerken L (1998) Differential regulation of interleukin-10 (IL-10) and IL-12 by glucocorticoids in vitro. Blood 91:4255–4264

252. Wang C, Leung A, Sinha-Hikim AP (1993) Reproductive aging in the male brown-Norway rat: a model for the human. Endocrinology 133:2773–2781

253. Wang C, Cunningham G, Dobs A, Iranmanesh A, Matsumoto AM, Snyder PJ, Weber T, Berman N, Hull L, Swerdloff RS (2004) Long-term testosterone gel (AndroGel) treatment maintains beneficial effects on sexual function and mood, lean and fat mass, and bone mineral density in hypogonadal men. J Clin Endocrinol Metab 89:2085–2098

254. Warren MP (2007) Historical perspectives in postmenopausal hormone therapy: defining the right dose and duration. Mayo Clin Proc 82:219–226

255. Weinstein Y, Ran S, Segal S (1984) Sex-associated differences in the regulation of immune responses controlled by the MHC of the mouse. J Immunol 132:656–661

256. Wichmann MW, Zellweger R, DeMaso CM, Ayala A, Chaudry IH (1996) Mechanism of immunosuppression in males following trauma-hemorrhage. Critical role of testosterone. Arch Surg 131:1186–1191; discussion 1191–1182

257. Wichmann MW, Ayala A, Chaudry IH (1997) Male sex steroids are responsible for depressing macrophage immune function after trauma-hemorrhage. Am J Physiol 273:C1335–C1340

258. Wilson ME, Rosewell KL, Kashon ML, Shughrue PJ, Merchenthaler I, Wise PM (2002) Age differentially influences estrogen receptor-alpha (ERalpha) and estrogen receptor-beta (ERbeta) gene expression in specific regions of the rat brain. Mech Ageing Dev 123:593–601

259. Wise PM (1982) Alterations in the proestrous pattern of median eminence LHRH, serum LH, FSH, estradiol and progesterone concentrations in middle-aged rats. Life Sci 31:165–173

260. Wu JM, Zelinski MB, Ingram DK, Ottinger MA (2005) Ovarian aging and menopause: current theories, hypotheses, and research models. Exp Biol Med (Maywood) 230:818–828

261. Yaffe K, Edwards ER, Lui LY, Zmuda JM, Ferrell RE, Cauley JA (2003) Androgen receptor CAG repeat polymorphism is associated with cognitive function in older men. Biol Psychiatry 54:943–946

262. Yamamoto Y, Saito H, Setogawa T, Tomioka H (1991) Sex differences in host resistance to Mycobacterium marinum infection in mice. Infect Immun 59:4089–4096

263. Yao J, Mackman N, Edgington TS, Fan ST (1997) Lipopolysaccharide induction of the tumor necrosis factor-alpha promoter in human monocytic cells. Regulation by Egr-1, c-Jun, and NF-kappaB transcription factors. J Biol Chem 272:17795–17801

264. Yoshikawa TT (2000) Epidemiology and unique aspects of aging and infectious diseases. Clin Infect Dis 30:931–933

265. Young DG, Skibinski G, Mason JI, James K (1999) The influence of age and gender on serum dehydroepiandrosterone sulphate (DHEA-S), IL-6, IL-6 soluble receptor (IL-6 sR) and transforming growth factor beta 1 (TGF-beta1) levels in normal healthy blood donors. Clin Exp Immunol 117:476–481

266. Zellweger R, Wichmann MW, Ayala A, Stein S, DeMaso CM, Chaudry IH (1997) Females in proestrus state maintain splenic immune functions and tolerate sepsis better than males. Crit Care Med 25:106–110

267. Zhang J, Pugh TD, Stebler B, Ershler WB, Keller ET (1998) Orchiectomy increases bone marrow interleukin-6 levels in mice. Calcif Tissue Int 62:219–226

268. Zhang X, Wang L, Zhang H, Guo D, Qiao Z, Qiao J (2001) Estrogen inhibits lipopolysaccharide-induced tumor necrosis factor-alpha release from murine macrophages. Methods Find Exp Clin Pharmacol 23:169–173

269. Zhou DH, Munster AM, Winchurch RA (1992) Inhibitory effects of interleukin 6 on immunity. Possible implications in burn patients. Arch Surg 127:65–68; discussion 68–69

270. Zitzmann M, Brune M, Kornmann B, Gromoll J, Junker R, Nieschlag E (2001) The CAG repeat polymorphism in the androgen receptor gene affects bone density and bone metabolism in healthy males. Clin Endocrinol (Oxf) 55:649–657

Glucocorticoids and DHEA: Do They Have a Role in Immunosenescence?

Moisés E. Bauer, Cristina M. Moriguchi Jeckel, Cristina Bonorino, Flávia Ribeiro and Clarice Luz

Contents

Abstract: This chapter summarizes recent work suggesting that human immunosenescence may be closely related to both psychological distress and stress hormones. The age-related immunological changes are also similarly found during chronic

M. E. Bauer (✉) · C. Bonorino
Faculdade de Biociências
Instituto de Pesquisas Biomédicas
Pontifícia Universidade Católica do Rio Grande do Sul (PUCRS)
Av. Ipiranga 6690, 2° andar
P.O. Box 1429. Porto Alegre, RS 90.610-000, Brazil
E-mail: mebauer@pucrs.br

C. M. Moriguchi Jeckel
Faculdade de Farmácia,
PUCRS, Av. Ipiranga, 6681.
Porto Alegre, RS 90619-900, Brazil

F. Ribeiro
Ageing and Tumour Immunology Group,
University of Tübingen,
Sektion Transplantionsimmunologie / Immunhämatologie,
Waldhörnle Strasse 22, D- 72072 Tübingen, Germany

C. Luz
LabVitrus, Rua Garibaldi,
659/502, Porto Alegre,
RS 90035-050, Brazil

T. Fulop et al. (eds.), *Handbook on Immunosenescence,*
DOI 10.1007/ 978-1-4020-9062-2_43, © Springer Science+Business Media B.V. 2009

stress or glucocorticoid exposure. It follows that endogenous glucocorticoids (cortisol) could be associated to immunosenescence. When compared with young subjects, healthy elders are emotionally distressed in parallel to increased cortisol/dehydroepiandrosterone (DHEA) ratio. Furthermore, chronic stressed elderly subjects may be particularly at risk of stress-related pathology because of further alterations in glucocorticoid-immune signaling. Although DHEA and its metabolites have been described with immune-enhancing properties, their potential use as hormonal boosters of immunity should be interpreted with caution. The psychoneuroendocrine hypothesis of immunosenescence is presented in which the age-related increase in the cortisol/DHEA ratio is major determinant of immunological changes observed during aging. We finally discuss that strictly healthy elders are largely protected from chronic stress exposure and show normal cortisol levels and T-lymphocyte function. This information adds a new key dimension on the biology of aging and stress.

Keywords: Aging • Immunosenescence • Glucocorticoids • Lymphocytes

1 Introduction

Aging is a continuous and slow process that compromises the normal functioning of various organs and systems in both qualitative and quantitative terms. The clinical consequences of immunosenescence may include increased susceptibility to infectious diseases, neoplasias and autoimmune disease (Castle 2000). This altered morbidity is not evenly distributed and should be influenced by other immune-modulating factors, including genetic background and chronic stress exposure (Bauer 2005). Indeed, several immunosenescence-related changes (e.g., thymic involution, lower counts of naïve T-cells and blunted T-cell proliferation) resemble those observed following chronic stress (McEwen et al. 1997; Selye 1936) or glucocorticoid (GC) treatment (Fauci 1975).

In addition to immunosenescence, the endocrine system also undergoes important changes during aging (endocrinosenescence). It has been demonstrated a decline in growth hormone (GH), sex hormones and dehydroepiandrosterone (DHEA) with aging (Roshan et al. 1999). DHEA is the major secretory product of the human adrenal and is synthesized from cholesterol stores (Fig. 1). The hormone is uniquely sulphated (DHEAS) before entering the plasma, and this prohormone is converted to DHEA and its metabolites in various peripheral tissues (Canning et al. 2000). Following secretion, total DHEA in the circulation consists mainly of DHEAS—the serum concentration of free DHEA is less than 1%. Serum DHEA levels decrease by the second decade of life reaching about 5% of the original level in the elderly (Migeon et al. 1957). It has been suggested that DHEAS/DHEA may antagonize many physiological changes of endogenous glucocorticoids (Hechter et al. 1997) including enhancing immunomodulatory properties.

There is also evidence suggesting that aging is associated with significant activation of the hypothalamic-pituitary-adrenal (HPA) axis (Halbreich et al. 1984; Heuser

Fig. 1 Adrenal steroidogenic pathways.

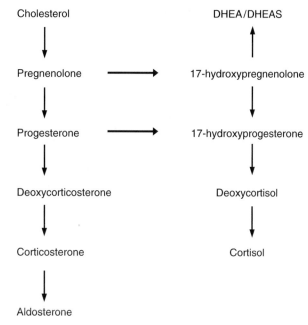

et al. 1998; Luz et al. 2003) in increased production of cortisol in the man. The HPA axis is pivotal for the homeostasis of the immune system and its dysregulation has been associated with several immune-mediated diseases. For instance, HPA axis over-activation, as occurs during chronic stress, can affect susceptibility to or severity of infectious disease through the immunosuppressive effect of the glucocorticoids (Kiecolt-Glaser et al. 1996); (Vedhara et al. 1999). In contrast, blunted HPA axis responses are associated with enhanced susceptibility to autoimmune inflammatory disease (Sternberg 2002). It is noteworthy to mention that elderly subjects are particularly at risk for both infectious and chronic inflammatory diseases. Furthermore, chronic inflammatory diseases may be associated with premature aging of the immune system and present several similarities of immunosenescence including shortening of cellular telomeres, decreased T-cell receptor specificities, loss of naïve T-cells and increased production of proinflammatory cytokines (Straub et al. 2003). Dysregulation of the HPA axis may contribute to but it is not solely responsible to immunosenescence. Chronic stressed elderly subjects may be at risk of stress-related pathology because of further alterations in GC immunoregulation (immune signaling).

The present chapter summarizes recent findings that suggest that immunosenescence may be closely related to both psychological distress and stress hormones. In particular, striking similarities of immunological changes are found during aging, stress exposure or GC treatment in vivo. The neuroendocrine hypothesis of immunosenescence is reconsidered in which both the psychological distress and increased cortisol/DHEA (C/D) ratio are thought to be major determinants of immunological changes observed during aging. We also discuss the protective effects of a strictly health status during chronic stress exposure during aging.

2 The SENIEUR Protocol

It remains controversial whether immunosenescence cause or are caused by underlying disease commonly observed in elderly populations. Therefore, strenuous efforts have been made to circumvent this problem by separating "disease" from "aging", as exemplified by the application of the SENIEUR protocol (Ligthart et al. 1984) that defines rigorous criteria for selecting healthy individuals in immunogerontological studies. The health conditions are checked accordingly to clinical investigations and to hematological and various biochemical parameters. The exclusion criteria includes: infections, acute or chronic inflammation, autoimmune diseases, heart disease, undernourishment, anemia, leucopenia, clinical depression, neurodegenerative disease, neoplasia and use of hormones and drugs. Based on this protocol, it is possible to select up to 10% of strictly healthy volunteers from elderly populations.

3 Healthy Aging is Associated with Emotional Distress and Increased Cortisol/DHEA Ratio

Psychological distress may be an important risk factor for immunosenescence. Human aging has been associated with several psychological and behavioral changes, including difficulty to concentrate, progressive cognitive impairments and sleep disturbances (Howieson et al. 2003; Piani et al. 2004). Although individually identified, these alterations may be associated with major depression. Indeed, depression is highly prevalent in several age-related chronic degenerative diseases, including cardiovascular diseases, Parkinson's disease, Alzheimer's dementia, cancer and rheumatoid arthritis (Dew et al. 1998). In addition, both aging (Gabriel et al. 2002) and major depression (Schiepers et al. 2005; Trzonkowski et al. 2004) have been associated to increased levels of proinflammatory cytokines and could thus contribute for further immunological diseases in the frail elderly.

We have recently demonstrated that healthy aging was associated with significant psychological distress. In particular, it was found that SENIEUR elders were significantly more stressed, anxious and depressed than young adults (Collaziol et al. 2004; Luz et al. 2003). Several stressors were ascribed to the healthy elders, including: feeling unable to work or having problems to perform their house work, sexual problems and reduced libido, loss of a relative or friend, and social exclusion. The literature regarding age-related psychological changes is controversial and others did not find these changes (Nolen-Hoeksema and Ahrens 2002). This could be due to methodological issues, since specific clinical interviews are required to assess depression in the elderly.

In parallel to psychological distress, we have also observed that SENIEUR elders had significantly higher (~45%) salivary cortisol production throughout the day compared to young adults (Luz et al. 2003). Cortisol peaked in the morning and presented a nadir at night, with a regular circadian pattern for both groups. These data further suggest that healthy aging is associated with significant activation of the HPA axis (Deuschle et al. 1997; Ferrari et al. 2000; Ferrari et al. 2004; Halbreich et al. 1984; Heuser et al. 1998; Van Cauter et al. 1996). However, some previous studies have also observed an flattened diurnal amplitude of ACTH and cortisol levels during aging (Deuschle et al. 1997; Ferrari et al. 2004). Increased cortisol levels are also seen in demented patients (Maeda et al. 1991), major depression (Gold et al. 1988) or during chronic stress (Bauer et al. 2000; Kirschbaum et al. 1995).

In addition, it was observed that healthy elders had lower DHEA levels (-54%) throughout the day compared to young adults (Luz et al. 2006). Furthermore, elders also displayed a flat circadian pattern for DHEA secretion. The morphological correlates of the age-related changes of DHEAS/DHEA secretion are progressive atrophy of the zona reticularis of adrenal glands (Ferrari et al. 2001). The lack of appropriate DHEA levels could be another detrimental factor during immunosenescence since this hormone has immune enhancing properties (as further discussed in this chapter).

The higher cortisol in parallel to lower DHEA levels will consequently lead to higher C/D ratios throughout the day. The assessment of molar concentrations constitute another way to evaluate the adrenal function in the organism (Butcher and Lord 2004; Ferrari et al. 2001; Straub et al. 2000). The measurement of isolated hormonal samples may be an oversimplification and the C/D ratio may contribute to the effective determination of functional hypercortisolemia. The impaired DHEA secretion, together with the increase of cortisol, results in an enhanced exposure of various bodily systems (including brain and immune system) to the cytotoxic and modulatory effects of GCs. Some brain cells (hypocampus) and lymphocytes are specially targeted by the cortisol because they express higher densities of mineralo receptors (MRs) and GC receptors (GRs) (McEwen et al. 1997). The peripheral tissues of elders may be thus more vulnerable to the GC actions in a milieu of low protective DHEA levels. The antagonist action of DHEA to cortisol in the brain suggests that measurement of cortisol alone may provide an incomplete estimate of hypercortisolemia.

In our previous study, psychological distress was positively related to salivary cortisol levels and negatively correlated to DHEA levels during aging (Luz et al. 2003). Therefore, it becomes difficult to dissociate these neuroendocrine changes observed in the elderly with those produced by psychological stimuli. It should be also pointed out that endocrinosenescence includes a substantial decline in several hormones, including growth hormone, testosterone, progesterone and aldosterone—all of which with reported immunomodulatory properties. Thus the endocrinosenescence may be considered as another risk factor for immunosenescence.

3.1   The Glucocorticoid Cascade Hypothesis

Cumulative neural damage produced by stressors during life may contribute to increased HPA function during aging. In this context, peripheral GCs may have an important role in damaging key brain areas involved with regulation of the HPA axis. Evidence for GC involvement in hippocampal aging led to the establishment of the "glucocorticoid cascade hypothesis" (Sapolsky et al. 1986). This hypothesis states that GCs participate in a fed-forward cascade of effects on the brain and body. In this case, progressive damage to the hippocampus, induced by GCs, promotes a progressive elevation of adrenal steroids (i.e. cortisol) and dysregulation (down-regulation of GC receptors) of the HPA axis (Sapolsky et al. 1986). The glucocorticoid cascade hypothesis of aging is a prime example of "allostatic load" (McEwen 1998; McEwen 2003) since it recognizes a mechanism that gradually wears down a key brain structure, the hippocampus, while the gradually dysregulated HPA axis promotes pathophysiology in tissues and organs throughout out the body. The net results of the age-related hippocampal damage are impairment of episodic, declarative, spatial, and contextual memory and also in regulation of autonomic, neuroendocrine, and immune responses. It should be mentioned that the effects of glucocorticoids on the hippocampus are reversible.

Sapolsky and col. (1986) have also proposed that several age-related pathologies are also observed following excessive glucocorticoid exposure and include muscle atrophy (Salehian and Kejriwal 1999), osteoporosis/hypercalcemia (Tamura et al. 2004), hyperglycemia/hyperlipidemia, atherosclerosis, type II diabetes and major depression (Juruena et al. 2003; Lee et al. 2002).

4 Similarities between Aging and Chronic Glucocorticoid Exposure

We have now discussed that healthy aging is associated with psychological distress in parallel to increased C/D ratio. All leucocytes exhibit receptors for the neuroendocrine products of the HPA and sympathetic-adrenal medullary axes. It seems reasonable to speculate that increased cortisol and lower DHEA may thus contribute to immunological changes observed during aging. This section will provide significant evidence that the immunological changes observed during aging are also similarly found during psychological stress or chronic GC exposure.

4.1 Changes in Cellular Trafficking

Trafficking or redistribution of peripheral immune cells in the body is of pivotal importance for effective cell-mediated immune responses. Aging is associated with several peripheral enumerative changes in leukocytes, including a decrease of naive (CD45RA+) and an increase of memory (CD45RO+) T-cells, an expansion of CD28- T-cells or an increase of natural killer (NK) cells (Gabriel et al. 1993; Globerson and Effros 2000; Hannet et al. 1992; Martinez-Taboada et al. 2002). Overall, cellular components of the innate immune system (e.g., monocytes, neutrophils and NK-cells) seems to be preserved during aging in contrast to several age-related decrements in adaptive immune responses—especially T-cells (Pawelec et al. 2002). However, T-cells are also especially targeted in the same direction during chronic stress exposure (Biondi 2001) or following GC treatment in vivo(Bauer et al. 2002; McEwen et al. 1997) (see Table1). Immunologists have recently characterized a new T-cell subset (CD4+C25+FoxP3+) with important regulatory role in suppressing excessive or misguided immune responses that can be harmful the host. These lymphocytes were called regulatory T (Treg) cells and are responsible for turning off immune responses against self antigens in autoimmune disease, allergy or commensal microbes in certain inflammatory diseases (Fontenot et al. 2003; Sakaguchi 2000). It was interestingly found that aging, glucocorticoid or chronic-stress can increase peripheral Treg cell numbers (Hoglund et al. 2006; Navarro et al. 2006; Trzonkowski et al. 2006). In spite of the several similarities among age- and stress-related immunological alterations, only a few studies have addressed the role of stress factors on human immunosenescence.

We have recently investigated the role of psychoneuroendocrine factors in regulating the distribution of peripheral T-cell subsets during healthy aging (Collaziol et al. 2004). The mechanisms underlying the regulation of the peripheral pool of lymphocytes are still largely unknown. It has been speculated that CD95 (APO1/Fas) may be involved in this process through engagement of apoptosis (Potestio et al. 1999). CD95 is a member of tumour necrosis factor (TNF) family and its ligand (CD95L) is found on activated T-cells (Nagata and Golstein 1995). The CD95-CD95L binding seems to play an important role in maintaining the cellular homeostasis of the immune system and may contribute to stress-related changes in cell trafficking (Yin et al. 2000). Confirming previous reports, we recently demonstrated that changes in lymphocyte distribution were noted in the elderly as demonstrated by a significant drop in naïve T-cells associated with higher expression

Table 1 Changes in cellular trafficking. Direction of arrows indicate increase (⇧), decrease (⇩) or no change (⇔) compared to corresponding control levels. ? = data not available; NK, natural killer; Treg = T-regulatory; CD3+CD45RA+, naïve T-cells; CD3+CD45RO+, memory T-cells. Based on references (Bauer et al. 2002; Biondi 2001; Fauci 1975; Globerson and Effros 2000; Hoglund et al. 2006; McEwen et al. 1997; Navarro et al. 2006; Trzonkowski et al. 2006)

Cell	Aging	Stress	GC treatment
Neutrophils	⇔	⇧	⇧
Monocytes	⇔	⇩	⇔
NK cells	⇧	⇧	⇧
B cells	⇩	⇩	⇩
CD4+ T cells	⇩	⇩	⇩
CD8+ T cells	⇩	⇩ or ⇧	⇩
Treg cells	⇧	⇧	⇧
CD3+CD45RA+	⇩	⇩	⇩
CD3+CD45RO+	⇧	⇩ or ⇧	⇩
CD3+CD28-	⇧	?	?

of CD95 in this subset (Collaziol et al. 2004). We have speculated this differential expression of CD95 may potentially select naive T-cells for apoptosis and could further explain age-related reductions in CD45RA+ (naïve) cells. Furthermore, healthy elders were significantly distressed and stress scores were found positively associated to CD95 expression on CD45RA+ cells.

Glucocorticoids may also contribute to the numerical cellular changes observed during aging. It has been demonstrated that GC-induced apoptosis on monocytes is at least partially mediated by the expression of both CD95 and CD95L (Schmidt et al. 2001). Another study showed that glucocorticoids may either induce T-cell apoptosis in a CD95-independent manner, or protect T-cells from CD95-mediated apoptosis (Zipp et al. 2000). Furthermore, there is some evidence that psychological stress may regulate the proportion of peripheral lymphocytes via the expression of CD95. It has been demonstrated that chronic stress may induce lymphocyte apoptosis in mice (Yin et al. 2000) or in man (Oka et al. 1996) via upregulation of CD95. Our results support the concept that age- or stress-related increase in cortisol levels may be preferentially altering the expression of CD95 on CD45RA+ cells. Preliminary data from our laboratory indicate that human CD45RA+CD95+ cells are in fact more sensitive to dexamethasone (DEX) treatment in vitro(unpublished results). There is some data suggesting that human naïve T CD4+ cells are more sensitive to DEX than memory T CD4+ cells (Nijhuis et al. 1995). Overall, our results suggest that there are complex psychoneuroendocrine interactions involved with the regulation of the peripheral pool of lymphocytes. In particular, it was shown that both psychological stress and GCs synergize during aging to produce alterations in T-cell trafficking.

4.2   Changes in Innate Immunity—Focus on DCs

To date, the effects of stress or aging on dendritic cells (DC) are largely unknown. These professional antigen presenting cells play a determinant role on the interface between innate and adaptive immunity (Steinman 2003). They sense pathogens through a myriad of toll-like receptors, endocytose them and produce immune mediators that lead to inflammation, such as TNF-α and nitric oxide (NO). They also secrete cytokines that are key to the development of specific, adaptive responses, such as type I interferons (IFN-α and $-\beta$), and IL-12. DC process antigens from pathogens and present them to T-cells and the concentration of antigen, the magnitude of co-stimulatory signals such as CD86 delivered, together with the cytokines produced, set up the stage for T-cell responses. Antigen presentation by mature DC leads to the initiation of immune responses, and the predominant cytokines produced can skew the response towards a TH1 or TH2 phenotype (Banchereau et al. 2000). Presentation by immature DC, however, can result in tolerance, in some situations even leading to the recruitment of regulatory, CD4+CD25+Foxp3+ T-cells (Luo et al. 2007; Yamazaki et al. 2006). Thus, DC play a fundamental regulatory role in immunity.

An intriguing aspect of dendritic cell biology is the existence of different subpopulations (Vremec and Shortman 1997). These can be distinguished by the expression of different surface markers, are distributed in different body compartments, and possess different functions. Also, some are derived from distinct precursors. Basically, both in human and mice, two subpopulations can be identified; tissue derived, and blood derived cells. Tissue derived DC include Langerhans cells (LC) and interstitial cells, that respectively reside in skin and tissues. They capture antigen in the periphery and migrate to lymph nodes, to interact with other DC and T-cells. Blood derived DC are replenished in lymphoid organs from the blood, and are generally designated as plasmacytoid (important for anti-viral immunity-(Banchereau et al. 2000), myeloid or lymphoid, these latter ones apparently responsible for cross-presentation (the ability to present endocytosed antigens in MHC Class I molecules—(Brossart and Bevan 1997). DC can be derived in vitro directly from bone marrow precursors (Inaba et al. 1992) and also from circulating monocytes, although the cells that arise from these cultures do not directly correspond to the same populations identified in vivo. Because so little is known about antigen presentation and T-cell activation by each subpopulation, it is important to identify the effects of stress on different DC populations, as well as how that relates to immunosenescence.

Probably, the most studied effect of chronic stress over dendritic cell function is the modulatory function of glucocorticoids. For example, in vitro studies show that murine bone marrow differentiated DC treated with DEX show downregulation of the costimulatory molecules CD86, CD40, CD54, as well as of MHC Class II, but not MHC Class I, molecules (Pan et al. 2001). This study also verified a decreased capacity of MHC class II presentation of antigens, but not of endocytic activity for DEX treated DC, and a reduction on their production of interleukin (IL)-1β and IL-12. It has also been reported that glucocorticoids can downregulate the production of TNF-α and IL-12, but not IL-10, by DC, and thus are able to affect skew T-cell responses towards a TH2 phenotype (Elenkov et al. 2000). Studies with glucocorticoids applied to skin in vivo for 7 days showed a reduction in the number of LC in situ, as well as a reduction in expression of costimulatory molecules, leading to reduced alloreactive stimulatory capacity (Ashworth et al. 1988). Accordingly, in transplant models, DEX has been shown to affect differentiation and reduce costimulatory function of DC (Abe and Thomson 2003) suppressing MHC Class II and CD86 expression (Muller et al. 2002), and consequently DC maturation in vitro. In the same study, treatment with DEX during graft procedure reduced DC, as well as T-cell, infiltration on the graft.

There are very few studies on DC function in experimental systems of psychological stress. One study found that the increase in corticosterone levels correlated with decreased processing of viral antigens and their presentation in MHC Class I molecules, leading to decreased antiviral immune responses (Truckenmiller et al. 2005). Their results pointed to an effect over the processing machinery of all cells, suggesting stress can profoundly affect the protein processing pathways. Finally, glucocorticoids can induce natural anti-inflammatory cells through DC. Studies with bone marrow derived DCs showed that glucocorticoids can not only impair development of immature DC into mature DC, but also that multiple restimulation of CD4+ T-cells with DEX treated DC can lead to the expansion of T-cells with the regulatory phenotype (CD4+CD25+) (Matyszak et al. 2000), which are vital for the control of inflammation and autoimmunity in vivo.

Curiously, DHEA and DEX appear to have somewhat opposing effects over the differentiation of dendritic cells from monocyte precursors. The only study comparing the 2 hormones (Canning et al. 2000) showed that continuous presence of DHEA on dendritic cell cultures from monocytes in the presence of GM-CSF and IL-4 leads to the accumulation of immature DC, although markers like CD80 or CD40 are only slightly altered compared to the control. Cultures of monocytes in the same conditions, only continuously supplemented with DEX, however, leads to their differentiation into macrophage-like cells, with high CD14 expression, and low surface CD80 and CD40, with almost no IL-12, but high IL-10 production.

Aging has been associated with similar changes in DC function. While some report no changes in surface expression of MHC Class II and CD86 in aged in vitro monocyte-derived DC (Agrawal et al. 2007b) or in vivo DC (Lung et al. 2000), others have observed a markedly reduced expression of HLA-DR (Pietschmann et al. 2000) for monocyte enriched, lymphocyte depleted peripheral blood cells of aged subjects. Also, the numbers of LC in gingival epithelium (Zavala and Cavicchia 2006) or and skin (Bhushan et al. 2002) appear to be diminished in aged individuals. A normal TNF-α and IL-12 production by monocytes-derived DC from aged subjects was reported (Lung et al. 2000), but an increased TNF-α and IL-6 response to LPS was found by others (Agrawal et al. 2007a), as well as a decreased migratory and phagocytic capacity. Monocyte-derived DC from elderly individuals were not impaired in their ability to induce T-cell responses (Grewe 2001) or proliferation of T-cell lines (Steger et al. 1997). However, the efficacy of autologous DC-based antitumor vaccines was impaired in aged individuals (Sharma et al. 2006).

In our laboratory, we compared the effects of stress induced glucocorticoids and aging on the differentiation of bone marrow derived DCs. Results are shown in Fig. 2. After seven days of culture with IL-4 and GM-CSF (Inaba et al. 1992), murine bone marrow cells consistently yield three distinct populations of DC, as determined by MHC Class II and CD86 expression (Fig. 2). The population in the upper right quadrant of the plots (Class II hi, CD86 hi) represents the mature DC, while the population in the middle (Class II lo, CD86 lo) contains the immature DC. The population in the bottom left quadrant is negative for both markers and has not yet started to differentiate. Bone marrow cultures from 6 month old mice yielded precisely these populations (in A and C). However, treatments with 10^{-7} M DEX (B) on day 5 of culture lead to an arrest of dendritic cell differentiation, leaving the cells mostly at the immature stage. A similar pattern was observed in D, when bone marrow of a 2 year old mouse was cultured in the same conditions as A and C. Consequently, aged bone marrow produced mostly immature DC.

Together, these results consistently point to an inhibitory effect of stress, aging and glucocorticoids over DC function. They also suggest that these GCs can affect immunoregulation, modulating the TH1/TH2 decision and also leading to the generation of regulatory T-cells. These are pleiotropic effects, and it is likely that a variety of mechanisms is involved.

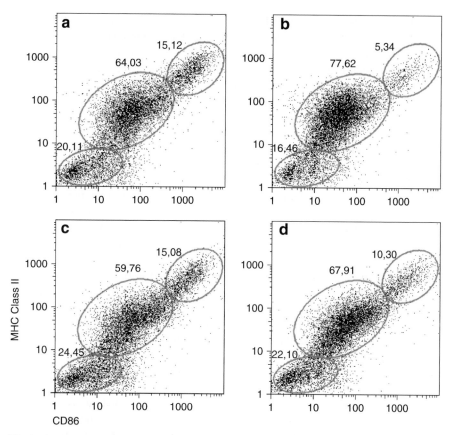

Fig. 2 Dexamethasone and aging lead to an arrest in the maturation phenotype of DC. Bone marrow cells from young (6 months: A, B and C) or aged (2 year old:D) mice were cultured in vitro with IL-4 and GM-CSF. In C, 10^{-7}M dexamethasone was added to the cultures on day 5. Numbers represent the percentages of gated populations.

4.3 Changes in Cell-mediated Immunity

Although many components of the immune system show age-related changes, T-cells show most consistent and largest alterations. T-cells are of pivotal importance for the generation of cell-mediated immunity. Cell-mediated immunity is a process that requires (1) recognition of antigens, (2) cell activation and proliferation, and (3) effector functions such as cellular cytotoxicity, phagocytosis, and immunoglobulin synthesis. Steps 2 and 3 seem to be particularly impaired during aging. Following antigen recognition, lymphocytes need to divide into several clones in order to mount effective cell-mediated immune responses. Cell division or proliferation can be readily assessed in vitroby stimulating lymphocytes with mitogens. When diseased subjects are excluded, immunosenescence involves impaired humoral responses and blunted T-cell proliferation to mitogens (Pawelec et al. 2002). The latter is one of the most documented age-related change observed during aging (Liu et al. 1997; Murasko et al. 1987). Yet, these changes are not exclusive of aging and stress or GC treatment are also associated with decrements of T-cell proliferation) (see Table 2). Indeed, we have observed that healthy SENIEUR elders were signifi-cantly more distressed, had activated HPA axis and had significant lower (-53.6%) T-cell proliferation compared to young adults (Luz et al. 2006) (Fig. 2). Interest-ingly, the HPA axis may be implicated with this change since salivary cortisol levels were found negatively correlated to T-cell proliferation.

Thymic involution is a common consequence of mammal aging and it precedes the malfunctioning of the immune system, resulting in a diminished capacity to gen-erate new T-cells. This thymic involution has been proposed to be due to changes in the thymic microenvironment resulting in its failure to support thymopoiesis (Henson et al. 2004). However, stress-related GCs (Selye 1936) or GC treatment (Fauci 1975) also atrophy the thymus and, to a lesser extent, other lymphoid tissues, triggering apoptotic death in immature T- and B-cell precursors and mature T-cells (Sapolsky et al. 2000). Therefore, thymic involution is not an exclusive phenom-enon of aging.

The effector phases of both innate and acquired immunity are in large part medi-ated by cytokines. Different subpopulations of CD4+ T-cells synthesize specific cytokines and have been designated Th1 (IFN-g, IL-2, lymphotoxin a) or Th2 (IL-4, IL-10) cells. Th1 cytokines provide help for cell-mediated responses and the IgG2a antibody class switching whereas Th2 cytokines help B cells and IgA, IgE and IgG1 antibody class switching. Both human and mouse models have demonstrated that aging is associated with a Th1 to Th2 shift in cytokine production (Ginaldi et al. 2001; Globerson and Effros 2000). However, this is not an age-specific phenom-enon but also seen during stress (Biondi 2001; Glaser et al. 2001) or GC treatment (Galon et al. 2002; Ramirez et al. 1996).

Recent work suggests that cytokines and hormones could be considered as possible links between endocrinosenescence and immunosenescence (Straub et al. 2000). Indeed, it has long been known that proinflammatory cytokines can readily activate the HPA axis during infection in animals (Besedovsky et al. 1977) or after administration in humans (Mastorakos et al. 1993). Another studies have linked the

Table 2 Changes in cell-mediated immunity. Direction of arrows indicate increase (⇧), decrease (⇩) or no change (⇔) compared to corresponding control levels. Based on references (Biondi 2001; Galon et al. 2002; Globerson and Effros 2000; Ramirez et al. 1996; Sapolsky et al. 2000)

Mechanism	Aging	Stress	GC treatment
Thymus	⇩	⇩	⇩
T-cell proliferation	⇩	⇩	⇩
Cytotoxicity	⇩	⇩	⇩
IL-2, IFN-γ	⇩	⇩	⇩
IL-4, IL-10	⇧	⇧	⇧
TNF-α, IL-1, IL-6	⇧ or ⇔	⇧	⇩

age-related decline in DHEA production to increased serum levels of IL-6 (Daynes et al. 1993; Straub et al. 1998). In addition, increased plasma TNF-α levels were correlated to major depression in the elderly (Vetta et al. 2001). However, we do not know exactly how the extent of these changes may be related to altered psychological and HPA axis functions in the elderly.

We have investigated whether psychoneuroendocrine status of healthy elders was associated with changes in lipopolysaccharide (LPS)-induced monocyte production of proinflammatory cytokines (TNF-α and IL-6) and soluble IL-2 receptor (sIL-2Ra) production by T-cells in vitro(Luz et al. 2003). Cellsofhealthyelders produced equivalent proinflammatory cytokines and soluble IL-2Rα when compared to cells of young adults. These data are in disagreement with previous work showing that human aging was associated to increased serum (Straub et al. 1998) or monocyte proinflammatory cytokines (Fagiolo et al. 1993; Gabriel et al. 2002). However, these data should be interpreted with caution because other cellular sources than monocytes can produce cytokines and thus increase serum levels. Considering that our cohort of elderly subjects was significantly distressed, we hypothesize this could have normalized the cytokines investigated in this study—due to antiinflammatory GC actions. On the other hand, there is also some evidence of increased proinflammatory cytokines during major depression (Schiepers et al. 2005; Trzonkowski et al. 2004; Vetta et al. 2001). Therefore, it becomes difficult to dissociate the cytokine changes observed in the elderly with those induced by psychological stimuli. Ghrelin, an endogenous ligand of the GH secretagogue receptor, has been recently demonstrated to inhibit the expression and production of proinflammatory cytokines (TNF-α, IL-1β and IL-6) (Dixit et al. 2004). This effect was mediated via binding on ghrelin receptors expressed on peripheral T-cells and monocytes. There is some evidence for increased stomach ghrelin production in the aged rat (Englander et al. 2004). Increased peripheral ghrelin levels may thus attenuate cytokine levels during aging. It remains to be investigated, however, whether psychological stress is capable of producing significant effects on stomach or immunoreactive ghrelin levels.

Previous studies have long demonstrated that serum growth hormone (hGH) levels are significantly reduced during aging (Corpas et al. 1993)—a process known as somatosenescence. However, hGH is not exclusively produced by pituitary gland and human immune cells are able to secrete several neuropeptides including GH (Hattori et al. 1994; Weigent et al. 1988). Immunoreactive GH has several immuno-enhancing proprieties and may be important in modulating both humoral and cellular immune function (Malarkey et al. 2002; Weigent et al. 1988). However, there is no data on the impact of aging on the production of GH by immune cells. In a recent study, we investigated whether somatosenescence could be associated with (a) related reduced production of immunoreactive GH and (b) psychological status of healthy SENIEUR elderly subjects (Luz et al. 2006). We found that elders had significantly lower (77%) serum hGH levels compared to young adults. In contrast, however, no changes in hGH production by activated monocytes or lymphocytes were observed between elders and adults (Luz et al. 2006). Interestingly, psychological distress (stress, anxiety and depression) was found negatively correlated to serum hGH levels only. No differences in serum hGH levels were observed between groups when controlling for psychological variables (partial correlation). We provided first line of evidence that age-related psychological distress may be implicated with somatosenescence. Finally, somatosenescence was not associated with reciprocal decline in immunoreactive GH.

5   Role of DHEA During Immunosenescence

The lack of appropriate DHEAS levels during aging could be another detrimental factor for immunosenescence. This androgen and its metabolites have reported immune enhancing properties in contrast to the immunosuppressive action of GCs. Indeed, this hormone may be considered as natural antagonist of GCs and the impaired DHEA secretion, together with the increase of cortisol, results in an enhanced exposure of lymphoid cells to the deleterious GC actions. Therefore, previous studies have evaluated the immunomodulatory DHEA(S) effects in vitroas well as its properties during in vivosupplementation. The immunomodulatory in vitroeffects include increased mitogen-stimulated IL-2 production (Daynes et al. 1990; Suzuki et al. 1991), increased rodent or human lymphocyte proliferation (Padgett and Loria 1994), stimulated monocyte-mediated cytotoxicity (McLachlan et al. 1996), diminished TNFa or IL-6 production (Di Santo et al. 1996; Straub et al. 1998) and enhanced natural killer cell activity (Solerte et al. 1999).

DHEA(S) replacement therapy has yielded significant beneficial effects for healthy elders, including increased well-being, memory performance, bone mineral density and altered immune function (Buvat 2003). It has been shown that DHEA supplementation significantly increased NK-cell counts and activity and decreased IL-6 production and T-cell proliferation of the elderly (Casson et al. 1993). These data highlight the potential use of DHEA(S) as antiaging hormone. However, there is lacking information concerning the clinical significance of those findings.

Because of its enhanced immunomodulatory properties, several studies investigated the potential of DHEA(S) as adjuvants in vaccine preparations. Initial studies reported increased adjuvant effects on the immunization of aged mice with recombinant Hepatitis B surface antigen (Araneo et al. 1993) or influenza (Danenberg et al. 1995). These studies reported increased antibody titers to vaccines or even effective protection against challenge with the influenza infection (Danenberg et al. 1995). More recently, we studied the adjuvant effects of DHEAS during immunization to *Mycobaterium tuberculosis* in mice (Ribeiro et al. 2007). Only young mice co-immunized with *M. tuberculosis* heat shock protein 70 (HSP70) and DHEAS showed an early increase in specific IgG levels compared to old mice. However, splenocytes of both young and old mice that received DHEAS showed increased IFN-g production following priming in vitro with HSP70. These data further highlight the importance of DHEAS as hormonal adjuvant because of the role of this cytokine in the cellular response against mycobacteria. However, these animal data are in contrast to previous studies reporting DHEA(S) with minor (Degelau et al. 1997) or no adjuvant effects (Ben-Yehuda et al. 1998; Danenberg et al. 1997; Evans et al. 1996) during immunization to influenza or tetanus in human elderly populations. Therefore, extrapolation from studies on murine models to the human should be regarded with caution—especially because of lower circulating DHEA(S) levels in rodents.

6 Aging Impairs Neuroendocrine-Immunoregulation

Most GC effects on the immune system are mediated via intracellular GC receptors (GR; genomic action) (McEwen et al. 1997). However, high concentration of GCs may also interact with membrane binding sites at the surface of the cells (nongenomic action) (Gold et al. 2001). The presence of these receptors indicates that the immune system is prepared for HPA axis activation and the subsequent elevation in endogenous GCs. However, the functional effect of a stress hormone will depend on the sensitivity of the target tissue for that particular hormone. For instance, the number and activity of specific receptors for these signaling molecules on the target organ will ultimately direct the physiologic effect of the stressor.

Recent findings suggest that GC sensitivity (a) may vary between different target tissues in the same organism, (b) shows large individual differences and (c) can be acutely changed in times of acute stress (Hearing et al. 1999; Rohleder et al. 2003). Furthermore and of special interest of this review, (d) GC sensitivity also changes during human ontogeny. Kavelaars and col. (1996) have shown that cord blood T-cells of newborns appear to be extremely sensitive to inhibition of the proliferative response. This high sensitivity of cells to DEX) can still be observed in the first two weeks after birth. Subsequently, the sensitivity to DEX inhibition of T-cell proliferation gradually decreases. At one year of age, the adult response pattern has been acquired. It is interesting that the increased sensitivity of the immune system to GC inhibition occurs at a period in life when the endogenous levels of glucocorticoids are low (Sippell et al. 1978). The increased sensitivity to glucocorticoids may serve as a compensatory mechanism, so that the important regulatory function of glucocorticoids is fully maintained despite low circulating levels.

In a recent study, we have also investigated the lymphocyte sensitivity to both synthetic (DEX) and natural occurring steroids (cortisol and DHEA) and so examined whether aging was associated with alterations in neuroendocrine-immunoregulation (Luz et al. 2006). It was found that healthy (SENIEUR) elders had a reduced (-19%) in vitrolymphocyte sensitivity to DEX (but not cortisol or DHEA) when compared to young adults. This phenomenon has previously been described during chronic stress (Bauer et al. 2000; Rohleder et al. 2002), major depression (Bauer et al. 2002; Bauer et al. 2003; Truckenmiller et al. 2005) or in clinical situations where GCs are administered, including treatment of autoimmune diseases, organ transplantation, and allergies. It has been recently shown (Rohleder et al. 2002) that aging is associated with changes in GC sensitivity of proinflammatory cytokine (TNF-α and IL-6) production following psychosocial (TRIER) stress test (Kirschbaum et al. 1993). In particular, monocytes of healthy (non-SENIEUR) elderly men had a higher sensitivity to DEX treatment in vitroat baseline and showed a reduced sensitivity to this steroid following acute stress exposure (speech coupled to mental arithmetic task). These data suggest that psychological factors may be implicated in regulating peripheral GC sensitivity during healthy aging.

A reduced sensitivity to GCs can also be demonstrated at the central level during aging. Indeed, higher cortisol levels in old than in young subjects have been described during some pharmacological challenges, such as the DEX suppression test, the stimulation by human or ovine corticotrophin-releasing hormone or by physostigmine (Ferrari et al. 2001; Raskind et al. 1994).

6.1   Potential Mechanisms of Impaired GC Signaling

The mechanisms underlying acquired steroid resistance are poorly understood. Based on our previous observations (Luz et al. 2003) we suggest that higher cortisol levels would render lymphocytes to be less sensitive to the effects of GCs in vitro. Indeed, there is some evidence in the literature suggesting that changes in GC sensitivity could be the result of chronic GC treatment (de Kloet et al. 1998; Silva et al. 1994). Several mechanisms may be implicated in this acquired steroid resistance (Juruena et al. 2003; Rohleder et al. 2003). Fig. 3 summarizes putative molecular mechanisms that may account for age-related changes in GC sensitivity. There is some evidence that aging is associated with reduced numbers of intracellular GRs (Grasso et al. 1997; Zovato et al. 1996) but changes in GR affinity cannot be ruled out. In addition, altered translocation of GC/GR complex to nucleus and altered acti vity of transcription factors may also explain acquired GC resistance. Alternatively, it has been shown that a non-ligand binding β-isoform of the human GR (hGRβ) may also be implicated in acquired steroid resistance (Castro et al. 1996). It was hypothesized that the hGRβ probably heterodimerises with ligand-bound hGRα and translocates into the nucleus to act as a dominant negative inhibitor of the classic receptor. However, there is no evidence for age-related changes in expression of GR isoforms. Furthermore, we cannot exclude the participation of mutations in the GR or changes in the GR transduction system (e.g., altered AP-1 and NF-kB expression, heat shock proteins) in promoting tissue sensitivity to glucocorticoids (reviewed in Bronnegard et al. 1996).

In addition, there is considerable evidence that cytokines may have a significant impact on GR expression and function. There is some evidence suggesting that local concentrations of cytokines produced during an inflammatory response may produce acquired GR resistance (Pariante et al. 1999a). Of note, the GR resistance in major depression has been associated with increased levels of proinflammatory cytokines (TNF-α, IL-1 and IL-6) and acute phase proteins (Maes et al. 1993; Schiepers et al. 2005; Trzonkowski et al. 2004). Furthermore, it has recently been shown that IL-13, a cytokine with similar properties to IL-4, reduces GR binding affinity in peripheral blood mononuclear cells (PBMCs) (Spahn et al. 1996). In summary, various mechanisms may mediate age-related changes in immune GC signaling, however, further research is required to fully understand the basis of the changes in altered lymphocyte sensitivity to steroid.

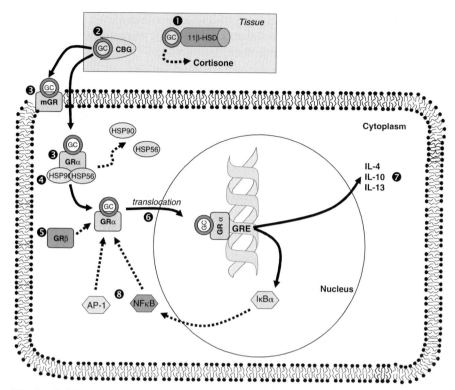

Fig. 3 Cellular sensitivity to glucocorticoids. Extracellular hormone availability can be determined by (1) differential expression of tissue-dependent expression of 11β-hydroxysteroid dehydrogenases that catalyze the interconversion of active glucocorticoids (cortisol) to inactive forms (cortisone) and vice versa (Zhang et al. 2005); and (2) levels of plasma corticosterone binding globulin (CBG) which delivers biologically active glucocorticoids (GCs) into peripheral tissues. Intracellular sensitivity to glucocorticoids can be modulated by several mechanisms, including: (3) altered densities of functional membrane or intracellular glucocorticoid receptor (GRα) as well as receptor affinity changes (Pereira et al. 2003); (4) altered expression of heat shock proteins (HSP90 and HSP56) which stabilizes GR and are dissociated following binding of GCs (Picard et al. 1990); (5) altered expression of GRβ which in turn antagonises GRα (Castro et al. 1996); (6) altered translocation of GR-GC complexes into the nucleus (Matthews et al. 2004); (7) altered expression of several cytokines (Kam et al. 1993; Pariante et al. 1999b); and (8) altered expression of transcription factors AP-1 (Adcock et al. 1995) and NFkB which in turn antagonise GRα. Dashed lines represent inhibitory actions on GRα Adapted from Bauer (2005).

7 The Impact of Chronic Stress on Strictly Healthy Aging— Damaging and Protecting Effects

The caregiving of demented patients is a recognized model to study the impact of chronic stress in elderly populations (Bauer et al. 2000; Kiecolt-Glaser et al. 1991; Vedhara et al. 1999). Care of the chronically ill is a demanding task that is associated with increased stress, depression, and poorer immune function (Redinbaugh et al. 1995). Furthermore, providing care for a relative with dementia typically falls on the partners who are themselves elderly and often ill prepared for the physical and emotional demands placed upon them.

The daily stress experienced by the caregivers of Alzheimer patients may accelerate many age-related changes, particularly on neuroendocrine and immune systems. We have previously demonstrated that caregivers of demented patients had a blunted T-cell proliferation in association with increased cortisol levels (Bauer et al. 2000) compared to nonstressed elders. Furthermore, lymphocytes of elderly caregivers were more resistant to GC treatment in vitrocompared to noncaregiver elders. When stressed elderly are compared to healthy elderly and young adults (see Fig. 4), these immunological changes are found in similar magnitude to increased cortisol levels. These data suggest that chronic stress and cortisol would thus accelerate human immunosenescence. Indeed, it has recently been observed that psychological stress (both perceived stress and chronicity of stress) was significantly associated with higher oxidative stress, lower telomerase activity, and shorter telomere length, which are known determinants of cell senescence and longevity (Epel et al. 2004).

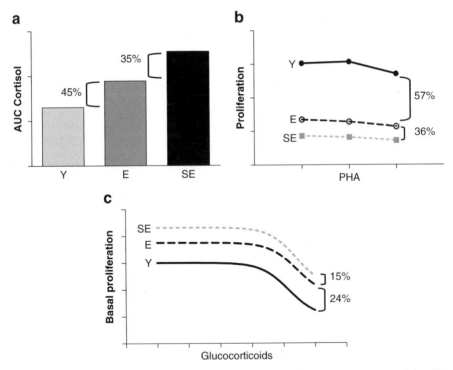

Fig. 4 Effects of chronic stress on cortisol and T-cell function during aging. Young adults (Y), elderly (E) or stressed elderly (SE) subjects were compared accordingly to area under the curve (AUC) cortisol production (A), T-cell proliferation to phytohemagglutinin(PHA) stimulation (B) or T-cell sensitivity to glucocorticoids in vitro(C). Data summarized from previous work (Bauer et al. 2000; Luz et al. 2003; Luz et al. 2002) and shown as the percentage of change between groups. Adapted from Bauer (2005).

Several studies have implicated caregiving as a risk factor for health of elderly populations. Compared with noncaregivers, subjects who provide care to a spouse with a stroke or dementia report more infectious illness episodes (Kiecolt-Glaser et al. 1991), they have poorer immune responses to influenza virus (Kiecolt-Glaser et al. 1996; Vedhara et al. 1999) and pneumococcal pneumonia vaccines (Glaser et al. 2000), they present a slow wound healing (Kiecolt-Glaser et al. 1995), they are at greater risk for developing mild hypertension (Shaw et al. 1999), and they may be at greater risk for coronary heart disease (Vitaliano et al. 2002). In addition, a prospective longitudinal study found that the relative risk for mortality among caregivers was significantly higher (63%) than noncaregiving controls (Schulz and Beach 1999). A recent study indicates that a proinflammatory cytokine (IL-6) may be involved with this increased morbidity in caregiving populations (Kiecolt-Glaser et al. 2003). It remains to be investigated, however, how the extent of these changes may be related to neuroendocrine alterations observed during aging.

Recent data produced by our laboratory have suggested that the maintenance of health status during aging may protect elders from chronic stress exposure. We have recruited strictly healthy (SENIEUR) elderly caregivers (n=41) from a large population of primary caregivers of demented patients (n=342). Only 12% of caregivers were considered "strictly healthy" accordingly to this stringent protocol and this may further confirm that chronic stress exposure is associated with increased morbidity in elderly populations. Therefore, we investigated whether a stringent health status would protect caregivers from chronic stress exposure and compared psychoneuroendocrine and immunological changes to nonstressed controls.

We observed that SENIEUR elderly caregivers were significantly distressed, as shown by increased stress, anxiety and depression scores as well as by higher systolic blood pressure compared to nonstressed elders (unpublished data). These data provide further support for this chronic stress model. However, salivary cortisol levels remained unchanged in healthy caregivers compared to nonstressed elders, contrasting to previous work (Bauer et al. 2000). Indeed, previous studies have linked the stress-related hypercortisolemia with blunted cellular and humoral immune responses (Bauer et al. 2000; Vedhara et al. 1999). This could be of beneficial value for the caregiver and may indicate that a stringent health status in the elderly can buffer the impact of chronic stress on neuroendocrine responses. Therefore, healthy caregivers would be protected from the deleterious effects of cortisol excess in the organism. The normalization of HPA axis function could be related to endocrine habituation associated to the development of coping strategies, cognitive and learning skills (Huether 1996). These results, taken together with our previous studies with nonstressed SENIEUR elders, may further indicate that a stringent health status may protect individuals from stress exposure but not from age-related increase in salivary cortisol (Luz et al. 2003). The peripheral lymphoid cells could be spared from the increased and deleterious cortisol signaling normally observed during chronic stress exposure.

The SENIEUR caregivers had increased T-cell proliferation when compared nonstressed healthy controls (unpublished data). We speculate that the intact HPA axis function may have spared the lymphocytes from the negative effects of cortisol excess. Peripheral lymphocytes of caregivers are thus expected to display a better GC signaling. Indeed, the lymphocytes of SENIEUR caregivers had a higher GC sensitivity when compared to non-stressed controls, as shown by the increased GC-induced suppression of lymphocyte proliferation in vitro(unpublished data). These data further highlight the close communication of neuroendocrine and immune systems during aging. In contrast to increased peripheral GC-immune signaling, the healthy caregivers were more resistant to central effects of glucocorticoids. Indeed, there were a higher proportion of SENIEUR caregivers (29.3%) who had failure to suppress cortisol levels through dexamethasone administration comparing to nonstressed controls (3%). The dexamethasone suppression test suggests that caregivers may have a dysfunction of the HPA axis related to chronic stress exposure but not to peripheral GC levels. These data are in partial contrast to previous work relating hypercortisolemia to reduced lymphocyte sensitivity to GCs in elderly British caregivers (Bauer et al. 2000). However, the central defect in HPA axis regulation may not necessarily be associated to endogenous GC levels since previous studies reported this change in patients with major depression without hypercortisolemia (Bauer et al. 2003).

Taken together, these results suggest that a strictly healthy (SENIEUR) aging may buffer or attenuate many deleterious neuroendocrine and immunological effects associated to chronic stress exposure.

8   The Psychoneuroendocrine Hypothesis of Immunosenescence

The studies reviewed here support the notion that immunological changes observed during healthy aging may be closely related to both psychological distress and stress hormones. Of note, changes cellular trafficking as well as cell-mediated immunity observed during aging are similarly found following stress or chronic GC exposure. These changes are mainly produced via engagement of specific intracellular adrenal receptors expressed on peripheral lymphocytes. Based on these data, the neuroendocrine hypothesis of immunosenescence is reconsidered here (see Fig. 5). During aging, cumulative neuronal damage produced by stress-related cortisol action in the brain (hippocampus and hypothalamus) is associated with decreased central sensitivity to cortisol (Ferrari et al. 2001; Raskind et al. 1994; Sapolsky et al. 1986). This will lead to increased cortisol levels (Deuschle et al. 1997; Ferrari et al. 2004; Halbreich et al. 1984; Heuser et al. 1998; Luz et al. 2003; Van Cauter et al. 1996) which in turn may produce more neuronal damage in the brain and promote thymic involution. These effects may be exacerbated by reduced DHEA/DHEAS levels frequently observed during aging. The impaired DHEAS secretion, together with the increase of cortisol, results in an enhanced exposure of various bodily systems (including brain and immune system) to the cytotoxic/immunomodulatory effects of GCs. These tissues are preferentially targeted by cumulative cortisol action because they express the greatest densities of MRs (hippocampus) and GRs (thymus) (McEwen et al. 1997). The critical consequence of thymic involution is reduced output of naïve T-cells—a hallmark of immunosenescence. It remains to be investigated, however, why peripheral T-cells are preferentially targeted during aging comparing to B or NK-cells. It

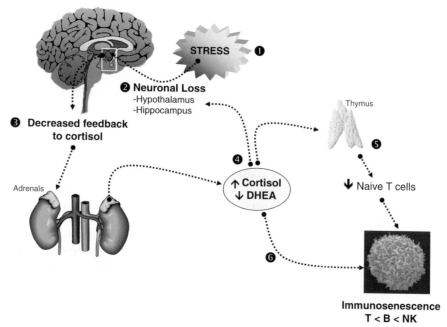

Fig. 5 The psychoneuroendocrine hypothesis of immunosenescence. During aging, cumulative neuronal damage produced by stress-related cortisol action in the brain (1 and 2) (Sapolsky et al. 1986) is associated with decreased central sensitivity to cortisol (3) (Ferrari et al. 2001; Raskind et al. 1994). This specific effect is associated with increased cortisol/DHEA ratio (4) (Ferrari et al. 2004; Luz et al. 2003) which in turn may produce more neuronal damage in the brain and further promote thymic involution (5). The latter may be related to immunosenescence via two ways: (a) indirectly reducing the output of central naïve T-cells and (b) directly acting at the level of peripheral lymphoid cells (6)(Luz et al. 2006). Adapted from Bauer (2005).

should be kept in mind this hypothesis is over simplistic and do not take into account other stress-related mediators (neuropeptides, noadrealine, GH, etc.) and intrinsic cellular mechanisms of aging, including oxidative stress and telomere shortening. Further studies are required to investigate whether cellular aging is associated with aging of neuroendocrine functions. In addition, the role of increased cortisol/DHEA ratio during immunosenescence may be over simplistic since many other important hormones also become lower during aging in relation to cortisol (Straub et al. 2001).

9 Conclusions and Outlook

When age-related diseases are controlled for, healthy aging is associated with changes in allostatic systems (endocrine and immune) that play major roles in the adaptation of organism to outside forces that are threatening the homeostasis of the internal milieu. In particular, healthy aging is associated with significant psychological distress and activation of the HPA axis (increased cortisol and reduced DHEA).

Over weeks, months, or years, exposure to increased secretion of stress hormones would result in allostatic load ("wear and tear") and its pathophysiologic consequences (McEwen 1998). Given the findings that even discrete HPA axis activation may impair cognitive function (Lupien et al. 1994) and induce sleep disturbances (Starkman et al. 1981), conditions frequently associated in the elderly, psychological or pharmacological strategies attenuating or preventing increased HPA function during aging might be of considerable benefit for the elderly.

Although the mechanisms underlying immunosenescence are still being unraveled, it is becoming increasingly clear that many of the physiologic changes associated with aging are characterized by deficient communication between neuroendocrine and immune systems. Data presented here suggest that aging is associated with reduced lymphocyte sensitivity to GCs. Glucocorticoid-induced acquired resistance may have an important physiological significance of protecting cells from the dangerous effects of prolonged GC-related immunosuppression. However, the significance of this adaptive phenomenon is questionable since T-cell proliferation is still profoundly suppressed during aging. Additionally, altered steroid immunoregulation may have important therapeutic implications in clinical situations where GCs are administered, including treatment of autoimmune diseases, organ transplantation, and allergies. Clinicians should consider both patient's age and psychological status in prescribing steroids as anti-inflammatory drugs.

Chronic stressed elderly subjects may be particularly at risk of stress-related pathology because of further alterations in GC-immune signaling. Elderly individuals who experience chronic stress exhibit poorer immune functions, and thus increased disease vulnerability, than their less stressed counterparts. Indeed, chronic stressed elderly populations are associated with increased morbidity and mortality rates. Therefore, stress management and psychosocial support should promote a better quality of life for the elderly as well as reducing hospitalization costs for the governments. In addition, the maintenance of health status during aging may protect elders from chronic stress exposure (Fig. 6). Further studies in systems biology are needed to analyze the role and relationships of health-related behaviors on immunity that might promote better coping with aging and stress exposure. We are currently entering a new era of investigation in biology of aging in which systemic approach will replace reductionism in order to explain how we age and get sick.

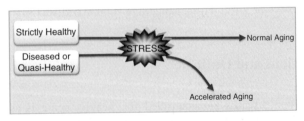

Fig. 6 Buffering effects of health status during chronic stress exposure. This picture presents two different scenarios of protective (upper line) or damaging (bottom line) stress-related effects during aging. Strictly healthy individuals will be protected from chronic stress and will have extended life span. Diseased or quasi-healthy subjects, however, will show accelerated aging.

Acknowledgments This study was supported by grants from CNPq (M.E.B, #470747/2006-4 and #305155/2006-7).

References

Abe M and Thomson AW (2003) Influence of immunosuppressive drugs on dendritic cells. Transpl Immunol 11:357–365

Adcock IM, Lane SJ, Brown CR, Lee TH and Barnes PJ (1995) Abnormal glucocorticoid receptor-activator protein 1 interaction in steroid-resistant asthma. J Exp Med 182:1951–1958

Agrawal A, Agrawal S, Cao JN, Su H, Osann K and Gupta S (2007a) Altered innate immune functioning of dendritic cells in elderly humans: a role of phosphoinositide 3-kinase-signaling pathway. J Immunol 178:6912–6922

Agrawal A, Agrawal S and Gupta S (2007b) Dendritic cells in human aging. Exp Gerontol 42:421–426

Araneo B, Woods M and Daynes R (1993) Reversal of the immunosenescent phenotype by dehydroepiandrosterone: hormone treatment provides an adjuvant effect on the immunization of aged mice with recombinant hepatitis B surface antigen. J Infect Dis 167:830–840

Ashworth J, Booker J and Breathnach SM (1988) Effects of topical corticosteroid therapy on Langerhans cell antigen presenting function in human skin. Br J Dermatol 118:457–69

Bancherau J, Briere F, Caux C, Davoust J, Lebecque S, Liu YJ, Pulendran B and Palucka K (2000) Immunobiology of dendritic cells. Annu Rev Immunol 18:767–811

Bauer ME (2005) Stress, glucocorticoids and ageing of the immune system. Stress 8:69–83

Bauer ME, Papadopoulos A, Poon L, Perks P, Lightman S, Checkley S and Shanks N (2002) Dexamethasone-induced effects on lymphocyte distribution and expression of adhesion molecules in treatment resistant major depression. Psychiatry Res 113:1–15

Bauer ME, Papadopoulos A, Poon L, Perks P, Lightman S, Checkley S and Shanks N (2003) Altered glucocorticoid immunoregulation in treatment resistant depression. Psychoneuroendocrinology 28:49–65

Bauer ME, Vedhara K, Perks P, Wilcock G, Lightman S and Shanks N (2000) Chronic stress in caregivers of dementia patients is associated with reduced lymphocyte sensitivity to glucocorticoids. J Neuroimmunol 103:84–92

Ben-Yehuda A, Danenberg H, Zakay-Rones Z, Gross D and Friedman G (1998) The influence of sequential annual vaccination and DHEA administration on the efficacy of the immune response to influenza vaccine in the elderly. Mech Ageing Dev 102:299–306

Besedovsky H, Sorkin E, Felix D and Haas H (1977) Hypothalamic changes during the immune response. Eur J Immunol 7:323–325

Bhushan M, Cumberbatch M, Dearman RJ, Andrew SM, Kimber I and Griffiths CE (2002) Tumour necrosis factor-alpha-induced migration of human Langerhans cells: the influence of ageing. Br J Dermatol 146:32–40

Biondi M (2001) Effects of Stress on Immune Functions: an overview. In Ader, R et al. (eds.), Psychoneuroimmunonology, Academic Press, San Diego, vol 2, pp 189–226

Bronnegard M, Stierna P and Marcus C (1996) Glucocorticoid resistant syndromes - molecular basis and clinical presentations. J Neuroendocrinol 8:405–415

Brossart P and Bevan MJ (1997) Presentation of exogenous protein antigens on major histocompatibility complex class I molecules by dendritic cells: pathway of presentation and regulation by cytokines. Blood 90:1594–1599

Butcher SK and Lord JM (2004) Stress responses and innate immunity: aging as a contributory factor. Aging Cell 3:151–160

Buvat J (2003) Androgen therapy with dehydroepiandrosterone. World J Urol 21:346–55

Canning MO, Grotenhuis K, de Wit HJ and Drexhage HA (2000) Opposing effects of dehydroe-piandrosterone and dexamethasone on the generation of monocyte-derived dendritic cells. Eur J Endocrinol 143:687–695

Casson PR, Andersen RN, Herrod HG, Stentz FB, Straughn AB, Abraham GE and Buster JE (1993) Oral dehydroepiandrosterone in physiologic doses modulates immune function in post-menopausal women. Am J Obstet Gynecol 169:1536–1539

Castle SC (2000) Clinical relevance of age-related immune dysfunction. Clin Infec Dis 31:578–585

Castro M, Elliot S, Kino T, Bamberger C, Karl M, Webster E and Chrousos G (1996) The non-ligand binding beta-isoform of the human glucocorticoid receptor (hGC-beta): tissue levels, mechanism of action, and potential physiologic role. Molec Med 2:597–607

Collaziol D, Luz C, Dornelles F, Cruz I and Bauer ME (2004) Psychoneuroendocrine correlates of lymphocyte subsets during healthy ageing. Mech Ageing Dev 125:219–227

Corpas S, Harman M and Blackmann MR (1993) Human Growth Hormone and Human Aging. Endocr Rev 14:20–39

Danenberg H, Ben-Yehuda A, Zakay-Rones Z and Friedman G (1995) Dehydroepiandrosterone (DHEA) treatment reverses the impaired immune response of old mice to influenza vaccination and protects from influenza infection. Vaccine 13:1445–1448

Danenberg HD, Ben-Yehuda A, Zakay-Rones Z, Gross DJ and Friedman G (1997) Dehydroepian-drosterone treatment is not beneficial to the immune response to influenza in elderly subjects. J Clin Endocrinol Metab 82:2911–2914

Daynes R, Araneo B, Ershler W, Maloney C, Li G-Z and Ryu S-Y (1993) Altered regulation of IL-6 production with normal aging—possible linkage to the age-associated decline in dehy-droepiandrosterone and its sulfated derivative. J Immunol 150:5219–5230

Daynes R, Dudley D and Araneo B (1990) Regulation of murine lymphokine production in vivo. II. Dehydroepiandrosterone is a natural enhancer of interleukin-2 synthesis by helper T cells. Eur J Immunol 20:793–802

de Kloet ER, Vreugdenhil E, Oitzl MS and Joels M (1998) Brain corticosteroid receptor balance in health and disease. Endocr Rev 19:269–301

Degelau J, Guay D and Hallgren H (1997) The effect of DHEAS on influenza vaccination in aging adults. J Am Geriatr Soc 45:747–751

Deuschle M, Gotthardt U, Schweiger U, Weber B, Korner A, Schmider J, Standhardt H, Lammers C and Heuser I (1997) With ageing in humans the activity of the hypothalamus-pituitary-adrenal system increases and its amplitude flattens. Life Sci 61:2239–2246

Dew MA, Reynolds CF, Frank E, Begley AE, Miller MD, Cornes C, Mazumdar S, Perel JM and Kupfer DJ (1998) Effects of age at onset of first lifetime episode of recurrent major depression on treatment response and illness course in elderly patients. Am J Psychiatry 155:759–799

Di Santo E, Sironi M and Mennini T (1996) A glucocorticoid receptor independent mechanism for neurosteroid inhibition of tumor necrosis factor production. Eur J Pharmacol 299:179–186

Dixit VD, Schaffer EM, Pyle RS, Collins GD, Sakthivel SK, Palaniappan R, Lillard JW, Jr. and Taub DD (2004) Ghrelin inhibits leptin- and activation-induced proinflammatory cytokine expression by human monocytes and T cells. J Clin Invest 114:57–66

Elenkov IJ, Chrousos GP and Wilder RL (2000) Neuroendocrine regulation of IL-12 and TNF-alpha/IL-10 balance. Clinical implications. Ann N Y Acad Sci 917:94–105

Englander EW, Gomez GA and Greeley GH, Jr. (2004) Alterations in stomach ghrelin produc-tion and in ghrelin-induced growth hormone secretion in the aged rat. Mech Ageing Dev 125:871–875

Epel ES, Blackburn EH, Lin J, Dhabhar FS, Adler NE, Morrow JD and Cawthon RM (2004) Accelerated telomere shortening in response to life stress. Proc Natl Acad Sci U S A 101:17312–17315

Evans TG, Judd ME, Dowell T, Poe S, Daynes RA and Araneo BA (1996) The use of oral dehy-droepiandrosterone sulfate as an adjuvant in tetanus and influenza vaccination of the elderly. Vaccine 14:1531–1537

Fagiolo U, Cossarizza A, Scala E, Fanales-Belasio E, Ortolani C, Cozzi E, Monti D, Franceschi C and Paganelli R (1993) Increased cytokine production in mononuclear cells of healthy elderly people. Eur J Immunol 23:2375–2378

Fauci A (1975) Mechanisms of corticosteroid action on lymphocyte subpopulations. Immunology 28:669–679

Ferrari E, Arcaini A, Gornati R, Pelanconi L, Cravello L, Fioravanti M, Solerte SB and Magri F (2000) Pineal and pituitary-adrenocortical function in physiological aging and in senile dementia. Exp Gerontol 35:1239–1250

Ferrari E, Cravello L, Muzzoni B, Casaritti D, Paltro M, Sorlete SB, Fioravanti M, Cuzzoni G, Pontiggia B and Magri F (2001) Age-related changes of the hypothalamic-pytuitary-adrenal axis: phathophysiological correlates. Eur J Endocrinol 144:319–329

Ferrari E, Mirani M, Barili L, Falvo F, Solerte SB, Cravello L, Pini L and Magri F (2004) Cognitive and affective disorders in the elderly: a neuroendocrine study. Arch Gerontol Geriatr Suppl:171–182

Fontenot JD, Gavin MA and Rudensky AY (2003) Foxp3 programs the development and function of CD4+CD25+ regulatory T cells. Nat Immunol 4:330–336

Gabriel H, Schmitt B and Kindermann W (1993) Age-related increase of CD45RO+ lymphocytes in physically active adults. Eur J Immunol 23:2704–2706

Gabriel P, Cakman I and Rink L (2002) Overproduction of monokines by leukocytes after stimulation with lipopolysaccharide in the elderly. Exp Gerontol 37:235–247

Galon J, Franchimont D, Hiroi N, Frey G, Boetner A, Ehrart-Bornstein M, O´Shea J, Chrousos GP and Bornstein S (2002) Gene profiling reveals unknown enhancing and suppressive actions of glucocorticoids on immune cells. FASEB J 16:61–71

Ginaldi L, Loreto MF, Corsi MP, Modesti M and De Martinis M (2001) Immunosenescence and infectious diseases. Microbes Infect 3:851–857

Glaser R, McCallum R, Laskowski BF, Malarkey WB, Sheridan J and Kiecolt-Glaser J (2001) Evidence for a shift in the Th-1 to Th-2 cytokine response associated with chronic stress and aging. J Gerontol Med Sci 56A:M477–M482

Glaser R, Sheridan J, Malarkey WB, MacCallum RC and Kiecolt-Glaser JK (2000) Chronic stress modulates the immune response to a pneumococcal pneumonia vaccine. Psychosom.Med. 62: 804-807.

Globerson A and Effros R (2000) Ageing of lymphocytes and lymphocytes in the aged. Immunol. Today 21:515–521

Gold P, Goodwin F and Chrousos G (1988) Clinical and biochemical manifestations of depression I. N Engl J Med 319:348–413

Gold R, Buttgereit F and Toyka KV (2001) Mechanism of action of glucocorticosteroid hormones: possible implications for therapy of neuroimmunological disorders. J Neuroimmunol 117:1–8

Grasso G, Lodi L, Lupo C and Muscettola M (1997) Glucocorticoid receptors in human peripheral blood mononuclear cells in relation to age and to sport activity. Life Sci 61:301–308

Grewe M (2001) Chronological ageing and photoageing of dendritic cells. Clin Exp Dermatol 26:608–12

Halbreich U, Asnis G, Zumoff B, Nathan R and Shindledecker R (1984) Effect of age and sex on cortisol secretion in depressives and normals. Psychiatry Res 13:221–229

Hannet I, Erkeller-Yuksel F, Lydyard P, Deneys V and DeBruyere M (1992) Developmental and maturational changes in human blood lymphocyte subpopulations. Immunol Today 13:215, 218

Hattori N, Ikekubo K, Ishihara T, Moridera K, Hino M and Kurahachi N (1994) Spontaneous Growth Hormone (GH) Secretion by Unstimulated Human Lymphocytes and the Effects of GH-Releasing Hormone and Somatostatin. J Clin Endocrinol Metab 79:1678–1680

Hearing SD, Norman M, Smyth C, Foy C and Dayan CM (1999) Wide variation in lymphocyte steroid sensitivity among healthy human volunteers. J Clin Endocrinol Metab 84:4149–4154

Hechter O, Grossman A and Chatterton RT (1997) Relationship of dehydroepiandrosterone and cortisol in disease. Med Hypotheses 49:85–91

Henson SM, Pido-Lopez J and Aspinall R (2004) Reversal of thymic atrophy. Exp Gerontol 39:673–678

Heuser I, Deuschle M, Luppa P, Schweiger U, Standhadt H and Weber B (1998) Increased diurnal plasma concentrations of dehydroepiandrosterone in depressed patients. J Clin Endocrinol Metab 83:3130–3133

Hoglund CO, Axen J, Kemi C, Jernelov S, Grunewald J, Muller-Suur C, Smith Y, Gronneberg R, Eklund A, Stierna P and Lekander M (2006) Changes in immune regulation in response to examination stress in atopic and healthy individuals. Clin Exp Allergy 36:982–992

Howieson DB, Camicioli R, Quinn J, Silbert LC, Care B, Moore MM, Dame A, Sexton G and Kaye JA (2003) Natural history of cognitive decline in the old old. Neurology 60:1489–1494

Huether G (1996) The central adaptation syndrome: psychosocial stress as a trigger for adaptive modifications of brain structure and brain function. Prog Neurobiol 48:569–612

Inaba K, Inaba M, Romani N, Aya H, Deguchi M, Ikehara S, Muramatsu S and Steinman RM (1992) Generation of large numbers of dendritic cells from mouse bone marrow cultures supplemented with granulocyte/macrophage colony-stimulating factor. J Exp Med 176:1693–1702

Juruena MF, Cleare AJ, Bauer ME and Pariante CM (2003) Molecular mechanisms of glucocorticoid receptor sensitivity and relevance to affective disorders. Acta Neuropsychiatr 15:354–367

Kam J, Szefler S, Surs W, Sher E and Leung D (1993) Combination of IL-2 and IL-4 reduces glucocorticoid receptor- binding affinity and T cell response to glucocorticoids. J Immunol 151:3460–3466

Kavelaars A, Cats B, Visser G, Zegers B, Bakker J, Van Rees E and Heijnen C (1996) Ontogeny of the response of human peripheral blood T cells to glucocorticoids. Brain Behav Immun 10:288–297

Kiecolt-Glaser J, Dura J, Speicher C, Trask J and Glaser R (1991) Spousal caregivers of dementia victims: longitudinal changes in immunity and health. Psychosom Med 53:345–362

Kiecolt-Glaser J, Glaser R, Gravenstein S, Malarkey W and Sheridan J (1996) Chronic stress alters the immune response to influenza virus vaccine in older adults. Proc Natl Acad Sci U S A 93:3043–3047

Kiecolt-Glaser J, Marucha P, Malarkey W, Mercado A and Glaser R (1995) Slowing of wound healing by psychological stress. Lancet 346:1194–1196

Kiecolt-Glaser JK, Preacher KJ, MacCallum RC, Atkinson C, Malarkey WB and Glaser R (2003) Chronic stress and age-related increases in the proinflammatory cytokine IL-6. Proc Natl Acad Sci USA 100:9090–9095

Kirschbaum C, Pirke KM and Hellhammer DH (1993) The 'Trier Social Stress Test'–a tool for investigating psychobiological stress responses in a laboratory setting. Neuropsychobiology 28:76–81

Kirschbaum C, Prussner J, Stone A, Federenko I, Gaab J, Lintz D, Schommer N and Hellhammer D (1995) Persistent high cortisol responses to repeated psychological stress in a subpopulation of healthy men. Psychol Med 57:468–474

Lee AL, Ogle WO and Sapolsky RM (2002) Stress and depression: possible links to neuron death in the hippocampus. Bipolar Disord 4:117–128

Ligthart G, Corberand J, Fournier C, Galanaud P, Humans W, Kennes B, Möller-Hermelink H and Steinmann G (1984) Admission criteria for immunogerontological studies in man: the SENIEUR protocol. Mech Ageing Dev 28:47–55

Liu J, Wang S, Liu H, Yang L and Nan G (1997) The monitoring biomarker for immune function os lymphocytes in the elderly. Mech Ageing Dev 94:177–182

Lung TL, Saurwein-Teissl M, Parson W, Schonitzer D and Grubeck-Loebenstein B (2000) Unimpaired dendritic cells can be derived from monocytes in old age and can mobilize residual function in senescent T cells. Vaccine 18:1606–1612

Luo X, Tarbell KV, Yang H, Pothoven K, Bailey SL, Ding R, Steinman RM and Suthanthiran M (2007) Dendritic cells with TGF-beta1 differentiate naive CD4+CD25- T cells into islet-protective Foxp3+ regulatory T cells. Proc Natl Acad Sci U S A 104:2821–2826

Lupien S, Lecours A, Lussier I, Schwartz G, Nair N and Meaney M (1994) Basal cortisol levels and cognitive deficits in human aging. J Neurosci 14:2893–2903

Luz C, Collaziol D, Preissler T, da Cruz IM, Glock L and Bauer ME (2006) Healthy Aging Is Associated with Unaltered Production of Immunoreactive Growth Hormone but Impaired Neuroimmunomodulation. Neuroimmunomodulation 13:160–169

Luz C, Dornelles F, Preissler T, Collaziol D, Cruz I and Bauer ME (2003) Impact of psychological and endocrine factors on cytokine production of healthy elderly people. Mech Ageing Dev 124:887–895

Luz C, Dornelles F, Scapini E, Collaziol D, Preissler T, Cruz I and Bauer ME (2002) Psychological and nutritional correlates of T-cell function in the healthy elderly. Stress 5:80–80

Maeda K, Tanimoto K, Terada T, Shintani T and Kakigi T (1991) Elevated urinary free cortisol in patients with dementia. Neurobiol Aging 12:161–163

Maes M, Scharp, S, Meltzer H, Bosmans E, Suy E, Calabrese J and Cosyns P (1993) Relationships between interleukin-6 activity, acute phase proteins, and function of the hypothalamic-pituitary-adrenal axis in severe depression. Psychiatry Res 49:11–27

Malarkey WB, Wang J, Cheney C, Glaser R and Nagaraja H (2002) Human lymphocyte growth hormone stimulates interferon gamma production and is inhibited by cortisol and norepinephrine. J Neuroimmunol 123:180–187

Martinez-Taboada V, Bartolome MJ, Amado JA, Blanco R, Garcia-Unzueta MT, Rodriguez-Valverde V and Lopez-Hoyos M (2002) Changes in peripheral blood lymphocyte subsets in elderly subjects are associated with an impaired function of the hypothalamic-pituitary- adrenal axis. Mech Ageing Dev 123:1477–1486

Mastorakos G, Chrousos GP and Weber J (1993) Recombinant IL-6 activates the hypothalamic-pituitary-adrenal axis in humans. J Clin Endocrinol Metab 77:1690–1694

Matthews JG, Ito K, Barnes PJ and Adcock IM (2004) Defective glucocorticoid receptor nuclear translocation and altered histone acetylation patterns in glucocorticoid-resistant patients. J Allergy Clin Immunol 113:1100–1108

Matyszak MK, Citterio S, Rescigno M and Ricciardi-Castagnoli P (2000) Differential effects of corticosteroids during different stages of dendritic cell maturation. Eur J Immunol 30:1233–1242

McEwen B (1998) Protective and damaging effects of stress mediators. New Engl J Med 338:171–179

McEwen B, Biron C, Brunson K, Bulloch K, Chambers W, Dhabhar F, Goldfarb R, Kitson R, Miller A, Spencer R and Weiss J (1997) The role of adrenocorticosteroids as modulators of immune function in health and disease: neural, endocrine and immune interactions. Brain Res Rev 23:79–133

McEwen BS (2003) Interacting mediators of allostasis and allostatic load: towards an understanding of resilience in aging. Metabolism 52:10–16

McLachlan JA, Serkin CD and Bakouche O (1996) Dehydroepiandrosterone modulation of lipopolysaccharide-stimulated monocyte cytotoxicity. J Immunol 156:328–35

Migeon C, Keller A, Lawrence B and Shepard T (1957) Dehydroepiandrosterone and androsterone levels in human plasma: effects of age, sex, day to day diurnal variations. J Clin Endocrinol Metab 17:1051

Muller DN, Shagdarsuren E, Park JK, Dechend R, Mervaala E, Hampich F, Fiebeler A, Ju X, Finckenberg P, Theuer J, Viedt C, Kreuzer J, Heidecke H, Haller H, Zenke M and Luft FC (2002) Immunosuppressive treatment protects against angiotensin II-induced renal damage. Am J Pathol 161:1679–1693

Murasko D, Weiner P and Kaye D (1987) Decline in mitogen induced proliferation of lymphocytes with increasing age. Clin Exp Immunol 70:440–448

Nagata S and Golstein P (1995) The Fas death factor. Science 267:1449–1456

Navarro J, Aristimuno C, Sanchez-Ramon S, Vigil D, Martinez-Gines ML, Fernandez-Cruz E and de Andres C (2006) Circulating dendritic cells subsets and regulatory T-cells at multiple sclerosis relapse: differential short-term changes on corticosteroids therapy. J Neuroimmunol 176:153–161

Nijhuis EW, Hinloopen B, van Lier RA and Nagelkerken L (1995) Differential sensitivity of human naive and memory CD4+ T cells for dexamethasone. Int Immunol 7:591–5

Nolen-Hoeksema S and Ahrens C (2002) Age differences and similarities in the correlates of depressive symptoms. Psychol Aging 17:116–124

Oka M, Hirazawa K, Yamamoto K, Iizuka N, Hazama S, Suzuki T and Kobayashi N (1996) Induction of Fas-mediated apoptosis on circulating lymphocytes by surgical stress. Ann Surg 223:434–440

Padgett DA and Loria R (1994) In vitro potentiation of lymphocyte activation by dehydroepian-drosterone, androstenediol, and androstenetriol. J Immunol 153:1544–1552

Pan J, Ju D, Wang Q, Zhang M, Xia D, Zhang L, Yu H and Cao X (2001) Dexamethasone inhibits the antigen presentation of dendritic cells in MHC class II pathway. Immunol Lett 76:153–161

Pariante C, Pearce B, Pisell T, Sanshez C, Po C, Su C and Miller A (1999a) The proinflammatory cytokine, interleukin-1a, reduces glucocorticoid receptor translocation and function. Endocrinology 140:4359–4366

Pariante CM, Pearce BD, Pisell TL, Sanchez CI, Po C, Su C and Miller AH (1999b) The proinflammatory cytokine, interleukin-1alpha, reduces glucocorticoid receptor translocation and function. Endocrinology 140:4359–4366

Pawelec G, Barnett Y, Forsey R, Frasca D, Globerson A, McLeod J, Caruso C, Franceschi C, Fulop T, Gupta S, Mariani E, Mocchegiani E and Solana R (2002) T cells and aging, January 2002update. Front Biosci 7:D1056–D1183

Pereira M, Traverse M, Barros D, Bianchini A and Martinez P (2003) The effects of aging on leukocyte glucocorticoid receptor concentration and response to dexamethasone in dogs. Exp Gerontol 38:989–995

Piani A, Brotini S, Dolso P, Budai R and Gigli GL (2004) Sleep disturbances in elderly: a subjective evaluation over 65. Arch Gerontol Geriatr Suppl:325–331

Picard D, Khursheed B, Garabedian MJ, Fortin MG, Lindquist S and Yamamoto KR (1990) Reduced levels of hsp90 compromise steroid receptor action in vivo. Nature 348:166–168

Pietschmann P, Hahn P, Kudlacek S, Thomas R and Peterlik M (2000) Surface markers and transendothelial migration of dendritic cells from elderly subjects. Exp Gerontol 35:213–224

Potestio M, Pawelec G, Di Lorenzo G, Candore G, D'Anna C, Gervasi F, Lio D, Tranchida G, Caruso C and Romano GC (1999) Age-related changes in the expression of CD95 (APO1/FAS) on blood lymphocytes. Exp Gerontol 34:659–673

Ramirez F, Fowell D, Puklavec M, Simmonds S and Mason D (1996) Glucocorticoids promote a Th2 cytokine response by CD4+ T cells in vitro. J Immunol 156:2406–2412

Raskind M, Peskind E and Wilkinson C (1994) Hypothalamic-pituitary-adrenal axis regulation and human aging. Ann N Y Acad Sci 746: 327–335

Redinbaugh E, McCallum R and Kiecolt-Glaser J (1995) Recurrent syndromal depression in caregivers. Psychol Aging:358–368

Ribeiro F, Lopes RP, Nunes CP, Maito F, Bonorino C and Bauer ME (2007) Dehydroepiandrosterone sulphate enhances IgG and Interferon-gamma production during immunization to tuberculosis in young but not aged mice. Biogerontology 8:209–220

Rohleder N, Kudielka BM, Hellhammer DH, Wolf JM and Kirschbaum C (2002) Age and sex steroid-related changes in glucocorticoid sensitivity of pro-inflammatory cytokine production after psychosocial stress. J Neuroimmunol 126:69–77

Rohleder N, Wolf JM and Kirschbaum C (2003) Glucocorticoid sensitivity in humans-interindividual differences and acute stress effects. Stress 6:207–222

Roshan S, Nader S and Orlander P (1999) Ageing and hormones. Eur J Clin Invest 29:210–213

Sakaguchi S (2000) Regulatory T cells: key controllers of immunologic self-tolerance. Cell 101:455–458

Salehian MB and Kejriwal MK (1999) Glucocorticoid-induced muscle atrophy: mechanisms and therapeutic strategies. Endocr Pract 5:277–281

Sapolsky RM, Krey LC and McEwen BS (1986) The neuroendocrinology of stress and aging: the glucocorticoid cascade hypothesis. Endocr Rev 7:284–301

Sapolsky RM, Romero LM and Munck AU (2000) How do glucocorticoids influence stress responses? Integrating permissive, suppressive, stimulatory, and preparative actions. Endocr Rev 21:55–89

Schiepers OJ, Wichers MC and Maes M (2005) Cytokines and major depression. Prog Neuropsychopharmacol Biol Psychiatry 29:201–217

Schmidt M, Lugering N, Lugering A, Pauels HG, Schulze-Osthoff K, Domschke W and Kucharzik T (2001) Role of the CD95/CD95 ligand system in glucocorticoid-induced monocyte apoptosis. J Immunol 166:1344–1351

Schulz R and Beach SR (1999) Caregiving as a risk factor for mortality: the caregiver health effects study. JAMA 282:2215–2219

Selye H (1936) Syndrome produced by diverse nocuous agents. Nature 138:32

Sharma S, Dominguez AL and Lustgarten J (2006) Aging affect the anti-tumor potential of dendritic cell vaccination, but it can be overcome by co-stimulation with anti-OX40 or anti-4-1BB. Exp Gerontol 41:78–84

Shaw WS, Patterson TL, Ziegler MG, Dimsdale JE, Semple SJ and Grant I (1999) Accelerated risk of hypertensive blood pressure recordings among Alzheimer caregivers. J Psychosom Res 46:215–227

Silva C, Powell-Oliver F, Jewell C, Sar M, Allgood V and Cidlowski J (1994) Regulation of the human glucocorticoid receptor by long-term and chronic treatment with glucocorticoid. Steroids 59:436–442

Sippell WG, Becker H, Versmold HT, Bidlingmaier F and Knorr D (1978) Longitudinal studies of plasma aldosterone, corticosterone, deoxycorticosterone, progesterone, 17-hydroxyprogesterone, cortisol, and cortisone determined simultaneously in mother and child at birth and during the early neonatal period. I. Spontaneous delivery. J Clin Endocrinol Metab 46:971–985

Solerte SB, Fioravanti M, Vignati G, Giustina A, Cravello L and Ferrari E (1999) Dehydroepiandrosterone sulfate enhances natural killer cell cytotoxicity in humans via locally generated immunoreactive insulin- like growth factor I. J Clin Endocrinol Metab 84:3260–3267

Spahn J, Szefler S, Surs W, Doherty D, Nimmagadda S and Leung D (1996) A novel action of IL-13: induction of diminished monocyte glucocorticoid receptor-binding affinity. J Immunol 157:2654–2659

Starkman M, Schteingart D and Schork M (1981) Depressed mood and other psychiatric manifestations of Cushing's syndrome: relationship to hormone levels. Psychosom Med 43:3–18

Steger MM, Maczek C and Grubeck-Loebenstein B (1997) Peripheral blood dendritic cells reinduce proliferation in in vitro aged T cell populations. Mech Ageing Dev 93:125–130

Steinman RM (2003) Some interfaces of dendritic cell biology. APMIS 111:675–697

Sternberg E (2002) Neuroendocrine regulation of autoimmune/inflammatory disease. J Endocrinol 169:429–435

Straub R, Miller L, Scholmerich J and Zietz B (2000) Cytokines and hormones as possible links between endocrinosenescence and immunosenescence. J Neuroimmunol 109:10–15

Straub R, Schölmerich J and Cutolo M (2003) The multiple facets of premature aging in rheumatoid arthritis. Arthritis Rheum 48:2713–2721

Straub RH, Cutolo M, Zietz B and Scholmerich J (2001) The process of aging changes the interplay of the immune, endocrine and nervous systems. Mech Ageing Dev 122:1591–1611

Straub RH, Konecna L, Hrach S, Rothe G, Kreutz M, Scholmerich J, Falk W and Lang B (1998) Serum dehydroepiandrosterone (DHEA) and DHEA sulfate are negatively correlated with serum interleukin-6 (IL-6), and DHEA inhibits IL-6 secretion from mononuclear cells in man in vitro: possible link between endocrinosenescence and immunosenescence. J Clin Endocrinol Metab 83:2012–2017

Suzuki T, Suzuki N, Daynes R and Engleman E (1991) Dehydroepiandrosterone enhances IL2 production and cytotoxic effector function of human T cells. Clin Immunol Immunop 61:202–211

Tamura Y, Okinaga H and Takami H (2004) Glucocorticoid-induced osteoporosis. Biomed Pharmacother 58:500–504

Truckenmiller ME, Princiotta MF, Norbury CC and Bonneau RH (2005) Corticosterone impairs MHC class I antigen presentation by dendritic cells via reduction of peptide generation. J Neuroimmunol 160:48–60

Trzonkowski P, Mysliwska J, Godlewska B, Szmit E, Lukaszuk K, Wieckiewicz J, Brydak L, Machala M, Landowski J and Mysliwski A (2004) Immune consequences of the spontaneous pro-inflammatory status in depressed elderly patients. Brain Behav Immun 18: 135–148

Trzonkowski P, Szmit E, Mysliwska J and Mysliwski A (2006) CD4+CD25+ T regulatory cells inhibit cytotoxic activity of CTL and NK cells in humans-impact of immunosenescence. Clin Immunol 119:307–316

Van Cauter E, Leproult R and Kupfer DJ (1996) Effects of gender and age on the levels and circadian rhythmicity of plasma cortisol. J Clin Endocrinol Metab 81:2468–2473

Vedhara K, Cox N, Wilcock G, Perks P, Lightman S and Shanks N (1999) Chronic stress in elderly carers of dementia patients and antibody response to influenza vaccination. Lancet 353:627–631

Vetta F, Ronzoni S, Lupatelli M, Novi B, Fabbriconi P, Ficconeri C, Cicconetti P, Russo F and Bollea M (2001) Tumor necrosis factor-alpha and mood disorders in the elderly. Arch Gerontol Geriatr Suppl 7:442

Vitaliano PP, Scanlan JM, Zhang J, Savage MV, Hirsch IB and Siegler IC (2002) A path model of chronic stress, the metabolic syndrome, and coronary heart disease. Psychosom Med 64:418–435

Vremec D and Shortman K (1997) Dendritic cell subtypes in mouse lymphoid organs: cross-correlation of surface markers, changes with incubation, and differences among thymus, spleen, and lymph nodes. J Immunol 159:565–573

Weigent DA, Baxter JB, Wear WE, Smith LR, Bost KL and Blalock JE (1988) Production of immunoreactive growth hormone by mononuclear leukocytes. FASEB J 2:2812–2818

Yamazaki S, Inaba K, Tarbell KV and Steinman RM (2006) Dendritic cells expand antigen-specific Foxp3+ CD25+ CD4+ regulatory T cells including suppressors of alloreactivity. Immunol Rev 212:314–329

Yin D, Tuthill D, Mufson RA and Shi Y (2000) Chronic restraint stress promotes lymphocyte apoptosis by modulating CD95 expression. J Exp Med 191:1423–1428

Zavala WD and Cavicchia JC (2006) Deterioration of the Langerhans cell network of the human gingival epithelium with aging. Arch Oral Biol 51:1150–1155

Zhang TY, Ding X and Daynes RA (2005) The expression of 11 beta-hydroxysteroid dehydrogenase type I by lymphocytes provides a novel means for intracrine regulation of glucocorticoid activities. J Immunol 174:879–889

Zipp F, Wendling U, Beyer M, Grieger U, Waiczies S, Wagenknecht B, Haas J and Weller M (2000) Dual effect of glucocorticoids on apoptosis of human autoreactive and foreign antigen-specific T cells. J Neuroimmunol 110:214–222

Zovato S, Simoncini M, Gottardo C, Pratesi C, Vampollo V and Spigariol A (1996) Dexamethasone suppression test: corticosteroid receptors regulation in mononuclear leukocytes of young and aged subjects. Aging Clin Exp Res 8:360–364

Mechanisms- Thymus

Thymic Involution and Thymic Renewal

Frances T. Hakim

Contents

Abbreviations

AIRE	Autoimmune regulator
CCL	Chemokine (C-C motif) ligand; CCL21 and CCL25
CCR	Chemokine (C-C motif) receptor; CCR9 and CCR7
CMJ	Cortical-medullary junction
cTEC	Cortical thymic epithelial cells
DN	Double negative (CD4$^-$ CD8$^-$) thymocyte
DP	Double positive (CD4$^+$CD8$^+$) thymocyte
ETP	Early thymocyte progenitor
FGF	Fibroblast growth factor
FGFR2-IIIb	Fibroblast growth factor receptor 2-IIIb
GH	Growth hormone
HAART	Highly active anti-retroviral therapy
HSC	Hematopoietic stem cell
IGF	Insulin-like growth factor 1
IL-7	Interleukin 7
KGF	Keratinocyte growth factor, also FGF7
LHRH	Luteinizing hormone releasing hormone
MPP	Multipotent progenitor cell
mTEC	Medullary thymic epithelial cells
PSGL1	P-selectin ligand
PVS	Perivascular space

F. T. Hakim (✉)
Experimental Transplantation and Immunology Branch
National Cancer Institute, NIH
10 Center Drive, CRC-3E-3330
Bethesda, MD, 20892-1203
Tel: 1 301-402-3627
Fax: 301-480-8146
E-mail: hakimf@mail.nih.gov

T. Fulop et al. (eds.), *Handbook on Immunosenescence*,
DOI 10.1007/978-1-4020-9062-2_44, © Springer Science+Business Media B.V. 2009

RAG2/γ_c	Recombination-activating gene/common γ chain
RTE	Recent thymic emigrant
SCZ	Subcapsular zone
sjTREC	Signal joint T cell receptor rearrangement excision circle
SP	Single positive (CD4$^+$ or CD8$^+$) thymocyte
TCR	T cell receptor
Treg	Regulatory T cell
VDJ	Variable, diversity and joiner elements of the TCR beta chain

Abstract: A primary factor in immunosenescence, the age-dependent deterioration in immune function, is the decline in the capacity to generate naïve T-cells due to thymic involution. The thymus reaches its greatest size and cellularity in the first year of life and undergoes a gradual involutional decline in both structure and thymopoietic productivity. Thymic involution results from the interplay of systemic factors and intrinsic changes in thymic epithelial cells and thymocyte progenitors themselves. In patients undergoing lymphodepletion, however, the thymus is capable of significant renewal through the fifth decade of life. This chapter will explore the factors regulating thymic growth, involution and renewal.

Keywords: Thymus • Thymocyte • Thymic epithelial cells • Cortex • Medulla • Hematopoietic stem cell • ETP • DN • Notch • IGF-1 • KGF • IL-7

1 Introduction: The Immunologic Consequences of Thymic Involution in the Elderly

Aging is associated clinically with a decline in adaptive immune system responses to vaccines, increases in the frequency and severity of infectious diseases, and an increased incidence of chronic inflammatory and autoimmune disorders. The alterations in immune competence underlying these disorders have been collectively termed immunosenescence. A primary cause of immunosenescence is the gradual decline in thymic generation of new naïve T-cells. When the thymus can no longer replace the naïve T-cells lost daily, the result is a steady decline in the levels of naïve T-cells.

This decline has profound consequences for immune function. The naïve T-cell population provides a reservoir of T-cell receptor (TCR) diversity that may be needed to respond to novel antigens. In young and even middle aged adults the repertoire diversity has been estimated at 20 million different TCRβ chains; in the elderly (greater than 70 years), the pool has severely contracted to 200,000 TCRβ specificities (Naylor et al. 2005). The 99% decline in TCR repertoire diversity in CD4 T-cells in the elderly may in itself be a critical factor in limiting functional response; a 2–10 fold decrease in repertoire has been found to abrogate T-cell mediated responses in mice (Nanda et al. 1991). Furthermore, studies in adults recovering from lymphopenia have demonstrated that both the capacity to respond to vaccines and the resistance to opportunistic infections correlate with the levels of naïve CD4$^+$ T-cells and the presence of broad TCR repertoire diversity (Lewin et al. 2002; Roux et al. 2000).

Since naïve cells provide the reservoir from which memory cells are drawn, a decline in the frequency of naïve cells impacts memory populations. The relative representation of different T-cell specificities remains relatively constant throughout life, due to a homeostatic balance between turnover and a steady influx of new T-cells (Tanchot et al. 2000). In the elderly, this balance is lost. The repertoire diversity of memory populations in the elderly declines concurrent with the decline in the frequency of naïve cells (Schwab et al. 1997). Analogously, the repertoire diversity of the memory CD4+ T-cell population in adult patients recovering from transplant-induced lymphopenia has been found to directly depend upon the extent of posttransplant thymic function (Hakim et al. 2005). Individuals lacking a strong recovery of thymic function had a limited oligoclonal repertoire in their memory T-cell populations even 2–5 years post transplant (Hakim et al. 2005). Chronic infection with CMV and to a lesser extent EBV may further alter the memory/effector repertoire by driving virus-reactive cells into oligoclonal expansions or even to replicative exhaustion (Fletcher et al. 2005). Oligoclonal expansions can by themselves limit overall immune function in the remainder of the T-cell population (Khan et al. 2004; LeMaoult et al. 2000; Messaoudi et al. 2004). Yet these expanded cells are often dysfunctional, responding poorly to stimulation by their target antigens (Ouyang et al. 2003). Thus the loss of a strong influx of 'replacement' cells into the memory/effector pool may contribute to immune deficits.

The decline in naïve CD4+ T-cell numbers may also affect humoral immune function. Much of the decline in vaccine responses in the elderly is due to reductions in the formation and function of germinal centers as compared to those in young individuals (Lazuardi et al. 2005). Germinal center formation depends upon the frequency of CCR7 and CD62L-bearing naïve and central memory CD4+ T-cells, which can enter lymph nodes and initiate germinal center formation. These CD4 populations decline in the elderly. Within germinal centers, cognate interaction between CD4+ T-cells and B-cells promotes somatic hypermutation of immunoglobulin chains, a process that increases the avidity of antibodies. Age-dependent deficits in CD4+ T-cells that reduce cognate B-T interactions may therefore contribute to the decline in antibody avidity observed in the elderly.

Finally the involutional changes in the thymus with age may result not only in immune deficits but also in dysfunctional increases in autoreactivity. The thymus contributes to the regulation of tolerance and the prevention of autoimmunity at many levels. First of all, auto-reactive CD4+ and CD8+ T-cells are clonally deleted during negative selection in the thymus, establishing central tolerance. The unique expression of the AIRE (autoimmune regulator) gene in medullary thymic epithelial cells (mTEC) results in expression of a broad array of tissue-specific antigens (Gallegos et al. 2004). Thymocytes bearing T-cell receptors (TCR) that bind to these tissue-specific antigens are clonally deleted. This process removes self-reactive T-cells from the repertoire before T-cells are exported into the periphery. Although the thymus is known to continue to support a low level of thymopoieis for many decades (Jamieson et al. 1999; Sempowski et al. 2000), the continued efficiency of negative selection in involuted thymuses has not been evaluated in man. With age, there is a decline in the level of mTEC expressing high levels of MHC II (Gray et al. 2006); these include the AIRE expressing cells critical in negative selection. Secondly, regulatory T-cells (Treg) are believed to play a critical role in the prevention of autoimmunity, suppression of inflammatory responses and the modulation of T-cell homeostasis. Treg develop in parallel with CD4$^+$ and CD8$^+$ effector T-cells in the thymus (Wing et al. 2002; Wing et al. 2005), but whether their production similarly declines in parallel with overall thymopoiesis has not been assessed. Since Treg development has been linked to Hassall's corpuscles of the human thymus (Watanabe et al. 2005), the loss of these medullary structures with aging may be problematic. Treg can also arise in the periphery from memory CD4 T-cell populations in adults (Walker et al. 2003), but such cells may turn over rapidly (Vukmanovic-Stejic et al. 2006). The numbers of circulating Treg cells have been found to actually increase with age, but regulatory function declined (Gregg et al. 2005; Zhao et al. 2007). Finally, productive thymopoiesis, in and of itself, may be a factor deterring autoimmunity. Under conditions of lymphopenia prolonged by inadequate thympopoiesis, compensatory peripheral expansion of T-cells occurs to maintain stable T-cell levels. This extended homeostatic proliferation has been proposed to provide the opportunity for T-cells reactive to self-antigens to expand, leading to autoimmune disorders (King et al. 2004). Both lymphopenia and elevated levels of cycling (Ki-67$^+$) peripheral T-cells are found in the elderly, consistent with such a model of autoimmune development (Naylor et al. 2005). In all of these respects, the thymus maintains immunologic tolerance to self. The gradual age-dependent decline in thymic cytoarchitecture and thympoietic productivity may therefore contribute to the development of autoreactivity and loss of self-tolerance.

2 Thymic Organogenesis and Thymopoiesis

The thymus is located in the superior mediastinum, just over the heart, and consists of two lobes, connected by areolar tissue and enclosed in a fibrous capsule. Each lobe is further subdivided into lobules containing immature thymocytes in a network of epithelial cells termed thymic stroma. The denser outer areas are termed cortex and the looser inner areas are termed medulla. Committed T-progenitors enter the thymus through the vasculature at the cortico-medullary junction (CMJ); as these cells proliferate and differentiate, they follow a migration path outwards through the cortex to the subcapsular zone (SCZ) (Fig. 1). Thymocytes then migrate back inwards through the cortex to complete maturation and selection in the medulla, before emigrating from the thymus as mature, naïve T-cells via the CMJ vasculature. Lying between the lobules are is the perivascular space of the thymus (PVS). While limited to narrow septa of connective tissue in the neonate, it is the PVS which expands and fills with adipocytes and fibroblasts during thymic involution.

   The thymus begins as an outpocketing of the third pharyngeal pouch endoderm which gives rise to thymic epithelial cells. Mesenchymal cells derived from neural crest contribute to the thymic capsule and PVS connective tissue at this early stage, but previously postulated ectodermal contributions to thymic anlage have recently been excluded (Gordon et al. 2004). When the thymic rudiment is subsequently colonized by a wave of hematopoietic progenitors, the progenitors of the thymic epithelial cells are still immature and capable of differentiation into both cortical and medullary thymic epithelial cells (cTEC and mTEC) (Rossi SW et al. 2006; Rossi SW et al. 2007). Thymocytes are not necessary for the initial development of the TEC, but are required for the subsequent development and maintenance of TEC (Klug et al. 2002). Mesenchymal production of the fibroblast growth factor family cytokine FGF10 is necessary, however, for proliferation and early expansion of the TEC (Jenkinson et al. 2003; Jenkinson et al. 2007). Failure to express the FGFR2-IIIb receptor for these mesenchymally derived factors blocks TEC expansion (Revest et al. 2001). Thus it is through the cooperative interactions of mesenchymal cells, endoderm-derived thymic epithelial cells and hematopoietic-derived T-cell progenitors that the fetal thymus is formed.

T-progenitors arise in the marrow from hematopoietic stem cells (HSC). HSC give rise to multipotent progenitors (MPP), which in turn are the source of myeloid and lymphoid cells. Progenitors may become committed to the T lineage upon interaction of the Notch ligand Delta-like-1 on supportive stroma with Notch expressed on lymphoid progenitors (Schmitt et al. 2002; Schmitt et al. 2004). This commitment step may occur in the marrow prior to emigration to the thymus, but when the early thymocyte progenitor (ETP) engrafts in the thymus the T lineage commitment is reinforced by Notch/Notch ligand interactions during thymopoiesis (Schmitt et al. 2004). Upon leaving the marrow, T-progenitors home to the thymus (Rossi FM et al. 2005). The most immature thymocytes are termed double negative cells (DN) due to a lack of expression of CD4 or CD8. In the DN stage, subdivided into DN1 through DN4, thymocytes increase in number, migrate outward through the cortex, and rearrange the variable (V), diversity (D) and joiner (J) segments of the TCRβ chain (see Fig. 1). During the DN3 stage, signaling through the rearranged TCRβ chain and an associated invariant preTα receptor chain triggers the main proliferative expansion of thymocytes. and differentiation into CD4 and CD8 double positive (DP) cortical thymocytes. Upon final rearrangement of the TCRα chain and surface expression of a complete TCRαβ, the DP-cells undergo positive selection, based on affinity for Class II or Class I MHC molecules, into single positive (SP) CD4$^+$ or CD8$^+$ T-cells, respectively. During this positive selection process, DP thymocytes migrate back inwards across the cortex. Finally, within the medulla, the SP-cells undergo a negative selection process in which autoreactive cells are clonally deleted. Mature SP CD4$^+$ and CD8$^+$ T-cells then leave the thymus through the cortical-medullary vasculature (See Fig. 1).

Interactions between developing thymocytes and surrounding thymic epithelia control all aspects of thymopoiesis. Entry of T-progenitors depends on interaction between chemokine and adhesion molecules on progenitors, such as CCR9 and PSGL1, and the corresponding ligands (CCL25 and P-selectin) expressed by thymic stroma (Jenkinson et al. 2007; Rossi FM et al. 2005; Schwarz et al. 2007; Scimone et al. 2006; Zediak et al. 2007). T-cell lineage commitment and differentiation is reinforced upon signaling through Notch receptors (on T-progenitor cells) triggered by delta-1-like ligand expressed on stromal cells (Ciofani et al. 2004; Schmitt and

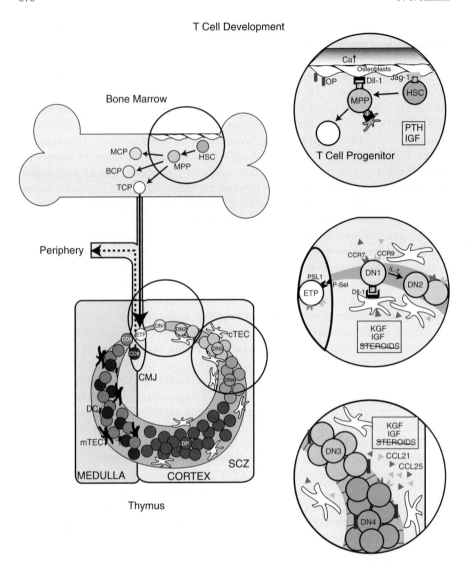

Fig. 1 An overview of T-cell maturation is shown at the left with expanded views on the right of the 3 areas of control of thymic productivity: the marrow compartment site of T-progenitor commitment, the CMJ vasculature and inner thymic cortex niches for progenitor engraftment, and the outer cortex and SCZ sites of thymocyte migration and expansion. Agents affecting each of these sites are noted in boxes.

In the bone marrow, pluripotent hematopoietic stem cells (HSC) with the capacity for self-renewal are supported in a calcium rich endosteal microenvironment. Proliferation is regulated by osteopontin (OP), secreted by osteoblasts, and by interaction of Notch (N, white box) on HSC with its ligand Jagged-1 on osteoblasts; osteoblast support for hematopoiesis in turn is regulated by levels of parathyroid hormone (PTH) and Insulin-like Growth Factor 1 (IGF) and IL-7. HSC give rise to Multipotent Progenitors (MPP), which cannot self-renew, but can expand and give rise to myeloid common progenitors (MCP), B-lymphoid and T-lymphoid progenitors. Commitment to the T

Zuniga-Pflucker 2002; Schmitt et al. 2004). Thymocyte migration across the thymus is controlled by chemokine signals in the stroma (Takahama 2006). Cytokines secreted by TEC, such as IL-7, support thymocyte survival at key checkpoints, such as the DN1–>DN2 transition (Phillips et al. 2004) and the positive selection process (Yu et al. 2003). Finally, thymic stroma is critical to the positive and negative selection processes. Cortical TEC expressing Class I and Class II MHC molecules support positive selection of cortical thymocytes into CD4 and CD8 SP T-cells. Medullary TEC and dendritic cells, expressing tissue antigens, support negative selection of autoreactive thymocytesand development of Treg (Gallegos and Bevan 2004; Watanabe et al. 2004). Thus all aspects of adult thymopoiesis depend upon interaction of thymocytes and TEC.

Yet this interaction is not unidirectional. After the fetal organogenesis period, the maintenance of TEC structure is strictly dependent upon on the presence of thymocytes. In mice in which the T-cell developmental pathway is blocked at its earliest stages, such as Ikaros mutant, CD3εtg26 mice and recombination-activating gene/common γ chain (RAG2/$γ_c$) deficient mice, immature TEC cells proliferate in the fetal thymus and develop characteristic cytokeratins (Jenkinson et al. 2005; Klug et al. 2002). The continued maintenance of cortical and medullary TEC in the adult, however, requires the presence of functional thymocytes. Thymuses in adult CD3εtg26 mice, in which T-cell development is blocked at the earliest DN1 stage, show an absence of both cortical and medullary TEC, with only immature TEC pro-

---

lineage results from Notch interactions with Delta-like ligand 1 (Dll). T-progenitors leave the bone marrow and home to the thymus, where they become early thymocyte progenitors (ETP).

The thymus is divided structurally and functionally into three main areas, the subcapsular epithelial zone (SCZ), the cortex (COR) and the medulla (MED). Distinct populations of cortical and medullary thymic epithelial cells (cTEC and mTEC) support T-cell maturational stages in each region. The migration path of thymocytes undergoing proliferative expansion and differentiation is symbolized by the gray band.

T-progenitor cells enter the thymus from the circulation via the vasculature at the cortico-medullary junction (CMJ). Uptake of ETP into the thymus is in part controlled by the interaction of P-Selectin Ligand 1 (PSGL1, black) expressed on the ETP with P-selectin (P-sel, black triangle) on CMJ vasculature. Upon entering the cortex, the earliest thymocytes, termed double negative cells (DN) due to a lack of expression of CD4 or CD8, strengthen commitment to the T lineage by repeated signaling through Notch (N, white box) and Delta-like ligand 1 on cTEC, and migrate outward toward the subcapsular zone. Migration depends upon adhesion of DN integrins (black box) to VCAM (black stripes) and is polarized by a gradient of cTEC secreted chemokines, including CCL21 (gray triangle) and CCL25 (dark gray triangle) which bind to chemokine receptors CCR7 and CCR9 on DN-cells. Based on the expression of surface markers (that correlate with the process of TCRβ chain rearrangement), the DN stage is subdivided into DN1 through DN4. During the outward migration and in the SCZ, the main proliferative expansion of DN cells occurs. Several factors, such as KGF and IGF-1 and gonadal steroids have regulatory effects on thymopoiesis, increasing the uptake of T-progenitors, the numbers of TEC and the associated expansion of DN thymocytes. Upon final rearrangement of the TCRα chain and expression of a complete TCRαβ, the CD4 and CD8 double positive (DP) thymocytes begin a migration back across the cortex and into the medulla. DP differentiate into single positive (SP) CD4+ or CD8+ T-cells, based on affinity for Class II or Class I MHC molecules, respectively. Finally, within the medulla, the SP cells undergo a negative selection process in which autoreactive cells are clonally deleted based on interaction with self peptides expressed on mTEC and dendritic cells (DC). Mature SP CD4+ and CD8+ T-cells then leave the thymus through the CMJ vasculature.

genitors present (Jenkinson et al. 2005). The interdependence between thymocytes and TEC is stepwise. Cortical TEC but not medullary TEC are present in RAG$^{-/-}$ mice, which have a block at the DN2/3 stage (Klug et al. 1998; van Ewijk et al. 2000). SCID mice, which similarly are unable to generate T-cell receptor-expressing thymocytes, have small thymuses with disorganized structure, with only scattered mTEC; yet when TCR-transgenic thymocytes expressing a full TCR are present in SCID mice, a medulla develops (Shores et al. 1991; Shores et al. 1994). These interactions between thymocytes and TEC are not limited to the early postnatal period of greatest thymic productivity. TEC populations are not static, but rather are continuously differentiating and turning over (Gray et al. 2006). Thymocytes are constantly being renewed by an input of T-progenitors. The interdependence of thymocytes and TEC may contribute to their mutual decline with aging. Yet this same interdependence may underlie the ability of thymuses to renew growth and expand.

3   Thymic Involution

The thymus attains its greatest size and cellularity in the late fetal and early neonatal period. The overall physical size of the thymus remains relatively constant after early childhood (Steinmann et al. 1985), but perivascular spaces containing connective tissue expand and thymic epithelial spaces are reduced, until thymic medullary and cortical tissues are limited to small islands surrounded by adipose and fibrous tissue (Gruver et al. 2007; Shiraishi et al. 2003). Thymocyte depletion begins in the subcapsular area and then declines throughout the cortex (Brelinska 2003). Cortical TEC markers gradually decline. The relative levels of thymocytes and stromal cells are reduced proportionately. By computerized tomography the large thymic profile and radiodense parenchyma evident in children dwindles into a much smaller profile in adults and appears merely as diffuse strands after middle-age (Hakim et al. 2005; Mackall et al. 1995; Sfikakis et al. 2005).

Despite the quantitative reductions in cortical and medullary tissue, thymopoiesis at some level continues throughout life (Haynes BF et al. 2000; Jamieson et al. 1999; Naylor et al. 2005). The thymus continues to generate new T-cells into the adult years and even into old age (Douek et al. 2000; Jamieson et al. 1999; Nasi et al. 2006; Naylor et al. 2005). The naïve T-cells that are newly generated in aged mice appear functionally normal, capable of germinal center formation and support of humoral immunity (Haynes L et al. 2005). In adoptive transfer studies into irradiated aged host mice, thymuses seem capable of supporting positive and negative selection (Mackall et al. 1998). Thus the main effect of thymic involution is quantitative—concomitant with involution, the level of productive thymopoiesis declines. By 40–50 years of age the thymus is producing only about 10% its maximal capacity (Flores et al. 1999). Phenotypically naive T-cells (CD45RA$^+$CD45RO$^-$ CD62L$^+$CCR7$^+$CD95$^-$) are present in the peripheral blood even in the elderly, but their numbers dwindle and fewer of these cells express markers of recent thymic emigrants (RTE)—CD31 in CD4+ T-cells and CD103 in CD8+ T-cells respectively

(Kimmig et al. 2002; McFarland et al. 2000; Nasi et al. 2006). This decline in naïve T-cells in the peripheral blood is paralleled by the decline in cells containing T-cell receptor rearrangement excision circles (TREC). TREC are non-replicating episomal DNA circles generated during V(D)J rearrangement in TCR β and α chain formation. The most commonly measured TREC, the signal joint TREC (sjTREC), is generated through the excision of the TCRδ locus during the rearrangement of the TCRα locus (Douek et al. 1998). Because most intrathymic expansion has been completed at this point, sjTREC are found in a high percentage of DP and SP thymocytes and in RTE in the peripheral blood. Because episomal DNA does not replicate, TREC frequencies are diluted by activation-induced or even homeostatic T-cell proliferation (Hazenberg et al. 2002). TREC frequencies in peripheral blood T-cells decline with age, reflecting both the decline in the level of thymopoiesis and the dilutional effects of T-cell proliferation (Douek et al. 1998; Gruver, Hudson and Sempowski 2007). Indeed the 2-log decline in TREC frequency between young adults and elderly is more extreme than the decline in phenotypically naïve T-cells; the numbers of phenotypically naïve cells are maintained by increased homeostatic cycling despite falling thymic production (Naylor et al. 2005; Wallace et al. 2004).

4 Capacity for Renewal of Thymopoiesis

Despite this gradual age-dependent decline in thymic productivity and structure, the adult thymus is remarkably capable of renewal of thymopoiesis after severe peripheral cytoreduction (Douek and Koup 2000; Hakim et al. 2005; Sfikakis et al. 2005). In a cohort of middle-aged to elderly patients undergoing autologous hematopoietic stem cell transplant for treatment of breast cancer, we were able to examine the frequency, timecourse and consequences of thymic recovery without the presence of confounding factors such as hematologic malignancy, immunosuppressive drugs or graft-versus-host disorder (Hakim et al. 2005).

We assessed thymic structural change during the post transplant period by evaluating serial thoracic CT scans using a 4 point thymic size index (Hakim et al. 2005; Kolte et al. 2002; McCune et al. 1998). The thymic profile was extremely reduced in size by the end of transplant conditioning (thymic index (TI) = 0) and in most patients thymic size remained minimal after transplant. In one third of the patients, however, thymic size gradually increased, attaining a maximum TI of at least 2, the size of the typical thymus in middle-aged adults (Hakim et al. 2005; McCune et al. 1998). Furthermore 7 of 32 patients achieved a TI of at least 3, a significantly larger thymic profile with moderate cellularity. This change in size and radiodensity is particularly remarkable in that only 2 of these patients had a TI of 3 prior to the start of therapy. Thus the development of a radiodense thymic profile post transplant in these patients represented not merely a return to the pretreatment status, but an increase over their previous status.

Two points are worth noting. The first is that the maximum thymic size attained correlated strongly with age. Whereas 4 out of 5 of the patients aged 30–39 showed a significant thymic enlargement, the incidence of thymic recovery dropped to only 6 of 13 patients among those aged 40–49, and only 2 of 14 over 50 years of age demonstrated any thymic enlargement from the treatment nadir (Hakim et al. 2005). Second the development of thymic enlargement proceeded very slowly, requiring 6–12 months in younger patients to reach maximal size and as long as 24 months in older patients showing thymic recovery.

The changes in thymic profiles represented a renewal of thymopoiesis. The recovery of radiodense thymic mass correlated strongly with the recovery of newly matured CD4$^+$ T-cells in the peripheral blood. Because more than 95% of naive CD4$^+$ T-cells are lost during transplant regimens, the reappearance and increase of phenotypically naïve T-cells post transplant can provide an estimate of recovery of newly matured cells and hence an assessment of thymic function (Hakim et al. 2005; Mackall et al. 1995). Following autologous HSC transplant, levels of naive (CD45RA$^+$CD62L$^+$) CD4$^+$+ T-cells remained low, returning to normal levels of naïve cells only in the second year, even in patients with the best thymic recovery (Hakim et al. 2005). Consistent with the pattern of thymic enlargement, the levels of naïve cells at the end of 2 years—whether assessed by phenotypic markers or by quantitative PCR of TREC—were strongly age-dependent and correlated with the maximum thymic expansion. Finally, a broad TCR repertoire diversity appeared within CD45RA$^+$ naïve CD4$^+$ T-cells within a few months after transplant. Hence the thymic role of generating broad TCR repertoire diversity was maintained in the restored thymus post transplant (Hakim et al. 2005).

In HIV seropositive patients, initiation of highly-active antiretroviral therapy (HAART) has similarly resulted (after a several month lag) in increased thymic volume and cellularity, and enhanced metabolic activity as assessed by PET imaging (Hardy et al. 2004; Hudson et al. 2007). Rapid early increases in CD4 numbers have occurred after HAART, but these were due to trafficking, increased T-cell survival and peripheral expansion (Bucy et al. 1999; Pakker et al. 1998). In contrast, the slow long-term increases in the total CD4 count after HAART were accompanied by increases in the numbers of naïve CD4 and sjTREC in the peripheral blood, indicative of a renewal of functional thymopoiesis (Dion et al. 2004; Dion et al. 2007; Douek et al. 1998; Hudson et al. 2007). As in the studies of transplant patients, however, the recovery of naïve populations required months to appear and the frequency of successful renewal of thymopoiesis declined with age (Dion et al. 2004; Dion et al. 2007; Hudson et al. 2007).

5 Control Points of Thymic Involution and Renewal

The capacity of the adult or even the aged thymus to expand and increase both thymocyte and TEC content is not limited to rebound from transplant or HIV infection. When aged porcine thymic lobes were placed in young swine as vascularized renal grafts, the thymuses were rejuvenated. Expanded TEC and thymocyte populations appeared, and became organized into densely cellular cortical and medullary structures (Nobori et al. 2006). Infusion of normal hematopoietic stem cells into IL-7Rα$^{-/-}$ mice resulted in not only an influx of normal thymocytes into the stunted thymus, but a marked increase in thymic size and cellularity (Prockop et al. 2004). Treatment with a variety of cytokines and systemic hormones has been found to enhance thymic recovery after transplant and to renew thymic size and productivity even in aged hosts, as described in section-6. Thus the adult thymus shows a remarkable ability to reverse involution, to increase thymic epithelial space and enhance productive thymopoiesis. Given this plasticity, therefore, it is important to identify the elements which control thymic size and productivity in involution and in renewal. The conditions of cytoreductive transplant regimens and the addition of various agents can impact the thymopoietic process at multiple levels. Current research points to 3 main control points determining the status of thymopoieisis: the number of functional T-progenitors that migrate to the thymus, the number of available "niches" for such cells to enter and initiate thymopoiesis, and the productive capacity of the thymopoietic maturational process itself (see Fig. 1).

5.1   Stem Cells

The capacity to generate T-cells is ultimately dependent upon the availability of functional T-progenitors. When marrow from normal mice was mixed with that from mice with T-cell maturational blocks, the final output of T-cells was directly dependent on the proportion of competent progenitors (Almeida et al. 2001). Conversely, when T-progenitors isolated from marrow or generated ex vivo by Notch signaling were infused into irradiated mice, the increased T-progenitor doses enhanced thymocyte numbers, TREC and peripheral T repopulation (Chen et al. 2004; Zakrzewski et al. 2006). Increasing evidence suggests that age-dependent declines in the levels of marrow-derived T-progenitors are a key element in decreased thymic productivity. When equivalent numbers of T-depleted marrow from young and old mice have been transplanted into irradiated young hosts, the aged marrow generated fewer peripheral T-cells (Mackall et al. 1998). Competitive thymic repopulation studies using mixtures of young and aged marrow have further determined that the aged marrow gave rise to only one tenth as many DP-thymocytes as the young marrow (Zediak, Maillard and Bhandoola 2007). The problem was not an engraftment failure; the aged marrow-derived progenitors were less productive even when injected directly into the thymus, or when cultured with Notch-ligand expressing stroma ex vivo (Zediak, Maillard and Bhandoola 2007).

These adoptive transfer and culture studies point to quantitative and qualitative changes in the marrow derived T-progenitor population. There is no evidence of a quantitative deficit in marrow of the long-term self-renewing HSC (LT-HSC). Earlier studies suggesting that LT-HSC increased 5 fold with age have been substantiated with current multiparameter cytometry (Rossi DJ et al. 2005; Rossi DJ et al. 2007; Sudo et al. 2000). The LT-HSC, which are mostly quiescent, give rise to MPP, that in turn become committed to myeloid and lymphoid lineages in response to ligand-receptor interactions and growth factors provided by the marrow microenvironment. In adoptive transfer experiments, the MPP in aged mice retained the capacity to generate myeloid populations, but lymphoid lineages were markedly reduced compared to MPP from young mice (Rossi DJ et al. 2005; Zediak, Maillard and Bhandoola 2007). It is this skewing away from lymphoid commitment that has been proposed to underlie declining lymphoid progenitor activity.

One unresolved question is whether the changes in lymphoid progenitors are due to intrinsic changes in the stem cells or to age-dependent changes in the marrow microenvironment. Rossi has argued persuasively for intrinsic changes. He determined that LT-HSC expressed a broad diversity of genes believed to be restricted to more mature and lineage-committed cell types, suggesting that transcription of lineage associated genes in stem cells occurred prior to full lineage commitment, if not as a requirement of that differentiation. When lineage-associated genes were compared in young and old HSC, marked changes in gene expression were observed, consistent with a pattern of reduced commitment toward lymphocytes and increased commitment to myeloid lineage. Genes consistent with lymphoid development such as IL-7R and Flt3 were reduced while myeloid genes were increased (Rossi DJ et al. 2005; Rossi DJ, Bryder and Weissman 2007). Since these changes occurred in the LT-HSC, preceding lineage commitment, these data support an intrinsic model of HSC decline. On the other hand, the marrow compartment undergoes aging-dependent changes that may well impact on stem cells. The most primitive long term HSC are maintained in the marrow in the calcium rich environment along the bone. In these endosteal niches, osteoblast cells producing osteopontin regulate HSC proliferation (Haylock et al. 2006). Osteoblasts provide growth factors and express Notch ligands such as Jagged-1 that shape HSC expansion and differentiation (Calvi et al. 2003; Weber et al. 2006). Administration of osteoblasts or bone fragments at the time of transplant has enhanced HSC engraftment (El-Badri et al. 1998). Furthermore administration of parathyroid hormone, which stimulates osteoblast growth, markedly increased the number of stem cells in intact mice and improved survival after transplant with limited HSC doses (Calvi et al. 2003). Finally, purified primary murine osteoblasts, cultured with parathyroid hormone, supported the full differentiation of HSC into mature B-cells whereas cytokines produced by nonosteoblast stroma shifted the cultures instead toward myeloid differentiation (Zhu et al. 2007). These last data would support a microenvironment model, one that suggests that declines in osteoblast and calcium-rich bone levels in the elderly skew the marrow microenvironment toward stromal elements favoring myeloid commitment.

Whether T-progenitor changes are intrinsic or marrow microenvironment-induced, these models would propose that a decline in committed T-progenitors would gradually starve the thymus of new progenitors and, in the absence of adequate numbers of developing thymocytes, the TEC would decline. Min et al. have determined that while thymic DN1 levels appeared to remain constant, the number of thymic ETP in unmanipulated aged mice was reduced 40-fold as compared to those in young mice (Min H et al. 2004). A gradual age-dependent decline in T-progenitors could therefore contribute to thymic decline.

5.2   Changes in Thymic Niches

The second control point for thymopoiesis is the entry or engraftment of T-progenitors into the thymus. The ability of progenitors to productively engraft is constrained by thymic elements. Much of the evidence for this is indirect. Entry of progenitors into the thymus is not a continuous process but rather a gated event; progenitor entry occurs in waves during embryogenesis and in adulthood, at least in mice, with a periodicity of 3–5 weeks in nonirradiated mice (Goldschneider 2006). Adoptive transplant experiments have shown that the number of progenitor binding sites in the thymus is limited and can be saturated (Foss et al. 2001). Treatments such as KGF (see below) can increase the number of engraftment sites, as measured by uptake of labeled progenitors (Rossi SW et al. 2007). Furthermore, functional and dysfunctional DN thymocytes can compete for these limited numbers of sites (Prockop and Petrie 2004). Capacity to productively mature into T-cells does not determine occupancy of progenitor niches; occupancy by Rag$^{-/-}$ thymocytes can block engraftment of normal progenitors (Prockop and Petrie 2004). This may be particularly relevant to aging given Min's findings that ETP in aged mice were not only severely reduced in number, but that these cells were less functional than ETP from young mice (Min H, Montecino-Rodriguez and Dorshkind 2004). If dysfunctional ETP occupying thymic niches accumulate (since they do not mature and "move on"), then productive thymopoiesis could be progressively reduced. This is an intriguing hypothesis, in that the ablation of dysfunctional (as well as functional) ETP by transplant irradiation or chemotherapy regimens could open up these niches for new engraftment. Such a general clearance of niches could contribute to the thymic renewal and expansion observed after transplant in man (Hakim et al. 2005).

The mechanisms determining progenitor engraftment "niches" remain unknown. Part may relate to expression (on progenitors or thymus) of the factors regulating T-progenitor homing. In the fetus thymus, T-progenitors depend on chemotaxis to migrate into the thymic anlaga. CC-chemokine ligands 21 (CCL21) and CCL25 on TEC interact with their corresponding receptors CCR7 and CCR9 on progenitors (Takahama 2006). Later, ETP enter through the vasculature at the CMJ (Lind et al. 2001). Although CCR9 deficiency reduces homing, it is unclear whether chemokines are specifically involved in homing or in drawing engrafted DN1 cells away from the CMJ (see 5.3 below) (Petrie et al. 2007; Takahama 2006). In contrast, the interaction of P-selectin on thymic endothelium and P-selectin ligand (PSL1) on circulating thymic progenitors plays a significant role in uptake through the CMJ vasculature (Rossi FM et al. 2005). Furthermore, the number of thymic progenitors present in the inner cortex can affect expression of P-selectin on the endothelial cells, a negative feedback loop which may play a role in gating entry of progenitors (Rossi FM et al. 2005).

5.3   Changes in Productive Expansion of DN Thymocytes

Thymic productivity is determined not only by progenitor engraftment in the thymus, but by the proliferative expansion of DN thymocytes, the process by which small numbers of progenitors can increase many thousand fold. Assessment of TREC provides evidence that the degree of expansion of DN cells during the process of thymic maturation declines with age. Although the overall number of thymocytes declines with age, the ratio of sjTREC per 10^5 thymocytes remains constant (Jamieson et al. 1999; Sempowski et al. 2000). This does not necessarily mean that increasing the supply of progenitors would increase thymopoiesis in a straightforward manner. The vast majority of thymocytes are DP cells that have just completed TCRα chain rearrangement and therefore most of these cells contain sjTREC. Dion has further analyzed thymic productivity by measuring the ratio of sjTREC (generated at the end of DN4 thymocyte proliferative expansion) to DβJβTREC (generated early in the TCR β-chain rearrangement process) (Dion et al. 2004). This ratio therefore measures the extent of proliferative expansion occurring during the main DN3/DN4 period of thymocyte increase. This ratio steadily declines with age (Dion et al. 2004). Dion's analysis of TREC ratios was particularly informative in the renewal of thymopoiesis with HAART therapy. The ratio of sjTREC to DβJβTREC increased after HAART therapy indicating an increase in the proliferative expansion of DN thymocytes during maturation, that is, an increase in thymic productivity (Dion et al. 2004; Dion et al. 2007).Thus the structural changes in the thymus are associated with a lower intrathymic proliferative expansion of progenitors, resulting in a lower thymic productivity.

The mechanisms regulating the extent of DN expansion are not fully resolved, but it is well supported that this process involves the close association of DN thymocytes with cortical TEC cells and the factors they produce during the DN migration from the CMJ vasculature outward to the SCZ of the cortex. T-cell commitment occurs in DN1 and DN2 thymocytes by recurrent signaling through Notch by its Delta-like-1 ligand on TEC-cells (Schmitt et al. 2004). TEC-cells produce IL-7, which provides a necessary survival signal during the DN1 transition to DN2 (Andrew et al. 2001; von Freeden-Jeffry et al. 1997). TEC-cells also produce the chemokines CCL21 and CCL25 that draw DN from the inner to the outer cortex and into the SCZ. Migration requires not only polarizing signals but a substrate for cell adhesion; TEC also produce the V-CAM1 that binds with the α4β1 integrins on DN-cells. The main expansion of DN occurs during this outward migration and in the SCZ, all in close association with TEC. It is recently been recognized that the TEC populations are not static but rather are maintained in a dynamic equilibrium with thymocytes (Gray et al. 2006). The wave of proliferative expansion of TEC produced by factors like keratinocyte growth factor (KGF), are immediately followed by a wave of expansion of thymocytes (Rossi SW et al. 2007). Thus factors that stimulate TEC expansion can result in expansion of thymocytes.

6 Factors Regulating Thymic Involution and Supporting Thymic Renewal

Over the last decade several factors have been identified that can effectively act on one or more of the control points in thymopoiesis (see Fig. 1). These factors can be broadly subdivided into those produced systemically in the body, those generated by the thymic stromal cells, and finally those intrinisic to the hematopoietic-lineage thymocytes themselves. Some of these factors may interact with thymopoiesis at multiple levels. Nevertheless examination of these 3 categories is useful in terms of suggesting potential avenues for thymic renewal.

6.1 Systemic Hormones

Thymopoiesis can be significantly affected by systemic hormones; age-related changes in these may therefore contribute to involution or support renewal. One candidate is the growth hormone (GH)/insulin-like growth factor 1 (IGF-1) axis. Pituitary growth hormone (GH) levels peak in man early in the third decade of life and decline with age. Most of the actions of GH are carried out by IGF-1, which is generated in the liver in response to GH, but is also produced by TEC (de Mello Coelho et al. 2002). Preclinical studies in aged mice as well as studies in lymphopenic HIV[+] patients have consistently found that treatment with either GH or IGF-1 can produce an increase in thymic cellularity and circulating naïve T-cell levels (Montecino-Rodriguez et al. 1998; Napolitano et al. 2002). Administration of IGF-1 or GH accelerates enhances hematopoietic and immune reconstitution after hematopoietic stem cell transplant in murine transplant models (Alpdogan et al. 2003; Chen et al. 2003). GH and IGF-1 may affect thymopoiesis at two levels. IGF-1 treatment increases lymphoid progenitors in the marrow, resulting in increases in pre and pro B-cells as well as increasing the supply of functional DN thymocytes (Alpdogan et al. 2003). IGF-1 also increases production of extracellular matrix by TEC and increases thymocyte adhesion to TEC (de Mello Coelho et al. 2002). Since the earliest T-progenitors migrate from the vasculature at the cortico-medullary junction to the outer subcapsular epithelium in the course of their proliferative expansion, factors that enhance DN interactions with TEC and accelerate this migration could enhance thymic productivity. Yet the level of GH is not the main determinant of involution. Thymic size is normal and involution rate is not significantly different in GH-deficient Little (*lit/lit*) mice and their normal littermates (Min H et al. 2006). Furthermore, while GH treatment can produce a doubling in thymic cellularity in old mice, just as in young ones, this increase does not reverse the much greater decline accompanying age-dependent involution (Montecino-Rodriquez et al. 2005).

While the declining levels of GH and IGF-1 may reduce lymphopoiesis, it is the converse, the post-pubertal rise in gonadal steroids—androgens, estrogens and progesterone—that may contribute to the involutional process. Gonadal steroid treatment induces involutional changes in the thymus, whereas castration or ovariectomy in rodents results in thymic enlargement, and increased thymic and peripheral T-cell populations, even in aged animals (Greenstein et al. 1986; Leposavic et al. 2001; Windmill et al. 1998). The effects of androgens on thymopoiesis are mediated through TEC, as demonstrated by experiments involving reciprocal marrow transplants between normal mice and those lacking expression of androgen receptors (Olsen et al. 2001). Drugs blocking testosterone production are equally as effective as surgical treatment. Treatment of aged rats with luteinizing hormone-releasing hormone (LHRH) analogue produced a significant increase in thymic weight (Kendall et al. 1990). Following autologous or allogeneic hematopoietic stem cell transplant, treatment with an LHRH agonist enhanced thymic recovery and increased the numbers of circulating naïve CD4$^+$+ T-cells (Goldberg et al. 2005; Goldberg et al. 2007; Heng et al. 2005; van den Brink et al. 2004). These data support the role of systemic levels of gonadal hormones in modulating thymopoiesis. It must be remembered however that progressive thymic decline in man begins in the first year of life, not at puberty. Hypogonadal mice do not have delayed thymic involution (Min H, Montecino-Rodriguez and Dorshkind 2006). Additional mechanisms must therefore contribute to thymic involution.

6.2   TEC Generated Cytokines—IL-7

Because of the critical role of TEC in all aspects of thymopoiesis, changes in TEC could regulate thymopoiesis. One mechanism proposed for thymic involution is a decline in TEC production of the cytokine IL-7, which is necessary for thymocyte maturation from DN1 to DN2. T-cell maturation was severely reduced in both IL-7 and IL-7Ra$^{-/-}$ mice(Peschon et al. 1994). In mice (although not in man), the level of IL-7 mRNA declined with age (Andrew et al. 2002). IL-7 therapy in vivo and in vitro reduced the apoptotic loss of thymocytes during the DN1->DN2 transition in aged mice (Andrew and Aspinall 2002; Phillips et al. 2004). Systemic IL-7 treatment also sped recovery of thymopoiesis following marrow transplant into irradiated hosts (Alpdogan et al. 2001; Bolotin et al. 1996). But IL-7 effects on thymopoiesis seemed to be greatest under conditions of TEC damage. IL-7 supplementation post transplant may have been replacing cytokine production lost by radiation damage to stromal cells (Chung et al. 2001). Supplemental IL-7 therapy has had only limited effects on thymopoiesis in intact hosts. IL-7 treatment did not increase thymic size or productivity in young mice (Chu et al. 2004), and short term IL-7 treatment in aged mice produced no increase in overall thymopoiesis (Sempowski et al. 2002). Marrow stroma also produce IL-7, which plays a significant role in early B-lymphoid development. Addition of IL-7 to IGF therapy had additive effects on marrow B-cell development, but did not further enhance thymopoiesis (Alpdogan et al. 2003). The strongest evidence of the limitations of IL-7 in contolling thymopoiesis come from studies of long-term IL-7 augmentation by injection of IL-7 producing stromal cells into the thymus in young mice (Phillips et al. 2004). When these mice with elevated intrathymic IL-7 production were monitored for up to 2 years, the levels of DN1 thymocytes transiting to the DN2 stage were maintained in aged mice, but structural involution of the thymus and the age-dependent decline in DP and SP thymocytes were not altered. The age-dependent decline in DN4 proliferative expansion continued unchanged despite elevated IL-7 (Phillips et al. 2004). Thus the decline in thymopoietic productivity is not dependent primarily on TEC IL-7 production.

6.3 Thymocyte Generated Cytokines—KGF

Keratinocyte growth factor, also known as fibroblast growth factor 7 (FGF-7), is produced in the mature thymus by DP- and SP-thymocytes (Erickson et al. 2002; Jenkinson et al. 2003). The TEC express the receptor (FGFR2IIIb), which binds KGF as well as the mesenchymally derived FGF-10 (Min D et al. 2002; Rossi SW et al. 2007). Unlike FGF-10. KGF is not necessary for initial thymic organogenesis, but plays an important role in the adult in renewing thymopoiesis post cytoreduction (Alpdogan et al. 2005). KGF treatment increased the uptake of labeled T-progenitors, that is the number of engraftment niches (Rossi SW et al. 2007). KGF treatment in adult mice also stimulated growth of TEC-precursors and expansion of TEC, resulting shortly afterwards in a wave of proliferative expansion in DN-thymocytes (Rossi SW et al. 2007). In aged mice or in *klotho* mice, an aging model showing early thymic involution, KGF treatment increased thymopoietic capacity and reversed involutional changes (Min D et al. 2007). Repeated monthly KGF treatments prolonged these effects and reversed involution in aged murine thymic structure, returning the thymuses to the size of those in young adults (Min D et al. 2007). The KGF results also point up the interconnections between thymocytes and TEC. RAG$^{-/-}$ thymocytes, perhaps because they are arrested prior to the DP stage, do not produce KGF (Erickson et al. 2002). The RAG$^{-/-}$ medullary region is rudimentary and disorganized in mice, but can be induced to develop either by transplant of normal hematopoietic stem cells (van Ewijk et al. 2000), or by treatment with KGF (Erickson et al. 2002).

Thus factors such as systemic hormonal shifts and intrinsic cytokine programs within thymocytes and TEC-cells can all affect thymopoiesis. The complex interactive web linking thymocyte and TEC survival and differentiation acts as an amplifying factor. Increasing the input of functional thymic progenitors can trigger an expansion of TEC, which create in turn new niches for T-cell lineage commitment and supports increased thymocyte proliferation. Alternatively, in aging, the decline in these factors may reinforce a downward spiral resulting in thymic involution.

7 Conclusions

Aging is associated with a progressive decline in the generation of new T-lymphocytes, with consequent losses in repertoire diversity and functional competence. The age-dependent involution of the thymus underlies this loss. Achieving its greatest size in the neonatal period, the thymus undergoes a steady lifelong decline in structure and productive thymopoiesis. Yet the presence of thymic renewal in adults—following autologous transplantation in cancer patients or HAART therapy in HIV+ individuals—demonstrates that the thymus is capable of regrowth. Multiple experiments in animal models have demonstrated dramatic increases in thymic size and productivity. Thus the decline in thymopoiesis is not irreversible.

Our understanding of the regulation of thymic structure and thymopoietic productivity is in a rapid state of flux. The availability of recombinant cytokines and transgenic and knockout mice have shaped our concepts of the cellular and cytokine factors regulating lymphocyte generation and homeostasis. Thymopoiesis is dependent upon a continuing supply of T-lymphoid progenitors, maintenance of open thymic niches for progenitor engraftment and support of DN migration and productive expansion by the cortical stromal microenvironment. All of these are regulated by reciprocal interactions between the marrow and thymic stromal elements and developing lymphocytes, involving both cytokine/chemokine signals and direct cell contact mediated signalling. Novel strategies have been tested to enhance progenitor numbers by supporting osteoblast growth (Ballen et al. 2007; Calvi et al. 2003; Zhu et al. 2007), or to directly stimulate early lymphoid progenitors with IGF or IL-7 (Alpdogan et al. 2003), or to bypass the marrow completely and expand committed T-progenitors ex vivo (Zakrzewski et al. 2006). On the thymic stromal side, factors such as IGF, KGF or LHRH agonists have produced increases in TEC and subsequent increases in productive thymopoiesis. Combinations of these therapies may provide the means to reverse thymic decline and renew the generation of naïve T-cells in adults or even in the aged. Although many questions remain, such treatments might provide a long-term benefit in reversing immunosenescence.

References

Almeida AR, Borghans JA and Freitas AA (2001) T cell homeostasis: thymus regeneration and peripheral T cell restoration in mice with a reduced fraction of competent precursors. J Exp Med 194:591–599

Alpdogan O, Schmaltz C, Muriglan SJ, Kappel BJ, Perales MA, Rotolo JA, Halm JA, Rich BE and Van Den Brink MR (2001) Administration of interleukin-7 after allogeneic bone marrow transplantation improves immune reconstitution without aggravating graft-versus-host disease. Blood 98:2256–2265

Alpdogan O, Muriglan SJ, Kappel BJ, Doubrovina E, Schmaltz C, Schiro R, Eng JM, Greenberg AS, Willis LM, Rotolo JA, O'Reilly RJ and Van Den Brink MR (2003) Insulin-like growth factor-I enhances lymphoid and myeloid reconstitution after allogeneic bone marrow transplantation. Transplantation 75:1977–1983

Alpdogan O, Eng JM, Muriglan SJ, Willis LM, Hubbard VM, Tjoe KH, Terwey TH, Kochman A and Van Den Brink MR (2005) Interleukin-15 enhances immune reconstitution after allogeneic bone marrow transplantation. Blood 105:865–873

Andrew D and Aspinall R (2001) IL-7 and not stem cell Factor Reverses both the increase in apoptosis and the decline in thymopoiesis seen in aged mice. J Immunol 166:1524–1530

Andrew D and Aspinall R (2002) Age-associated thymic atrophy is linked to a decline in IL-7 production. Exp Gerontol 37:455–463

Ballen KK, Shpall EJ, Avigan D, Yeap BY, Fisher DC, McDermott K, Dey BR, Attar E, McAfee S, Konopleva M, Antin JH and Spitzer TR (2007) Phase I trial of parathyroid hormone to facilitate stem cell mobilization. Biol Blood Marrow Transplant 13:838–843

Bolotin E, Smogorzewska M, Smith S, Widmer M and Weinberg K (1996) Enhancement of thymopoiesis after bone marrow transplant by in vivo interleukin-7. Blood 88:1887–1894

Brelinska R (2003) Thymic epithelial cells in age-dependent involution. Microsc Res Tech 62:488–500

Bucy RP, Hockett RD, Derdeyn CA, Saag MS, Squires K, Sillers M, Mitsuyasu RT and Kilby JM (1999) Initial increase in blood CD4(+) lymphocytes after HIV antiretroviral therapy reflects redistribution from lymphoid tissues. J Clin Invest 103:1391–1398

Calvi LM, Adams GB, Weibrecht KW, Weber JM, Olson DP, Knight MC, Martin RP, Schipani E, Divieti P, Bringhurst FR, Milner LA, Kronenberg HM and Scadden DT (2003) Osteoblastic cells regulate the haematopoietic stem cell niche. Nature 425:841–846

Chen BJ, Cui X, Sempowski GD and Chao NJ (2003) Growth hormone accelerates immune recovery following allogeneic T-cell-depleted bone marrow transplantation in mice. Exp Hematol 31:953–958

Chen BJ, Cui X, Sempowski GD, Domen J and Chao NJ (2004) Hematopoietic stem cell dose correlates with the speed of immune reconstitution after stem cell transplantation. Blood 103:4344–4352

Chu YW, Memon SA, Sharrow SO, Hakim FT, Eckhaus M, Lucas PJ and Gress RE (2004) Exogenous IL-7 increases recent thymic emigrants in peripheral lymphoid tissue without enhanced thymic function. Blood 104:1110–1119

Chung B, Barbara-Burnham L, Barsky L and Weinberg K (2001) Radiosensitivity of thymic interleukin-7 production and thymopoiesis after bone marrow transplantation. Blood 98:1601–1606

Ciofani M, Schmitt TM, Ciofani A, Michie AM, Cuburu N, Aublin A, Maryanski JL and Zuniga-Pflucker JC (2004) Obligatory role for cooperative signaling by pre-TCR and Notch during thymocyte differentiation. J Immunol 172:5230–5239

de Mello Coelho V, Villa-Verde DM, Farias-de-Oliveira DA, de Brito JM, Dardenne M and Savino W (2002) Functional insulin-like growth factor-1/insulin-like growth factor-1 receptor-mediated circuit in human and murine thymic epithelial cells. Neuroendocrinology 75:139–150

Dion ML, Poulin JF, Bordi R, Sylvestre M, Corsini R, Kettaf N, Dalloul A, Boulassel MR, Debre P, Routy JP, Grossman Z, Sekaly RP and Cheynier R (2004) HIV infection rapidly induces and maintains a substantial suppression of thymocyte proliferation. Immunity 21:757–768

Dion ML, Bordi R, Zeidan J, Asaad R, Boulassel MR, Routy JP, Lederman MM, Sekaly RP and Cheynier R (2007) Slow disease progression and robust therapy-mediated CD4+ T-cell recovery are associated with efficient thymopoiesis during HIV-1 infection. Blood 109:2912–2920

Douek DC, McFarland RD, Keiser PH, Gage EA, Massey JM, Haynes BF, Polis MA, Haase AT, Feinberg MB, Sullivan JL, Jamieson BD, Zack JA, Picker LJ and Koup RA (1998) Changes in thymic function with age and during the treatment of HIV infection. Nature 396:690–695

Douek DC and Koup RA (2000) Evidence for thymic function in the elderly. Vaccine 18:1638–1641

El-Badri NS, Wang BY, Cherry and Good RA (1998) Osteoblasts promote engraftment of allogeneic hematopoietic stem cells. Exp Hematol 26:110–116

Erickson M, Morkowski S, Lehar S, Gillard G, Beers C, Dooley J, Rubin JS, Rudensky A and Farr AG (2002) Regulation of thymic epithelium by keratinocyte growth factor. Blood 100:3269–3278

Fletcher JM, Vukmanovic-Stejic M, Dunne PJ, Birch KE, Cook JE, Jackson SE, Salmon M, Rustin MH and Akbar AN (2005) Cytomegalovirus-specific CD4+ T cells in healthy carriers are continuously driven to replicative exhaustion. J Immunol 175:8218–8225

Flores KG, Li J, Sempowski GD, Haynes BF and Hale LP (1999) Analysis of the human thymic perivascular space during aging. J Clin Invest 104:1031–1039

Foss DL, Donskoy E and Goldschneider I (2001) The importation of hematogenous precursors by the thymus is a gated phenomenon in normal adult mice. J Exp Med 193:365–374

Gallegos AM and Bevan MJ (2004) Central tolerance to tissue-specific antigens mediated by direct and indirect antigen presentation. J Exp Med 200:1039–1049

Goldberg GL, Sutherland JS, Hammet MV, Milton MK, Heng TS, Chidgey AP and Boyd RL (2005) Sex steroid ablation enhances lymphoid recovery following autologous hematopoietic stem cell transplantation. Transplantation 80:1604–1613

Goldberg GL, Alpdogan O, Muriglan SJ, Hammett MV, Milton MK, Eng JM, Hubbard VM, Kochman A, Willis LM, Greenberg AS, Tjoe KH, Sutherland JS, Chidgey A, Van Den Brink MR and Boyd RL (2007) Enhanced Immune Reconstitution by Sex Steroid Ablation following Allogeneic Hemopoietic Stem Cell Transplantation. J Immunol 178:7473–7484

Goldschneider I (2006) Cyclical mobilization and gated importation of thymocyte progenitors in the adult mouse: evidence for a thymus-bone marrow feedback loop. Immunol Rev 209:58–75

Gordon J, Wilson VA, Blair NF, Sheridan J, Farley A, Wilson L, Manley NR and Blackburn CC (2004) Functional evidence for a single endodermal origin for the thymic epithelium. Nat Immunol 5:546–553

Gray DH, Seach N, Ueno T, Milton MK, Liston A, Lew AM, Goodnow CC and Boyd RL (2006) Developmental kinetics, turnover, and stimulatory capacity of thymic epithelial cells. Blood 108:3777–3785

Greenstein BD, Fitzpatrick FT, Adcock IM, Kendall MD and Wheeler MJ (1986) Reappearance of the thymus in old rats after orchidectomy: inhibition of regeneration by testosterone. J Endocrinol 110:417–422

Gregg R, Smith CM, Clark FJ, Dunnion D, Khan N, Chakraverty R, Nayak L and Moss PA (2005) The number of human peripheral blood CD4+ CD25high regulatory T cells increases with age. Clin Exp Immunol 140:540–546

Gruver AL, Hudson LL and Sempowski GD (2007) Immunosenescence of ageing. J Pathol 211:144–156

Hakim FT, Memon SA, Cepeda R, Jones EC, Chow CK, Kasten-Sportes C, Odom J, Vance BA, Christensen BL, Mackall CL and Gress RE (2005) Age-dependent incidence, time course, and consequences of thymic renewal in adults. J Clin Invest 115:930–939

Hardy G, Worrell S, Hayes P, Barnett CM, Glass D, Pido-Lopez J, Imami N, Aspinall R, Dutton J, Gazzard B, Peters AM and Gotch FM (2004) Evidence of thymic reconstitution after highly active antiretroviral therapy in HIV-1 infection. HIV Med 5:67–73

Haylock DN and Nilsson SK (2006) Osteopontin: a bridge between bone and blood. Br J Haematol 134:467–474

Haynes BF, Markert ML, Sempowski GD, Patel DD and Hale LP (2000) The role of the thymus in immune reconstitution in aging, bone marrow transplantation, and HIV-1 infection. Annu Rev Immunol 18:529–560

Haynes L, Eaton SM, Burns EM, Randall TD and Swain SL (2005) Newly generated CD4 T cells in aged animals do not exhibit age-related defects in response to antigen. J Exp Med 201:845–851

Hazenberg MD, Otto SA, de Pauw ES, Roelofs H, Fibbe WE, Hamann D and Miedema F (2002). T-cell receptor excision circle and T-cell dynamics after allogeneic stem cell transplantation are related to clinical events. Blood 99:3449–3453

Heng TS, Goldberg GL, Gray DH, Sutherland JS, Chidgey AP and Boyd RL (2005) Effects of castration on thymocyte development in two different models of thymic involution. J Immunol 175:2982–2993

Hudson LL, Louise Markert M, Devlin BH, Haynes BF and Sempowski GD (2007) Human T cell reconstitution in DiGeorge syndrome and HIV-1 infection. Semin Immunol 19:297–309

Jamieson BD, Douek DC, Killian S, Hultin LE, Scripture-Adams DD, Giorgi JV, Marelli D, Koup RA and Zack JA (1999) Generation of functional thymocytes in the human adult. Immunity 10:569–575

Jenkinson WE, Jenkinson EJ and Anderson G (2003) Differential requirement for mesenchyme in the proliferation and maturation of thymic epithelial progenitors. J Exp Med 198:325–332

Jenkinson WE, Rossi SW, Jenkinson EJ and Anderson G (2005) Development of functional thymic epithelial cells occurs independently of lymphostromal interactions. Mech Dev 122:1294–1299

Jenkinson WE, Rossi SW, Parnell SM, Agace WW, Takahama Y, Jenkinson EJ and Anderson G (2007) Chemokine receptor expression defines heterogeneity in the earliest thymic migrants. Eur J Immunol 37:2090–2096

Jenkinson WE, Rossi SW, Parnell SM, Jenkinson EJ and Anderson G (2007) PDGFRalpha-expressing mesenchyme regulates thymus growth and the availability of intrathymic niches. Blood 109:954–960

Kendall MD, Fitzpatrick FT, Greenstein BD, Khoylou F, Safieh B and Hamblin A (1990) Reversal of ageing changes in the thymus of rats by chemical or surgical castration. Cell Tissue Res 261:555–564

Khan N, Hislop A, Gudgeon N, Cobbold M, Khanna R, Nayak L, Rickinson AB and Moss PA (2004) Herpesvirus-specific CD8 T cell immunity in old age: cytomegalovirus impairs the response to a coresident EBV infection. J Immunol 173:7481–7489

Kimmig S, Przybylski GK, Schmidt CA, Laurisch K, Mowes B, Radbruch A and Thiel A (2002) Two subsets of naive T helper cells with distinct T cell receptor excision circle content in human adult peripheral blood. J Exp Med 195:789–794

King C, Ilic A, Koelsch K and Sarvetnick N (2004) Homeostatic expansion of T cells during immune insufficiency generates autoimmunity. Cell 117:265–277

Klug DB, Carter C, Crouch E, Roop D, Conti CJ and Richie ER (1998) Interdependence of cortical thymic epithelial cell differentiation and T-lineage commitment. Proc Natl Acad Sci U S A 95:11822–11827

Klug DB, Carter C, Gimenez-Conti IB and Richie ER (2002) Cutting edge: thymocyte-independent and thymocyte-dependent phases of epithelial patterning in the fetal thymus. J Immunol 169:2842–2845

Kolte L, Dreves AM, Ersboll AK, Strandberg C, Jeppesen DL, Nielsen JO, Ryder LP and Nielsen SD (2002) Association between larger thymic size and higher thymic output in human immunodeficiency virus-infected patients receiving highly active antiretroviral therapy. J Infect Dis 185:1578–1585

Lazuardi L, Jenewein B, Wolf AM, Pfister G, Tzankov A and Grubeck-Loebenstein B (2005) Age-related loss of naive T cells and dysregulation of T-cell/B-cell interactions in human lymph nodes. Immunology 114:37–43

LeMaoult J, Messaoudi I, Manavalan JS, Potvin H, Nikolich-Zugich D, Dyall R, Szabo P, Weksler ME and Nikolich-Zugich J (2000) Age-related dysregulation in CD8 T cell homeostasis: kinetics of a diversity loss. J Immunol 165:2367–2373

Leposavic G, Obradovic S, Kosec D, Pejcic-Karapetrovic B and Vidic-Dankovic B (2001) In vivo modulation of the distribution of thymocyte subsets by female sex steroid hormones. Int Immunopharmacol 1:1–12

Lewin SR, Heller G, Zhang L, Rodrigues E, Skulsky E, Van Den Brink MR, Small TN, Kernan NA, O'Reilly RJ, Ho DD and Young JW (2002) Direct evidence for new T-cell generation by patients after either T-cell-depleted or unmodified allogeneic hematopoietic stem cell transplantations. Blood 100:2235–2242

Lind EF, Prockop SE, Porritt HE and Petrie HT (2001) Mapping precursor movement through the postnatal thymus reveals specific microenvironments supporting defined stages of early lymphoid development. J Exp Med 194:127–134

Mackall CL, Fleisher TA, Brown MR, Andrich MP, Chen CC, Feuerstein IM, Horowitz ME, Magrath IT, Shad AT, Steinberg SM and et al. (1995) Age, thymopoiesis, and CD4+ T-lymphocyte regeneration after intensive chemotherapy. N Engl J Med 332:143–149

Mackall CL, Punt JA, Morgan P, Farr AG and Gress RE (1998) Thymic function in young/old chimeras: substantial thymic T cell regenerative capacity despite irreversible age-associated thymic involution. Eur J Immunol 28:1886–1893

McCune JM, Loftus R, Schmidt DK, Carroll P, Webster D, Swor-Yim LB, Francis IR, Gross BH and Grant RM (1998) High prevalence of thymic tissue in adults with human immunodeficiency virus-1 infection. J Clin Invest 101:2301–2308

McFarland RD, Douek DC, Koup RA and Picker LJ (2000) Identification of a human recent thymic emigrant phenotype. Proc Natl Acad Sci U S A 97:4215–4220

Messaoudi I, Lemaoult J, Guevara-Patino JA, Metzner BM and Nikolich-Zugich J (2004) Age-related CD8 T cell clonal expansions constrict CD8 T cell repertoire and have the potential to impair immune defense. J Exp Med 200:1347–1358

Min D, Taylor PA, Panoskaltsis-Mortari A, Chung B, Danilenko DM, Farrell C, Lacey DL, Blazar BR and Weinberg KI (2002) Protection from thymic epithelial cell injury by keratinocyte growth factor: a new approach to improve thymic and peripheral T-cell reconstitution after bone marrow transplantation. Blood 99:4592–4600

Min D, Panoskaltsis-Mortari A, Kuro OM, Hollander GA, Blazar BR and Weinberg KI (2007) Sustained thymopoiesis and improvement in functional immunity induced by exogenous KGF administration in murine models of aging. Blood 109:2529–2537

Min H, Montecino-Rodriguez E and Dorshkind K (2004) Reduction in the developmental potential of intrathymic T cell progenitors with age. J Immunol 173:245–250

Min H, Montecino-Rodriguez E, and Dorshkind K (2006) Reassessing the role of growth hormone and sex steroids in thymic involution. Clin Immunol 118:117–123

Montecino-Rodriguez E, Clark R and Dorshkind K (1998) Effects of insulin-like growth factor administration and bone marrow transplantation on thymopoiesis in aged mice. Endocrinology 139:4120–4126

Montecino-Rodriquez E, Min H and Dorshkind K (2005) Reevaluating current models of thymic involution. Semin Immunol 17:356–361

Nanda NK, Apple R and Sercarz E (1991) Limitations in plasticity of the T-cell receptor repertoire. Proc Natl Acad Sci U S A 88:9503–9507

Napolitano LA, Lo JC, Gotway MB, Mulligan K, Barbour JD, Schmidt D, Grant RM, Halvorsen RA, Schambelan M and McCune JM (2002) Increased thymic mass and circulating naive CD4 T cells in HIV-1-infected adults treated with growth hormone. AIDS 16:1103–1111

Nasi M, Troiano L, Lugli E, Pinti M, Ferraresi R, Monterastelli E, Mussi C, Salvioli G, Franceschi C and Cossarizza A (2006) Thymic output and functionality of the IL-7/IL-7 receptor system in centenarians: implications for the neolymphogenesis at the limit of human life. Aging Cell 5:167–175

Naylor K, Li G, Vallejo AN, Lee WW, Koetz K, Bryl E, Witkowski J, Fulbright J, Weyand CM and Goronzy JJ (2005) The influence of age on T cell generation and TCR diversity. J Immunol 174:7446–7452

Nobori S, Shimizu A, Okumi M, Samelson-Jones E, Griesemer A, Hirakata A, Sachs DH and Yamada K (2006) Thymic rejuvenation and the induction of tolerance by adult thymic grafts. Proc Natl Acad Sci U S A 103:19081–19086

Olsen NJ, Olson G, Viselli SM, Gu X and Kovacs WJ (2001) Androgen receptors in thymic epithelium modulate thymus size and thymocyte development. Endocrinology 142:1278–1283

Ouyang Q, Wagner WM, Wikby A, Walter S, Aubert G, Dodi AI, Travers P and Pawelec G (2003) Large numbers of dysfunctional CD8+ T lymphocytes bearing receptors for a single dominant CMV epitope in the very old. J Clin Immunol 23:247–257

Pakker NG, Notermans DW, de Boer RJ, Roos MT, de Wolf F, Hill A, Leonard JM, Danner SA, Miedema F and Schellekens PT (1998) Biphasic kinetics of peripheral blood T cells after triple combination therapy in HIV-1 infection: a composite of redistribution and proliferation. Nat Med 4:208–214

Peschon JJ, Morrissey PJ, Grabstein KH, Ramsdell FJ, Maraskovsky E, Gliniak BC, Park LS, Ziegler SF, Williams DE, Ware CB and et al. (1994) Early lymphocyte expansion is severely impaired in interleukin 7 receptor-deficient mice. J Exp Med 180:1955–1960

Petrie HT and Zuniga-Pflucker JC (2007) Zoned out: functional mapping of stromal signaling microenvironments in the thymus. Annu Rev Immunol 25:649–679

Phillips JA, Brondstetter TI, English CA, Lee HE, Virts EL and Thoman ML (2004) IL-7 gene therapy in aging restores early thymopoiesis without reversing involution. J Immunol 173:4867–4874

Prockop SE and Petrie HT (2004) Regulation of thymus size by competition for stromal niches among early T cell progenitors. Journal of Immunology 173:1604–1611

Revest JM, Suniara RK, Kerr K, Owen JJ and Dickson C (2001) Development of the thymus requires signaling through the fibroblast growth factor receptor R2-IIIb. J Immunol 167:1954–1961

Rossi DJ, Bryder D, Zahn JM, Ahlenius H, Sonu R, Wagers AJ and Weissman IL (2005) Cell intrinsic alterations underlie hematopoietic stem cell aging. Proc Natl Acad Sci U S A 102:9194–9199

Rossi DJ, Bryder D and Weissman IL (2007) Hematopoietic stem cell aging: mechanism and consequence. Exp Gerontol 42:385–390

Rossi FM, Corbel SY, Merzaban JS, Carlow DA, Gossens K, Duenas J, So L, Yi L and Ziltener HJ (2005) Recruitment of adult thymic progenitors is regulated by P-selectin and its ligand PSGL-1. Nat Immunol 6:626–634

Rossi SW, Jenkinson WE, Anderson G and Jenkinson EJ (2006) Clonal analysis reveals a common progenitor for thymic cortical and medullary epithelium. Nature 441:988–991

Rossi SW, Chidgey AP, Parnell SM, Jenkinson WE, Scott HS, Boyd RL, Jenkinson EJ and Anderson G (2007) Redefining epithelial progenitor potential in the developing thymus. Eur J Immunol 37:2411–2418

Rossi SW, Jeker LT, Ueno T, Kuse S, Keller MP, Zuklys S, Gudkov AV, Tkahama Y, Krenger W, Blazar BR and Hollander GA (2007) Keratinocyte growth factor (KGF) enhances postnatal T-cell development via enhancements in proliferation and function of thymic epithelial cells. Blood 109

Roux E, Dumont-Girard F, Starobinski M, Siegrist CA, Helg C, Chapuis B and Roosnek E (2000) Recovery of immune reactivity after T-cell-depleted bone marrow transplantation depends on thymic activity. Blood 96:2299–2303

Schmitt TM and Zuniga-Pflucker JC (2002) Induction of T cell development from hematopoietic progenitor cells by delta-like-1 in vitro. Immunity 17:749–756

Schmitt TM, Ciofani M, Petrie HT and Zuniga-Pflucker JC (2004) Maintenance of T cell specification and differentiation requires recurrent notch receptor-ligand interactions. J Exp Med 200:469–479

Schmitt TM, de Pooter RF, Gronski MA, Cho SK, Ohashi PS and Zuniga-Pflucker JC (2004) Induction of T cell development and establishment of T cell competence from embryonic stem cells differentiated in vitro. Nat Immunol 5:410–417

Schwab R, Szabo P, Manavalan JS, Weksler ME, Posnett DN, Pannetier C, Kourilsky P and Even J (1997) Expanded CD4+ and CD8+ T cell clones in elderly humans. J Immunol 158:4493–4499

Schwarz BA, Sambandam A, Maillard I, Harman BC, Love PE and Bhandoola A (2007) Selective thymus settling regulated by cytokine and chemokine receptors. J Immunol 178:2008–2017

Scimone ML, Aifantis I, Apostolou I, von Boehmer H and von Andrian UH (2006) A multistep adhesion cascade for lymphoid progenitor cell homing to the thymus. Proc Natl Acad Sci U S A 103:7006–7011

Sempowski GD, Hale LP, Sundy JS, Massey JM, Koup RA, Douek DC, Patel DD and Haynes BF (2000) Leukemia inhibitory factor, oncostatin M, IL-6, and stem cell factor mRNA expression in human thymus increases with age and is associated with thymic atrophy. J Immunol 164:2180–2187

Sempowski GD, Gooding ME, Liao HX, Le PT and Haynes BF (2002) T cell receptor excision circle assessment of thymopoiesis in aging mice. Mol Immunol 38:841–848

Sfikakis PP, Gourgoulis GM, Moulopoulos LA, Kouvatseas G, Theofilopoulos AN and Dimopoulos MA (2005) Age-related thymic activity in adults following chemotherapy-induced lymphopenia. Eur J Clin Invest 35:380–387

Shiraishi J, Utsuyama M, Seki S, Akamatsu H, Sunamori M, Kasai M and Hirokawa K (2003) Essential microenvironment for thymopoiesis is preserved in human adult and aged thymus. Clin Dev Immunol 10:53–59

Shores EW, Van Ewijk W and Singer A (1991) Disorganization and restoration of thymic medullary epithelial cells in T cell receptor-negative scid mice: evidence that receptor-bearing lymphocytes influence maturation of the thymic microenvironment. Eur J Immunol 21:1657–1661

Shores EW, Van Ewijk W and Singer A (1994) Maturation of medullary thymic epithelium requires thymocytes expressing fully assembled CD3-TCR complexes. Int Immunol 6:1393–1402

Steinmann GG, Klaus B and Muller-Hermelink HK (1985) The involution of the ageing human thymic epithelium is independent of puberty. A morphometric study. Scand J Immunol 22:563–575

Sudo K, Ema H, Morita Y and Nakauchi H (2000) Age-associated characteristics of murine hematopoietic stem cells. J Exp Med 192:1273–1280

Takahama Y (2006) Journey through the thymus: stromal guides for T-cell development and selection. Nat Rev Immunol 6:127–135

Tanchot C, Fernandes HV and Rocha B (2000) The organization of mature T-cell pools. Philos Trans R Soc Lond B Biol Sci 355:323–328

Van Den Brink MR, Alpdogan O and Boyd RL (2004) Strategies to enhance T-cell reconstitution in immunocompromised patients. Nat Rev Immunol 4:856–867

van Ewijk W, Hollander G, Terhorst C and Wang B (2000) Stepwise development of thymic microenvironments in vivo is regulated by thymocyte subsets. Development 127:1583–1591

von Freeden-Jeffry U, Solvason N, Howard M and Murray R (1997) The earliest T lineage-committed cells depend on IL-7 for Bcl-2 expression and normal cell cycle progression. Immunity 7:147–154

Vukmanovic-Stejic M, Zhang Y, Cook JE, Fletcher JM, McQuaid A, Masters JE, Rustin MH, Taams LS, Beverley PC, Macallan DC and Akbar AN (2006) Human CD4+ CD25hi Foxp3 +regulatory T cells are derived by rapid turnover of memory populations in vivo. J Clin Invest 116:2423–2433

Walker MR, Kasprowicz DJ, Gersuk VH, Benard A, Van Landeghen M, Buckner JH and Ziegler SF (2003) Induction of FoxP3 and acquisition of T regulatory activity by stimulated human CD4+CD25- T cells. J Clin Invest 112:1437–1443

Wallace DL, Zhang Y, Ghattas H, Worth A, Irvine A, Bennett AR, Griffin GE, Beverley PC, Tough DF and Macallan DC (2004) Direct measurement of T cell subset kinetics in vivo in elderly men and women. J Immunol 173:1787–1794

Watanabe N, Hanabuchi S, Soumelis V, Yuan W, Ho S, de Waal Malefyt R and Liu YJ (2004) Human thymic stromal lymphopoietin promotes dendritic cell-mediated CD4+ T cell homeostatic expansion. Nat Immunol 5:426–434

Watanabe N, Wang YH, Lee HK, Ito T, Wang YH, Cao W and Liu YJ (2005) Hassall's corpuscles instruct dendritic cells to induce CD4+CD25+ regulatory T cells in human thymus. Nature 436:1181–1185

Weber JM, Forsythe SR, Christianson CA, Frisch BJ, Gigliotti BJ, Jordan CT, Milner LA, Guzman ML and Calvi LM (2006) Parathyroid hormone stimulates expression of the Notch ligand Jagged1 in osteoblastic cells. Bone 39:485–493

Windmill KF and Lee VW (1998) Effects of castration on the lymphocytes of the thymus, spleen and lymph nodes. Tissue Cell 30:104–111

Wing K, Ekmark A, Karlsson H, Rudin A and Suri-Payer E (2002) Characterization of humanCD25 +CD4+ T cells in thymus, cord and adult blood. Immunology 106:190–199

Wing K, Larsson P, Sandstrom K, Lundin SB, Suri-Payer E and Rudin A (2005) CD4+ CD25+ FOXP3 +regulatory T cells from human thymus and cord blood suppress antigen-specific T cell responses. Immunology 115:516–525

Yu Q, Erman B, Bhandoola A, Sharrow SO and Singer A (2003) In vitro evidence that cytokine receptor signals are required for differentiation of double positive thymocytes into functionally mature CD8+ T cells. J Exp Med 197:475–487

Zakrzewski JL, Kochman AA, Lu SX, Terwey TH, Kim TD, Hubbard VM, Muriglan SJ, Suh D, Smith OM, Grubin J, Patel N, Chow A, Cabrera-Perez J, Radhakrishnan R, Diab A, Perales MA, Rizzuto G, Menet E, Pamer EG, Heller G, Zuniga-Pflucker JC, Alpdogan O and Van Den Brink MR (2006) Adoptive transfer of T-cell precursors enhances T-cell reconstitution after allogeneic hematopoietic stem cell transplantation. Nat Med 12:1039–1047

Zediak VP, Maillard I and Bhandoola A (2007) Multiple prethymic defects underlie age-related loss of T progenitor competence. Blood 110:1161–1167

Zhao L, Sun L, Wang H, Ma H, Liu G and Zhao Y (2007) Changes of CD4+CD25+Foxp3+ regulatory T cells in aged Balb/c mice. J Leukocyte Biol 81:1386–1394

Zhu J, Garrett R, Jung Y, Zhang Y, Kim N, Wang J, Joe GJ, Hexner E, Choi Y, Taichman RS and Emerson SG (2007) Osteoblasts support B-lymphocyte commitment and differentiation from hematopoietic stem cells. Blood 109:3706–3712

Mechanisms- Inflammation

Inflamm-Aging

L. Bucci, R. Ostan, M. Capri, S. Salvioli, E. Cevenini, L. Celani, D. Monti
and C. Franceschi

Contents

1 Introduction

The function of immune system depends on a subtle and well tuned network of humoral mediators, collectively called cytokines, responsible for differentiation, proliferation and survival of lymphoid cells. They include colony stimulating factors, and cytokines such as interferons and tumor necrosis factors (TNFs). These molecules constitute a complex network: cytokines, such as IL-2, have a particular importance for the proliferation and differentiation of T, B, and NK cells. IL-2 and IL-10 lead to an increased production of IgM, IgG and IgA, whereas IL-4 and IL-13 induce IgE and IgG4 synthesis. Other cytokines, such as IL-1, IL-6 and TNF-α are considered proinflammatory agents, and play an important role in the immune response and inflammation.

C. Franceschi (✉) · L. Bucci · M. Capri · S. Salvioli
Department of Experimental Pathology
University of Bologna, Via San Giacomo 12
I-40126 Bologna, Italy
Tel.: +39 051 209 4743
Fax: +39 051 209 4747
E-mail: claudio.franceschi@unibo.it

R. Ostan · D. Monti
Department of Experimental Pathology and Oncology
University of Florence, Viale Morgagni 50
I-50134 Florence, Italy

M. Capri · S. Salvioli · E. Cevenini · L. Celani · C. Franceschi
CIG-Interdepartmental Center "L. Galvani"
University of Bologna, Via San Giacomo 12
I-40126 Bologna, Italy

T. Fulop et al. (eds.), *Handbook on Immunosenescence,*
DOI 10.1007/ 978-1-4020-9062-2_45, © Springer Science+Business Media B.V. 2009

It's widely accepted that many of the most important age-associated diseases, such as cardiovascular diseases, atherosclerosis, Alzheimer's disease, arthrosis and arthritis, sarcopenia and diabetes share a common inflammatory background (Appay and Rowland-Jones 2002; Boren and Gershwin 2004; Cappola et al. 2003; Licastro et al. 2003; Roubenoff et al. 2003a,b; Szmitko et al. 2003; Zanni et al. 2003). Inflammatory reactions are a complex series of physiological events designed to limit insult and promote repair. During aging it has been observed a complex remodelling of the immune system responsible for a series of age-related phenomena, among which a profound modification within the cytokine network. The typical feature of this phenomenon is a general increase in plasmatic levels and cell capability to produce proinflammatory cytokines. The first evidence of this age-associated modification in the balance of cytokine network was described by Fagiolo et al. (1993) who found an increase of IL-6 plasma levels and a decrease of IL-2 production in healthy elderly subjects (Fagiolo et al. 1993; Franceschi et al. 1995). Moreover, the authors described a significant increase of IL-6, TNF-α and IL-1β levels in mitogen-stimulated cultures from aged donors. These data indicated that the cellular machinery for the production of these cytokines is well preserved in aging, and also that cells from old people are able to up-regulate their production in response to appropriate stimuli. The well established increase with age of IL-1, IL-6 and TNF-α plasma levels appears to be unexpectedly present either in persons who enjoyed successful aging and those who suffered age-associated pathologies. This increase continues with age, until the extreme limit of human life, and high levels of IL-6 are found in healthy centenarians (Baggio et al. 1998). In these exceptional individuals other inflammatory factors, such as acute phase proteins, lipoprotein a [Lp(a)], fibrinogen, coagulation factors, and other proinflammatory cytokines are similarly increased (Baggio et al. 1998; Bruunsgaard et al. 1999; Mannucci et al. 1997; Mari et al. 1995). Thus, even if high levels of IL-6 have been indicated as one of the most powerful predictors of morbidity and mortality in the elderly (Ferrucci et al. 1999; Harris et al. 1999), an inflammatory status is compatible with extreme longevity and paradoxically proin-flammatory condition have been documented in centenarians in relatively good health (category A and B as in Franceschi et al. 2000a). Another proinflamma-tory cytokine, IL-18, increases with age and centenarians display significant higher serum levels compared to people of younger ages. However, higher levels of IL-18-binding protein, a protein which binds and neutralizes IL-18, is also increased, suggesting that compensatory mechanisms capable of quenching the proinflam-matory activity of IL-18 likely occur with age (Gangemi et al. 2003). In addition, the reshaping of the cytokine network in aging is extended to chemokines and proinflammatory molecules regulating monocyte and T lymphocyte recruitment towards sites of inflammation. The production of chemokines such as RANTES, MIP-1α, IL-8 and MCP-1 is increased in the elderly with clear consequences for the inflammatory mechanisms and the recirculation of lymphocyte subsets (Gerli et al. 2000; Mariani et al. 2002).

This chronic, low grade, proinflammatory condition was named *inflamm-aging* (Franceschi et al. 2000b,c) and it is characterized by a general increase in the production of inflammatory cytokines and a subsequent rise of the main inflammatory markers, such as C-reactive protein (CRP) and serum amyloid A. It is at the present unknown whether the derangement in the regulation of inflammatory reactions is a cause or rather an effect of the aging process as a whole. Nevertheless, an altered inflammatory response can probably be the result of the chronic exposure to stressors, such as antigens, leading to a progressive activation of macrophages and related cells in most organs and tissues of the body, but also to chemical and physical agents that threaten the integrity of the organism (Franceschi et al. 2000b). The chronic proinflammatory status can be in some cases an important cause of damage, by itself or by interacting with other pathological molecular mechanisms, thus contributing to the acceleration of the onset of different diseases or their severity. Indeed, it has been demonstrated that a proinflammatory status is related to mortality risk for all causes in older persons (Bruunsgaard et al. 2001) rendering the subjects more prone to a variety of infectious and noninfectious diseases (cardiovascular diseases, neurodegenerative disorders, osteoporosis, sarcopenia and diabetes, among others; De Martinis et al. 2005).

2 Memory Cells and Filling of Immunological Space

Immunosenescence is not accompanied by an unavoidable and progressive deterioration of the immune function, but is rather the result of a remodelling where some functions are reduced, others remain unchanged or even increased. Both humoral and cell-mediated specific immune response are modified and remodelled by aging. The ancestral/innate compartment of the immune system appears relatively preserved during aging in comparison to the more recent and sophisticated adaptive compartment that exhibit more profound modifications. Clinical evidence indicates that with advancing age, immune responses against recall antigens may still be conserved (Ahmed et al. 1996), but the ability to mount primary immune responses against novel antigens declines significantly (Weigle 1989). The impaired ability to mount immune responses to new antigens may result in an higher susceptibility to infectious diseases and may limit the efficacy of vaccination strategies in elderly people.

In fact, one of the main characteristics of immunosenescence is the process termed *thymic involution*, responsible for a progressive, age-related reduction in size of the thymus, due to profound changes in its anatomy, associated with loss of thymic epithelial cells and a decrease in thymopoiesis. This decline in the output of newly developed T-cells results in a diminished number of circulating naïve T-cells and an impaired cell mediated immunity (Fagnoni et al. 2000). A major consequence of thymic involution is a profound age-related change in T lymphocyte subpopulations (Nasi et al. 2006).

The rate of naïve T-cell output from the thymus dramatically declines, and memory T-cells proliferate in the periphery to replace the loss of thymic output, a phenomenon called *homeostatic expansion* (or *proliferation*; Aspinall et al. 2000, Berzins et al. 2002).

Thus, the loss of naïve T-cells, able to cope with new antigens, leads to the accumulation of memory and effector cells, a phenomenon described as "filling of the immunological space" (Franceschi et al. 2000b,c; Luciani et al. 2001). Indeed, we demostrated that aging is accompanied by an increase of memory T-cells, and this phenomenon is different in CD4+ and CD8+ T-cells (Cossarizza et al. 1996). The concomitant occurrence of these two phenomena, i.e., decrease of virgin T-cells and increase of memory T-cells, related to thymic involution and lifelong antigenic load, respectively, is the most important characteristics of immunosenescence and of its clinical correlates.

The exhaustion of thymic output occurring during aging is also confirmed by phenotypic analysis, and this phenomenon is more rapid and evident in CD8+ T-cells (Fagnoni et al. 1996, 2000; Franceschi et al. 1995; Zanni et al. 2003). Recently, CD31-CD4+ T-cells were identified as an autonomously regulated subset, characterized by a highly restricted oligoclonal TCR repertoire, which constitutes a pool of naïve T-cells not affected by thymic decline, likely playing a central role in adaptive immunity and providing sufficient number of naïve CD4+ T-cells in the elderly, even in the presence of a drastically reduced thymic function (Kohler et al. 2005). T-cells accumulating with age are mainly CD28- T lymphocytes in both CD8+ and CD4+ subsets (Fagnoni et al. 1996; Valenzuela et al. 2002; Zhang et al. 2002). CD28 serves both as a costimulatory molecule for T-cell activation (Krause et al. 1998; Sepulveda et al. 1999) and as a signal for glucose transport (Frauwirth et al. 2002). CD28- T-cells display several aspects of senescence, including oligoclonal expansion (Batliwalla et al. 1996), shortened telomeres (Effros 1997; Valenzuela et al. 2002), limited proliferative potential (Effros 1997; Valenzuela et al. 2002, Vallejo et al. 2001), production of TNF-α and IL-6 (Zanni et al. 2003), and resistance to apoptosis (Brzezinska et al. 2004; Posnett et al. 1999). Many studies indicate that the memory pool is composed of different subsets based on the expression of chemokine receptors, selectins, and costimulatory receptors. *Central memory T-cells* (TCM) bear lymph node homing receptors (L-selectin, CD62L, and CC-chemokine receptor 7 [CCR7]) and costimulatory molecules, such as CD27 and CD28. These cells show a scarce effector function, but can have extensive replicative response to their specific antigen (Maus et al. 2004). *Effector memory* T-cells (TEM) have the capability to exert immediate effector functions (cytokines secretion and/or cytotoxic activity) and are characterized by the lack of CCR7 and by a heterogeneous expression of CD62L. Both the mentioned cell subsets have down-regulated the CD45RA, a marker of virgin T lymphocytes. Moreover, *terminally differentiated T-cells* (TTD), characterized by the expression of CD45RA (as naïve cells), the lack of CCR7 and CD62L, and usually of CD28-, accumulate with age, particularly in CD8+ T-cells (Pawelec et al. 2005). These profound age-related changes at the cellular level are accompanied by the peculiar, chronic, low grade proinflammatory status (inflamm-aging) suggesting that immunosenescence is mainly driven by a chronic antigenic load which not only induces an enormous expansion of CD28- T-cells, but also increases their functional activity, confirmed by an high frequency of cells positive for proinflammatory cytokines.

Indeed, a general trend towards an increase of both type 1 and type 2 cytokine-positive cells in naïve, memory and effector/cytotoxic CD8 T-cells was found. The increase of type 1 intracellular cytokines is particularly marked in memory and effector T CD8⁺ lymphocytes. In old subjects, IFN-γ and TNF-α producing cells account for more than 60% of the CD8⁺ T-cells. The increase of type 2 cytokines producing cells is lower when compared to type 1 and it results more evident in CD8⁺ memory cells (Zanni et al. 2003).

The increased proinflammatory cytokines can be regarded as a double edged sword that at one side could be beneficial and protective in amplifying, via IFN-γ, the immune response against internal or external pathogens (Guidotti et al. 1996), and, on the other side, could be detrimental, later in life, via an excessive TNF-α and IFN-γ production capable of sustaining chronic inflammatory or autoimmune processes (Feldmann et al. 1997) that negatively correlate with human longevity.

Within this scenario, we can surmise that the continuous attrition caused by clinical and subclinical infections, as well as the continuous exposure to other types of antigens (food, allergens), is likely responsible for the chronic immune system activation and inflammation (De Martinis et al. 2004; Franceschi et al. 1999).

Emerging data suggest a possible contribution of CMV infection to this progressive, systemic, low grade proinflammatory status characteristic of immunosenescence. The age-dependent expansion of CD8⁺CD28⁻ T-cells, mostly positive for proinflammatory cytokines and including the majority of Cytomegalovirus (CMV)-epitope-specific cells, underlines the importance of chronic antigenic stimulation in the pathogenesis of the main immunological alterations of aging and may favor the appearance of several inflammatory pathologies (arteriosclerosis, dementia, osteoporosis, cancer; Sansoni et al. 2008).

Large clonal expansion of peripheral CD8⁺ T-cells carrying receptors for single epitopes of CMV and Epstein-Barr Virus, detected using tetramer technology, are common in the elderly and are associated with a loss of effector memory cells, an increase of terminally differentiated CD8⁺ cells and a gradual reduction of the immunological space (Franceschi et al. 2000c).

Functional T-cell responses to pp65 and IE-1 peptides, two CMV immunogenic proteins, performed on humans of different ages indicate that the pp65 is the major antigen against which aged people target their T-cells effector function with massive production of Th1 cytokines and increased presence of potential cytotoxic cells exhibiting degranulation markers (CD107a). Indeed, both CMV antigens are able to increase the production of IFN-γ and TNF-α in old subject in comparison with younger even if the CD4 and CD8 T- responses are not so similar. In fact, these two lymphocyte subsets respond differently to the same antigen and an inverse correlation exists between anti pp65-INF-γ⁺ CD4⁺ and CD8⁺ T-cells (Vescovini et al. 2007).

On the whole, the existing literature suggests that CMV could represent one of the most important agent of effector T-cell expansion and a possible main mechanism underlying the persistent activation of the immune system in the elderly. This stable load of effector helper and cytotoxic T-cells producing IFN-γ and TNF-α and having a potential cytolytic activity may be necessary to protect elderly people from CMV endogenous reactivation but, at the same time, may also became detrimental at the systemic and tissue levels. Finally, we can say that the expansion of functional effector T-cell producing high amounts of inflammatory cytokines may be considered as a general age-related phenomenon in CMV seropositive donors, that might give a substantial contribution to inflamm-aging (Vescovini et al. 2007).

Indeed, the number of functional CMV-specific CD8 cells is quite similar in young and old individuals. This is consistent with suggestion that these cells may contribute to the proinflammatory status often observed in the elderly and may contribute to frailty and mortality. Furthermore, in the elderly there is an accumulation of CMV-specific CD8 cells negative for CD28 and positive for the KLRG-1 and CD57. The presence of these two markers identifies dysfunctional CD8 T-cells that were not able to proliferate (Koch et al. 2007). In CMV seropositive individuals an accumulation of CMV-specific CD4 cells during aging is present. These cells are characterized by an effector phenotype (CD28⁻, IFN-γ⁺ and IL-2; Pourgheysari et al. 2007).

Moreover, the production of type 1 or type 2 cytokines by CD4⁺ T-cells appears to be differently affected by aging process. Precisely, the percentage of INF-γ⁺ cells decreases in virgin CD4⁺ and in activated/memory T-cells from aged subjects in comparison with young subjects. The percentage of TNF-α⁺ cells increases in activated/memory CD4⁺ T subsets from nonagenarians. Concerning type 2 cytokines, IL-4⁺ cells increased in activated/memory CD4⁺ subset from nonagenarians suggesting a shift towards type 2 cytokines (Alberti et al. 2006).

3   Shrinkage of T-Cell Repertoire

Both quantitative and qualitative changes of T lymphocyte subsets are implicated in the age-related remodelling of the immune response (Miller et al. 1996). Antigen-independent mechanisms such as different survival of T-cell clones or decreased thymic generation of new naïve T-cells may also influence the clonal composition of peripheral T-cells. These factors may eventually lead to the narrowing of the clonal repertoire and to the appearance of predominant clones in aged people. Both in CD4 and in CD8 T-cells, clonal expansion comprises several TCR V$_\beta$ families suggesting that a multiplicity of antigenic stimulations are involved in the selection of the expanded clones. The CD4⁺ T-cell repertoire remains largely polyclonal throughout life, since CD4⁺ expanded clones accumulate predominantly in the CD45R0⁺ compartment of exceptionally individuals (centenarians; Wack et al. 1998). On the other hand, CD8⁺ T-cell subsets contain expanded clones which are already detectable in young adults and become very frequent in older donors both in CD45RA⁺ and in CD45R0⁺ compartments. The presence of expanded clones in the CD45RA⁺ compartment implies that this age-related phenomenon starts earlier, and it is more pronounced in CD8⁺ than in the CD4⁺ T-cell subsets indicating that in these two subsets the clonal expansion is controlled by substantially different mechanisms. Besides, while the finding of expanded CD45R0$^+$ T-cell clones is explained by antigen-driven proliferation, the detection of expanded clones both in CD45RA$^+$ and in CD45R0$^+$ subsets support the idea of reversion from the CD45R0$^+$ to the CD45RA$^+$ phenotype after antigen encounter (Wack et al. 1998). Moreover, TCR V$_\beta$ repertoire of T lymphocytes was studied in healthy, long-living people and centenarians using a spectra typing method, and expansion of TCR Vβ1, Vβ8, and Vβ20 in long-living people compared with young people was found. In addition these expanded clones were mainly negative for CD28 (Pennesi et al. 1999, 2001) moderate. Indeed, human aging markedly reduces diversity in both CD45RA$^+$ and CD45R0$^+$ CD8$^+$ T lymphocytes thus affecting the cytotoxic compartment in elderly where several compensatory mechanisms may contribute to alleviate the restricted CD8$^+$ T-cell repertoire (increased cross-reactivity of primed CTL clones, increased number of cytolytic CD28$^-$ T-cells or finally increased number of NK cells). Furthermore CD4+ T cell clones derived from centenarians produce mainly Th0 type cytokines with wide effector functions (Wack et al. 1998).

4 Systemic Inflamm-Aging

The inflammatory scenario that characterizes inflamm-aging constitutes a highly complex response to various subtle internal and environmental inflammatory stimuli mediated mainly by the increased circulating levels of pro-inflammatory cytokines. This condition is able to continuously generate Reactive Oxygen Species (ROS) causing both oxidative damage and eliciting an amplification of the cytokines' release, thus perpetuating a vicious cycle resulting in a chronic systemic proinflammatory state where tissue injury and healing mechanisms proceed simultaneously and damages accumulate slowly and asymptomatically over decades. Accordingly inflamm-aging is at the same time a major determinant both of the aging process and of the development of age-associated diseases (Candore et al. 2006; De Martinis et al. 2005; Franceschi et al. 1995; Giunta, 2006; Lio et al. 2003; Vasto et al. 2007). Moreover, the shift of cytokine production toward a pro-inflammatory profile is accompanied by endocrine and metabolic alterations (Paolisso et al. 2000) that could explain some age-related processes such as sarcopenia, obesity, metabolic syndrome and diabetes, among others.

Sarcopenia, i.e. the age-associated decline in skeletal muscle mass, strength and power resulting in physical disfunctioning, contributes to physical inactivity, functional disability and mortality. The specific mechanisms underlying age-related muscle wasting are still largely unknown, although a decreased anabolic state in combination with an increased catabolic state results in a progressive loss of lean tissue. In recent years, the role of inflammatory cytokines in the progression of muscle wasting has been focused (Roth et al. 2006). Recent data support the association between elevated IL-6 levels with in advancing age increased physical decline and mortality. For example, muscle performance measures are significantly lower in hospitalized geriatric patients with high levels of CRP and IL-6 compared with matched patients with normal levels of inflammation (Bautmans et al. 2005). We evaluated the joint effect of IGF-I and IL-6 on muscle function in a population-based sample of 526 persons with a wide age range (20–102 years). After adjusting for potential confounding factors (age, sex, body mass index), IL-6 receptor, IL-6 promoter polymorphism, IL-6, IGF-I, and their interaction were significant predictors of muscle power. In analyses stratified by IL-6 tertiles, IGF-I was an independent predictor of muscle function only in subjects in the lowest IL-6 tertile, suggesting that the effect of IGF-I on muscle function depends on IL-6 levels. This mechanism may explain why IL-6 is a strong risk factor for disability (Barbieri et al. 2003a). Giresi and colleagues (2005) reported a "molecular signature" of sarcopenia, coming from microarray analyses of young versus old skeletal muscle response. An increased expression of genes involved in the inflammatory was noted within this signature, providing some of the first direct evidence of the role of inflammation in aged muscle changes.

Several papers show data about the importance of TNF-α in muscle wasting. Roubenoff et al. (2003b) reported an association between higher levels of TNF-α and IL-6 with increased mortality in community dwelling elderly, while Yende et al. (2006) observed lower quadriceps strength in older man and woman with high IL-6 and TNF-α levels. Importantly, an interplay between an increase of inflammatory signals and a reduction of opposite growth factors signals may have the most relevance for the progression of muscle wasting. For example, elevated levels of TNF-α and IL-6 have been associated with an increased risk of sarcopenia, frailty and mortality, whereas elevated IGF-I levels have generated opposite associations (Leng et al. 2004; Payette et al. 2003; Roubenoff et al. 2003b).

Recent data on animals and humans indicate a possible more complex role of IL-6. It has been suggested that muscle-derived IL-6 contributes to mediate the beneficial metabolic effects of exercise and may contribute to inhibit TNF-production and thereby insulin resistance (Pedersen and Bruunsgaard 2003). Indeed experimental data indicate that IL-6 is released from skeletal muscle during acute exercise, and its production can result in an increase of antiinflammatory cytokines such as IL-1ra and IL-10 and in a concomitant inhibition of TNF-α (Petersen and Pedersen 2006).

Several studies have investigated the potential relationship between muscle mass and body fatness. How these two components of body composition change with aging, and their combined effects on functional performance and development of frailty, has led to the concept of "sarcopenic obesity" (Baumgartner et al. 2004; Dominguez and Barbagallo 2007; Roubenoff et al. 2004; Zoico et al. 2004). Weight changes are associated with the loss both of fat and lean mass, with the greatest proportion being fat. Individuals with an obesity state associated with high levels of body fat and low levels of muscle mass have an increased risk of functional decline (Baumgartner et al. 2004; Newman et al. 2003; Visser et al. 2002; Zoico et al. 2004) and mortality.

Obesity itself is associated with an elevation of inflammatory markers, and adipose tissue evolved from being identified as a mere deposit of fat as highly metabolically active organ with a critical role in the inflammatory process. In fact, the current view of adipose tissue is that of a dynamic secretory organ, sending out and responding to signals that modulate appetite, energy eaxpenditure, insulin sensivity, endocrine and reproductive systems, bone metabolism, inflammation and immunity. Mature adipocytes are involved in endocrine, paracrine and autocrine regulatory processes trough the secretion of a large number of multifunctional molecules collectively termed as "adipokines" (Yudkin et al. 1999). In addition to playing roles in the regulation of lipid and glucose homeostasis, adipokines modify some physiological processes, such as hematopoiesis reproduction, feeding behavior and may mediate the genesis of the multiple pathologies associated with increased fat mass (Chaldakov et al. 2003; Rajala et al. 2003). In humans, the development of adipose tissue has been associated with an increased production of inflammatory markers, including adhesion molecules (P-selectin, intercellular adhesion molecule-1, and plasma E-selectin) and inflammatory cytokines (TNF-α, IL-6, IL-8 and MCP-1; Loffreda et al. 1998; Takahashi et al. 2003). It has also been shown that macrophages residing in the adipose tissue may also be a source of proinflammatory factors, such as IL-6 and TNF-α, and that they also may modulate the secretory activity of adipocytes (Xu et al. 2003). It is therefore tempting to speculate that adipocytes, via the production of adipokines, are directly involved in the genesis of systemic and vascular inflammation.

The effects of adipocytokines on vascular function, immune regulation and adipocyte metabolism make them key players in the pathogenesis of metabolic syndrome. Obesity and inflammation have also been associated with the presence of the metabolic syndrome (Aronson et al. 2004; Florez et al. 2006), a cluster of clinical symptoms associated with increased risk of developing cardiovascular disease, diabetes, mortality, and other important adverse health outcomes. The prevalence of metabolic syndrome increases dramatically with age and comprises five cardiovascular risk factors including abdominal obesity, hypertriglyceridemia, low high-density lipoprotein (HDL) levels, hypertension, and hyperglycemia. Insulin resistance is at the basis of most of the features of this syndrome. Given the role of insulin in suppressing several proinflammatory transcription factors, such as NF-kB, Egr-1 and AP-1 (Aljada et al. 2002), an impairment of the action of insulin would result in the activation of these proinflammatory transcription factors, explaining why an insulin-resistant state may be considered proinflammatory (Dandona et al. 2005). High levels of inflammation increase the risk of developing diabetes and atherosclerosis and are thought to be a possible mechanism for the adverse consequence of metabolic syndrome (Barzilay et al. 2001; Pradhan et al. 2001). Whether inflammation leads to metabolic syndrome or vice versa is unclear. Most likely, inflammation and metabolic syndrome are related in a circular process (inflammation leads to metabolic syndrome, and metabolic syndrome increases inflammation; Dandona et al. 2005). In addition, markers of inflammation and several individual components of the metabolic syndrome have been associated with an increased risk of developing dementia and cognitive decline (McGeer EG and McGeer PL 1999, 2004; Yaffe et al. 2003). Most likely, the metabolic syndrome contributes to accelerate atherosclerosis associated with inflammatory response and, in turn, either atherosclerosis or inflammation or both contribute to the cognitive decline (Yaffe 2007; Grundy 2003; Ridker and Morrow 2003). Insulin resistance and/or hyperinsulinemia associated with metabolic syndrome, increasing systemic inflammatory responses and oxidative stress (Caballero 2004; Parrott and Greenwood 2007), play a central role in increasing central nervous system (CNS) inflammatory markers (Fishel et al. 2005). We showed that independently of age, sex, body mass index, waist-to-hip ratio, triglycerides, drug intake, diastolic blood pressure, smoking habit, and carotid atherosclerotic plaques, higher IL-6 serum concentrations were associated with higher insulin resistance, whereas sIL-6R levels were associated with lower insulin resistance. Furthermore, IL-1ra concentrations were associated with insulin-resistance syndrome, and higher sIL-6R plasma levels continued to correlate negatively with insulin-resistance syndrome (Abbatecola et al. 2004).

Interestingly, increased CNS inflammation has been positively correlated with amyloid-beta (Aβ) levels and insulin-resistant individuals with the highest inflammation exhibit more serious cognitive deficits (Yaffe et al. 2004). This synchronous hyperinsulinemia-induced increase of Aβ and inflammation may represent an important pathway through which insulin resistance promotes both cognitive deterioration and Alzheimer's disease pathology (AD; Craft 2007). Thus, inflammation has been demonstrated to play a role in AD pathogenesis and IL-1 and IL-6 are two of the most important cytokines involved in AD neuro-inflammation (Akiyama et al. 2000; Franceschi et al. 2001; Griffin et al. 2000). In this context, it is important to remember that the biological role of these cytokines in the brain is quite complex, and that their release may directly affect neuronal survival and injury response. In fact, IL-1 and IL-6 may have either trophic or toxic effects. In particular, IL-1 can induce the over-expression of S100β, a neurite growth-promoting cytokine markedly elevated in the brain of AD patients, by reactive astrocytosis. IL-1 can stimulate excessive synthesis, translation and processing of Aβ and plaque associated proteins, and it was shown to lead to over-expression and increased phosphorylation of TAU, thus contributing to an acceleration of degenerative cascades. This cytokine can activate astrocytes and their production of neurotoxic molecules, being astrogliosis a hallmark of AD in the cortex and hippocampus. Concerning IL-6, it appears that microglia, astroglia, neurons and endothelial cells are capable injury response this cytokine, which in turn can induce acute phase proteins. Elevated levels of IL-6 cause significant CNS damage and behavioral deficits (Akiyama et al. 2000). In AD patients, the expression of IL-6 mRNA is increased in brain areas where amyloid deposition and astroglia activation are more prominent (Strauss et al. 1992) and increased IL-6 levels in the brain have been implicated in plaque formation (Huell et al. 1995). Two different polymorphic regions of the IL-6 gene were investigated in patients with AD and nondemented controls (Licastro et al. 2003). The -174 C allele in the promoter region of IL-6 gene was over-represented in AD patients compared to controls, significantly increasing the risk of AD. Moreover, the -174 CC genotype was associated with a high risk of the disease in women. The D allele of a variable number of tandem repeat (VNTR) was in strong linkage disequilibrium with the -174 C allele and slightly increased AD risk. On the other hand, the frequency of the VNTR C allele decreased in patients with AD and was negatively associated with the risk of developing AD. Both the -174 CC and VNTR DD genotypes were also associated with increased IL-6 levels in blood and brain from AD patients. These findings suggest that IL-6 may play a multifaceted role in AD affecting the turnover of the cytokine.

However, at present, the sources of inflammatory stimuli underpinning and sustaining inflamm-aging are not completely cleared. In addition to the age-related increase of inflammatory compounds occurring the brain (Licastro et al. 2003), adipose tissue, and muscle, it is becoming more and more evident the possible and until now unexplored contribution of other organs or districts, such as gut and liver (Hotamisligil 2006).

The distal human intestine represents an anaerobic bioreactor provided with an enormous population of bacteria (gut microbiota, GM; Eckburg et al. 2005; Rajilic-Stojanovic et al. 2007; Zoetendal et al. 2006). The size of this ecosystem, up to 100 trillion, far exceeds that of all other microbial communities associated with the human body, and is around 10 times greater than the total number of our somatic and germ cells. The human distal gut microbiota is estimated to contain >100 times as many genes as our 2.85 billion bp human genome (Backhed et al. 2005; Gill et al. 2006; Ley et al. 2006). GM has a profound impact on human health, influencing nutritional, physiological and immunological status of the host (Guarner and Malagelada 2003; Hooper and Gordon 2001). A well balanced GM composition is essential in minimizing the production of potentially toxic compounds (xenobiotics) either ingested with the food or locally produced as a consequence of microbial metabolism (Nicholson et al. 2005). Furthermore, recent studies indicate that specific aspects of the GM affect various physiological characteristics of the host, such as fat storage, obesity (Gore et al. 2008; Ley et al. 2005; Turnbaugh et al. 2006), and intestinal disorders, including inflammatory bowel diseases (Sokol et al. 2007). In particular, accumulating evidences indicate the requirement of intimate interaction between GM and host defense mechanisms to maintain intestinal homeostasis and balanced immune function, avoiding exaggerated responses to luminal antigens while protecting from pathogens (Collier-Hyams et al. 2005; MacDonald and Monteleone 2005; Macpherson & Harris 2004; Stecher and Hardt 2008). Nevertheless, the data on the correlation between microbiota composition and function and specific metabolic and/or immune diseases are very fragmented and have not yet been addressed by large-scale and consistent molecular analyses. It is important to note that despite its potential importance as a major source of chronic immunological stimuli, likely contributing to inflamm-aging, the knowledge on GM composition in people of different ages, including long-lived people, is in its infancy. Notably, aging has been associated with changes of the GM (van Tongeren et al. 2005), albeit on basis of small groups of individuals and mostly using classical culture-dependent methodologies of limited capability to grasp the complexity of GM.

In conclusion, inflamm-aging involves a complex cross-talk among the different cell types, tissues and organs, and thus must be considered a systemic process that should be approached and analyzed with the emerging tools of Systems Biology.

5 Evolutionary Perspective

Apart from difference in their genomes, a major difference between humans and laboratory animals used to study aging and longevity is the quantity and quality of antigenic exposure. Typical laboratory organisms are usually housed in "artificially clean" environments and thus underexposed to pathogens, or even completely protected from them, except for limited period of time (acute infections) that can be required for experimental reasons. These animals are quite different from those living in the wild and spending their life exposed to a plethora of different microrganisms that, on the long run, cause the wear and tear of the immune system. On the contrary, humans do not live literary "in the wild" but in an environment full of microbes.

In order to cope with and survive, lower creatures are equipped with an "innate" immune system, based on macrophage as central cell type, which together with Pattern Recognition Receptors and a variety of small antimicrobial molecules, is capable of protecting invertebrates from all type of invasors (Ottaviani and Franceschi 1997).

Starting from teleostean fishes, a much more sophisticated immune system appeared, characterized by the presence of large repertoire of clonally distributed lymphocytes, each of them capable of recognizing a defined antigenic determinant present on a given microrganism and covering the entire universe of possible antigens.

Why did this new and extremely complex immune system emerge? A reasonable hypothesis suggests that a major force was to take under control the intestinal microflora characterized by an enormous variety of bacterial species (Pancer and Cooper 2006). On the basis of data on comparative and phylogenetic studies from invertebrates to fishes, reptiles, birds and mammals, we proposed a unifying hypothesis according to which the immune response, centered on the macrophage, ispart of an integrated and evolutionary conserved set of response crucial for survival and aimed to counteract all kind of stressor (Ottaviani and Franceschi 1997, 1998). We collected a variety of data in favour of the hypothesis of the common evolutionary origin of natural immunity, inflammation and stress response. These phenomena seem to be mediated by a common pool of molecules (POMC-derived peptides, cytokines, biogenic amines, glucocorticoids, and nitric oxide). Macrophages are able to release all the above mentioned molecules. They play a primary role in defense mechanisms and we argued that this cell can be considered as the eye-witness of the common evolutionary origin of the immune and neuroendocrine systems. On the basis of evolutionary studies, we argued that immune and stress responses are equivalent and antigens can be considered particular types of stressors. We also proposed to return macrophage to its rightful place as central actor not only in the inflammatory response and immunity, but also in the stress response. Accordingly, within such an evolutionary perspective, the age-related activation of macrophage, that constitutes the core of inflamm-aging, may be interpreted as the result of the capability of such cell to be a major cellular target, where all type of stressors, including the immunological ones, converge. We surmise that the macrophage has maintained throughout evolution its ancestral capability to receive, integrate and deliver a large variety of inflammatory stimuli, owing to not only to its presence in most tissues and organs of the body, but also to its specific and marked locomotory and migratory capability towards chemiotactic stimuli and stress signals (Franceschi et al. 2000b).

6 Inflamm-Aging and the Centenarian Paradox

We proposed that the rate of reaching the threshold of proinflammatory status over which diseases/disabilities ensue and the individual capacity to cope with and adapt to stressors should be considered as a complex trait(s) with a genetic component (Franceschi et al. 2000a). We also argued that the persistence of inflammatory stimuli over time represents the biologic background (first hit) favouring the susceptibility to age-related diseases/disabilities. A second hit (absence of robust gene variants and/or presence of frail gene variants) is likely necessary to develop overt organ-specific age-related diseases having an inflammatory pathogenesis, such as atherosclerosis, Alzheimer's disease, osteoporosis, and diabetes (Franceschi et al. 2000a). Following this perspective, several paradoxes of healthy centenarians (increase of plasma levels of inflammatory cytokines, acute phase proteins, and coagulation factors) can be explained.

How is it possible to explain the fact that low grade chronic inflammation, considered a reliable marker of high risk morbidity and mortality is still present in centenarians who largely escaped from major age-related diseases having a strong inflammatory pathogenetic component? These extraordinary subjects have a complex mix of pro and antiinflammatory characteristics both phenotypically and genetically. From a phenotypic point of view, they show high plasma levels of IL-6 (Baggio et al. 1998), increased levels of IL-18 and IL-15 (Gangemi et al. 2003) a reduction of proinflammatory and proatherosclerotic properties of platelets (Mutus et al. 2000), low serum levels of Hsp70 (also present in offspring of centenarians), increased plasma levels of TGF-β (Carrieri et al. 2004) a pleiotropic cytokine with strong suppressor activity on a variety of inflammatory and immune responses (Li et al. 2006) and increased levels of cortisol (Ostan et al. 2008; Troiano et al. 1999).

From a genetic point of view, centenarians are characterized by the -174C polymorphism in the promoter of IL-6 (Bonafè et al. 2001) associated with higher body mass index and insulin resistance (Barbieri et al. 2005). Moreover centenarians show an increased frequency of TLR4+896 polymorphism (Balistreri et al. 2004), an increased frequency of IL-10 -1082GG genotype associated with high production of this antiinflammatory cytokine (Lio et al. 2002) and an increased frequency of CCR5 Δ32+ genotypes (Candore et al. 2006). The 32pb (Δ32+) deletion appears to halve the receptor molecule number at the cell surface decreasing the recruitment of monocyte and macrophage cells at the vascular wall.

All these characteristics indicate that in centenarians pro and antiinflammatory responses are well balanced and optimized, likely as a result of a peculiar genetic background (Franceschi et al. 2006).

7 Antagonistic Pleiotropy

The aging of the immune system is not a random process without rules or directions, but rather it is subject to evolutionary constraints (Hughes et al. 2002). The immune system has been probably selected to serve individuals living until reproduction. The trend of thymic ontogenesis and involution likely supports this hypothesis (Ginaldi and Sternberg 2003). Our ancestors lived until 30–50 years of age. Nowadays, the immune system must serve the soma of individuals living 80–120 years, an enormous amount of time longer than that predicted by evolutionary forces.

Negative selection against mutations causing harmful effects late in life fails because, in the wild, most organisms do not live long enough to experience the harmful effects of such mutations. Thus, the negative effects of aging are not selected traits, but rather the consequence of alleles fixed in evolution by their reproductive advantage early in life, with harmful effects in the postreproductive period, a process Williams called antagonistic pleiotropy (Williams 1957). According to this theory, the somatic decline associated with aging would be an inevitable late-life result of adaptations that increase fitness early in life. In line with this reasoning, the cellular responses, apoptosis, and cellular senescence may have antagonistically pleiotropic effects on cancer and life span, as these protect individuals from cancer early in life, but may promote aging phenotypes, including late life cancer, in older individuals.

Within an "antagonistic pleiotropy" perspective we can assume that efficient inflammatory responses can confer high resistance to infections, but also an increased susceptibility to inflammation-based diseases later in life. On the other side, low inflammatory responses, while rendering more susceptible to infectious pathologies, can confer a survival advantage in old age. If this hypothesis is correct, the oldest people and centenarians should pay the price of being more susceptible and prone to infections. In this view longevity could be, at least in part, the positive counterpart of unsuccessful aging.

Thus, aging is a sort of side-effect of genes playing an important role during juvenile age. As an example, it is possible that a genetic variant that increases reproductive fitness can have a detrimental effect on longevity. Thus, it is evident that, if a genetic variant confers a selective advantage during young age, it will be selected even if it is unfavourable for longevity (for example by conferring a higher risk for age-related diseases). This seems to be the case for the inflammatory gene polymorphisms responsible for a higher responder status that were selected to fight infections in young age (Licastro et al. 2005).

8   Antiinflamm-Aging Strategies

In recent years, it has been proposed that inflammation resolves not merely because of the absence of proinflammatory signals, but rather because of the activation of specific inhibitory pathways, involving a series of molecules such as annexin 1, galectins, adrenocorticotropic hormone (ACTH) and melanocortins, adenosine, prostanoids, lipoxin A_4, heparin, nitric oxide, known to have potent antiinflammatory effects and able to modulate and eventually turn off the inflammatory process (Perretti and D'Acquisto 2006). Thus, antiinflammation should be considered an active phenomenon. One of the most important examples of such inflammation/antiinflammation circuit is represented by the induction of the Hypothalamus-Pituitary- Adrenal (HPA) axis by proinflammatory cytokines leading to the production of the antiinflammatory hormone cortisol.

Indeed, an important response to inflammation is a neuroendocrine stimulation, since neuronal cells possess specific receptors for a number of cytokines able to activate the HPA axis (Turnbull and Rivier 1999). A chronic proinflammatory state is also systemic and it has been showed that cytokines can readily pass through leaky areas in the blood–brain barrier (BBB) at any time, and that transcellular, saturable transport mechanisms afford a mean of cytokine entry into the brain even when the BBB integrity is not compromised (Banks et al. 1995). Moreover, nonneuronal brain cells also produce cytokines, and can stimulate and regulate the HPA axis resulting in the release of Corticotropin Releasing Hormone (CRH; Banks et al. 1995). Therefore, we can infer that, just like in acute inflammation, CRH-secreting neurons are likely to be the targets of cytokines also during inflamm-aging, where these immune signals may persistently activate the HPA axis, finally resulting in a cortisol-mediated restraint of the immune-inflammatory response (antiinflamm-aging).

The age-associated cytokine derangement is observed in "normal" aged people. Thus, if strong inflammatory response is associated with higher risk of life-threatening diseases, longevity should be correlated to the capability to maintain a low intensity inflammatory status. Moreover, the individual genetic background and the possible influence of counteracting cytokines could play a crucial role in the onset of age-related diseases. Lifelong, acute, or chronic exposure to bacteria, viruses and other pathogens or antigens are at the basis of the progressive increase of the inflammatory status during aging. In this context, any procedure aimed to avoid immunological extra burden is highly recommended for elderly individuals. First of all, careful attention should be paid to neglected sources of antigenic stimulation, such as chronic, subclinical infections in the oral cavity and the gastrointestinal and urogenital tracts among others, which probably represent a major source of chronic antigenic stimulation. From this point of view, a systematic search for chronic infections and setup of safe procedures to eradicate them would likely have a strong beneficial impact on health status and functional capability and on the overall survival and life span in the elderly (Capri et al. 2006). Recent advances indicate that a marked alteration of the composition of gastrointestinal microflora occurs in old people, and it is associated with frailty (van Tongeren et al. 2005). This derangement of the intestinal microflora likely represents an important source of continuous antigenic stimulation. Tools for large scale monitoring of such age-associated derangement and specific strategies to reconstitute the normal microflora in the elderly should represent a priority in aging research. Data from animal models testing the efficacy of probiotic treatment for inflammatory bowel disease seems to be very promising (Sartor 2005) and data obtained in vitro experiments suggest that Bifidobacterium genomic DNA and other probiotic bacteria are able to modulate the secretion of pro and antiinflammatory cytokines, such as TNF-α, IL-1β and IL-10, by peripheral blood mononuclear cells (Helwig et al. 2006; Lammers et al. 2003).

Another strategy to counteract inflamm-aging is to reduce the antigenic load represented by common infectious agents such as influenza virus and CMV, among others. Strategies of specific vaccination should be applied to prevent morbidity, mortality and any additional persistent stimulation of the immune system in the elderly (Armstrong et al. 2004). However the antibody response to influenza vaccine in the elderly is considerably lower than in younger adults (Goodwin et al. 2006). In addition, some published data suggest a correlation between CMV-seropositivity, chronic proinflammatory activity and nonresponsiveness to antiinfluenza vaccine. This phenomenon appears more pronounced in the elderly subjects (Trzonkowski et al. 2003). Therefore, because CMV seems to be one of the main driving force of immunosenescence and because the number of CMV$^+$ subjects increases with age, the possibility to administrate large scale vaccination against CMV early in life should be investigated.

On one hand, it is reasonable to assume that antiinflammatory treatment could be useful to counteract and to reduce inflamm-aging, but, on the other hand, a decrease in the rate of inflamm-aging should prevent the activation of the immune system to levels that favour age-related diseases and the persistence of pathogens such as CMV. Moreover, aspirin has been proposed as an antiaging agent for its antiinflammatory and antioxidant properties with positive effects on immune system and cardiovascular health (Phillips and Leeuwenburgh 2004).

Another crucial topic is to provide elderly subjects with a correct dietary intake. It is important to underline that elderly individuals often have an unbalanced diet, which can cause malnutrition, frailty, and weakening of the immune system. Thus, it is fundamental to prevent malnutrition and sometimes to add minerals or vitamins to the diet. Actually, it was shown that the dietary supplementation with the recommended daily intakes of zinc for 1 or 2 months decreases the incidence of infections and increases the rate of survival to further infections in the elderly (Mocchegiani et al. 2000). Moreover, a number of observational studies have found that the dietary profile benefiting cognitive function with aging contains weekly serving of fish and multiple daily servings of cereals, darkly or brightly colored fruits and leaf vegetables. In particular, studies on animal models of aging and AD have found that dietary plant polyphenols reduce neuro-inflammation and stimulate the activity of phosphotidylinositol-3 kinase (PI3K), a ubiquitous enzyme involved in many cellular responses with a particular importance to insulin signaling, resulting in improved neuronal survival and memory (Joseph et al. 2003, 2005; Parrot and Greenwood 2007). Similarly, omega-3 fatty acids, in addition to their role in supporting membrane-bound protein functions and neurotransmission, may have antiinflammatory and prosurvival capabilities by modulating cytokine activity and antiapoptotic pathways, including those influenced by PI3K (Horrocks and Farooqui 2004; Lukiw et al. 2005; Marcheselli et al. 2003; Parrot and Greenwood 2007).

In addition, nutritional supplementation with vitamin D in the elderly should be a recommended strategy to prevent bone fractures. A recent study about bone status and metabolism in 104 subjects over 89 years of age evaluated possible interventions able to avoid fragility fractures and disability (Passeri et al. 2003). Vitamin D was undetectable in 99 out of 104 subjects, while serum IL-6 was elevated in 81% of the subjects and it was positively correlated with parathormone and negatively correlated with serum calcium. Thus, extreme decades of life seem characterized by a pathophysiological sequence of events linking vitamin D deficiency, low serum calcium and secondary hyperparathyroidism with an increase in bone resorption, severe osteopenia and inflammation (Passeri et al. 2003). These data offer a rational for the possible prevention of elevated bone turnover, bone loss and the consequent reduction of osteoporotic fractures and fractures-induced disability, in the oldest old, through the simple supplementation with calcium and vitamin D (Passeri et al. 2008). Immune system contributes to the development of osteoporosis. In this context, inflamm-aging could play an important role through the chronic up-regulation of proinflammatory cytokines superimposed to the effects of vitamin D and hormones such as estrogens (Clowes et al. 2005). Thus, the supplementation with vitamin D could have a general effect on inflamm-aging and immunosenescence, besides the specific effect on bone metabolism. In addition, new evidences in animal models suggest that vitamin D3 acts as an antiinflammatory agent, thus being useful for different age-associated diseases, such as AD (Moore et al. 2005).

In addition, cross-sectional studies demonstrate an association between physical inactivity and low-grade systemic inflammation in elderly people (Bruunsgaard et al. 2003). On the contrary, it has been demonstrated that regular exercise induces antiinflammatory effects with elevated levels of antiinflammatory cytokines and suppression of TNF-α production (Pedersen and Bruungaard 2003; Petersen and Pedersen 2006). Moreover, the finding in two longitudinal studies that regular training induces a reduction in CRP level (Fallon et al. 2001) suggests that physical activity may suppress systemic low-grade inflammation. Given that the atherosclerotic process is characterized by inflammation, regular moderate exercise in aged people could offer protection against vascular inflammation and it could reduce the risk of atherosclerosis (Petersen and Pedersen 2006).

In this context, it is becoming more and more evident that all the strategies able to reduce the low, chronic, and systemic inflammatory status in elderly people could play a fundamental role in the decrease of the incidence of the most important age-related pathologies.

References

Abbatecola AM, Ferrucci L, Grella R, Bandinelli S, Bonafe` M, Barbieri M, Corsi AM, Lauretani F, Franceschi C, Paolisso G (2004) Diverse effect of inflammatory markers on insulin resistance and insulin-resistance syndrome in the elderly. J Am Geriatr Soc 52:399–404

Ahmed R, Gray D (1996) Immunological memory and protective immunity: understanding their relation. Science 272:54–60

Akiyama H, Barger S, Barnum S, Bradt B, Bauer J, Cole GM, Cooper NR, Eikelenboom P, Emmerling M, Fiebich BL, Finch CE, Frautschy S, Griffin WS, Hampel H, Hull M, Landreth G, Lue L, Mrak R, Mackenzie IR, McGeer PL, O'Banion MK, Pachter J, Pasinetti G, Plata-Salaman C, Rogers J, Rydel R, Shen Y, Streit W, Strohmeyer R, Tooyoma I, Van Muiswinkel FL, Veerhuis R, Walker D, Webster S, Wegrzyniak B, Wenk G, Wyss-Coray T (2000) Inflammation and Alzheimer's disease. Neurobiol Aging 21(3):383–421

Alberti S, Cevenini E, Ostan R, Capri M, Salvioli S, Bucci L, Ginaldi L, De Martinis M, Franceschi C, Monti D (2006) Age-dependent modifications of Type 1 and Type 2 cytokines within virgin and memory CD4+ T cells in humans. Mech Ageing Dev 127(6):560–566

Aljada A, Ghanim H, Mohanty P, Kapur N, Dandona P (2002) Insulin inhibits the pro-inflammatory transcription factor early growth response gene-1 (Egr)-1 expression in mononuclear cells (MNC) and reduces plasma tissue factor (TF) and plasminogen activator inhibitor-1 (PAI-1) concentrations. J Clin Endocrinol Metab 87(3):1419–1422

Appay V, Rowland-Jones SL (2002) Premature ageing of the immune system: the cause of AIDS? Trends Immunol 23(12):580–585

Armstrong BG, Mangtani P, Fletcher A, Kovats S, McMichael A, Pattenden S, Wilkinson P (2004) Effect of influenza vaccination on excess deaths occurring during periods of high circulation of influenza: cohort study in elderly people. BMJ 329(7467):660

Aronson D, Bartha P, Zinder O, Kerner A, Markiewicz W, Avizohar O, Brook GJ, Levy Y (2004) Obesity is the major determinant of elevated C-reactive protein in subjects with the metabolic syndrome. Int J Obes Relat Metab Disord 28(5):674–679

Aspinall R, Andrew D (2000) Thymic involution in aging. J Clin Immunol 20:250–256

Bäckhed F, Ley RE, Sonnenburg JL, Peterson DA, Gordon JI (2005) Host-bacterial mutualism in the human intestine. Science 307(5717):1915–1920

Baggio G, Donazzan S, Monti D, Mari D, Martini S, Gabelli C, Dalla Vestra M, Previato L, Guido M, Pigozzo S, Cortella I, Crepaldi G, Franceschi C (1998) Lipoprotein(a) and lipoprotein profile in healthy centenarians: a reappraisal of vascular risk factors. FASEB J 12(6):433–437

Balistreri CR, Candore G, Colonna-Romano G, Lio D, Caruso M, Hoffmann E, Franceschi C, Caruso C (2004) Role of Toll-like receptor 4 in acute myocardial infarction and longevity. JAMA 292:2339–2340

Banks WA, Kastin AJ, Broadwell RD (1995) Passage of cytokines across the blood-brain barrier. Neuroimmunomodulation 2(4):241–248

Barbieri M, Rizzo MR, Papa M, Acampora R, De Angelis L, Olivieri F, Marchigiani F, Franceschi C, Paolisso G (2005) Role of interaction between variants in the PPARG and interleukin-6 genes on obesity related metabolic risk factors. Exp Gerontol 40:599–604

Barbieri M, Ferrucci L, Ragno E, Corsi A, Bandinelli S, Bonafe` M, Olivieri F, Giovagnetti S, Franceschi C, Guralnik JM (2003a) Chronic inflammation and the effect of IGF-I on muscle strength and power in older persons. Am J Physiol Endocrinol Metab 284:481–487

Barzilay JI, Abraham L, Heckbert SR, Cushman M, Kuller LH, Resnick HE, Tracy RP (2001) The relation of markers of inflammation to the development of glucose disorders in the elderly: the Cardiovascular Health Study. Diabetes 50(10):2384–2389

Batliwalla F, Monteiro J, Serrano D, Gregersen PK (1996) Oligoclonality of CD8+ T cells in health and disease: aging, infection, or immune regulation? Hum Immunol 48:68–76

Baumgartner RN, Wayne SJ, Waters DL, Janssen I, Gallagher D, Morley JE (2004) Sarcopenic obesity predicts instrumental activities of daily living disability in the elderly. Obes Res 12(12):1995–2004

Bautmans I, Njemini R, Lambert M, Demanet C, Mets T (2005) Circulating acute phase mediators and skeletal muscle performance in hospitalized geriatric patients. J Gerontol A Biol Sci Med Sci 60(3):361–367

Berzins SP, Uldrich AP, Sutherland JS, Gill J, Miller JF, Godfrey DI, Boyd RL (2002) Thymic regeneration: teaching an old immune system new tricks. Trends Mol Med 8(10):469–476

Bonafe M, Olivieri F, Cavallone L, Giovagnetti S, Marchegiani F, Cardelli M, Pieri C, Marra M, Antonicelli R, Lisa R, Rizzo MR, Paolisso G, Monti D, Franceschi C (2001) A gender-dependent genetic predisposition to produce high levels of IL-6 is detrimental for longevity. Eur J Immunol 31:2357–2361

Boren E, Gershwin ME (2004) Inflamm-aging: autoimmunity, and the immune-risk phenotype. Autoimmun Rev 3(5):401–406

Bruunsgaard H, Ladelund S, Pedersen AN, Schroll M, Jørgensen T, Pedersen BK (2003) Predicting death from tumour necrosis factor-alpha and interleukin-6 in 80-year-old people. Clin Exp Immunol 132(1):24–31

Bruunsgaard H, Pedersen M, Pedersen BK (2001) Aging and proinflammatory cytokines. Curr Opin Hematol 8(3):131–136

Bruunsgaard H, Andersen-Ranberg K, Jeune B, Pedersen AN, Skinhøj P, Pedersen BK (1999) A high plasma concentration of TNF-alpha is associated with dementia in centenarians. J Gerontol A Biol Sci Med Sci 54(7):M357–M364

Brzezinska A, Magalska A, Szybinska A, Sikora E (2004) Proliferation and apoptosis of human CD8 (+) CD28 (+) and CD8 (+) CD28 (–) lymphocytes during aging. Exp Gerontol 39:539–544

Caballero AE (2004) Endothelial dysfunction, inflammation, and insulin resistance: a focus on subjects at risk for type 2 diabetes. Curr Diab Rep 4(4):237–246

Candore G, Balistreri CR, Grimaldi MP, Listi F, Vasto S, Caruso M, Caimi G, Hoffmann E, Colonna-Romano G, Lio D, Paolisso G, Franceschi C, Caruso C (2006) Opposite role of proinflammatory alleles in acute myocardial infarction and longevity: results of studies performed in a Sicilian population. Ann N Y Acad Sci 1067:270–275

Cappola AR, Xue QL, Ferrucci L, Guralnik JM, Volpato S, Fried LP (2003) Insulin-like growth factor I and interleukin-6 contribute synergistically to disability and mortality in older women. J Clin Endocrinol Metab 88(5):2019–2025

Capri M, Monti D, Salvioli S, Lescai F, Pierini M, Altilia S, Sevini F, Valensin S, Ostan R, Bucci L, Franceschi C (2006) Complexity of anti-immunosenescence strategies in humans. Artif Organs 30(10):730–742

Carrieri G, Marzi E, Olivieri F, Marchegiani F, Cavallone L, Cardelli M, Giovagnetti S, Stecconi R, Molendini C, Trapassi C, De Benedictis G, Kletsas D, Franceschi C (2004) The G/C915 polymorphism of transforming growth factor beta1 is associated with human longevity: a study in Italian centenarians. Aging Cell 3(6):443–448

Chaldakov GN, Stankulov IS, Hristova M, Ghenev PI (2003) Adipobiology of disease: adipokines and adipokine-targeted pharmacology. Curr Pharm Des 9:1023–1031

Clowes JA, Riggs BL, Khosla S (2005) The role of the immune system in the pathophysiology of osteoporosis. Immunol Rev 208:207–227

Collier-Hyams LS, Neish AS (2005) Innate immune relationship between commensal flora and the mammalian intestinal epithelium. Cell Mol Life Sci 62(12):1339–1348

Cossarizza A, Ortolani C, Paganelli R, Barbieri D, Monti D, Sansoni P, Fagiolo U, Castellani G, Bersani F, Londei M, Franceschi C (1996) CD45 isoforms expression on CD4+ and CD8+ T cells throughout life, from newborns to centenarians: implications for T cell memory. Mech Ageing Dev 86(3):173–195

Craft S (2007) Insulin resistance and Alzheimer's disease pathogenesis: potential mechanisms and implications for treatment. Curr Alzheimer Res 4(2):147–152

Dandona P, Aljada A, Chaudhuri A, Mohanty P, Garg R (2005) Metabolic syndrome: a comprehensive perspective based on interactions between obesity, diabetes, and inflammation. Circulation 111(11):1448–1454

De Martinis M, Franceschi C, Monti D, Ginaldi L (2005) Inflamm-ageing and lifelong antigenic load as major determinants of ageing rate and longevity. FEBS Lett 579(10):2035–2039

De Martinis M, Modesti M, Ginaldi L (2004) Phenotypic and functional changes of circulating monocytes and polymorphonuclear leucocytes from elderly persons. Immunol Cell Biol 82:415–420

Dominguez LJ, Barbagallo M (2007) The cardiometabolic syndrome and sarcopenic obesity in older persons. J Cardiometab Syndr 2(3):183–189

Eckburg PB, Bik EM, Bernstein CN, Purdom E, Dethlefsen L, Sargent M, Gill SR, Nelson KE, Relman DA (2005) Diversity of the human intestinal microbial flora. Science 308(5728):1635–1638

Effros RB (1997) Loss of CD28 expression on T lymphocytes. A marker of replicative senescence. Dev Comp Immunol 21:471–478

Fagiolo U, Cossarizza A, Scala E, Fanales-Belasio E, Ortolani C, Cozzi E, Monti D, Franceschi C, Paganelli R (1993) Increased cytokine production in mononuclear cells of healthy elderly people. Eur J Immunol 23(9):2375–2378

Fagnoni FF, Vescovini R, Passeri G, Bologna G, Pedrazzoni M, Lavagetto G, Casti A, Franceschi C, Passeri M, Sansoni P (2000) Shortage of circulating naive CD8(+) T cells provides new insights on immunodeficiency in aging. Blood 95:2860–2868

Fagnoni FF, Vescovini R, Mazzola M, Bologna G, Nigro E, Lavagetto G, Franceschi C, Passeri M, Sansoni P (1996) Expansion of cytotoxic CD8+CD28– T cells in healthy ageing people, including centenarians. Immunology 88:501–507

Fallon KE, Fallon SK, Boston T (2001) The acute phase response and exercise: court and field sports. Br J Sports Med 35(3):170–173

Feldmann M, Elliott MJ, Woody JN, Maini RN (1997) Anti-tumor necrosis factor-alpha therapy of rheumatoid arthritis. Adv Immunol 64:283–350

Ferrucci L, Harris TB, Guralnik JM, Tracy RP, Corti MC, Cohen HJ, Penninx B, Pahor M, Wallace R, Havlik RJ (1999) Serum IL-6 level and the development of disability in older persons. J Am Geriatr Soc 47(6):639–646

Fishel MA, Watson GS, Montine TJ, Wang Q, Green PS, Kulstad JJ, Cook DG, Peskind ER, Baker LD, Goldgaber D, Nie W, Asthana S, Plymate SR, Schwartz MW, Craft S (2005) Hyperinsulinemia provokes synchronous increases in central inflammation and beta-amyloid in normal adults. Arch Neurol 62(10):1539–1544

Florez H, Castillo-Florez S, Mendez A, Casanova-Romero P, Larreal-Urdaneta C, Lee D, Goldberg R (2006) C-reactive protein is elevated in obese patients with the metabolic syndrome. Diabetes Res Clin Pract 71(1):92–100

Franceschi C, Capri M, Monti D, Giunta S, Olivieri F, Sevini F, Panourgia MP, Invidia L, Celani L, Scurti M, Cevenini E, Castellani GC, Salvioli S (2007) Inflammaging and anti-inflammaging: a systemic perspective on aging and longevity emerged from studies in humans. Mech Ageing Dev 128(1):92–105

Franceschi C, Valensin S, Lescai F, Olivieri F, Licastro F, Grimaldi LM, Monti D, De Benedictis G, Bonafè M (2001) Neuroinflammation and the genetics of Alzheimer's disease: the search for a pro-inflammatory phenotype. Aging (Milano) 13(3):163–170

Franceschi C, Motta L, Valensin S, Rapisarda R, Franzone A, Berardelli M, Motta M, Monti D, Bonafè M, Ferrucci L, Deiana L, Pes GM, Carru C, Desole MS, Barbi C, Sartoni G, Gemelli C, Lescai F, Olivieri F, Marchegiani F, Cardelli M, Cavallone L, Gueresi P, Cossarizza A, Troiano L, Pini G, Sansoni P, Passeri G, Lisa R, Spazzafumo L, Amadio L, Giunta S, Stecconi R, Morresi R, Viticchi C, Mattace R, De Benedictis G, Baggio G (2000a) Do men and women follow different trajectories to reach extreme longevity? Italian Multicenter Study on Centenarians (IMUSCE). Aging (Milano) 12(2):77–84

Franceschi C, Bonafè M, Valensin S, Olivieri F, De Luca M, Ottaviani E, De Benedictis G. Inflamm-aging (2000b) An evolutionary perspective on immunosenescence. Ann N Y Acad Sci 908:244–254

Franceschi C, Bonafè M, Valensin S (2000c) Human immunosenescence: the prevailing of innate immunity, the failing of clonotypic immunity, and the filling of immunological space. Vaccine 18(16):1717–1720

Franceschi C, Valensin S, Fagnoni F, Barbi C, Bonafè M (1999) Biomarkers of immunosenescence within an evolutionary perspective: the challenge of heterogeneity and the role of antigenic load. Exp Gerontol 34(8):911–921

Franceschi C, Monti D, Sansoni P, Cossarizza A (1995) The immunology of exceptional individuals: the lesson of centenarians. Immunol Today 16(1):12–16

Frauwirth KA, Riley JL, Harris MH, Parry RV, Rathmell JC, Plas DR, Elstrom RL, June CH, Thompson CB (2002) The CD28 signaling pathway regulates glucose metabolism. Immunity 16(6):769–777

Gangemi S, Basile G, Merendino RA, Minciullo PL, Novick D, Rubinstein M, Dinarello CA, Lo Balbo C, Franceschi C, Basili S, D'Urbano E, Davi G, Nicita-Mauro V, Romano M (2003) Increased circulating Interleukin-18 levels in centenarians with no signs of vascular disease: another paradox of longevity? Exp Gerontol 38:669–672

Gerli R, Monti D, Bistoni O, Mazzone AM, Peri G, Cossarizza A, Di Gioacchino M, Cesarotti ME, Doni A, Mantovani A, Franceschi C, Paganelli R (2000) Chemokines, sTNF-Rs and sCD30 serum levels in healthy aged people and centenarians. Mech Ageing Dev 121(1–3):37–46

Gill SR, Pop M, Deboy RT, Eckburg PB, Turnbaugh PJ, Samuel BS, Gordon JI, Relman DA, Fraser-Liggett CM, Nelson KE (2006) Metagenomic analysis of the human distal gut microbiome. Science 312(5778):1355–1359

Ginaldi L, Sternberg H (2003) The immune system. In: Timiras PS (ed) Physiological basis of aging and geriatrics, 3rd edn. CRC Press, New York, pp 265–283

Giresi PG, Stevenson EJ, Theilhaber J, Koncarevic A, Parkington J, Fielding RA, Kandarian SC (2005) Identification of a molecular signature of sarcopenia. Physiol Genomics 21(2):253–263

Giunta S (2006) Is inflammaging an auto[innate]immunity subclinical syndrome? Immun Ageing 3:12

Goodwin K, Viboud C, Simonsen L (2006) Antibody response to influenza vaccination in the elderly: a quantitative review. Vaccine 24(8):1159–1169

Gore C, Munro K, Lay C, Bibiloni R, Morris J, Woodcock A, Custovic A, Tannock GW (2008) Bifidobacterium pseudocatenulatum is associated with atopic eczema: a nested case-control study investigating the fecal microbiota of infants. J Allergy Clin Immunol 121(1):135–140

Griffin WS, Nicoll JA, Grimaldi LM, Sheng JG, Mrak RE (2000) The pervasiveness of interleukin-1 in alzheimer pathogenesis: a role for specific polymorphisms in disease risk. Exp Gerontol 35(4):481–487

Grundy SM (2003) Inflammation, hypertension, and the metabolic syndrome. JAMA 290(22):3000–3002

Guarner F, Malagelada JR (2003) Gut flora in health and disease. Lancet 361(9356):512–519

Guidotti LG, Ishikawa T, Hobbs MV, Matzke B, Schreiber R, Chisari FV (1996) Intracellular inactivation of the hepatitis B virus by cytotoxic T lymphocytes. Immunity 4(1):25–36

Harris TB, Ferrucci L, Tracy RP, Corti MC, Wacholder S, Ettinger WH Jr, Heimovitz H, Cohen HJ, Wallace R (1999) Associations of elevated interleukin-6 and C-reactive protein levels with mortality in the elderly. Am J Med 106(5):506–512

Helwig U, Lammers KM, Rizzello F, Brigidi P, Rohleder V, Caramelli E, Gionchetti P, Schrezenmeir J, Foelsch UR, Schreiber S, Campieri M (2006) Lactobacilli, bifidobacteria and E. coli nissle induce pro- and anti-inflammatory cytokines in peripheral blood mononuclear cells. World J Gastroenterol 12(37):5978–5986

Hooper LV, Gordon JI (2001) Commensal host-bacterial relationships in the gut. Science 292(5519):1115–1118

Horrocks LA, Farooqui AA (2004) Docosahexaenoic acid in the diet: its importance in maintenance and restoration of neural membrane function. Prostaglandins Leukot Essent Fatty Acids 70(4):361–372

Hotamisligil GS (2006) Inflammation and metabolic disorders. Nature 444(7121):860–867

Hughes KA, Alipaz JA, Drnevich JM, Reynolds RM (2002) A test of evolutionary theories of aging. Proc Natl Acad Sci 99:14286–14291

Huell M, Strauss S, Volk B, Berger M, Bauer J (1995) Interleukin-6 is present in early stages of plaque formation and is restricted to the brains of Alzheimer's disease patients. Acta Neuropathol 89(6):544–551

Joseph JA, Shukitt-Hale B, Casadesus G, Fisher D (2005) Oxidative stress and inflammation in brain aging: nutritional considerations. Neurochem Res 30(6–7):927–935

Joseph JA, Denisova NA, Arendash G, Gordon M, Diamond D, Shukitt-Hale B, Morgan D (2003) Blueberry supplementation enhances signaling and prevents behavioral deficits in an Alzheimer disease model. Nutr Neurosci 6(3):153–162

Koch S, Larbi A, Ozcelik D, Solana R, Gouttefangeas C, Attig S, Wikby A, Strindhall J, Franceschi C, Pawelec G (2007) Cytomegalovirus infection: a driving force in human T cell immunosenescence. Ann N Y Acad Sci 1114:23–35

Kohler S, Wagner U, Pierer M, Kimmig S, Oppmann B, Möwes B, Jülke K, Romagnani C, Thiel A (2005) Post-thymic in vivo proliferation of naive CD4+ T cells constrains the TCR repertoire in healthy human adults. Eur J Immunol 35(6):1987–1994

Krause A, Guo HF, Latouche JB, Tan C, Cheung NK, Sadelain M (1998) Antigen-dependent CD28 signaling selectively enhances survival and proliferation in genetically modified activated human primary T lymphocytes. J Exp Med 188(4):619–626

Lammers KM, Brigidi P, Vitali B, Gionchetti P, Rizzello F, Caramelli E, Matteuzzi D, Campieri M (2003) Immunomodulatory effects of probiotic bacteria DNA: IL-1 and IL-10 response in human peripheral blood mononuclear cells. FEMS Immunol Med Microbiol 38(2):165–172

Leng SX, Cappola AR, Andersen RE, Blackman MR, Koenig K, Blair M, Walston JD (2004) Serum levels of insulin-like growth factor-I (IGF-I) and dehydroepiandrosterone sulfate (DHEA-S), and their relationships with serum interleukin-6, in the geriatric syndrome of frailty. Aging Clin Exp Res 16(2):153–157

Ley RE, Peterson DA, Gordon JI (2006) Ecological and evolutionary forces shaping microbial diversity in the human intestine. Cell 124(4):837–848

Ley RE, Bäckhed F, Turnbaugh P, Lozupone CA, Knight RD, Gordon JI (2005) Obesity alters gut microbial ecology. Proc Natl Acad Sci U S A 102(31):11070–11075

Licastro F, Candore G, Lio D, Porcellini E, Colonna-Romano G, Franceschi C, Caruso C (2005) Innate immunity and inflammation in ageing: a key for understanding age-related diseases. Immun Ageing 2:8

Licastro F, Grimaldi LM, Bonafè M, Martina C, Olivieri F, Cavallone L, Giovanietti S, Masliah E, Franceschi C (2003) Interleukin-6 gene alleles affect the risk of Alzheimer's disease and levels of the cytokine in blood and brain. Neurobiol Aging 24(7):921–926

Li MO, Sanjabi S, Flavell RA (2006) Transforming growth factor-beta controls development, homeostasis, and tolerance of T cells by regulatory T cell-dependent and -independent mechanisms. Immunity 25(3):455–471

Lio D, Scola L, Crivello A, Colonna-Romano G, Candore G, Bonafe M, Cavallone L, Marchegiani F, Olivieri F, Franceschi C, Caruso C (2003) Inflammation, genetics, and longevity: further studies on the protective effects in men of IL-10 -1082 promoter SNP and its interaction with TNF- -308 promoter SNP. J Med Genet 40:296–299

Lio D, Scola L, Crivello A, Colonna-Romano G, Candore G, Bonafe M, Cavallone L, Franceschi C, Caruso C (2002) Gender-specific association between -1082 IL-10 promoter polymorphism and longevity. Genes Immun 3:30–33

Loffreda S, Yang SQ, Lin HZ, Karp CL, Brengman ML, Wang DJ, Klein AS, Bulkley GB, Bao C, Noble PW, Lane MD, Diehl AM (1998) Leptin regulates proinflammatory immune responses. FASEB J 12:57–65

Luciani F, Valensin S, Vescovini R, Sansoni P, Fagnoni F, Franceschi C, Bonafè M, Turchetti G (2001) A stochastic model for CD8(+)T cell dynamics in human immunosenescence: implications for survival and longevity. J Theor Biol 213(4):587–597

Lukiw WJ, Cui JG, Marcheselli VL, Bodker M, Botkjaer A, Gotlinger K, Serhan CN, Bazan NG (2005) A role for docosahexaenoic acid-derived neuroprotectin D1 in neural cell survival and Alzheimer disease. J Clin Invest 115(10):2774–2783

Mannucci PM, Mari D, Merati G, Peyvandi F, Tagliabue L, Sacchi E, Taioli E, Sansoni P, Bertolini S, Franceschi C (1997) Gene polymorphisms predicting high plasma levels of coagulation and fibrinolysis proteins. A study in centenarians. Arterioscler Thromb Vasc Biol 17(4):755–759

Marcheselli VL, Hong S, Lukiw WJ, Tian XH, Gronert K, Musto A, Hardy M, Gimenez JM, Chiang N, Serhan CN, Bazan NG (2003) Novel docosanoids inhibit brain ischemia-reperfusion-mediated leukocyte infiltration and pro-inflammatory gene expression. J Biol Chem 278(44):43807–43817

Mari D, Mannucci PM, Coppola R, Bottasso B, Bauer KA, Rosenberg RD (1995) Hypercoagulability in centenarians: the paradox of successful aging. Blood 85(11):3144–3149

Mariani E, Pulsatelli L, Neri S, Dolzani P, Meneghetti A, Silvestri T, Ravaglia G, Forti P, Cattini L, Facchini A (2002) RANTES and MIP-1alpha production by T lymphocytes, monocytes and NK cells from nonagenarian subjects. Exp Gerontol 37(2–3):219–226

Maus MV, Kovacs B, Kwok WW, Nepom GT, Schlienger K, Riley JL, Allman D, Finkel TH, June CH (2004) Extensive replicative capacity of human central memory T cells. J Immunol 172:6675–6683

Macdonald TT, Monteleone G (2005) Immunity, inflammation, and allergy in the gut. Science 307(5717):1920–1925

McGeer EG, McGeer PL (1999) Brain inflammation in Alzheimer disease and the therapeutic implications. Curr Pharm Des 5(10):821–836

McGeer PL, McGeer EG (2004) Inflammation and the degenerative diseases of aging. Ann N Y Acad Sci 1035:104–116

Macpherson AJ, Harris NL (2004) Interactions between commensal intestinal bacteria and the immune system. Nat Rev Immunol 4(6):478–485

Miller RA (1996) The aging immune system: primer and prospectus. Science 273(5271):70–74

Mocchegiani E, Muzzioli M, Giacconi R (2000) Zinc and immunoresistance to infection in aging: new biological tools. Trends Pharmacol Sci 21(6):205–208

Moore ME, Piazza A, McCartney Y, Lynch MA (2005) Evidence that vitamin D3 reverses age-related inflammatory changes in the rat hippocampus. Biochem Soc Trans 33(Pt 4):573–577

Mutus B, Rabini RA, Franceschi C, Paolisso G, Rizzo MR, Ragno E, Rappelli A, Braconi M, Mazzanti L (2000) Cellular resistance to homocysteine: a key for longevity. Atherosclerosis 152:527–528

Nasi M, Troiano L, Lugli E, Pinti M, Ferraresi R, Monterastelli E, Mussi C, Salvioli G, Franceschi C, Cossarizza A (2006) Thymic output and functionality of the IL-7/IL-7 receptor system in centenarians: implications for the neolymphogenesis at the limit of human life. Aging Cell 5(2):167–175

Newman AB, Kupelian V, Visser M, Simonsick E, Goodpaster B, Nevitt M, Kritchevsky SB, Tylavsky FA, Rubin SM, Harris TB (2003) Health ABC Study Investigators. Sarcopenia: alternative definitions and associations with lower extremity function. J Am Geriatr Soc 51(11):1602–1609

Nicholson JK, Holmes E, Wilson ID (2005) Gut microorganisms, mammalian metabolism and personalized health care. Nat Rev Microbiol 3(5):431–438

Ostan R, Bucci L, Capri M, Salvioli S, Scurti M, Pini E, Monti D, Franceschi C (2008) Immunosenescence and immunogenetics of human longevity. Neuroimmunomodulation (in press)

Ottaviani E, Franceschi C (1998) A new theory on the common evolutionary origin of natural immunity, inflammation and stress response: the invertebrate phagocytic immunocyte as an eye-witness. Domest Anim Endocrinol 15(5):291–296

Ottaviani E, Franceschi C (1997) The invertebrate phagocytic immunocyte: clues to a common evolution of immune and neuroendocrine systems. Immunol Today 18:169–174

Paolisso G, Barbieri M, Bonafè M, Franceschi C (2000) Metabolic age modelling: the lesson from centenarians. Eur J Clin Invest 30(10):888–894

Pancer Z, Cooper MD (2006) The evolution of adaptive immunity. Annu Rev Immunol 24:497–518

Parrott MD, Greenwood CE (2007) Dietary influences on cognitive function with aging: from high-fat diets to healthful eating. Ann N Y Acad Sci 1114:389–397

Passeri G, Pini G, Troiano L, Vescovini R, Sansoni P, Passeri M, Gueresi P, Delsignore R, Pedraz-zoni M, Franceschi C (2003) Low vitamin D status, high bone turnover, and bone fractures in centenarians. J Clin Endocrinol Metab 88(11):5109–5115

Passeri G, Vescovini R, Sansoni P, Galli C, Franceschi C, Passeri M (2008) The Italian Multicentric Study on Centenarians (IMUSCE). Calcium metabolism and vitamin D in the extreme longevity. Exp Gerontol 43(2):79–87

Pawelec G, Akbar A, Caruso C, Solana R, Grubeck-Loebenstein B, Wikby A (2005) Human immu-nosenescence: is it infectious? Hum Immunol 205:257–268

Payette H, Roubenoff R, Jacques PF, Dinarello CA, Wilson PW, Abad LW, Harris T (2003) Insulin-like growth factor-1 and interleukin 6 predict sarcopenia in very old community-living men and women: the Framingham Heart Study. J Am Geriatr Soc 51(9):1237–1243

Pedersen BK, Bruunsgaard H (2003) Possible beneficial role of exercise in modulating low-grade inflammation in the elderly. Scand J Med Sci Sports 13(1):56–62

Pennesi G, Morellini M, Lulli P, Cappellacci S, Brioli G, Franceschi C, Trabace S (2001) TCR V> repertoire in an italian longeval population including centenarians. J Am Aging Assoc 24:63–70

Pennesi G, Liu Z, Ciubotariu R, Jiang S, Colovai A, Cortesini R, Suciu- Foca N, Harris P (1999) TCR repertoire of suppressor CD8 + CD28-T cell populations. Hum Immunol 60:291–304

Perretti M, D'Acquisto F (2006) Novel aspects of annexin 1 and glucocorticoid biology: intersection with nitric oxide and the lipoxin receptor. Inflamm Allergy Drug Targets 5(2):107–114

Petersen AM, Pedersen BK (2006) The role of IL-6 in mediating the anti-inflammatory effects of exercise. J Physiol Pharmacol 57 Suppl 10:43–51

Phillips T, Leeuwenburgh C (2005) Muscle fiber specific apoptosis and TNF-alpha signaling in sarcopenia are attenuated by life-long calorie restriction. FASEB J 19(6):668–670

Phillips T, Leeuwenburgh C (2004) Lifelong aspirin supplementation as a means to extending life span. Rejuvenation Res 7(4):243–251

Posnett DN, Edinger JW, Manavalan JS, Irwin C, Marodon G (1999) Differentiation of human CD8 T cells: implication for in vivo persistence of CD8+ CD28– cytotoxic effector clones. Int Immunol 11:229–41

Pourgheysari B, Khan N, Best D, Bruton R, Nayak L, Moss PA (2007) The cytomegalovirus-spe-cific CD4+ T-cell response expands with age and markedly alters the CD4+ T-cell repertoire. J Virol 81(14):7759–7765

Pradhan AD, Manson JE, Rifai N, Buring JE, Ridker PM (2001) C-reactive protein, interleukin 6, and risk of developing type 2 diabetes mellitus. JAMA 286(3):327–334

Rajala MW, Scherer PE (2003) Minireview: the adipocyte: at the crossroads of energy homeosta-sis, inflammation, and atherosclerosis. Endocrinology 144(9):3765–3773

Rajili>-Stojanơi> M, Smidt H, deVos WM (2007) Diversity of the human gastrointestinal tract m icrobiota revisited. Environ Microbiol 9(9):2125–2136

Ridker PM, Morrow DA (2003) C-reactive protein, inflammation, and coronary risk. Cardiol Clin 21(3):315–325

Roth SM, Metter EJ, Ling S, Ferrucci L (2006) Inflammatory factors in age-related muscle wast-ing. Curr Opin Rheumatol 18(6):625–630

Roubenoff R (2004) Sarcopenic obesity: the confluence of two epidemics. Obes Res 12(6):887–888

Roubenoff R, Parise H, Payette HA, Abad LW, D'Agostino R, Jacques PF, Wilson PW, Dinarello CA, Harris TB (2003a) Cytokines, insulin-like growth factor 1, sarcopenia, and mortality in very old community-dwelling men and women: the Framingham Heart Study. Am J Med 115(6):429–435

Roubenoff R (2003b) Catabolism of aging: is it an inflammatory process? Curr Opin Clin Nutr Metab Care 6(3):295–299

Sansoni P, Vescovini R, Fagnoni F, Biasini C, Zanni F, Zanlari L, Telera A, Lucchini G, Passeri G, Monti D, Franceschi C, Passeri M (2008) The immune system in extreme longevity. Exp Gerontol 43(2):61–65

Sartor RB (2005) Probiotic therapy of intestinal inflammation and infections. Curr Opin Gastroenterol 21(1):44–50

Sepulveda H, Cerwenka A, Morgan T, Dutton RW (1999) CD28, IL-2-independent costimulatory pathways for CD8 T lymphocyte activation. J Immunol 163:1133–1142

Sokol H, Lepage P, Seksik P, Doré J, Marteau P (2007) Molecular comparison of dominant microbiota associated with injured versus healthy mucosa in ulcerative colitis. Gut 56(1):152–154

Stecher B, Hardt WD (2008) The role of microbiota in infectious disease. Trends Microbiol 16(3):107–114

Strauss S, Bauer J, Ganter U, Jonas U, Berger M, Volk B (1992) Detection of interleukin-6 and alpha 2-macroglobulin immunoreactivity in cortex and hippocampus of Alzheimer's disease patients. Lab Invest 66(2):223–230

Szmitko PE, Wang CH, Weisel RD, de Almeida JR, Anderson TJ, Verma S (2003) New markers of inflammation and endothelial cell activation. Circulation 108(16):1917–1923

Takahashi K, Mizuarai S, Araki H, Mashiko S, Ishihara A, Kanatani A, Itadani H, Kotani H (2003) Adiposity elevates plasma MCP-1 levels leading to the increased CD11b-positive monocytes in mice. J Biol Chem 278:46654–46660

Troiano L, Pini G, Petruzzi E, Ognibene A, Franceschi C, Monti D, Masotti G, Cilotti A, Forti G (1999) Evaluation of adrenal function in aging. J Endocrinol Invest 22(10 Suppl):74–75

Trzonkowski P, My>liwska J, Szmit E, Wieckiewicz J, Lukaszuk K, Brydak LB, Machała M, My>liwski A(2003) Association between cytomegalovirus infection, enhanced proinflammatory response and low level of anti-hemagglutinins during the anti-influenza vaccination—an impact of immunosenescence. Vaccine 21(25–26):3826–3836

Turnbaugh PJ, Ley RE, Mahowald MA, Magrini V, Mardis ER, Gordon JI (2006) An obesity-associated gut microbiome with increased capacity for energy harvest. Nature 444(7122):1027–1031

Turnbull AV, Rivier CL (1999) Sprague-Dawley rats obtained from different vendors exhibit distinct adrenocorticotropin responses to inflammatory stimuli. Neuroendocrinology 70(3):186–195

Valenzuela HF, Effros RB (2002) Divergent telomerase and CD28 expression pattern in human CD4 and CD8 T cells following repeated encounters with the same antigenic stimulus. Clin Immunol 105:117–125

Vallejo AN, Weyand CM, Goronzy JJ (2001) Functional disruption of the CD28 gene transcriptional initiator in senescent T cells. J Biol Chem 2736:2565–2570

van Tongeren SP, Slaets JP, Harmsen HJ, Welling GW (2005) Fecal microbiota composition and frailty. Appl Environ Microbiol 71(10):6438–6442

Vasto S, Candore G, Balistreri CR, Caruso M, Colonna-Romano G, Grimaldi MP, Listi F, Nuzzo D, Lio D, Caruso C (2007) Inflammatory networks in ageing, age-related diseases and longevity. Mech Ageing Dev 128(1):83–91

Vescovini R, Biasini C, Fagnoni FF, Telera AR, Zanlari L, Pedrazzoni M, Bucci L, Monti D, Medici MC, Chezzi C, Franceschi C, Sansoni P (2007) Massive load of functional effector CD4+ and CD8+ T cells against cytomegalovirus in very old subjects. J Immunol 179(6):4283–4291

Visser M, Kritchevsky SB, Goodpaster BH, Newman AB, Nevitt M, Stamm E, Harris TB (2002) Leg muscle mass and composition in relation to lower extremity performance in men and women aged 70 to 79: the health, aging and body composition study. J Am Geriatr Soc 50:897–904

Wack A, Cossarizza A, Heltai S, Barbieri D, D'Addato S, Fransceschi C, Dellabona P, Casorati G (1998) Age-related modifications of the human alphabeta T cell repertoire due to different clonal expansions in the CD4+ and CD8 +subsets. Int Immunol 10(9):1281–1288

Weigle WO (1989) Effects of aging on the immune system. Hosp Prac 24(12):112–119

Williams GC (1957) Pleiotropy, natural selection and the evolution of senescence. Evolution 11:398–411

Xu H, Barnes GT, Yang Q, Tan G, Yang D, Chou CJ, Sole J, Nichols A, Ross JS, Tartaglia LA, Chen H (2003) Chronic inflammation in fat plays a crucial role in the development of obesity-related insulin resistance. J Clin Invest 112(12):1821–1830

Yaffe K (2007) Metabolic syndrome and cognitive disorders: is the sum greater than its parts? Alzheimer Dis Assoc Disord 21(2):167–171

Yaffe K, Kanaya A, Lindquist K, Simonsick EM, Harris T, Shorr RI, Tylavsky FA, Newman AB (2004) The metabolic syndrome, inflammation, and risk of cognitive decline. JAMA 292(18):2237–2242

Yaffe K, Lindquist K, Penninx BW, Simonsick EM, Pahor M, Kritchevsky S, Launer L, Kuller L, Rubin S, Harris T (2003) Inflammatory markers and cognition in well-functioning African-American and white elders. Neurology 61(1):76–80

Yende S, Waterer GW, Tolley EA, Newman AB, Bauer DC, Taaffe DR, Jensen R, Crapo R, Rubin S, Nevitt M, Simonsick EM, Satterfield S, Harris T, Kritchevsky SB (2006) Inflammatory markers are associated with ventilatory limitation and muscle dysfunction in obstructive lung disease in well functioning elderly subjects. Thorax 61(1):10–16

Yudkin JS, Stehouwer CD, Emeis JJ, Coppack SW (1999) C-reactive protein in healthy subjects: associations with obesity, insulin resistance, and endothelial dysfunction: a potential role for cytokines originating from adipose tissue? Arterioscler Thromb Vasc Biol 19(4):972–978

Zanni F, Vescovini R, Biasini C, Fagnoni F, Zanlari L, Telera A, Di Pede P, Passeri G, Pedrazzoni M, Passeri M, Franceschi C, Sansoni P (2003) Marked increase with age of type 1 cytokines within memory and effector/cytotoxic CD8+ T cells in humans: a contribution to understand the relationship between inflammation and immunosenescence. Exp Gerontol 38(9):981–987

Zhang X, Fujii H, Kishimoto H, Le Roy E, Surh CD, Sprent J (2002) Aging leads to disturbed homeostasis of memory phenotype CD8+ T cells. J Exp Med 195(3):283–293

Zoetendal EG, Vaughan EE, de Vos WM (2006) A microbial world within us. Mol Microbiol 59(6):1639–1650

Zoico E, Di Francesco V, Guralnik JM, Mazzali G, Bortolani A, Guariento S, Sergi G, Bosello O, Zamboni M (2004) Physical disability and muscular strength in relation to obesity and different body composition indexes in a sample of healthy elderly women. Int J Obes Relat Metab Disord 28(2):234–241

Molecular and Cellular Aspects of Macrophage Aging

Carlos Sebastián, Jorge Lloberas and Antonio Celada

Contents

Abbreviations

AML1/CFB	acute myeloid leukaemia/core-binding factor
Atm	ataxia telangiectasia mutated
BMP	bone morphogenetic protein
C/EBP	CCAAT/enhancer-binding protein
CBP	CREB-binding factor
CCR	CC chemokine receptor
dsRNA	double-stranded RNA
EGF	epithelial growth factor
FcγRI	Fc-γ receptor I
GEMM-CFU	granulocyte-erythrocyte-megakariocyte-macrophage colony-forming unit
GM-CFU	granulocyte-macrophage colony-forming unit
GM-CSF	granulocyte-macrophage colony-stimulating factor
HSC	hematopoietic stem cell
IFN-γ	interferon gamma
IκB	inhibitor of NF-κB
IL	interleukin
LPS	lipopolysaccharide
MAPK	mitogen-activated protein kinase
MCAF	macrophage chemotactic and activating factor
M-CFU	macrophage colony-forming unit

A. Celada (✉) · C. Sebastián · J. Lloberas
Institute for Research in Biomedicine- University of Barcelona
Josep Samitier 1-5, E-08028 Barcelona, Spain
Tel.: +34-93-403 71 65
Fax: +34-93-403 47 47
E-mail: acelada@ub.edu

T. Fulop et al. (eds.), *Handbook on Immunosenescence,*
DOI 10.1007/978–1-4020–9062–2_46, © Springer Science+Business Media B.V. 2009

M-CSF	macrophage colony-stimulating factor
MDC	macrophage-derived chemokine
MHC	major histocompatibility complex
MIP-1	macrophage inflammatory protein-1
MR	mannose receptor
NER	nucleotide excision repair
NF-κB	nuclear factor-kappa B
NHEJ	non-homologous end-joining
NOS2	inducible nitric oxide synthase
OPG	osteoprotegerin
PASG	proliferation-associated SNF2-like gene
PBMC	peripheral blood mononucleated cell
PKC	protein kinase C
RANKL	soluble receptor activator of NF-κB ligand
ROS	reactive oxygen species
Sir2	silent information regulator 2
SIRT	sirtuin
TARDC	thymus and activation regulated chemokine
TGF	tumor growth factor
TLR	toll-like receptor
TNF-α	tumour necrosis factor alpha
TRAF	TNF-receptor-associated factor
VEGF	vascular endothelial growth factor

Abstract: Macrophages are key cells in innate and adaptive immune function. These cells are involved in the destruction of bacteria, parasites, viruses and tumor cells and lead to the initiation of the inflammatory process. In addition, macrophages are responsible for processing antigens and presenting digested peptides to T-lymphocytes initiating the adaptive immune response. Finally, macrophages participate in the resolution of the inflammatory process by promoting tissue repair. Macrophage functions are affected by aging, thereby contributing to the immunosenescence of adaptive and innate immunity. Here, we summarize data about the effects of aging on macrophages and we discuss the molecular events that could be involved in this process.

Keywords: Aging • DNA damage • Immunosenescence • Inflammation • Macrophages

1 Introduction

Aging can be defined as the time-related deterioration of the physiological functions required for survival and fertility. Among these, immune function has been shown to be dysregulated with advancing age, thus leading to increased susceptibility to viral and bacterial infections, reactivation of latent viruses and decreased response to vaccines (Miller, 1996; Effros, 2001). This impairment of the immune system, called immunosenescence, is associated with increased mortality and major incidence of immune diseases and cancer in the elderly.

Innate and adaptive immunity are compromised by aging. T-cell-dependent and T-cell-mediated functions, such as proliferation, cytotoxicity, cytokine secretion and capacity to respond to novel antigens, are impaired in old age (Fabris et al. 1997; George and Ritter, 1996; Miller, 1996; Pawelec and Solana, 1997). Alterations in B-cells during aging have also been reported. In mice, a progressive decline in germinal centre formation is observed with age (Zheng et al. 1997); the number of circulating CD27[+] memory B-cells is reduced in the elderly (Breitbart et al. 2002; Colonna-Romano et al. 2003), and CD40 expression in B-cells is also impaired. Similar to the decline of the adaptive immune system, the functions of NK cells, macrophages and neutrophils also decrease with age (Butcher et al. 2001; Garg et al. 1996; Lloberas and Celada, 2002; Solana and Mariani, 2000), which may explain the increased incidence of bacterial and viral gastrointestinal and skin infections.

Macrophages are key cells in innate and adaptive immune function. These cells may act directly, by destroying bacteria, parasites, viruses and tumor cells, or indirectly, by releasing mediators such as interleukin-1 (IL-1), tumor necrosis factor-α (TNF- α), etc, which can regulate other cells. Macrophages are also responsible for processing antigens and presenting digested peptides to T-lymphocytes, as well as for tissue damage repair. Macrophage functions are altered in old age in humans, mice and rats, thereby contributing to the immunosenescence of adaptive and innate immunity (Lloberas and Celada, 2002). Phagocytic activity, cytokine and chemokine secretion, antibacterial defenses such as the production of reactive oxygen and nitrogen intermediates, infiltration and wound repair function in the late phase of inflammatory response, and antigen presentation, are altered in aged macrophages (Donnini et al. 2002; Herrero et al. 2002; Plowden et al. 2004), which lead to impairment in the first line of immune defense and a decreased capacity to contribute to the development of specific immune responses by presenting antigens to T-cells and by producing regulatory cytokines. Since macrophage activity is essential for the proper function of the immune system, studies regarding the effects of aging on the biology of these phagocytic cells and the molecular mechanisms involved in this process may contribute to a greater understanding of aging and immunosenescence. In addition, it would be of great interest to distinguish between the indirect (i.e., interactions with other cells) and the direct (i.e., genome modifications) effects of aging on macrophage biology to fully understand the macrophage aging process.

2   Macrophages

Macrophages are phagocytic cells involved in a number of complex functions in disease and health. They are critical to the establishment of the immune response against invading pathogens and to the maintenance of homeostasis, by promoting angiogenesis and tissue remodeling and repair. In addition, these cells are responsible for scavenging cellular debris and apoptotic cells (Mantovani et al. 2002).

Under the effect of growth factors, macrophages proliferate but the presence of microbial agents, cytokines or inflammatory molecules blocks this proliferation and induces functional activities (Xaus et al. 1999). This activation leads to the release of toxic metabolites and to the elimination of microbes by phagocytosis (Schroder et al. 2004).

Macrophages, as all blood cells, originate from hematopoietic stem cells (HSCs) in bone marrow under the presence of some growth factors and cytokines. The combined action of interleukin (IL)-1, IL-3 and/or IL-6 induces stem cell division, giving rise to a new stem cell and a pluripotent myeloid cell, also referred to as granulocyte-erythrocyte-megakariocyte-macrophage colony-forming unit (GEMM-CFU). In the presence of IL-1 and/or IL-3, this precursor is committed to becoming a progenitor of both macrophages and granulocytes known as the granulocyte-macrophage colony-forming unit (GM-CFU), which is also committed to the macrophage colony-forming unit (M-CFU) by action of the macrophage colony stimulating factor (M-CSF), the granulocyte-macrophage colony stimulating factor (GM-CSF) and IL-3. The M-CFU differentiates, in the presence of M-CSF, into monoblast, promonocyte, monocyte and, finally, into differentiated macrophages.

The differentiation process is regulated by the combined action of several transcription factors (Valledor et al. 1998); among these, PU.1, C/EBP and AML1/CFBβ play a crucial role in regulating the myeloid-specific expression of the M-CSF and GM-CSF receptors required for differentiation, proliferation and survival of mac-

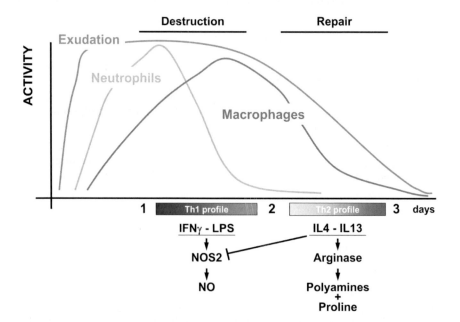

Fig. 1 Macrophages originate from HSC in bone marrow and migrate to body tissues where they become differentiated. Once in the tissues, macrophages may proliferate or become activated during an inflammatory process. However, when not activated, most macrophages die by apoptosis

rophages (Hohaus et al. 1995; Lloberas et al. 1999; Smith et al. 1996). Once in the blood, these cells can migrate to body tissues and differentiate, under the influence of cytokines and depending on the tissue type, into cell types with different functional activities such as osteoclasts (bone), Kupffer cells (liver), microglia (brain), etc. However, when not activated, most macrophages die by apoptosis (Fig. 1).

2.1 Macrophage Functions

Macrophages play a key role in both innate and adaptive immunity. They recognize and destroy invading pathogens and apoptotic cells and modulate the immune response by producing cytokines and chemokines. Moreover, macrophages, as antigen presenting cells, are involved in the regulation of the differentiation and activation of T-cells by the antigen presentation process. In addition to these functions, macrophages play a crucial role in the resolution of inflammation and in tissue repair by promoting synthesis of the extracellular matrix, fibroblast proliferation, angiogenesis and elimination of cellular debris (Rosmarin et al. 1995). Lastly, macrophages eliminate modified proteins, oxidized low density lipoproteins, apoptotic cells and other components from the tissues by expressing scavenger receptors.

Macrophages arriving at the inflammatory loci in the early steps kill remaining microorganisms, remove cell debris and apoptotic bodies and, in a second step, these cells reconstitute damaged tissues (Arnold et al. 2007; Fig. 2). Under the effect of

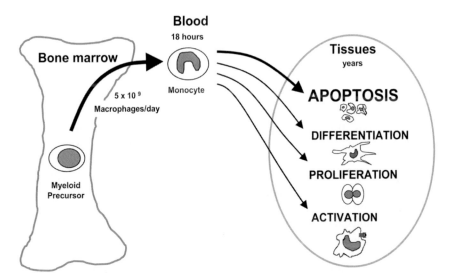

Fig. 2 Macrophages play a key role during the inflammatory process. In the initial phase they are activated in a Th1 context, leading to the release of inflammatory mediators (proinflammatory cytokines and chemokines, nitric oxide, ROS, etc.). In the resolution phase, macrophages become alternatively activated by Th2-type cytokines and participate in tissue repair and remodeling through the production of polyamines and proline

cytokines or bacterial products, macrophages become activated and undergo a series of biochemical, morphological and functional modifications. Th1-type cytokines such as interferon-gamma (IFN-γ) that interacts with its specific receptor, or bacterial products such as lipopolysaccharide (LPS), Gram-positive bacteria and yeast cell wall components, dsRNAs, bacterial flagellin and CpG oligodeoxynucleotides, induce classical activation of macrophages. These molecules are recognized by specific receptors called Toll-like receptors (TLRs; Akira et al. 2001; Alexopoulou et al. 2001; Gewirtz et al. 2001; Hemmi et al. 2002). This activation leads to inflammation and elimination of the pathogen. In addition to this classical activation, also known as M1, it has been reported that several cytokines such as IL-4 and IL-13 induce a distinct alternative activation programme (M2; Gordon, 2003). Recently, it has been shown that IL-21, Activin A and Chitin also mediate alternative macrophage activation (Ogawa et al. 2006; Pesce et al. 2006; Reese et al. 2007). Classical activation is characterized by the expression of inducible nitric oxide synthase (NOS2) and by the biosynthesis and release of proinflammatory cytokines, including tumor necrosis factor (TNF)-α, IL-1 and IL-6. In the alternative activation, the expression of arginase 1 is induced, together with the upregulation of the mannose receptor (MR) and several other markers (Mantovani et al. 2004). Curiously enough, arginine is the substrate for NOS2 and for arginase 1 and the system that transports this amino acid is induced by both types of cytokines providing more arginine inside the cell (Yeramian et al. 2006a, b). NOS2 degrades arginine to produce NO while arginase produces ornithine and polyamines. Alternatively activated macrophages exert immunoregulatory functions, drive type II responses and participate in tissue remodeling.

2.2 Activation of Macrophages

The main activators of macrophages are LPS and IFN-γ. These molecules induce microbicidal and proinflammatory functions in macrophages and, therefore, the destruction of the invading pathogen.

IFN-γ is a type II interferon mainly produced by activated T and NK cells (Imai et al. 1999; Yoshimoto et al. 1998). However, other cell types such as professional antigen presenting cells can also release it (Frucht et al. 2001; Pestka et al. 2004). IFN-γ induces an antiproliferative and antiviral response and is critical to the establishment of the immune response as it promotes the recruitment of lymphocytes at the inflammation site by inducing the production of chemokines and the expression of adhesion molecules (Puddu et al. 1997). Moreover, IFN-γ leads to the expression of several genes that regulate many aspects of macrophage biology. It induces the expression of the Fc high affinity receptors (FcγRI) in the cell surface leading to increased antibody-dependent cytotoxicity (Vaday et al. 2001); it increases the phagocytic activity of macrophages; it induces a respiratory burst (generation of nitric oxide and reactive species of oxygen) and the expression of lysosomal enzymes promoting the destruction of the pathogen (Capsoni et al. 1994). IFN-γ inhibits M-CSF-dependent proliferation and protects macrophages from apoptosis induced by glucocorticoids or M-CSF withdrawal. This protective effect of IFN-γ is mediated by p21[waf1] expression and blockade of the cell cycle at the G1/S boundary (Xaus et al. 1999). We have observed that in granulomas, where macrophages need to survive for a longer time, there are increased levels of IFN-γ correlating with increased levels of p21[waf-1] (Xaus et al. 2003). In addition to modulating the innate immunity, IFN-γ regulates the adaptive immunity by regulating the expression of the major histocompatibility complex (MHC) class II genes at several levels (Cullell-Young et al. 2001; Gonalons et al. 1998), which are crucial for presenting antigens to T-lymphocytes and for initiating an immune response.

The effect of LPS on macrophage function is mediated by the interaction with its receptor, the Toll-like receptor 4 (TLR4). Activation of macrophages by LPS leads to an increase in mRNA synthesis and to the secretion of proinflammatory cytokines such as TNF-α, IL-6, IL-1β, IL-8, IL-12, TGF-β and the macrophage inhibitory factor (MIF). Moreover, in response to LPS macrophages release arachidonic acid metabolites (e.g., platelet-activating factor, prostaglandin and leukotriens), proteases, eicosanoids, nitric oxide and other reactive oxygen species (ROS; Miller et al. 2005; Muzio et al. 1997). All these cytokines and mediators are critical to the initiation of inflammatory response and contribute to the efficient control of growth and dissemination of invading pathogens.

In addition to this classical activation, macrophages can be activated by Th2 cytokines acquiring an M2 phenotype. Alternative activation of macrophages by IL-4 and IL-13 produces M2-type responses, particularly in allergic, cellular and humoral responses to parasitic and extracellular pathogens. This alternative activation results in the up-regulation of the expression of the MR and MHC class II molecules, which stimulates endocytosis and antigen presentation, respectively. These cytokines also induce the expression of selective chemokines such as macrophage-derived chemokine (MDC, also known as CCL22) and thymus and activation regulated chemokine (TARDC, CCL17), and intracellular enzymes, such as arginase, that are involved in cell recruitment and repair of granuloma formation, thereby counteracting the effects of the inducible NOS2 activation and nitric oxide release (Gordon, 2003). Moreover, the induction of arginase down-regulates the expression of NOS2 at the translational level (Lee et al. 2003). The catabolism of arginine by arginase produce l-ornithine and ultimately polyamines that induce fibroblasts proliferation and collagen production.

3 Aged Macrophages

Macrophages from aged humans and mice display several defects in their function. Many studies have focused on the effects of aging on macrophage biology but have yielded conflicting, and sometimes opposing, results. This may be due to factors such as the strain and sex of experimental subjects, distinct macrophage origin (bone-marrow, peritoneum, spleen, or alveolus) and differences in experimental conditions (culture, stimulant used, etc.). Furthermore, in the case of humans, it is difficult to define the term ``healthy elderly subject,'' which implies careful screening for health. Furthermore, most studies on humans have been performed with monocytes, which generally provide a limited view of tissue macrophages. In addition, the majority of studies on macrophage aging have shown modifications in their functional activities; however, in few cases these studies have provided an explanation of the basis of this dysfunction.

3.1   Differentiation and Maturation of Macrophages

The immune system is maintained by the generation of immune cells from HSCs. These cells reside in the bone marrow and provide lifelong production of progenitors and peripheral blood cells. Simultaneously, HSCs must be able to maintain the stem cell pool by selfrenewal divisions. Increasing experimental evidence supports the premise that HSCs become aged and have a limited functional lifespan (Geiger and Van Zant, 2002). The first studies to suggest stem cell aging involved serial transplantation of whole bone marrow that supported only 4 to 5 rounds of transplantation (Harrison and Astle, 1982; Van Zant and Liang, 2003). Given that the HSC compartment facilitates this regeneration, these findings suggested an exhaustion of the stem cell pool. In fact, there is ample evidence that stem cell quality decreases with each selfrenewal division (Van Zant et al. 1997). Mouse experiments revealed that the number of HSCs increased while their proliferative capacity decreased with age (de Haan and Van Zant, 1999; Morrison et al. 1996). Results from studies comparing HSCs in different mouse strains indicate that HSC functional decline can be correlated with lifespan. In addition, a negative correlation has also been shown between lifespan and proliferative capacity (de Haan et al. 1997; Geiger and Van Zant, 2002). Progenitor cells from long-lived C57BL/6 mice have a relatively low cycling activity, whereas the stem cell pool increases with age and is relatively small. In contrast, DBA/2 mice have a shorter lifespan than C57BL/6 mice, their progenitors show increased cycling activity, and their stem cell pool decreases upon aging and is relatively large (de Haan et al. 1997). All this suggests that rapidly dividing cells exhaust faster.

But, how does the aging of HSCs affect the generation of macrophages? To date, it is not clear whether the generation of macrophages from their precursors is impaired with aging. In humans, there is a reduction of CD68-positive cells, which are markers of macrophage population (Ogawa et al. 2000). The percentage of CD68-positive cells is high in children (first and second decades) and then decreases as the individual gets older. Moreover, it has been hypothesized that this reduction in the macrophage population may have an influence on the reduction of HSC proliferation and on the induction of apoptosis in the bone marrow of elderly people, probably via reduced production of growth factors and cytokines (Arkins et al. 1993; Kelley et al. 1996; Minshall et al. 1997). By contrast, macrophages increase in density in myeloproliferative disorders suggesting that there was a correlation between macrophage density and myelopoietic activity (Sadahira et al. 1999). In mice there are conflicting data. According to Wang et al. (1995), the macrophage population is enhanced in bone marrow, as shown by an increase in Mac1-positive cells. This is reflected as an increase with age in the macrophage colony forming unit (M-CFU). Moreover, macrophages from bone marrow of old mice generate less TNF-α than macrophages from young mice suggesting that the increase in the number of macrophages may reflect a compensation for their reduced function. However, we have found that the number, size, DNA content and cell surface markers expressed during macrophage maturation, such as Mac1, were similar in macrophages from aged and young mice (Herrero et al. 2001). Recently, Rossi et al. (2007) have demonstrate that accumulation of DNA damaged has a profound impact on the functional capacity of HSCs with age, leading to loss of reconstitution and proliferative potential, diminished selfrenewal, increased apoptosis and, ultimately, functional exhaustion. In transplantation experiments, it has been shown that recipients transplanted with HSCs from mice deficient in several genomic maintenance pathways have a marked decrease in reconstitution of B-cells, T-cells and myeloid cells. Moreover, these authors provide evidence that endogenous DNA damage accumulates with age in wild-type stem cells. This suggests that an impaired functional capacity of HSCs accumulating DNA damage may derive in a deficient generation of blood cells.

3.2   Effects of Aging on Macrophage Functions

A great number of macrophage functions including phagocytosis, antibacterial defenses, chemotaxis, wound repair and activation have been reported to be altered in human, rats and mice during aging, thereby contributing to the immunosenescence of adaptive and innate immunity (Table 1).

Table 1 Effect of aging on macrophage function

Function	Change with aging
IFN-g activation	
Production of ROS	Decreased
Production of NO	Decreased
Activation of MAPK	Decreased
Expression of MHC II	Decreased
Production of PGE2	Increased
LPS activation	
Production of proinflammatory citokines	Decreased
Production of chemokines	Decreased
Production of ROS	Decreased
Production of NO	Decreased
Expression of TLR4	Decreased or no change
Activation of MAPK	Decreased
Phagocytosis	Decreased
Wound repair	Decreased
Chemotaxis	Decreased

3.2.1 Phagocytosis

Phatocytosis constitutes the first step of immune defense against invading pathogens. Tissue macrophages, alveolar macrophages and polymorphonuclear leucocytes in the blood have all phagocytic activity. However, the data available addressing the effect of aging on the phagocytic function of macrophages and monocytes is unclear. An age-related decline in phagocytosis by neutrophils but not by alveolar macrophages was observed in rats (Mancuso et al. 2001). However, several reports using murine models indicate a decline in the adherence, opsonization, tumor cell killing and phagocytosis by peritoneal macrophages (De La Fuente, 1985; De la Fuente et al. 2000; Khare et al. 1996). In addition, it is observed that the phagocytic activity of macrophages from aged individuals declines in parallel with reduced production of macrophage-derived chemokines (Swift et al. 2001). Altered expression and function of receptors involved in the phagocytic process and their signal transduction may explain the observed reduced phagocytic ability in aging models. However, the effect of aging on these proteins has not been reported.

3.2.2 Chemotaxis

To eliminate invading pathogens macrophages must migrate toward the inflammation site in a process controlled by chemotactic stimuli. The main chemotactic factors are chemokines secreted by the endothelium, neutrophils, T-cells, monocytes and macrophages, such as macrophage chemotactic and activating factor (MCAF), macrophage inflammatory protein (MIP)-1α, MIP-1β, RANTES and IL-8 as well as complement products such as C5a, C3a and C4a. A reduction in the production of MIP-1α and MIP-1β by macrophages from aged mice has been described (Ashcroft et al. 1998). Moreover, the chemotactic response of macrophages to complement-derived factors is impaired in elderly individuals (Fietta et al. 1993). Aschroft et al. (1998) collected coetaneous punch biopsies of the wounds from 138 healthy subjects, aged 19–96 years at fixed time-points from day 1 up to 3 months postwounding. Using quantitative imaging, they demonstrated that monocyte/macrophage and lymphocyte appearance was delayed in the aged individuals. Thus, these data suggest that aged macrophages show an impaired chemotactic response that may contribute to delayed pathogen clearance in healthy elderly individuals.

3.2.3 Activation of Macrophages

The different aspects of macrophage classical activation is the most studied effect of aging on macrophages. IFN-γ activation is impaired in aged macrophages. Studies using rats have demonstrated a 75% decrease in the capacity of macrophages from aged animals to produce superoxide anion after incubation with IFN-γ or opsonized zymosan (Davila et al. 1990). Furthermore, the production of peroxide and nitric oxide in response to IFN-γ by peritoneal macrophages is diminished in aged mice (Ding et al. 1994). This was explained by a reduced IFN-γ induced mitogen-activated protein kinase (MAPK) phosphorylation in macrophages from aged mice.

In addition to microbicidal activities, IFN-γ induces the expression of MHC class II molecules that are involved in the initiation of the adaptive immune response. Antigen presentation by macrophages is decreased with age, possibly due to diminished expression of MHC class II molecules both in human and mice (Herrero et al. 2001; Plowden et al. 2004). We have found that bone marrow macrophages from aged mice express half of the MHC class II antigen IA molecules at the cell surface when stimulated with IFN-γ (Herrero et al. 2001). IAβ mRNA expression is also lower in aged macrophages because there is a smaller amount of transcription factors that bind to the W and X boxes of MHC class II gene promoter. In addition, it has been shown that human monocytes express decreased levels of HLA-DR/DP (Villanueva et al. 1990). Moreover, activated macrophages from aged humans and mice produce higher amounts of prostaglandin E2 than younger individuals, which inhibits surface expression of MHC class II, thus contributing to the decreased capacity of antigen presentation of macrophages observed with age (Plowden et al. 2004).

Activation by LPS is also altered in aged macrophages. Although inflammatory cytokines are elevated in the plasma of aged animals and humans (Franceschi et al. 2000; Saurwein-Teissl et al. 2000), the production of inflammatory cytokines by peritoneal macrophages from rats and mice decreases with age. Stimulation of macrophages from aged rodents with LPS results in significantly lower production of IL-1, TNF-α, and IL-6 (Inamizu et al. 1985; Plackett et al. 2004; Wallace et al. 1995), as well as lower production of chemokines, such as MIP-1α and MIP-1β (Swift et al. 2001). The production of oxidative radicals in response to LPS also appears to decline with age, and the expression of NOS2 and the production of nitric oxide are reduced in macrophages from aged rodents (Alvarez et al. 1996; Khare et al. 1996; Kissin et al. 1997; Plackett et al. 2004).

There is some controversy concerning the basis for the decline in the production of inflammatory cytokines and oxidative radicals in response to LPS stimulation. Renshaw et al. (2002) found that expression of a variety of TLRs, including TLR4, was decreased in the aged, which could be the reason for a decreased response of macrophages from aged mice to LPS. Conversely, Boehmer et al. (2004) did not find a reduction in TLR expression and they attributed the impaired cytokine production to a decrease in c-jun N-terminal kinase (JNK) and p38 MAPK activation in macrophages from aged mice. In humans, the decreased response of monocytes to LPS has been associated with deficiencies in the activation of protein kinase C (PKC)-α, PKC-βI and PKC-βII, MAPK and deficient expression of c-Fos and c-Jun (Delpedro et al. 1998). Using a microarray analysis on RNA from resting and LPS-stimulated macrophages from aged and control mice, Chelvarajan et al. (2006) demonstrated that immune response (proinflammatory chemokines, cytokines and their receptors) and signal transduction genes (TLR and MAPK pathways) were specifically reduced in aged mouse macrophages. In addition to reduced levels of IL-1β, IL-6, IL-12 and TNF-α, they found a decrease in IFN-γ, M-CSF, GM-CSF and bone morphogenetic protein-1 (BMP-1) production in aged macrophages. Moreover, many chemokines involved in innate immunity and inflammation are reduced in macrophages from aged mice, such as CCL4, CXCL1, CCL6, CCL9 and CCL24, as well as the receptors CC chemokine receptor 3 (CCR3) and CCR5, involved in chemotaxis of neutrophils, macrophages and eosinophils (Chelvarajan et al. 2006). All this correlates with the reduction in the overall inflammatory response in spleens from aged mice. Furthermore, a variety of chemokines and receptors (CXCL9, CXCL10, CXCL11, CCR7), which affect CD4 and CD8 T-cell migration and T helper cell type 1 (Th1) development, are reduced in macrophages from aged mice (Chelvarajan et al. 2006). This is in agreement with an age-associated decrease in T-cell function and in particular, Th1 cell function. Several components of the TLR pathway [TNF-receptor-associated factor 6 (TRAF6), CD14, Rel, RelB and some of the subunits of the NF-κB transcription factor] have reduced levels in LPS-stimulated aged macrophages. As this pathway is known to be critical for the production of chemokines and proinflammatory cytokines, these authors conclude that reduced levels of the components of TLR pathway could explain the impaired production of several cytokines and chemokines in LPS-stimulated macrophages from aged mice. In addition to TLR pathway, they also found an increase in the expression and phosphorylation of p38 MAPK in aged macrophages. Low doses of a p38 MAPK inhibitor enhanced proinflammatory cytokine production by macrophages indicating that p38 MAPK activity has a role in cytokine dysregulation in aged mouse macrophages. This is in contrast with the results of Boehmer et al. (2004; See above). This discrepancy could be the result of the use of thioglycollate-induced peritoneal macrophages in the Boehmer study versus macrophages from spleen in the Chelvarajan study.

There are few data regarding the way in which aging may affect the alternative activation of macrophages. However, alterations in cytokine secretion by T-cells could affect this process. In mice infected with *S. mansoni*, the production of Th2 cytokines is lower in aged BALB/c animals compared to young ones (Smith et al. 2001). Moreover, older IL-4-/- BALB/c mice express a transient resistance to *L. major* infection, indicating that these animals have a lower capacity for Th2 response (Kropf et al. 2003). Arginase expression, which may play a crucial role in M1/M2 polarization, is also affected by age. Total arginase activity in the postrhinal cortex and in some regions of the hippocampus decreases in aged mice (Liu et al. 2003a, b). However, it has been shown that insulin augments alternative activation of macrophages by IL-4 (Hartman et al. 2004; Liang et al. 2004). As insulin blood levels and insulin resistance increase with age (Petersen et al. 2003), it is tempting to speculate that alternative activation of macrophages may increase during aging. Moreover, the insulin pathway regulates the lifespan in worms, flies and mammals (Tatar et al. 2003). Mutations in some of the components of this pathway leads to an extension of the lifespan of these species (Kenyon, 2005) suggesting that increased insulin signaling may be related to aging. However, further studies are required to examine whether changes in macrophage polarization with aging are responsible for some aspects of immunosenescence.

3.2.4   Wound Repair

In addition to their crucial role in the initial phases of the inflammatory response, macrophages develop important functions in the removal and regeneration of the damaged tissue by secreting angiogenic and fibrogenic growth factors. Studies in human and rodent species have shown an age-related decline in the coetaneous wound repair process, which impacts on the inflammatory response and the growth phase of the repair process (Gosain and DiPietro, 2004; Thomas, 2001). These changes include enhanced platelet aggregation, delayed re-epithelialization, delayed agiogenesis, delayed collagen deposition, turnover and remodeling, delayed healing strength, decreased wound strength, and delayed infiltration and function of macrophages. Using a murine model of excision wound repair, Danon et al. (1989) demonstrated that repair and re-epithelialization processes were delayed significantly in aged mice and that the rate of wound repair could be partially restored by the addition of peritoneal macrophages from young mice. In addition, the rates of collagen synthesis and angiogenesis [attributed to a decrease in the secretion of vascular endothelial growth factor (VEGF)] were delayed. TLRs 2, 4, 7, and 9 and adenosine A (2A) receptors mediates the production of VEGF and other angiogenic factors by macrophages (Olah and Caldwell, 2003; Pinhal-Enfield et al. 2003). Hence, the observed decrease in TLR function in aging may contribute to delayed wound healing. Furthermore, the expression of cell adhesion molecules on the vascular endothelium is decreased in the elderly (Ashcroft et al. 1998), and responsiveness (receptor expression) to VEGF and epithelial growth factor (EGF) is reduced (Ashcroft et al. 1997; Kraatz et al. 1999). Thus, the communication between tissue cells and the innate immune system appears impaired, contributing to the observed functional deficiencies in tissue repair.

3.3 Effect of Aging on Tissue-Specific Macrophages

In addition to studies regarding the effect of aging on macrophage biology, many reports have focused on the impact of aging on some tissue-specific macrophages. Thus, alteration in the function of these macrophages may contribute to the pathologies observed in these tissues during the aging process.

Macrophages are dispersed throughout the body. Some take up residence in particular tissues becoming fixed macrophages which serve different functions in different tissues and are named to reflect their tissue location: alveolar macrophages in the lung, thymic macrophages in the thymus, histiocytes in connective tissues, Kupffer cells in the liver, mesangial cells in the kidney, osteoclasts in bones, Langerhans' cells (LCs) in the skin and microglia in the brain.

LCs were originally described as an epidermal macrophage population containing large granules and capable of phagocytosis (Hume et al. 1983; Ralfkiaer et al. 1985). Later, LCs were typed as immature dendritic cells since they can migrate after activation from the skin to regional lymph nodes, a hallmark characteristic of dendritic cells (Cumberbatch and Kimber, 1992; Yamazaki et al. 1998; Wang et al. 1999). Although both macrophages and LCs belong to myeloid lineage, the precise lineage relationship between them is not yet clear. The number of epidermal LCs and their function is diminished as a result of the aging process in humans and mice (Bhushan et al. 2002; Thiers et al. 1984). However, it is not clear whether this defect is a consequence of diminished bone marrow precursor production. These age-related changes may contribute to altered coetaneous immune function, such as poor or variable contact hypersensitivity to allergens in the elderly.

The functional capacity of Kupffer cells is also impaired in aged mice. They have a substantial reduction in their respiratory burst activity, lessened endocytic capacity and enhanced oxidative stress (Videla et al. 2001).

Among the most striking changes that occur with age is thymic involution, which correlates with the observed impairment of T-cell immunity. This decrease in thymus size is also associated with alterations in thymus architecture (Aspinall, 1997; Bertho et al. 1997). However, little information is available on macrophages during age-dependent thymus involution. In mice, relatively early in the involution process, the number of macrophages and their phagocytic activity increases, with these cells appearing to have a large number of phagolysosomes containing cellular material at various stages of lysis (Hirokawa, 1977; Nabarra and Andrianarison, 1996). This correlates with the decrease in thymocyte numbers (Aspinall, 1997). Over time the number of thymic macrophages diminishes gradually (Nabarra and Andrianarison, 1996; San Jose et al. 2001), in correlation with a reduction in the total number of macrophage precursors and their capacity to proliferate (Zeira and Gallily, 1990). In addition, Varas et al. (2003) demonstrated that the thymic macrophages phenotype (expression of cell surface markers and chemokine receptors) is unaltered in the elderly suggesting that their functional properties on T-cell stimulation, adhesion and migration would also be unimpaired.

Microglia cells are the small, highly ramified immune sentinels of the brain. These cells are distributed throughout the brain parenchyma and are continuously sensing the microenvironment in search for injuries or pathogens (Davalos et al. 2005; Nimmerjahn et al. 2005). After activation, microglia initiate an innate immune response by producing proinflammatory cytokines. Different lines of evidence from humans and mice suggest that senescence of microglia does occur leading to neurodegeneration. Proliferation of microglia during activation is not impaired by old age. In fact, microglia appear to proliferate even more vigorously in older rats after a facial nerve lesion (Conde and Streit, 2006). Moreover, human and rodent microglia show signs of aging-related structural and morphological deterioration (Streit, 2006). The incidence of dystrophic microglia increases in older individuals, supporting the idea that dystrophy is a reflection of cell aging. It is suggested that the deterioration of microglia may be involved in the pathogenesis of neurodegenerative disease, perhaps through progressive loss of microglial neuroprotective capacity (Streit, 2002). In addition to this structural alteration, microglia from healthy aging brains show an increased expression of proinflammatory cytokines (TNF-α, IL-1β, IL-6 and IL-12; Sierra et al. 2007). The higher levels of these cytokines produce tissue degeneration (Aloisi, 2005), and thus the increased levels in aging microglia could contribute to brain damage during aging, and even contribute to the onset of neurodegenerative diseases (Mrak and Griffin, 2005).

There are few data regarding how aging affects the function of osteoclasts. Bone mass is maintained by a delicate balance between formation and resorption. At cell level, the rates of bone formation and resorption reflect the number and activity of stromal/osteoblastic cells and osteoclasts, cells of macrophage origin. Stromal/osteoblastic cells regulate the number and activity of osteoclasts through expression of the soluble receptor activator of NF-κB ligand (RANKL), M-CSF and osteoprotegerin (OPG; Cao et al. 2005). With advancing age, expression of RANKL in whole bone and in culture marrow cells from both, humans and animals, gradually increases, and expression of OPG either decreases or remains unchanged. RANKL expression is also increased in early stromal/osteoblastic cells from aged mice (Cao et al. 2003; Fazzalari et al. 2001; Ikeda et al. 2001; Makhluf et al. 2000). Furthermore, the osteo-clast progenitor pool is reported to increase with advancing age in mice (Perkins et al. 1994). Cao et al. (2005) showed that aging significantly increases stromal/osteob-lastic cell-induced osteoclastogenesis, promotes expansion of the osteoclast precur-sor pool and alters the relationship between osteoblasts and osteoclasts. Coincident with these changes, the efficacy of osteoclasts to form bone is also impaired. All these modifications may contribute to the osteoporosis associated with aging.

In summary, the aging process has an impact on the function of macrophages and tissue-specific macrophages, thus leading not only to an impaired immune response but also to the development of several pathologies in the tissues where they reside.

4 Molecular Mechanisms Involved in Macrophage Aging

The data presented so far indicates an age-associated malfunction of macrophages. Most of these publications describe the events but do not shed light on the origin of this malfunction. Many theories have been formulated to explain the aging process. Because immunosenescence is a hallmark of aging, these theories may also explain the changes that occur in the immune system as a result of maturation (Fig. 3).

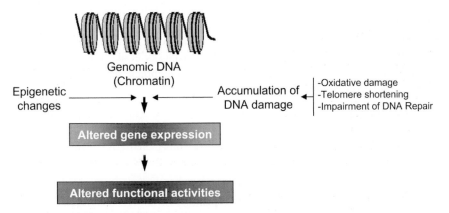

Fig. 3 Molecular view of macrophage aging. Altered gene expression caused by accumulation of DNA damage and by epigenetic changes may, in part, explain the altered functional activities observed in aged macrophages

4.1   Aging and Altered Gene Expression

Aging has been associated with changes in gene expression (Kanungo, 1975). Many genes show an altered expression in several cell types contributing to the observed modification of some functional activities during aging. Loss of the expression of several genes occurs in immune cells. For instance, in T-cells, loss of expression of CD28 (Effros et al. 1994) and IL-2 receptor is related to a deficient co-stimulatory signal and poor proliferative responses. As discussed above, aged macrophages also have altered expression of many genes (TLRs, proinflammatory cytokines, chemokines, MHC class II molecules, signal transduction molecules, transcription factors, etc), which may explain the loss of some functional activities. The molecular basis of the altered expression of some of these genes is related to an impaired signal transduction (MAPK, PKC; Boehmer et al. 2004; Delpedro et al. 1998). In other cases, changes in gene expression result from age-related modifications of one or more transcriptional factors. For example, we have demonstrated that loss of MHC class II expression in aged macrophages was due to lower levels of transcription factors that bind to the promoter of these genes, indicating reduced binding efficiency (Herrero et al. 2001). Moreover, changes in gene expression may be due to epigenetic mechanisms. It has been reported that methylation of CpG islands decreases during cellular senescence and aging (Hornsby et al. 1992; Singhal et al. 1987) and that the activity of the DNA-methyl transferase is also lower in senescent cells (Vertino et al. 1994). In addition, disruption of PASG (lsh), a SNF2-like factor that facilitates DNA methylation, causes premature aging in mice (Sun et al. 2004), which suggests that DNA methylation is essential to maintain the expression patterns required for normal growth and longevity. Furthermore, acetylation and deacetylation of histones are involved in cell senescence (Howard, 1996; Ogryzko et al. 1996; Villeponteau, 1997). In mammals, the histone acetyl transferase activity of p300/CBP is reduced in several tissues in aged mice (Li et al. 2002) and its expression is impaired in neurons of aged rats (Matsumoto, 2002). Moreover, the histone deacetylase Sir2 and its homologs in mammals SIRT1 and SIRT6 are involved in regulation of genomic stability and aging in yeast, worms and mice (Chua et al. 2005; Hekimi and Guarente, 2003; Mostoslavsky et al. 2006). On the basis of these observations, it is of interest to study the epigenetic regulation of gene expression during aging in macrophages.

4.2   Telomere Shortening

Telomeres are chromatin structures that cap and protect the end of chromosomes. In vertebrates, they are formed by tandem repeats of hexamer sequences (TTAGGG) that are associated with various specific proteins (Blackburn, 2001; Chan and Blackburn, 2002; de Lange, 2002) involved in the maintenance and regulation of telomere length. With selfreplication, telomeres lose TTAGGG repeats because conventional DNA polymerases are not able to completely replicate linear chromosomes (Lansdorp, 2005). Progressive telomere shortening has detrimental implications; chromosome caps are unprotected leading to genomic instability and cell death (Blackburn, 2001; McEachern et al. 2000). However, in normal cells, telomere erosion initiates a cell senescence program which prevents further divisions, thereby protecting cells from excessive telomere loss and cell death (Blackburn, 2001; McEachern et al. 2000).

Telomere shortening has been involved in the aging process and in the regulation of replicative lifespan (Iwama et al. 1998). Late generations of the telomerase KO mice, Terc$^{-/-}$, show severe telomere dysfunction characterized by critically short telomeres and end-to-end fusions. These mice suffer from various age-related diseases that affect highly proliferative tissues (Blasco, 2002). Among these, the generation and function of immune cells has been shown to be affected by telomere attrition. Numerous studies have confirmed that loss of telomeric DNA with progressive telomere shortening occurs in cells of the hematopoietic system as a function of normal replicative aging. Age-dependent loss of telomeric DNA was demonstrated in both neutrophils and lymphocytes (Hastie et al. 1990; Vaziri et al. 1993). Moreover, reduced proliferative capacity of T- and B cells has been described in Terc$^{-/-}$ mice (Blasco, 2002). However, no direct assessment of aged-induced changes in telomere length in monocytes and macrophages has been performed to date. Several studies using peripheral blood mononucleated cells consisting of 10–15% monocytes, 60–70% lymphocytes and 30–15% granulocytes, have shown that these structures shorten with age at a rate comparable to that of purified lymphocytes (Weng, 2001). Mature monocytes do not undergo further cell division after activation. Thus, the variations in telomere length in monocytes as the aging process advances may reflect changes in telomere length in hematopoietic progenitor cells. In fact, HSCs show telomere shortening during in vitro culture and in vivo aging (Engelhardt et al. 1997; Vaziri et al. 1994; Zimmermann et al. 2004). HSCs derived from human and mice lose telomeric DNA with age despite the presence of detectable telomerase activity (Allsopp et al. 2001; Vaziri et al. 1994). Moreover, telomere shortening occurs during serial transplantation of HSCs, coinciding with impaired function (Allsopp et al. 2001). This suggests that telomere attrition may alter the HSC capacity to generate blood cells. In support of this notion, HSCs from telomerase-deficient mice whith short telomeres show a reduced ability to repopulate irradiated mice (Allsopp et al. 2003; Samper et al. 2002).

4.3 DNA Damage

Accumulation of DNA damage may also explain the aging process. Increasing experimental data suggest that somatic mutations accumulate during aging (Curtis and Crowley, 1963; Ramsey et al. 1995; Tucker et al. 1999) and that this accumulation increases exponentially (Martin et al. 1996). This may be due to an increase in the number of mutations or to a deficient repair activity. DNA damage produced by these mutations may cause an alteration in gene expression patterns, the generation of modified proteins and the alteration of some cellular functions. To repair this DNA damage, cells have developed a DNA damage response which includes the detection of the lesion, the activation of cell cycle checkpoints and the activation of several repair mechanisms to eliminate the damage (Sancar et al. 2004). Deficiencies in some of the components of the DNA damage response leads to senescence and premature aging (Lieber and Karanjawala, 2004) supporting the idea that accumulation of DNA damage is involved in the aging process.

An important mechanism that leads to a wide spectrum of intracellular damage during aging is extended exposure to ROS generated by cellular metabolism (Kregel and Zhang, 2007). It has been long recognized that high levels of ROS can inflict direct damage on macromolecules such as lipids, nucleic acids and proteins impairing their function (Blumberg, 2004). In the hematopoietic system, stem cell functional capacity is severely affected by accumulation of DNA damage (Nijnik et al. 2007; Rossi et al. 2007). Alterations in telomere length maintenance and in the nucleotide excision repair (NER) and non-homologous end-joining (NHEJ) repair pathways limit stem cell function in an age-dependent manner by intrinsically diminishing selfrenewal and proliferative capacity of HSCs. Moreover, elevated levels of ROS are involved in the impairment of HSC function. Studies in mice deficient for the ataxia telangiectasia mutated (*Atm*) gene show that the selfrenewal capacity of HSCs depends on *Atm*-mediated inhibition of oxidative stress. *Atm*-deficient mice show progressive bone marrow failure resulting from a defect in HSC function that is associated with elevated ROS (Ito et al. 2004). Therefore, DNA damage- and ROS-dependent HSC failure may lead to an impaired generation of blood cells and, among these, macrophages during the aging process.

Few reports have assessed the direct influence of DNA damage and ROS on macrophage biology. Activation of macrophages leads to an increase in ROS and nitric oxide production as well as many proinflammatory cytokines that result in the clearance of the invading pathogen. However, this pro-oxidant environment may also cause DNA damage in macrophages themselves, including the induction of apoptosis (Xaus et al. 2000), suggesting that having very efficient antioxidant defenses could be very important for these cells. In this regard, it has been shown that the levels of antioxidant defenses, such as superoxide dismutase activity, decrease with aging in macrophages (de la Fuente et al. 2004), although no data about DNA damage in these cells has been reported.

In addition, elevated levels of ROS modulate some redox-sensitive transcription factors (Kregel and Zhang, 2007). Among these, NF-κB is very relevant because it is a key regulator of macrophage biology. It is thought that the phosphorylation of IκB, the inhibitory subunit of NF-κB, is the key step in NF-κB redox activation. ROS-mediated phosphorylation of IκB, leading to its ubiquitination and degradation, allows the NF-κB complex to be translocated to the nucleus and act as a transcriptional activator (Piette et al. 1997). On the other hand, direct oxidation of critical cysteine residues in the p50 subunit of NF-κB decreases its DNA binding activity (Piette et al. 1997). It has been reported that macrophages suffer from oxidative stress with aging as reflected by an increase in the oxidized glutathione/reduced glutathione ratio (de la Fuente et al. 2004). Thus, alteration of redox status in macrophages during aging may alter the activity of NF-κB and the expression of its target genes which may lead to the loss of some functional activities.

5   Conclusions and Perspectives

Macrophages are a key component of both innate and adaptive immunity and are of outmost importance in the elimination of an invading pathogen, the initiation of an immune response by activating T-cells and in the resolution of inflammation and tissue repair. Among the physiological functions that are affected by aging, the deterioration of the immune system, called immunosenescence, represents a hallmark of the aging process and contributes to the increased mortality and major incidence of immune diseases and cancer observed in the elderly. Because of the importance of macrophages in the immune system, the altered functions of these cells as a result of the aging process may play a key role in immunosenescence.

Here, we have summarized increasing experimental data about how aging affects macrophage functions. We, and many other authors, have described that most of these functions are altered in aged humans, rats and mice suggesting that dysfunctional macrophages may be involved in the deterioration of the immune system with aging. However, most of these studies have used peritoneal macrophages or blood monocytes which may be influenced by their interaction with other cell types that are also affected by aging, thereby providing a limited view of macrophage aging. On the other hand, the use of bone-marrow derived macrophages represents an extraordinary model to study the effect of aging on the genomic expression of macrophages without the influence of other cell types but does not reflect the precise function of macrophages in vivo in the tissues. Therefore, the integration of data from all macrophage models provides the best strategy to assess how aging affects macrophage function and the molecular mechanisms involved in this process.

Many theories have been postulated to explain the aging process. Even though these theories have been demonstrated in many cell types, very few data are available regarding the cellular and molecular mechanisms involved in macrophage aging. It would be of great interest to study telomere shortening and telomerase activity in aged macrophages as well as the influence of accumulation of ROS and DNA damage in these cells with aging because these studies could probably shed light on the origin of macrophage dysfunction with aging. In summary, a great amount of data demonstrates that macrophage functions are altered by aging contributing to immunosenescence. However, an integrative model which includes all macrophages subsets and a more profound study of the molecular mechanisms involved in this process would be necessary to gain further insight into macrophage aging and immunosenescence.

References

Akira S, Takeda K, Kaisho T (2001) Toll-like receptors: critical proteins linking innate and acquired immunity. Nat Immunol 2:675–680

Alexopoulou L, Holt AC, Medzhitov R, Flavell RA (2001) Recognition of double-stranded RNA and activation of NF-kappaB by Toll-like receptor 3. Nature 413:732–738

Aloisi F (2005) Cytokine production. In: Kettenmann HRRB (ed) Neuroglia. Oxford University Press, New York, pp 285–301

Alvarez E, Machado A, Sobrino F, Santa Maria C (1996) Nitric oxide and superoxide anion production decrease with age in resident and activated rat peritoneal macrophages. Cell Immunol 169:152–155

Allsopp RC, Cheshier S, Weissman IL (2001) Telomere shortening accompanies increased cell cycle activity during serial transplantation of hematopoietic stem cells. J Exp Med 193:917–924

Allsopp RC, Morin GB, DePinho R, Harley CB, Weissman IL (2003) Telomerase is required to slow telomere shortening and extend replicative lifespan of HSCs during serial transplantation. Blood 102:517–520

Arkins S, Rebeiz N, Biragyn A, Reese DL, Kelley KW (1993) Murine macrophages express abundant insulin-like growth factor-I class I Ea and Eb transcripts. Endocrinology 133:2334–2343

Arnold L, Henry A, Poron F, Baba-Amer Y, van Rooijen N, Plonquet A, Gherardi RK, Chazaud B (2007) Inflammatory monocytes recruited after skeletal muscle injury switch into antiinflammatory macrophages to support myogenesis. J Exp Med 204:1057–1069

Ashcroft GS, Horan MA, Ferguson MW (1997) The effects of ageing on wound healing: immunolocalisation of growth factors and their receptors in a murine incisional model. J Anat 190(Pt 3):351–365

Ashcroft GS, Horan MA, Ferguson MW (1998) Aging alters the inflammatory and endothelial cell adhesion molecule profiles during human cutaneous wound healing. Lab Invest 78:47–58

Aspinall R (1997) Age-associated thymic atrophy in the mouse is due to a deficiency affecting rearrangement of the TCR during intrathymic T cell development. J Immunol 158:3037–3045

Bertho JM, Demarquay C, Moulian N, Van Der Meeren A, Berrih-Aknin S, Gourmelon P (1997) Phenotypic and immunohistological analyses of the human adult thymus: evidence for an active thymus during adult life. Cell Immunol 179:30–40

Bhushan M, Cumberbatch M, Dearman RJ, Andrew SM, Kimber I, Griffiths CE (2002) Tumour necrosis factor-alpha-induced migration of human Langerhans cells: the influence of ageing. Br J Dermatol 146:32–40

Blackburn EH (2001) Switching and signaling at the telomere. Cell 106:661–673

Blasco MA (2002) Immunosenescence phenotypes in the telomerase knockout mouse. Springer Semin Immunopathol 24:75–85

Blumberg J (2004) Use of biomarkers of oxidative stress in research studies. J Nutr 134:3188S–3189S

Boehmer ED, Goral J, Faunce DE, Kovacs EJ (2004) Age-dependent decrease in Toll-like receptor 4-mediated proinflammatory cytokine production and mitogen-activated protein kinase expression. J Leukoc Biol 75:342–349

Breitbart E, Wang X, Leka LS, Dallal GE, Meydani SN, Stollar BD (2002) Altered memory B-cell homeostasis in human aging. J Gerontol A Biol Sci Med Sci 57:B304–B311

Butcher SK, Chahal H, Nayak L, Sinclair A, Henriquez NV, Sapey E, O'Mahony D, Lord JM (2001) Senescence in innate immune responses: reduced neutrophil phagocytic capacity and CD16 expression in elderly humans. J Leukoc Biol 70:881–886

Cao J, Venton L, Sakata T, Halloran BP (2003) Expression of RANKL and OPG correlates with age-related bone loss in male C57BL/6 mice. J Bone Miner Res 18:270–277

Cao JJ, Wronski TJ, Iwaniec U, Phleger L, Kurimoto P, Boudignon B, Halloran BP (2005) Aging increases stromal/osteoblastic cell-induced osteoclastogenesis and alters the osteoclast precursor pool in the mouse. J Bone Miner Res 20:1659–1668

Capsoni F, Minonzio F, Ongari AM, Bonara P, Pinto G, Carbonelli V, Lazzarin A, Zanussi C (1994) Fc receptors expression and function in mononuclear phagocytes from AIDS patients: modulation by IFN-gamma. Scand J Immunol 39:45–50

Colonna-Romano G, Bulati M, Aquino A, Scialabba G, Candore G, Lio D, Motta M, Malaguarnera M, Caruso C (2003) B cells in the aged: CD27, CD5, and CD40 expression. Mech Ageing Dev 124:389–393

Conde JR, Streit WJ (2006) Effect of aging on the microglial response to peripheral nerve injury. Neurobiol Aging 27:1451–1461

Cullell-Young M, Barrachina M, Lopez-Lopez C, Gonalons E, Lloberas J, Soler C, Celada A (2001) From transcription to cell surface expression, the induction of MHC class II I-A alpha by interferon-gamma in macrophages is regulated at different levels. Immunogenetics 53:136–144

Cumberbatch M, Kimber I (1992) Dermal tumour necrosis factor-alpha induces dendritic cell migration to draining lymph nodes, and possibly provides one stimulus for Langerhans' cell migration. Immunology 75:257–263

Curtis H, Crowley C (1963) Chromosome aberrations in liver cells in relation to the somatic mutation theory of aging. Radiat Res 19:337–344

Chan SW, Blackburn EH (2002) New ways not to make ends meet: telomerase, DNA damage proteins and heterochromatin. Oncogene 21:553–563

Chelvarajan RL, Liu Y, Popa D, Getchell ML, Getchell TV, Stromberg AJ, Bondada S (2006) Molecular basis of age-associated cytokine dysregulation in LPS-stimulated macrophages. J Leukoc Biol 79:1314–1327

Chua KF, Mostoslavsky R, Lombard DB, Pang WW, Saito S, Franco S, Kaushal D, Cheng HL, Fischer MR, Stokes N, Murphy MM, Appella E, Alt FW (2005) Mammalian SIRT1 limits replicative life span in response to chronic genotoxic stress. Cell Metab 2:67–76

Danon D, Kowatch MA, Roth GS (1989) Promotion of wound repair in old mice by local injection of macrophages. Proc Natl Acad Sci U S A 86:2018–2020

Davalos D, Grutzendler J, Yang G, Kim JV, Zuo Y, Jung S, Littman DR, Dustin ML, Gan WB (2005) ATP mediates rapid microglial response to local brain injury in vivo. Nat Neurosci 8:752–758

Davila DR, Edwards CK 3rd, Arkins S, Simon J, Kelley KW (1990) Interferon-gamma-induced priming for secretion of superoxide anion and tumor necrosis factor-alpha declines in macrophages from aged rats. FASEB J 4:2906–2911

de Haan G, Van Zant G (1999) Dynamic changes in mouse hematopoietic stem cell numbers during aging. Blood 93:3294–3301

de Haan G, Nijhof W, Van Zant G (1997) Mouse strain-dependent changes in frequency and proliferation of hematopoietic stem cells during aging: correlation between lifespan and cycling activity. Blood 89:1543–1550

De La Fuente M (1985) Changes in the macrophage function with aging. Comp Biochem Physiol A 81:935–938

De la Fuente M, Medina S, Del Rio M, Ferrandez MD, Hernanz A (2000) Effect of aging on the modulation of macrophage functions by neuropeptides. Life Sci 67:2125–2135

de la Fuente M, Hernanz A, Guayerbas N, Alvarez P, Alvarado C (2004) Changes with age in peritoneal macrophage functions. Implication of leukocytes in the oxidative stress of senescence. Cell Mol Biol (Noisy-le-grand) 50 Online Pub:OL683–OL690

de Lange T (2002) Protection of mammalian telomeres. Oncogene 21:532–540

Delpedro AD, Barjavel MJ, Mamdouh Z, Faure S, Bakouche O (1998) Signal transduction in LPS-activated aged and young monocytes. J Interferon Cytokine Res 18:429–437

Ding A, Hwang S, Schwab R (1994) Effect of aging on murine macrophages. Diminished response to IFN-gamma for enhanced oxidative metabolism. J Immunol 153:2146–2152

Donnini A, Argentati K, Mancini R, Smorlesi A, Bartozzi B, Bernardini G, Provinciali M (2002) Phenotype, antigen-presenting capacity, and migration of antigen-presenting cells in young and old age. Exp Gerontol 37:1097–1112

Effros RB (2001) Ageing and the immune system. Novartis Found Symp 235:130–139; discussion 139–145, 146–139

Effros RB, Boucher N, Porter V, Zhu X, Spaulding C, Walford RL, Kronenberg M, Cohen D, Schachter F (1994) Decline in CD28+ T cells in centenarians and in long-term T cell cultures: a
possible cause for both in vivo and in vitro immunosenescence. Exp Gerontol 29:601–609

Engelhardt M, Kumar R, Albanell J, Pettengell R, Han W, Moore MA (1997) Telomerase regulation, cell cycle and telomere stability in primitive hematopoietic cells. Blood 90:182–193

Fabris N, Mocchegiani E, Provinciali M (1997) Plasticity of neuroendocrine-thymus interactions
during aging. Exp Gerontol 32:415–429

Fazzalari NL, Kuliwaba JS, Atkins GJ, Forwood MR, Findlay DM (2001) The ratio of messenger
RNA levels of receptor activator of nuclear factor kappaB ligand to osteoprotegerin correlates
with bone remodeling indices in normal human cancellous bone but not in osteoarthritis. J
Bone Miner Res 16:1015–1027

Fietta A, Merlini C, De Bernardi PM, Gandola L, Piccioni PD, Grassi C (1993) Non specific
immunity in aged healthy subjects and in patients with chronic bronchitis. Aging (Milano)
5:357–361

Franceschi C, Bonafe M, Valensin S, Olivieri F, De Luca M, Ottaviani E, De Benedictis G (2000)
Inflamm-aging. An evolutionary perspective on immunosenescence. Ann N Y Acad Sci
908:244–254

Frucht DM, Fukao T, Bogdan C, Schindler H, O'Shea JJ, Koyasu S (2001) IFN-gamma production
by antigen-presenting cells: mechanisms emerge. Trends Immunol 22:556–560

Garg M, Luo W, Kaplan AM, Bondada S (1996) Cellular basis of decreased immune responses to
pneumococcal vaccines in aged mice. Infect Immun 64:4456–4462

Geiger H, Van Zant G (2002) The aging of lympho-hematopoietic stem cells. Nat Immunol
3:329–333

George AJ, Ritter MA (1996) Thymic involution with ageing: obsolescence or good housekeeping? Immunol Today 17:267–272

Gewirtz AT, Navas TA, Lyons S, Godowski PJ, Madara JL (2001) Cutting edge: bacterial flagellin
activates basolaterally expressed TLR5 to induce epithelial proinflammatory gene expression.
J Immunol 167:1882–1885

Gonalons E, Barrachina M, Garcia-Sanz JA, Celada A (1998) Translational control of MHC class
II I-A molecules by IFN-gamma. J Immunol 161:1837–1843

Gordon S (2003) Alternative activation of macrophages. Nat Rev Immunol 3:23–35

Gosain A, DiPietro LA (2004) Aging and wound healing. World J Surg 28:321–326

Harrison DE, Astle CM (1982) Loss of stem cell repopulating ability upon transplantation. Effects
of donor age, cell number and transplantation procedure. J Exp Med 156:1767–1779

Hartman ME, O'Connor JC, Godbout JP, Minor KD, Mazzocco VR, Freund GG (2004) Insulin
receptor substrate-2-dependent interleukin-4 signaling in macrophages is impaired in two models of type 2 diabetes mellitus. J Biol Chem 279:28045–28050

Hastie ND, Dempster M, Dunlop MG, Thompson AM, Green DK, Allshire RC (1990) Telomere
reduction in human colorectal carcinoma and with ageing. Nature 346:866–868

Hekimi S, Guarente L (2003) Genetics and the specificity of the aging process. Science
299:1351–1354

Hemmi H, Kaisho T, Takeuchi O, Sato S, Sanjo H, Hoshino K, Horiuchi T, Tomizawa H, Takeda
K, Akira S (2002) Small anti-viral compounds activate immune cells via the TLR7 MyD88-
dependent signaling pathway. Nat Immunol 3:196–200

Herrero C, Marques L, Lloberas J, Celada A (2001) IFN-gamma-dependent transcription of MHC
class II IA is impaired in macrophages from aged mice. J Clin Invest 107:485–493

Herrero C, Sebastian C, Marques L, Comalada M, Xaus J, Valledor AF, Lloberas J, Celada A
(2002) Immunosenescence of macrophages: reduced MHC class II gene expression. Exp Gerontol 37:389–394

Hirokawa K (1977) The thymus and aging. In: Immunology and aging. In: Makinodan TJJE (ed).
Plenum Press, New York, pp 51–76

Hohaus S, Petrovick MS, Voso MT, Sun Z, Zhang DE, Tenen DG (1995) PU.1 (Spi-1) and C/EBP
alpha regulate expression of the granulocyte-macrophage colony-stimulating factor receptor
alpha gene. Mol Cell Biol 15:5830–5845

Hornsby PJ, Yang L, Gunter LE (1992) Demethylation of satellite I DNA during senescence of bovine adrenocortical cells in culture. Mutat Res 275:13–19

Howard BH (1996) Replicative senescence: considerations relating to the stability of heterochromatin domains. Exp Gerontol 31:281–293

Hume DA, Robinson AP, MacPherson GG, Gordon S (1983) The mononuclear phagocyte system of the mouse defined by immunohistochemical localization of antigen F4/80. Relationship between macrophages, Langerhans cells, reticular cells, and dendritic cells in lymphoid and hematopoietic organs. J Exp Med 158:1522–1536

Ikeda T, Utsuyama M, Hirokawa K (2001) Expression profiles of receptor activator of nuclear factor kappaB ligand, receptor activator of nuclear factor kappaB, and osteoprotegerin messenger RNA in aged and ovariectomized rat bones. J Bone Miner Res 16:1416–1425

Imai T, Nagira M, Takagi S, Kakizaki M, Nishimura M, Wang J, Gray PW, Matsushima K, Yoshie O (1999) Selective recruitment of CCR4-bearing Th2 cells toward antigen-presenting cells by the CC chemokines thymus and activation-regulated chemokine and macrophage-derived chemokine. Int Immunol 11:81–88

Inamizu T, Chang MP, Makinodan T (1985) Influence of age on the production and regulation of interleukin-1 in mice. Immunology 55:447–455

Ito K, Hirao A, Arai F, Matsuoka S, Takubo K, Hamaguchi I, Nomiyama K, Hosokawa K, Sakurada K, Nakagata N, Ikeda Y, Mak TW, Suda T (2004) Regulation of oxidative stress by ATM is required for self-renewal of haematopoietic stem cells. Nature 431:997–1002

Iwama H, Ohyashiki K, Ohyashiki JH, Hayashi S, Yahata N, Ando K, Toyama K, Hoshika A, Takasaki M, Mori M, Shay JW (1998) Telomeric length and telomerase activity vary with age in peripheral blood cells obtained from normal individuals. Hum Genet 102:397–402

Kanungo MS (1975) A model for ageing. J Theor Biol 53:253–261

Kelley KW, Arkins S, Minshall C, Liu Q, Dantzer R (1996) Growth hormone, growth factors and hematopoiesis. Horm Res 45:38–45

Kenyon C (2005) The plasticity of aging: insights from long-lived mutants. Cell 120:449–460

Khare V, Sodhi A, Singh SM (1996) Effect of aging on the tumoricidal functions of murine peritoneal macrophages. Nat Immun 15:285–294

Kissin E, Tomasi M, McCartney-Francis N, Gibbs CL, Smith PD (1997) Age-related decline in murine macrophage production of nitric oxide. J Infect Dis 175:1004–1007

Kraatz J, Clair L, Rodriguez JL, West MA (1999) Macrophage TNF secretion in endotoxin tolerance: role of SAPK, p38, and MAPK. J Surg Res 83:158–164

Kregel KC, Zhang HJ (2007) An integrated view of oxidative stress in aging: basic mechanisms, functional effects, and pathological considerations. Am J Physiol Regul Integr Comp Physiol 292:R18–R36

Kropf P, Herath S, Weber V, Modolell M, Muller I (2003) Factors influencing Leishmania major infection in IL-4-deficient BALB/c mice. Parasite Immunol 25:439–447

Lansdorp PM (2005) Major cutbacks at chromosome ends. Trends Biochem Sci 30:388–395

Lee J, Ryu H, Ferrante RJ, Morris SM, Jr., Ratan RR (2003) Translational control of inducible nitric oxide synthase expression by arginine can explain the arginine paradox. Proc Natl Acad Sci U S A 100:4843–4848

Li Q, Xiao H, Isobe K (2002) Histone acetyltransferase activities of cAMP-regulated enhancer-binding protein and p300 in tissues of fetal, young, and old mice. J Gerontol A Biol Sci Med Sci 57:B93–B98

Liang CP, Han S, Okamoto H, Carnemolla R, Tabas I, Accili D, Tall AR (2004) Increased CD36 protein as a response to defective insulin signaling in macrophages. J Clin Invest 113:764–773

Lieber MR, Karanjawala ZE (2004) Ageing, repetitive genomes and DNA damage. Nat Rev Mol Cell Biol 5:69–75

Liu P, Smith PF, Appleton I, Darlington CL, Bilkey DK (2003a) Regional variations and age-related changes in nitric oxide synthase and arginase in the sub-regions of the hippocampus. Neuroscience 119:679–687

Liu P, Smith PF, Appleton I, Darlington CL, Bilkey DK (2003b) Nitric oxide synthase and arginase in the rat hippocampus and the entorhinal, perirhinal, postrhinal, and temporal cortices: regional variations and age-related changes. Hippocampus 13:859–867

Lloberas J, Celada A (2002) Effect of aging on macrophage function. Exp Gerontol 37:1325–1331

Lloberas J, Soler C, Celada A (1999) The key role of PU.1/SPI-1 in B cells, myeloid cells and macrophages. Immunol Today 20:184–189

Makhluf HA, Mueller SM, Mizuno S, Glowacki J (2000) Age-related decline in osteoprotegerin expression by human bone marrow cells cultured in three-dimensional collagen sponges. Biochem Biophys Res Commun 268:669–672

Mancuso P, McNish RW, Peters-Golden M, Brock TG (2001) Evaluation of phagocytosis and arachidonate metabolism by alveolar macrophages and recruited neutrophils from F344xBN rats of different ages. Mech Ageing Dev 122:1899–1913

Mantovani A, Sozzani S, Locati M, Allavena P, Sica A (2002) Macrophage polarization: tumor-associated macrophages as a paradigm for polarized M2 mononuclear phagocytes. Trends Immunol 23:549–555

Mantovani A, Sica A, Sozzani S, Allavena P, Vecchi A, Locati M (2004) The chemokine system in diverse forms of macrophage activation and polarization. Trends Immunol 25:677–686

Martin GM, Ogburn CE, Colgin LM, Gown AM, Edland SD, Monnat RJ, Jr. (1996) Somatic mutations are frequent and increase with age in human kidney epithelial cells. Hum Mol Genet 5:215–221

Matsumoto A (2002) Age-related changes in nuclear receptor coactivator immunoreactivity in motoneurons of the spinal nucleus of the bulbocavernosus of male rats. Brain Res 943:202–205

McEachern MJ, Krauskopf A, Blackburn EH (2000) Telomeres and their control. Annu Rev Genet 34:331–358

Miller RA (1996) The aging immune system: primer and prospectus. Science 273:70–74

Miller SI, Ernst RK, Bader MW (2005) LPS, TLR4 and infectious disease diversity. Nat Rev Microbiol 3:36–46

Minshall C, Arkins S, Straza J, Conners J, Dantzer R, Freund GG, Kelley KW (1997) IL-4 and insulin-like growth factor-I inhibit the decline in Bcl-2 and promote the survival of IL-3-deprived myeloid progenitors. J Immunol 159:1225–1232

Morrison SJ, Wandycz AM, Akashi K, Globerson A, Weissman IL (1996) The aging of hematopoietic stem cells. Nat Med 2:1011–1016

Mostoslavsky R, Chua KF, Lombard DB, Pang WW, Fischer MR, Gellon L, Liu P, Mostoslavsky G, Franco S, Murphy MM, Mills KD, Patel P, Hsu JT, Hong AL, Ford E, Cheng HL, Kennedy C, Nunez N, Bronson R, Frendewey D, Auerbach W, Valenzuela D, Karow M, Hottiger MO, Hursting S, Barrett JC, Guarente L, Mulligan R, Demple B, Yancopoulos GD, Alt FW (2006) Genomic instability and aging-like phenotype in the absence of mammalian SIRT6. Cell 124:315–329

Mrak RE, Griffin WS (2005) Glia and their cytokines in progression of neurodegeneration. Neurobiol Aging 26:349–354

Muzio M, Ni J, Feng P, Dixit VM (1997) IRAK (Pelle) family member IRAK-2 and MyD88 as proximal mediators of IL-1 signaling. Science 278:1612–1615

Nabarra B, Andrianarison I (1996) Ultrastructural study of thymic microenvironment involution in aging mice. Exp Gerontol 31:489–506

Nijnik A, Woodbine L, Marchetti C, Dawson S, Lambe T, Liu C, Rodrigues NP, Crockford TL, Cabuy E, Vindigni A, Enver T, Bell JI, Slijepcevic P, Goodnow CC, Jeggo PA, Cornall RJ (2007) DNA repair is limiting for haematopoietic stem cells during ageing. Nature 447:686–690

Nimmerjahn A, Kirchhoff F, Helmchen F (2005) Resting microglial cells are highly dynamic surveillants of brain parenchyma in vivo. Science 308:1314–1318

Ogawa K, Funaba M, Chen Y, Tsujimoto M (2006) Activin A functions as a Th2 cytokine in the promotion of the alternative activation of macrophages. J Immunol 177:6787–6794

Ogawa T, Kitagawa M, Hirokawa K (2000) Age-related changes of human bone marrow: a histometric estimation of proliferative cells, apoptotic cells, T cells, B cells and macrophages. Mech Ageing Dev 117:57–68

Ogryzko VV, Hirai TH, Russanova VR, Barbie DA, Howard BH (1996) Human fibroblast commitment to a senescence-like state in response to histone deacetylase inhibitors is cell cycle dependent. Mol Cell Biol 16:5210–5218

Olah ME, Caldwell CC (2003) Adenosine receptors and mammalian toll-like receptors: synergism in macrophages. Mol Interv 3:370–374

Pawelec G, Solana R (1997) Immunosenescence. Immunol Today 18:514–516

Perkins SL, Gibbons R, Kling S, Kahn AJ (1994) Age-related bone loss in mice is associated with an increased osteoclast progenitor pool. Bone 15:65–72

Pesce J, Kaviratne M, Ramalingam TR, Thompson RW, Urban JF, Jr., Cheever AW, Young DA, Collins M, Grusby MJ, Wynn TA (2006) The IL-21 receptor augments Th2 effector function and alternative macrophage activation. J Clin Invest 116:2044–2055

Pestka S, Krause CD, Walter MR (2004) Interferons, interferon-like cytokines, and their receptors. Immunol Rev 202:8–32

Petersen KF, Befroy D, Dufour S, Dziura J, Ariyan C, Rothman DL, DiPietro L, Cline GW, Shulman GI (2003) Mitochondrial dysfunction in the elderly: possible role in insulin resistance. Science 300:1140–1142

Piette J, Piret B, Bonizzi G, Schoonbroodt S, Merville MP, Legrand-Poels S, Bours V (1997) Multiple redox regulation in NF-kappaB transcription factor activation. Biol Chem 378:1237–1245

Pinhal-Enfield G, Ramanathan M, Hasko G, Vogel SN, Salzman AL, Boons GJ, Leibovich SJ (2003) An angiogenic switch in macrophages involving synergy between Toll-like receptors 2, 4, 7, and 9 and adenosine A(2A) receptors. Am J Pathol 163:711–721

Plackett TP, Boehmer ED, Faunce DE, Kovacs EJ (2004) Aging and innate immune cells. J Leukoc Biol 76:291–299

Plowden J, Renshaw-Hoelscher M, Engleman C, Katz J, Sambhara S (2004) Innate immunity in aging: impact on macrophage function. Aging Cell 3:161–167

Puddu P, Fantuzzi L, Borghi P, Varano B, Rainaldi G, Guillemard E, Malorni W, Nicaise P, Wolf SF, Belardelli F, Gessani S (1997) IL-12 induces IFN-gamma expression and secretion in mouse peritoneal macrophages. J Immunol 159:3490–3497

Ralfkiaer E, Stein H, Ralfkiaer N, Hou-Jensen K, Mason DY (1985) Normal and neoplastic Langerhans cells: phenotypic comparison with other types of macrophages. Adv Exp Med Biol 186:1009–1015

Ramsey MJ, Moore DH 2nd, Briner JF, Lee DA, Olsen L, Senft JR, Tucker JD (1995) The effects of age and lifestyle factors on the accumulation of cytogenetic damage as measured by chromosome painting. Mutat Res 338:95–106

Reese TA, Liang HE, Tager AM, Luster AD, Van Rooijen N, Voehringer D, Locksley RM (2007) Chitin induces accumulation in tissue of innate immune cells associated with allergy. Nature 447:92–96

Renshaw M, Rockwell J, Engleman C, Gewirtz A, Katz J, Sambhara S (2002) Cutting edge: impaired Toll-like receptor expression and function in aging. J Immunol 169:4697–4701

Rosmarin AG, Caprio DG, Kirsch DG, Handa H, Simkevich CP (1995) GABP and PU.1 compete for binding, yet cooperate to increase CD18 (beta 2 leukocyte integrin) transcription. J Biol Chem 270:23627–23633

Rossi DJ, Bryder D, Seita J, Nussenzweig A, Hoeijmakers J, Weissman IL (2007) Deficiencies in DNA damage repair limit the function of haematopoietic stem cells with age. Nature 447:725–729

Sadahira Y, Wada H, Manabe T, Yawata Y (1999) Immunohistochemical assessment of human bone marrow macrophages in hematologic disorders. Pathol Int 49:626–632

Samper E, Fernandez P, Eguia R, Martin-Rivera L, Bernad A, Blasco MA, Aracil M (2002) Longterm repopulating ability of telomerase-deficient murine hematopoietic stem cells. Blood 99:2767–2775

San Jose I, Garcia-Suarez O, Hannestad J, Cabo R, Gauna L, Represa J, Vega JA (2001) The thymus of the hairless rhino-j (hr/rh-j) mice. J Anat 198:399–406

Sancar A, Lindsey-Boltz LA, Unsal-Kacmaz K, Linn S (2004) Molecular mechanisms of mammalian DNA repair and the DNA damage checkpoints. Annu Rev Biochem 73:39–85

Saurwein-Teissl M, Blasko I, Zisterer K, Neuman B, Lang B, Grubeck-Loebenstein B (2000) An imbalance between pro- and anti-inflammatory cytokines, a characteristic feature of old age. Cytokine 12:1160–1161

Schroder K, Hertzog PJ, Ravasi T, Hume DA (2004) Interferon-gamma: an overview of signals, mechanisms and functions. J Leukoc Biol 75:163–189

Sierra A, Gottfried-Blackmore AC, McEwen BS, Bulloch K (2007) Microglia derived from aging mice exhibit an altered inflammatory profile. Glia 55:412–424

Singhal RP, Mays-Hoopes LL, Eichhorn GL (1987) DNA methylation in aging of mice. Mech Ageing Dev 41:199–210

Smith LT, Hohaus S, Gonzalez DA, Dziennis SE, Tenen DG (1996) PU.1 (Spi-1) and C/EBP alpha regulate the granulocyte colony-stimulating factor receptor promoter in myeloid cells. Blood 88:1234–1247

Smith P, Dunne DW, Fallon PG (2001) Defective in vivo induction of functional type 2 cytokine responses in aged mice. Eur J Immunol 31:1495–1502

Solana R, Mariani E (2000) NK and NK/T cells in human senescence. Vaccine 18:1613–1620

Streit WJ (2002) Microglia as neuroprotective, immunocompetent cells of the CNS. Glia 40:133–139

Streit WJ (2006) Microglial senescence: does the brain's immune system have an expiration date? Trends Neurosci 29:506–510

Sun LQ, Lee DW, Zhang Q, Xiao W, Raabe EH, Meeker A, Miao D, Huso DL, Arceci RJ (2004) Growth retardation and premature aging phenotypes in mice with disruption of the SNF2-like gene, PASG. Genes Dev 18:1035–1046

Swift ME, Burns AL, Gray KL, DiPietro LA (2001) Age-related alterations in the inflammatory response to dermal injury. J Invest Dermatol 117:1027–1035

Tatar M, Bartke A, Antebi A (2003) The endocrine regulation of aging by insulin-like signals. Science 299:1346–1351

Thiers BH, Maize JC, Spicer SS, Cantor AB (1984) The effect of aging and chronic sun exposure on human Langerhans cell populations. J Invest Dermatol 82:223–226

Thomas DR (2001) Age-related changes in wound healing. Drugs Aging 18:607–620

Tucker JD, Spruill MD, Ramsey MJ, Director AD, Nath J (1999) Frequency of spontaneous chromosome aberrations in mice: effects of age. Mutat Res 425:135–141

Vaday GG, Franitza S, Schor H, Hecht I, Brill A, Cahalon L, Hershkoviz R, Lider O (2001) Combinatorial signals by inflammatory cytokines and chemokines mediate leukocyte interactions with extracellular matrix. J Leukoc Biol 69:885–892

Valledor AF, Borras FE, Cullell-Young M, Celada A (1998) Transcription factors that regulate monocyte/macrophage differentiation. J Leukoc Biol 63:405–417

Van Zant G, Liang Y (2003) The role of stem cells in aging. Exp Hematol 31:659–672

Van Zant G, de Haan G, Rich IN (1997) Alternatives to stem cell renewal from a developmental viewpoint. Exp Hematol 25:187–192

Varas A, Sacedon R, Hernandez-Lopez C, Jimenez E, Garcia-Ceca J, Arias-Diaz J, Zapata AG, Vicente A (2003) Age-dependent changes in thymic macrophages and dendritic cells. Microsc Res Tech 62:501–507

Vaziri H, Dragowska W, Allsopp RC, Thomas TE, Harley CB, Lansdorp PM (1994) Evidence for a mitotic clock in human hematopoietic stem cells: loss of telomeric DNA with age. Proc Natl Acad Sci U S A 91:9857–9860

Vaziri H, Schachter F, Uchida I, Wei L, Zhu X, Effros R, Cohen D, Harley CB (1993) Loss of telomeric DNA during aging of normal and trisomy 21 human lymphocytes. Am J Hum Genet 52:661–667

Vertino PM, Issa JP, Pereira-Smith OM, Baylin SB (1994) Stabilization of DNA methyltransferase levels and CpG island hypermethylation precede SV40-induced immortalization of human fibroblasts. Cell Growth Differ 5:1395–1402

Videla LA, Tapia G, Fernandez V (2001) Influence of aging on Kupffer cell respiratory activity in relation to particle phagocytosis and oxidative stress parameters in mouse liver. Redox Rep 6:155–159

Villanueva JL, Solana R, Alonso MC, Pena J (1990) Changes in the expression of HLA-class II antigens on peripheral blood monocytes from aged humans. Dis Markers 8:85–91

Villeponteau B (1997) The heterochromatin loss model of aging. Exp Gerontol 32:383–394

Wallace PK, Eisenstein TK, Meissler JJ Jr, Morahan PS (1995) Decreases in macrophage mediated antitumor activity with aging. Mech Ageing Dev 77:169–184

Wang B, Amerio P, Sauder DN (1999) Role of cytokines in epidermal Langerhans cell migration. J Leukoc Biol 66:33–39

Wang CQ, Udupa KB, Xiao H, Lipschitz DA (1995) Effect of age on marrow macrophage number and function. Aging (Milano) 7:379–384

Weng N (2001) Interplay between telomere length and telomerase in human leukocyte differentiation and aging. J Leukoc Biol 70:861–867

Xaus J, Cardo M, Valledor AF, Soler C, Lloberas J, Celada A (1999) Interferon gamma induces the expression of p21waf-1 and arrests macrophage cell cycle, preventing induction of apoptosis. Immunity 11:103–113

Xaus J, Besalduch N, Comalada M, Marcoval J, Pujol R, Mana J, Celada A (2003) High expression of p21 Waf1 in sarcoid granulomas: a putative role for long-lasting inflammation. J Leukoc Biol 74:295–301

Xaus J, Comalada M, Valledor AF, Lloberas J, Lopez-Soriano F, Argiles JM, Bogdan C, Celada A (2000) LPS induces apoptosis in macrophages mostly through the autocrine production of TNF-alpha. Blood 95:3823–3831

Yamazaki S, Yokozeki H, Satoh T, Katayama I, Nishioka K (1998) TNF-alpha, RANTES, and MCP-1 are major chemoattractants of murine Langerhans cells to the regional lymph nodes. Exp Dermatol 7:35–41

Yeramian A, Martin L, Arpa L, Bertran J, Soler C, McLeod C, Modolell M, Palacin M, Lloberas J, Celada A (2006a) Macrophages require distinct arginine catabolism and transport systems for proliferation and for activation. Eur J Immunol 36:1516–1526

Yeramian A, Martin L, Serrat N, Arpa L, Soler C, Bertran J, McLeod C, Palacin M, Modolell M, Lloberas J, Celada A (2006b) Arginine transport via cationic amino acid transporter 2 plays a critical regulatory role in classical or alternative activation of macrophages. J Immunol 176:5918–5924

Yoshimoto T, Wang CR, Yoneto T, Waki S, Sunaga S, Komagata Y, Mitsuyama M, Miyazaki J, Nariuchi H (1998) Reduced T helper 1 responses in IL-12 p40 transgenic mice. J Immunol 160:588–594

Zeira M, Gallily R (1990) Effect of strain and age on in vitro proliferation of murine thymus-derived macrophages. Thymus 15:1–13

Zheng B, Han S, Takahashi Y, Kelsoe G (1997) Immunosenescence and germinal center reaction. Immunol Rev 160:63–77

Zimmermann S, Glaser S, Ketteler R, Waller CF, Klingmuller U, Martens UM (2004) Effects of telomerase modulation in human hematopoietic progenitor cells. Stem Cells 22:741–749

Subject Index